Immunology, Infection, and Immunity

Immunology, Infection, and Immunity

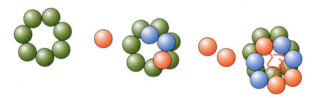
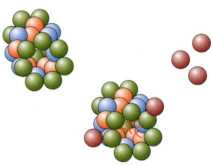
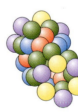
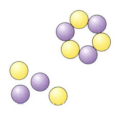

EDITED BY

Gerald B. Pier

Channing Laboratory, Brigham and Women's Hospital
and
Harvard Medical School, Boston, Massachusetts

Jeffrey B. Lyczak

Channing Laboratory, Brigham and Women's Hospital
and
Harvard Medical School, Boston, Massachusetts

Lee M. Wetzler

Evans Biomedical Research Center
and
Division of Infectious Diseases, Department of Medicine,
Boston University School of Medicine
and
Boston Medical Center, Boston, Massachusetts

ASM PRESS

WASHINGTON, D.C.

Address editorial correspondence to ASM Press, 1752 N St. NW, Washington, DC
20036-2904, USA

Send orders to ASM Press, P.O. Box 605, Herndon, VA 20172, USA
Phone: (800) 546-2416 or (703) 661-1593
Fax: (703) 661-1501
E-mail: books@asmusa.org
Online: www.asmpress.org

Library of Congress Cataloging-in-Publication Data

Immunology, infection, and immunity / edited by Gerald B. Pier, Jeffrey
 B. Lyczak, Lee M. Wetzler.
  p. ; cm.
 Includes bibliographical references and index.
  ISBN 1-55581-246-5 (hardcover)
 1. Immunology. 2. Infection.
 [DNLM: 1. Immune System. 2. Immunity, Cellular. 3. Immunologic
Diseases. 4. Infection. QW 504 I333 2004] I. Pier, Gerald Bryan. II.
Lyczak, Jeffrey B. III. Wetzler, Lee M. IV. Title.
 QR181.I443 2004
 616.07'9—dc21

               2003002554

10 9 8 7 6 5 4 3 2 1

For all of their wonderful support and help, I dedicate this book to my wife, Susan Bennett; my two children, Danielle and Elizabeth Pier; members of my laboratory research group, both past and present; and my colleagues at the Channing Laboratory who have made the research and teaching effort all worthwhile

Gerald B. Pier

To my wife, Karen Yates, for always offering her support and for sharing in the successes and the trials of research; to my parents, Bernard and Lorraine Lyczak, for encouraging my learning and curiosity; to my teachers and mentors, for showing me the way and for their patience; and lastly to my students, who, by questioning, have taught me so much

Jeffrey B. Lyczak

To my wife, Hilde-Kari Guttormsen, and my three children, Gabrielle, Isabel, and Andrea, and to my parents, who always encouraged me; to my colleagues at the Boston University School of Medicine in the Division of Infectious Diseases and the Department of Microbiology; to the past and present members of my laboratory; and to my mentor, Emil Gotschlich, whose support allowed me to become a better scientist

Lee M. Wetzler

Contents

SECTION **III**

CELLULAR IMMUNITY 259

chapter 18

Immunity to Bacterial Infections 425

Gerald B. Pier

chapter 19

Immunity to Viruses 453

Edward Barker

chapter 20

Immunity to Parasitic and Fungal Infections 469

Judith E. Allen and Leo X. Liu

chapter 21

Vaccines and Vaccination 497
Gerald B. Pier

SECTION V

IMMUNE SYSTEM DYSFUNCTION: DEFICIENCIES 529

chapter 22

Immunology and AIDS 531
Saskia Boisot and Gerald B. Pier

Contributors

Judith E. Allen
Institute of Cell, Animal and Population Biology, University of Edinburgh, Edinburgh EH9 3JT, United Kingdom

Edward Barker
Department of Microbiology and Immunology, State University of New York/Syracuse, Syracuse, NY 13210

Steven A. Bogen
Department of Pathology and Laboratory Medicine, Boston University School of Medicine, Boston, MA 02118

Saskia Boisot
School of Medicine, University of California at San Diego, San Diego, Calif.

Lisa H. Butterfield
Departments of Medicine and Surgery, University of Pittsburgh, Pittsburgh, PA 15213

Carolyn L. Cannon
Division of Allergy and Pulmonary Medicine, Washington University School of Medicine, St. Louis, MO 63110

Howard Ceri
Department of Biological Sciences, University of Calgary, Calgary, Alberta T2N 1N4, Canada

Anil Chandraker
Transplant Research Center, Brigham and Women's Hospital, 75 Francis St., Boston, MA 02115

Ronald B. Corley
Department of Microbiology, Boston University School of Medicine, Boston, MA 02118

William R. Green
Department of Microbiology and Immunology, Dartmouth Medical School, Lebanon, NH 03576

Hilde-Kari Guttormsen
Channing Laboratory, Brigham and Women's Hospital and Harvard Medical School, 181 Longwood Ave., Boston, MA 02115

Johannes Huebner
Channing Laboratory and Department of Medicine, Brigham and Women's Hospital and Harvard Medical School, Boston, MA 02115

Elinor M. Levy
Department of Microbiology, Boston University School of Medicine, Boston, MA 02118

Leo X. Liu
Cambria Biosciences LLC, 8A Henshaw St., Woburn, MA 01801

Jeffrey B. Lyczak
Channing Laboratory, Brigham and Women's Hospital and Harvard Medical School, 181 Longwood Ave., Boston, MA 02115

Jeff M. Milunsky
Clinical Genetics, Center for Human Genetics, and Department of Pediatrics, Boston University School of Medicine, Boston, MA 02118

Chris Mody
Department of Microbiology and Infectious Diseases, University of Calgary, Calgary, Alberta T2N 1N4, Canada

Francis Moore, Jr.
Department of Surgery, Brigham and Women's Hospital, Boston, MA 02115

Stephen I. Pelton
Department of Pediatrics, Boston University School of Medicine, and Section of Pediatric Infectious Diseases, Boston Medical Center, Boston, MA 02118

Gerald B. Pier
Channing Laboratory and Department of Medicine, Brigham and Women's Hospital and Harvard Medical School, Boston, MA 02115

Michael Preston
Channing Laboratory and Department of Medicine, Brigham and Women's Hospital, Boston, MA 02115

Mohamed H. Sayegh
Transplant Research Center, Brigham and Women's Hospital, 75 Francis St., Boston, MA 02115

Stephen P. Schoenberger
Division of Immune Regulation, La Jolla Institute for Allergy and Immunology, 10355 Science Center Dr., San Diego, CA 92121

Michael K. Shaw
Department of Immunology and Microbiology, Wayne State University School of Medicine, Detroit, MI 48201

Scott Simpson
Evans Biomedical Research Center and Division of Infectious Diseases, Department of Medicine, Boston University School of Medicine and Boston Medical Center, 650 Albany St., Boston, MA 02118

Guillermo E. Taccioli
Department of Microbiology, Boston University School of Medicine, Boston, MA 02118

Harley Y. Tse
Department of Immunology and Microbiology, Wayne State University School of Medicine, Detroit, MI 48201

Arthur O. Tzianabos
Channing Laboratory, Brigham and Women's Hospital and Harvard Medical School, 181 Longwood Ave., Boston, MA 02115

Lee M. Wetzler
Evans Biomedical Research Center and Division of Infectious Diseases, Department of Medicine, Boston University School of Medicine and Boston Medical Center, 650 Albany St., Boston, MA 02118

J. Patrick Whelan
AIDS Research Center, Massachusetts General Hospital, CN4, Building 149, 149 13th St., Charlestown, MA 02129

Karen E. Yates
Department of Orthopedic Surgery, Brigham and Women's Hospital and Harvard Medical School, 75 Francis St., Boston, MA 02115

Preface

If one looks around the medical scene in North America or Australia, the most important current change he sees is the rapidly diminishing importance of infectious diseases. The fever hospitals are vanishing or being turned to other uses. With full use of the knowledge we already possess, the effective control of every important infectious disease, with the one outstanding exception of poliomyelitis, is possible.

Sir Frank Macfarlane Burnet
Director of the Walter and Eliza Hall
Institute of Medical Research
May 1951

Sir Frank Macfarlane Burnet was one of the greatest immunologists of the 20th century. He won the Nobel Prize in physiology and medicine for his discoveries related to the phenomenon of immunological tolerance. His work was carried out at a time when the disciplines of microbiology and immunology were completely entwined, and his prophecy in 1951 came at a time following the emergence in the 1930s and 1940s of effective antibiotics for bacterial infections. These drugs, along with continued use and development of vaccines, caused dramatic changes in medicine, particularly in the field of infectious diseases. Yet, over half a century later, his prophecy has not come to pass, and indeed it is poliovirus, and not other infectious agents, that is mostly controlled and likely will be eliminated as a cause of human disease in the near future.

There are many reasons why microbes have outwitted humans' ability to control infectious diseases. But at the center of this struggle between microbes and humans is the immune system. Functionally, it exists for one major purpose: to prevent and control infections with pathogenic microbes and eliminate the pathogens and their harmful products from multicellular hosts. Without an immune system, there is only a short period of survival, terminated by overwhelming infection. Without an immune system but with complete environmental elimina-

tion of microbes, as occurred with the famous "bubble boy," David Vetter, a human can grow and survive. Immune function is generally not needed for the successful function of other body organs and physiologic systems. Similarly, many genetically manipulated strains of mice lacking functional immune systems can grow and survive if kept in environments that exclude pathogenic microbes. It is with the acknowledgment of this centrality of function of the immune system that we proudly publish this textbook, *Immunology, Infection, and Immunity*, bringing the basic molecular and cellular components of the immune system into close juxtaposition to the pathogenesis and prevention of infectious diseases.

This is not to exclude the other important areas where the immune system is of central importance to human health and disease. In addition to the emphasis on infectious diseases, the book focuses strongly on those areas where the immune system does not act when it should (primary and acquired immunodeficiency and the failure to control cancer) as well as areas where the overactivity or dysregulation of the immune system is a cause of pathology (hypersensitivity reactions, including allergy and asthma; autoimmunity; and the unwanted immune responses to transplanted tissues and organs). These topics are all part of the study of the basic biology of the immune system and represent important areas where the centrality of the immune system function affects health. But even in these areas, the root cause of the pathology can often be tied to the central function of the immune system in preventing and controlling infections. In immunodeficiency states, the affected individual most often struggles with infections, which are often the cause of death. Individuals with serious diseases due to cancer are dealing with pathologic events with many parallels to those that occur in dealing with an infectious pathogen:

an out-of-control progression of the growth of an undesired living entity. In the case of cancer, a cell derived from one's own body causes disruption of the normal function of tissues and organs. Disease, and all too often death, is the outcome of the uncontrolled growth of microbial or cancerous cells. Even for the overreactive immune diseases, the basic immunologic process that is used to fight infection—inflammation—goes out of control and harms one's own tissues. The various manifestations and functions of the cellular and molecular components of the immune system that have evolved to control and prevent infectious diseases are inextricably linked with the pathology of other diseases.

Immunology is admittedly not the easiest subject to teach and learn, but it is one of the most fascinating, challenging, and important areas of biology. A few immunologists can be obtuse and circular. In teaching students basic immunology, we often have had to encourage patience in students when they can encounter definitions such as "An antibody is a substance made by a mammal in response to an encounter with a foreign antigen. A foreign antigen is a substance that induces an antibody response in an animal." True, accurate, but not highly informative. To bring the full flavor and excitement of immunology to new students, we have assembled an outstanding group of contributors with expertise in the multiple areas of immunology to provide up-to-date information in a field that moves all too rapidly. There are a variety of presentation styles, but all of the chapters have thematic and structural aspects standardized to provide critical information in a comprehensible style. Importantly, this text is intended to complement traditional views and dogmas about immunology with today's cutting-edge ideas and experimental data describing how the immune system works, some of which are challenging and changing some long-held beliefs about immunology.

While there are other excellent basic textbooks of immunology, most have different organizations and emphases from that in *Immunology, Infection, and Immunity*. To teach both basic and applied aspects of immunology, we have used, where feasible, examples and illustrations depicting basic immunologic processes in conjunction with their role in infectious or other diseases. The foundation concepts of immunology are among the most exciting in modern biology and medicine, but their application to the real world of diseases and health is a concept never far from the intent of researchers—even those concepts that define the most detailed (some might even say arcane) molecular and cellular functions of the immune system. It is to this goal of scientific inquiry that we have focused the information and content in this book.

Acknowledgments

We thank Matthew Fenton for figure suggestions for chapter 2, Michael Ross for micrographs of large granular lymphocytes in chapter 3, John Warner for the mouse thymus and mouse intestine photographs in chapter 4, and Walter Pieciak, Andrew Onderdonk, and the Clinical Microbiology Laboratory of Brigham and Women's Hospital for the photographs of Gram-stained bacteria in chapter 18. We also thank Nancy Voynow for editorial assistance with many chapters of this book.

About the Editors

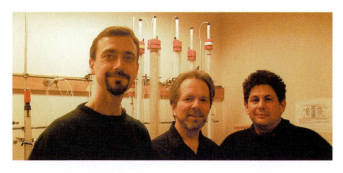

Gerald B. Pier (middle editor in photo) received his bachelor's degree in liberal arts from the now-defunct Raymond College cluster college at the University of the Pacific in Stockton, Calif., followed by a Ph.D. in microbiology from the University of California at Berkeley. He received a National Research Council postdoctoral fellowship award to work in the Department of Bacterial Diseases at the Walter Reed Army Institute of Medical Research, where he started a research program on pathogenesis and immunity to *Pseudomonas aeruginosa*. He moved to the Channing Laboratory in the Department of Medicine at Brigham and Women's Hospital and Harvard Medical School and is now a professor of medicine (microbiology and molecular genetics) at Harvard Medical School. His primary research interests encompass pathogenesis and immunity to *P. aeruginosa, Staphylococcus aureus,* and *Staphylococcus epidermidis,* with major goals focused on understanding basic and applied aspects of immunity to pathogenic microbes. He started teaching a two-semester immunology course to undergraduate and graduate students in 1980, and compiling and editing *Immunology, Infection, and Immunity* are among the major culminations of this teaching effort.

Jeffrey B. Lyczak (left) received his bachelor of science degree in biology from Saint Joseph's University in Philadelphia, Pa. He then studied at the Department of Microbiology and Molecular Genetics of the University of California at Los Angeles, where he performed his dissertation research on the function of the antibody immunoglobulin E. He moved to the Channing Laboratory in the Department of Medicine at Brigham and Women's Hospital and Harvard Medical School to do a postdoctoral fellowship studying corneal infection by *P. aeruginosa*. Upon completion of his fellowship, he remained at the Channing Laboratory as a junior faculty member to expand his research to the field of gastrointestinal infection by *Salmonella enterica*. He also began teaching introductory-level immunology courses offered to graduate and undergraduate students at Harvard University.

Lee M. Wetzler (right) received his bachelor of science degree at the State University of New York at Binghamton and his doctorate in medicine at the State University of New York at Syracuse/Upstate Medical Center. He performed his medical residency at the University of Michigan. Then he became a postdoctoral fellow in the Laboratory of Bacterial Pathogenesis and Immunology at the Rockefeller University, studying the vaccine potential of neisserial outer membrane proteins, and was eventually promoted to assistant professor. He then moved to the Division of Infectious Diseases in the Department of Medicine at the Boston University School of Medicine, where he is now an associate professor in both the Department of Medicine and the Department of Microbiology. He studies innate immunity to bacteria and its relationship to immune protection and vaccine development.

FUNCTION AND COMPOSITION OF THE IMMUNE SYSTEM

SECTION I

chapter 1

Overview of Immunity

Karen E. Yates and Jeffrey B. Lyczak

topics covered

- ▲ Definitions and key concepts
- ▲ Cell types that carry out immune function
- ▲ The innate immune response
- ▲ The adaptive (or specific) immune response
- ▲ Organs and tissues essential for immune function
- ▲ Interactions between innate and acquired immune functions

- ▲ Modes of protection against various forms of disease
- ▲ Immune system dysfunction: immunodeficiency
- ▲ Diseases caused by undesirable immune responses: hypersensitivity and autoimmunity
- ▲ Role of the immune system in organ transplantation

Overview of Immunology

Definitions of Immunology and Immunity

Immunology is the study of the biologic mechanisms that constitute the cellular, molecular, and functional properties of the *immune system*. The principal biologic role of the immune system is to protect us from microbial infection. To accomplish this, the immune system produces molecular and cellular factors that can eliminate harmful microbes, often by having these factors bind directly to the microbe to promote its killing and eradication. The term for this protection, *immunity,* is derived from the Latin word *immunis* ("exempt").

The principal function of the immune system is to protect against infection. The modern appreciation of the physiologic function of the immune system is barely more than 100 years old. However, dating back to antiquity, it was known that for many diseases individuals were affected only once, after which they were immune or exempt from further bouts of the specific disease. In 430 B.C., the historian Thucydides, writing of a plague in Athens, noted that the ill could be nursed only by recovered plague victims, who would not contract the disease again. Even without any insight into the way in which the immune system worked, Edward Jenner was able in 1796 to expand on observations made by local farmers that their milkmaids who had a bout of cowpox, a mild disease, did not get the much more serious disease smallpox. Jenner took pustular material from a woman with cowpox and deliberately inoculated it into a young boy and subsequently challenged him with pustular material from someone with smallpox. The boy did not get the disease, and Jenner disseminated this finding to the physicians of the day, paving the way for understanding the immune system in modern terms and manipulating it to improve health—in this case, by vaccination.

Concurrent with the understanding of the germ theory of disease that emerged in the late 1800s, when microbial causes of infection and disease were first discovered, was the initial understanding that factors that mediated immunity were present in the blood. Both the noncellular or "humoral" fraction of the blood and the cells within the blood were found to have important functions in protecting against infection and mediating immunity. Early immunologists debated the relative importance of the humoral and cellular factors in carrying out immunity until it was realized that both played important roles in resistance to infection. But even rudimentary knowledge was sufficient to spur major advances in medicine. In the 1890s a German, Emil von Behring, and a Japanese colleague, Shibasaburo Kitasato, developed serum therapies for diseases known to be caused by toxins. In the presentation speech in 1901 for the first Nobel Prize in physiology or medicine award to von Behring, Count K. A. H. Mörner, rector of the Royal Caroline (now Karolinska) Institute in Sweden and professor of medicine, stated: "Blood fluid—or blood serum—from an individual who has been immunized with poisons from a certain bacterium can, namely, when introduced into the organs of another individual, confer resistance upon him against the bacterium in question. Upon this fact modern serum therapy is based." Von Behring's and Kitasato's serum therapy was one of the first demonstrations of how the careful scientific investigations pioneered by Louis Pasteur in France could be used as a basis for developing medical treatments that saved lives. Today, the foundation of biomedical scientific discoveries leading to advances in medical therapies is based on the value and importance of achieving a basic understanding of the molecular and cellular factors that are essential to the manifestation of a physiologic or pathologic process.

Whereas the 19th century saw the explosive start of the field of immunology, our current understanding of immunology has come mainly from work done in the last century wherein the molecular and cellular mechanisms that constitute the complex functions of the immune system have been uncovered. Thus, there is a sophisticated understanding of how the immune system works to mount a response to a microbial pathogen, rid the body of the agent, and become immune to further infection with the same agent through the development of *immunologic memory*. Advances in immunology have had

a widespread impact on health care. But typical of all current knowledge about biology, our information is incomplete, and many of the exact processes or mechanisms contributing to an immune response are not fully elucidated. Overall, there are many fine, detailed delineations of the functional aspects of immunity, but there are also many unknowns, giving rise to important questions that remain to be answered.

The Immune System: Key Definitions and Concepts

If immunity is defined as protection from infectious diseases, the immune system then consists of the molecules, cells, tissues, and organs that mediate this protection. The major primary organs of the immune system are the *bone marrow* and the *thymus,* where the cells of the immune system develop into functional cells (Fig. 1.1). Since the immune system must be ready to respond to infection anywhere in the body, its principal components are the cells that carry out responses to infection. These cells are concentrated in immune tissues, which include the blood, spleen, and lymphatic tissues, but the cells can go anywhere in the body to respond to and fight off infection.

Figure 1.1 Organs and tissues of the immune system.

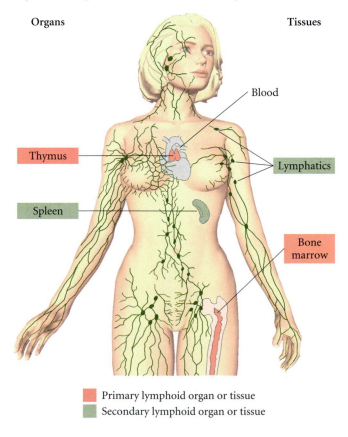

Organs   Tissues

Blood

Thymus

Lymphatics

Spleen

Bone marrow

■ Primary lymphoid organ or tissue
■ Secondary lymphoid organ or tissue

Blood is an important component of the immune system. It contains the *hematopoietic cells,* proteins, and liquid that circulate throughout the body. Hematopoietic cells are classified into *myeloid* (monocytes, macrophages, neutrophils, basophils, mast cells, and eosinophils), *lymphoid* (B cells and T cells), and *erythroid* lineages (red cells or erythrocytes). Each type of hematopoietic cell serves one or more immunologic functions (Fig. 1.2).

Plasma, the liquid component of blood, contains clotting factors. When blood clots, the hematopoietic cells are bound up in a web of protein created by clotting factors. The liquid that remains after the clot is formed is called *serum.* Many proteins in the blood also play an important role in immune responses (Fig. 1.2).

The major protein found in the blood and on mucosal surfaces such as the respiratory, gastrointestinal, and urogenital tracts that mediates immune system function is *antibody.* Antibodies, also called *immunoglobulins* (Ig), are distinguished by their ability to bind to foreign cells or molecules, termed *antigens,* in a highly specific manner. Antigens, most simply, are substances that an individual animal or human sees as foreign or *nonself* and mounts an immune response. These substances are distinguished from an individual's own biologic structures, representing *self* antigens, which should not provoke an immune system response against one's own body components. Thus, another hallmark of the immune system is the ability to discriminate between self and nonself antigens.

Often, but not always, the immune response involves production of antibodies. One end of an antibody molecule recognizes and binds to antigens in what can generally be conceptualized as a "lock-and-key" model, with the antigen-binding site on the antibody showing specificity for the antigen in the same way a key fits into a specific lock. This process is slightly more complex on an operational level, but it describes a basic hallmark of the immune system known as *immunologic specificity.* Practically, what this means is that the part of the antibody that recognizes and binds an antigen recognizes and binds only antigens or substances that are closely related in terms of their structure in three-dimensional space.

The lymphatic system is a network of vessels and nodes that circulate *lymph,* a plasma-derived fluid, throughout the body. Interstitial fluids (extracellular fluids that bathe many tissues of the body) drain into the lymphatic tissues, where they are filtered before returning to the bloodstream. The fluid-filtering structures (*lymph nodes*) are important immune tissues; here the cells of the immune system can survey the lymph for the presence of foreign agents brought there by cells that normally reside in the tissues and are programmed to identify and trans-port foreign antigens to the lymphatics. Many immune responses are initiated by cellular interactions that occur in the lymph nodes.

Hematopoietic cells are produced in the bone marrow. These cells originate from a single type of cell, called a *stem cell,* which has the potential to develop into any of the hematopoietic cells. The development of hematopoietic cells occurs in many stages. Cells that have completed the process of development are described as mature or *terminally differentiated.* Cells that mediate the immunologic reactions that lead to killing and elimination of harmful microbes or other harmful substances are said to be *effector cells.*

Most types of blood cells undergo the entire process of maturation in the bone marrow. One of these in particular is a central cell of the immune system, the *B cell* or *B lymphocyte.* This cell will produce the antibody molecule when the cell has been activated in an immunologically specific fashion by an antigen. Another type of lymphoid cell, called *T cell* or *T lymphocyte,* begins its development in the bone marrow but completes its maturation in the thymus. The final stages in the maturation of lymphoid cells therefore occur in both the bone marrow and thymus, and thus these tissues are called *primary lymphoid organs* or *tissues.* Mature lymphocytes leave the primary lymphoid organs and circulate through the blood and lymphatics, spending much of their time in lymph nodes. Activation of lymphocytes by antigen occurs at sites in the body called *secondary lymphoid organs* or *tissues.* These organs are specialized to support the activation of the mature immune cells. Secondary lymphoid tissues include the spleen and lymph nodes (Fig. 1.1), as well as the *mucosa-associated lymphoid tissue,* which is located in the gastrointestinal tract, respiratory tract, and urogenital tract and protects these barrier sites that are in constant contact with the microbe-filled environment.

T cells also recognize foreign antigens in an immunologically specific manner, but the form of the antigen recognized by the T cell is different from the form recognized by the B cell. As it turns out, the T cells have on their surface a specialized recognition structure known as the *T-cell receptor* (TCR). But for the TCR to bind to an antigen, the antigen first has to be derived from another parental protein molecule and broken down into small peptides by proteases. These small peptides are produced inside specialized cells called *antigen-presenting cells* (APCs). Once the small peptide is generated within the APC, it is complexed to another molecule made by the APCs termed a *major histocompatibility complex* (MHC) class II molecule. The complexing of the peptide and MHC class II occurs in vacuoles within the cytoplasm of

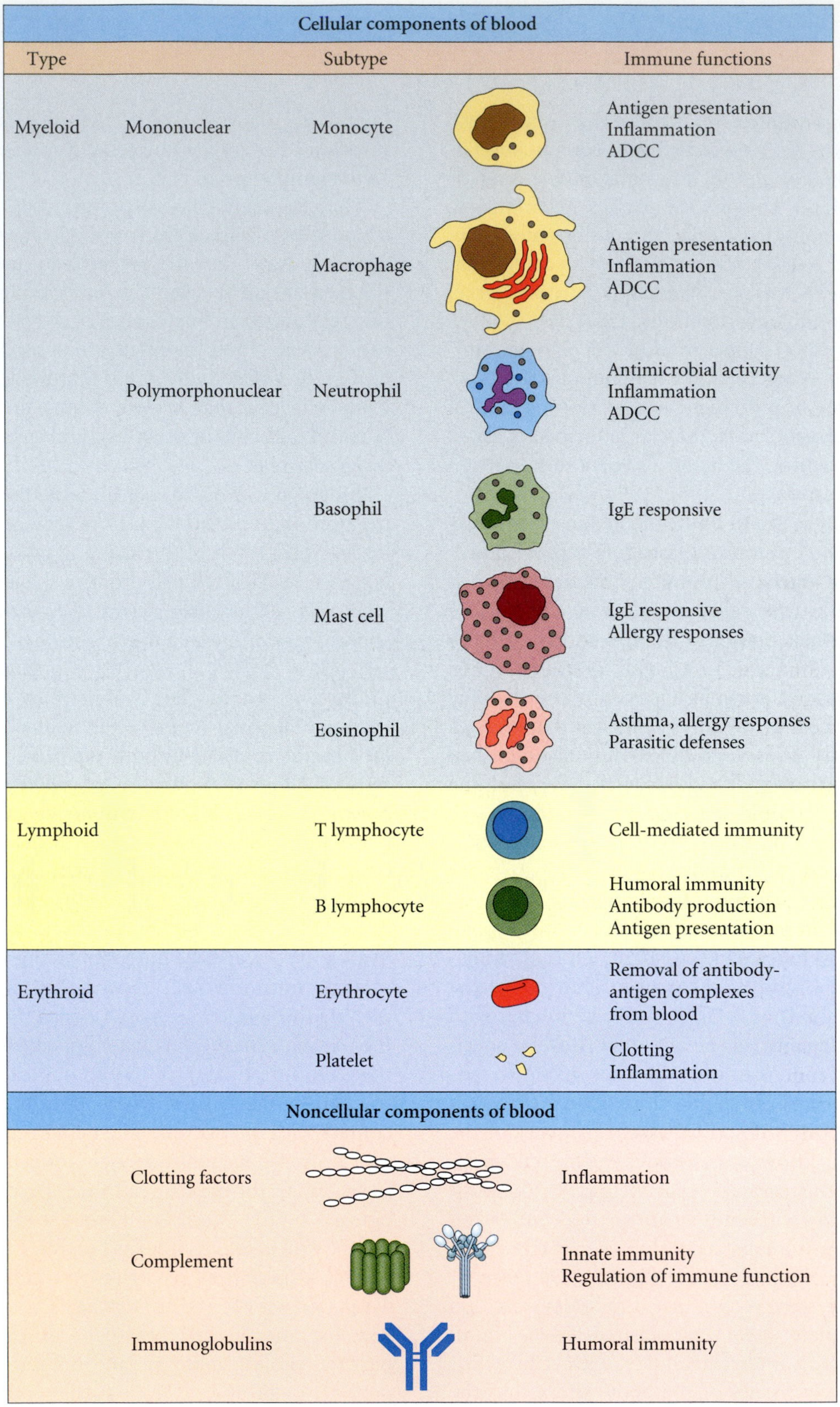

Figure 1.2 Components of blood and their immune functions. The hematopoietic cells are divided into myeloid, lymphoid, and erythroid lineages. These classifications are based both on developmental events and on specific functions of the mature effector cells. Each type of hematopoietic cell serves a distinct immune function(s). There is some overlap in the functions of different cell types. The noncellular components of blood are proteins that also serve immune functions. ADCC, antibody-dependent cell-mediated cytotoxicity.

the APCs, and the complex is then placed on the surface of the APCs. The TCR does not recognize the individual MHC class II or the individual peptide, but the complex of these two together. Cells that are not APCs can also produce small peptides and complex them to a different MHC molecule, termed the MHC class I molecule, for recognition by the TCR on T cells. In addition to peptide fragments complexed to MHC molecules, some T cells can recognize glycolipid antigens complexed to MHC-like molecules. Finally, those T cells that recognize peptides complexed to MHC class II have on their surface a specific molecule termed CD4, giving rise to *CD4+ T cells,* whereas those T cells that recognize peptides complexed to MHC class I have on their surface a specific molecule termed CD8, giving rise to *CD8+ T cells.*

Categories of Immune System Functions

Two broad categories of immune system function have been defined: *innate immunity* and *adaptive immunity* (Table 1.1). Innate immune mechanisms are nonspecific, meaning that the cells and molecules of the innate immune system respond in a general fashion to a broad array of foreign stimuli such as proteins, nucleic acids, carbohydrates, and microbial surface structures. These stimuli are made by a broad array of pathogens. Many of the response factors of the innate immune system are said to be always "on," meaning they are constitutive factors and present in the body at a basal level at all times. Some of these factors increase in number or amount during the initial response to antigenic stimuli, but the factors return to basal or homeostatic levels once the immune stimulus is removed. Factors of the innate immune system function well against many different disease-causing microorganisms (a microbe that can cause disease is termed a *pathogen*) because the factors recognize and respond to conserved molecules and structures produced by pathogens. Thus, they are generally *nonspecific* in the sense that conserved structures are produced by divergent microbial sources. In contrast, *adaptive* (also called *acquired* or *specific*) immune mechanisms are at rest until they encounter a particular pathogen expressing a specific antigen. Adaptive immunity can be subdivided into *humoral* and *cell-mediated* immune mechanisms.

Humoral immunity involves the activation of B lymphocytes and the production of antibodies by these B lymphocytes. Antibodies are found as soluble proteins in various body fluids, once called *humors,* and thus the name. Cell-mediated immunity involves activation of T lymphocytes by binding of antigenic peptides or glycolipids complexed to MHC molecules. T lymphocytes work by either activating other cell types to enhance their ability to kill and eliminate foreign microbes or directly killing a cell in the body infected with a foreign microbe, due to the property of *cytotoxicity.*

Adaptive immune responses are generally made to any foreign antigen, whether part of a living microbe or not. In addition, adaptive immune responses can be made to harmful cells like cancer cells and can potentially mediate resistance to cancer. In the cases where the antigen is not necessarily harmful, undesirable adaptive immune responses can occur. This happens with *allergy* or *hypersensitivity* when the immune response to something usually harmless like pollen or peanuts can be life-threatening instead of protective. Similarly, in modern medicine where lives can be saved by surgical transplantation of tissues, the immune system of the recipient of the transplant will see the transplanted tissue as foreign and mount an undesirable destructive response. And at times the immune system loses its normal refractivity to responding to self antigens and mounts an attack on an individual's own cells and tissues, leading to *autoimmune disease.*

Innate Immunity

Mechanisms of Innate Immunity

Innate immunity prevents pathogens from establishing themselves in the host's body (by convention, the animal being invaded, colonized, or infected by a foreign agent is called the *host*). This objective is achieved through diverse mechanisms (Table 1.2). Innate immune defenses range from physical barriers that keep pathogens out of the host's body to some enzymes that kill microorganisms that have gained access to the body. Innate immune

Table 1.1 Types of immunity

Innate	Adaptive	
Nonspecific; always on	Pathogen specific; induced	
	Humoral	Cell mediated
	Activation of B cells	Activation of T cells
	Production of antibody	Generation of cytokines

Table 1.2 Mechanisms of innate immunity

Mechanism	Example
Anatomic barriers	Skin, mucous membranes, mucus
Clearance mechanisms	Phagocytosis
Physiologic variables	pH, temperature, iron-binding proteins (lactoferrin, transferrin)
Enzymatic proteins	Lysozyme, complement
Chemical defenses	Superoxide, nitric oxide
Antimicrobial peptides	Defensins

mechanisms do not specifically target any particular pathogen, but rather molecules with similar structures expressed by a range of pathogens, and therefore work well against many different microorganisms. This quality is useful, considering the wide variety of microorganisms that are common in the environment.

Anatomic barriers prevent pathogens from entering the host's tissues. The host's exterior is protected by skin, and interior body spaces exposed to the outside environment (such as the digestive, excretory, and reproductive tracts) are protected by *mucous membranes.* The mucus produced by these membranes also acts as an anatomic barrier by trapping foreign microorganisms, bacteria, and particles, thus preventing them from gaining access to the underlying tissue where they can cause destruction and disease.

Physiologic barriers also include normal conditions in a host that create an environment unfavorable for the growth of microorganisms. For example, some pathogens such as the organism that causes leprosy infect body extremities because their growth is inhibited by the normal body temperature of humans (37°C [98.6°F]). In contrast, the growth of other pathogens is inhibited by temperatures above normal, as occurs during a fever. The low (acidic) pH in the stomach also inhibits the growth of most microorganisms, making the gastrointestinal route of infection a challenging one for most microbes. Sebum, an oily secretion produced by sebaceous glands in the dermal layer of the skin, helps maintain the pH of the skin surface between 3 and 5, limiting the range of microbes that can grow there.

Other innate immune mechanisms involve the killing of microorganisms by enzymatic, chemical, or antimicrobial activities of small peptides. *Lysozyme* is one such enzyme. Lysozyme is present in mucous secretions, tears, and saliva. Its substrate is peptidoglycan, a component of bacterial cell walls. Degradation of peptidoglycan by lysozyme damages the integrity of the bacterial cell, and the organism cannot survive.

Chemical killing of microorganisms can occur intracellularly or extracellularly. Phagocytic cells release chemicals (nitric oxide, hypochlorous acid, and superoxide) into the phagosome, where they destroy engulfed bacteria (Fig. 1.3). When macrophages are activated, these chemicals also are released into the extracellular space, killing any nearby bacteria.

Antimicrobial peptides are small proteins present on many mucosal surfaces that have potent bactericidal activity. One such type of peptide is called a *defensin.* These are small peptides produced by phagocytic cells that are stored in subcellular organelles called *granules.* When these cells are activated, the granules fuse with the

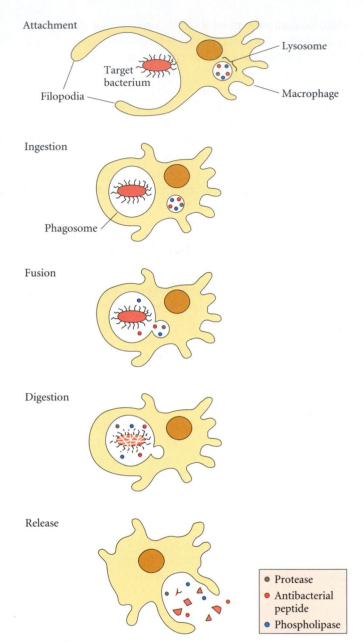

Figure 1.3 Phagocytosis. The phagocytic cell adheres to a microorganism by extrusions of the cell membrane called *filopodia.* The cell surrounds the microorganism and engulfs, or ingests, it into a subcellular structure called the phagosome. Other membrane-bound organelles, called *lysosomes,* contain enzymes and cytotoxic chemicals. The lysosome fuses with the phagosome and releases its contents. The engulfed microorganism is digested, and the debris is released from the cell by fusion of the phagosome to the cell membrane.

cellular plasma membrane and release their contents into the extracellular space, where they are thought to act primarily by damaging the membranes of the bacteria they encounter. Defensins also are produced by certain cells in the lining of the intestine (intestinal crypts), where they are called *cryptdins.*

Some components of the innate immune response are aimed at depriving bacteria of essential nutritional materials. For example, bacterial growth requires iron since this element is commonly utilized by bacterial enzymes as a cofactor. The mammalian host, therefore, produces proteins such as *lactoferrin* and *transferrin* that tightly bind iron and make it unavailable for bacterial utilization. In addition, these iron-binding proteins also have some intrinsic antibacterial properties associated with production of cleavage products that act like antimicrobial peptides and disrupt bacterial membranes, resulting in killing.

Another central component of innate immunity is the family of serum proteins called the *complement system*. Complement proteins are synthesized in an inactive state awaiting activation by any of a number of stimuli. Although complement can be activated by the binding of antibodies to their antigens, it can also be activated directly by some antigens. This is possible because the surfaces of many microbial cells contain a number of molecular structures that do not exist on animal cells. When complement proteins bind to such foreign cells, they are able to undergo activation and thus alert the host to the presence of a nonself substance. Most members of the complement family of proteins are enzymes that, when activated, partake in a chain reaction that culminates in several immunologically important events. One such event is the formation of a *membrane attack complex* (MAC) on the surface of a microbial cell or virus. The MAC can protect the host by directly destroying the microbe or virus. Other events caused by complement activation include enhanced phagocytosis due to attachment of complement proteins to the microbe (*opsonization*) and attraction of several immune cell types to the location of complement activation.

Although the innate immune system is designed to deal with a wide array of bacterial, fungal, viral, and protozoan microorganisms, it requires multiple means of identifying its targets as foreign and potentially harmful. In addition to complement activation, the innate immune system has other means to recognize microbial *molecular patterns*, structural components or motifs that are present on a wide variety of microorganisms but are not found among the host's own cells or tissues. An example of a molecular pattern associated with bacterial infection is the lipopolysaccharide (LPS), also called endotoxin, that comprises the outer leaflet of the outer membrane of gram-negative bacteria. This structure is not produced by mammalian cells, and its presence in the tissues of a mammal, therefore, heralds the presence of gram-negative bacteria. Molecular patterns such as LPS are rec-

ognized by a class of cell surface receptors termed *pattern recognition receptors* or *pattern recognition molecules*. In the case of LPS, the molecular pattern is recognized by the receptor called Toll-like receptor 4 that is present on the surface of several immune cell types. Some components of the complement family of protein can also be classified as pattern recognition molecules and serve to activate the complement system when microbe-associated patterns are detected.

Cellular Effectors of Innate Immunity

Phagocytes

Patrolling the body, particularly on mucosal surfaces and in the blood, are cells that can readily recognize foreign antigens, often tagged with activated complement components, and ingest the antigen in a process call *phagocytosis*. Phagocytosis is a clearance mechanism that serves to remove and kill microbial pathogens that have gained access to normally sterile tissues (Fig. 1.3). Phagocytic cells recognize foreign microorganisms and ingest (or engulf) them. The ingested organism is held within a subcellular organelle called the *phagosome*. The cell releases into the phagosome toxic compounds that digest and kill the microorganism.

The major types of phagocytes, often referred to as "professional phagocytes," are the *monocyte/macrophage* and the *polymorphonuclear neutrophil* (PMN). Monocytes are found in the blood and migrate into different tissues where they further differentiate to become *tissue-fixed macrophages*. These are referred to by older anatomical names such as alveolar macrophages found in the lung, Kupffer cells found in the liver, and mesangial cells found in the kidney. The network of tissue-fixed macrophages forms the basis for the *mononuclear phagocyte system*, which has been referred to in older literature as the *reticuloendothelial system*. These phagocytes look for foreign substances in the blood or tissues and ingest them via phagocytosis for neutralization and elimination.

PMNs are principally found in the blood and live only 12 to 24 hours. Therefore, a prodigious amount of new PMNs are made each day by an individual. However, early after an antigenic stimulus is detected, the PMNs leave the blood and travel to the site of infection, ready to ingest antigens and kill those that are living. On their surface PMNs express receptors for antibody molecules and for factors of the complement system that have bound to a foreign antigen. Such tagged antigens are even more readily ingested and, if appropriate, killed by the PMNs. Individuals who undergo cancer chemotherapy often have a major decline in their PMN level, which leaves them susceptible to infection from bacteria and fungi. This type of clinical experience provides crucial insight to support the role of PMNs in resistance to these infections.

Natural killer cells

The *natural killer* (NK) cell is a type of lymphocyte with cytotoxic activity. One major function of NK cells is to patrol the body looking for aberrant cells that have reduced or eliminated expression of MHC class I. This occurs during intracellular microbial infection or with some tumor cells. NK cells have a default program to kill target cells they encounter. To prevent killing of healthy cells, NK cells have receptors for MHC-class I; engagement of the receptor by a self-MHC inhibits the NK cells' killing activity. Therefore, these cells identify and destroy cells that are identified as aberrant by their lack of proper MHC expression. NK cells are effective in destroying tumors and virus-infected cells, both of which may have a decreased expression of MHC class I proteins and therefore escape killing by CTLs.

Most of the time the mechanisms of innate immunity function exceedingly well to protect an animal against a constant onslaught of potential pathogens and toxic and harmful substances. However, problems can arise quickly when innate mechanisms of immunity do not function properly or are subverted by microorganisms that have developed means to evade innate immune defenses. Disruption of an anatomic barrier can provide microorganisms with easy access to a normally sterile environment. For example, a break in the skin may allow microorganisms to enter the blood, or a breakdown of clearance mechanisms may enable microorganisms to gain access to the body. When such situations arise, it is the role of the adaptive immune system to mount a response to protect the host from infection and disease.

Cooperation among Innate Immune Mechanisms

Several types of innate defenses act in concert with other physiologic events to produce the body's response to tissue damage (*inflammation*). The first event in inflammation is the release of factors affecting blood vessel diameter (*vasoactive factors*). Histamine is a vasoactive factor released by several types of cells in response to tissue damage. It causes capillaries and venules to increase in diameter (*vasodilation*) and increases their permeability. Kinin, another vasoactive factor, is a small plasma protein that is activated by tissue injury.

Capillaries within the damaged tissue vasodilate and vessels that lead away from the damaged tissue vasoconstrict (decrease in diameter), resulting in the entry of more blood into the injured site and the departure of less blood from the site. Thus, the local capillary network becomes engorged, creating redness (*erythema*) and increasing the temperature in the tissue. Capillary permeability increases, which allows fluid (*exudate*) and cells to enter the damaged tissue. The exudate contains blood-clotting proteins and enzymes, and its accumulation leads to swelling of the tissue (*edema*).

At this site of inflammation, phagocytic cells exit the circulation and move into the damaged tissue (*emigration*) to survey it for possible infection. This occurs in several steps. First, the phagocytic cells adhere to endothelial cells that line the blood vessel (*margination*). This adherence is enhanced when endothelium is activated to express additional "cell-adhesion" molecules. Next, the phagocytic cells enter the tissue by squeezing between the epithelial cells (*diapedesis* or *extravasation*). Finally, the phagocytic cells migrate to the site of the inflammation (*chemotaxis*) (Fig. 1.4). When the phagocytic cells arrive at the site of damage, they engulf bacteria that are present. As noted above, phagocytosis triggers the release of enzymes and chemicals that can damage the nearby host tissue. Thus, the killing of bacteria may be accompanied by some damage to normal host cells and tissues. The accumulated detritus of dead cells, digested material, and fluid is called *pus*.

Figure 1.4 The inflammatory response. The black arrows show the path of the monocyte from its initial location in the blood circulation to its final destination at the site of injury or infection.

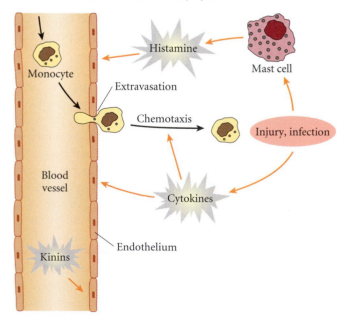

The exudate contains blood-clotting enzymes and proteins. The blood-clotting cascade is activated, resulting in the deposit of a netlike web of *fibrin* (the major protein in blood clots). The blood clot serves to wall off the injured area and helps prevent the spread of infection.

Later events in inflammation occur at sites remote from the active inflammatory process. The so-called *acute-phase proteins* are released. For example, the liver produces C-reactive protein. This protein binds to a conserved structure called the C-polysaccharide found in the cell wall of a number of bacteria and fungi. Binding of C-reactive protein activates the complement system, enhancing clearance of the microorganisms by lysis or phagocytosis. The acute-phase response also increases the synthesis of complement proteins.

Repair and regeneration begin when phagocytic cells have cleared most of the debris away and the inflammatory response has subsided. Capillaries grow into the blood clot. As the clot dissolves, connective tissue cells (fibroblasts) replace the fibrin with a matrix that is primarily collagen. The repair tissue is usually scar tissue (except in the liver, which can regenerate, and bone, which undergoes remodeling).

Innate immune mechanisms collaborate in other ways. The complement system, in particular, enhances and activates other innate immune mechanisms. For example, activated complement proteins coat bacteria, and the bacteria are opsonized as a result. Complement also activates the fibrinolytic system. Finally, the activated complement proteins are chemotactic for neutrophils and eosinophils.

Mechanisms of Adaptive Immunity

Self/Nonself Discrimination

The concept of acquired immunity (i.e., resistance to subsequent infection) is based on the development of immunity *after* an individual is exposed to a particular microorganism. A key element of adaptive immunity is the concept of self and the discrimination between self and nonself antigens. For acquired immune responses to be appropriately activated, the immune system must be able to differentiate between something of the individual's own body (self) and something that is not (nonself). The MHC proteins, expressed on the surface of all cells in the body, serve to provide the immune system with the information to discriminate self from nonself. There are two types of MHC proteins: class I proteins are expressed on all cells, and class II proteins are expressed only on APCs. APCs include cells known as macrophages, B cells, and dendritic cells. During maturation of the T cells of the immune system the MHC proteins present peptides derived from self antigens to the maturing cells, and this serves as one means to eliminate any lymphocytes that could react to self antigens. Similarly, maturing B lymphocytes in the bone marrow that encounter self antigens during this early phase are eliminated. If this mechanism allows a potentially self-reactive lymphocyte to mature, other mechanisms exist to prevent one's own lymphocytes from reacting to one's own antigens. Some immunologists have proposed that nonself reactivity is maintained by making it difficult for an immune response to be initiated unless there is some damage to the tissue, resulting in production of a *danger signal*. Under these circumstances the immune system is activated to respond to the antigens initiating the damage.

Self and nonself recognition is essential to the health of an individual. If foreign invaders are not recognized as nonself, the acquired immune responses are not triggered. Similarly, inappropriate triggering of the immune response by self antigens can lead to the host's being attacked by the very immune effectors intended to protect it.

Cellular Effectors of Adaptive Immunity

Adaptive immunity can be subdivided into cell-mediated and humoral immunity (Fig. 1.5; Table 1.3), labels that can be somewhat confusing, since both types of immunity involve cells—the lymphocytes. Cell-mediated

Figure 1.5 Effectors of the acquired immune response. The lymphocytes (T cells and B cells) are the mediators of acquired immune responses. T cells express the TCR, coreceptors (CD4 or CD8), and other cell surface proteins (CD3, Thy1). Activated T cells produce cell-mediated acquired immune responses (either cytotoxic or helper functions, depending on the type of T cell stimulated). B cells express mIg or BCR and other cell surface proteins with immune functions (Ig-α/β, B220). Activated B cells produce humoral acquired immune responses (production of antibodies).

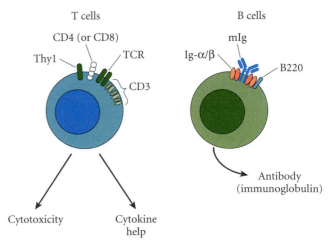

Table 1.3 Lymphocytes and proteins involved in acquired immune response

Acquired immune mechanism	Type of lymphocyte	Proteins produced
Cell mediated	T cell	Cytokines
Humoral	B cell	Antibodies

immunity involves activation of T lymphocytes and other cells capable of cytotoxic activity against foreign agents. Humoral immunity involves activation of B lymphocytes and the production of antibodies.

The capacity of the acquired immune system to respond to any type of invading organism depends on an elegant network of cells and cell products. In brief, specialized immune cells (lymphocytes) circulate throughout the body. Each lymphocyte leaves the bone marrow or thymus programmed to respond to a single foreign antigen. Before these cells encounter their antigens, they are called *naive*. When a lymphocyte encounters the antigen for which it is specific, the lymphocyte is activated and its immune functions are initiated. Activated lymphocytes

proliferate (divide) and then differentiate into either effector cells or memory cells (Fig. 1.6). Memory cells are strategically placed throughout an individual's body to await subsequent encounters with the same antigen and are more readily activated by that antigen. Memory cells are long-lived, and their persistence explains, in part, why frequently we do not become ill from the same disease twice. The memory response makes acquired immunity well suited for repeated encounters with a given foreign agent and for responding to large threats (e.g., large doses of bacteria). One mechanism whereby pathogenic microbes counter adaptive immunity is by varying the antigens on their surface such that an immune response to one form of the microbe does not protect against another form. For example, only one antigenic variant of tetanus toxin exists so immunity to this single protein, provided by vaccination, is sufficient to protect against tetanus no matter which strain of the tetanus-causing bacterium is encountered. On the other hand, the common cold virus comes in over 200 different antigenic variants, so humans suffer colds throughout their lives, usually with a different variant causing disease each time.

Figure 1.6 The acquired immune response involves the activation of lymphocytes upon their encounter with specific antigen. Before encountering its antigen, the lymphocyte (then referred to as a naive lymphocyte) is quiescent. Upon encountering antigen, the lymphocyte undergoes a two-step activation process that first involves rapid cell division (proliferation) and then differentiation into a mature cell type. Each activated lymphocyte that results from the period of proliferation differentiates into either an effector cell (which can carry out immune functions) or a memory cell. The memory cell reenters a resting state to await encounter with the same antigen.

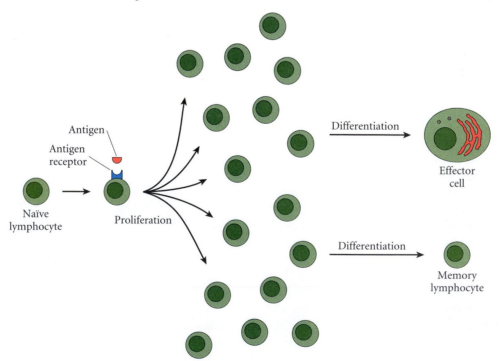

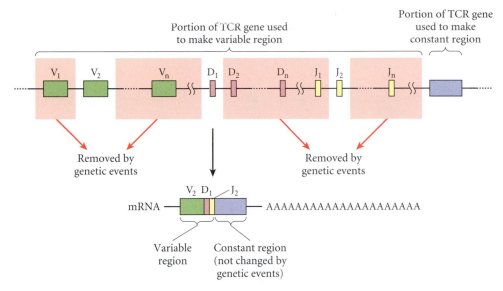

Portion of TCR gene used to make variable region

Portion of TCR gene used to make constant region

Removed by genetic events

Removed by genetic events

mRNA

Variable region

Constant region (not changed by genetic events)

Figure 1.7 Generation of TCRs by gene rearrangement. The gene that eventually encodes the TCR originally consists of many *gene segments*. Some of these gene segments, called *V, D,* and *J* segments, are randomly combined with each other to produce a combination of segments that confers a unique antigenic specificity on the TCR (due to the variable region). Another portion of the TCR gene (called the constant region) is not altered by the gene rearrangements. This portion of the TCR gene is the same for all TCRs in each of the four TCR classes (α, β, γ, and δ).

T lymphocytes

T lymphocytes are generated in the bone marrow and move to the thymus to complete their development. They express cell surface proteins called TCRs (receptors found *on* T cells as opposed to receptors *for* T cells) (Fig. 1.5). TCRs are encoded by special genes that undergo genetic changes during the development of the T cell (Fig. 1.7). During these genetic changes (called *rearrangements*), segments of these genes are spliced out of the cellular genomic DNA. The proteins encoded by the rearranged genes are unique to each T cell. It has been estimated that there are 10^{12} possible combinations of genes to generate TCR proteins, meaning that an enormous number of antigens can potentially be recognized by T cells.

The TCR is like one piece of a puzzle and the antigen engaged by that TCR is like the matching puzzle piece. Interaction of the TCR with its specific antigen leads to activation of the T cell (Fig. 1.8). The TCR-antigen interactions shown in Fig. 1.8 are simplified to illustrate this concept. In reality, the antigen must be presented to the T cell by an APC (Fig. 1.9). For antigen presentation to occur, the antigen must first be processed by the APC. During processing, the antigen, usually a protein, is broken down into smaller peptide fragments and noncovalently loaded onto an MHC molecule. Part of the MHC molecule contains a pocket or groove for loading of peptide fragments. In order to bind a large variety of peptides many different forms of MHC molecules exist, and a small subset of these are expressed by one individual. The subset is usually sufficient to complex a wide variety of antigenic peptides that can be transported to the surface of the APC. The TCR recognizes the complex, not the individual peptide alone or the MHC alone or the two independently. Thus the matching "puzzle piece" recognized by the TCR is in reality the peptide-MHC complex.

Figure 1.8 Simplified view of antigen recognition by a T cell. The T cell recognizes not a whole, intact antigen, but a small peptide fragment of a protein antigen complexed to an MHC protein. For the T cell to become activated, its antigen receptor must be able to recognize both the MHC and the antigenic peptide.

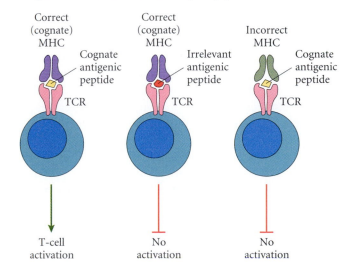

Correct (cognate) MHC

Correct (cognate) MHC

Incorrect MHC

Cognate antigenic peptide

Irrelevant antigenic peptide

Cognate antigenic peptide

TCR

TCR

TCR

T-cell activation

No activation

No activation

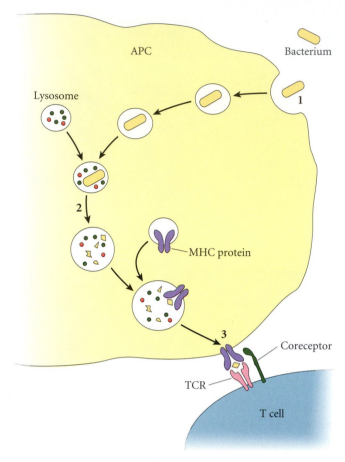

Figure 1.9 Simplified view of antigen presentation. A microorganism (in this case, a bacterium) is phagocytosed (**1**) and killed (**2**) by an APC. The green and red circles represent hydrolytic enzymes that are stored in vesicles known as lysosomes. Portions of the digested bacterium are displayed on the surface of the phagocytic cell by MHC proteins (**3**). The TCR recognizes the antigen, and the coreceptor recognizes the MHC.

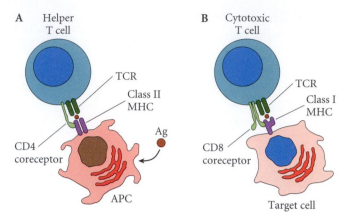

Figure 1.10 Interactions between a helper or cytotoxic T cell and an APC. (**A**) TH cells express the CD4 coreceptor, which interacts with MHC class II on a professional APC. TH cells enhance the functions of other immune cells (phagocytic or B cells). (**B**) Cytotoxic T cells express the CD8 coreceptor, which interacts with MHC class I on any cell (called a target cell). Cytotoxic T cells lyse target cells presenting the antigen (Ag) for which the T cell is specific.

Along with the TCR, the T cell expresses other proteins known as coreceptor proteins (termed CD4 and CD8) that interact with the MHC on the surface of APCs. However, CD4, which binds to MHC class II, and CD8, which binds to MHC class I, bind to conserved portions of the MHC molecule, not the portion containing the antigen-MHC complex.

Several types of T lymphocytes serve specific and somewhat different immune functions. Helper T cells (TH cells), so-called because they help to increase the activity of other immune cells by producing signaling molecules called *cytokines,* are identified by the presence of the CD4 coreceptor (CD4$^+$ T cells) on their surface. Thus, CD4$^+$ T cells specifically interact with peptides bound to MHC class II on professional APCs (Fig. 1.10A). A subclass of TH cells, TH1, produces a certain pattern of signaling cytokines that often results in

immune responses that combat intracellular pathogens that are able to reside in host phagocytic cells and prevent the cells from killing them. The cytokines produced by stimulated TH1 cells enhance intracellular killing of pathogens residing in phagocytic cells. In contrast, TH2 cells produce a pattern of signaling cytokines resulting in antibody production that is mostly effective at mediating opsonization and killing of extracellular antigens that do not normally survive within host cells. Often activated TH1 cells produce cytokines that inhibit TH2 responses and vice versa.

The second major population of T cells is the CTLs that express the CD8 coreceptor (CD8$^+$ T cells). This molecule interacts with MHC class I, which is present on all nucleated cells of the body although with varying levels of expression (Fig. 1.10B). The MHC class I molecule on a cell is also complexed to a peptide, but normally this peptide is derived from a self antigen. Under these circumstances the cell is recognized as self and left alone by the immune system. However, if a foreign, replicating pathogen such as a virus infects the cell, then the MHC class I will display peptides derived from the foreign invader since these peptides are derived from viral proteins being synthesized within the infected cell in the same manner as self proteins. CD8$^+$T cells can recognize the complex of self-MHC class I and microbial peptide as foreign and respond by becoming activated. The activated CTLs induce lysis of the target cell, thereby destroying the cell that harbored the pathogen. This prevents further replication of the pathogen. In addition, CTLs may also express antimicrobial factors that directly kill the intracellular parasites released, preventing them from infecting other cells. CD8$^+$ CTLs are not only effective in mediating protection against intracellular pathogens but can also serve to eliminate aberrant self cells such as those that could give rise to cancers.

B lymphocytes

Like T cells, B cells have unique cell surface proteins (B-cell receptors [BCRs]) that bind antigen (Fig. 1.5). Unlike T cells, however, B cells produce secreted forms of the BCR, and this is antibody or Ig. The BCR, therefore, is often referred to as membrane immunoglobulin (mIg). A schematic diagram of a basic antibody monomer is shown in Fig. 1.11. The antibody monomer is a heterotetramer and is composed of two large, identical *heavy chains* and two smaller, identical *light chains.* Both the heavy and light chains have regions that are similar in many antibodies (called the *constant region*) and other regions that are unique to each antibody (called the *variable region*). The variable regions confer the antibody's specificity for its antigen and bind directly to the antigen (the antigen-binding region of the antibody molecule). Some antibodies, such as IgM, are made up of multiple monomers. However, each monomer still has two identical heavy chains and two identical light chains.

The diversity of antibodies for binding to a large array of different antigens is generated through gene rearrangement similar to the process used to generate the T cell's antigen receptor (Fig. 1.7). This gene-rearrangement process occurs during B-cell development in the bone mar-row. By relatively random rearrangements, two or three genes (also called genetic segments) encoding for the variable regions of light and heavy chains, respectively, are brought together to form a new gene that encodes the amino acids that make up the variable region of the antibody molecule. By these random associations many more combinations of antigen-binding regions can be generated from a limited number of variable-region genes. For example, if there were 10 genes for each of the 2 light-chain antigen-binding segments that could combine together randomly, then out of 20 genes there are 100 possible combinations (10 × 10). Similarly, if there were 10 genes for each of the 3 heavy-chain antigen-binding segments, then out of 30 genes there are 1,000 possible combinations (10 × 10 × 10). And because heavy and light chains can combine more or less randomly, then out of the 50 genes for antigen-binding segments in this hypothetical example, there are 100,000 (100 light chains × 1,000 heavy chains) possible combinations. The genetic basis for generating diversity in antibodies, discovered in the 1980s, showed that BCR, and later, TCR are not produced by the one-to-one relationship previously thought to exist between genes and proteins.

When B cells finish their maturation in the bone marrow, they are said to be *immunocompetent* and leave the marrow and migrate to the lymphatic system. They circulate throughout the body by spending time migrating between the lymph nodes of the lymphatics and also spend time being distributed throughout the body via the blood circulation. This provides B cells access to vascular secondary lymphoid organs such as the spleen and also places them at other body sites if they are needed to respond to an antigenic stimulus. B cells not only have the capacity to produce antibody in response to antigen, but they can also function as APCs due to expression of MHC class II molecules, albeit not as well as other APCs such as dendritic cells. But if a circulating B cell captures foreign antigen on its surface BCR, it will migrate to a local lymphoid tissue and present the antigen to TH cells. The lymphoid tissues are the sites of interaction between lymphocytes that have encountered antigens.

Activation of B cells generally requires two signals (Fig. 1.12). The first signal is initiated by binding of mIg molecules to the specific or *cognate* antigen, resulting in *crosslinking* of the mIg. The mIg-antigen complex is internalized into the B cell, the antigen processed and presented for interaction with TCR on a T cell that recognizes antigen-MHC complexes. The TH cell also provides a second set of stimulatory signals mediated by binding of additional, non-antigen-specific receptors and ligands on T and B cells and by soluble factors released by the TH

Figure 1.11 Structural diagram of an antibody. Antibodies are tetramers consisting of four peptides: two heavy chains and two light chains. Both the heavy and light chains have constant regions (blue), where the amino acid sequence is conserved (similar) among all antibodies, and variable regions (green), where the amino acid sequence is unique to that particular antibody. Antibodies may be secreted or may be "tethered" to the cell surface by a short, transmembrane domain added to the amino acid sequence of the heavy chain.

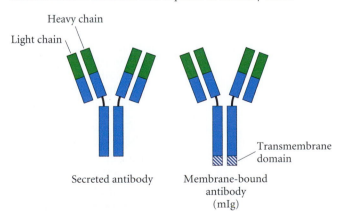

Heavy chain
Light chain
Transmembrane domain
Secreted antibody
Membrane-bound antibody (mIg)

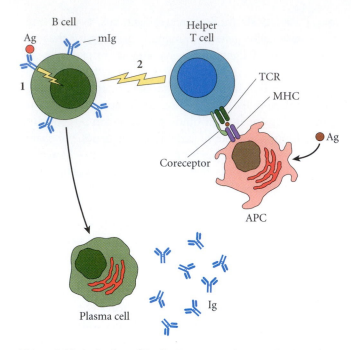

Figure 1.12 Activation of B cells. For most antigens, activation of B cells requires two signals. Signal 1 is delivered by the binding of the antigen to the mIg on the B cell. Signal 2 is delivered to the B cell by a TH cell that is also stimulated by antigenic fragments bound to MHC molecules. Activation of a B cell in this manner leads to differentiation of the B cell into an antibody (Ig)-secreting plasma cell. This figure also highlights the fact that B cells and T cells recognize the same antigen by two different mechanisms—the B cell by "directly" binding to the intact antigen and the T cell by recognizing a peptide fragment of the antigen complexed to an MHC protein.

cell. These activated B cells then develop into two types of cells: the *plasma cell,* which is the source of synthesis of large amounts of specific antibody, and the *memory B cell,* which will participate in rapid responses to subsequent encounters with its specific antigen.

Plasma cells are specialized for the production and secretion of large quantities of soluble antibodies. The first type of antibody produced by a newly activated plasma cell is of the class called IgM (Table 1.4). This initial production of antibody is part of the *primary immune response.* As the B cell matures, the specificity of its antibody for the stimulating antigen stays the same, but the class of antibody changes through a process called *class switching.* Different classes of antibodies perform different immunologic and biologic functions in the body. For example, antibodies of the IgM class are very efficient in activating the complement system. Antibodies of the IgG class also activate complement, although not as well as IgM. However, IgG antibodies are bound by specialized cell surface receptors expressed by macrophages and other immune cells, triggering phagocytosis and killing of the antibody-bound microbes. Typically, anti-

bodies produced early after the initial activation of a B cell are low-affinity antibodies (meaning the interaction between antibody and antigen is not very strong). During B-cell maturation after antigenic activation, a second process, called *affinity maturation,* can alter the antigen-binding site of the antibody, which through a complex process increases the affinity for antigen but without changing the specificity in any significant way.

Memory B cells also develop from mature B cells after an initial or primary antigenic stimulation and, once established in the body, rapidly produce large amounts of antibody, not of the IgM class but of other classes, upon subsequent or secondary antigenic stimulation. Memory B cells usually develop to produce either IgG, IgA, or IgE when activated by additional encounters with an antigen to which there has been a previous response. Memory B cells act as sentinels that can rapidly produce antibodies to neutralize a harmful foreign microbe or toxin. The rapid and enhanced synthesis of antibodies by memory B cells comprises the *secondary immune response,* which is also the molecular basis for immunologic memory.

There are, however, certain antigens, called *T-cell-independent antigens,* that can bypass the two-signal mechanism shown in Fig. 1.12 and stimulate B cells directly without the assistance of TH cells (Fig. 1.13). Type 1 T-cell-independent antigens are *mitogenic,* meaning that they have an intrinsic ability to stimulate proliferation of B cells. Thus, in addition to binding to mIg on specific B cells that recognize the antigen, T-cell-independent antigens also send a proliferative signal through other receptors, bypassing the need for T-cell help (Fig. 1.13A). Also, these type 1 T-cell-independent antigens

Table 1.4   Immunoglobulin classes

Subtype	Cell type	Characteristics
IgM	Newly activated B cells	Indicates primary exposure to antigen
		Forms pentamers in serum
		Effectively fixes complement proteins
IgD	Naive B cells	Expressed as mIg (with IgM)
IgG	Memory B cells	Indicates reexposure to antigen
		Monomeric in serum
		Effectively fixes complement proteins
		Can cross the placental barrier
IgE	Memory B cells	Mediates allergic and asthmatic responses
IgA	B cells in mucosa	Dimeric (J chain binds constant regions)
		High concentrations in mucosal secretions

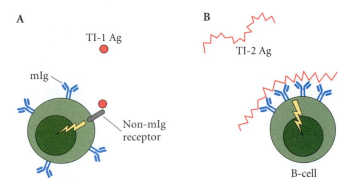

Figure 1.13 T-cell-independent antigens. (A) Type 1 T-cell-independent antigens (TI-1 Ag) are mitogenic for B cells, regardless of the antigenic specificities of the B cell. (B) Type 2 T-cell-independent antigens (TI-2 Ag) engage many BCRs of the same specificity on a single B-cell surface at the same time, effectively cross-linking the mIg and activating the B cell in a manner that does not depend on activational signals from a TH cell.

can stimulate the proliferation of many different B cells, not just those that are specific for the antigen, because the mitogenic property of the antigen is able to initiate activation of many B cells in what is referred to as *nonspecific activation*. An example of such an antigen is endotoxin, a glycolipid also commonly called LPS that is found in the cell wall of gram-negative bacteria. In contrast, type 2 T-cell-independent antigens extensively cross-link mIg in a specific fashion on the surface of B cells recognizing the antigen in a classic fashion, and this provides a type of costimulatory signal in the absence of T-cell help (Fig. 1.13B). These type 2 T-cell-independent antigens are typically very large with a highly repetitive structure, such as polysaccharides found in and on bacterial cell surfaces.

Organs That Support the Acquired Immune Response

The antigen receptors that are expressed by T and B lymphocytes recognize a wide array of antigenic structures and do so in a highly discriminating fashion. Although diversity and specificity allow lymphocytes the flexibility to respond to an incredible chemical and structural array of foreign antigens, this situation leads to having only a few lymphocytes existing in the body at one time point that can respond to a given antigen. How is it that one of these antigen-specific lymphocytes is able to *find* its antigen after the antigen enters the host's body? This problem is partially addressed through the existence of specialized tissues termed secondary lymphoid tissues such as the spleen and lymph nodes that serve to maximize the efficiency with which lymphocytes encounter their antigens. What generally happens is that foreign antigens are recognized and ingested at or close to sites of entry by a

highly effective APC termed a *dendritic cell*. The dendritic cell is immature at this point, but as it migrates toward a local secondary lymphoid tissue with its cargo of antigen, it begins to change and mature. The secondary lymphoid tissues are loaded with B cells and T cells that arrive there in high numbers due to a specialized vasculature that serves to recruit lymphocytes to the secondary lymphoid tissue. This process brings antigens associated with the dendritic cells and lymphocytes together in relatively high concentrations such that interactions are more likely to occur. Dendritic cells have long arms or processes (i.e., dendrites) so that one dendritic cell bearing antigen can interact with many different lymphocytes at once. Thus, the rapid movement of the lymphocytes around the arms of the dendritic cells facilitates their ability to find the correct antigen or antigen-MHC complex.

Cytokines: Regulators of Immune Function

Virtually every aspect of both innate and acquired immune function requires careful regulation. Such regulation enhances the effectiveness of the immune response and ensures that the immune response occurs only under appropriate conditions, lasts for an appropriate duration, and has an appropriate magnitude. In most cases, regulation of the immune response is mediated by cytokines, small proteins that are produced by one cell and have a biological effect on another cell (although, in some circumstances, a cytokine can affect the same cell that produced it). Whereas TH cells have the distinction of being dedicated to the production of cytokines, many cell types, immune and nonimmune, have the ability to secrete cytokines. The cell that is affected by the cytokine bears a cell surface receptor that binds specifically to that one cytokine. The greater that cell's expression of the cytokine receptor, the more sensitive the cell is to the presence of the cytokine.

Cytokines have numerous cellular effects that result in stimulation, suppression, and/or modification of the immune response. The cytokine interleukin-2 (IL-2) is usually produced by TH cells and binds to a receptor on cytotoxic T cells. The binding of IL-2 to its receptor is essential for activation of the cytotoxic T cell. Cytokines with immunosuppressive activity include IL-10 and transforming growth factor beta. Cytokines such as interferon-gamma and IL-4 can help guide a developing acquired immune response, deciding whether the host response will entail predominantly antibody production or cytotoxic T-cell activation. Thus, the presence of cytokines can determine not only *whether* an immune response will occur but also *what kind* of immune response develops. Another family of cytokines, the *chemokines,* seems largely responsible for the regulation of chemotaxis and cell trafficking through the body. For example, during a localized inflammatory response (Fig. 1.4), the chemokine IL-8 is a critical signal for instructing leukocytes in the bloodstream to leave the circulation and enter the surrounding tissue near the site of injury or infection.

Interactions between Acquired and Innate Immunity

Innate and acquired immune systems are two means of defending against infection and, together, provide high levels of protection for an individual. The features of the acquired immune response make it useful for dealing with a repeated exposure to a specific microbial pathogen. However, using this system all of the time to respond to the continuous, low-level exposure to diverse microorganisms encountered by a typical mammal from day to day would be inefficient. For example, airborne bacteria typically number 100 to 500 per cubic meter, such that an animal inhales many bacteria each day, but only in small doses at a given time. Urban water supplies (even those purified through modern sanitation methods) can contain many bacterial organisms per milliliter, meaning that an individual, by drinking a glass of water, may be exposed to a large oral dose of bacteria. Even showering exposes a human to an inhaled inoculum of bacteria as the water aerosolizes microbes found in the water and trapped within the sink drain, allowing these microbes access to the normally sterile lungs. The time lag required for the acquired immune response to react to any one specific bacterial species makes this an impractical defense against continuous exposure to a wide array of bacteria. Moreover, the innate immune response is characterized by a rapid response to an antigenic challenge, followed by a rapid return to basal levels, making this type of response most effective against a continuous and broad array of microbial species, rendering these typical, everyday exposures harmless.

Typically, innate immune mechanisms are the first response to injury and/or infection, and acquired immune mechanisms are the second response (Fig. 1.14A). Immune responses, however, do not occur in isolation. As we have seen, all defense mechanisms can cooperate, and an immune response involves components of both the innate and acquired arms (Fig. 1.14B). For example, phagocytosis (an innate mechanism) is optimal in the presence of both complement (another component of innate immunity) and antibody, produced during

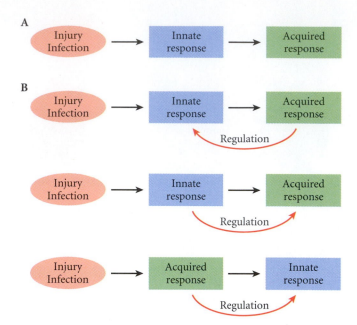

Figure 1.14 Sequence of innate and acquired events in an immune response. **(A)** Typically, innate responses are immediate and are followed by acquired responses. **(B)** The acquired immune responses, however, can regulate innate responses and vice versa.

the acquired response (Fig. 1.15). Likewise, cytokines secreted by activated TH cells (an acquired mechanism) can enhance phagocytic and cytotoxic activities of several innate immune cell types (Fig. 1.16).

The Primary Role of the Immune System: Protection against Infection and Disease

The human body is continuously challenged by infection with a staggering array of bacterial, viral, protozoan, and fungal microorganisms. In the vast majority of cases, such infection is effectively dealt with by the immune system, such that the infection does not result in disease (in fact, in most cases, a person is never aware that the microorganism was encountered). In the 1970s and 1980s, the entire world became acutely aware of the vital role of the immune system in protection against infection, as it followed the life of David Joseph Vetter. Born via cesarean section on September 21, 1971, and immediately placed in a sterile incubator, David was afflicted with an inherited form of immunodeficiency called *X-linked severe combined immunodeficiency.* This disorder is caused by a failure of lymphocyte maturation, resulting in an absence of T cells and B cells. In the 1990s the molecular basis for this disease was discovered: affected males carry a mutant gene that fails to produce a functional protein that is a necessary component of the receptor for five different cytokines. Without this functional receptor B and T cells do not mature in the thymus and bone marrow. Being extremely

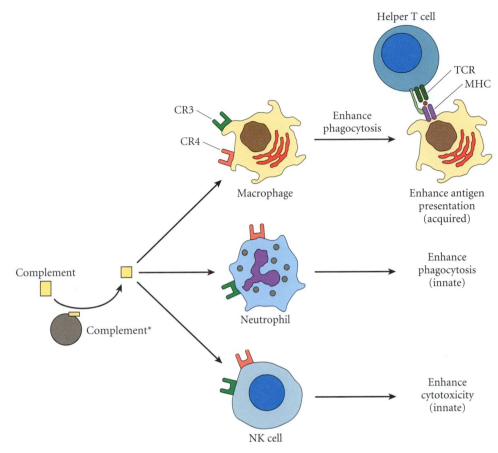

Figure 1.15 Example of innate responses regulating innate and acquired mechanisms. Activated (*) complement can interact with macrophages or neutrophils to enhance phagocytic killing or with NK cells to enhance cytotoxicity. This is possible because macrophages, neutrophils, and NK cells possess cell surface receptors (CR3 and CR4) for activated complement. While this enhances the innate immune response in neutrophils and NK cells, it also affects the acquired immune response, since the enhancement of phagocytosis by macrophages leads to higher levels of antigen presentation to T cells.

susceptible to infections of all kinds, David was required to live his life within the confines of a sterile plastic environment (prompting the press to dub him "the bubble boy"). David grew and lived for $12\frac{1}{2}$ years within his sterile environment, documenting that as long as he was protected from contact with microbes he was able to survive. His life was dramatic testimony to the central role of the immune system in protection against infection.

While this sterile environment protected David from infectious disease, social and economic reasons forced doctors to attempt to correct his immunodeficiency. The attempt was unsuccessful, and David died in February 1984 following an unsuccessful bone marrow transplant from his sister. David's immune system was not reconstituted by the transplant and, as it turned out, could not protect him from a viral infection that was latent in the transplanted marrow. His sister had this infection as well, but with her

intact immune system, she suffered no ill effects from the infection and was not aware of it. All individuals with intact immune systems are likewise protected from, and usually completely unaware of, countless attempts by microorganisms to take up residence within their bodies.

Protection against bacterial infection

Being resistant to environmental damage and flexible in their ability to use sparse nutrients, bacteria are able to exist throughout the environment, often in numbers much higher than one would estimate. Bacterial pathogens cause disease in human hosts for a number of reasons, depending on the bacterial species. Some bacteria cause disease by virtue of a toxic protein they produce and secrete. Others cause disease simply because they are able to grow in a certain tissue of their host, where their growth impedes the normal function of that tissue.

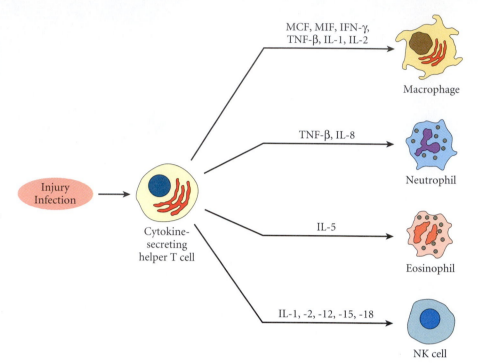

Figure 1.16 Example of acquired response influencing innate mechanisms. The cytokines produced by cells of the acquired immune response (mostly TH cells) influence activation of cells of the innate immune response, such as macrophages, neutrophils, eosinophils, and NK cells. Several particular cytokines are named as examples: MCF, macrophage chemotactic factor; MIF, migration inhibitory factor; IFN-γ, interferon-gamma; TNF-β, tumor necrosis factor beta; IL, interleukin.

The immune mechanisms that are needed to successfully combat bacterial infection vary, depending on the route of infection, the structure of the bacterial cell, and the mechanisms by which the bacterium causes disease. Extracellular bacteria can usually be killed by phagocytes aided by specific antibodies and activation of the complement system, whereas these same immune effectors are ineffective against bacteria that reside within cells of their host. *Gram-negative bacteria,* characterized by the presence of an *outer membrane* surrounding a rigid cell wall, can also be susceptible to the lytic action of the complement MAC (Fig. 1.17A). In contrast, *gram-positive bacteria* do not have an outer membrane, just a rigid cell wall impermeable to the MAC. These bacteria can only be killed by phagocytosis (Fig. 1.17B). Bacteria that cause disease by growing in the tissues of their host must be killed to prevent or reverse disease. In contrast, disease caused by a toxin-producing bacterium can frequently be prevented simply by antibody-mediated neutralization of the toxin.

Protection against viral infection

Viruses are intracellular pathogens consisting of a nucleic acid genome (either single- or double-stranded DNA or RNA) surrounded by a protective protein *capsid.* In addition, some viruses possess a membrane *envelope* that surrounds the capsid. Lacking their own biosynthetic enzymes and organelles, viruses must use their host cells' machinery to replicate the viral genome, synthesize viral proteins, and assemble new viral proteins and genetic material into com-

plete, new virus particles. This replication process can lead to death of the host cell, to tissue damage, and eventually to disease. Some viruses, however, can cause disease by means other than bringing about the lysis of the cells they infect. For example, certain human T-lymphotropic viruses can cause a latent infection that is associated with an increase in the incidence of some forms of cancer. *Human immunodeficiency virus,* the agent of *acquired immunodeficiency syndrome* (AIDS), is capable of both residing latently in cells and causing death of a host cell (usually a CD4⁺ T cell) by lysis to release new virus particles.

The need of the virus to carry out its replicative cycle within the cells of its host renders viruses resistant to some forms of immune recognition (for example, an intracellular virus is not available for binding by antibody after it is in the cell although it can readily be bound before entering a host cell). At the same time, this intracellular lifestyle renders the virus susceptible to some forms of intervention by the immune system. In response to viral infection, the host produces a type of cytokine called *interferon,* which can signal a nearby uninfected host cell that there is a virus present and render the neighboring, uninfected cell resistant to infection. Antibodies also provide an antiviral response (Fig. 1.18). The action of antibodies can also prevent viruses from entering the host cells and can sometimes prevent viruses from uncoating their nucleic acids even if they have entered a cell. Last, antibodies can destroy virus-infected cells to reduce the level of virus replication. This

A

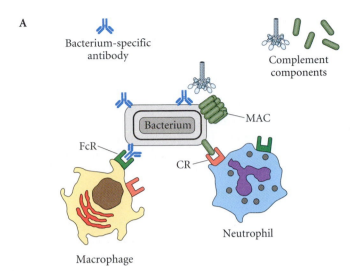

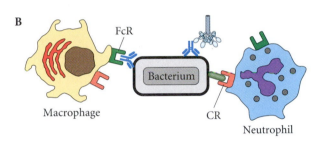

Bacterium-specific antibody

Complement components

MAC

FcR

CR

Neutrophil

Macrophage

B

FcR

Bacterium

FcR

CR

Macrophage

CR

Neutrophil

Figure 1.17 Examples of antibody-mediated effector mechanisms that combat bacterial infection. (**A**) Gram-negative bacteria are susceptible to a number of effector mechanisms. Antibody can trigger complement activation, leading to the formation of a MAC on the bacterium's outer membrane. In addition, both antibody and complement proteins that bind to the bacterium can target the bacterium for macrophages and neutrophils, which express antibody Fc receptors (FcR) and complement receptors (CR). These cells can kill the bacterium through either phagocytosis or the release of toxic mediators (ADCC). (**B**) Gram-positive bacteria have no outer membrane and are therefore not susceptible to MAC formation. However, they are still susceptible to opsonization and ADCC after antibody binding and/or complement activation.

can occur when viral proteins are inserted into the infected cell's membrane, making them available for binding of antiviral antibody, which can lyse the infected cell if complement proteins are recruited to mediate a cytolytic activity. Also, cytotoxic cells with their own intrinsic ability to lyse infected cells are composed of several types of immune cells and can bind antibody via specific receptors on their surface to mediate antibody-dependent cell-mediated cytotoxicity (ADCC) killing of the infected cell.

Protection against parasites and fungi

Eukaryotic parasites include protozoa and multicellular helminth worms and have life cycles that can require residence within a host organism. Some parasites are intra-

cellular, residing within host cells such as macrophages, whereas others are extracellular, living in various tissues of their host, such as the gut. To survive within their host for a time sufficient to allow their propagation, parasites have evolved numerous elaborate strategies to circumvent or forestall their host's immune responses. These strategies include rapid change of surface antigens to avoid preexisting immune responses, seclusion within the cells of their host, mimicking the surface structures of their host's cells to make themselves appear to be a self tissue, inactivation of immune effector molecules, and dysregulation of the host's cytokine network. Because of these evasion tactics, effective immune responses against

Figure 1.18 Examples of antibody-mediated effector mechanisms that combat viral infection. (**A**) Enveloped viruses are susceptible to MACs and antibody- and complement-mediated opsonization for phagocytosis by macrophages and neutrophils, which express antibody Fc receptors (FcR) and complement receptors (CR). (**B**) Nonenveloped viruses have no membrane and are therefore not susceptible to MAC formation. However, they are still susceptible to opsonization after antibody binding and/or complement activation (**left**). In addition, antibodies and activated complement proteins can enshroud a virus in a thick layer of protein (**right**). Although this does not kill the virus, it can render it noninfectious.

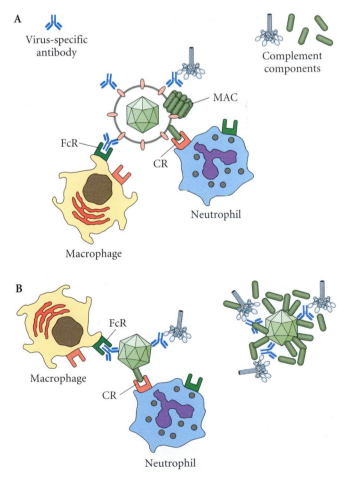

A

Virus-specific antibody

Complement components

MAC

FcR

CR

Neutrophil

Macrophage

B

FcR

Macrophage

CR

Neutrophil

parasites often arise only after long-term or chronic exposure.

Fungal pathogens are also eukaryotic microbes that can cause infection. However, fungal pathogens do not usually require a mammalian host for the completion of their life cycle. Many pathogenic fungi are dimorphic, meaning they can exist as both single cells and as multicellular structures. Most of the medically important fungal pathogens cause disease when they are in a single-cell state, although there are exceptions. In normal immunocompetent hosts, fungal pathogens are effectively dealt with by T-cell-mediated immune mechanisms, although it is becoming increasingly appreciated that antibodies can be effective mediators of immunity to some fungi. The importance of T cells in the normal control of these pathogens can be seen by the frequent occurrence of fungal opportunistic infections in patients with AIDS who have an impairment of the CD4$^+$ T cells due to infection with human immunodeficiency virus.

Protection against Cancer

Although the primary role of the immune system is to protect against pathogenic microbes, it also has a potential role in helping to control aberrant cells that can give rise to cancer. Cancer or tumor cells have acquired the ability to divide in a dysregulated fashion and are termed *transformed cells*. Such cells are also sometimes called *malignant cells*. Cancerous cells can cause disease for several reasons. When a cell becomes cancerous, it frequently does not perform its normal physiological function, at least, not at the normal physiological level. If this function is essential to health (which is usually the case), then disease will ensue from tissue or organ failure. In addition, the physical expansion of the growing cancer cells will frequently impinge upon nearby healthy cells and tissues, thus impairing their normal function by disrupting blood flow, the local environment, and so forth. The overall similarity of cancer cells to the host's normal healthy cells makes it difficult for the acquired immune response to detect these cells. Indeed, it may be a given that for a cancer cell to grow and become pathologic it must be able to avoid recognition as an antigenic cell by the immune system. Moreover, even if the acquired immune system is able to effectively recognize tumor cells, the cells' rapid proliferation and genetic instability greatly increase the likelihood that "escape variants" of the cancer cells will emerge that are resistant to immune recognition or killing.

Despite these obstacles, the immune system is able at times to recognize tumor cells as different from normal healthy cells and under these circumstances is able to selectively destroy the tumor cells. Several components of the immune system have activity against tumor cells. These include antibodies, which can target tumor cells for complement-mediated or ADCC reactions, and CTLs, which can directly kill tumor cells that present altered tumor antigens on MHC class I proteins. Whether the antitumor immune response is mediated by antibodies or CTLs, this response is optimal when the tumor cells express antigens that are not expressed by normal healthy cells of the host. For example, the antigen might be a mutated portion of a host protein that is only changed in the cells of the tumor. Such antigens are termed *tumor-specific antigens*. In most practical cases, however, tumors do not express tumor-specific antigens, either because they never expressed one in the first place or because they lost expression of them due to the tumor's genetic instability. In such cases, the immune system can sometimes recognize tumor cells on the basis of another type of antigen termed *tumor-associated antigens* (TAAs). TAAs are not entirely unique to the tumor but are antigens aberrantly expressed by the tumor cells for one of the following reasons: (i) the TAA is a host protein that is expressed by the tumor cells, but among healthy nontumor cells is expressed only during fetal development; (ii) the TAA is expressed by tumor cells, but among healthy nontumor cells is only expressed in rare portions of the body where it is sequestered from the immune cells of the host (these rare anatomic locations are termed *sites of immune privilege*); or (iii) the TAA is expressed in large quantities by tumor cells, but only in minuscule quantities by healthy nontumor cells.

Even if a tumor expresses an antigen that can be recognized by the cells of the immune system, it still might not be targeted by CTLs for a number of other reasons. As tumor cells expand and become genetically unstable, variants of the tumor frequently arise that have reduced expression of MHC class I on their surface. This can result in an inability of CD8$^+$ CTLs to recognize the tumor's antigens. In some cases, such MHC class I-deficient tumor cells can be killed by NK cells, which have the ability to sense abnormal MHC class I expression on target cells (Fig. 1.19).

Pathology Related to the Immune Response

For all of the importance of the immune system in protecting against disease, it sometimes can fail to function or can produce unwanted reactions that lead to pathology and disease. Failure to function leads to a state of *immunodeficiency*. This can be generalized, leading to a failure to respond adequately to many antigens, or some-

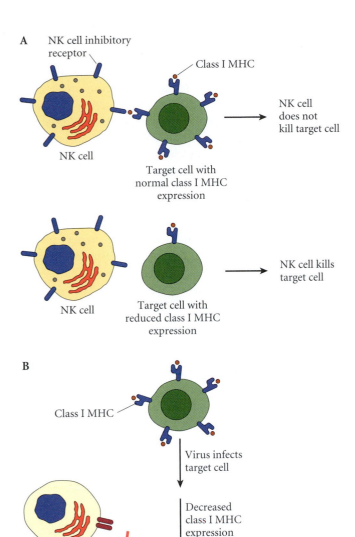

Figure 1.19 NK cells are able to kill host cells that exhibit abnormal expression of MHC class I proteins. (**A**) If a target cell expresses normal levels of MHC class I (**top**), an inhibitory receptor on the NK cell binds the MHC and prevents the NK cell from killing the target. If the target cell expresses reduced amounts of MHC class I (**bottom**), the inhibitory receptor does not deliver this inhibitory signal and the NK cell kills the target cell. (**B**) Some tumors demonstrate reduced expression of MHC class I and are thus poorly recognized by CTLs. This reduced expression of MHC class I may allow NK cells to kill the tumor cell. Therefore, NK cells can function as a "backup" killing mechanism.

times selective, with an affected individual unable to respond to a subset of antigenic stimuli or mount a specific type of immune response such as cell-mediated immunity. Alternately, the immune system can be overactive, producing unwanted responses. When an overactive response is made to an antigen that is usually harmless, but the reaction itself causes unwanted symptoms or pathology, then a state of hypersensitivity is produced. Hypersensitivity reactions can also extend to unwanted and inappropriate immune responses to self antigens, leading to pathologic *autoimmunity*. Finally, in the past 100 years or so surgeons have had the technical capability of transplanting tissues and organs between different individuals, but unfortunately, the immune system of the recipient usually recognizes the MHC antigens of the donor as foreign. In this setting the transplanted donor tissue is the target of the recipient's immune system, which can lead to destruction of the transplant. Understanding the basis for this and finding ways to avoid transplant rejection are encompassed in the study of *transplantation immunology*.

Immunodeficiency

Immunodeficiency refers to a large number of conditions in which the immune response is impaired by a block in either the development or the function of immune cells. The vast majority of these cases, in both children and adults, are classified as *secondary immunodeficiencies*, meaning they are acquired during the lifetime of the affected individual and are not due to a primary genetic deficiency. Secondary immunodeficiencies are usually due to malnutrition, malignancy, taking of cytotoxic drugs, or chronic disease. *Primary immunodeficiencies*, in contrast, are immunodeficiencies caused by inherited genetic defects. The hallmark of both primary and secondary immunodeficiency syndromes is enhanced susceptibility to infection, as manifested by more frequent illness, disease due to uncommon pathogens (or even to microorganisms that are normally nonpathogenic such as weakened vaccine strains of microorganisms), or clinical disease that is less responsive to standard antimicrobial therapy. Immunodeficient individuals are also at greater risk for some but not all malignancies.

The past two decades have seen the identification and detailed investigation of a new immunodeficiency state, AIDS. Not only has this epidemic immunodeficiency syndrome heightened public awareness of immunodeficiency in general, it has also expanded our understanding and appreciation of the delicate regulatory balances that interconnect the various cellular effectors of the immune system.

The past two decades have also seen the coming of age of molecular genetic research techniques. This technology has enabled immunologists to characterize many immunodeficiency syndromes at the level of a specific gene that is defective in each situation. This, in turn, has expanded our understanding of the molecular and cellular bases of immunodeficiency and, by extension, has broadened our comprehension of the normal molecular and genetic function of the immune system. Many of the proteins crucial for proper function of the immune system have been discovered when a mutant form of a gene encoding the protein has been determined to be the basis of an immunodeficiency disease. For example, for the cells of the immune system to develop properly, they need to respond to a set of specific growth factors. The cellular response is dependent on expression of a proper receptor for the growth factor. Importantly, understanding the molecular genetic basis for immunodeficiency disease can lead to new therapeutic options based on molecular correction of the specific genetic lesions that give rise to a large number of human diseases. In 2002, some of the first reports of long-term correction of immunodeficiency by gene therapy were published, potentially heralding an era wherein genetic diseases can be permanently corrected.

Hypersensitivity

The term hypersensitivity was first used to denote a pathological condition characterized by exaggerated immune responses. Although this is sometimes true, it is more accurate to define hypersensitivity as a condition brought about by an *inappropriate* immune response, rather than an exaggerated one. In general, hypersensitive reactions often represent immune reactions that occur in response to antigens that, in and of themselves, pose no serious threat to the individual. The irony of this situation is that, while the antigen posed no threat to the host, the inappropriate immune response *to* that antigen *does* pose a threat to the host.

Hypersensitivity reactions can occur as a result of an inappropriate humoral or cell-mediated immune response. Most people are familiar with some forms of hypersensitivity in the form of allergies leading to hay fever, asthma, and reactions to food, perfumes, and so forth. When the hypersensitive response occurs via a humoral response, the symptoms of the reaction can be obvious within minutes to hours of exposure to the antigen (sometimes called an *allergen* to denote that the antigen can give rise to hypersensitive, or allergic, responses). The exact timeframe depends on the isotype of antibody that mediates the reaction. If the reaction is mediated by antibodies of the IgE class, then the reaction occurs via

the activation of leukocytes called *mast cells*. This reaction is very quick (minutes), and the resulting reaction is termed an *immediate-type hypersensitivity* reaction (Fig. 1.20, top). If, on the other hand, the reaction is mediated by antibodies of the IgG class, then the reaction occurs via the activation of complement proteins, which generate an ensuing inflammatory response. This reaction is not as quick as mast cell activation, requiring several hours (usually 4 to 6 hours) to develop. Reactions of this type are usually classified as immediate-type hypersensitivity reactions, although the term *intermediate-type hypersensitivity reaction* is sometimes also used to describe them (Fig. 1.20, middle and bottom). Last, some hypersensitive reactions are mediated not by antibodies, but by the activation of cytokine-secreting TH cells that draw macrophages to the site of activation. This process requires several days to occur and so is termed *delayed-type hypersensitivity*. An example of this type of response is the rash that develops 1 to 2 days after exposure to poison oak or poison ivy.

It is important that the immune effector mechanisms that are operative during hypersensitive responses are identical to those mechanisms that occur during appropriate and protective immune responses in other circumstances. For example, the cell-mediated delayed-type hypersensitivity response to antigens in poison oak is mechanistically identical to the protective immune response against the intracellular bacterial pathogen *Mycobacterium tuberculosis.* What distinguishes the protective response from the hypersensitive response is that the protective reaction is occurring in response to a bacterial pathogen, which, if left unchecked, would cause serious or lethal disease. In contrast, the hypersensitive reaction occurs in response to an antigen that, in and of itself, is not dangerous to the host. Therefore, there is nothing intrinsically pathological about these immune responses, except for the circumstances under which they are occurring.

Autoimmunity

The cells of the acquired immune response are normally subjected to a series of overlapping regulatory mechanisms that prevent them from recognizing and attacking the host's own normal, healthy cells and tissues. Collectively, this phenomenon of nonresponsiveness to self antigens is termed *tolerance*. Tolerance influences the development of lymphocytes and their function. In a minority of individuals, however, there is a failure of self-tolerance, leading to immune attack against the host's own healthy tissues. This pathological condition is termed autoimmunity. In a broad sense, autoimmunity can be considered to be akin to hypersensitivity, since both con-

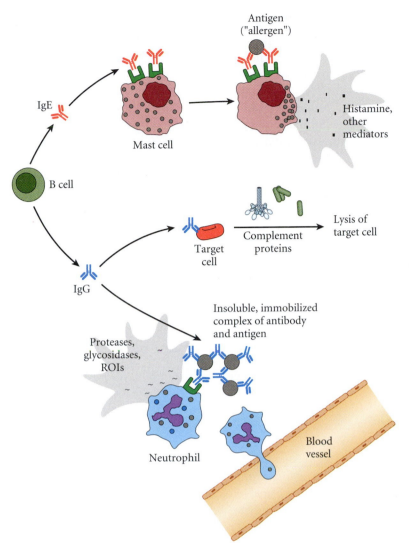

Figure 1.20 Antibody-mediated hypersensitive reactions occur by different mechanisms, depending in part on which isotype of antibody is produced. (**Top**) IgE antibodies mediate immediate-type hypersensitivity by binding to Fc receptors on the surface of mast cells. Subsequent binding of this IgE by an antigen (called an allergen) results in mast cell activation and the release of compounds such as histamine that cause the allergic response. (**Middle**) IgG antibodies can cause a form of hypersensitivity brought about by destruction of a normal host cell by complement activation, phagocytosis, or ADCC. The example shown depicts antibody-mediated hemolysis of a red blood cell (RBC) such as might occur after transfusion of incompatible blood into a patient. (**Bottom**) IgG antibodies can also cause hypersensitivity if they form immune complexes with antigen that become immobilized or lodged in tissues such as vascular beds. In this case, localized complement activation draws neutrophils to the site that bind the immune complexes and release toxic substances such as proteases, glycosidases, and reactive oxygen intermediates (ROIs), causing *innocent bystander damage* to the nearby tissues.

ditions entail an inappropriate immune response. In the case of autoimmunity, however, the eliciting antigens arise from within one's own body and the sequelae are usually more grave since the autoimmune response almost always results in damage to critical organs or systems of the host that in many cases is irreversible.

Autoimmunity tends to occur in individuals during early adult life and, for reasons that are not entirely understood, frequently affects women more than men. The autoimmune response can be mediated by self-reactive antibodies, self-reactive T cells, or both. Self-reactive antibodies can cause pathology by triggering complement- or ADCC-mediated damage to normal host cells, can trigger localized inflammation following complement activation, or can bind to cell surface receptor proteins, interfering with their normal function. Self-reactive T cells can cause disease either by direct cytotoxicity against normal host

cells or by production of cytokines that recruit and activate other host immune cells to the affected tissue.

In most cases, treatment options for autoimmunity are limited to various regimens of immunosuppressive agents. These regimens yield variable degrees of success, depending on the form of autoimmunity. All of them have in common, though, that they render the patient more susceptible to infectious disease. Treatment of the autoimmune condition must therefore be carefully balanced with maintaining the maximum possible immune function of the patient.

Transplantation immunology

The negative effects of many diseases and injuries can potentially be alleviated by replacing a damaged organ with a functional organ. Over the past century, great strides have been made toward increasing the success of organ transplantation. The earliest successes (and highest success rates) in this field were and still are achieved by transplanting tissues or organs from one site to another within the same individual (this process is termed an *autograft*). This occurs when healthy skin is transplanted to a site of skin damage arising from burns or trauma. Early research indicated that similar high success rates could also be achieved with transplants between different animals *as long as the donor and recipient animal were genetically identical to each other* (for example, identical twins; this is called an *isograft*). This led to the appreciation that rejection of transplanted tissue was mediated by immune recognition of the transplanted tissue as different from the host's own tissues. Since it is rare to have two human subjects who are genetically identical to each other, in clinical practice "transplantation" usually refers to transfer of tissue or an organ between genetically nonidentical individuals (termed an *allograft*).

Although early attempts at allografts almost invariably ended in failure, short-term (and in some instances, long-term) success has been achieved in some cases. Similar to what is observed with other forms of undesired immune reactions, transplant rejection can be mediated by both donor-specific antibodies and donor-specific T cells. It was the development of these transplant-rejection reactions that led to the initial identification of the MHC genes, with subsequent work showing their role and importance in the normal immune response. Increased success in the field of clinical transplantation is due to progress in the development of immunosuppressive treatment protocols. Some forms of immunosuppression have been developed that can suppress some particular aspects of immune function, without globally suppressing the patient's immune system. These advances have made it possible to maintain immunosuppression more aggressively and for longer periods without rendering the transplant recipient totally susceptible to all forms of infectious disease. Such treatment protocols have made it feasible to begin considering the clinical usefulness of *xenotransplantation* (transplantation from one species to another). Since a xenograft is highly dissimilar to the human graft recipient, xenografts are usually typified by intense rejection reactions (indeed, long-term success has yet to be achieved with a xenograft). However, further research in the area of specific immunosuppression or genetically engineering animals such as pigs to minimize recognition of their tissues as foreign may help realize xenografts as a viable therapeutic option in the future.

Summary

The principal function of the immune system is to protect us against infectious disease. Such protection is mediated by a system of cells, tissues, and organs that provide both general protection against microorganisms (innate immunity) and pathogen-specific responses (acquired immunity). Innate immune mechanisms include barriers such as skin that physically exclude microorganisms from the host's body, as well as a number of enzymes, proteins, and nonprotein factors that either damage microbes or inhibit their growth. Pathogen-specific defenses are classified as humoral (B cells and antibodies) or cell-mediated (cytotoxic cells). Innate immunity has the advantage that it can act rapidly following the initiation of an infection and is active against a wide variety of microbial pathogens. However, pathogenic microbes are often able to thwart the innate immune defenses, requiring a response from the acquired immune system. The acquired immune system has the advantage that B cells and T cells have the ability to expand exponentially during an immune response and to specifically target a particular strain of a microorganism for killing and elimination. Furthermore, the acquired immune response demonstrates the important characteristic of *memory,* allowing it to reply faster and more robustly against subsequent encounters with the same pathogen or antigen. The innate and acquired responses supplement and enhance each other to provide maximal protection for the host.

For the host to remain healthy in a microbe-filled environment, the innate and acquired immune responses must deal with continuous encounters with bacteria, viruses, protozoans, parasitic worms, and fungi. All of these forms of microorganisms present the immune system with a unique set of challenges. Some bacteria produce toxic proteins that need to be neutralized. Viruses reside within the cells of their host, where they remain hidden from their host's antibodies. Parasitic worms have devised clever ways to make themselves appear to be their host's own normal tissue. To carry out its protective role, the immune system must use various combinations of effectors in its arsenal against these threats.

Pathologic consequences ensue when the immune system fails to function as it should. This can occur if the immune system is incapable of responding as a result of an immunodeficient state and also when the immune system responds inappropriately. The latter situations include hypersensitivity reactions such as allergic reactions to house dust or pollen as well as serious or even fatal immune responses to the host's own cells and tissues. The study of these pathological conditions has taught us a great deal about the normal function of the immune system and has pointed the way to some potential future therapies that are currently under development.

Suggested Reading

Delves, P. J., and I. M. Roitt. 2000. The immune system. Part I. *N. Engl. J. Med.* **343**:37–49.

Delves, P. J., and I. M. Roitt. 2000. The immune system. Part II. *N. Engl. J. Med.* **343**:108–117.

Foss, F. M. 2002. Immunologic mechanisms of antitumor activity. *Semin. Oncol.* **29**(3 Suppl. 7):5–11.

Leng, Q., and Z. Bentwich. 2002. Beyond self and nonself: fuzzy recognition of the immune system. *Scand. J. Immunol.* **56**:224–232.

Maddox, L., and D. A. Schwartz. 2002. The pathophysiology of asthma. *Annu. Rev. Med.* **53**:477–498.

Medzhitov, R., and C. Janeway, Jr. 2000. Innate immunity. *N. Engl. J. Med.* **343**:338–344.

Rotrosen, D., J. B. Matthews, and J. A. Bluestone. 2002. The immune tolerance network: a new paradigm for developing tolerance-inducing therapies. *J. Allergy Clin. Immunol.* **110**:17–23.

Smith, J. B., and M. K. Haynes. 2002. Rheumatoid arthritis—a molecular understanding. *Ann. Intern. Med.* **136**:908–922.

Innate Immunity

Jeffrey B. Lyczak

Throughout their lives individuals are challenged with a variety of microbial and toxic substances and need to protect themselves from these agents with a rapid and effective response. The *innate immune response* has such a function. The innate defenses consist of a large group of partially overlapping mechanisms that act at many steps in the infection process either to prevent pathogens from gaining access to an individual's tissues or to limit the extent of an infection (Fig. 2.1). The innate defenses include physical barriers, which prevent microbes from gaining access to tissues; physiologic barriers, which impede microbial growth; various enzymatic and cellular effectors that kill or inactivate foreign agents; and nonspecific defenses tailored to prevent viral infections. These barriers and effectors, which are produced by an individual continuously, can act on a pathogen immediately after it gains access to the tissues. This response stands in marked contrast to the acquired response, which is activated only 1 to 2 weeks after a foreign antigen gains access to an individual's tissues and is encountered by lymphocytes. The innate defenses are either constitutively active or rapidly mobilized and are effective against many types of microbial agents (Fig. 2.2), whereas the acquired immune response is activated slowly, depends on the entry of an antigenic stimulus into an individual's tissues, and is specific to a particular foreign material. This is not to say that innate responses are superior to acquired responses. The innate response cannot expand exponentially upon encountering a foreign agent and can be overwhelmed by a large challenge (e.g., a large bacterial inoculum) and lacks the attribute of *memory*, making it incapable of mounting a more rapid and robust response to a frequently encountered antigen. The acquired and the

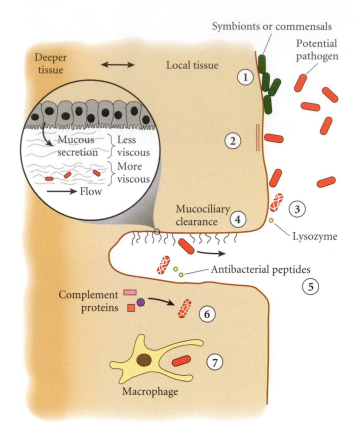

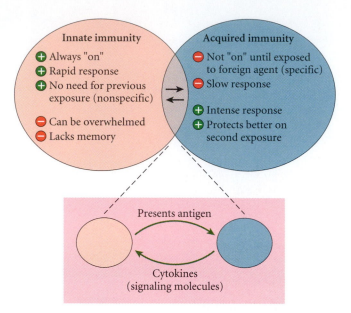

Figure 2.1 Mechanisms of innate immunity against bacterial infection at a physical barrier such as the skin or mucosal surfaces. (**1**) Symbiotic or commensal bacteria residing on the skin occupy limiting attachment sites on the skin and consume limiting nutrients, making colonization by potentially pathogenic microorganisms unlikely. (**2**) If pathogens do attach, the skin is an effective physical barrier and bacterial growth is retarded by the low pH of lactic acid-containing sebum secreted by sebaceous glands. (**3**) Secretions on the mucosal surfaces contain destructive enzymes such as lysozyme that degrade the cell walls of bacteria. (**4**) The respiratory tract is protected by the mucociliary escalator (**inset**), by which a mucus layer is continuously propelled upward toward the nasopharynx by the motion of epithelial cell cilia. The mucus layer is biphasic, with a less viscous layer where epithelial cilia beat and a more viscous layer that entraps bacteria (red). Bacteria caught in the more viscous layer are carried with the mucus and thus removed from the airways. (**5**) The mucosal secretions of the respiratory and digestive tracts contain antimicrobial peptides that can kill infectious agents directly. (**6 and 7**) A potential pathogen that manages to penetrate these barriers to the tissue below can be killed by complement proteins forming MACs and ingestion by phagocytes such as macrophages.

Figure 2.2 Comparison of innate immunity and acquired immunity. Overlap of the two arms of immunity where cross-regulation occurs is shown where the ovals intersect.

innate immune responses supplement each other and stimulate and regulate each other's activity (Fig. 2.2).

Physical and Physiologic Barriers

An individual's primary defense against infectious agents is the physical barrier separating it from its environment (Fig. 2.1). The skin covering most of the outer surfaces of mammals provides a first line of defense against infection. Several attributes of the skin make it an effective barrier against infection, the most obvious being its ability to prevent access to deeper tissues. Epithelial cells in the skin are constantly being replaced by cell division in the underlying basal epithelial cell layer, with new layers being formed and the outermost layers being sloughed off. In addition, as the skin cells move outward toward the surface, they produce the protein *keratin,* which makes the epithelial cell layer tough and water resistant. The low pH of the skin also contributes to its efficacy as a barrier against infection, since most bacteria grow optimally at pH values near neutrality. Small glands in the dermal layer of the skin called *sebaceous glands* secrete *sebum,* a component of sweat that contains lactic acid, which lowers the pH of the skin to about 4.

Sebum inhibits the growth of most, but not all, microbes. Several bacterial species, including staphylococci, utilize sebum as a nutrient, allowing them to colonize the skin surface. This colonization usually does not have negative effects (unless a break in the skin allows them access to deep tissues and the bloodstream). In contrast, these colonizing bacteria, together called the *normal flora,* either have no direct effect on an individual (i.e., they are classified as *commensal organisms*) or actually benefit the individual (and are classified as *symbiotic organisms*). The microbes of the normal flora benefit their host because they compete with other, potentially pathogenic, bacteria for space (physical attachment sites) and nutrients on the skin surface (Fig. 2.1).

The skin represents a small part of an individual's surface area. Most of the surface (about 99%) comprises a different type of physical barrier, the *mucosal surfaces.* These surfaces consist of an epithelial cell layer, generally only one-cell-layer thick, that forms the *mucous membrane.* In contrast to the epithelial cells of the skin, the epithelial cells of mucous membranes do not become keratinized and are therefore not nearly as durable as skin. However, mucosal surfaces possess glandular cells (*goblet cells*) that secrete a viscous solution called mucus. Mucus is fairly adhesive and serves as an innate defense by trapping bacteria and preventing them from moving to deeper tissues. Mucus is also one component of the *mucociliary escalator* that protects the respiratory tract from infection. This clearance mechanism requires two anatomic features: the ciliated apical membrane of the airway epithelium and a biphasic layer of mucus secreted by goblet cells lining the airway lumen. The phase of the mucous layer closer to the epithelial cells (the *periciliary* layer) is less viscous than the outer phase to allow the cilia to beat freely, whereas the outer phase is more viscous to entrap inhaled particles. The airway cilia beat synchronously, continually moving the mucous layer upward toward the pharynx. When functioning normally, this system traps foreign particles in the mucus and subsequently carries them to the pharynx (along with the mucus), where they are expelled by coughing or swallowed and thus removed from the airway (Fig. 2.1).

The epithelial areas of some areas of the body cannot be classified as either skin or mucosal surface. For example, the cornea covering the outer surface of the eye consists of multiple layers of epithelial cells that resemble the layers of epithelial cells in the skin. However, because the corneal epithelium must remain translucent for the eyes to function, the outer layers of epithelial cells remain alive and do not become keratinized. In terms of innate immunity, there are other differences between the cornea and the skin. Although the skin is well populated with normal bacterial flora, the cornea is kept relatively free of bacteria by the continuous blinking of the eyelids and the flow of tears from tear ducts.

Physical conditions such as temperature and pH act as innate barriers to infection at many anatomic sites besides epithelial surfaces. Pathogens grow optimally within a certain temperature range and are less active at temperatures above or below this range. One feature of the systemic innate response, the *acute-phase response,* is an elevation of body temperature. This fever response elevates the temperature often to one that is outside the optimal temperature for growth of a pathogen. Barriers provided by pH are also excellent defenses that provide a large degree of protection to the gastrointestinal tract, since ingested material must pass through the stomach (with a pH of ~2) before reaching the small intestine, which is often a site of entry into deeper tissues. Last, the urinary tract is protected by the frequent flow of urine. *Urea,* a small molecule that is the principal nitrogen waste product of mammalian species, is also a powerful denaturant that destroys the secondary, tertiary, and quaternary structures of proteins, thus killing or inactivating microbes that reside for too long in the urinary tract.

Enzymatic and Protein Effectors

Individuals also possess a large battery of enzymes that can damage bacteria, viruses, and other even nonviable foreign antigens. These enzymatic effectors of innate immunity generally function by damaging the structural integrity of the microbial surface, although the different effectors accomplish this in different ways.

Enzymatic and Protein Effectors at Mucosal Surfaces

Lysozyme
Many of the enzymatic effectors of innate immunity are present in mucosal secretions such as tears and saliva. One antibacterial enzyme called *lysozyme* is such an effector (Fig. 2.1). Gram-positive bacteria rely on their rigid cell wall to protect them from osmotic shock and lysis when they are in a hypotonic environment, and removal or degradation of this cell wall renders them susceptible to injury. The bacterial cell wall consists of linear "backbones" comprising alternating residues of the monosaccharides *N*-acetylglucosamine (NAG) and *N*-acetylmuramic acid (NAM), which are cross-linked via tetrapeptide and pentapeptide "cross-bridges" to form a strong three-dimensional lattice. Lysozyme degrades this lattice structure by specifically cleaving the $\beta(1 \rightarrow 4)$ glycosidic linkage between the NAG and NAM saccharides (Fig. 2.3).

Proteases
Proteases are enzymatic effector molecules that contribute to innate immunity at mucosal surfaces. Microbial pathogens have many surface proteins that are important for their survival or their attachment to mammalian cells and tissues. The outer membrane proteins of gram-negative bacteria, for example, frequently serve to transport nutrients or raw materials into the cell or bacterial biosynthetic products out of the cell. Destruction of these outer membrane proteins has a profound negative effect on bacterial viability. Viral pathogens frequently use their

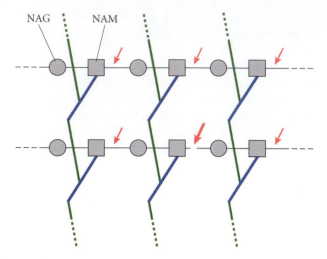

Figure 2.3 Diagram of the peptidoglycan of bacterial cell walls. Horizontal lines represent alternating molecules of NAG (circles) and NAM (squares). Blue and green lines represent peptide cross-bridges that join the NAG-NAM copolymers into a three-dimensional matrix. Red arrows represent potential target sites for cleavage of peptidoglycan by lysozyme. The heavy red arrow shows a site where lysozyme has cleaved the backbone of the NAG-NAM copolymer.

outer capsid proteins or envelope proteins as a means of docking with mammalian cells, and proteolytic degradation of these viral proteins, although it usually does not completely destroy the viral particle, can render the virus incapable of infecting mammalian cells. Potentially harmful antigens such as toxic proteins can also be inactivated by these proteases.

Antimicrobial peptides

Antimicrobial peptides are another type of effector in mucosal secretions. These are short peptides (20 to 45 amino acids) capable of inserting into phospholipid bilayers and disrupting the permeability barrier. This barrier function is important for maintaining an osmotic balance between the microbial cell and its environment, and disruption of lipid bilayers by antimicrobial peptides can result in death of the affected microbe. Antimicrobial peptides are highly effective against pathogens that have an external membrane, such as enveloped viruses surrounded by a mammalian cell-derived membrane and gram-negative bacteria, which have an outer membrane as their outermost layer. These peptides are sometimes less effective against gram-positive bacteria, which have a thick peptidoglycan cell wall surrounding the single-membrane layer, but there are peptides that have a good degree of killing activity against gram-positive bacteria.

Antibacterial peptides have been widely conserved in evolution and are important components of host defenses in many species. Some of the earliest characterized peptides were from the skin of frogs and named magainins or from silk moths and named cecropins. The antibacterial peptides of humans have been grouped into three categories on the basis of their amino acid sequence homology and overall three-dimensional topology: α-defensins, β-defensins, and the recently identified θ-defensins. Some immune cell types also store large amounts of antibacterial peptides in cytoplasmic granules; e.g., neutrophils store β-defensins, which they use to kill microbes they have ingested by phagocytosis. Defensins are synthesized as inactive precursor molecules containing an additional peptide sequence that inactivates the membrane-disrupting function of the defensin, ensuring that the defensin will not damage the cell that synthesizes it. When the defensin is activated to destroy a pathogen, a protease removes the precursor peptide.

Iron-sequestering proteins

Iron plays several important roles in biologic systems, usually as a cofactor for enzymatic reactions. In addition, almost all bacteria require iron to regulate the activity of specific transcription factors and transport proteins, and the availability of iron is a critical determinant of microbial growth during infection. It is therefore not surprising that mammals have developed proteins that prevent microbes from acquiring iron from their environment. Transferrin and lactoferrin are two examples of these *iron-sequestering proteins.* Transferrin is the chief iron-transporting protein in the blood, and lactoferrin serves a similar role in mucosal secretions. These proteins provide a convenient way of transporting iron selectively to an anatomic site where it is needed (e.g., cells expressing transferrin receptor proteins can capture transferrin, and thus capture iron atoms, originating from the blood). Additionally, these iron-sequestering proteins lower the concentration of free iron, making it unavailable to invading microorganisms. In this respect, iron-sequestering proteins serve an innate immune function. This function becomes more important during overt infection, when plasma iron (bound to transferrin) is internalized by hepatocytes in the liver. The iron inside the hepatocyte is shifted from its transferrin carrier to a lactoferrin carrier and is retained within the hepatocyte rather than being returned to the plasma. This rapid diminution in levels of iron in the plasma that accompanies infection (called *induced hypoferremia*) is part of the systemic innate response to infection in mammals.

Besides being present in secretions, lactoferrin also is found in the granules of neutrophils, where it has an important antibacterial role. The antibacterial activity of lactoferrin was long presumed to be a function of its ability to deprive microorganisms of essential iron. However, although depriving bacteria of iron inhibits their growth, it usually does not kill them. Research on the bactericidal activities of lactoferrin and transferrin has determined that they may have a biologic function in addition to their iron-sequestering function: the ability to disrupt the outer membrane of gram-negative bacteria. The membrane-disrupting activity of lactoferrin seems to reside in a cationic peptide fragment called *lactoferricin.* Electron microscopic images of bacteria exposed to lactoferricin show that the bacteria rapidly develop electron-dense "membrane blisters." Since intact lactoferrin does not have this bactericidal activity, some immunologists have questioned the relevance of this activity to real infections. Perhaps lactoferrin is cleaved by an individual's own proteolytic enzymes to produce a fragment similar to lactoferricin, which can then disrupt bacterial membranes.

Enzymatic and Protein Effectors in the Blood: the Complement System

The complement system is a family of about 30 serum proteins that serve many effector and regulatory functions in both the innate and the acquired immune responses. The proteins of the complement system normally circulate in the blood in an inactive precursor state (as *proenzymes* or *zymogens*) but, when activated, are capable of directly killing target cells and of regulating other immune functions. The complement system can be activated in many ways (Fig. 2.4). The three main activating stimuli are (i) antibody-antigen complexes; (ii) strongly ionic biologic surfaces such as the outer membranes of gram-negative bacteria and the cell walls of gram-positive bacteria and fungi; and (iii) carbohydrates with a high mannose content, which are unlike the complex carbohydrates produced by most mammalian species. These three mechanisms of activation are, respectively, termed the *classical, alternative,* and *lectin* pathways of activation. The first of these mechanisms usually, but not always, requires the production of antigen-specific antibody by B lymphocytes. This activator mechanism is relevant to innate immunity in only a limited context. The other two activation mechanisms are excellent examples of innate immunity. In both cases, the complement system is activated by a very general stimulus usually indicative of a microbial presence. In addition, the chemical nature of one of the central components of the complement system, the C3 component, allows it to be slowly

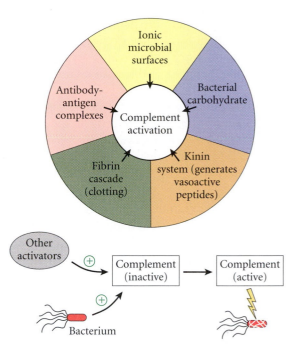

Figure 2.4 Activators of the complement system. (**Top**) Many different entities can activate the complement system. (**Bottom**) Simplified sequence of events leading to killing of a bacterium by the complement system. Note that the complement system can kill a bacterium even if the original activator was completely unrelated to the bacterium, as long as the microbe is close to the site of complement activation.

but spontaneously activated in the fluid or plasma phase of blood. This spontaneous activation recruits some additional components and forms an enzymatic complex that acts on other C3 molecules to yield a breakdown product of the C3 component, termed C3b, that can attach itself to nonself components and promote their elimination or destruction.

The ability of the complement system to become activated in response to high-mannose carbohydrates is attributable to the complement protein called *mannose-binding protein* (MBP) or *mannose-binding lectin* (MBL). MBP binds directly to high-mannose carbohydrates and activates other proteins of the complement system. Moreover, MBP is capable of distinguishing these high-mannose carbohydrates from carbohydrates normally found on the surface of mammalian cells. Thus, MBP recognizes high-mannose carbohydrates as a "molecular pattern" indicative of bacterial infection. MBP belongs in a category of immune proteins called *pattern-recognition receptors.* Because these activating stimuli are nonspecific, multiple regulatory mechanisms are necessary to prevent the complement system from being activated accidentally by an individual's own cells and tissues.

Other innate immune mechanisms for activating the complement system involve the *clotting cascade,* which is activated by tissue injury and ultimately forms fibrin blood clots and fibrin "scaffolds," which are essential for tissue remodeling and the growth of new blood vessels. Two proteolytic enzymes involved in this process, kallikrein and factor XII, are capable of acting directly on components of the complement system and activating complement. Given the potent antibacterial activities of the complement system, its activation during the clotting process is easily understandable, since sites of tissue injury frequently serve as entry points for infectious microorganisms.

Once activated, the complement system generates many active proteins that mediate several immunologic functions (Fig. 2.4). One mechanism by which complement directly kills microorganisms is the *membrane attack complex* (MAC), a multiprotein complex that inserts into the membrane of its target cell, creating a large transmembrane pore. Not all microorganisms, however, are susceptible to the MAC. Gram-positive bacteria, for example, have a thick cell wall surrounding their membrane, preventing the insertion of the MAC. In such cases, the complement system mobilizes other biologic activities to protect an individual from infection. Immune cell types such as neutrophils and macrophages are capable of ingesting and killing microorganisms through a process known as *phagocytosis.* Some of the activated complement products become covalently attached to a microbe, enhancing the ability of neutrophils and macrophages to phagocytose the bacterium. This enhancement of phagocytosis, called *opsonization,* results from the expression of cell surface complement receptors by neutrophils and macrophages. Some complement products also are able to activate and regulate the *inflammatory response,* a mechanism for coordinating many biologic functions to maximize the efficacy of the innate immune response.

Cellular Effectors of Innate Immunity

Several types of white blood cells (leukocytes) participate in the innate immune response. Among them are neutrophils (also called *polymorphonuclear leukocytes* [PMNs]), monocytes, macrophages, and a type of lymphocyte known as a natural killer (NK) cell. PMNs, monocytes, and macrophages are all capable of *pinocytosis, endocytosis,* and phagocytosis, i.e., engulfing and internalizing particulates (whether microbial cells, viruses, or inert particles). NK cells are important for recognizing damaged or altered cells such as virally infected cells or tumor cells. NK cells mediate *cytotoxicity* against these target cells and cause them to die, usually via *apoptosis,* or

programmed cell death (Fig. 2.5). This event is characterized by condensation of the cytoplasm and nucleus. The host's chromosomal DNA is cleaved by endogenous nonspecific endonucleases into 200-base-pair units corresponding to the length of DNA between consecutive histones. This is followed by the breaking apart of the cell into *apoptotic bodies,* which are later removed from the host by phagocytic cells such as macrophages. Viable microbial cells that are phagocytosed usually are killed and/or degraded within the leukocyte (see Fig. 1.3). Monocytes, macrophages, and PMNs all possess dense vesicular structures called *granules* or *lysosomes* in their cytoplasm. These contain numerous cytotoxic proteins, such as proteases, glycosidases, antimicrobial peptides, and lysozyme. These proteins degrade substances that have been phagocytosed by the leukocyte. In addition, the contents of these granules can be extruded from the leukocyte to kill foreign microorganisms that have not yet been internalized by the blood cell.

Not all of the cytotoxic agents possessed by monocytes, macrophages, and PMNs are proteins or stored in granules. Some are synthesized upon activation of the leukocyte. After taking up foreign material by phagocytosis, monocytes, macrophages, and PMNs initiate a process called the *oxidative burst.* Several enzymatic pathways are activated during this process, producing highly reactive products. These products (Table 2.1) comprise ions, free radicals, and reactive oxides, which kill foreign microorganisms by damaging their proteins, carbohydrates, and nucleic acids.

NK cells have also been referred to as null cells or third-population cells, as they represent a lineage of lymphocytes that is neither a T cell nor a B cell. NK cells were first discovered because of their ability to mediate cytotoxic killing of transformed tumor cells, even when taken from individuals with no known history of cancer. NK cells might play a role in identifying and eliminating potentially cancerous cells before they have a chance to grow into a pathologic tumor. However, support for a role of NK cells in this aspect of mammalian physiology and homeostasis is inconclusive. NK cells are potent sources of cytokines, and their ability to produce these factors is considered to be important in their role in fighting tumors. Similarly, NK cells are able to identify and kill virally infected cells. They are likely critical for an early response to viral infection. NK cells are potent sources of interferon-gamma (IFN-γ), which has a potent ability to confer resistance to viral infection to potential target cells. Both tumor cells and virally infected cells often have altered surfaces, particularly in regard to the reduced expression of major histocompatibility complex (MHC)

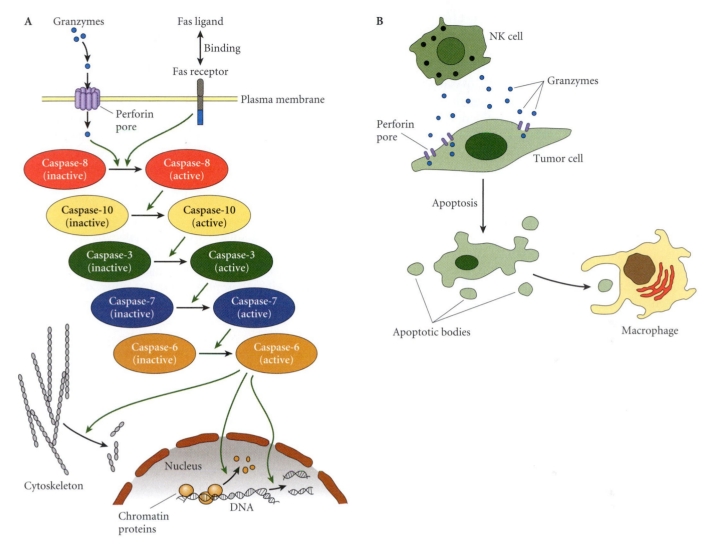

Figure 2.5 NK cells and other cytotoxic cells can kill target cells by causing the target cells to undergo programmed cell death or apoptosis. (**A**) Apoptosis can be triggered by either proteases called *granzymes* or the membrane protein *Fas ligand*. Granzymes enter the target cell through transmembrane pores generated by the protein *perforin*. Fas ligand delivers its cell death signal by binding to its receptor protein, called *Fas*. In either case, a protease cascade is initiated, resulting in the activation of a family of cytoplasmic proteases called *caspases*. The caspase cascade ultimately results in the cleavage of critical molecules such as cytoskeletal elements, DNA, and chromatin proteins, bringing about the death of the target cell. (**B**) A target cell that is triggered to undergo apoptosis undergoes characteristic morphological changes, including compaction of the cell, condensation of the chromatin, and the formation of membrane-bound cellular fragments called *membrane blebs* or apoptotic bodies. These apoptotic bodies are recognized and phagocytosed by nearby macrophages.

Table 2.1 Products of the oxidative burst

Reactive oxygen intermediates	Reactive nitrogen intermediates
O_2^- (superoxide)	NO (nitric oxide)
OH· (hydroxyl)	NO_2 (nitrogen dioxide)
H_2O_2 (hydrogen peroxide)	HNO_2 (nitrous acid)
$HClO^-$ (hypochlorite)	

class I molecules. Receptors present on the surface of NK cells can recognize target cells with reduced MHC class I expression as part of the cytotoxic process.

Finally, a type of NK cell has a role in maintaining normal pregnancy. They are the major population of lymphocytes present in the lining of the pregnant uterus, and loss of NK cell function in knockout mice results in 64%

fetal loss, a situation that can be corrected by transplanting normal NK cells. The role of NK cells in pregnancy seems related to their ability to promote fetal implantation and maintenance of the integrity of the uterus during pregnancy. NK cell-derived IFN-γ produced in the uterus is a key mediator of maintenance of uterine integrity during pregnancy. Also, as the developing fetus expresses paternal MHC antigens that the mother could recognize as foreign and induce an immune attack against the fetus, NK cells may have a role in preventing maternal rejection of the growing fetus.

Mast cells are another type of white blood cell involved in innate immunity. These cells also possess cytoplasmic granules; however, their granules contain vasoactive compounds such as histamine. Although histamine is widely known for its role in allergic reactions, mast cells and the vasoactive substances they release also are important in the regulation of inflammatory processes.

Signal Transduction

When cells of the immune system encounter either external antigens or molecules secreted by other cells with which they are communicating, a signal needs to be sent to the interior of the cell that an external binding event has occurred. This notification involves *signal transduction,* a process by which the binding of a stimulatory ligand to its receptor on the cell surface results in potent changes in the cytoplasm that are ultimately transmitted to the nucleus to influence gene expression. This process is initiated, for example, when neutrophils or macrophages bind to bacterial cell wall components. Signal transduction events are frequently initiated in discrete areas of the plasma membrane called *lipid rafts* or *microdomains* (Fig. 2.6A). These are areas in the plasma membrane rich in sphingolipids and cholesterol and underneath them in the cellular cytoplasm are concentrations of signal transduction molecules. Signal transduction also requires proteins that contain tyrosine, serine, threonine, or histidine that can be enzymatically phosphorylated or dephosphorylated (Fig. 2.6B)—changes that alter their energy state, induce other enzymatic activities, and allow for binding of the protein to other ligands. The proteins that phosphorylate other proteins are referred to as *kinases* such as protein tyrosine kinases or protein serine/threonine kinases, while those that dephosphorylate other proteins are referred to as *phosphatases.* The phosphorylation or dephosphorylation of one protein can lead to the phosphorylation or dephosphorylation of an entire cascade of proteins, ultimately resulting in changes in the subcellular localization or activity of one or more DNA-binding proteins, which in turn influence gene expression. Overall, the balance between protein tyrosine kinases and protein tyrosine phosphatases is a critical factor in regulating cell activation.

Another key aspect of the phosphorylation or dephosphorylation events is that new sites are created that allow cytoplasmic proteins to bind to the altered protein (Fig. 2.6B). The altered protein itself may not acquire a new activity, but the proteins that bind to the phosphorylated or dephosphorylated sites become concentrated within the cell and can now efficiently mediate further signaling events. Also, some of these proteins become activated when they bind to a phosphorylated amino acid.

Important contributors to the interaction of membrane-associated kinases with other proteins are adaptor proteins that bind together proteins involved in the signaling cascade (Fig. 2.6C). When the signaling molecules are bound together, their enzymatic and other activities are concentrated, amplifying their effects. Often the action of a tyrosine kinase results in a phosphotyrosine that can bind to proteins that express a specific domain referred to as Src homology domain 2 (SH2). The SH2 was first described as part of the Src family of protein kinases. Another domain, SH3, is found in many signaling proteins and interacts with proline-rich areas of other proteins.

To control signaling, a family of proteins known as protein phosphatases exists that can remove phosphate substituents from tyrosines and other phosphorylated amino acids. This control mechanism limits the amount of activation a cell can undergo and returns the signaling molecules to their basal state. Control of cellular activation allows further stimuli to activate the cell, if appropriate, and also prevents an uncontrolled response from occurring.

Mechanisms of Recognition by Cells of the Innate Immune Response

The innate immune response, although it lacks the specificity of the acquired immune response (Fig. 2.2), still requires a mechanism(s) for identifying when a cell or particle should be targeted for a response if these innate effectors are not to damage an individual's healthy cells and tissues. One means of identifying potential targets has already been discussed: the attachment of complement proteins to a foreign surface (which enhances phagocytosis). Similarly, attachment of antibodies to a microorganism, although requiring the participation of the acquired immune response, opsonizes the microorganism for enhanced phagocytosis.

Toll-like receptors

The innate immune system has recently been found to possess a family of receptors known as the Toll-like recep-

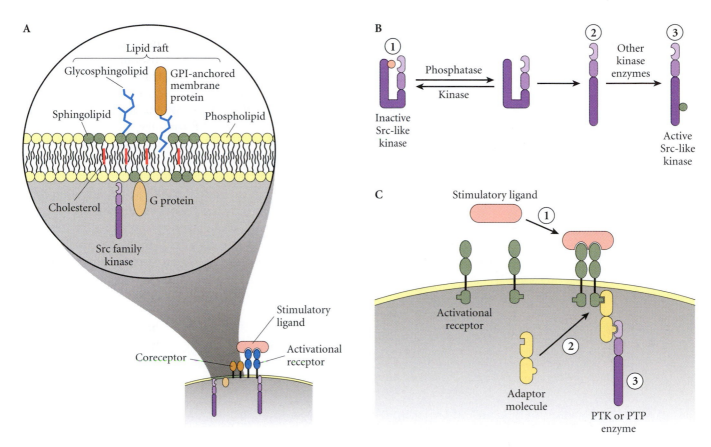

Figure 2.6 General principles and components of signal transduction. (**A**) Representation of the composition of lipid rafts, also known as microdomains, detergent-insoluble glycolipid-rich membranes or glycolipid-enriched membrane fractions. Sphingolipids and cholesterol aggregate together within the plasma membrane. On the outer side of the cell there is enrichment for glycophosphatidylinositol-anchored proteins and glycosphingolipids. On the cytoplasmic side, membrane-anchored signal transduction molecules are found. When a cell binds to stimulatory ligand, lipid rafts are recruited to the receptor complex via a raft-associated coreceptor protein. Localization of the lipid raft to the receptor complex results in recruitment of signaling molecules such as G proteins and Src family kinases. (**B**) Activation of signal transduction molecules. In the resting state there is a balance between the protein tyrosine kinases (PTKs) and protein tyrosine phosphatases (PTPs) such that the Src-like kinases are held mostly in an inactive form (**1**). When acted upon by a PTP, the dephosphorylated Src-like kinase can open up into an active form (**2**). Other PTK enzymes then phosphorylate a tyrosine residue to produce an enzymatically active molecule (**3**). Since the Src-like kinase is itself a PTK, it will act on other phosphate groups to promote cell activation. (**C**) Ligation of membrane receptors by stimulatory ligands allows adaptor molecules to bind to the aggregated receptors, promoting their interaction with PTK or PTP enzymes.

tors (TLRs). So far, 10 TLRs have been identified. Most of the TLRs interact with microbial factors that are seldom or never found in mammalian cells or tissues and are termed pathogen-associated molecular patterns (PAMP). The known ligands recognized by TLRs 1 through 10 and microorganisms that possess the ligand are listed in Table 2.2. TLR1 and TLR6 do not recognize a PAMP directly but seem to regulate TLR2-mediated responses to bacterial lipoteichoic acids.

It is not clear yet if the ligands recognized by TLRs bind directly to the TLR. Binding of some PAMPs to cells with

TLR response elements requires participation of a coreceptor protein such as CD14 for bacterial lipopolysaccharide (LPS) (Fig. 2.7). CD14 is not a transmembrane protein but is tethered to the outer leaflet of the cell's plasma membrane by a glycosylphosphatidylinositol linkage. Also, there is a fair amount of soluble CD14 found in blood. LPS must bind to CD14 in order for TLR4 to activate cells. In addition, the binding of LPS to CD14 is enhanced by the participation of two other proteins: LPS-binding protein (LBP) and CD55 (also called decay-accelerating factor). LBP and CD55 are thought to play a role in binding

Table 2.2 TLRs and their ligands

Receptor	Ligand (found in/on)
TLR1	Regulates TLR2
TLR2	Lipoarabinomannan (mycobacteria)
	Lipoteichoic acid (gram-positive bacteria)
	Peptidoglycan (gram-positive bacteria)
TLR3	?
TLR4	LPS (gram-negative bacteria)
TLR5	Flagellin (many bacteria)
TLR6	Regulates TLR2
TLR7	?
TLR8	?
TLR9	DNA CpG motifs[a]
TLR10	?

[a]DNA fragment in which a cytosine is followed immediately by a guanine. GT/ACGTT is the optimal DNA motif recognized by TLR9.

LPS and then transferring the LPS to CD14, which then associates with TLR4. Another membrane factor, MD-2, can be found associated with TLR4 and, to a lesser extent, with TLR2. MD-2 confers upon TLR4 the ability to recognize LPS and is thought to bind to the lipid portion of LPS, even in the absence of LBP, thus assisting in the interaction of LPS with the TLR complex.

After responding to its cognate ligand, a TLR delivers activation signals to the cell. Signaling proceeds via several biochemical pathways; the best characterized of these pathways results in activation of the nuclear factor-κB (NF-κB) pathway (Fig. 2.7). Ligand binding triggers *dimerization* of a TLR, meaning that two ligand-bound TLRs associate with each other. This event recruits additional signaling molecules to the receptor complex in the

Figure 2.7 Activation of a macrophage by bacterial lipoarabinomannan (LAM), lipoteichoic acid (LTA), or LPS. In each case, the bacterial product interacts with a macrophage TLR, sometimes requiring the participation of the proteins CD14 and MD-2. The bacterial product triggers homodimerization of the TLR. This dimerization event recruits the adaptor molecules MyD88 and MAL to the receptor complex, which in turn recruits the serine kinases IRAK or IRAK-2. In the cytoplasm, IRAK is associated with the protein Tollip, which appears to assist the recruitment of IRAK to the TLR complex. The IRAKs activate the kinases NIK (NF-κB-inducing kinase) or TAK-1 (transforming growth factor-β-activated kinase 1). Activation of NIK and TAK-1 requires the assistance of the cofactor protein TRAF6 (tumor necrosis factor receptor-associated factor 6). NIK or TAK-1 phosphorylates the protein IKK (inhibitor of κB kinase), which in turn phosphorylates the protein inhibitor of κB (IκB), resulting in the degradation of IκB. This releases the transcription factor NF-κB, which can then translocate to the nucleus to participate in gene transcription.

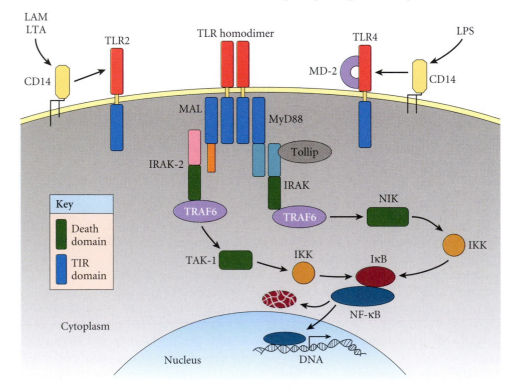

cytoplasm of the activated cell. Recruitment is achieved through multimerization events between two different protein domain types: the *TIR domain* and the *death domain*. The TIR domain (named for its importance in signaling by the toll and the interleukin-1 receptors) is present on the cytoplasmic tails of the TLRs and at the C terminus of the MyD88 protein. Death domains (named for the early observation of domains in proteins that mediate a cell suicide pathway called programmed cell death) are present on the N terminus of the MyD88 protein and on the protein kinase called interleukin-1 receptor-associated kinase (IRAK). Thus, MyD88 possesses both a TIR domain and a death domain and serves as a bridge between the TLR complex and signaling enzymes (Fig. 2.7). MyD88 is frequently referred to as an *adapter protein*. Another adapter protein, MyD88 adaptor-like protein (MAL) or TIR domain-containing adapter protein, transduces signals from TLR4 following interaction of TLR4 with bacterial LPS and is part of a signaling cascade that is distinct from (but similar to) that mediated by MyD88. The signaling cascade activated within the cell involves a number of kinases and other enzymes and culminates in the activation and nuclear translocation of transcription factors such as NF-κB, which results in transcription of immunologically important molecules such as cytokines.

The signaling pathway used by the TLR family of receptors is widely conserved in an evolutionary respect, and orthologs of this signaling pathway are found in numerous mammalian, insect, and plant species. In insects, the orthologous signaling pathway is also responsible for mediating dorsal-ventral patterning during embryogenesis (Fig. 2.8). This same signaling pathway mediates the production of antifungal peptides (similar to antibacterial peptides) in fruit flies. Thus, the TLR signaling pathway may be derived from an evolutionarily ancient response to infection.

Endocytic pattern-recognition receptors

Some cell surface receptors of the innate immune system do not activate transcription but stimulate endocytosis or phagocytosis. The mannose receptor/scavenger protein is expressed on the plasma membrane of macrophages and dendritic cells (DCs) and binds to high-mannose carbohydrates typically found on bacterial surfaces. The complement receptor 3 (CR3), which normally mediates phagocytosis of complement-coated antigens by neutrophils and macrophages, has recently been found to bind directly to zymosan, the principal component of fungal cell walls. Thus, CR3 serves a secondary role as a pattern-recognition receptor.

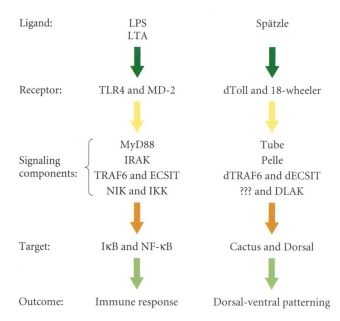

Figure 2.8 Evolutionary conservation of the Toll/TLR signaling pathway. The left side shows signaling via TLR4 in response to bacterial LPS, generating an innate immune response. The right side shows an orthologous signaling pathway in *Drosophila melanogaster* that leads to dorsal-ventral patterning during embryogenesis. TRAF, tumor necrosis factor receptor-associated factor; ECSIT, evolutionarily conserved signaling intermediate in Toll pathways; NIK, NF-κB-inducing kinase; IKK, inhibitor of κB kinase; IκB, inhibitor of κB; DLAK, *Drosophila* LPS-activated kinase. "d" preceding an acronym (e.g., dECSIT) indicates the *Drosophila* ortholog of the component. "???" indicates a component hypothesized to exist but not yet positively identified. Adapted from T. K. Means et al., *Cytokine Growth Factor Rev.* 11:219–232, 2000, with permission.

Soluble collectins: pattern-recognition receptors with many modes of action

Collectins are a family of pattern-recognition molecules that also recognize high-mannose carbohydrates common on bacterial surfaces. They are named for their long collagen-like "stalk" region and globular, lectin-type "head" region. The head region of the collectin binds carbohydrate. A growing number of soluble collectins have been experimentally studied. These include the proteins conglutinin; collectin-43 (CL-43); MBL; and two lung-specific proteins, surfactant proteins A and D (SP-A and SP-D). Although all of the soluble collectins are specific for high-mannose carbohydrates, they have subtle differences in binding specificities and the effector functions they activate. MBL has already been described as an activator of the complement cascade. Recent evidence suggests that CL-43 may also have this activity although CL-43 seems to bind to different complement components than MBL. MBL, conglutinin, and SP-A all bind to the surface of influenza virus, inhibiting the ability of the virus to infect host cells.

C-type lectins: surface-bound recognition molecules on DCs and Langerhans cells

Throughout the body are cells specialized for very early recognition of the presence of pathogens that collectively make up a group of diverse cells referred to as DCs and Langerhans cells (LCs) (see chapter 3). The LCs are found predominantly in the skin and are thought by some to be a form of skin-based DC whereas other types of DCs are found on mucosal sites and in the blood. These cells are now known to be the most potent cells in the immune system for recognizing antigen and for bringing it to lymph nodes in a form that initiates activation and differentiation responses by T and B cells.

One mechanism for recognizing foreign antigens, particularly infectious microbes, is the *C-type lectins* prominently displayed on DCs and LCs (Table 2.3). C-type lectins require Ca^{2+} ions for binding to carbohydrate residues on the surfaces of microbes using the lectin's carbohydrate recognition domain (CRD). Some of the soluble collectins are also C-type lectins: lung SP-A and SP-D and MBP, for example. Other C-type lectins are bound to the surface of DCs as transmembrane proteins. Two categories of cell-bound C-type lectins are known and are distinguished from each other on the basis of the orientation of the amino terminus (Fig. 2.9). Type I C-type lectins have their amino termini outside the cell, whereas type II C-type lectins have an intracellular amino terminus. The type I molecules have multiple CRDs, whereas the type II molecules have only a single CRD. The CRDs may also bind to microbial peptides and lipids. Full documentation of the range of ligands for the C-type lectins is not yet available, but they are known to bind microbial carbohydrates rich in mannose or galactose residues.

The C-type lectins function to capture antigen and deliver it into the cytoplasm of the DCs and LCs. Inside the cell the pathogen is targeted for destruction, and if this is as far as the reaction goes, then an effective innate immune response has occurred. However, if the antigenic stimulus is sufficient, the microbial constituents will be targeted to be processed and presented by the DC or LC to the lymphocytes of the immune system. This will lead to an acquired immune response. The C-type lectins also mediate interactions of DCs and LCs with other cells, notably endothelial cells that line blood vessels and cells within the lymph node where immune responses are taking place. An emerging recognition of the importance of C-type lectins in the immune system comes from findings that the human immunodeficiency virus uses C-type lectins to enter DCs on mucosal surfaces where the virus can then be transported to lymph nodes and enter T cells to initiate infection. In this instance, the pathogen has co-opted the normal role of the C-type lectin in immunity to establish infection.

Table 2.3 Characteristics of C-type lectins produced by DCs and LCs

C-type lectin	Type	Amino acids	Chromosomal location	Production[a]	Ligand[a]	Function	Key antibodies
MMR (CD206)	I	1,456	10p13	DCs, LCs, Mo, M·, DMECs	Mannose, fucose, sLeX	Antigen uptake	MG38, antihuman
DEC-205 (CD205)	I	1,722	2q24	DCs, LCs, high on actDCs, thymic ECs	?	Antigen uptake	
Dectin 1	II	247	12p13	DCs, LCs	β-Glucan	T-cell interaction	
Dectin 2	II	209	2p13	DCs, LCs	?	Antigen uptake	
Langerin (CD207)	II	328	2p13	LCs	?	Formation of Birbeck granules	DCGM4, antihuman
DC-SIGN (CD209)	II	404	19p13	DCs	HIV-1 (gp120), SIV, mannan, ICAM-2, ICAM-3	T-cell interaction, HIV-1 pathology, migration antigen uptake	AZN-D1, antihuman
BDCA-2	II	?	?	Plasmacytoid DCs	?	Antigen uptake?	AC-144, antihuman
DCIR (LLIR)	II	237	12p13	DCs, Mo, M·, PMN, B	?	?	
DLEC		231	12p13				
CLEC-1	II	280/229	12	DCs	?	?	

[a]actDCs, activated dendritic cells; B, B cells; DMECs, dermal microvascular endothelial cells; HIV-1, human immunodeficiency virus 1; ICAM, intercellular adhesion molecule; Mo, monocytes; M·, macrophages; SIV, simian immunodeficiency virus; sLeX, sialyl Lewis X; thymic ECs, thymic endothelial cells. Used with permission from C.G. Figdor et al., *Nat. Rev. Immunol.* 2:77–84, 2002.

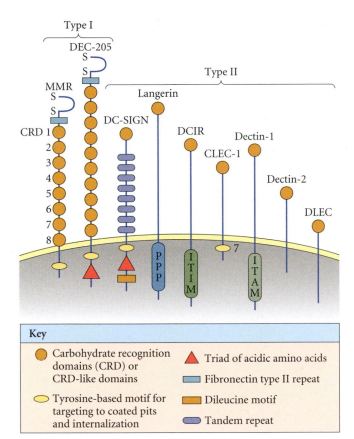

Figure 2.9 C-type lectins on DCs and LCs. Within the type I C-type lectins such as macrophage mannose receptor (MMR) and DEC-205 is a cysteine-rich repeat (S–S) in the amino terminus, a repeat domain for binding type II fibronectin (FN), and between 8 and 10 CRDs. The type II C-type lectins have an intracellular amino terminus and express only one CRD in the extracellular carboxy terminus. Within the cytoplasm are portions of the C-type lectins that express some important properties: a domain with tyrosines involved in the intracellular targeting of the lectin and targeting it to endocytic vesicles known as coated pits, and other motifs known by the presence of a triad of acidic amino acids and a dileucine motif. Transmembrane molecules involved in immune responses also contain portions involved in signaling such as the immunoreceptor tyrosine-based activation motif (ITAM) and immunoreceptor tyrosine-based inhibitory motif (ITIM) and proline-rich regions (PPP). CLEC-1, C-type lectin receptor 1; DCIR, dendritic cell immunoreceptor; DC-SIGN, dendritic-cell specific ICAM-3 grabbing nonintegrin; DLEC, dendritic cell lectin. Used with permission from C. G. Figdor et al., *Nat. Rev. Immunol.* 2:77–84, 2002.

Innate Responses to Viral Infection

The immune system must deal with many different pathogens, including fungal, viral, and protozoan pathogens and large, multicellular parasites such as worms. Viruses are ubiquitous in the environment and present the immune system with many interesting challenges. Unlike most bacteria, viruses can propagate only inside living cells. Once intracellular, a virus is resistant to many extracellular immune effector mechanisms such as antibodies and complement. The life cycle of the virus makes it dependent on the metabolic machinery of the host cell. This metabolic dependence is the basis of many innate defense strategies against viral infections.

Type I Interferons

Many innate defenses against viruses are mediated by a class of cytokine termed *interferons* (named for their ability to interfere with viral propagation). Most important in innate immunity to viruses are the type I interferons, IFN-α and IFN-β. During viral infection, these cytokines are secreted by lymphocytes, monocytes, and macrophages and bind to a receptor (IFN-α and IFN-β bind to the same receptor) expressed by almost all cell types (Fig. 2.10A). When a type I interferon binds to its receptor, the cell enters an "antiviral state" during which viral replication is inhibited by interference with protein synthesis within the infected cell. Synthesis of viral proteins necessary for assembly of virus particles is prevented. Interferons induce synthesis of a protein within the host cells called *double-stranded RNA-activated inhibitor of translation* (DAI). When DAI binds to double-stranded RNA (dsRNA) (common in the genomes of many viruses but not normally encountered in mammalian cells), DAI becomes activated and acquires the ability to phosphorylate and inactivate initiation factor 2, which is required for protein synthesis (Fig. 2.10B). Thus, DAI prevents viral replication at the expense of normal protein synthesis. Some viruses are able to circumvent this innate defense by inhibiting the activity of DAI. For example, adenovirus produces a small RNA called VA RNA L that binds to DAI and locks DAI in an inactive conformation. With DAI inactivated, synthesis of viral proteins can proceed. Epstein-Barr virus produces a small RNA called EBER-1 (Epstein-Barr-encoded small RNA 1) that functions similarly to VA RNA L.

A connection between the TLR signaling molecules and type I interferons has recently been made. TLR3 responds to dsRNA, which is the genetic information for many types of viruses. TLR gene expression is activated by type I interferons, and TLR3 expression in epithelial and endothelial cells was notably enhanced by interferons. As these cells are usually the first to be infected by pathogenic viruses, the role of interferons in antiviral protection appears to be multifaceted. Also, TLR3 response to dsRNA stimulates type I interferon production, indicating a potential amplification loop in innate immunity to viral infections.

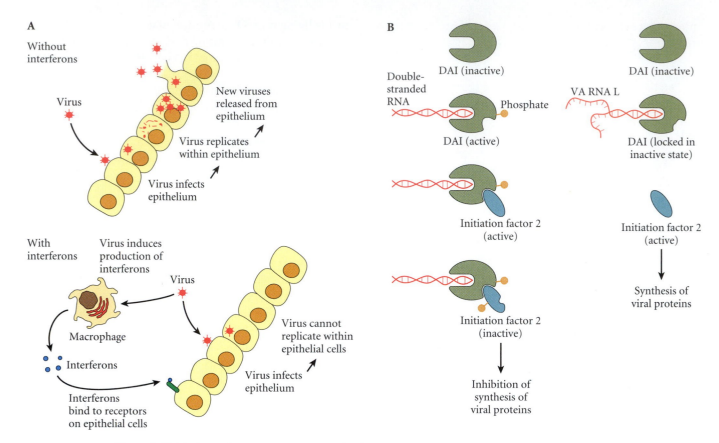

Figure 2.10 The innate immune response to viral infection is mediated by the cytokines called type I interferons. (**A**) Without interferons (**top**), a virus can infect a host cell, replicate within the infected cell by producing new viral nucleic acid and protein, and spread progeny viruses from the infected cell to other host cells. When type I interferons are produced in response to infection (**bottom**), the interferons bind to receptors on the surface of most host cells, terminating protein synthesis. This prevents synthesis of new viral proteins and thus the replication of viruses. (**B**) Interferons act by inducing the synthesis of the protein DAI. (**Left**) DAI is activated upon binding to dsRNA, which is common in the genomes of many viruses. Active DAI phosphorylates and inactivates eukaryotic initiation factor 2, shutting down protein synthesis. (**Right**) Some viruses, e.g., adenovirus and Epstein-Barr virus, are able to inhibit the activity of DAI with small RNAs, e.g., adenovirus VA RNA L.

A newly discovered member of the type I interferon family, IFN-κ, is expressed by keratinocytes of the skin. While differing in its expression pattern, IFN-κ seems to function by binding to the same receptor as IFN-α and IFN-β and possesses the same antiviral properties as the other type I interferons.

Complement as an Antiviral Agent

Although complement proteins usually are thought of in terms of their bactericidal activity, they also are active against viral particles. However, since the main lytic mechanism of the complement cascade is the MAC, the extent of the activity of complement against a specific virus depends on whether the virus has a membrane. Viruses that exit a mammalian cell by lysing it usually do not possess a membrane and are generally resistant to MAC-mediated killing. However, viruses that exit a mammalian cell by *budding* take a portion of their host cell membrane with them as an *envelope* that surrounds their protein core. Enveloped viruses can be targets of MAC activity, and insertion of enough MACs disrupts the envelope, rendering the virus noninfectious. Although nonenveloped viruses are resistant to the effects of the MAC, complement proteins can still inactivate these viruses if enough complement protein becomes activated. Activated complement proteins can attach to the virus and enshroud it in a thick protein layer that effectively blocks viral receptors from interacting with counter-receptors of their host cell. In such cases, the virus is not destroyed by the complement protein but is merely rendered incapable of initiating infection.

Inflammation: Orchestrating the Innate Effectors

Innate immune effector mechanisms usually do not act alone but rather participate in a larger, concerted response known as the inflammatory response. Inflammation can be thought of as a regulatory event aimed at mobilizing various innate immune effectors and trafficking them to the anatomic location where they can be most effective. The inflammatory response can occur as a localized or as a systemic phenomenon. Each type of inflammation has its own mechanisms and unique purposes.

Localized Inflammatory Responses

The localized inflammatory response is familiar to all who have had a splinter lodged deep in their skin or have had a similar injury. Very soon, the skin surrounding the injury becomes red, swollen, warm, and painful to touch. These four symptoms are the chief signs of localized inflammation and, in fact, are the basis for the name of this phenomenon, derived from the Latin word *inflammare*, meaning "to set on fire." Such injuries are a possible route of entry of microbes into an individual's tissues. Therefore, local inflammation quickly recruits many innate immune cells (such as macrophages and neutrophils) from the local blood vessels to the extravascular tissue at the site of injury (Fig. 2.11). This is achieved through regulated changes in the blood vessels near the site of injury or infection. Blood vessels in the injured tissue rapidly constrict, causing an increase in blood pressure inside the local vessels. At the same time, the vascular endothelium at the site of injury becomes "leaky," and the elevated pressure inside the blood vessels results in seepage of plasma into the extravascular tissue. This plasma is rich in complement proteins. The loosening of the tight junctions between endothelial cells also makes it easier for white blood cells to leave the blood vessel by squeezing between the endothelial cells, a process called *extravasation*.

One of the molecular signals that initiate and regulate localized inflammation is the complement cascade (Fig. 2.11), which gives rise to proteins that bind receptors on cells such as neutrophils, summoning them via a chemotactic concentration gradient to the infection site. Other signals initiate local inflammation. The kinin and plasmin systems are two enzymatic cascades activated in response to tissue injury. The kinin system (Fig. 2.12) pro-

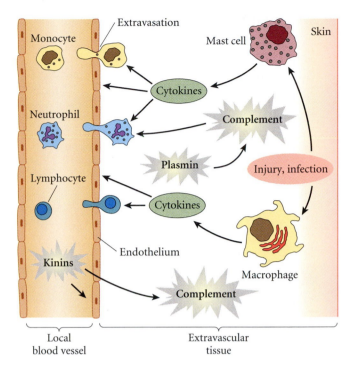

Figure 2.11 The localized inflammatory response. Injury or infection can result in the activation of the plasmin and kinin cascades. The kinin cascade produces vasoactive peptides that act on vascular endothelium to increase vascular permeability; the enzymes of the kinin cascade also can activate the complement cascade. The plasmin cascade is important in the remodeling of extracellular matrix that accompanies wound healing; the enzymes of the plasmin cascade also can activate the complement cascade. Once activated, complement proteins cause leukocytes such as PMNs, lymphocytes, and monocytes to leave the blood circulation (*extravasate*) and home to the site of infection or injury. Extravasation and homing of leukocytes also are regulated by cytokines produced by local mast cells (activated by complement proteins) and macrophages (activated by bacterial products).

duces the vasoactive peptides *kallidin* and *bradykinin*, which increase vascular permeability at the site of injury. The kinin system serves a second role as an activator of complement. The plasmin system plays a central role in remodeling the extracellular matrix during wound repair. The protease plasmin, a component of this enzymatic cascade, is also an activator of the complement cascade (Fig. 2.13). Not all of the regulators of localized inflammation result from protease cascades; some are cytokines produced locally by mast cells and macrophages that are activated by complement proteins or bacterial products (Fig. 2.11). The cytokines tumor necrosis factor alpha, interleukin-1 (IL-1), and IL-6 have all been found to regulate inflammation in various tissues, although the importance of these various cytokines varies from tissue to tissue.

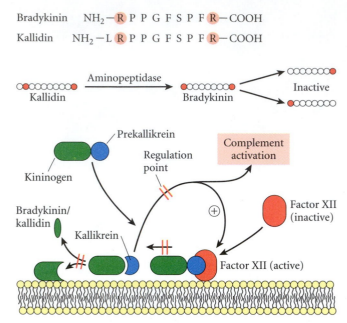

Bradykinin NH₂—R P P G F S P F R—COOH

Kallidin NH₂—L R P P G F S P F R—COOH

Figure 2.12 The kinin system (also called the kallikrein system) produces the vasoactive peptides bradykinin and kallidin, which regulate inflammation. (**Top**) Diagrams of the vasoactive peptides bradykinin and kallidin. Amino acids are indicated in the one-letter code (see inside front cover). Essential arginine amino acids, which are required for biological activity, are highlighted. After its generation, kallidin can be converted to bradykinin by the action of aminopeptidase enzyme. Further cleavage of bradykinin leads to a loss of biological activity. (**Bottom**) The enzymes of the kinin system (kallikrein and factor XII) become activated during blood clotting and wound repair. Activated factor XII cleaves the proenzyme prekallikrein to its active form, kallikrein. Active kallikrein then acts on its substrate, kininogen, to form the vasoactive peptides bradykinin and kallidin. This process is negatively regulated at several steps, indicated by double red lines. In addition to the generation of bradykinin and kallidin, kallikrein can also activate the complement cascade, resulting in a stimulation of innate immunity. In this way, the innate immune system is set to become activated at wound sites, which are likely entry points for microbes.

Systemic Inflammatory Responses: the Acute-Phase Response

Other aspects of the innate response require participation of organs and tissues that are remote from the site of injury. Body temperature is regulated in the hypothalamus. Replacement of white blood cells lost while combating infection (e.g., neutrophils and macrophages) requires increased hematopoiesis in the bone marrow, and replacement of complement proteins consumed by the response requires de novo synthesis within hepatocytes in the liver. All of these responses are triggered by cytokines that are produced locally at the site of injury or infection and that enter the blood circulation to cause systemwide effects. This systemic arm of the inflammatory response is collectively termed the acute-phase response (Fig. 2.14).

Cross-Talk between the Innate and Acquired Arms of Immunity

Although it is convenient to discuss the innate and acquired responses as separate processes, in reality these two types of responses interact to protect an individual from infection, stimulating and regulating each other's activities (Fig. 2.2; see Fig. 1.15). For example, phagocytosis is an innate immune mechanism; however, antigens that are engulfed by a macrophage or DC frequently are presented to helper T cells on MHC class II molecules on the cell surface, thus stimulating an acquired immune response. Similarly, although type I interferons can prevent intracellular viruses from replicating, they also stimulate higher expression of MHC class I by a virus-infected cell, increasing the likelihood of a virus-specific cytotoxic T lymphocyte becoming activated by the infected cell. Complement proteins either can kill a microbial cell via MAC formation or can opsonize the bacterium for phagocytosis—both innate immune mechanisms. Complement proteins on an antigenic surface also promote the activation of B cells that respond to the foreign antigen. These are all examples of how an innate response stimulates an acquired response.

Figure 2.13 The plasmin cascade can be initiated by a number of proteases (e.g., elastase, kallikrein, cathepsin G, and thrombin) normally found at a site of injury or infection. The cascade results in the production of the active protease plasmin from the precursor plasminogen. Plasmin functions in the remodeling of extracellular matrix during wound repair and also can activate the complement cascade.

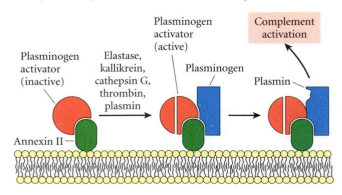

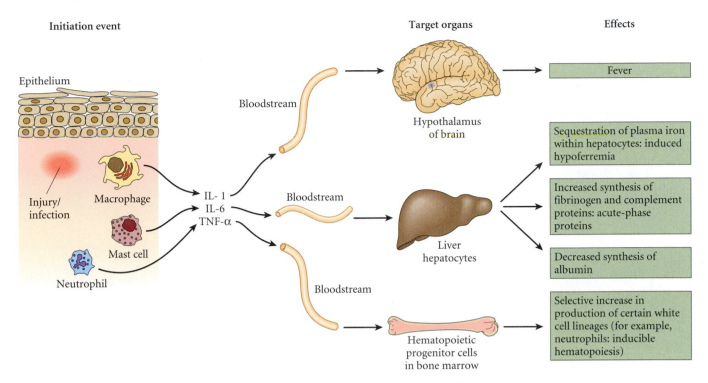

Figure 2.14 The systemic inflammatory response: the acute-phase response. The acute-phase response increases production of effectors consumed during inflammation (PMNs, complement components) and induces increases in body temperature to inhibit microbial growth. The acute-phase response is initiated by cytokines produced at the site of infection that travel to distant tissues via the circulation. The most crucial cytokines appear to be IL-1, tumor necrosis factor alpha (TNF-α), IL-6, leukemia inhibitory factor, and oncostatin M. Targets of these cytokines include the hypothalamus of the brain (which produces prostaglandins, resulting in the fever response), the liver (which begins to synthesize immunologically important proteins at the expense of the synthesis of some housekeeping proteins), and bone marrow (which increases production of leukocytes such as neutrophils—a reaction called *inducible hematopoiesis*). The proteins whose synthesis is stimulated within the liver during the acute-phase response include many components of the complement cascade and are commonly referred to as *acute-phase proteins*.

Cross-regulation between innate and acquired responses also flows in the other direction, with acquired responses regulating innate immune mechanisms. Cytokines produced by T cells during an acquired immune response can enhance the phagocytic function of macrophages and stimulate other activities of these innate immune cells, such as the oxidative burst. Last, antibodies can opsonize microorganisms and other antigens, making them more readily phagocytosed.

Summary

The innate immune response represents the first line of defense against infection, possessing properties that enable it to deal effectively with a continuous onslaught of microbial agents. Thus, the innate response is activated rapidly but is generally nonspecific in order to be capable of responding equally to a diverse array of potential pathogens. Many of the effectors of innate immunity are highly conserved in an evolutionary sense, representing ancient defense mechanisms carried through evolutionary history. In mammals, these mechanisms now function in concert with the acquired immune response. The mechanisms of the innate response integrate with the acquired response, helping regulate the overall immune response while also accepting regulatory cues from the acquired response. Together, the innate and the acquired immune responses provide individuals with more complete protection than that provided by either the innate or acquired response alone.

Suggested Reading

Caamaño, J., and C. A. Hunter. 2002. NF-κB family of transcription factors: central regulators of innate and adaptive immune functions. *Clin. Microbiol Rev.* **15**:414–429.

Devine, D. A., and R. E. Hancock. 2002. Cationic peptides: distribution and mechanisms of resistance. *Curr. Pharm. Des.* 8:703–714.

Figdor, C. G., Y. van Kooyk, and G. J. Adema. 2002. C-type lectin receptors on dendritic cells and Langerhans cells. *Nat. Rev. Immunol.* 2:77–84.

Ganz, T. 2001. Fatal attraction evaded: how pathogenic bacteria resist cationic polypeptides. *J. Exp. Med.* 193:F31–F34.

Modlin, R. L. 2002. Mammalian toll-like receptors. *Ann. Allergy Asthma Immunol.* 88:543–547.

Uthaisangsook, S., N. K. Day, S. L. Bahna, R. A. Good, and S. Haraguchi. 2002. Innate immunity and its role against infections. *Ann. Allergy Asthma Immunol.* 88:253–264.

Yang, D., A. Biragyn, L. W. Kwak, and J. J. Oppenheim. 2002. Mammalian defensins in immunity: more than just microbicidal. *Trends Immunol.* 23:291–296.

Cells of the Immune System

Elinor M. Levy

Hematopoiesis and Generation of Cells of the Immune System

Stem Cells, Myeloid Cells, and Lymphoid Cells

The cells of the immune system are produced throughout life from a common pluripotent stem cell by a process called hematopoiesis. These cells include the granulocytes (neutrophils, eosinophils, and basophils), mast cells, monocytes, dendritic cells, lymphocytes, and platelets. During ontogeny the pluripotent stem cell is first found in the para-aortic splanchnopleura but later moves to the yolk sac, then to the fetal liver, and finally to the fetal spleen. In adults, hematopoiesis normally takes place in the bone marrow. Here the pluripotent stem cell reproduces either in a process of self-renewal or to give rise to progeny that differentiate into cells of the erythroid, myeloid, or lymphoid lineage (Fig. 3.1). The stem cell and the lineage precursors it produces are influenced to follow these different pathways by the stromal cells and soluble factors in the surrounding microenvironment. The myeloid precursor is the source of granulocytes (neutrophils, eosinophils, basophils, and mast cells), monocytic cells, and megakaryocytes. Megakaryocytes fragment to give rise to platelets. The lymphoid precursor gives rise to cells called T lymphocytes, B lymphocytes, and null lymphocytes. In adult mammals, most immune cells mature to a competent (i.e., functional) stage in the bone marrow. However, T-lymphocyte precursors leave the bone marrow in an immature form and generally require passage through the thymus to progress from this progenitor stage to a mature, immunocompetent stage. Mast cells and dendritic cells also enter the circulation in an immature form.

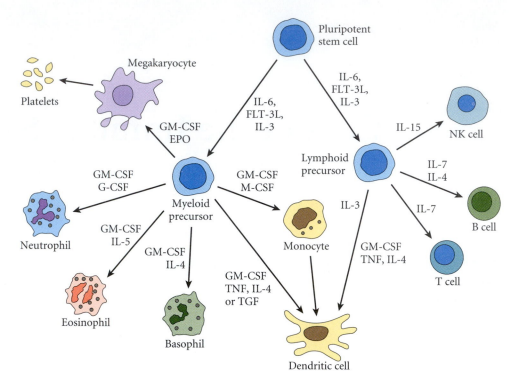

Figure 3.1 White blood cell hematopoiesis and role of key cytokines in this process. Stem cells either self-renew or produce progeny that are more committed to a particular differentiation path. The process is influenced both by factors produced within the bone marrow and by factors produced outside the bone marrow in response to stressors such as infections. Some cells, such as dendritic cells, can be produced by alternative pathways. Note that dendritic cells can arise from several different progenitor cells, some myeloid and some lymphoid. EPO, erythropoietin.

Growth Factors and Genesis of Cells of the Immune System

Hematopoiesis is regulated both by factors produced by stromal cells within the bone marrow and by factors produced outside the bone marrow. The latter usually are synthesized in response to infection. The body produces factors that signal the precursor cells to produce more immune cells of an appropriate type; this directed generation of a specific subpopulation(s) of leukocytes is referred to as *inducible hematopoiesis*. As indicated in Fig. 3.1, numerous *cytokines* are involved in hematopoiesis, with some stimulating more than one lineage and influencing the process at more than one developmental stage. Cytokines are small proteins made by cells, particularly those of the immune system, that influence the production, growth, or differentiation of other cells. Because some cytokines function to promote and direct the growth and development of blood cells, these particular cytokines are often referred to as *growth factors*. In some cases, the growth factors have overlapping functions such that any one of several factors is sufficient to promote development. The pluripotent stem cell divides in response to stem cell factor, interleukin-3 (IL-3), IL-6, and the flt-3 ligand.

Granulocyte-macrophage colony-stimulating factor (GM-CSF) and IL-3 act on the myeloid precursor to induce differentiation of other precursors specific for the myeloid cell lineage. Additional factors such as granulocyte colony-stimulating factor then induce the production of mature neutrophils. IL-5 directs the production of eosinophils, and IL-4 directs the production of basophils. Mast-cell development is a little more complicated. Mast cells share many characteristics with basophils and once were thought to arise from basophils. Although their developmental pathway is still not entirely understood, mast cells have been found to enter the blood in a precursor form and then move into the tissues, where they complete their development under the influence of local growth factors. It is thought that the extreme phenotypic heterogeneity observed among mast cells of different tissues reflects differences in the local cytokine environments in these tissues.

In a similar stepwise process, the lymphoid precursor can be stimulated by IL-3 and IL-7 to become a B-cell progenitor, which is further stimulated by IL-2, IL-4, IL-5, and IL-6 to develop into a mature B cell. Alternatively, IL-7 acts on a T-cell progenitor, which leaves the bone marrow and travels to the thymus to become a thymocyte. Thymocytes are further stimulated by the thymic microenvironment and by the factors IL-2, IL-4, and IL-7 to develop into mature T cells. The unique hematopoietic function of IL-7 was first suggested by the results of experiments employing antibodies that blocked IL-7. These results have more recently been verified by experiments with mice genetically deficient in either IL-7 or its receptor. Development of B and T cells is severely restricted in each of these types of mice, and the few B and T cells found are unable to function normally. IL-15 directs the development of natural killer (NK) cells in the bone marrow.

Identification of Cells via Surface Markers

The Concept of the Use of Cell Surface Antigens To Generate Antibodies

The lymphocytes are a diverse group of cells functionally but are similar morphologically. This morphologic similarity would be a great barrier to the study of these cells were it not possible to tell the various lineages apart. Much of the progress that has been made in understanding lymphocyte function has followed from the realization that each of these cell lineages can be distinguished on the basis of its expression of a unique set of membrane protein molecules. These distinguishing surface molecules are referred to as *markers* and can be detected with the use of marker-specific antibodies. Differences in the expression of these surface molecules as detected by such antibodies have been especially useful for the designation, isolation, and characterization of lymphocyte subsets (Fig. 3.2A). Other hematopoietic cells are distinguished on the basis of their surface markers and their distinctive morphologic features.

Given the general utility of marker-specific antibodies in the characterization of immune cells, a brief discussion of the preparation of such antibodies would be beneficial. Since most organisms do not routinely produce antibodies specific for self proteins, marker-specific antibodies must be produced by cross-species immunization with the marker of interest. For example, an antibody that recognizes the human CD4 protein marker could be made by first purifying human CD4 and then using the human CD4 to immunize mice. Serum from an immunized mouse will contain a collection of antibodies directed at the foreign protein (in this case, human CD4). These antibodies will bind to different portions (antigenic determinants) of the human CD4 molecule. Because these marker-specific antibodies are derived from many diverse B lymphocytes, the antibody is referred to as *polyclonal antibody*. Similarly, the serum that contains the antibody is called *polyclonal antiserum*.

Alternatively, one can immunize a mouse against human CD4 protein and then use the mouse's splenic lymphocytes as a source of antigen-specific B cells. These splenic B cells can be fused with a myeloma cell drived from a B-cell tumor. This fusion product is called a *hybridoma*. It is possible to isolate individual hybridoma cells by diluting suspensions of hybridoma cells such that a culture vessel is seeded with a single hybridoma cell! These individual (i.e., cloned) hybridoma cells and their progeny produce antibody referred to as *monoclonal antibody,* which refers to the fact that all of the marker-specific antibody-producing B cells are the progeny of one original parent cell. Unlike polyclonal antibodies, a monoclonal antibody will recognize a single antigenic determinant. The ability to identify and isolate cell lineages of interest has been enhanced enormously by the availability of monoclonal antibodies that can be produced reliably in great quantities.

Use of Monoclonal and Polyclonal Antibodies To Identify Cells via Expressed Markers

As of early 2000, more than 160 markers had been defined by antibodies. The markers are designated either by names indicating their function or, more often, by a cluster-of-differentiation (or CD) designation arrived at by scientists at annually held workshops. Some markers are expressed by multiple cell types; others are specific for a cell type (or lineage) (Fig. 3.2B). In some cases, a marker is expressed transiently during differentiation (and is therefore referred to as *differentiation marker*) or following cell activation (in which case it is referred to as an *activation marker*). CD1, which is expressed by thymocytes but not by mature T cells, is an example of a differentiation marker; CD25, which functions as an IL-2 receptor on activated T cells but is not expressed by resting T cells, is an example of an activation marker. By using multiple markers, one not only can identify a cell type but also can understand something about its current status (Table 3.1).

Morphology and Function of Myeloid Cells

Monocytes, Macrophages, and Other Antigen-Presenting Cells

Identification by morphologic means

Monocytic cells (Fig. 3.3) carry out a diverse set of functions in the immune response (Fig. 3.4) and take part in both the innate and the specific arms of the immune system. Cells of this lineage include monocytes, which circulate in the blood, and macrophages, which are located in the

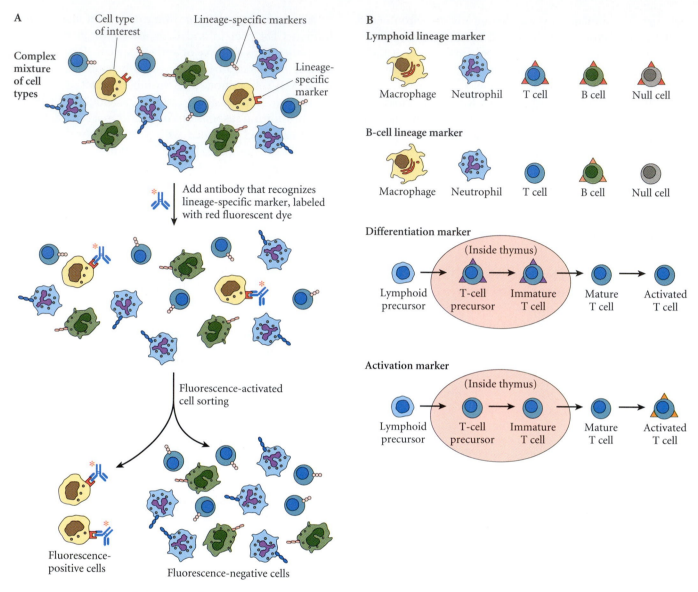

Figure 3.2 The use of antibodies to specific cell surface markers to characterize different types of cells. (**A**) Monoclonal antibodies specific for lineage-specific markers can be used to identify one cell type of interest in a complex mixture of cell types. Through the use of fluorescently labeled monoclonal antibodies and a process called fluorescence-activated cell sorting, cells of a particular lineage can be physically separated from a complex mixture of irrelevant cell types. (**B**) Cell-specific markers can be used to identify cells within a broad lineage (such as lymphocytes) or to identify cells of a single particular lineage (such as B cells). Some markers are only expressed at certain developmental stages (differentiation markers) or are only expressed after cell activation (activation markers), and are useful for identifying cells that are in a particular developmental or activational stage. A triangle indicates a cell that can be identified within a particular group of cells.

Table 3.1 Immune cell markers

Type	Examples	Expressed on
Activation	CD25, CD38	Activated T cells
Differentiation	CD1	Thymocytes
	CD38	Early T and B cells
Lineage specific	CD3	T cells
	CD19	B cells

tissues. Monocytes are about 10 to 18 micrometers (μm) in diameter and are 1 to 6% of the circulating white blood cells. Monocytes can move into the tissues and differentiate into macrophages. Alternatively, monocytes can develop into another cell type referred to as dendritic cells. Macrophages can survive in the tissues for several months. Some macrophages have a relatively fixed location and take on distinguishing characteristics depending on the organs isms. Additional markers and their associated function are noted below.

Functions

Phagocytosis

Monocytic cells are also referred to as *mononuclear phagocytic cells,* a designation reflecting their important ability to engulf and phagocytose large particulate bodies. During phagocytosis, the macrophage sends out long cytoplasmic extensions (called *pseudopodia*) to surround and engulf particulate matter. In the past, the system of tissue macrophages, together with endothelial cells and granulocytes, was called the *reticuloendothelial system.* This collection of cells removes foreign particulate matter, dead cells, and debris from the circulation. Phagocytes also can move to sites of inflammation or injury throughout the body to remove debris and to attack invading organisms.

Monocytes and macrophages often use CD14, a receptor for the lipopolysaccharide (LPS) component of the gram-negative bacterial cell wall, to identify these microbes. Since LPS is not found on mammalian cells, its presence is a good indicator of bacterial infection. Similarly, macrophages use mannose receptors and scavenger receptor type I for microbial recognition. Some of these scavenger receptors also take up modified low-density lipoprotein cholesterol particles and contribute to the formation of lesions called atherogenic plaques that can lead to heart disease.

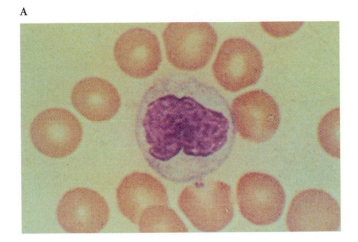

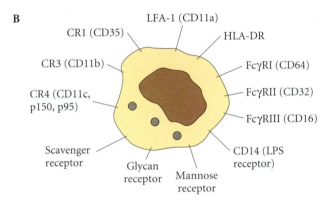

Figure 3.3 (**A**) Photomicrograph of a monocyte or macrophage. (**B**) Schematic diagram of a monocytic cell indicating characteristic surface molecules. Receptors such as the mannose and LPS receptors allow monocytic cells to be broadly reactive with microbes. When microbes are coated with antibody or complement, Fc and complement receptors promote a much more vigorous phagocytic response.

in which they reside. In the lung, these cells are called *alveolar macrophages;* in the liver, *Kupffer cells;* in the kidney, *intraglomerular mesangial cells;* and in the brain, *microglial cells.* That these different populations of macrophages have different names is a historical artifact, in that the cells were identified histologically before they were known to represent cells of the same lineage. Monocytic cells generally have a kidney-shaped nucleus and contain faint azurophilic granules (Fig. 3.3A) similar to the primary granules of neutrophils. They have a ruffled membrane, and their cytoplasm contains many lysosomes and a well-developed Golgi apparatus. The macrophage or monocyte also is characterized by several surface molecules (Fig. 3.3B), including complement receptor 3 (CR3; also called the C3bi receptor, CD11b, or MAC-a), the adhesion molecule LFA-1 (also called CD11a), and CR4 (also called p150,95 and CD11c). These molecules help stabilize interactions between monocytic cells and other cells or microorgan-

Figure 3.4 Functions of monocytic cells. Monocytic cells are versatile cells, being important in both innate and acquired immune responses. Not only do these cells attack microbes and cancer cells and act as APCs, they also produce cytokines that mobilize defenses in response to an infection. Cytokines such as IL-1, IL-6, and TNF-α induce fever, induce the production of acute-phase reactants by the liver, modulate the circulation of zinc and copper, induce production of adrenal corticotropic hormone in the brain, and influence metabolism. As phagocytic scavenger cells, monocytic cells also are involved in tissue remodeling and repair. In addition, monocytes are important sources of several components of the complement system.

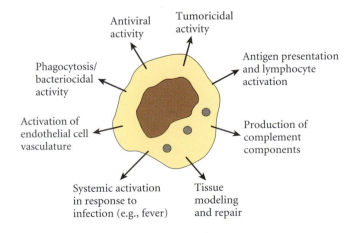

In addition, phagocytosis is greatly facilitated (*opsonized*) when phagocytic targets are first bound by antibodies or complement proteins present in the host's serum. Macrophages have receptors for the complement component C3b (called CR1 or CD35) as well as for the Fc portion of immunoglobulin molecules. Examples of such Fc receptors (FcRs) are FcγRI (CD64), FcγRII (CD32), FcγRIII (CD16), and FcεRII (CD23). C3b is an activated form of complement component C3, which is generated upon the initiation of the complement cascade. In contrast, the Fc portion of an antibody is always present as part of the antibody molecule but binds the FcRs efficiently only when the antibody is complexed with its antigen.

Macrophages constantly monitor their environment using pinocytosis, a process in which vesicles invaginate from the cell membrane and bring any fluids that are adjacent to the cell membrane into the cell. When macrophages encounter an activating stimulus, their metabolism, motility, and phagocytosis increase rapidly. Activated macrophages are somewhat larger than resting macrophages and are more efficient at killing pathogens. Following phagocytosis, mononuclear phagocytes digest or otherwise destroy ingested particles with acid hydrolases and peroxidases contained within their lysosomes. Monocytic cells are less efficient than neutrophils at destroying phagocytized particles, probably because the monocytes have fewer hydrolytic enzymes per cell. Activated monocytic cells also can kill pathogens through the production of reactive oxygen products such as hydrogen peroxide, hydroxyl radicals, superoxide anion, and nitric oxide generated in a process referred to as *respiratory* or *oxidative burst* (Fig. 3.5). Macrophages can be activated by a broad range of stimuli, including contact with particulate matter and exposure to bacterial products (particularly LPS), activated components of the complement or coagulation system, and cytokines, particularly interferon-gamma (IFN-γ).

Antigen presentation

The second major role of monocytic cells is antigen presentation. Activation of helper T (TH) lymphocytes in response to an antigen cannot occur until that antigen is displayed (on an antigen-presenting cell [APC]) in a context that helper T cells can recognize (i.e., as an antigenic peptide complexed to a major histocompatibility complex (MHC) class II protein). The ability of any cell to function as an APC requires the cell to have the ability to carry out several molecular mechanisms: (i) to "process" a protein antigen by cleaving the original protein antigen into a series of small peptides (13 to 18 amino acids) and

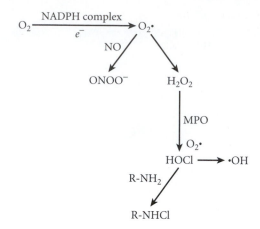

Figure 3.5 Reactive oxygen products generated in a respiratory burst can kill microorganisms. The reduced nicotinamide adenine dinucleotide phosphate (NADPH) oxidase complex at the phagocyte surface or adjoining a phagosome can be activated by phagocytosis, by bacterial products such as LPS or formylated peptides, and by certain cytokines. The oxidase transfers electrons to oxygen to produce superoxide, which can further react to produce hydrogen and nitrogen peroxide, hypochlorous acid, and hydroxyl radicals and related toxic molecules. MPO, myeloperoxidase; $O_2 \cdot$, superoxide; ONOO, nitrogen peroxide; H_2O_2, hydrogen peroxide; HDCL, hyperchlorous acid; OH, hydroxyl radical; R-NHCl, reactive nitrogen.

then loading these short peptides into the antigen-binding groove of a MHC class II protein; (ii) to "present" or display this antigen-MHC complex to an appropriate, antigen-specific TH cell; and (iii) to provide that TH cell with other activational signals that, together with the antigen, stimulate the TH cell to become activated.

Production of cytokines

When they encounter certain stimuli, particularly those of bacterial origin, monocytic cells are activated and produce a variety of cytokines. These cytokines are capable of causing systemic and local effects. The cytokines produced include IL-1, IL-6, IL-8, IL-10, IL-12, IL-15, tumor necrosis factor alpha (TNF-α), IFN-α, IFN-β, and transforming growth factor beta (TGF-β). IL-1, IL-6, and TNF-α are referred to as *inflammatory cytokines*. They can induce systemic changes such as fever and the acute-phase response (see Fig. 2.12) and stimulate the function of cytotoxic cells. IL-12 is important in determining the direction of a T-lymphocyte response, preferentially inducing a cell-mediated (cytotoxic) response. IL-10, on the other hand, inhibits such a cytotoxic response. Activated macrophages also produce the colony-stimulating factors GM-CSF, macrophage colony-stimulating factor, and granulocyte colony-stimulating factor, which increase the production of granulocytes and macrophages (inducible hematopoiesis) to further assist in combating infections.

Table 3.2 Granulocytes

Type	Neutrophil	Eosinophil	Basophil
Blood count/mm^2	3,500–5,000	5–20	<5
Major functions	Phagocytosis	ADCC against parasites	Allergic reactions
	Inflammation	Asthma effectors	

Effectors of immunity

In addition to its role as a phagocytic cell, the macrophage can act as a killer cell to destroy target cells and pathogens without ingesting them. Macrophages bind to and kill certain tumor cells and cells perceived to be foreign and also kill antibody-coated cells by a process known as *antibody-dependent cell-mediated cytotoxicity* (ADCC). Cytotoxic mediators include nitric oxide and the cytokine TNF-α; in addition, the cytokines IFN-α and IFN-β can inhibit viral infections directly (see Fig. 2.8). Some of the products of activated macrophages can suppress the functions of lymphocytes. These products include nitric oxide, prostaglandin E$_2$, and phosphatidyl serine. Macrophages also are the source of a number of complement products and coagulation factors and are therefore important effectors of wound healing and homeostasis.

Granulocytes: Neutrophils, Eosinophils, and Basophils

Identification by morphologic means

Granulocytes make up 60 to 70% of circulating white blood cells (Table 3.2) and rapidly leave the blood circulation by a process called extravasation at inflammatory sites. Extravasation uses the ability of these cells to *diapedis* or crawl between adjacent endothelial cells that make up the lining of the blood vessels (see Fig. 2.9). Granulocytes are generally short-lived cells, surviving for several hours in the blood or for up to several days in tissues after leaving the bone marrow.

The major subclass of granulocytes is the neutrophils, which make up more than 90% of circulating granulocytes (Fig. 3.6A and B). They are 10 to 20 μm in diameter and have a characteristic multilobed nucleus. The cytoplasm of a neutrophil contains three types of granules (Table 3.3). The primary granules, also called the *azurophilic* granules because they stain a clear blue or azure color with certain biological dyes, contain acid hydrolases, myeloperoxidase, elastase, cathepsin, and lysozyme. The secondary or *specific* granules contain lysozyme, collagenase, and lactoferrin. The third type of granules contains gelatinase. Similar to monocytes, neutrophils express several different receptors (including CD32 and CD16) that bind to the Fc portion of antibody.

Eosinophils have a bilobed nucleus, are 12 to 17 μm in diameter, and make up 2 to 4% of circulating leukocytes in healthy persons. They also are stored in the bone marrow and in connective tissue throughout the body. Their granules include major basic protein, cationic protein, and an eosinophil peroxidase. Major basic protein binds the red dye eosin, which causes these granules to stain intensely after treatment with hematoxylin and eosin stain (Fig. 3.6D), the characteristic that gives the eosinophil its name. Eosinophils express the high-affinity FcR for IgE (FcεRI) and a low-affinity receptor (CD32) for immunoglobulin G (IgG) (Fig. 3.6C). They are thought to play an important role in defense against parasitic organisms and are also key mediators of both the inflammatory response and the late-phase response of immediate-type hypersensitivity reactions.

Basophils make up less than 0.2% of circulating white blood cells. They are 5 to 7 μm in diameter with an eccentric round or oval nucleus (Fig. 3.6F). Their many granules stain a dark blue-purple with hematoxylin stains. These granules contain histamine, neutral proteases, heparin, chondroitin sulfate, and the cytokine TNF-α. Basophils express FcεRI (Fig. 3.6E) and release their granule contents upon cross-linking of receptor-bound IgE. Thus, basophils

Table 3.3 Granulocyte products

Product(s)	Neutrophils	Eosinophils	Basophils
Granule contents	Myeloperoxidase, lysozyme, defensins, acid hydrolases, elastase, cathepsin G, collagenase G, azurocidin, collagenase, gelatinase, lactoferrin, bacterial permeability-increasing proteins	Eosinophil peroxidase, Charcot-Leyden crystal protein (lyophosphatase), major basic protein, eosinophil cationic protein	Histamine, chondroitin sulfate, neutral proteinases, major basic protein, Charcot-Leyden crystal protein
Effector molecules synthesized after activation	Oxidative products (O$_2$, OH, H$_2$O$_2$, NO)		Leukotriene C$_4$, prostaglandins
Cytokines	IL-1, IL-6, IL-8, IL-12, TNF-α, MIP-1α[a]	IL-3, IL-4, IL-5, IL-10, IL-12, GM-CSF, IFN-γ	IL-4, IL-5, IL-6, IL-13, TNF-α

[a]MIP, macrophage inflammatory protein.

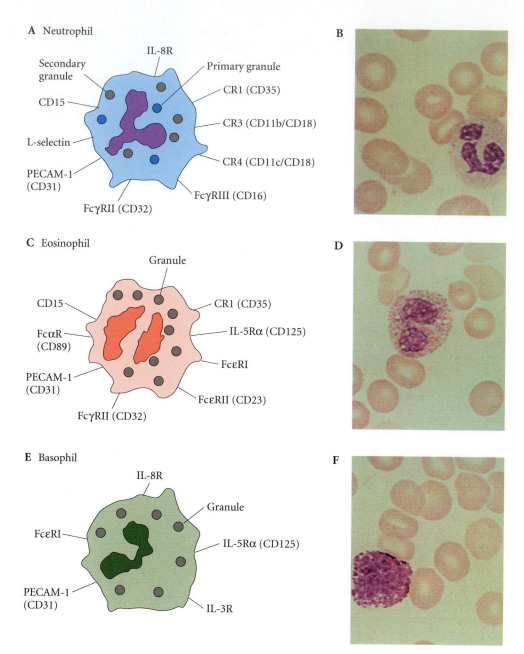

A Neutrophil

Secondary granule
IL-8R
Primary granule
CD15
CR1 (CD35)
L-selectin
CR3 (CD11b/CD18)
PECAM-1 (CD31)
CR4 (CD11c/CD18)
FcγRIII (CD16)
FcγRII (CD32)

C Eosinophil

Granule
CD15
CR1 (CD35)
FcαR (CD89)
IL-5Rα (CD125)
PECAM-1 (CD31)
FcεRI
FcεRII (CD23)
FcγRII (CD32)

E Basophil

IL-8R
Granule
FcεRI
IL-5Rα (CD125)
PECAM-1 (CD31)
IL-3R

Figure 3.6 The granulocytes. (**A**) Schematic diagram of a neutrophil. The neutrophil is characterized by a number of adhesion molecules, FcRs, and receptors for complement. The primary, or azurophilic, granules contain acid hydrolases, myeloperoxidase, elastase, cathepsin, and lysozyme. Secondary, or specific, granules contain lysozyme, collagenase, and lactoferrin. (**B**) Photomicrograph of a neutrophil. Note the irregularly shaped nucleus. (**C**) Schematic diagram of an eosinophil. Eosinophils express FcRs for IgA, IgE, and IgG and for several adhesion molecules. Their granules contain major basic protein, cationic protein, and an eosinophil peroxidase. (**D**) Photomicrograph of an eosinophil. (**E**) Schematic diagram of a basophil. Basophils express a high-affinity FcR for IgE, which allows them to degranulate in response to IgE-containing immune complexes. Basophil granules contain histamine, neutral proteases, heparin, chondroitin sulfate, and the cytokine TNF-α. (**F**) Photomicrograph of a basophil.

play an important role in type I immediate hypersensitivity reactions, commonly referred to as allergic or atopic responses.

Mast cells are similar to basophils in many ways. However, unlike basophils, mast cells are found along mucosal surfaces or in connective tissues. They are 10 to 15 μm in diameter with a lobed nucleus. The granules of mast cells include the above-noted contents of basophil granules and several additional components. For example, the granules of mast cells along mucosal surfaces contain tryptase. On its surface, the mast cell expresses FcεRI as well as CD88, a receptor for a split product of the complement cascade derived from component C5 and designated C5a. Therefore, a mast cell can be triggered by cross-linking of its FcεRI-bound IgE by an *allergen* (a type of antigen that stimulates an allergic response). Mast cells are thus mediators of immediate-type hypersensitivity and can also be activated by products of complement activation. By this latter mechanism, mast cells play an important role in regulating vascular permeability during inflammation events (see Fig. 2.9). The mast cells found in connective tissues contain both tryptase and chymotryptase in their granules and are thought to be involved primarily with tissue remodeling.

Functions

Phagocytosis

All of the granulocytes are phagocytic cells, although the neutrophil is the most numerous and important phagocyte. When particles are phagocytized by neutrophils, the phagosome containing the ingested particle fuses with the lysosome containing digestive enzymes to produce a structure called the *phagolysosome*. Storage granules are fused with the phagolysosome, and it is there that the ingested material is digested. In addition to the enzymes listed above, the neutrophil releases peptides called *defensins* that render the bacterial or fungal membranes permeable. Also, the neutrophil oxidases create highly toxic reactive oxygen species, as described for macrophages. As with macrophages, engagement of the complement and/or Fc receptors on granulocytes greatly enhances the uptake of particles and the activation events that follow. The spillover of degradative enzymes and toxic products from activated granulocytes can result in damage to surrounding tissues, as seen in chronic inflammation.

Antigen processing and presentation

It has recently been reported that eosinophils express the costimulatory molecules CD80 and CD86 needed for antigen presentation. Furthermore, when stimulated by GM-CSF, eosinophils are induced to express MHC class II molecules. In vitro, these cells can present antigens to T lymphocytes. This, together with their ability to produce cytokines, including IL-4, suggests that eosinophils have important influences on the initiation of T-cell immunity, particularly in tissues and at mucosal surfaces, and also may play an important role in determining the type of TH cell that develops during an immune response.

Production of cytokines

Only recently has it been appreciated that cytokines produced by granulocytes are important not only in innate immunity but also in directing the type of response produced by lymphocytes. Neutrophils produce the proinflammatory cytokines TNF-α, IL-1β, IL-6, and IL-8 and the immunomodulating IL-1 receptor antagonist and TGF-β. However, these cytokines may be short-lived; e.g., IL-8 is degraded by elastase released from neutrophil granules. Eosinophils are able to produce factors that further stimulate eosinophil differentiation, i.e., IL-3, GM-CSF, and IL-5, as well as cytokines that stimulate lymphocytes. These include IL-4, IL-5, and IL-10, which are produced by one subset of eosinophils, and IFN-γ, which is produced by another subset. Basophils and mast cells produce IL-4, IL-5, IL-6, IL-13, and TNF-α. Unlike lymphocytes, basophils constitutively contain IL-4 and IL-13 and release these cytokines when stimulated. Similarly, mast cells contain preformed cytokines, including IL-4. This suggests that, in addition to being important mediators of allergic inflammation, basophils and mast cells may also be important in influencing the type of acquired immune response that develops. For example, in releasing IL-4, basophils could direct the differentiation of TH cells along the TH type 2 (TH2) pathway. TH2 cells secrete cytokines that cause B cells to produce antibody of the isotype IgE.

Effectors of immunity

Neutrophils are the most numerous leukocytes in the blood and the most important cellular component of the innate immune system for destroying bacteria and fungi via phagocytosis. As such, neutrophils are a major first line of defense against such infections. They are also the most abundant cells participating in the early stages of inflammation. In such situations, neutrophils not only kill pathogens but also release digestive enzymes and oxidative products into the surrounding tissues, making neutrophils an important cause of damage to "innocent bystander" cells.

Although eosinophils are capable of phagocytosis, they are better known for attaching themselves to a target via complement receptors or FcRs and releasing granules to expose the target to the granules' toxic contents. The number of eosinophils is increased in parasitic diseases, and these cells are thought to play a major role in clearing extracellular parasites. Eosinophils are also important in the pathogenesis of asthma and other chronic inflammatory diseases, particularly in the late phases of such responses.

Cross-linking of the FcεRI with IgE and its antigen leads to degranulation of mast cells or basophils and the synthesis and release of a number of factors responsible for the symptoms of an allergic reaction, including vasodilation, contraction of smooth muscle, and secretion of mucus. Together, these effects result in the swelling, redness, and irritation that are the hallmarks of an allergic response. These factors include histamine, the major preformed effector molecule in these cells, and prostaglandins and leukotrienes synthesized following activation.

Platelets and Their Role in Immunity

Relationship to myeloid cells

Platelets are small (~2 μm in diameter) anucleate blood elements that arise from the fragmentation of megakaryocytes, which in turn are derived from a common myeloid precursor. Platelets have a circulating life span of about 10 days and are involved in blood clotting and inflammation. Production of platelets is increased in response to IL-6 or IL-11. Megakaryocytes and platelets characteristically have a complex on their surface called *glycoprotein IIb/IIIa,* which is a receptor for fibrinogen and is involved in platelet aggregation. They also have receptors for a specific type of chemokine, termed the CXCR4 receptor, and for other extracellular matrix proteins, as well as for the complement component C3b and the Fc portions of IgG and IgE. CXCR4 and the C3b receptor are involved in the ability of platelets to respond to inflammatory stimuli.

Response to cytokines

Platelets can be activated by a variety of stimuli, including antigen-antibody complexes and platelet-activating factor (PAF) produced by neutrophils, basophils, and macrophages. When activated, platelets release a variety of factors that initiate or increase inflammatory or allergic reactions (Fig. 3.7). The factors are either preformed or released from the cell membrane when it is perturbed. Preformed factors include the chemokines TGF-β and RANTES, which recruit neutrophils or monocytes and eosinophils, respectively. Other factors that directly activate leukocytes include PAF and platelet factor 4 (PF4), which causes granulocytes to degranulate and increases expression of surface adhesion molecules and FcRs for IgG and IgE.

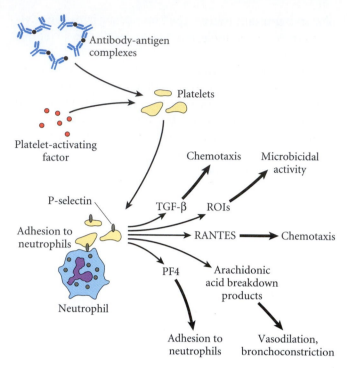

Figure 3.7 Immune function of platelets. Platelets that have been activated by PAF or immune complexes express P-selectin on their surface and can release a number of mediators that influence immunity. Activated neutrophils can bind to the P-selectin. PF4 also induces expression of adhesion molecules on monocytes and neutrophils. Platelets also can release several chemotactic factors, including PF4, platelet-derived growth factor, PAF, RANTES, TGF-β, IL-6, IL-8, and the lipoxygenase products 12-HETE and LT4B. Histamine, serotonin, and cationic proteins induce vasodilation, whereas serotonin, PAF, and thromboxane cause bronchoconstriction. In addition, platelets that are stimulated through their FcRs can be directly cytotoxic to bacteria and parasites, in part through the production of reactive oxygen intermediates (ROIs) such as hydrogen peroxide and superoxide.

The cytokines IL-6 and IL-8 activate platelets and increase their expression of the adhesion molecule P-selectin. The binding of neutrophils to P-selectin on activated platelets may be an early step in the formation of atherosclerotic plaques that contribute to heart disease. IL-6 also increases the sensitivity of platelets to activation by thrombin and PAF. In addition, the factors neutrophilin and nitric oxide released by neutrophils can activate platelets. The c-kit ligand upregulates FcγRIIA on megakaryocytes.

Role of coagulation in inflammation and immunity

Coagulation with fibrin deposition is frequently associated with inflammatory diseases. Fibrin is responsible for the induration (firmness) associated with CD4+ T-cell mediated delayed-type hypersensitivity reactions and is presumed to be important in restricting the inflammatory reaction to a discrete location. Macrophage-derived tissue factor can initiate the extrinsic clotting cascade. Products of the coagulation cascade can also enhance inflammatory reactions; thus, the cross-regulation of inflammation and coagulation is bidirectional. For instance, fibrin break-down products increase vascular permeability and act as chemoattractants for neutrophils and macrophages. Thrombin activates macrophages, is chemotactic for poly-morphonuclear leukocytes, and induces neutrophils to release PAF. Coagulation is accompanied by production of IL-8 and IL-6, which increase platelet activation.

Dendritic Cells

Relationship to myeloid cells

Dendritic cells are the most potent of the APCs. Dendritic cells arise either from the myeloid stem cell in the bone marrow or from a monocyte precursor in the blood or even from monocytes themselves. An alternative dendritic cell precursor in the thymus that can give rise to dendritic cells, T cells, and NK cells has recently been identified.

Morphology and anatomic occurrence

Dendritic cells are named for the fine stellate cytoplasmic projections (or dendrites) that characterize their plasma membranes (Fig. 3.8). Dendritic cells are found in very small numbers (<0.1%) in the blood and are called *veiled cells* at this stage because of their extensively ruffled membrane. Dendritic cells in the skin are known as *Langerhans cells.* These cells can migrate rapidly to the draining lymph nodes to become *interdigitating cells* carrying antigen to the T-cell regions of the node (it is thought that these migrating Langerhans cells are identical to veiled cells). Interdigitating cells, also called *interdigitating reticular cells,* are found in the T-cell regions of other lymphoid organs as well.

Role in antigen presentation

Dendritic cells are the most efficient APCs in the body. To fulfill this role, dendritic cells phagocytose foreign antigens, process the antigens they take up, and present those

Figure 3.8 Schematic diagram of a dendritic cell highlighting cell surface molecules important to its function as an APC. These include MHC class II for antigen presentation; CD80 (B7-1) and CD86 (B7-2), which are important costimulatory molecules for activating T cells; and several adhesion molecules.

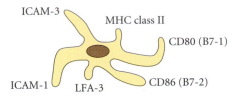

antigens to T cells on MHC class II proteins. It should be noted, however, that although immature dendritic cells are phagocytic, mature dendritic cells are not. Thus, in the normal sequence of events, an immature dendritic cell phagocytoses an antigen and then homes to a secondary immune tissue such as a lymph node to present its processed antigens to T cells that reside in the lymphoid tissue. During transit to a secondary lymphoid tissue, the dendritic cell progresses to become a mature dendritic cell. This mature dendritic cell cannot process new antigens but rather presents to T cells the antigens it has already internalized. Mature dendritic cells can endocytose soluble antigens even though these cells are generally incapable of phagocytosis.

The high constitutive expression of MHC class II molecules and costimulatory molecules CD80 and CD86 by dendritic cells accounts for their powerful antigen-presenting abilities. Dendritic cells also express CD1 (a non-classical MHC class I protein) and several accessory molecules such as CD40, LFA-3, ICAM-1, and ICAM-3. Like classical MHC class I proteins, CD1 functions as a platform for the presentation of foreign antigens to T lymphocytes. However, unlike classical MHC class I, CD1 can present lipid, glycolipid, and phosphoprotein antigens to T cells. Presentation of such antigens by CD1 appears particularly important in stimulating immunity to mycobacterial infection (the cause of tuberculosis).

Dendritic cells in the thymus are important in the process of negative selection, the deletion of thymocytes expressing a T-cell receptor with a high affinity for self antigens. In addition, dendritic cells are particularly good at presenting antigen to naive T cells. Dendritic cells are very efficient in presenting viral antigens and are also capable of presenting certain exogenous antigens on MHC class I molecules. The latter is a unique ability, since exogenous antigens (antigens brought into a cell by endocytosis or phagocytosis) are normally presented only on MHC class II proteins.

In addition to their antigen-presentation functions, activated dendritic cells also serve important immuno-regulatory roles. One way that dendritic cells carry out this function is through the production of the immune-activating cytokines IL-1β, TNF-α, and IL-12. Also, dendritic cells perform a pivotal regulatory role through their activation of TH1 and TH2 cells. It has been proposed by Marie-Clotilde Rissoan and coworkers that naive, undifferentiated TH0 precursor cells are induced to become either TH1 cells or TH2 due to interaction with one of two types of dendritic cells called DC1 cells and DC2 cells, respectively (Fig. 3.9A). Furthermore, these workers propose that TH1 cells and TH2 cells negatively

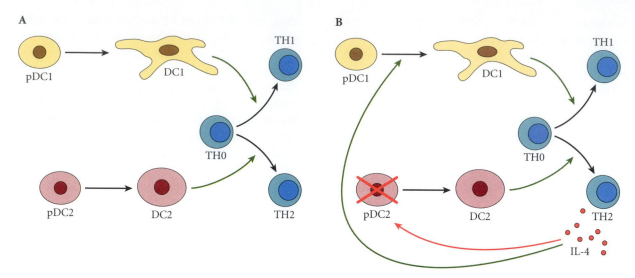

Figure 3.9 (**A**) The activity of two different subsets of dendritic cells (DC1 and DC2), arising from precursor cells (pDC1 and pDC2), regulates the maturation of TH cells into either TH1 or TH2. (**B**) Cytokines produced by mature TH cells (such as IL-4) exert feedback regulation on the development of DC1 and DC2 cells. Therefore, if TH2 cells become the predominant type of TH cell in a given host animal, IL-4 secreted by the TH2 cells will preferentially induce the maturation of TH1 cells. Thus, this feedback regulation ensures a balance of TH1 and TH2 cells within the host.

regulate each other indirectly through regulation of the development of DC1 and DC2 cells. For example, cytokines produced by TH2 cells were found to stimulate the development of DC1 cells and to inhibit the development of DC2 cells (Fig. 3.9B). This ensures that, when needed, a balance is maintained between TH1- and TH2-type responses. Although DC1 cells and DC2 cells carry out similar functions in the immune system, they appear to arise from different lineages. DC1 cells are descendants of the monocyte or macrophage lineage, whereas DC2 cells (characterized by the lineage marker phenotype CD4$^+$ CD3$^-$ CD11b$^-$) descend from a lymphoid precursor that resides in the blood or tonsils.

Follicular dendritic cells (FDCs) are a cell type found in follicles and germinal centers of lymphoid tissues that are involved in antigen presentation to B cells. Despite their name, FDCs are not related to dendritic cells. Their name stems from their cellular morphology, which includes stellate cytoplasmic projections similar to those present on conventional dendritic cells. FDCs are nonphagocytic cells and do not express MHC class II proteins. However, FDCs are able to present antigens to B cells because of their extensive surface processes decorated with antigen-antibody complexes that bind via the FcRs and complement receptors (such as CD21) of the FDC. The antigen-antibody complexes present on the processes of the FDC are important in presenting antigen to B cells during affinity maturation. Since these antigen-antibody complexes per-

sist for very long periods, they also are thought to play a role in maintenance of immunologic memory.

Morphology and Function of Lymphoid Cells

Lymphoid Cells

Identification by morphologic means

Lymphoid cells are morphologically the simplest and functionally the most diverse cells of the immune system (Fig. 3.10). The lymphocytes are generally round cells 6 to 10 μm in diameter with a large nucleus-to-cytoplasm ratio (Fig. 3.10A). The large majority of lymphocytes are either bone marrow derived (B cells) (Fig. 3.10B) or thymus derived (T cells) (Fig. 3.10C). The nucleus most often appears to be round. About 5% of lymphocytes have somewhat more cytoplasm with azurophilic granules and are called *large granular lymphocytes* or NK cells (Fig. 3.10D and E).

Identification by cell surface markers

Because of the paucity of distinguishing morphologic features among different types of lymphocytes, molecular surface markers have been extremely important in quantifying and studying lymphocyte subsets (Fig. 3.2). Over time, functions have been ascribed to many of these molecules so that, in addition to identifying subsets of lymphocytes, many of these markers have helped to explain how the cell that bears them carries out its unique activities. The appendixes of this text contain tables that list cell markers by their CD designation and give the markers' common (pre-CD) designations, their tissue distributions, and when known, their functions. In addition, some lineage-specific markers are expressed in a develop-

mentally regulated fashion or are expressed only during certain cell-activation states. For example, the markers CD2, CD3, and TCR are found on all T cells (and are therefore referred to as *pan-T-cell markers*), whereas other markers, such as CD1, are differentiation markers and are

Figure 3.10 (**A**) Photomicrograph of a lymphocyte. Lymphocytes appear as small round cells that contain a relatively large nucleus and a small amount of cytoplasm. (**B and C**) Schematic diagrams of B and T lymphocytes. (**B**) B lymphocytes are characterized by the expression of surface immunoglobulin (BCR) and the markers CD19 and CD20. The BCR is flanked by the signal transduction molecules Ig-α and Ig-β. In addition, B cells constitutively express MHC class II molecules, several complement receptors, and a receptor of the Fc portion of immunoglobulin. (**C**) T cells are characterized by the expression of a TCR in association with the signal transduction complex CD3. T cells also express the CD28 molecule, which functions as a receptor for a costimulatory signal. CD2 is a pan-T-cell marker expressed on all T cells that also can provide an activation signal when engaged. Mature T cells are subdivided into those that express CD4 and those that express CD8. (**D**) Photograph of a large granular lymphocyte. These cells are several micrometers larger than normal lymphocytes and have cytoplasmic granules containing lytic enzymes, perforin, and the cytokine TNF-α. Courtesy of Michael H. Ross. (**E**) Schematic diagram of NK cell. NK cells express a number of markers shared with other cells with killer function. These include CD7, CD11b, CD16, CD57, and CD94. NK cells also express the IL-2R α chain. The killer inhibitor receptor (KIR) molecule inhibits killer function when it is engaged by MHC on the potential target cell.

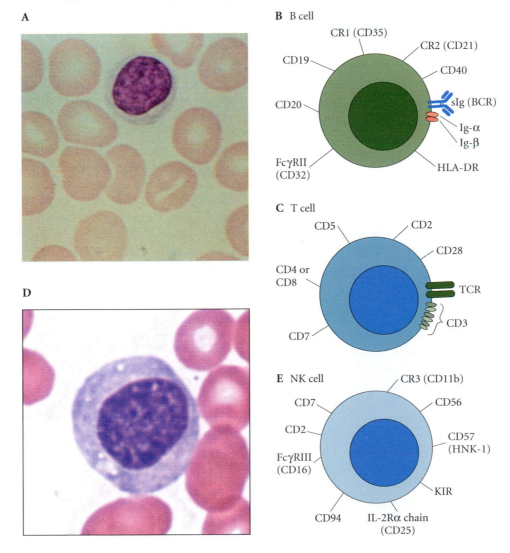

expressed transiently. CD1 is expressed by thymocytes at an early stage of their development. Markers such as the IL-2 receptor (CD25) and CD69 (which seems to play a role in biochemical events such as calcium flux) are associated with lymphocyte activation. The nicotinamide adenine dinucleotide glycohydrolase CD38 is both an activation and a differentiation marker for T cells, being expressed not only on thymocytes but also following activation of mature T cells. Most T cells express the surface marker CD45 (a protein tyrosine phosphatase important in T-cell activation). CD45 exists in several isoforms, which are variants of a protein usually formed by alternative RNA splicing. Naive T cells generally express the CD45RA isoform, whereas activated T cells and memory cells generally express the CD45RO isoform. In summary, lymphoid cell surface markers can be used to provide not only information about a lymphocyte's lineage but also specific information about a lymphocyte's maturation and activational state.

Major Populations and Subpopulations of Lymphocytes

T Lymphocytes

Although all T lymphocytes bear a TCR and share a common mechanism of antigen recognition, they comprise a functionally heterogeneous group of cells. As such, T lymphocytes are commonly categorized into subpopulations based on their function or their expression of various surface proteins.

CD4$^+$ versus CD8$^+$ T cells

CD4 and CD8 are cell surface proteins that function as important antigen coreceptors and are usually expressed in mature T cells in a mutually exclusive fashion (Fig. 3.10C). The earliest T-cell progenitors in the thymus express neither CD4 nor CD8 (and are therefore called *double-negative cells*) and make up approximately 10% of thymocytes. As these T-cell progenitors mature, the genes encoding the TCR are rearranged to give a functional antigen receptor, which is then expressed on the cell surface in conjunction with the CD3 complex. As the thymocyte successfully completes the first stage of TCR gene rearrangement, both CD4 and CD8 become expressed, with the majority of immature thymocytes (~75%) being CD4$^+$CD8$^+$ (called *double-positive cells*). These cells reside in the cortical region of the thymus. On further maturation, the thymocytes become CD4$^+$CD8$^-$ or CD4$^-$CD8$^+$ (and are called *single-positive cells*) and are found primarily in the thymus medulla. In the blood, approximately 65 to 70% of T cells are CD4$^+$, 25 to 30% are CD8$^+$, and 1% are CD4$^+$ CD8$^+$.

CD4 and CD8 are important in determining which MHC molecule is recognized by the TCR. CD4 binds to MHC class II molecules, helping the TCR to recognize antigen presented by MHC class II molecules. In contrast, CD8 binds to MHC class I molecules and CD8$^+$ cells recognize antigen presented by MHC class I molecules. The CD8 molecule is actually a disulfide-linked dimer, with most CD8 being composed of one α chain and one β chain (i.e., an αβ heterodimer); however, a minor subset of CD8 cells found primarily along mucosal surfaces are CD8 αα homodimers. These mucosal T cells constitute a separate lineage of lymphocytes and appear to serve a unique function, which seems to include the recognition of antigens presented by CD1-bearing APCs.

T cells expressing the αβ versus the γδ form of the TCR

T cells can be further subdivided into subclasses on the basis of the type of TCR they express. TCRs exist in two different forms, each of which is a heterodimer of two transmembrane protein chains. The vast majority of circulating T cells express a TCR composed of α and β chains (and are thus called αβ T cells) and are generally CD4$^+$ CD8$^-$ or CD4$^-$ CD8$^+$. αβ T cells are enormously diverse in their antigenic specificities. A minor subset of T cells that express the αβ TCR also express a marker associated with NK cells, the NK1 marker, and designated as NK T cells. These cells express a very restricted subset of TCRs, bind to antigens presented by the CD1 MHC-like molecules, and like NK cells, seem to be part of the innate immune system. They have a propensity to recognize autoantigens, including proteins expressed by cells under stress. Unlike conventional T cells, these cells produce IL-4 on primary stimulation.

A small minority of circulating T cells (~5%), but a substantial majority of T cells in the skin (as well as a portion of T cells located along mucosal surfaces), express a different antigen receptor comprising γ and δ protein chains (and are called γδ T cells). γδ T cells are generally CD4$^-$CD8$^-$ or CD4$^-$CD8$^+$. Early in fetal development, γδ T cells are the predominant type of T cells that arise in the thymus. However, later in life these T cells develop in a thymus-independent fashion, i.e., they do not require a thymus to mature and are produced in normal numbers in animals that lack a thymus. The heterogeneity of γδ TCRs is limited compared with the enormous diversity of αβ TCRs on traditional T cells. Some γδ T cells interact with CD1 as an antigen-presenting molecule rather than with *classical* MHC class I or class II molecules. The γδ T cells are also unusual in recognizing nonpeptide antigens such as phosphorylated nucleotides and prenyl pyrophosphates. They can act as cytotoxic cells and also can produce cytokines upon activation.

TH1 versus TH2 cells

TH cells have been categorized according to the cytokines they produce when activated. Naive T cells produce a mixture of cytokines when stimulated but can differentiate to produce a restricted cytokine pattern. CD4$^+$ T cells that secrete IL-2, IFN-γ, and TNF-β are TH1 cells. Cells that secrete IL-4, IL-5, IL-6, IL-9, IL-10, and IL-13 are TH2 cells. In addition, both subsets can produce IL-3, TNF-α, and GM-CSF. TH1 cells preferentially stimulate T-cell immunity and are proinflammatory, whereas TH2 cells stimulate antibody production by promoting B-cell growth and differentiation. Production of IgG1, IgE, and IgA is favored by TH2 cytokines. Production of IgG2a and IgG3 is favored by TH1 cytokines. CD8 T cells can be similarly divided into type 1 and type 2 patterns of cytokine secretion. In humans, the division between TH1 and TH2 cells is less definitive, with both cell types making IL-2, IL-10, and IL-13. Nevertheless, the TH1 versus TH2 phenotype has important clinical implications for patients with certain infectious diseases, allergies, and autoimmune diseases, in which the predominance of one or the other phenotype determines the presentation and severity of the disease.

The developmental pathways and activation of TH1 and TH2 lymphocytes are mutually antagonistic. IFN-γ produced by TH1 cells inhibits differentiation of TH2 cells, whereas IL-4 and IL-10 produced by TH2 cells inhibit differentiation of TH1 cells. The cytokine IL-12, which is produced by dendritic cells, macrophages, and neutrophils, favors the development of TH1 cells, whereas the cytokine IL-4 favors the induction of TH2 cells. This means that the cytokines that are present when naive T cells are stimulated by antigen have an important influence on the type of immune responses these cells develop.

B Lymphocytes

B lymphocytes make up about 5 to 15% of circulating lymphocytes (Fig. 3.10B). Transmembrane immunoglobulin is a primary lineage marker for B cells and serves as the B-cell antigen receptor. Immunoglobulin molecules are divided into classes called *isotypes* on the basis of the amino acid sequence of their heavy-chain constant region. Immunoglobulin isotypes include IgG, IgA, IgM, IgD, and IgE. The different isotypes have distinct biologic properties, but all isotypes can be produced as transmembrane proteins that serve as a part of the B-cell antigen receptor. Newly produced mature B cells express both IgM and IgD molecules on their membrane, whereas previously activated B cells can express other isotypes on their surface.

B cells constitutively express MHC class II. Other B-cell markers include the complement receptors CD35 and CD21, the IgG FcR CD32, the IgE FcR CD23, and B220, which is a B-cell-specific isoform of the protein tyrosine phosphatase CD45. CD40 is expressed on B cells and is important in antigen-driven interactions between B cells and T cells. Interactions between CD40 and CD40L on T cells provide a costimulatory signal for the B cells. In addition to their role as immunoglobulin-producing cells, B cells can present antigen to T cells.

CD5$^+$ and CD5$^-$ cells

B cells can be subdivided on the basis of the presence or absence of the CD5 marker. The large majority of B cells are CD5$^-$. The small subset that is CD5$^+$ is of interest, however, as they are the principal source of autoantibodies. In the mouse, these cells are found primarily in the peritoneal cavity. The immunoglobulins expressed by CD5$^+$ cells are much less diverse than those found on CD5$^-$ cells.

Antigen presentation by myeloid and dendritic cells

The TCR recognizes antigenic peptide that is bound to an MHC molecule. Antigenic peptides may arise from exogenous or endogenous antigens, including self antigens. Generally, exogenous antigens are phagocytosed or endocytosed by APCs, degraded, and presented on MHC class II molecules to CD4$^+$ T cells. Antigens produced inside the cell, such as self antigens or viral antigens produced within infected cells, are degraded in the cytoplasm and presented on MHC class I molecules to CD8$^+$ cells.

TCR engagement by peptide and MHC is only the first signal in the productive activation of T cells. In fact, if the TCR is engaged without further stimulation, the T cell becomes anergic or unresponsive to activation by antigen. Usually the second signal comes from binding of the T-cell protein CD28 with CD80 or CD86 on the APC. Additional interactions between adhesion molecules and other receptor-ligand pairs on the T cell and APC help strengthen the bond between the two cells and can provide additional activation signals. Interaction between the T cell and the APC also induces the APC to produce cytokines such as IL-1, which can further stimulate the T cell.

Antigen presentation by B cells

B cells also are able to function as APCs. In this case, antigen that binds to the B-cell receptor (BCR) (i.e., surface immunoglobulin) is endocytosed, degraded, and presented on MHC class II molecules on the surface of the B cell. B cells are limited in their ability to take up and degrade particulate antigens or antigens for which they do not have a specific antigen receptor. However, the high-affinity interaction between the BCR and its ligand allows B cells to internalize and process antigen even when the amount of antigen is minute, giving B cells an advantage over other APCs in such circumstances. Engagement of the TCR induces the T cell to express CD40 ligand (CD40L) on its surface, which then interacts with CD40 on the surface of the B cell.

Interaction of T cells and B cells

Although B cells can bind soluble antigens directly via their antigen receptor, they too require additional signals to become productively activated. It is particularly advantageous for the B cell to present antigen to the T cell, since this puts the B cell in position to receive the additional signals it requires from the TH cell. Activated T cells express CD40L. Binding of CD40L by CD40 receptors on B cells provides B cells with a costimulatory signal. In response to CD40 ligation, the B cell increases expression of CD80 and CD86, which bind to CD28 on the T cell to deliver the needed second signal to the T cell. This signaling then stimulates the production of cytokines by T cells that the B cells require to proliferate, to switch their immunoglobulin isotype, to secrete antibody, and to become memory cells. In particular, these include the TH2 cytokines IL-4, IL-5, and IL-6.

Interaction of T cells and T cells

Similarly, in addition to recognizing an MHC-antigen complex on an APC, the T cell requires help from other T cells for proliferation and further differentiation. Following activation through the TCR and a costimulatory signal, the T cell is induced to express new gene products, including IL-2 and the IL-2 receptor. IL-2 is an important cytokine that stimulates proliferation of T cells that have been activated to express an IL-2 receptor. Since the stimulated T cell simultaneously expresses both IL-2 and its receptor, the T cell can stimulate itself toward complete activation (this action of a cytokine on the very cell that produced it is termed *autocrine* activity). IL-2 also induces the production of other cytokines, such as IFN-γ, which leads to further T-cell differentiation. IFN-γ induces differentiation of cytotoxic T cells to an effector stage and enhances cytotoxic activity. As previously mentioned, the cytokines IFN-γ and IL-4 induce differentiation of TH cells toward TH1 and TH2 phenotypes, respectively, whereas IFN-γ inhibits differentiation of TH2 cells. CD4 helper cells are most proficient at producing cytokines and stimulating other T cells, although other T-cell subsets can also produce cytokines.

Interaction of T cells and macrophages

Although macrophages are capable of considerable activity on their own, this activity can be boosted by interaction with T cells. This additional boost in activity is critical to the ability of macrophages to fight off organisms that have become adapted to grow inside macrophages after phagocytosis (e.g., the bacterium *Mycobacterium tuberculosis*). IFN-γ, produced by CD8+ T cells or proinflammatory CD4+ cells, causes macrophages to become more efficient at lysosome fusion and enhances their oxidative burst, especially increasing production of nitric oxide, which enhances cytotoxic activity. The activation of macrophages also requires a second signal, which can be provided by LPS or TNF, particularly the membrane-associated form of TNF (TNF-β).

Cellular effectors of immunity

Cytotoxic T cells are important in the killing of infected cells and tumor cells. Both CD8+ and CD4+ T cells can carry out cytotoxic activity, although cytotoxic T cells are usually of the CD8+ variety. CD8+ cells generally kill their targets through the use of the protein *perforin,* which forms pores in the plasma membrane of a target cell. The pores allow entry of the *granzymes,* which are serine proteases that induce apoptosis. Within minutes of binding to the target cell, the activated CD8+ killer cells direct exocytosis of preformed perforin and other cytotoxic mediators toward the target cell. TNF-β and NK cytotoxic factor are additional cytotoxic effector molecules produced by CD8+ cells.

Killing by activated CD4+ T cells is accomplished by membrane molecules referred to as Fas (CD95) and Fas ligand (FasL or CD95L). Cross-linking of Fas receptors on target cells to be killed by FasL on the activated cytotoxic T cells induces apoptosis in the target cells. T cells themselves can become targets for apoptosis if they express both Fas and FasL. This situation occurs following complete activation of a T cell and has been termed *activation-induced cell death.* Such induced apoptotic killing of activated T cells once they have completed their job is an important regulatory pathway for limiting immune activation and controlling the function of effector T cells. Thus, continued exposure to antigen would ideally lead to productive activation and clonal expansion of reactive cells, followed by the elimination of responder cells once they are no longer needed.

Null or Third-Population Cells

Null cells are lymphoid cells that have neither a TCR nor a BCR. They account for 15% of circulating lymphocytes. The most abundant of these cells is the NK cell. NK cells can be found circulating in the blood but also are found in the liver, in lungs, and along the intestinal mucosa.

Identification by morphologic and histochemical methods

NK cells are the major population of null lymphocytes (i.e., lymphocytes that are neither B cells nor T cells). Morphologically, NK cells are large granular lymphocytes (Fig. 3.10D and E) and can be identified by the presence of CD56, an adhesion molecule, and CD16 (FcγRIII). In addition, NK cells express CD2 and CD7, which are also found on T cells. However, unlike T cells, NK cells are thymus independent (i.e., they do not require the thymus for development). Some NK cells also express CD8 and CD57, two markers associated with cytotoxic activity in T cells. Unlike resting T cells, resting NK cells express a surface protein that is part of the receptor for IL-2 and is designated the α chain (CD25). The expression of the IL-2R α chain results in constitutive surface expression of receptors with a high affinity for IL-2, a situation that allows resting NK cells to proliferate in response to low concentrations of IL-2. Culturing NK cells with IL-2 broadens their target-cell range and increases their cytotoxic activity. These IL-2-activated killers, which can include both NK cells and T cells, are termed *lymphokine-activated killer* cells.

Functions

NK cells are part of the innate immune system and are able to act rapidly, within several hours of challenge. They are the first line of defense against viral infections and also play a role in certain bacterial infections. They can kill virus-infected cells directly. The receptor molecules that NK cells use to recognize intact versus infected or debilitated cells have recently been defined. Some of these receptors respond to decreases in expression of MHC-class I on an infected cell or cancer cell. Others respond to less well-characterized products of infected cells that may be encoded by the infecting virus. NK cells have also been shown to be capable of recognizing alterations in the spectrum of MHC-bound peptides on a target cell (which may occur when viral antigens or tumor antigens are overexpressed in the target cell). NK cells also produce IFN-γ, which has multiple direct antiviral effects, stimulates the cytotoxic activity of T cells and macrophages, and influences naive T cells to differentiate into TH1 cells. NK cells also kill cancer cells and are thought by some to kill newly transformed cells, preventing tumor growth, a function termed *immune surveillance.*

The receptors on the surface of an NK cell are critically important in determining whether the target cell to which the NK cell is bound will be killed or not. Inhibitory receptors prevent the NK cell from destroying a target cell; these receptors generally contain a cytoplasmic domain known as an immunoreceptor tyrosine-based inhibitory motif, whose activation prevents cytotoxic activity. NK cells that can kill their targets do so using surface molecules that associate with adaptor proteins that contain an immunoreceptor tyrosine-based activating motif. Three types of inhibitory receptors are known: one is called Ly-49 and is found in mice and rats; the second is referred to as killer-cell immunoglobulin-like receptor, which appears to be a primate-specific molecule; and the third type of molecule shared among rodents and primates is termed the CD94-NKG2A heterodimers. The first two receptors bind to MHC class I molecules. The third type binds to a conserved, MHC class I-like molecule known as HLA-E in humans and Qa-1 in mice. When these receptors are engaged, the NK cell is inhibited. Because infected cells and cancer cells often have decreased levels of MHC class I molecules, they are unable to bind with sufficient strength to the inhibitory receptor, thus allowing the NK cell to complete its cytotoxic activity. Some viruses counter this strategy by inducing an infected cell to produce more surface MHC proteins; human cytomegalovirus increases HLA-E expression to avoid destruction by NK cells.

NK-cell receptors that contribute to the killing of infected cells by giving a positive signal to destroy the target cell are just beginning to be defined. What they can recognize to determine whether a cell should be destroyed is poorly defined. One type of receptor is known as Ly-49H in the mouse, and it associates with an adaptor protein, DAP 12, that contains an immunoreceptor tyrosine-based activating motif. Presumably when Ly-49H recognizes an appropriate ligand on a target cell, it activates the NK cell. The genes for activating and inhibiting receptors on NK cells appear to be tightly linked, suggesting they have co-evolved to regulate the function of NK cells.

NK cells and other cells with FcRs, such as eosinophils and macrophages, also can kill by ADCC. In ADCC, effector cells recognize their target by virtue of the antibody bound to the target cell (Fig. 3.11). The ADCC effector cells bind to the Fc portion of target-bound antibody by means of an FcR. Under these circumstances the antibody serves as the specific recognition entity that promotes and mediates cytotoxic killing of target cells.

NK cells are activated in response to cytokines produced by other innate immune cells early during infection. They respond to IFN-α produced by macrophages and other NK cells and to IL-12 produced by macrophages and dendritic cells. NK cells are also stimulated to differ-

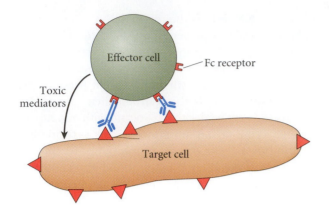

Figure 3.11 ADCC. Antibody bound to target cells can bind to effector cells via an FcR expressed by the effector cell. The effector cell is then activated to kill the target cell. Effector cells include NK cells, macrophages, and eosinophils. Effector cells can also be pre-armed by binding to antibody before their encounter with the target cell.

entiate and become activated in response to IFN-γ produced by T cells and other NK cells.

NK cells, like CD8$^+$ cytotoxic T cells, kill via perforin, granzyme, and NK cytotoxic factor. Following binding of NK cells to still-undefined targets, killing is rapid, occurring within hours. In addition to their cytotoxic function, NK cells may perform certain regulatory functions. The production of IFN-γ by NK cells early in a response may also be important in directing T-cell immunity away from a TH2 pathway.

Summary

The cells of the immune system include the granulocytes (neutrophils, eosinophils, and basophils), mast cells, monocytes, dendritic cells, lymphocytes, and platelets. They are produced throughout life from a common pluripotent stem cell by a process known as hematopoiesis. Hematopoiesis is regulated by growth factors produced by stromal cells within the bone marrow as well as by factors produced outside the bone marrow, particularly cytokines such as IL-3, IL-7, and GM-CSF. Some of these factors stimulate production of specific cell lineages, whereas others work more generally. Much of the progress made in understanding how these processes work has followed from the recognition that the set of membrane proteins expressed on the surface of a given cell can be used to characterize the lineage and physiologic state of that cell.

Hematopoietic cells can be divided broadly into myeloid and lymphoid lineages. Cells of the myeloid lineage perform important functions both in the innate and the specific arms of the immune system and include

monocytes/macrophages, granulocytes, platelets, and dendritic cells. Monocytes (which circulate in the bloodstream) and macrophages (which are present in solid tissues) are important APCs and important effectors of innate immune responses through their cytotoxic activity. Granulocytes are the most abundant class of myeloid cells and include the phagocytic neutrophils and eosinophils, as well as the basophils, which play a role in allergic reactions. Neutrophils are the most common white blood cell and are vital for protecting the host from bacterial infection. Platelets are anucleate blood elements involved in clotting and are derived from an early myeloid progenitor. Dendritic cells are specialized APCs, most often of myeloid origin, that are found particularly in the skin (where they are called Langerhans cells) and in the T-cell zones of various immune organs (where they are referred to as interdigitating cells). Dendritic cells express a variety of MHC molecules and accessory molecules and are the most powerful of the APCs.

Lymphocytes are perhaps the most diverse class of immunocyte. They are the effector cells of acquired immunity and can be subdivided according to surface markers and cell function. T cells express a T-cell antigen receptor, which recognizes antigenic peptides displayed on MHC molecules. T cells can be functionally divided into TH cells and cytotoxic T cells. Functionally, TH cells can be divided on the basis of the cytokines they produce into those that preferentially stimulate antibody production, TH2 cells, and those that stimulate inflammatory responses, TH1 cells. Cytotoxic T cells bind to and kill their targets through the release of perforin and granzymes and, in some instances, through a Fas-FasL interaction.

B lymphocytes are the source of antibodies. Each B cell has a surface immunoglobulin molecule expressed in association with a signal transduction complex. Following engagement of the BCR with its cognate antigen, the B cell differentiates into an antibody-producing cell. B cells can also present antigen to T cells.

NK cells are a third subset of lymphocytes that share some characteristics with cytotoxic T cells but differ in that they have a much broader target range and preferentially attack cells with low levels of MHC class I molecules. NK cells can also kill antibody-coated cells via ADCC.

Suggested Reading

Arock, M., E. Schneider, M. Boissan, V. Tricottet, and M. Dy. 2002. Differentiation of human basophils: an overview of recent advances and pending questions. *J. Leukoc. Biol.* **71:**557–564.

Austen, K. F., and J. A. Boyce. 2001. Mast cell lineage development and phenotypic regulation. *Leuk. Res.* **25:**511–518.

Bonnet, D. 2002. Haematopoietic stem cells. *J. Pathol.* **197:** 430–440.

Friedman, A. D. 2002. Transcriptional regulation of granulocyte and monocyte development. *Oncogene* **21:**3377–3390.

Guermonprez, P., J. Valladeau, L. Zitvogel, C. Thery, and S. Amigorena. 2002. Antigen presentation and T cell stimulation by dendritic cells. *Annu. Rev. Immunol.* **20:**621–667.

Kaushansky, K., and J. G. Drachman. 2002. The molecular and cellular biology of thrombopoietin: the primary regulator of platelet production. *Oncogene* **21:**3359–3367.

Moretta, L., C. Bottino, D. Pende, M. C. Mingari, R. Biassoni, and A. Moretta. 2002. Human natural killer cells: their origin, receptors and function. *Eur. J. Immunol.* **32:**1205–1211.

Robinson, D. S., and A. O'Garra. 2002. Further checkpoints in TH1 development. *Immunity* **16:**755–758.

Schebesta, M., B. Heavey, and M. Busslinger. 2002. Transcriptional control of B-cell development. *Curr. Opin. Immunol.* **14:**216–223.

Shortman, K., and Y. J. Liu. 2002. Mouse and human dendritic cell subtypes. *Nat. Rev. Immunol.* **2:**151–161.

chapter 4

Organs and Tissues of the Immune System

Steven A. Bogen

The various cell types comprising the immune system and their functions are distributed throughout the body but are concentrated within the organs and tissues that support the development and function of these immune cells. In general, the organs and tissues of the immune system can be categorized according to the role they play in the immune response (Fig. 4.1). The *primary lymphoid organs* (also called the *generative* or *central lymphoid organs*) are those that support the development of immune cells; in mammals, these include the bone marrow and thymus. The *secondary lymphoid organs* (also called the *peripheral lymphoid organs*) support the function of cells of the lymphoid lineage by maximizing the likelihood that these cells will encounter their cognate antigens. These organs include the spleen and lymph nodes; they are interconnected by two circulatory systems: the blood and the lymph circulatory systems. Immune cells travel through the body via these two circulatory systems, surveying the tissues for signs of infection. Foreign antigens can also circulate through these systems, passing through the secondary lymphoid organs along the way. Last, some tissues in the body (e.g., skin) can support immune functions under certain circumstances but not regularly. Under normal circumstances, the immune function of the skin is minimal; however, under certain circumstances (e.g., intense, chronic inflammation), the skin can become an active immune tissue. It is important to note that although the skin does not normally support lymphoid function, it is regularly populated with cells with immune function, such as dendritic cells and some varieties of lymphocyte.

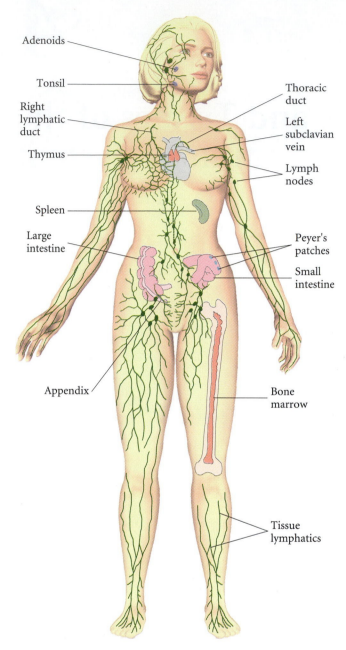

Figure 4.1 Organs and tissues of immunologic importance. In humans, the bone marrow and the thymus are the generative lymphoid organs where the various white blood cells develop and mature. The spleen, lymph nodes, tonsils, Peyer's patches, and appendix are peripheral lymphoid organs, which are highly specialized tissues designed to optimize the efficiency with which lymphocytes encounter their cognate antigens. The lymph nodes are interconnected by an elaborate network of vessels called lymphatics through which lymphocytes and antigens circulate.

Generative Lymphoid Organs

The generative organs are those that produce hematopoietic cells involved in host defense. In most mammals, these organs are the bone marrow and the thymus. Because most immunologic research focuses on immunity in

rodents and humans, those two organs are usually considered the only generative organs. However, in some species some of these functions are relegated to other organs. For example, in birds, the organ called the *bursa of Fabricius* is an obligatory site of B-lymphocyte maturation. In cattle and sheep, B-cell maturation takes place in a specialized lymphoid organ called the *ileal Peyer's patch*. In rabbits, much of the maturation of B cells takes place in the appendix.

Bone Marrow

The bone marrow is the most important source of hematopoiesis-derived cells in adult mammals. In humans, the bone marrow begins to assume its role as a generative organ at approximately 5 months of gestational age. At that time, the major bones begin to ossify. The marrow microenvironment develops concurrently and serves as a site where hematopoietic stem cells gather and proliferate.

The bone marrow is organized into two major compartments: vascular and hematopoietic (Fig. 4.2). The vascular compartment comprises large, thin-walled veins—vascular sinuses—that drain into a central vein. The central vein exits the marrow and drains into the general blood circulation. The hematopoietic compartment of the marrow is located in the perivenular space of the bone marrow. It contains the hematopoietic colonies, arterial vasculature, and accessory stromal cells. Hematopoietic cells originate from an undifferentiated type of stem cell that yields progeny committed to all of the hematopoietic lineages. Once hematopoietic cells differentiate into mature leukocytes, they exit the hematopoietic compartment by crossing into the vascular sinuses of the marrow. Mature leukocytes then migrate out of the marrow via the central vein.

The hematopoietic compartment of the bone marrow comprises, in large part, a network of *stromal cells* (also called *adventitial cells*). Typically, these are elongated cells that form a three-dimensional matrix in which the hematopoietic cells divide and differentiate. Although stromal cells are not themselves hematopoietic, they carry out several functions crucial to creating a microenvironment favorable for hematopoiesis. In vitro studies have shown that the bone marrow stroma is made up primarily of fibroblasts. Cultured stromal cells are characterized by their ability to synthesize extracellular matrix components including fibronectin, laminin, and type I and IV collagen. A small fraction of the cultured cells synthesize blood-clotting factor VIII-associated antigen typical of cells of endothelial origin. Some stromal cells secrete cytokines; the most important appear to be colony-stimulating factors; interleukin-7 (IL-7), IL-8, and IL-11; and stem cell factor (also called c-kit ligand). At least

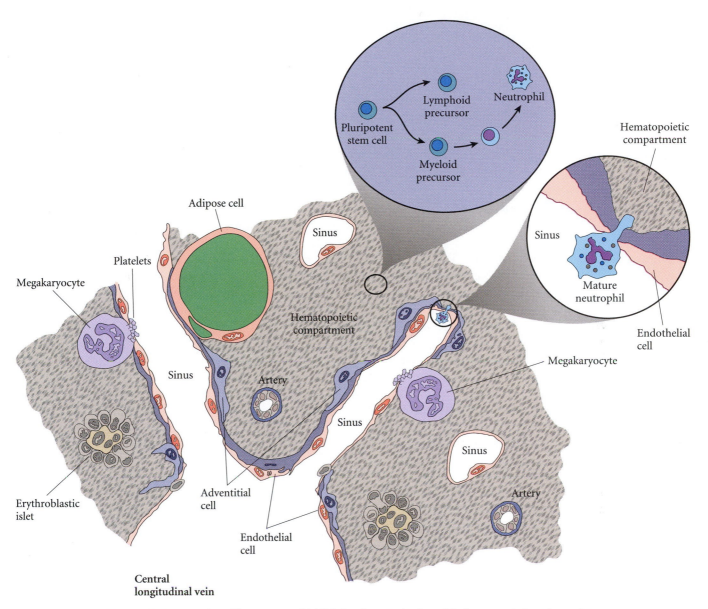

Figure 4.2 Cross-section of bone marrow highlighting the organization of the hematopoietic and vascular compartments of the tissue. Blood cells arise in the hematopoietic compartments, which are segregated into regions producing different types of blood cells (e.g., the erythroblastic islets where red blood cells are generated). Hematopoiesis is supported by soluble and contact-dependent factors produced by adventitial cells. When mature blood cells are generated, they migrate through the endothelium and enter the vascular sinuses, through which they leave the bone marrow. Some cell types (e.g., T lymphocytes and macrophages) enter the sinus while they are still immature. These cell types complete their maturation outside the bone marrow. Megakaryocytes can frequently be seen bordering the sinuses. From this location they continuously produce platelets, which are immediately deposited in the vascular sinus for immediate export from the marrow.

some of these stromal cells are capable of differentiating into cells that form bone, cartilage, fat, or muscle. Adipocytes (fat cells) also are present in bone marrow, and their numbers increase proportionally with age. Various possible functions for adipocytes in the marrow environment have been proposed: (i) a simple mechanical function, whereby these cells, by filling physical space, support the marrow reticular framework; (ii) as a possi-

ble energy depot for other cells; and (iii) involvement in systemic lipid and steroid metabolism.

Thymus

Like several other types of blood cells (basophils and monocytes), T lymphocytes do not complete their maturation process in the bone marrow. Instead, T-cell precursors exit the bone marrow and migrate to the thymus. The thymus is an important site of T-lymphocyte growth and maturation. When precursor T lymphocytes enter the thymus, they are not yet functionally competent, i.e., they are incapable of mounting an immune response. They do not express the T-cell receptor (TCR) complex or other cell surface accessory molecules (such as CD4 or CD8) that are conventionally associated with mature, functionally competent T lymphocytes. Once inside the thymus, precursor T lymphocytes (thymocytes) undergo a selection process in which more than 90% of the T-lymphocyte precursors are destined to die. A small percentage of the entering T-lymphocyte precursors are stimulated to proliferate, differentiate, and ultimately exit the thymus as mature T lymphocytes.

The thymic selection process includes (i) positive selection of T lymphocytes that are capable of recognizing foreign antigens in association with molecules encoded by the major histocompatibility complex (MHC) gene complex and (ii) negative selection of T lymphocytes that avidly bind to self antigens (in association with MHC molecules). The process of positive selection ensures that the lymphocytes that ultimately emerge from the thymus are capable of recognizing antigens complexed to molecules of the MHC. The process of negative selection eliminates potentially autoreactive T-lymphocyte clones with the potential to cause an autoimmune disorder. Thymocytes that fail either positive or negative selection are induced to undergo apoptosis.

The thymus is located in the anterior mediastinum, near the base of the neck. Histologically, it consists of an outer lymphocyte-rich region (the cortex) and an inner, less cellular region (the medulla) (Fig. 4.3). Precursor T lymphocytes enter the thymus just below the thymic capsule, high in the cortex. These primitive thymocytes actively proliferate, as detected by the preferential labeling seen in autoradiographs of thymocyte cultures labeled with [^{3}H]thymidine. At least some of these proliferating precursors come into contact with a specialized type of epithelial cell, the epithelial "nurse" cell. Contact with nurse cells promotes continued proliferation and differentiation of at least some of the progeny cells. As the proliferating thymocytes differentiate, they acquire new cell surface markers, notably the TCR complex, CD4, and CD8. Concurrently, the differentiating thymocytes migrate inward toward the corticomedullary junction. In addition to thymic nurse cells, the thymus contains bone marrow-derived dendritic cells and macrophages. Through their contact with these cells, differentiating thymocytes encounter a range of self antigens in association with MHC gene products. These diverse self antigens provide stimulatory signals for further thymocyte growth and differentiation or, alternatively, negative signaling that results in thymocyte apoptosis.

As lymphocyte differentiation is completed in the thymus, mature T lymphocytes exit the thymic cortex. Some thymocytes are believed to exit the thymus at the corticomedullary junction. These thymocytes then enter the bloodstream and seed peripheral lymphoid organs. Alternatively, some thymocytes may migrate directly from the thymic cortex to the thymic medulla.

Although the maturational processes of the thymic cortex are well documented, the function of the thymic medulla is not as clear. In addition to mature T lymphocytes, the thymic medulla contains epithelial cells, macrophages, and dendritic cells. In some places, the epithelial cells are arranged in round, lamellated whorls called *Hassall's corpuscles*. The function of these distinctive structures is unclear. Lymphocytes are believed to enter the medulla from one of two sources: they may arrive directly from the thymic cortex or populate the thymic medulla after seeding from the bloodstream.

The Anatomy of Immune Responses

One of the marvels of lymphoid organs is their ability to help lymphocytes find both antigen and other lymphocytes specific for the same antigen. This is an important function because antigen-specific lymphocytes must interact to mount most types of immune responses. This interaction includes the delivery of intercellular signals both by direct physical contact and via secreted cytokines.

How are antigen-specific lymphocytes that are randomly distributed throughout the body able to find each other to initiate an immune response? Generally, each lymphocyte is capable of recognizing a different antigen. The immune system is able to recognize a diverse array of antigens because of the presence of millions of different lymphocytes, each displaying a unique antigen-receptor specificity. The frequency of precursor cells specific to any single antigen is typically quite low. For example, in a healthy individual, only 1 in 10,000 to 100,000 lymphocytes may be capable of recognizing any particular antigen.

The importance and function of lymphoid organs can be appreciated by considering the likelihood of the following events. It is likely that, at most, T lymphocytes specific for a particular antigen are present in blood at a precursor frequency of 0.001 (1 per 1,000) and that B lymphocytes specific for the same antigen have approximately the same precursor frequency. In actuality, the precursor frequency to most protein antigens is typically even lower than 0.001. For an immune response to be generated, these two rare cells must find one another. If lymphocytes were randomly mixed in blood or a lymphoid organ, only 1 in 1 million combinations (1/1,000 × 1/1,000) of cells would

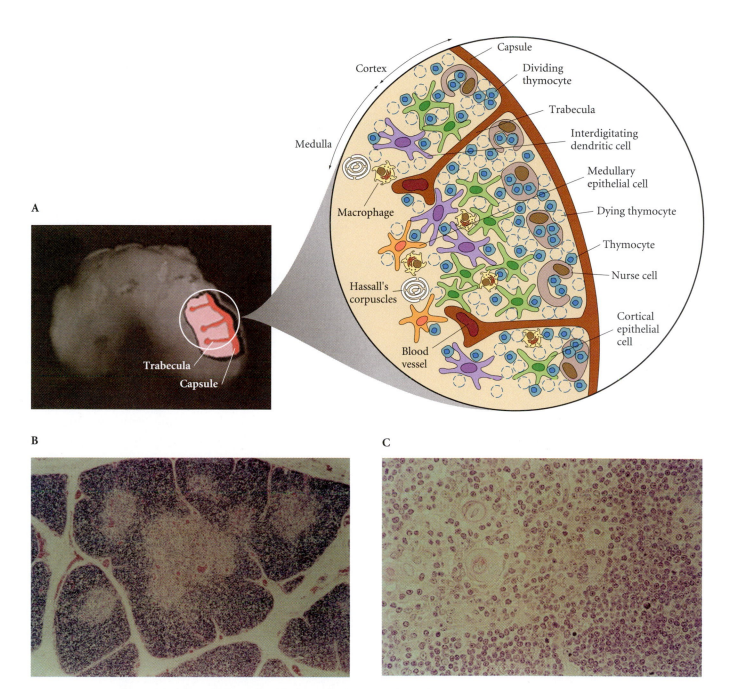

Figure 4.3 (A) Located just above the heart, the thymus is a bilobed, encapsulated organ that contains a stromal matrix (consisting of epithelial cells and dendritic cells) that supports the development of T lymphocytes. (**Inset**) In cross-section, the thymus can be seen to consist of two layers: the outer cortex and the inner medulla. Outside the cortex is a capsule that forms the boundary of the organ. Projections of connective tissue called *trabeculae* divide the stroma into compartments. The cortex is populated with T-lymphocyte precursors called *thymocytes* and with nurse cells and cortical epithelial cells. The latter two cell types create an environment that promotes thymocyte development. The medulla contains thymocytes (albeit fewer than in the cortex), macrophages, and medullary epithelial cells. Numerous IDCs reside at the interface of the cortex and medulla. These cells are essential for thymocyte development. (B) Low-power photomicrograph of a cross-section of thymus, showing the thymic cortex and medulla. (C) High-power photomicrograph of an involuting adult thymic medulla, showing several Hassall corpuscles.

yield the proper combination of antigen-specific T and B lymphocytes. Other cellular interactions that appear equally improbable also must occur. For example, antigen-presenting cells (APCs) bearing processed antigen must find antigen-specific T lymphocytes. Moreover, soluble antigen must find its way to antigen-specific B lymphocytes. Peripheral lymphoid organs are designed to facilitate these interactions.

Several features of the immune system facilitate these cellular interactions.

1. Lymphocytes do not recirculate through the body randomly but are guided through lymphoid organs by specific homing receptors that have organ or tissue specificity. Consequently, lymphocytes primed to an antigen in a particular anatomic site will home to the organs or tissues where they initially contacted antigen, increasing the likelihood of interaction between antigen-specific lymphocytes and sites of likely antigen entry.
2. Lymphocytes enter lymph nodes or Peyer's patches via specialized postcapillary blood venules. The lymphoid parenchyma or tissue around this site of entry, within the T-cell-rich zone of the lymph node, is a likely place where naive antigen-specific T and B lymphocytes initially interact. Activated lymphocytes are ini-

tially retained around postcapillary venules (i.e., the perivascular area) in a primary immune response. Activated T lymphocytes secreting lymphokines can be found immediately adjacent to antigen-specific B lymphocytes in the perivasculature of the lymph node. Moreover, lymphocyte-tracking experiments reveal that antigen-specific T lymphocytes initially reside in the T-cell zone of the lymph node, an area where postcapillary venules are prevalent. During active immune responses, some of these T lymphocytes later migrate into nearby lymph node germinal centers.
3. Lymphoid organs are designed to channel antigens to sites of lymphocyte activation. They accomplish this by an elaborate system of lymphatics (in most body tissues and organs) and lymphoid sinusoids (within lymph nodes).
4. Lymphoid tissues create specialized microenvironments for fostering the growth and differentiation of antigen-specific lymphocytes. The best characterized of these microenvironments is the germinal center.

Lymphocyte Recirculation

Lymphocytes recirculate continuously through the body following well-defined migration pathways from the blood to lymphoid and nonlymphoid organs (Fig. 4.4).

Figure 4.4 Lymphocytes recirculate through the body via well-defined pathways that depend on both the maturational and activation states of the lymphocyte. Red lines indicate the route of lymphocytes through the bloodstream, solid blue lines indicate the route through the lymph, and dashed blue lines indicate the course of lymphocytes through the interstitial space. (**A**) Naive lymphocytes. The recirculation of resting, naive lymphocytes occurs primarily through lymph nodes and spleen. The figure shows a representative pathway whereby lymphocytes leave the blood and enter the pelvic lymph node. After a time in the lymph node, the lymphocyte leaves the node through an efferent lymphatic and travels through the lymphatic circulation until it rejoins the blood at the thoracic duct. (**B**) Memory lymphocytes. Activated or memory lymphocytes tend to prefer recirculating through barrier organs such as the gut mucosa. In the gut mucosa, the lymphocyte enters lymphoid follicles or samples antigen being transported from the intestinal lumen. (**C**) The recirculation of lymphocytes also demonstrates tissue specificity. In the example shown, lymphocytes activated at the site of infection in the skin leave the site of infection to recirculate. After recirculation, the effector and memory lymphocytes preferentially home back to the skin.

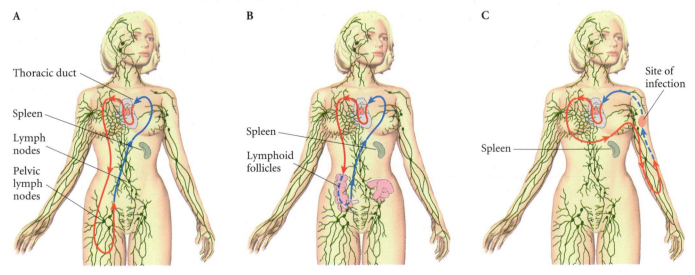

Circulating in this fashion allows lymphocytes to patrol their route for the presence of foreign antigens. Lymphocytes enter the lymph nodes and mucosa-associated lymphoid tissue (MALT) at specialized vascular beds called *postcapillary venules*. These postcapillary venules often are called *high endothelial venules* (HEV) because their activated endothelium often assumes a cuboidal instead of a flattened shape (Fig. 4.5). Postcapillary venules in other nonlymphoid tissues and organs also often assume a "high" endothelial morphology during times of inflammatory stress. The shape reflects cellular activation of the endothelium, a change associated with the synthesis of specific cytokines and adhesion molecules that mediate increased lymphocyte flux across the vessel wall. In a resting, antigenically unstimulated lymph node, comparatively few lymphocytes enter the

node. During times of antigenic stimulation, the entry rate can increase manyfold. In experimental animals, for example, the number of cells in lymph nodes can increase 100-fold relative to the number during the resting condition. Increases in cell number result in an enlarged lymph node (lymphadenopathy) that can often be clinically detected by physical exam or by X ray.

Lymphocytes reside in lymphoid tissues for various periods of time, the duration depending largely on whether the lymphocytes are activated by antigen. If naive lymphocytes are activated following encounter with antigen in a lymphoid organ, they are retained in the lymphoid organ and proliferate. If unactivated, these lymphocytes exit the lymphoid organ via the medulla and flow into the efferent lymph. Unactivated lymphocytes can traverse a lymph node within a day, whereas activated lymphocytes often are retained in a lymph node for days or weeks. Lymphocytes within the lymphatics ultimately reenter the bloodstream at the thoracic duct, the point where the lymphatics merge into the bloodstream. The recirculation process is then ready to start anew.

Lymphocyte-HEV interactions also include antigen-independent recognition mechanisms that control the types of tissues or organs through which lymphocytes migrate. For example, there is a distinction between the recirculation patterns of naive and memory T lymphocytes. Naive T lymphocytes preferentially recirculate through lymphoid organs (Fig. 4.4A), whereas memory T lymphocytes preferentially recirculate through barrier organs such as the skin or gut mucosa (Fig. 4.4B).

Lymphocytes also have an organ- or tissue-specific homing capability (Fig. 4.4C). For example, lymphocytes derived from MALT tend to home back to MALT tissues. Similarly, lymphocytes derived from lymph nodes will, when adoptively transferred into a syngeneic host, preferentially migrate back to lymph nodes (as compared with MALT or skin). The molecular mechanisms regulating this homing capacity are partly understood. Lymphocyte interaction with lymph node HEV is mediated by the interaction of L-selectin on the lymphocyte with both GlyCAM-1 and CD34 receptors on the blood vessel endothelium (Fig. 4.6A). L-selectin binds to a carbohydrate epitope on the receptor molecules. It is interesting that L-selectin does not mediate binding to ectopically expressed GlyCAM-1 and CD34. Moreover, L-selectin does not bind to CD34 expressed by other vascular endothelia. It is believed that L-selectin on lymphocytes has a specific affinity for carbohydrate epitopes that are added only to GlyCAM-1 and CD34 expressed by lymph node HEV.

Lymphocytes migrating to other sites use other ligand receptor pairs that confer their homing specificity. Binding of lymphocytes to Peyer's patches is initiated by

Figure 4.5 (A) A cross-section of a postcapillary venule in a lymph node, showing HEV and naive lymphocytes extravasating to leave the blood and enter the node. (B) Scanning electron micrograph of a blood vessel wall within a lymph node. Several lymphocytes are attached to the inner endothelial lining of the blood vessel in apparent transit across the vessel wall.

A

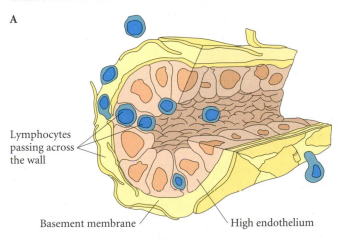

Lymphocytes passing across the wall

Basement membrane   High endothelium

B

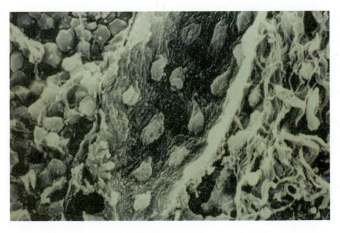

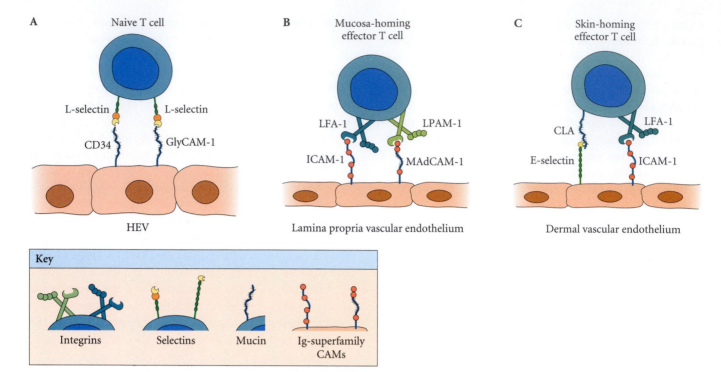

Figure 4.6 (A) The specificity of naive lymphocytes for the HEV of postcapillary venules is determined by the expression of specific adhesion molecules by both the lymphocyte and the HEV. (**B and C**) Other patterns of adhesion molecules are present on the surface of memory and effector lymphocytes and on the endothelium of other tissues.

the binding of ICAM-1 to αLβ2 integrin and further amplified by the interaction of MAdCAM-1 to α4β7 integrin (Fig. 4.6B). Skin-homing lymphocytes express cutaneous lymphocyte-associated antigen (CLA), which is structurally related to a blood group antigen present on erythrocytes known as sialyl Lewis a- and x-related antigens (Fig. 4.6C). CLA is capable of binding to E-selectin, which is inducibly expressed by some vascular endothelia, including those of skin. CLA is structurally similar to P-selectin glycoprotein ligand-1 (PSGL-1), the difference residing only in the carbohydrate component of the glycoprotein. Recent data have suggested that PSGL-1 also may mediate the skin-homing property of some lymphocytes; namely, PSGL-1 on lymphocytes can interact with P-selectin on vascular endothelia of skin.

Germinal Centers

Once the relevant cellular interactions have occurred, many lymphocytes migrate into specialized microenvironments found in peripheral lymphoid organs that support their differentiation. Probably the best known of these microenvironments is the germinal center, an important site of B-lymphocyte differentiation. Germinal centers, also called *secondary follicles*, arise from primary

follicles after lymphocyte stimulation by antigen. Primary follicles are present in all organized peripheral lymphoid organs or tissues: spleen, lymph nodes, Peyer's patches, and MALTs.

Primary follicles primarily contain a pool of recirculating B lymphocytes (Fig. 4.7A). Most of these lymphocytes express cell surface immunoglobulins M and D (IgM and IgD). Follicular dendritic cells (FDCs) are another important cell type within follicles. FDCs take up native antigen by virtue of immunoglobulin receptors that are distributed on their extensive dendritic cytoplasmic extensions. Cell surface immunoglobulin receptors thereby capture antigens in immune complexes, retaining them for months or years. FDCs, therefore, act as an antigen trap, focusing antigen for continued presentation to follicular B lymphocytes and supporting differentiation of B lymphocytes into memory cells and plasma cells.

After their exposure to an immunogenic form of antigen, primary follicles undergo a transformation. The small, resting B lymphocytes of the primary follicle are displaced to the periphery, forming a follicular mantle. The central portion of the follicle becomes a germinal center. This structure is also termed a secondary follicle (Fig. 4.7B). Germinal centers have two areas that may be visible by conventional light microscopy (Fig. 4.7C). A "dark zone" contains numerous densely packed large lymphocytes, many of which are actively proliferating. These large proliferating lymphocytes are termed *centroblasts*. The germinal center also contains a "light zone," where the lymphocytes are smaller and generally not proliferating. An extensive network of FDC cytoplasmic extensions surrounds the lymphocytes of the light zone. These light zone lymphocytes are termed *centrocytes*.

Germinal centers are important sites for B-lymphocyte differentiation. The initial activation of B lymphocytes most likely occurs outside the germinal center. The activated B lymphocyte then migrates to a primary follicle and undergoes clonal expansion. Microdissection studies of germinal centers have demonstrated that germinal center B lymphocytes are generally either monoclonal or oligoclonal in origin. Therefore, any single germinal center relates to one or, at most, only a few different antigens at any one time. Active proliferation of these blast-transformed B lymphocytes (centroblasts) gives rise to the germinal center dark zone. Labeling studies using [3H]thymidine indicate that centroblasts divide approximately once every 7 hours, a surprising finding that has been confirmed by different methods. Over time, a percentage of centroblasts cease dividing and migrate to the periphery of the dark zone, becoming centrocytes. Accumulation of centrocytes gives rise to the germinal center light zone.

The germinal center provides an important microenvironment for isotype switching of immunoglobulin production. Most germinal center B lymphocytes initially bear surface IgM. However, after prolonged stimulation with antigen, the majority of germinal center cells bear surface IgG (in lymph nodes) or surface IgA (in Peyer's patches). These changes suggest that the germinal center microenvironment provides a signal or signals for switching of heavy-chain class during B-lymphocyte responses.

Besides undergoing clonal amplification, germinal center B lymphocytes undergo extensive mutation (hypermutation) of their immunoglobulin genes in a process known as somatic hypermutation (Fig. 4.8). Some of these mutations result in germinal center B lymphocytes with an increased affinity for the stimulating antigen. These subclones with increased affinity for the antigen are preferentially stimulated to grow because of their increased capacity to bind the limited amount of antigen being displayed on the cell membrane of FDCs in the light zone of the germinal center (Fig. 4.8). Within the germinal center, these high-affinity B lymphocytes are induced to differentiate into memory B lymphocytes and plasma cells. Some mutations also result in a decreased rather than an increased affinity for the stimulating antigen. Because of the lower affinity, antigen on FDCs is less capable of cross-linking B-lymphocyte cell surface immunoglobulins, leading to B-lymphocyte apoptosis. In

Figure 4.7 Lymphoid follicles are the simplest example of organized lymphoid tissue containing lymphocytes and APCs. (**A**) Photomicrograph of primary follicle. Primary follicles contain primarily a pool of recirculating B lymphocytes. FDCs are another important cell type within follicles and act as "antigen traps" by binding antigen-antibody complexes via antibody Fc receptors. (**B**) Photomicrograph of germinal center. Following exposure to an antigen, a primary follicle is transformed into a secondary follicle, where intense lymphocyte proliferation takes place (gc, germinal center; m, mantle zone). (**C**) Germinal centers have three areas that can sometimes be discerned by conventional light microscopy. A dark zone contains numerous densely packed large lymphocytes (centroblasts) that are actively proliferating. The germinal center also contains a basal light zone, where the lymphocytes (centrocytes) are smaller and not proliferating. An extensive network of cytoplasmic extensions from FDCs surrounds the lymphocytes of the light zone. The centrocytes in the basal light zone are being selected for high affinity for antigen. Centrocytes that survive through this period of selection proceed to the apical light zone, where they differentiate into either memory cells or plasma cells. These areas are not always seen and depend on the age and state of activation of the germinal center.

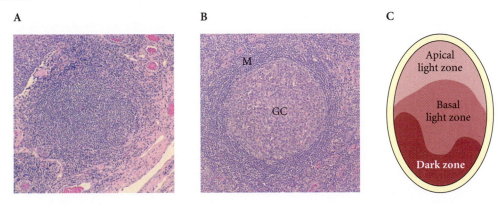

A   B   C

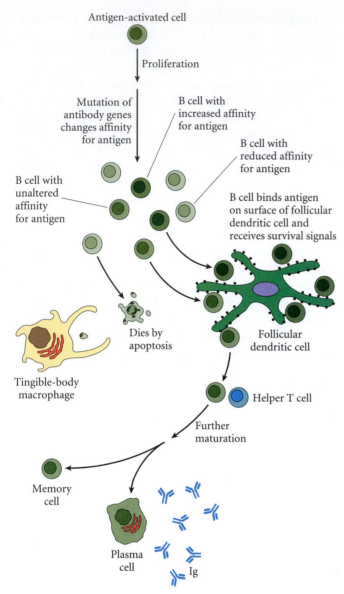

Antigen-activated cell

Proliferation

Mutation of antibody genes changes affinity for antigen

B cell with increased affinity for antigen

B cell with reduced affinity for antigen

B cell with unaltered affinity for antigen

B cell binds antigen on surface of follicular dendritic cell and receives survival signals

Dies by apoptosis

Follicular dendritic cell

Tingible-body macrophage

Helper T cell

Further maturation

Memory cell

Plasma cell

Ig

Figure 4.8 Affinity maturation. During B-lymphocyte proliferation in the germinal center, centrocytes (expanded B cells that have undergone the process of somatic hypermutation) must compete with each other for a limited amount of antigen that is being displayed by FDCs in the light zone of the germinal center. Only centrocytes with the highest affinity for antigen successfully interact with FDCs and receive survival signals from them. B cells with reduced affinity for antigen die by apoptosis, and the apoptotic bodies are engulfed by tingible-body macrophages present in the germinal center. The result is that only centrocytes bearing the highest-affinity receptors for antigen survive.

fact, many centrocytes undergo apoptosis, presumably as a result of affinity-driven apoptosis. Apoptotic lymphocytes are phagocytosed by germinal center macrophages. The engulfed cellular material can often be identified within the macrophages, leading to the so-called *tingible body macrophages*.

Peripheral Lymphoid Organs

The spleen and lymph nodes are the principal sites for the initiation of most primary immune responses. In general, lymph nodes drain specified anatomic regions of the body, whereas the spleen is the site of immunity to blood-borne pathogens. Both organs contain regions rich in T and B lymphocytes, including germinal centers, and are also capable of producing similar types of cellular and humoral immune reactions. Despite these superficial similarities, the types of anatomic pathways through which lymphocytes and antigen flow are distinct.

The Spleen

The spleen has two major functions. It serves as a filtration bed, filtering blood for pathogens and old or damaged blood cells; this filtration function occurs primarily in the splenic red pulp. The splenic white pulp, on the other hand, comprises an important immunologic organ. An estimated 25% of the body's mature lymphocytes reside in the spleen at any one time. If a pathogen, such as a bacterium, enters the blood circulation, it will generally be removed in the splenic red pulp, whereas a host immune response will be mounted in the white pulp.

The spleen receives blood through a single splenic artery. In humans, approximately 5% of the total cardiac output is directed through the spleen. Once the splenic artery enters at the splenic hilum, it divides into progressively smaller branches (Fig. 4.9). The distal branches are termed *trabecular arteries*. The trabecular arteries send off yet smaller arterial branches, called the *central arterioles*. Lymphocytes aggregate around the central arterioles, forming lymphocytic periarterial "cuffs." These cuffs are predominantly T lymphocytes and form an important part of the white pulp. The cuffs are termed the *periarterial lymphatic sheath* (PALS). The PALS also contains interdigitating dendritic cells, which are important APCs common to T-lymphocyte-rich lymphoid zones. B lymphocytes also aggregate adjacent to the central arterioles, often just beyond the PALS, forming discrete lymphocytic follicles. FDCs are present in the follicles. These cells serve as an antigen depot, supporting clonal expansion and differentiation of B lymphocytes.

Although the PALS and the follicles form right next to and around the central arterioles, these vessels do not supply the PALS and follicles with blood directly. Instead, the central arterioles further divide into smaller capillaries that project into the border of the white and red pulp. The blood circulation empties into a vascular sinus-like space termed the *marginal zone*. The marginal zone is an elaborate branching network of channels that separates the white and red pulp. It comprises a series of filtration beds that are lined with reticular cells, probably of fibroblastic origin, and macrophages. Many blood cells are processed in the marginal zone. Damaged erythrocytes are phagocytosed, senescent granulocytes are destroyed, and platelets are stored. Through as yet ill-defined mechanisms, neutrophils and erythrocytes are channeled directly into the red pulp, whereas at least some mononuclear cells (lymphocytes and monocytes) are directed to the white pulp.

The marginal sinus is a somewhat distinct sinusoidal space positioned immediately between the marginal zone and the white pulp. Several studies indicate that the marginal sinus also receives blood directly from distal branches of the central artery. However, white cells predominate in the marginal sinus, with only scant numbers of red cells. Therefore, the cellular composition of the marginal sinus is more like the white pulp than the red pulp. Although the function of the marginal sinus is less clear, it likely serves as a transit point, controlling the flow of mononuclear cells in and out of the white pulp.

The red pulp is the most distal vascular component of the spleen. The red pulp forms an indistinct boundary with the marginal zone. Like the marginal zone, the red pulp is composed of an extensive series of anastomosing filtration beds that ultimately coalesce into splenic veins. The filtration beds are lined with reticular (fibroblastic) cells and macrophages. Like the marginal zone, the red pulp has the capacity to clear the blood circulation of pathogens and old or damaged blood cells. The filtered blood ultimately exits the spleen via the splenic vein located at the splenic hilum.

Lymph Nodes

Lymph is a plasma filtrate that can include mononuclear cells. The cellular content is usually quite low except when there is inflammation. Lymphatics are thin-walled vessels that converge as they approach the heart, transporting lymph back to the blood circulation. Lymphatic vessels originate beneath epithelial surfaces throughout the body. The lymphatics ultimately coalesce into the thoracic duct, which, in turn, empties into the great veins at the base of the neck. Lymph nodes are interposed at key points along the way, forcing the lymph from a specific region of the body through the node (Fig. 4.10).

Lymph nodes are encapsulated collections of lymphocytes and accessory cells. They are found throughout the body, most commonly adjacent to vascular bifurcations, alongside major blood vessels, or near articular joints. Lymph nodes sample the lymph as it passes on its way back to the thoracic duct, continuously monitoring the lymph for the presence of foreign antigens or pathogens. Inflammatory responses in a particular region of the

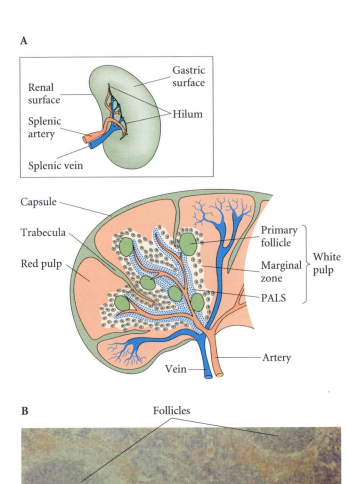

Figure 4.9 (A) The spleen is divided into red pulp and white pulp. The red pulp primarily contains erythrocytes, including numerous dying red blood cells as well as macrophages that contain engulfed red blood cells. The white pulp can be subdivided into the PALS (a T-lymphocyte-rich area that also contains IDCs), follicles (containing B lymphocytes and FDCs), and the marginal zone. Blood entering through the splenic artery percolates through the vascular endothelium at the splenic sinus (B) to enter the marginal zone. B cells stimulated by antigens migrate to the PALS to collaborate with T cells that reside in the PALS. If B-cell–T-cell collaboration is successful, activated B and T cells migrate into a primary follicle, which then becomes a secondary follicle. (**Inset.**) An external view of the entire spleen. (B) Hematoxylin-and-eosin-stained section of spleen. Three follicles are readily evident at this low magnification as being rich in lymphocytes and essentially devoid of erythrocytes. Numerous PALSs are also apparent and assume a rather serpentine shape that follows the course of various arterioles. The red pulp comprises the areas that are rich in erythrocytes and that stain predominantly with eosin, a red dye.

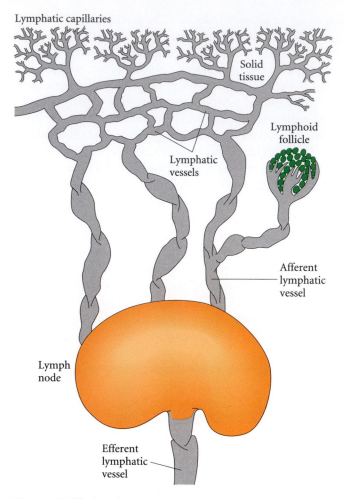

Lymphatic capillaries

Solid tissue

Lymphoid follicle

Lymphatic vessels

Afferent lymphatic vessel

Lymph node

Efferent lymphatic vessel

Figure 4.10 The lymphatics are a circulatory system that gathers lymph fluid (a plasma filtrate) from various tissues and returns that fluid to the bloodstream. Lymph enters the lymphatics at small, open-ended lymphatic capillaries and proceeds through progressively larger vessels. As the lymph makes its way through this circulatory system, it encounters various collections of organized lymphoid tissue. The most rudimentary of these are simple lymphoid follicles. At other places (usually at the junction of several lymphatics), the lymph will enter a lymph node. Eventually, the lymph reaches the largest lymphatic vessel (the thoracic duct), where it combines with the blood.

body will therefore usually be reflected by changes in the draining lymph node.

Lymph nodes are a site for the convergence of two distinct, nonoverlapping circulatory systems. Namely, both blood vessels and lymphatic vessels enter lymph nodes. In a primary immune response, antigen generally arrives via the lymph, whereas recirculating naive lymphocytes arrive via the bloodstream. Antigen is transported (from a peripheral site of inflammation to the draining lymph node) in lymph either as a soluble protein or carried by mononuclear cells after phagocytosis. Unlike mononuclear cells, polymorphonuclear leukocytes do not recirculate to a draining lymph node.

The afferent (incoming) lymphatic vessels penetrate the lymph node capsule and deliver their contents to a comparatively large sinusoidal space termed the *cortical sinus* (Fig. 4.11). The cortical sinus is an open space located at the outer edge of the lymph node. Lymph and draining mononuclear cells initially collect in the cortical sinus. The *cortical sinusoids* are conduits that exit the cortical sinus and penetrate into the lymph node parenchyma. As lymph enters the lymphoid parenchyma through the cortical sinusoids, it percolates through the reticular meshwork that forms the lymph node framework. The cortical sinusoids deliver lymph in proximity to follicles and postcapillary venules. This feature is important in facilitating the interaction of antigen, transported by lymph, with B and T lymphocytes. Proximity to postcapillary venules—the site of lymphocyte entry from the blood—facilitates the interaction of incoming lymphocytes with antigen. Proximity to follicles facilitates the delivery of antigen to FDCs for long-term retention of antigen. The cortical sinusoids ultimately coalesce into the larger medullary sinusoids found at the base of the lymph node. Numerous macrophages and plasma cells often are found in the medullary sinusoids. Lymphocytes exiting the lymph node also migrate into the medullary sinusoids. The medullary sinusoids converge into a single efferent lymphatic vessel through which lymph exits.

Lymph nodes are segregated into distinct B- and T-lymphocyte zones. The follicles are largely, although not exclusively, a B-lymphocyte region. As previously noted, they are the sites of germinal center formation. T lymphocytes are found between the follicles, in the interfollicular region of the lymph node. Just as the follicle contains an FDC, the T-cell zone has its own type of dendritic cell, the interdigitating dendritic cell (IDC). The IDC is usually found in close physical association with T lymphocytes in other lymphoid organs as well. The IDC expresses cell surface MHC class II gene products and is important for antigen presentation to $CD4^+$ T lymphocytes. The same or closely related cell type also is found in blood (veiled cell) and in stratified squamous epithelium such as skin (Langerhans cell).

MALT

The mucosal surfaces of the gastrointestinal, respiratory, and urogenital tracts have their own uniquely adapted immune system termed MALT. The mucosal immune system is designed to protect against microbial invasion along a considerably large perimeter. In an adult, the mucosal surfaces of the gastrointestinal, respiratory, and

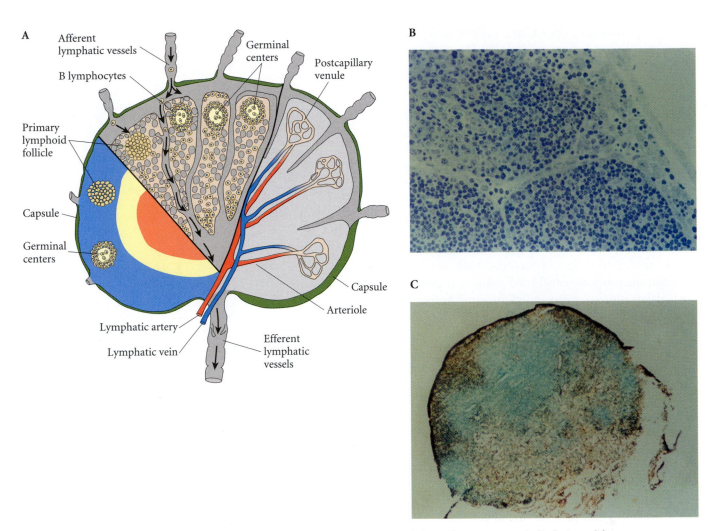

Figure 4.11 (A) Structure of a lymph node. The diagram is divided into three sectors, each displaying a different level of detail. The left sector demonstrates the arrangement of the three layers of each node. The outermost layer, the cortex (shown in blue in the left sector), contains mostly B cells and FDCs in primary lymphoid follicles. The middle layer, the paracortex (shown in yellow in the left sector), is enriched for T cells and IDCs. The innermost layer, the medulla (shown in red in the left sector), is enriched for antibody-secreting plasma cells. The middle sector of the figure shows the cellular detail and architecture of the node. Lymph that contains foreign antigens enters the nodes via the afferent lymphatics and is deposited beneath the capsule. The lymph percolates through the node to interact with T cells in the paracortex and with B cells in the cortex. Lymph exits the node through the single efferent lymphatic. The right sector displays the blood vasculature of the node. Each node is fed by a single lymphatic artery, which branches out to a number of arterioles. Each arteriole ends in a postcapillary venule that then empties into a lymphatic vein. Lymphocytes extravasate at the postcapillary venules to enter a lymph node. (B) Photomicrograph of lymph node cortex, showing the cortical sinus immediately underneath the lymph node capsule. Cortical sinusoids originate from the cortical sinus and penetrate the lymph node parenchyma. (C) Low-power photomicrograph of a naive lymph node, immunostained for IgM. IgM-positive cells are colored brown. IgM-negative cells are counterstained blue. The photomicrograph shows the segregation of T- and B-cell zones, as B lymphocytes (brown cells) are located in primary follicles toward the periphery of the lymph node. Some IgM staining is also seen in the medulla, a site where plasma cells can often be found.

urogenital tracts have a combined surface area of at least 400 square meters (m²). MALT is composed of three components: (i) the mucosal barrier, (ii) organized lymphoid tissues dispersed along the length of the gastrointestinal tract, and (iii) dispersed lymphoid cells within the epithelium and lamina propria.

The Mucosal Barrier

The epithelial linings of various mucosae present different types of barriers to microbial invasion. The mouth, pharynx, esophagus, urethra, and vagina all contain stratified squamous epithelium. The intestine is lined by a columnar epithelium that is one cell layer thick. The respiratory lining is composed of pseudostratified or simple cuboidal or columnar epithelium. From an immune perspective, each of these epithelial linings must prevent microbial invasion and, at the same time, internalize exogenous antigens for priming of immune cells.

Stratified squamous epithelia lack the tight junctions characteristic of intestinal epithelia. Nonetheless, many stratified squamous epithelia, such as that from the oral cavity, are largely impenetrable to protein tracers and large cations because of the tight packing of cells and a secreted glycolipoprotein. Other stratified squamous epithelia, such as that from the vagina, are somewhat permeable to proteins, depending on the stage of the hormonal cycle. However, such epithelia have no mechanism for directional transport of proteins. Thus, neither proteins nor microbes are capable of completely penetrating through stratified squamous epithelium. Antigen sampling in such epithelia is accomplished by a specialized type of dendritic cell, the Langerhans cell. Langerhans cells are professional APCs; they express MHC class II gene products. Langerhans cells are located between and among epithelial cells, facilitating intimate contact for complete antigen sampling (Fig. 4.12), and are motile. After a brief sojourn in the epithelium of 1 to 4 days, most Langerhans cells emigrate from the epithelium to the draining lymph node. There they can present antigens (derived from the epithelial microenvironment) to CD4$^+$ T lymphocytes and initiate immune responses. Therefore, antigens that may diffuse weakly into the epithelial layer are transported into the immune system by a system of motile, professional APCs (Langerhans cells) dispersed among epithelial cells.

Most of the gastrointestinal and respiratory tracts is lined with a columnar epithelium that forms tight junctions and defines the tissue's epithelial barrier. Since tight junctions exclude proteins and macromolecules from passage below the apical border (the epithelial cell membrane that delineates the epithelial surface from the cavity or lumen of these tubular tracts), specialized mechanisms have evolved for communicating samples of antigen found in the lumen to the associated immune cells below the epithelial barrier. In addition to the usual enterocytes, intestinal epithelium contains specialized antigen-transporting cells called *M cells* (an abbreviation for *microfold* or *multifenestrated cells*—a name describing the appearance of their apical plasma membrane). M cells are located only above subepithelial lymphoid aggregates. M cells transport macromolecules, and even microorganisms, directly to the underlying mucosal lymphoid tissue. Samples of the intestinal lumen are endocytosed across the apical surface of the M cell into a basolateral cellular "pocket." Lymphocytes and macrophages migrate in and

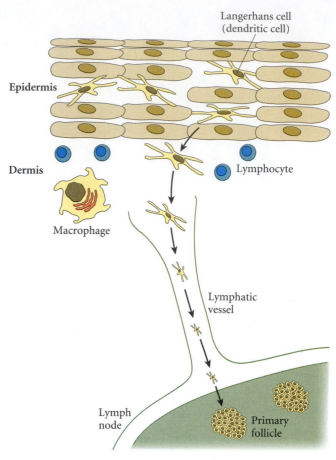

Figure 4.12 Antigen sampling in the skin is carried out by APCs known as Langerhans cells. Langerhans cells reside in the epidermal layer, where they serve in antigen capture. After antigen uptake, the Langerhans cells leave the skin, migrate to the draining lymph node, home to the node's paracortex, and display antigen to T cells. The skin also contains many different types of lymphocytes, some of which reside in the epidermis and others in the dermis.

out of M-cell pockets, sampling the antigenic contents of the transcytosed intestinal lumen (Fig. 4.13). It is likely that this specialized mode of antigen entry serves to anatomically focus incoming antigen with APCs and lymphocytes. Given their probable importance in initiating immune responses in the gut, the regions containing M cells and their underlying lymphoid follicles are sometimes referred to as *inductive sites.*

Anatomic Organization of Mucosal Lymphoid Tissues

Mucosal lymphocytes are scattered along the entire length of the gastrointestinal tract. These lymphocytes can be found both in organized lymphoid structures, such as in follicles or Peyer's patches, and dispersed singly or in small aggregates within the epithelium and lamina propria.

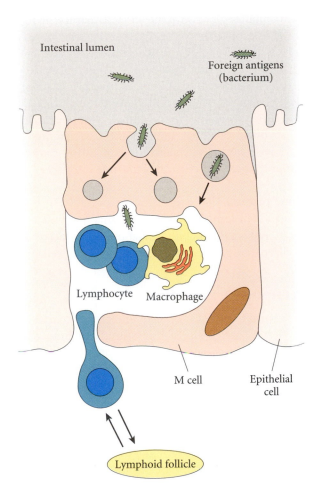

Intestinal lumen

Foreign antigens (bacterium)

Lymphocyte

Macrophage

M cell

Epithelial cell

Lymphoid follicle

Figure 4.13 Antigen sampling across the intestinal barrier occurs at so-called inductive sites by specialized antigen-transporting cells known as M cells. M cells have a unique morphology in that their basolateral membrane contains a large pocket, which is occupied by lymphocytes and macrophages. The M cell continuously transcytoses antigen from the intestinal lumen to the immune cells residing in the basolateral pocket. Lymphocytes or macrophages that encounter antigen in this manner leave the M cell and travel to the underlying lymphoid follicles.

Organized mucosal lymphoid tissues

Mucosal lymphoid follicles can be found along the entire length of the gastrointestinal tract. Oftentimes, these follicles are present singly, as in the colon and rectum. In the small intestine, oro- and nasopharynx, and appendix, aggregates of follicles comprise the Peyer's patches, tonsils, and appendiceal lymphoid tissue, respectively.

Peyer's patches are composed of approximately 30 to 40 lymphoid follicles. The follicles are subjacent to the intestinal epithelium in association with M cells (Fig. 4.14). The M cells are believed to be the sites for antigen penetration of intestinal epithelium. As in the spleen and lymph nodes, the follicles are B-lymphocyte-rich areas that often contain germinal centers. The follicles are sep-

arated by a T-lymphocyte-rich interfollicular region. The histologic organization of the tonsils is similar. The tonsils play a role in defense against antigens of the oro- or nasopharynx. There are actually three sets of tonsils: lingual tonsils, located at the base of the tongue; palatine

Figure 4.14 (**A**) A Peyer's patch is visible macroscopically as a small bulge in the side of the small intestine. Photo by John Warner. (**B**) Antigens transported across the intestinal epithelium by M cells will be delivered to large aggregates of lymphoid follicles known as Peyer's patches. Each Peyer's patch contains approximately 30 to 40 lymphoid follicles.

A

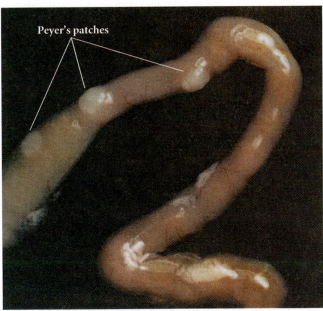

Peyer's patches

B

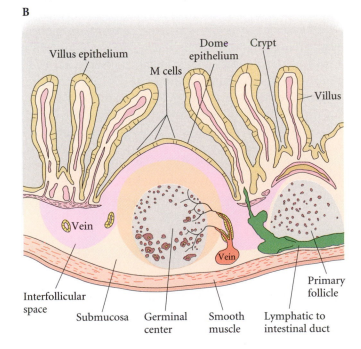

Villus epithelium

Dome epithelium

Crypt

M cells

Villus

Vein

Vein

Interfollicular space

Submucosa

Germinal center

Smooth muscle

Lymphatic to intestinal duct

Primary follicle

tonsils, on the side of the back of the mouth; and adenoids, in the roof of the nasopharynx.

MALT executes its defense function in part through the production of IgA antibodies. IgA is an immunoglobulin subtype that can be efficiently transported across epithelial boundaries (see chapters 6 and 17). Once within the lumen, IgA antibodies can bind to potential pathogens and toxins, preventing them from crossing the mucosal barrier. Although IgA is a minor immunoglobulin isotype in plasma, it is the predominant isotype secreted by mucosal B lymphocytes. In fact, the total production of IgA, secreted across epithelia, is believed to exceed the total production of IgG and IgM produced elsewhere in the body.

Although IgA that is present in the blood is largely monomeric in structure, secretory IgA is synthesized as a dimer, the two IgA monomers being held together by a J-chain polypeptide. Once within the epithelial lamina propria, dimeric IgA is shuttled across the mucosal epithelium by receptor-mediated transcytosis, using the so-called *polymeric immunoglobulin receptor* (pIgR). The pIgR is an immunoglobulin superfamily protein, approximately 100 kilodaltons (kDa) in size, that is synthesized by intestinal epithelial cells. Dimeric IgA binds to the pIgR on the basal surface of epithelial cells and is endocytosed and transported in vesicles across the cell to the luminal surface. During transcytosis across the epithelial cell, the pIgR is proteolytically cleaved to liberate the bound IgA from the vesicle membrane. The portion of the pIgR that physically binds to IgA remains associated with IgA after this cleavage event and is thereafter referred to as *secretory component*. The complex of IgA and secretory component is stabilized by a single disulfide bond that forms between IgA and the fifth immunoglobulin-like domain of secretory component. It is thought that secretory component plays an important role in protecting IgA from proteolytic cleavage after it is released from mucosal secretions. This protection of IgA is thought to occur by steric hindrance of proteases, as the presence of secretory component may physically block their access to the protease-sensitive hinge region of IgA. The pIgR also is responsible for the secretion of IgA into saliva, milk, and bile.

Dispersed mucosal lymphocytes
Individual lymphocytes that are not part of an organized lymphoid tissue can be found within the epithelium and lamina propria.

Epithelium
Intraepithelial lymphocytes (IELs) are predominantly T lymphocytes, most of which express CD8 in humans. A unique feature of intraepithelial T lymphocytes is their dis-

proportionately high use of the γδ TCR. In mice, up to 50% of the IELs express the γδ TCR rather than the more commonly used αβ TCR. The IELs also use fewer variable (V) genes in the formation of the γδ TCR than is commonly observed for most T lymphocytes in other parts of the body. This suggests that the IELs have a more limited array of antigenic specificities than do the T lymphocytes found in spleen or lymph nodes. It is hypothesized that these IELs may have evolved especially for combating pathogens commonly encountered at the intestinal interface.

Lamina propria
The intestinal lamina propria contains a mixed assortment of leukocytes, including T and B lymphocytes, plasma cells, macrophages, eosinophils, and mast cells.

Cutaneous Immunity

Skin is continuously exposed to an extraordinary variety of environmental antigens and stimuli, including living microorganisms, chemicals, direct trauma, and ultraviolet (UV) irradiation. In response, the skin has several novel features that help it carry out its dual roles as protective barrier and immune organ. These features include the ability of keratinocytes to trigger and support immune responses and the presence of epidermal Langerhans cells and dermal and intraepidermal lymphocytes.

Keratinocytes, the epithelial cells of the epidermis, are part of a stratified squamous epithelium. Keratinocytes have the ability to transduce noxious stimuli into a signal, in the form of cytokines. Two of these cytokines, IL-1 and tumor necrosis factor alpha, are capable of directly stimulating cutaneous inflammation. IL-1α is stored within keratinocytes and is rapidly released following the injury of keratinocytes. IL-1β and tumor necrosis factor alpha are synthesized de novo, and their release following cellular injury occurs later than that of IL-1α. These three cytokines have the ability to upregulate the expression of adhesion molecules on dermal endothelial cells and to induce release of chemotactic factors such as chemokines.

Keratinocytes are also capable of modulating the T-lymphocyte response by secreting IL-10 or IL-12. These cytokines are capable of polarizing the T-cell response toward the helper T-cell (TH1 or TH2) pathways (see chapter 14). IL-12 fosters the differentiation of T lymphocytes toward the TH1 pathway. TH1 lymphocytes secrete interferon-gamma, causing activation of nearby phagocytes. IL-10, on the other hand, inhibits TH1 cell development by preventing secretion of IL-12 by macrophages. Additional evidence implicates IL-10 in the suppression of local immune responses. Mice deficient in IL-10, for example, exhibit exaggerated cutaneous inflammatory reactions, suggesting that IL-10 normally down-regulates local immune responses. This may be an important protective response limiting inflammatory damage following UV irradiation, as indicated by the increase in production of IL-10 in response to UV light.

Keratinocytes secrete a number of chemokines, such as monocyte chemoattractant protein 1, IL-8, IL-10, Gro-α, Gro-β, and Gro-γ. In general, chemokines are capable of acting as chemotactic agents, directing different types of leukocytes to extravasate from the bloodstream to the adjacent cutaneous tissue. Keratinocytes have also been documented to synthesize IL-7 and IL-15, both of which promote the growth of T lymphocytes or T-lymphocyte precursors. Other keratinocyte-derived cytokines include granulocyte-macrophage colony-stimulating factor, transforming growth factor alpha, IL-6, and IL-3.

Langerhans cells are morphologically and functionally similar to dendritic cells and normally reside within the epidermis of the skin (Fig. 4.12). Langerhans cells serve a surveillance function; they are capable of initiating immune responses to cutaneous foreign antigens. They constitutively express MHC class II gene products and are the main type of cutaneous professional APC. Langerhans cells exist in the skin in an immature state in which they actively internalize and process antigens. Once foreign antigen is encountered, Langerhans cells leave the skin and travel through the lymphatics to the regional lymph nodes. During this period of transit, Langerhans cells complete their maturation process. This maturation involves an increase in the number of costimulatory molecules they express (rendering them even more potent at stimulating the activation of antigen-specific naive T lymphocytes) and in the cessation of antigen processing. Thus, migrating Langerhans cells "freeze" their current state of antigen presentation. This cessation of antigen-processing activity is important if the Langerhans cells are to present lymph node T cells with the same antigen they encountered in the skin (otherwise, the antigen encountered in the skin would be largely replaced with new antigen by the time the Langerhans cells reached the lymph nodes). Once in the draining lymph nodes, the Langerhans cells present the antigen to the resident T lymphocytes, possibly initiating an immune response to the captured antigen. Many T lymphocytes activated in such a way subsequently home to the skin, where they will reside in the dermal layer (presumably to protect against future encounters with the same antigen).

The epidermis also contains small numbers of lymphocytes, predominantly T lymphocytes. In mice, intraepidermal T lymphocytes assume a dendritic morphology and express the $\gamma\delta$ form of the TCR. These lymphocytes, termed *dendritic epidermal T cells,* express an invariant TCR comprising $V_\gamma 5$ and $V_\delta 1$ chains without any junctional diversity. Dendritic epidermal T cells of the tongue, vagina, and uterus express the same δ chain paired with $V_\gamma 6$. $\gamma\delta$ T cells are also highly represented in the intestinal mucosa. This strikingly restricted pattern of TCR usage suggests that $\gamma\delta$ T cells have a unique role in cutaneous or mucosal immune responses. A homologous population of intraepidermal $\gamma\delta$ T cells does not exist in humans.

The dermis is the layer of connective tissue immediately subjacent to the epidermis. Small numbers of lymphocytes, primarily T lymphocytes and macrophages, often are found within the dermis. These mononuclear cells are located predominantly around small postcapillary venules. During cutaneous immune responses, such as following contact sensitization, the dermal postcapillary venules may be surrounded by an intense cellular infiltrate, comprising primarily lymphocytes and macrophages. A population of dendritic cells, similar to the intraepidermal Langerhans cells, also is found in the dermis. These dermal dendritic cells have received far less attention than have the closely related intraepidermal Langerhans cells. Nonetheless, dermal dendritic cells share most of their cell surface markers with epidermal Langerhans cells. Dermal dendritic cells are often closely associated with dermal postcapillary venules and are capable of antigen presentation.

Summary

Immune responses occur in a complex, three-dimensional organ framework. That framework is usually essential for proper lymphocyte growth, differentiation, and effector function.

The growth and maturation of lymphocyte precursors occur within specialized organs, most prominently the bone marrow and thymus. In the bone marrow, lymphocyte precursors are one of the several hematopoietic lineages that can be found in the perivenular marrow space. The bone marrow microenvironment supports hematopoietic cell growth both through intercellular contacts (such as from stromal cells) and via the high local concentration of certain cytokines. T-lymphocyte precursors further differentiate in the thymus. In addition to lymphocytes, the thymic cortex contains a variety of nonlymphocyte cell types: epithelial nurse cells, bone marrow-derived dendritic cells, and macrophages. Through contact with these cells, thymic lymphocytes are both positively and negatively selected.

Peripheral lymphoid organs, such as the spleen and lymph nodes, direct antigen-reactive lymphocytes into specialized microanatomic compartments. These compartments are important for promoting the activation of antigen-reactive lymphocytes. For example, germinal centers support the ability of B lymphocytes to differentiate into memory B lymphocytes or plasma cells. Peripheral lymphoid organs are also designed to maximize the probability of contact between antigen and antigen-reactive lymphocytes. This is accomplished in a variety of ways: distinct lymphocyte recirculation pathways, channeling of antigen through lymphatics and sinusoids, and distinct antigen "traps" for long-term antigen retention (such as by FDCs).

Epithelial organs and tissues in contact with the external environment, such as MALT and skin, demonstrate adaptations related to specific anatomic needs. For example, intestinal antigens are focused to Peyer's patches by specialized M cells. Stratified squamous epithelia such as skin, on the other hand, focus antigens to draining lymph nodes by virtue of specialized Langerhans cells. In addition, IgA is produced by MALT. IgA is adapted for transport across mucosal epithelium.

Suggested Reading

Askin, D. F., and S. Young. 2001. The thymus gland. *Neonatal Netw.* 20:7–13.

Fabbri, M., E. Bianchi, L. Fumagalli, and R. Pardi. 1999. Regulation of lymphocyte traffic by adhesion molecules. *Inflamm. Res.* 48:239–246.

Fu, Y.-X., and D. D. Chaplin. 1999. Development and maturation of secondary lymphoid tissues. *Annu. Rev. Immunol.* 17:399–433.

Guy-Grand, D., and P. Vassalli. 2002. Gut intraepithelial lymphocyte development. *Curr. Opin. Immunol.* 14:255–259.

Kucharzik, T., N. Lugering, K. Rautenberg, A. Lugering, M. A. Schmidt, R. Stoll, and W. Domschke. 2000. Role of M cells in intestinal barrier function. *Ann. N. Y. Acad. Sci.* 915:171–183.

Kupper, T. S. 2000. T cells, immunosurveillance, and cutaneous immunity. *J. Dermatol. Sci.* 24(Suppl. 1):S41–S54.

Loy, A. L., and C. C. Goodnow. 2002. Novel approaches for identifying genes regulating lymphocyte development and function. *Curr. Opin. Immunol.* 14:260–265.

McHeyzer-Williams, L. J., D. J. Driver, and M. G. McHeyzer-Williams. 2001. Germinal center reaction. *Curr. Opin. Hematol.* 8:52–59.

Moser, B., and P. Loetscher. 2001. Lymphocyte traffic control by chemokines. *Nat. Immunol.* 2:123–128.

chapter 5

Complement

Francis Moore, Jr.

topics covered

- ▲ Proteins of the complement family

- ▲ Activation of complement by antibody-antigen complexes

- ▲ Spontaneous activation of complement on microbial surfaces

- ▲ Activation of complement by microbial carbohydrates

- ▲ Other mechanisms of complement activation

- ▲ Immunological functions of complement proteins and complement receptors

- ▲ Regulation of the complement system

- ▲ Synthesis of complement proteins

- ▲ Pathological disorders of the complement system

The term *complement* designates a family of proteins and proteolytic fragments derived from them that serve many roles in the both the innate and acquired immune response. These roles include both the direct killing of foreign cells and the regulation of many other effectors of the immune response. As a regulatory mechanism, the complement proteins have the ability to influence virtually every step in the immune response, from the initial recognition of a foreign antigen to its final elimination. Because of its central role in host defense, the complement system has survived long periods of evolution with surprisingly little change.

Complement was discovered in the late 19th century, first as a bacteriolytic activity and later as a hemolytic activity of serum. The name complement derives from the original observation, made by Jules Bordet, that the bacteriocidal activity of immune serum actually required two serum components: one antigen-specific and relatively heat-stable (which we now know to be antibody) and another antigen-nonspecific and heat-labile. Experiments at the time demonstrated that without this second component, antigen-specific antibody was incapable of killing bacteria. This second component was thus an essential complement to the biologic activity of antibodies. The bacteriocidal and cytolytic activity of complement occurs through the formation of large pores (called *membrane attack complexes* [MACs]) in the membrane of the target cell, resulting in the collapse of all chemical gradients across the membrane. For most eukaryotic target cells, this results in a massive influx of water and almost immediate lysis. Although bacteria are more resistant than eukaryotic cells to lysis because of their cell wall and (in gram-negative bacteria) lipopolysaccharide

(LPS) layer, the activation of complement on a bacterial surface can still serve to recruit numerous immune effector mechanisms that can destroy the bacterium.

The immunoregulatory role of complement was suggested just after the turn of the 20th century by the finding that complement partly mediates anaphylaxis (also called *hypersensitivity* or *allergy*). Nevertheless, until recently the lysis of bacteria was widely considered to represent the primary function of complement. The immunoregulatory functions of complement require, in addition to the complement proteins themselves, a family of complement receptor proteins, which are expressed by numerous cells in the host. Most of these receptors bind specifically to certain proteolytic fragments of complement proteins (called *split products*) generated during the process of complement activation. The effects of the binding of complement to its receptors, which vary with the cell type bearing the receptor, include chemotaxis of immune cells, regulation of vascular permeability, opsonization, and lymphocyte activation.

Complement Proteins

Complement proteins fall into three broad categories, although some complement proteins may actually fit into two of these categories. This first category (Table 5.1) encompasses the complement serum proteins, which react with foreign bodies in either an antibody-dependent or antibody-independent manner. Most of the proteins in this group are named with a C and a number, although the naming of a few (e.g., factor B) does not follow this convention. Unfortunately, the sequential numbers given to the complement proteins (e.g., C1, C2, and C3) do not reflect the actual sequence of their activity during complement activation because they were identified and named before the elucidation of the biochemical pathways of complement activation.

The proteins of the complement activation sequence participate in a series of well-defined steps that generate activated forms of each complement protein as the sequence proceeds (Fig. 5.1). Each protein in the complement activation sequence is said to be a *zymogen* or *proenzyme* (i.e., an enzyme that usually exists in an inactive precursor state). Activation of each zymogen usually involves proteolysis of the zymogen to remove a small inhibitory fragment. Generally these proteolytic fragments (split products) are named according to the original complement component from which they are derived, followed by a lowercase "a" or "b" (e.g., cleavage of the C3 component yields the C3a and C3b fragments). By convention, the larger of the two fragments, which is usually the fragment that acquires enzymatic activity upon cleavage, is termed the "b" fragment (e.g., C3b), and the small fragment, which usually diffuses away, is termed the "a" fragment. The exception is C2, with the names of the "a" and "b" fragments reversed. Thus, the complement activation sequence can be envisioned as a chain reaction in which each complement component is cleaved and activated by

Table 5.1 Primary proteins of the complement cascade

Protein	Active form	Function
C1	C1	Recognizes antibody-antigen complexes to initiate classical pathway
C2	C2a	Serine protease of C4b2a C3 convertase
	C2b	Unknown
C3	C3a	Anaphylatoxin; regulates antibody production
	C3b	Opsonin, component of C5 convertase
	C3(H_2O)	Component of C3(H_2O)Bb C3 convertase
	iC3b	Clearance of immune complexes
	C3d	Enhances immunogenicity of B-cell antigens
C4	C4a	Anaphylatoxin
	C4b	Component of C4b2a C3 convertase
C5	C5a	Anaphylatoxin
	C5b	Initiates MAC
C6	C6	Component of MAC
C7	C7	Component of MAC
C8	C8	Component of MAC
C9	C9	Pore-forming component of MAC
Factor B	Ba	Inhibits proliferation of B cells
	Bb	Serine protease of C3(H_2O)Bb C3 convertase
Factor D	D	Serine protease; cleaves B bound to C3b or C3(H_2O)
Properdin	Properdin	Stabilizes C3(H_2O)Bb C3 convertase

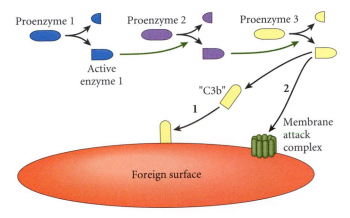

Figure 5.1 Diagram of the complement cascade, which consists of enzymatic steps involving a number of inactive proenzymes (or zymogens). Each step involves the activation of a given proenzyme, usually by proteolytic cleavage. Upon activation, the enzyme acts on a substrate, which is usually another proenzyme in the cascade. The sequence of activation events culminates with two end effects on the foreign surface: (**1**) deposition of complement proteins (e.g., component C3b) on a foreign surface, which has the ability to target the foreign surface for a number of immune effector functions, such as phagocytosis; and (**2**) formation on the foreign surface of a large transmembrane pore, called the MAC.

a preceding complement component and, when activated, attains the ability to cleave (and thus activate) a subsequent complement component (Fig. 5.1). This chain reaction leads first to the covalent attachment of a complement split product (known as C3b) to the foreign body (complement fixation) and eventually to the formation of the MAC (comprising complement proteins C5b, C6, C7, C8, and C9).

The second group of complement proteins are regulatory proteins present in serum or on the membranes of host cells. These complement proteins protect the host's own cells from accidental self-inflicted damage. These proteins also inhibit portions of the complement-activation sequence and thus are also considered to be involved in complement activation. The third group of complement proteins are cell surface receptors that bind to the products of complement activation and signal host cells to participate in inflammatory and immune reactions. The interaction of the various components of the complement system is a key factor in ensuring that there is minimal destruction to host tissues when the complement system is activated.

Activation of Complement

The complement system is designed to mobilize a large number of immune effector mechanisms when it detects infected or injured self tissues. Three pathways of com-

plement activation are now known: the alternative pathway, the classical pathway, and the lectin pathway (Fig. 5.2). The alternative and lectin pathways of activation are considered part of the innate immune system and are evolutionarily older. However, the first pathway to be defined was the *classical pathway,* which relies on the highly specific interaction of host antibody with target-cell antigens to direct complement activation efficiently to nonself cells and tissues. To carry out this function, the complement system must be able to differentiate uninjured, healthy self tissues from both nonself tissue and injured self tissue. Once activated, the complement system labels its activator for destruction by cellular immune

Figure 5.2 The three activation pathways of complement: the alternative pathway, classical pathway, and lectin pathway. Ag-Ab, antigen-antibody.

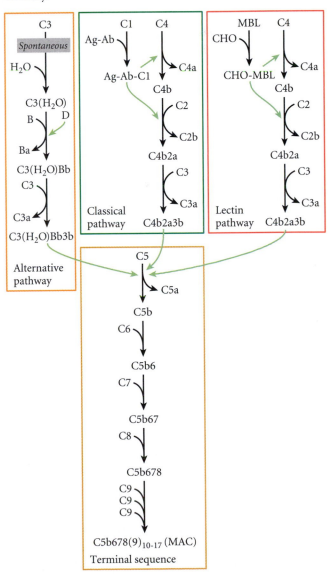

effectors. This labeling is accomplished by covalent attachment of the complement split product C3b to the organism or tissue responsible for complement activation. A second important function of C3b deposition is to serve as a crucial initiating event leading to subsequent formation of the MAC on the target-cell membrane. Given the importance of C3b, the immune system has multiple mechanisms for generating this split product.

The Classical Pathway of Complement Activation

Given the potent immunoregulatory roles of complement and the great destructive power of the MAC, selective activation of the complement system is essential to the host's well-being. The classical pathway of activation exploits the exquisite specificity of antibodies to ensure such discrimination and is made possible by complement component C1, which converts an initial signal (antibody-antigen binding) into a complement-activation event. C1 is a macromolecular complex consisting of three separate proteins—C1q, C1r, and C1s—in a molecular ratio of 1:2:2 (Fig. 5.3A). C1q comprises six globular domains attached by flexible strands to a central collagenous stalk, where C1q interacts with C1r and C1s (Fig. 5.3A). Each of the globular domains is capable of binding a single antibody Fc domain. Since a single C1q has six globular heads, each C1q is capable of binding multiple Fc regions simultaneously. However, a single C1q usually does not bind to more than four Fc regions simultaneously, probably because of steric constraints created by juxtaposition of so many immunoglobulin molecules. Not only is a single C1 *capable* of binding multiple Fc regions simultaneously, it actually *requires* such simultaneous interactions to activate the classical pathway. Because of this feature of complement activation by the classical pathway, the complement-activating abilities of the various antibody isotypes are radically different, due to differences in the amino acid residues in the constant part of the immunoglobulin heavy chain that interact with the C1q component.

Associated with the C1q protein are two molecules each of components C1r and C1s. C1r and C1s, like many other complement components, are proenzymes or zymogens. Both C1r and C1s have two domains: an interaction domain and a catalytic domain (Fig. 5.3B). The interaction domains help C1r and C1s to bind to each other, and the catalytic domains acquire serine protease activity when the complement cascade is initiated. Before C1 binds to an antigenic surface, C1r and C1s are in an inactive state in an elongated, end-to-end configuration (Fig. 5.3B). Binding of C1q to antibody alters the C1q collagenous stalk, permitting C1r and C1s to assume a figure

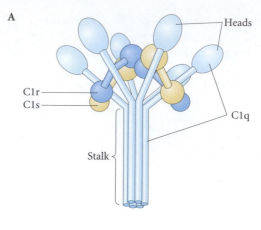

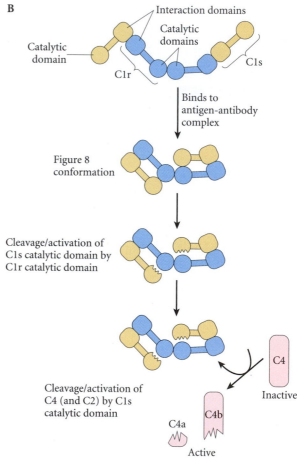

Figure 5.3 Complement component C1. (**A**) C1 contains three separate components: one component is C1q, which is composed of six identical protein units that interact with the other two components, C1r and C1s. There are two molecules each of C1r and C1s. C1q is able to bind to Fc regions of antibody when the antibody binds to antigen. C1r and C1s are serine proteases with the enzymatic activity necessary to initiate the complement cascade. (**B**) Before complement activation, C1r and C1s are associated in an extended conformation, intertwining between the C1q stalks. Binding to an antigen-antibody complex changes the conformation of C1r and C1s to a so-called figure 8 conformation. In this conformation, the catalytic domains of C1r are close enough to the catalytic domains of C1s to permit C1r to cleave (and activate) C1s. Cleaved, the activated C1s is then able to cleave and activate the next two components in the classical pathway: C4 and C2.

8 conformation (Fig. 5.3B), which brings the catalytic domains of C1r in close juxtaposition with those of C1s. These conformational changes induced by antigen binding by C1q also cause C1r to become an active serine protease. Activated C1r catalytic domains cleave the catalytic domains of C1s, thus activating C1s.

C1s, like C1r, becomes a serine protease when activated. However, the substrates of activated C1s are the complement components C4 and C2. Cleavage of C4 by C1s results in the generation of a small, readily diffusable split product, C4a, and of a larger fragment, C4b (Fig. 5.3B). The C4a fragment diffuses away from the activator and subsequently serves as a signal for leukocyte chemotaxis and mediates many of the events associated with inflammation. Since many of these events are a part of allergic or hypersensitivity reactions (also called *anaphylaxis*), C4a is commonly referred to as an *anaphylatoxin*. The larger fragment of C4, called C4b, becomes covalently bound to the activator surface at a site adjacent to the antibody that initiated activation (Fig. 5.4). Actually, two circulating isoforms of C4 originate from two distinct C4 genes. C4b of the A isoform preferentially fixes to proteins, while C4b of the B isoform usually interacts with carbohydrates. Since the reactive site of C4b also reacts rapidly with water, the half-life of reactive C4b is less than 1 second. This time constraint, which limits the binding of C4b to within 40 nanometers (nm) of the immunoglobulin-C1 complex, is an important biologic consideration because of the spatial constraints placed on C4b in the next phase of the complement cascade.

C4b, now covalently bound beside the immunoglobulin-C1 complex, next binds to complement component C2 (Fig. 5.4). Once bound to C4b, C2 is in position to be cleaved by the still-active C1s component of the immunoglobulin-C1 complex. As mentioned earlier, the terminology for C2 split products is inconsistent with that used for other C fragments; the small, readily diffusible fragment of C2 is called C2b and the larger fragment is called C2a. Because of disagreements among immunologists involved in the characterization of C2, some literature refers to the small fragment as C2a and the large fragment as C2b. Although this usage is more consistent with the rest of the complement nomenclature, modern immunologists follow the convention of calling the larger fragment C2a. The enzymatic activity acquired by C2a upon cleavage of C2 persists only as long as C2a remains associated with C4b. This complex of C4b and C2a serves a pivotal role in complement activation and is termed a *C3 convertase* (also called the *C4b2a complex*) for its ability to cleave component C3. The cleavage of C3 is a critical step in complement activation, since it represents a potential *amplification step* of the process, i.e.,

each C4b2a complex acts enzymatically and is capable of cleaving multiple C3 components in an iterative fashion. Cleavage of C3 generates multiple split products, one of which is the C3b fragment. C3b is able to label the surface of a nonself or injured self tissue for recognition by the immune system and is necessary for the next step of the complement activation cascade. Because C3b is such a potent immune regulator and because a single C4b2a complex is capable of generating many C3b fragments, the activity of the C4b2a complex is tightly regulated. The main point of regulation is the spontaneous and rapid decay of the C3 convertase by dissociation of C2a from C4b. Several circulating and membrane-bound regulatory factors assist in this event by facilitating the dissociation of the C3 convertase.

The ability of C4b and C3b to bind to the surface of an activator depends on the presence of a highly labile internal thioester linkage (Fig. 5.5), originally described by Margrett Hostetter and colleagues in 1982. Upon activation, this internal thioester linkage is destabilized and becomes capable of forming a covalent bond with any available hydroxy or amino group. Thus, if activation of C3 occurs in an aqueous solution, most C3b and C4b will bind the hydroxyl radical from water to form a product with no known biologic activities. However, if activation of C3 or C4 occurs in proximity to the activator's surface (such as the outer membrane of a gram-negative bacterium) or a protein conglomerate (such as an immune complex), the C3b or C4b will bind covalently to exposed amide or hydroxyl groups on proteins and carbohydrates on those surfaces. Attachment of C4b to the activator's surface is important for its recruitment of component C2 to the activator's surface. C3b that binds to the activator has multiple roles in the immune response.

One fate of the C3b fragment is direct binding to the C4b2a complex (the C3 convertase). When C3b interacts directly with C4b, the C3 convertase is transformed into a *C5 convertase* (also called the *C4b2a3b complex*) (Fig. 5.4), which is named for its ability to cleave the C5 component to yield the C5a and C5b fragments, the last of the proteolytic steps in the classical pathway. Similar to C4, the small fragment of C5 (C5a) is a diffusible fragment that can function as an anaphylatoxin. C5b, the larger fragment of C5, is labile (half-life of less than 2 minutes) and attaches to the activator membrane only transiently before becoming inactive. While attached to the activator surface, C5b becomes the site for the subsequent assembly of the MAC, which ultimately consists of C5b, C6, C7, C8, and C9. Binding of C6 to C5b stabilizes the latter, preventing its rapid inactivation. Next, C7 binds to the C5b6 complex, resulting in a conformational shift in C5b. This shift, termed a *hydrophobic transition,* results in the exposure of

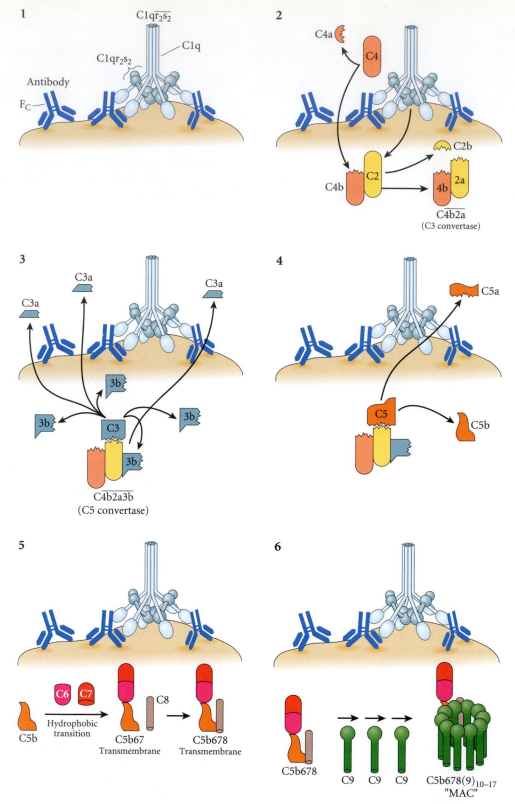

Figure 5.4 Diagram of the classical pathway of complement activation. (1) Binding of C1q to antibody alters the C1q collagenous stalk, permitting C1r and C1s to assume active forms. (2) Cleavage of C4 by C1s generates a small, readily diffusable split product, C4a, and a larger fragment, C4b. C4b next binds to complement component C2. C2 can be cleaved by the still-active C1s component of the immunoglobulin-C1 complex, yielding the soluble product C2b and the larger product C2a, which remains associated with C4b. This complex of C4b and C2a is a C3 convertase. (3) The cleavage of C3 is an amplification step. Interaction of C3b directly with C4b transforms the C3 convertase into a C5 convertase. In addition, many molecules of C3 are cleaved, with the 3b fragment binding to the antigenic surface, where it can serve as an opsonin. (4) The C4b2a3b C5 convertase generates two fragments from C5. The small fragment of C5 (C5a) is diffusible. C5b attaches to the activator membrane. (5) Binding of C6 to C5b stabilizes C5b, preventing its rapid inactivation. Next, C7 binds to the C5b6 complex, resulting in a hydrophobic transition in C5b. The C5b67 complex is then bound by a single molecule of C8. (6) Multiple copies of C9 bind to C5b678. C8 and C9 also undergo hydrophobic transitions as they bind to the growing MAC. The C9 components (~10 to 17) form a circular pore in the activator membrane.

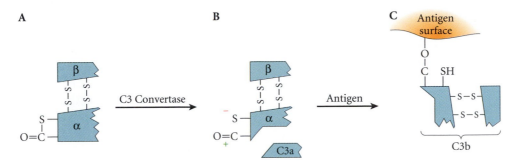

Figure 5.5 Activation of components C3 and C4 involves cleavage of an unstable thioester bond (O=C—S) in the α chain of the protein. This cleavage event can be spontaneous (possibly initiating the alternative pathway of activation) or triggered by proteolytic cleavage of C3 by the C3 convertases [C4b2a or C3(H₂O)Bb]. Cleavage of the thioester linkage generates a highly reactive carbon on the α chain, which can become covalently coupled to proteins or carbohydrates on an antigenic surface.

hydrophobic amino acid residues on the surface of C5b. This shift allows C5b to become embedded in the activator membrane (Fig. 5.4). Following this event, the C5b67 complex is bound by a single molecule of the C8 component, followed by multiple copies of the C9 component. The C8 and C9 components also undergo hydrophobic transitions as they bind to the growing MAC. The multiple (approximately 10 to 17) C9 components form a circular pore in the membrane of the activator.

The formation of the MAC is the basis for the hemolytic activity of complement. C5b-9 hemolysis may be the basis of some types of hemolytic autoimmune anemia and may be important in the lysis of certain bacteria, such as *Neisseria* spp. Although C5b-9 is ineffective in the lysis of nucleated cells, its insertion into a nucleated cell has membrane-perturbing effects of clinical relevance. For instance, the insertion of the MAC into an endothelial cell causes endothelial activation, possibly leading to irreversible cell injury, not by lysis but by the attraction of activated neutrophils.

Relative abilities of different antibody isotypes to activate complement

The classical pathway is initiated when complement component C1q binds simultaneously to the Fc regions of one multimeric immunoglobulin M (IgM) molecule or two or more IgG antibodies that are bound to the surface of an antigen. Because of the dependence of this process on the interaction of C1q and antibody, the efficiency of complement activation by a given antibody is affected by how well C1q binds to the Fc region of that antibody isotype. Antibodies of isotypes IgD, IgE, and IgA do not activate complement by the classical pathway because their Fc regions are not capable of binding to complement component C1q. Although some past

reports claimed that these isotypes are capable of low-level complement activation, it is now generally accepted that this weak activation was artifactual and that IgD, IgE, and IgA do not activate complement by the classical pathway.

There is a large difference in the complement-activating capabilities of IgM and IgG antibodies. IgM antibodies are approximately 1,000-fold more effective in activating complement activation than are IgG antibodies (i.e., for a given quantity of antigen, the amount of IgM required for complement activation is only 0.1% the amount of IgG required). This disparity is related to the structures of these isotypes. Each IgG molecule that binds antigen is capable of binding to a single globular head of C1q via its Fc region. For C1q to bind avidly to this antigen-bound IgG, two IgG molecules must be immobilized in close proximity on the antigenic surface. This is usually only possible when the antigen density is high and there is a large amount of antigen-specific antibody (Fig. 5.6B). In contrast, IgM contains five or six Fc regions per immunoglobulin molecule (depending on whether the IgM is a pentamer or a hexamer). Therefore, even if only a single IgM molecule binds to the antigenic surface (Fig. 5.6C), the IgM is capable of triggering the classical pathway of complement activation because the multimeric structure of IgM ensures that multiple adjacent Fc regions on the antigen surface are available for binding to C1q.

The multimeric nature of IgM antibodies, although allowing highly efficient complement activation upon binding to antigen, presented a troubling question to early immunologists. Since IgM is always secreted by B cells as a polymer (pentamer or hexamer), why does IgM not activate complement all of the time (i.e., why does IgM require antigen to activate complement)? Solving

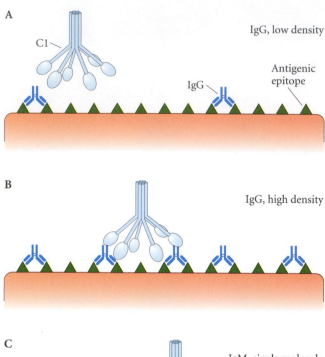

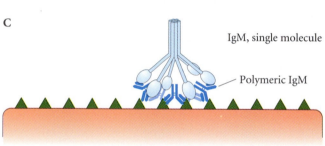

Figure 5.6 IgG antibodies are weaker activators of complement than are IgM antibodies. IgG binds to complement component C1q via a single C1q-binding site on its Fc region, which binds C1q with low affinity. (**A**) When the amount of IgG bound to an antigenic surface is low, C1q is unable to bind to the surface with sufficient avidity. (**B**) When the amount of surface-bound IgG is high, simultaneous binding by C1q to two or more IgG molecules is possible, increasing the avidity of C1q binding and allowing activation of C1. (**C**) IgM antibodies can activate the complement cascade even if a single IgM molecule is bound to an antigen, since each IgM molecule contains five or six C1q-binding sites, a number sufficient for avid C1q binding.

this puzzle required a detailed structure-function analysis of IgM antibodies. Mapping of the C1q-binding site on the Fc region of IgM revealed that this binding site is not exposed on the IgM surface when IgM is in its unbound "planar" configuration (Fig. 5.7A). However, when IgM binds to antigen, multiple V-region binding sites start to attach to the exposed epitopes (Fig. 5.7B to E). As more epitopes are bound, IgM undergoes a conformational shift (Fig. 5.7F and G) to assume a "staple" conformation, which exposes the C1q-binding sites in the Cμ3 domain of the IgM Fc region. These are then available for C1q binding (Fig. 5.7H).

Although it is true that IgG antibodies are approximately 1,000-fold less effective than IgM in activating complement, the various subclasses of IgG differ in their complement-activating potential. These subtle differences in complement activation are due in large part to the slight difference between the amino acid sequences of the various IgG subclasses in specific regions of the heavy chains that contain the C1q-binding site. These differences determine the ability of IgG molecules to associate with C1q. The hierarchy of complement activation among the human IgG subclasses is IgG3>IgG1>>IgG2. IgG4 cannot activate complement at all. Thus, the antibody isotype produced against an antigen will ultimately determine the degree of complement activation possible. For example, an immune response in which most of the antibody produced is IgG3 will have a high potential for activating complement, whereas a response producing IgG4 will result in no complement activation by the classical pathway.

The Alternative Pathway of Complement Activation

The classical pathway of complement activation has the benefit of being capable of directing the activation of complement components toward a foreign antigen with a high level of specificity. Although antibodies impart such a fine specificity to the classical pathway, they also confer a drawback, i.e., their inability to activate complement unless the target antigen has previously been encountered by the host and the host has produced antibodies to this antigen. This drawback prevents complement activation in response to a foreign antigen under certain circumstances (e.g., if the antigen has low immunogenicity). Also, it would be useful to utilize the complement system without relying on preformed antibody. Indeed, before the evolution of a means to integrate the acquired immune system and complement activation via the classical pathway, a mechanism of complement activation that does not require previous formation of antibody-antigen complexes—the *alternative pathway*—was well established.

The ability of the complement cascade to be activated in the absence of antibody is attributable to the inherent instability, residing in the thioester linkage, of complement component C3. This linkage is normally cleaved during activation by the C4b2a complex but can also break spontaneously, thus allowing a small amount of the C3 in the soluble or fluid phase of serum or mucosal secretions to be converted into the active molecule C3(H_2O) via a condensation reaction (Fig. 5.5 and Fig. 5.8, step 1). Therefore, fluid-phase C3 exhibits slow,

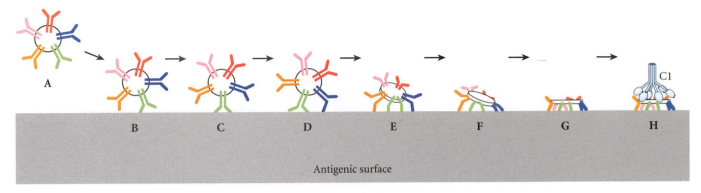

Antigenic surface

Figure 5.7 IgM-mediated complement activation can be explained by the conformation that the IgM polymer assumes upon antigen binding. (A) Free IgM before binding to antigen. (**B to D**) IgM antibody makes initial contact with one to three binding sites on the antigen. (**E to F**) Further stability of the antigen-IgM antibody complex due to increased attachment to antigen via multiple antigen-binding sites on IgM. (**G**) Formation of a staple binding conformation of IgM, which leads to exposure of the C1q binding sites. (**H**) High-affinity binding of C1 to the staple conformation of IgM.

but continuous, spontaneous activation. If such activation of C3 occurs near an appropriate surface (such as a biologic membrane), the resulting active $C3(H_2O)$ fragment can attach covalently to the surface.

Membrane-bound $C3(H_2O)$ fragments are able to bind to a complement component called *factor B* in a magnesium-dependent manner. When complexed to membrane-bound $C3(H_2O)$, factor B becomes a proteolytic substrate for a complement component called *factor D* (Fig. 5.8, step 3). Cleavage of factor B yields two split products, Ba and Bb. Fragment Ba, like split products C3a, C4a, and C5a, is a small, biologically active, and readily diffusable peptide. The larger split product of factor B (Bb) associates with the membrane-bound $C3(H_2O)$ to form the complex $C3(H_2O)$Bb, which has C3 convertase activity (Fig. 5.8, step 4). Like the C4b2a complex, $C3(H_2O)$Bb is able to cleave additional molecules of C3 to yield more C3a and C3b. Although most of these C3b molecules become inactivated by reacting with water, a few bind to nearby surfaces (Fig. 5.8, step 7). Thus, $C3(H_2O)$Bb performs a function analogous to that of complex C4b2a in the classical pathway by serving as an amplification step in the complement cascade. Since membrane-fixed C3b also is produced during the classical pathway of complement activation, activation of the alternative pathway can serve to amplify the classical pathway.

Although the $C3(H_2O)$Bb complex can function as an amplifier of the alternative pathway of complement activation, whether amplification occurs depends on several factors, most notably the half-life of the $C3(H_2O)$Bb enzyme. $C3(H_2O)$Bb, like the C4b2a complex, has a rapid rate of spontaneous dissociation. The stability of the

$C3(H_2O)$Bb complex, and hence its activity as a cascade amplifier, is regulated simultaneously by two complement factors, *properdin* and *factor H*. Properdin binds to $C3(H_2O)$Bb and stabilizes the complex (Fig. 5.8, step 5b), preventing the dissociation of Bb. Conversely, the plasma protein factor H, which also binds to C3b, can accelerate the release of Bb (Fig. 5.8, step 5a). Thus, activation of the amplified alternative pathway occurs only when factor H is prevented from triggering the dissociation of $C3(H_2O)$Bb.

The activation of the alternative pathway, although a spontaneous and random process, has been shown to be much more likely on microbial than on mammalian membranes and thus can be said to have a mild specificity for microbial membranes. This slight preference is related to the differences in carbohydrate content of their membranes. In particular, mammalian membranes are relatively rich in the carbohydrate heparin and in the monosaccharide sialic acid, whereas microbial membranes usually lack these structures. These two carbohydrate structures in mammalian membranes promote the binding of factor H to $C3(H_2O)$Bb and thereby prevent alternative pathway activation. Factor H also serves as the cofactor for the proteolytic inactivation of $C3(H_2O)$ by factor I (C3b-C4b inactivator). Mammalian cell surfaces also possess protective proteins that are structurally homologous to factor H and serve the same purpose.

A small portion of the C3 cleaved by the $C3(H_2O)$Bb complex associates with $C3(H_2O)$Bb to form the complex $C3(H_2O)$Bb3b (Fig. 5.8, step 8), which has C5 convertase activity. Thus, the $C3(H_2O)$Bb3b complex is analogous to the C4b2a3b complex of the classical pathway. The manner in which component C5 is activated and subsequent-

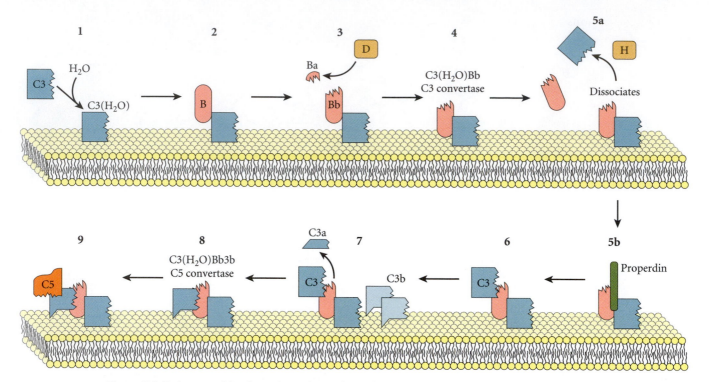

Figure 5.8 Early steps of the alternative pathway of complement activation leading to the activation of component C5. (**1**) C3 can be activated spontaneously through breakage of the thioester linkage in the α chain of C3 and reaction with water to yield C3(H_2O). C3 can also be activated to C3b by proteolytic cleavage (not shown) by preexisting C3 convertases (such as C4b2a). Activated C3 binds to the antigenic surface. (**2**) Surface-bound C3(H_2O) binds factor B. (**3**) C3(H_2O)-bound factor B is a substrate for factor D, which cleaves factor B, generating soluble fragment Ba and C3(H_2O)-bound fragment Bb. (**4**) The C3(H_2O) Bb complex functions as a C3 convertase. (**5**) The fate of the C3 convertase is decided by the relative activities of two other complement components: factor H and properdin. (**5a**) Factor H can bind to and dissociate the C3 convertase. (**5b**) Alternatively, properdin can bind to and stabilize the C3 convertase, permitting subsequent activation steps. (**6**) The C3 convertase binds to an additional molecule of C3. (**7**) The Bb component of the C3 convertase is able to bind and cleave multiple molecules of C3, most of which bind directly to the antigenic surface. (**8**) A small portion of the C3 cleaved by C3(H_2O)Bb remains associated with C3(H_2O)Bb to form the C5 convertase C3(H_2O)Bb3b. (**9**) The C5 convertase binds and cleaves component C5. Not shown: The cleaved, activated C5 then associates with the antigenic surface, associates with components C6 to C8, inserting into the target membrane, and ultimately forms poly-C9 MACs (i.e., containing multiple copies of the C9 component). These terminal steps of the alternative pathway are exactly the same as in the classical pathway.

ly assembled with components C6 through C9 to form the MAC is essentially identical to the process that occurs during complement activation by the classical pathway.

Sites of trauma and microbial invasion are typically observed to be the points of complement activation by the classical or alternative pathways. Known activators of complement at sites of injury and infection include microbes (with or without antibody affixed), denatured nucleic acids, denatured proteins, injured tissue, and antigen-antibody complexes. The distinction between the alternative pathway and the classical pathway is not complete, as the alternative pathway can be activated by antibody in some circumstances. Also, once C3b has been deposited by the classical pathway, it may well be bound to factor B and form an alternative pathway C3 conver-

tase, C3bBb [which functions like C3(H_2O)Bb], resulting in the further activation of the alternative pathway.

The Lectin Pathway

A third pathway of complement activation, the *lectin pathway,* has recently been defined but, like the alternative pathway of complement activation, likely arose during evolution prior to the classical pathway. The lectin pathway is initiated by binding of the protein called *mannan-binding lectin* (MBL), also called *mannose-binding protein,* to mannose or *N*-acetylglucosamine residues on foreign surfaces such as microbes (mammalian carbohydrates usually lack mannose-rich structures). MBL is structurally related to C1q and is part of the *collectin* protein family. The collectins are structurally conserved proteins that contain

NH$_2$-terminal regions that polymerize individual sub-units, a collagen-like domain, a "neck region," and a region for binding to the sugars on microbial surfaces (Fig. 5.9A). A second set of proteins termed *ficolins,* consisting of L-ficolin, M-ficolin, and H-ficolin, has also been recently found to have lectin activity and to activate the third pathway of complement. The ficolins use a fibrinogen-like domain in place of the C-type lectin domain. Three serine proteases called *MBL-associated serine proteases (MASPs)* are bound by MBL or ficolins. MASP-1 and MASP-3 are derived from the same gene due to alternative splicing, and they contain a polypeptide chain termed the A chain which is the same in MASP-1 and MASP-3. However, each has a distinct second polypeptide chain termed the B chain. The gene for MASP-2 can also be alternatively spliced into a protein termed MAp19, but MAp19 does not have enzymatic activity. The MASPs are closely related to the C1r and C1s subcomponents of C1, and thus the MBL–MASP-1/3–MASP-2 complex is closely related structurally and functionally to intact C1 (Fig. 5.9B).

Binding of the MBL–MASP-1–MASP-2 complex to an activating surface results in acquisition by the MASPs of proteolytic activity and the cleavage of complement components C4 and C2. This, in turn, results in the formation of the C4b2a C3 convertase, followed by formation of the C4b2a3b C5 convertase. The manner of activation of complement component C5 and its subsequent assembly with components C6 to C9 are analogous to the activation of the classical and alternative pathways.

Other Mechanisms of Complement Activation

C-reactive protein

C-reactive protein (CRP) is a serum protein produced by hepatocytes. In 1974, M. H. Kaplan and J. E. Volanakis showed that CRP is capable of activating the complement cascade in response to a bacterial surface component called the *C-polysaccharide* or *C-substance.* The mechanism by which CRP activates complement is thought to resemble the classical pathway, since CRP-mediated activation requires complement component C1q. The interaction of CRP with C1q is dependent on the biochemical nature of the target membrane, since modification of the membrane composition influences the degree of complement activation.

CRP also plays a second role as a regulator of the alternative pathway of complement activation. The mechanism of this interaction is through enhancement of the activity of factor H, a negative regulator of complement activation.

The kallikrein/kallidin system

The kallikrein system is a group of serum proteins involved in the generation of kallidin and bradykinin, two vasoac-

Figure 5.9 The lectin pathway of complement activation is initiated by a multisubunit complex resembling C1. (**A**) MBL (also called mannose-binding protein) is a member of the collectin family of proteins, which are composed of several identical subunits, each of which has a collagen-like stalk and a globular head which functions as a lectin (i.e., binds carbohydrates). The globular head domain binds to mannose-rich carbohydrates common on microbial surfaces. Ficolins have a collagen-like stalk but a fibrinogen-like carbohydrate recognition unit. (**B**) MBL or ficolin forms a complex with two serine proteases called MASP-1/3 and MASP-2, which become activated when MBL binds to carbohydrate. The MBL-MASP complex is therefore structurally and functionally homologous to the C1 complex. Although the MBL-MASP complex is depicted as having six MBL or ficolin subunits to emphasize the homology of this complex with C1, the actual number of MBL or ficolin subunits in the complex is variable.

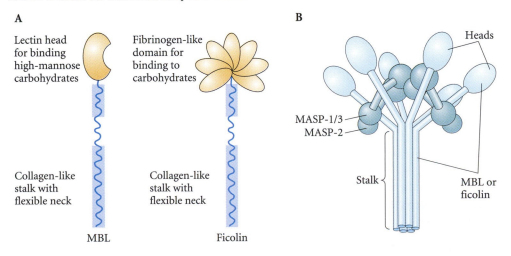

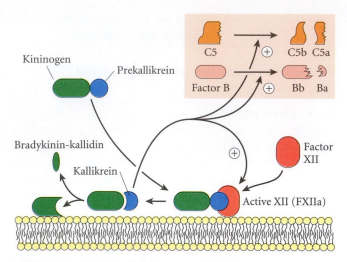

Figure 5.10 The kallikrein system is a group of serum proteins important in the inflammatory response. The inactive precursor form of kallikrein (prekallikrein) forms a complex with its substrate, kininogen. This complex then binds to activated factor XII, which cleaves prekallikrein to its active form, kallikrein. Activated kallikrein can then cleave kininogen to form the vasoactive peptides bradykinin and kallidin. Kallikrein is also capable of cleaving and activating C5 and factor B, possibly activating or amplifying the complement cascade during inflammation.

tive peptides important in the regulation of the inflammatory response. The inactive precursor form of kallikrein (prekallikrein) forms a complex with its substrate kininogen (Fig. 5.10). This complex then binds to activated blood-clotting factor XII, which cleaves prekallikrein to its active form, kallikrein. Activated kallikrein can then cleave kininogen to yield bradykinin or kallidin.

Work conducted in the 1980s by several research groups demonstrated that kallikrein also functions as an activator of complement, which occurs via direct activation of factor B by kallikrein (Fig. 5.10, top). In addition, R. C. Wiggins, in 1981, showed that incubation of purified kallikrein with component C5 resulted in production of the anaphylatoxin C5a, suggesting that kallikrein can activate C5. Thus, it appears that the complement system is activated as a result of the general inflammatory process. The role of complement activation in this context may be to generate chemotactic signals (such as C5a) to summon immune cells to the inflamed tissue as a defense against future infections.

Microbial products and surfaces

Several mechanisms of complement activation seem to be geared toward the nonspecific activation of complement near the surface of microbial agents that allows binding of C3b to the microbe. The spontaneous activation of complement via the alternative pathway along

with the lectin pathway is the major mechanism to achieve this. It is also apparent, however, that the complement system has the ability to be activated in response to other molecular signals that herald a microbial infection. These signals have different levels of specificity; in some cases the activating signal is present on virtually all microbial agents of a given class (e.g., the signal may be present on all gram-negative bacteria) and in others the signal appears to be specific to a given species or strain of microbe.

The ability of bacterial surfaces to activate complement has been well characterized since the 1970s (Table 5.2). Although the surfaces of gram-positive and gram-negative bacteria are different, both contain structures capable of activating the complement cascade. On gram-positive bacteria, complement activation can be triggered by both peptidoglycan and teichoic acids and can occur by both the classical and alternative pathways. On gram-negative bacteria, in which the peptidoglycan layer is hidden from the immune system by the outer membrane of the bacteria, the LPS present on the outer membrane can activate the complement system. The lipid A portion of the LPS of some bacterial strains can activate the classical pathway, whereas the polysaccharide portion of the LPS can activate either the alternative or the lectin pathways (depending on the monosaccharide composition of the LPS polysaccharide). Bacteria are not the only microorganisms capable of activating the complement system. Zymosan, the principal component of fungal cell walls, is capable of activating the alternative pathway.

Complement activation has also been observed in viral infection, although the precise molecular species that triggers activation is not always known. In 1989, T. G. Kimman and coworkers showed that epithelial cells

Table 5.2 Microbial surface structures capable of activating the complement system

Surface component	Complement pathway activated
Gram-negative bacteria	
LPS lipid A	Classical
LPS oligosaccharide	Alternative
LPS with mannose	Alternative or lectin
Homopolysaccharide	Lectin
Gram-positive bacteria	
Teichoic acid	Alternative
Peptidoglycan	Classical and alternative
Fungi	
Zymosan	Alternative
Viruses	
HIV gp120	Classical

infected with bovine respiratory syncytia virus were capable of activating complement by the classical pathway, whereas similar cells not infected with virus were incapable of activating complement. This activation, although it proceeded via the classical pathway, did not require the presence of virus-specific antibody. The following year, a similar phenomenon was reported with cells coinfected with human immunodeficiency virus (HIV) and human T-lymphotropic virus type 1. Once again, virus-specific antibody was not necessary for complement activation, since both nonimmune serum and agammaglobulinemic serum supported complement activation. Despite these findings, no complement activation was observed in this experimental system when the serum was from C4-deficient animals, strongly implying activation via the classical pathway. A possible clue to this mechanism of complement activation was the finding that the binding of shed HIV gp120 protein to uninfected host cells could trigger complement activation on the surface of the host cell. Perhaps the gp120 protein, once bound to the host cell surface, is capable of binding to component C1 or C4 and thus initiating the classical pathway.

Functions of Complement

Complement activation that ultimately leads to the formation of a MAC on the activator surface is a central function of the complement system. There are, however, many other consequences of complement activation of relevance to the immune response. Most of these effects depend on the interaction of various complement split products with receptor proteins expressed on the surface of many immune cell types.

Complement Receptors

Through their interaction with complement split products, complement receptor proteins (Table 5.3) utilize the proteolytic by-products of complement activation as a means of regulating several key aspects of the immune response (Fig. 5.11). The best characterized of these receptors are the C5a receptor (C5aR, also called CD88), which binds the soluble C5a fragment generated during the cleavage of C5 by C5 convertase, and complement receptors (CR) 1, CR2, and CR3, which bind to C3b fragments (and to smaller subfragments of C3b) that covalently bind to complement-activating surfaces. Each of these receptors has a distinct range of functions.

Inflammation is mediated in large part by C5aR, which is present on all cells of the myeloid lineage and possibly also on vascular endothelium (Fig. 5.12). C5aR binds C5a with high affinity ($K_d \sim 10^{-9}$ M) and is responsible for the biologic effects of the C5a anaphylatoxin, including directed migration (or *chemotaxis*) of myeloid cells (especially neutrophils) to the site of C5a production. At the same time, adhesiveness of myeloid cells to endothelium is increased. C5a ligation by C5aR causes degranulation of these myeloid cells and the activation of the reduced nicotinomide adenine dinucleotide phosphate (NADPH) oxidase of neutrophils, resulting in the respiratory burst that generates oxidative, microbicidal toxins such as superoxide, hypochlorite, and nitric oxide.

The vascular effects of C5a are diverse and may be influenced by coproduction of other inflammatory mediators. C5a increases vascular permeability directly through effects on endothelial and smooth-muscle cells and indirectly through activation of mast cells, which release histamine, prostaglandins, and leukotrienes and can increase vascular permeability. In the presence of tumor necrosis factor (a cytokine found at sites of inflammation and macrophage activation), C5a causes hemorrhagic necrosis of tissues, a phenomenon possibly reflecting an effect on the procoagulant capability of C5a-activated endothelial cells. Monolayers of endothelial cells incubated with C5a release heparin sulfate, a natural inhibitor of intravascular coagulation. The result of these activities is the local accumulation of leukocytes, plasma

Table 5.3 Complement receptors

Receptor	Binds to	Activity	Cells expressing receptor
CR1 (CD35)	C3b, C4b	Binds antigen-bound C3b for opsonization, assists degradation of C3b	Erythrocytes, neutrophils, monocytes, macrophages, eosinophils, B cells, T cells
CR2 (CD21)	iC3b, C3d, C3dg	Component of B-cell coreceptor	B cells, T cells
CR3 (CD11b/CD18)	iC3b	Binds antigen-bound iC3b for opsonization, regulates extravasation	Monocytes, macrophages, neutrophils, natural killer cells, T cells
CR4 (CD11c/CD18)	iC3b	Binds antigen-bound iC3b for opsonization, regulates extravasation	Monocytes, macrophages, neutrophils, natural killer cells, T cells
C3aR, C4aR	C3a, C4a	Induces degranulation	Mast cells, basophils
C5aR	C5a	Induces degranulation	Mast cells, basophils, monocytes, macrophages, platelets, endothelium, neutrophils

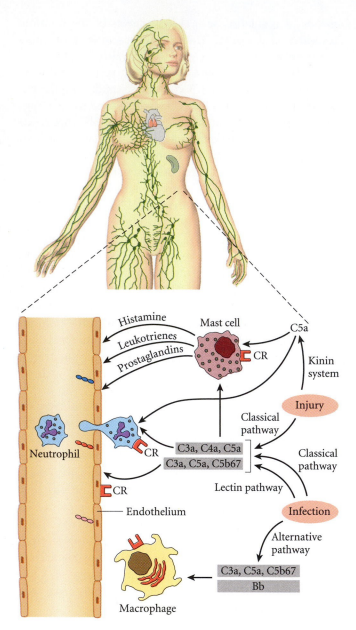

Figure 5.11 The various activities of complement proteins are mediated by cell surface complement receptors present on the membranes of immune cells (such as neutrophils, mast cells, and macrophages) and vascular endothelial cells. Injury or infection can trigger activation of the complement cascade, producing numerous complement split products. Some of these split products (e.g., C5a) can act directly on the vascular endothelium to enhance extravasation of leukocytes, and others can act on leukocytes (e.g., neutrophils). Extravasation is also enhanced by changes in vascular permeability induced by histamine, leukotrienes, and prostaglandins released by mast cells following stimulation by C3a and C5a.

proteins, and secondary mediators of inflammation at sites of complement activation.

Engagement of C5a by C5aR results in movement of the C5a-C5aR complex into the interior of the cell, with a consequent decrease in the number of cell surface C5aR

molecules. Cells exposed to relatively high concentrations of C5a are transiently deficient in cell surface C5aR and are therefore unresponsive to further stimulation with C5a. For this reason, neutrophils previously exposed to C5a (e.g., in a patient with ongoing complement activation) do not respond to C5a in a chemotaxis assay, a phenomenon termed *desensitization*.

The C5aR protein weaves through the plasma membrane seven times and is coupled to a guanine nucleotide-binding protein complex. In these respects, this protein resembles other members of a family that includes the receptors for formylated peptides, interleukin 8, thrombin, platelet-activating factor, MIP-1a, and RANTES, all of which promote inflammation. The binding of C5a to C5aR results in intracellular signaling with activation of several intracellular enzymes, including phospholipase C. In another situation, immune complex-mediated inflammation in the lung, lack of C5aR leads to markedly decreased inflammation and tissue damage, whereas immune complex-mediated inflammatory damage in the skin and peritoneum of C5aR-deficient mice is lessened but not totally absent. Thus, depending on the inflammatory stimulus and tissue site, the C5a-C5aR interaction can play a dominant role in inflammation or a synergistic one that involves other components of inflammation.

Figure 5.12 Signaling through the C5a receptor (C5aR). The receptor is linked to a G protein and following binding of C5a activates signaling transduction pathways leading to production of such factors as ERK and NF-AT.

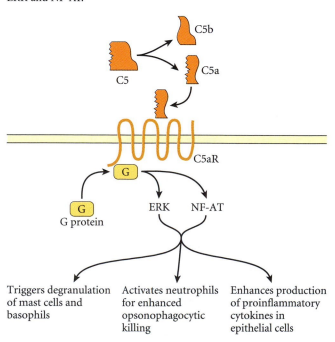

Although the type 1 complement receptor (CR1 or CD35) is thought to function primarily in opsonization and intracellular signaling, it also plays an important role in complement regulation (Fig. 5.13). CR1 is a cell surface receptor for C3b and C4b and is present on the plasma membranes of erythrocytes, neutrophils, monocytes, macrophages, eosinophils, B cells, some T cells, and epithelial cells in the kidney. As a receptor, CR1 promotes cellular uptake of complement-containing immune complexes by CR1-expressing phagocytes such as macrophages and neutrophils. As a regulator of complement activation, CR1 reduces complement activation on host membranes by assisting in the proteolytic cleavage (by factor I) of target-bound C3b to smaller C3 fragments such as iC3b, C3dg, and C3d. These smaller fragments can serve as ligands for two other complement

receptors, CR2 (CD21) and CR3 (CD11b/CD18). This function of CR1 is the basis for the development of a recombinant soluble form of CR1 for therapeutic prevention of complement activation. The concentration of a naturally occurring soluble form of CR1 detected in plasma is too low to be expected to regulate plasma complement activation. Likewise, the number of cell membrane CR1 molecules is insufficient to regulate plasma complement activation. The restriction of CR1 to a relatively few cell types and the low concentration of its soluble form in plasma indicate that its natural regulatory role may be limited to the processing of C3b- and C4b-containing immune complexes.

The structure of CR1 is shared by other complement-regulatory proteins. CR1 contains similar domains termed *short consensus repeats* or *complement-control protein repeats*. These repeats also are found in C1r, C1s, factor H, CR2, decay-accelerating factor (DAF), membrane cofactor protein (MCP), and C4-binding protein. Each repeat is a sequence of 60 to 70 amino acids that forms coils like a roll of barbed wire. CR1 contains 30 tandemly aligned short consensus repeats grouped into four long homologous repeats (LHR-A, -B, -C, and -D) and has a molecular mass of 200,000 daltons. This extremely long, filamentous molecule extends from the plasma membrane by approximately 90 nm. In contrast, more common phagocyte and lymphocyte surface proteins, such as membrane antibody and major histocompatibility complex molecules, extend only about 12 nm. LHR-A binds to C4b, and LHR-B and LHR-C bind strongly to C3b and weakly to C4b. A C1q-binding site has been localized to LHR-D and two additional short consensus repeat units. LHR-D shares a high homology with the repeats on C1r and C1s that anchor these enzymes to C1q. This repeat sequence may therefore represent a common dimerization motif among complement proteins. The presence of multiple binding sites for complement proteins gives CR1 molecules the advantage of increased binding to antigens coated with multiple C1q, C4b, and/or C3b molecules.

The importance of CR1 in immune responses is seen in transgenic CR1-knockout mice. These animals have deficient antibody responses to T-cell-dependent antigens. This defect emphasizes the need for CR1 in priming the T-cell immune response and most likely represents the role of CR1 in opsonizing antigens for phagocytosis and subsequent presentation to T cells. Most of the CR1 in a given cell is stored in cytoplasmic granules, with only 10% present on the membrane at any one time. When the cell is activated by C5a or other activators (e.g., endotoxin, cytokines, or bacterial cell wall products), the remain-

Figure 5.13 Structure of CR1 and CR3. CR1 contains 30 tandemly aligned short consensus repeats grouped into four LHRs (A, B, C, and D) and extends from the plasma membrane by about 90 nm. LHR A binds to C4b, and LHR B and C bind strongly to C3b and weakly to C4b. LHR D and two membrane-proximal short consensus repeats (gray ovals) can bind C1q. The presence of multiple binding sites for complement proteins gives CR1 molecules the advantage of increased binding to antigens coated with multiple C1q, C4b, and/or C3b molecules. Structure at upper left redrawn from M. Krych-Goldberg and J. P. Atkinson, *Immunol. Rev.* **180:**112–122, 2001, with permission.

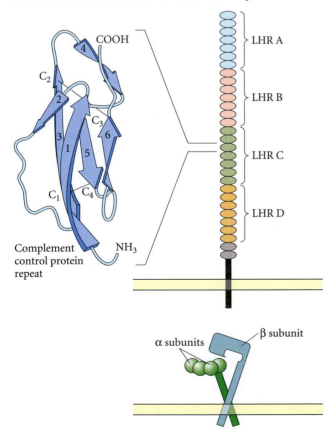

ing 90% of the protein is rapidly translocated to the cell surface, presumably increasing the level of CR1 as well as its biologic functions. In this way, complement activation both attracts leukocytes to the site of complement activation and increases the functional activity of those cells.

CR2 (CD21) is similar to CR1 in structure but not in specificity. Its binding of C3d (as opposed to C3b) is responsible for its distinct biologic activity. Like CR1, CR2 has a single transmembrane domain and a short cytoplasmic tail; however, CR2 has only half as many short consensus repeats as CR1 (15 versus 30). The expression of CR2 is restricted to B lymphocytes, in which CR2 plays a key role in the antigen-induced activation and antibody responses. CR2 is complexed on the cell membrane with molecules of either CR1 or CD19.

CR3 (CD11b/CD18) is the final member of the major C3 receptor family (Fig. 5.13). Its structure is completely unlike that of CR1 or CR2. A member of the β_2-integrin family of membrane proteins, CR3 has two separate chains. One is specific to CR3 (CD11b) and the other is common to all members of this integrin family (CD18). CR3 is found on the plasma membrane of all cells of myeloid lineage and, like CR1, the percentage of the CR3 molecules found on the membrane at any one time is small. Exposure of the cell to activators, such as C5a, produces a rapid increase in cell surface CR3. This response parallels that documented for CR1 in terms of magnitude, rapidity, and specificity to activators. The use of monoclonal antibodies directed to different portions of CR3 has elucidated two main functions for this receptor. The first is to bind intracellular adhesion molecules, especially on endothelial cells. Thus, an increase in number of cell surface CR3 molecules translates into increased cellular adhesiveness to vascular endothelium, with initiation of the extravasation of neutrophils and myeloid cells from the circulation into the inflamed interstitium. The second function is to promote phagocytosis by ligation to iC3b, which is an intermediate breakdown product of target-bound C3b that has been acted on by CR1 and factor I. The capacity of myeloid cells to phagocytose antigen-antibody complexes is significantly enhanced by the presence of CR3 on the myeloid cell and of iC3b on the target. This effect is so important that individuals born deficient in CR3 are as susceptible to infection as those born deficient in C3. Indeed, for the majority of pathogens that cause serious infections in humans, CR1- and CR3-mediated phagocytosis of microbes coated with C3b and iC3b appears to be the key immune effector involved in host resistance to infection. Anything that compromises this mechanism vastly increases the susceptibility of the affected host to infection.

Functions Associated with Surface-Bound Split Products

Virus neutralization

Viruses are infectious particles with a particularly simple structure consisting of nucleic acid surrounded by a modest number of proteins. Although virus particles are small, viruses that have been coated with antibodies directed to their repetitive surface proteins can form large immune complexes that are very potent activators of complement. Most viruses activate complement by the classical pathway through the large number of antibody molecules bound to their repetitive surface structures. However, influenza virus and Epstein-Barr virus can activate the alternative pathway independently of antibody (although the presence of antiviral antibody can augment this response). In addition to free virions, virus-infected host cells can be subject to complement-mediated lysis, frequently because proteins of the virus are expressed on the surface of the host cells they have infected. These cells can then activate the classical pathway.

Activation of complement by a virus particle does not necessarily lead to disruption of the virus. Only viruses that are surrounded by a lipid bilayer membrane (i.e., an *envelope*) are susceptible to disruption by the C5b-9 MAC. However, complement activation can result in virus neutralization, even if the virus is nonenveloped. One mechanism is by coating the particle with antibody and C3 so thoroughly that the thick coating of antibody and complement sterically blocks the viral proteins responsible for attachment to or entry into a target cell. A second important mechanism is the opsonization of the virus for phagocytic killing.

Opsonization

Opsonization is a broad term referring to the enhancement of phagocytosis resulting from the coating of foreign bodies with host proteins. Serum opsonins include antibody, complement, fibronectin, and CRP. Host phagocytes, such as neutrophils and macrophages, have receptor proteins on their cell surfaces that specifically recognize portions of the antibody molecule (Fc receptors), fragments of complement (C3 receptors), and fibronectin. Engagement of these receptors by their ligand provides a signal to the cell that opsonized material is attached and that ingestion should proceed. Antibody stays firmly fixed to foreign and injured targets by virtue of the very high affinity of antibody-combining sites for the engaged antigen. The process by which complement becomes attached to this antigen-antibody complex is termed *complement fixation*. The ability to bind covalently to the target is an important feature of complement fixation. Given the central role that C3 plays in this basic immune mechanism, it is not surprising that it has been highly conserved over evolutionary history. Indeed, C3 or C3 homologs can be found in such diverse groups as mammals, sharks, amphibians, and worms. Once C3 split products are fixed to the antigen-antibody complex, a broad array of cell surface receptor proteins can interact with the C3 fragments.

C3d: the "molecular adjuvant"

In 1996 D. Fearon and colleagues showed that an antigen linked to three molecules of the complement split product C3d was 1,000 to 10,000 times more immunogenic than the same antigen without the C3d fragments. The mechanism of this enhanced antibody response to C3d-coupled antigen is due to the expression of CR2 on the surface of B cells. In the membrane of the B cell, CR2 associates with CR1 and with the proteins CD19 and CD81. As C3b-containing immune complexes bind to these receptors, CR1 recruits the complement regulator factor I to cleave C3b to form C3d. The C3d-containing immune complex then binds to CR2, which delivers a costimulatory signal through CD19 (Fig. 5.14). CD19, a membrane protein of B cells, has an extracellular region composed of immunoglobulin-like domains and a long intercellular tail. The tail of CD19 can interact with the src-related kinases Fyn and Lyn. Thus, a complement-coated antigen might bind simultaneously to both the B-cell receptor (BCR) and to a CR2-CD19 complex on the surface of a B lymphocyte, resulting in cross-linking of the CR2-CD19 complex to the membrane immunoglobulin. Experimentally, one complex of membrane

Figure 5.14 CR1 and CR2 work together to enhance the immunogenicity of B-cell antigens. (1) An antigen coated with complement split product C3b binds to the B cell via both the BCR and CR1. (2) CR1 presents C3b to factor I, which cleaves C3b to generate the split product C3d. (3) Conversion of C3b to C3d results in the dissociation of CR1 and the association of CR2. (4) CD19, complexed with CR2, delivers a costimulatory signal to the B cell via the src-related kinases Lyn and Fyn. This costimulatory signal, together with an activational signal delivered through the BCR, activates the B cell.

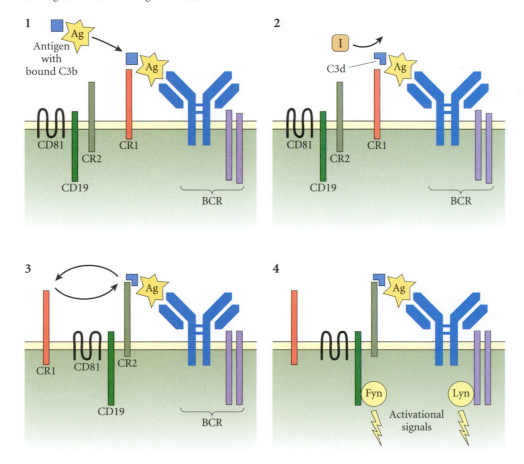

immunoglobulin cross-linked to one, two, or three complexes of CR2-CD19 is as effective as 10, 100, or 1,000 BCR complexes alone in activating a B cell. The function of this CR2-dependent enhancement of antigen signaling seems to be important in two situations: CR2 binding of C3d-coated antigen enhances immunogenicity when a nonimmune individual is exposed to a new antigen, and binding of small amounts of C3d-coated antigen to memory B cells facilitates a secondary response in an immune individual. No CR2-deficient patients have been described, but CR2-deficient transgenic mice have been produced. These animals have impaired, but not totally absent, antibody responses to antigen. Also consistent with the known function of CR2, coadministration of recombinant soluble CR2 with an antigen renders experimental immunization almost useless. Thus, the ligation of CR2 by antigen-bound C3d is of fundamental importance in the production of antibody.

Functions Associated with Soluble Split Products

Chemotaxis and cellular activation

A general principle governing the activation pathways of complement is that inactive serum complement proteins are cleaved into two fragments during activation. The larger fragment usually becomes covalently attached to the antigen, where it participates further in the activation cascade and, as described in the preceding section, can serve as an opsonin or as a costimulatory signal. The smaller, more easily diffusible peptide possesses immunoregulatory activity. Three such peptides, C3a, C4a, and C5a, are collectively known as the anaphylatoxins because they can trigger degranulation of mast cells typical of anaphylactic reactions. Each of these peptides has the capacity to cause smooth muscle either to relax or contract, depending on both the dose of peptide and the site of the smooth muscle. In an inflammatory site, the net effect is vasodilatation with increased local blood flow. In addition, capillary permeability increases and local mast cells release histamine. C5a causes expression of more opsonic membrane receptors such as CR1 and CR3 by neutrophils where opsonized material can be attached and ingested at the site of inflammation. For monocytes and macrophages, C5a also induces the production of proinflammatory cytokines, with further amplification of the inflammatory process and inflammatory infiltrate.

The biologic functions of the other complement split products are just beginning to be better understood with the identification and study of the cellular receptors for the split products. The C3a receptor, like the C5a receptor, is a G-protein-linked receptor with seven membrane-spanning domains. The activity of all three anaphylatoxins is negatively regulated by the activity of serum carboxypeptidase-N, which rapidly removes the carboxy-terminal arginine from each, producing less active forms designated C4a desArg, C3a desArg, and C5a desArg.

Regulation of Complement Activation

Intrinsic Biochemical Properties of Complement Proteins That Regulate Complement Activation

Several steps of the complement activation cascade have the characteristic of *amplification;* thus, complement has an intrinsic capacity for uncontrolled activation. Given that the products of complement activation induce vascular permeability and general inflammatory responses and can permeabilize biologic membranes, the consequences of such uncontrolled activation would be disastrous for the host. Complement activation is regulated on several levels to ensure that activation occurs only under appropriate circumstances. The first level of regulation is the inherent instability of many of the active forms of complement proteins. For example, the reactive thioester sites in freshly activated C4b and C3b react very quickly with water if no biologic surface with which they can interact is available. This rapid reactivity spatially limits the distance from the site of activation in which these proteins can form covalent attachments to become fixed and to perpetuate complement activation. Once bound to a biologic surface, complement protein complexes also are regulated by dissociation and concomitant inactivation. A rapid spontaneous molecular dissociation of the C3 convertases C4b2a and C3(H$_2$O)Bb provides the primary mechanism for keeping complement activation in check. In addition to their regulation by intrinsic molecular properties, complement components can also be regulated by the molecular properties of the biologic surface to which they become fixed. For example, when C3(H$_2$O) produced by the alternative pathway (i.e., spontaneous activation) interacts with a normal host cell, sialic acid present on the membrane of the host cell prevents the assembly of a C3 convertase. If, however, the C3(H$_2$O) attaches to a surface that does not exhibit the proper chemistry (e.g., a bacterial cell wall), the C3(H$_2$O) is free to interact with the other proteins of the alternative pathway and deposit more C3b adjacent to the original activating nidus, forming more sites of C3 cleavage until full-scale activation ensues.

Attenuation of Complement Activation by Dedicated Regulatory Proteins

Complement-control proteins are found both in serum and on membranes of host cells (Fig. 5.15). Serum proteins that inhibit the classical pathway include C1 esterase inhibitor (C1inh) and C4-binding protein (C4BP). C1inh is a member of a class of proteins termed *serpins* that have variable inhibitory activity against serum serine proteases. As its name implies, C1inh suppresses spontaneous activation of C1 and also inactivates C1r and C1s by triggering the dissociation of the C1 complex, causing C1r and C1s to be released from C1q. These effects limit the duration of classical pathway activation by a given immunoglobulin-C1 complex. A hereditary deficiency in

C1inh (manifested as hereditary angioneurotic edema) results in severe recurrences of classical pathway activation in response to minor trauma and in the absence of a defined antigen-antibody interaction. These attacks result in the release of soluble complement split products, which is thought to be responsible for the localized edema of the face, neck, and larynx that characterizes this disorder. These observations indicate that C1inh preserves the specificity of the classical pathway by ensuring that its activation takes place only in response to the engagement of antigen by antibody.

Although C1inh plays an important role in regulation of the first step of the classical pathway, perhaps the most important regulatory steps are those of the C3 convertases [C4b2a and C3(H_2O)Bb], since these are the first amplification steps of the classical and alternative pathways, respectively. Regulation of the C3 convertases is achieved in two ways. The first is through a triggered dissociation of the convertase by factor H or C4BP, and the second mechanism is enzymatic degradation of C3 and C4 by the protein called factor I (Fig. 5.16). Factor I is unusual among complement proteases, circulating in the serum in an enzymatically active state rather than requiring cleavage for activation. The activity of factor I appears to regulated by the availability of proper substrate orientation. The cleavage of C3(H_2O) into iC3b and C3dg and of C4b into C4c and C4d by factor I is dependent on the complexing of these substrates to cofactors, a process that results in presentation to factor I required for cleavage. The cofactors for factor I-mediated cleavage of C4b are C4BP, CR1 (CD35), and MCP, and for C3(H_2O), factor H, CR1, and MCP. The importance of factor I in complement regulation is underscored by examples of genetic deficiency in factor I, which leads to the uncontrolled formation of C3 enzymes, with the production of a second-

Figure 5.15 Regulatory proteins of the complement system. Most complement regulatory proteins act by preventing assembly of activated complement components or by inducing their dissociation. CR1, C4BP, DAF, MCP, and factor H are capable of both types of activity, inducing dissociation of preformed C3 and preventing association of new C3 convertases (double red bars). Factor I is capable of proteolytically cleaving and inactivating C3(H_2O) and C4b. Factor I requires CR1, C4BP, MCP, or factor H as a cofactor for this activity.

Regulator(s)	Mechanism	Pathway(s) affected
C1 inhibitor	Dissociates C1 complex	Classical
C4BP, CR1, decay-accelerating factor (DAF), membrane cofactor protein (MCP)	Dissociates C3 convertase	Classical, lectin
Factor H, CR1, DAF, MCP	Dissociates C3 convertase	Alternative
Factor I	Cleaves, inactivates C3b, C4b	All
S protein, clusterin	Prevents MAC formation	All
CD59, homologous restriction factor (HRF)	Blocks MAC assembly	All

Figure 5.16 Regulation of C3 by factor H. The diagram shows the structure of factor H, with each complement control protein repeat (CCP) represented as a red or pink oval. CCPs 1 to 4 are essential for both dissociation of the C3 convertase and recruitment of factor I.

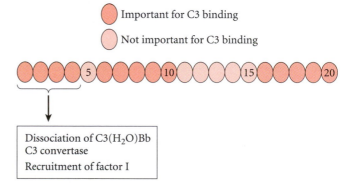

Important for C3 binding

Not important for C3 binding

Dissociation of C3(H_2O)Bb C3 convertase

Recruitment of factor I

ary deficiency of C3 because of excess turnover in the serum. This circumstance produces severe susceptibility to bacterial infection and is clinically identical to a congenital deficiency in C3 itself.

The regulation of factor I depends on its being presented with $C3(H_2O)$ or C4b substrates by a family of cofactor proteins. For alternative pathway complement activation, the most important of the cofactor proteins is factor H, which binds to the alternative pathway C3 convertase [$C3(H_2O)Bb$] and enhances dissociation of Bb from $C3(H_2O)$ in certain biochemical microenvironments. Although this has the effect of temporarily inhibiting complement activation, factor H is then capable of presenting the bound C3b to factor I for further proteolytic degradation, thus permanently inactivating the cascade.

Serum C4BP is structurally and functionally related to factor H and has the same function in the classical pathway as factor H has in the alternative pathway. C4BP blocks the C2a-binding site on C4b, preventing the formation of the classical pathway C3 convertase, C4b2a. In addition, when C4b is associated with C4BP, the C4b is susceptible to degradation by factor I into the inactive C4c and C4d fragments [just as $C3(H_2O)$ associated with factor H is degraded by factor I into inactive fragments].

Some membrane proteins display functional similarity to C4BP and factor H that protects the eukaryotic cell from damage due to "bystander lysis" when they are in the neighborhood of a complement-activation reaction. DAF (CD55) has a glycophosphatidylinositol (GPI) membrane anchor and is present on the surface membrane of many types of cells. It dissociates the C3-cleaving enzymes of the classical and alternative pathways, thereby combining the functions of C4BP and factor H. Unlike C4BP and factor H, however, DAF cannot serve as a cofactor for the cleavage of $C3(H_2O)$ and C4b by factor I. Instead, MCP (CD46) performs this function and, like DAF, dissociates C3 convertases, but then it presents $C3(H_2O)$ to factor I for proteolysis. Like DAF, MCP is widely distributed on the surface of many cell types. Of interest are several reports indicating that MCP is a receptor used by pathogenic bacteria (*Neisseria* spp.) and viruses (measles virus) to anchor themselves to cells and/or gain entry into the cells.

Several serum and membrane proteins interfere with the terminal stages of complement activation (the assembly of the MAC). Among such proteins are clusterin, S protein, homologous restriction factor (HRF), and CD59 (formerly called MIRL, for membrane inhibitor of reactive lysis). S protein acts by binding to the C5b67 complex in the target cell membrane and inducing the complex to undergo a *hydrophilic transition,* a structural shift that makes the complex incapable of remaining buried in

the target cell membrane (Fig. 5.15). S protein therefore removes the terminal complement complex from the target-cell membrane before the MAC is completely formed. It has been postulated that clusterin acts by a similar mechanism in regulating the complement system. Similarly, HRF and CD59 act by binding to the C5b678 complex and blocking association of C9 with the complex. This also has the effect of preventing MAC formation. A deficiency of CD59 on erythrocyte membranes makes the cells unusually susceptible to complement-mediated lysis. Like DAF, CD59 has a GPI anchor. Deficiencies in both of these proteins are found in patients with a mutation of the X-linked gene regulating the synthesis of the GPI anchor. The clinical result of the combined deficiencies is paroxysmal nocturnal hemoglobinuria, which is characterized by uncontrolled episodes of spontaneous lysis of red cells by host complement. In this condition, the hemoglobin released into the blood results in the production of red urine. Thus, defects in the regulation of virtually any stage of the complement cascade can have dire consequences for the host.

Evasion by Pathogenic Microorganisms of Complement-Mediated Killing

The complement system can be activated by multiple triggers, most of which are sensitive indicators of bacterial or viral infection. In addition, once activated, the complement system is capable of mobilizing a startling array of immune effector mechanisms aimed at neutralizing or destroying the foreign microbe. That so many microorganisms are capable of establishing infection in mammalian hosts despite these defense mechanisms suggests that these microbes have evolved countermeasures to avoid being killed by the complement system (Table 5.4). These countermeasures fall into three broad classes. The first of these encompasses microbial factors that protect against complement-mediated killing by enzymatically inactivating one or more protein components of the complement system. One example is the production of the enzyme *elastase* by the bacterium *Pseudomonas aeruginosa*. Elastase is a protease capable of cleaving multiple host proteins, including the anaphylatoxins C3a and C5a. Since these complement split products are important in the stimulation of inflammation and the concomitant recruitment of host leukocytes to the site of infection, cleavage of C3a and C5a by elastase results in a reduction in the local immune response to *P. aeruginosa,* thus favoring the establishment of infection. Another example of a microbial protein that cleaves and inactivates its host's complement proteins is the vaccinia complement control protein (VCP) produced by vaccinia virus. VCP binds to

Table 5.4 Microbial factors that inactivate or divert the complement system to protect against complement-mediated killing

Factor	Possessed by	Mechanism
Enzymatic		
Elastase	*P. aeruginosa*	Cleaves and inactivates C3a and C5a
VCP	Vaccinia virus	Cleaves and inactivates C4b and C3bBb
Affect complement regulation		
Surface proteins	Group A streptococcus	Bind factor H and inactivate C3b
	Neisseria spp.	Bind C4BP to block C4 activity
Surface sialic acid	*Neisseria* spp., group B streptococcus	Decease complement activation near cell surface
Steric		
Capsule	Various bacteria	Prevents C3b bound to bacterial membrane or cell wall from binding to complement receptors
Cell wall	Gram-positive bacteria	Prevents complement proteins that activate on cell wall peptidoglycan from inserting into bacterial membrane
O-side chain	Gram-negative bacteria	Prevents complement proteins that activate on O-side chain from inserting into bacterial membrane
HVSCD59	Herpesviruses	Binds C5b678 and prevents final MAC assembly

both the classical and alternative C3 convertases [C4b2a and C3(H_2O)Bb] and cleaves them to inactive forms.

A second class of countermeasures employed by microbes is to produce structural homologs of proteins the host uses to regulate complement activation or to create microbial surfaces that modulate complement activation. One such factor is the CD59-like protein HVSCD59 produced by herpesvirus saimiri. This viral protein seems to function just like the host's own CD59, binding to C5b678 and preventing the final assembly of the MAC. Various pathogens bind C4BP to decrease activation of complement on their surface. Other strategies include permitting factor H to bind to the microbial surface to dissociate the C3 convertase and sialylation of surface carbohydrates to make the microbial surface mimic the surface of a human cell. Also, sialylation decreases the ability of mannose-binding lectin and other complement factors to bind to the microbial cell surface.

A third class of factors that help microbes evade the complement system prevents complement-mediated killing for spatial or steric reasons (Table 5.4). These defense mechanisms act not by preventing activation of complement proteins but by causing the activated forms of complement proteins to be deposited in places where they are unable to effect bacterial killing. For example, the thick peptidoglycan layer surrounding gram-positive bacteria, the capsular polysaccharide surrounding gram-negative bacteria, and/or the long LPS O-side chains that also protrude from the surface of some gram-negative bacteria efficiently bind to activated C3 [C3b and C3(H_2O)]. However, this binding protects the bacterium from MAC-mediated lysis, since most of the activated C3 binds to the peptidoglycan or LPS on the outermost portion of the bacterial cell rather than to the cell membrane of the bacterium beneath. Such activated C3 on the outer peptidoglycan or LPS layers of a bacterium still could serve as an opsonin for phagocytic killing by neutrophils or macrophages. Many bacteria (e.g., *Streptococcus* and *Klebsiella* spp.) also inhibit opsonization through the production of a thick carbohydrate capsule outside the bacterial cell. Although the capsule cannot prevent C3b from becoming fixed to the underlying cell surface layer, C3b that is fixed to these subcapsular antigens cannot be bound by a neutrophil's complement receptors because the capsule physically blocks the neutrophil from accessing the bound C3b. Capsules have also been shown to protect bacteria from complement in the same manner as LPS or peptidoglycan by causing activated C3 to become fixed on the bacterium at a distance from the bacterial membrane and thus preventing insertion of the MAC into the bacterial cell membrane.

Synthesis of Complement Proteins

Constitutive synthesis of complement proteins is active, even under normal, healthy conditions, probably because many complement proteins are inherently unstable, resulting in their continuous, low-level spontaneous activation followed by inactivation. Most constitutive synthesis occurs in the liver, with lower levels of constitutive synthesis by monocytes, macrophages, and some types of epithelial cells. Continuous production of complement proteins is dependent on constant, low-level transcription of many complement genes.

Although constitutive synthesis of complement proteins produces sufficient quantities of protein to replenish components that spontaneously hydrolyze during alternative pathway activation and are consumed during low-level immune responses to common environmental pathogens, a faster rate of synthesis is required during and immediately after a systemic or severe infection. This temporary increase in complement synthesis is part of the systemic inflammatory response known as the *acute-phase response.* This response involves the elaboration of cytokines by immune and nonimmune cells during infection. Chief among these cytokines are interleukin-1 (IL-1) and IL-6 and tumor necrosis factor alpha. These cytokines bind to receptors on liver hepatocytes and induce a number of transcription factors that influence complement synthesis.

The most well-characterized of the transcription factors that regulate complement synthesis are members of the leucine zipper family, C/EBPα (CCAAT/enhancer binding protein), C/EBPδ, and NF-IL6 (nuclear factor associated with IL-6), which influence transcription by binding to a target *cis*-acting recognition site called bZIP1 located in the enhancers of complement genes, upstream of the transcriptional start site (Fig. 5.17). T. S. Juan and coworkers reported that alternative binding of C/EBP-α and C/EBP-δ to the bZIP1 enhancer element is important for constitutive and inducible transcription of the gene for complement component C3. According to their results, constitutive expression of C3 involves binding of C/EBPα to the bZIP1 element. However, IL-1-inducible transcription of C3 (as observed during the acute-phase response) requires binding of C/EBPδ to the same element. A few years earlier, H. Isshiki and coworkers (1991) had reported that induction of acute-phase proteins (such as complement proteins) is correlated with a decrease in synthesis of C/EBPα and an increase in synthesis of NF-IL6. Since NF-IL6 is responsible for the induction of acute-phase proteins and C/EBPα is essential for the constitutive production of complement and noncomplement liver proteins, it is likely that the shift from C/EBPα production to NF-IL6 production is central to the acute-phase response in hepatocytes.

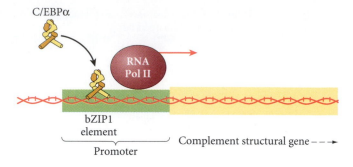

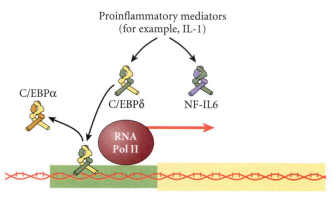

Figure 5.17 Transcriptional regulation of complement protein synthesis. Inflammatory cytokines such as IL-1 trigger the synthesis of transcription factors C/EBPδ and NF-IL6, which in turn mediate enhanced complement transcription.

A similar mechanism helps regulate the production of many complement regulatory proteins. G. J. Moffat and coworkers demonstrated that the same cytokines responsible for induction of complement proteins, such as C3 (IL-1, IL-6, and tumor necrosis factor alpha), also are able to induce expression of the complement regulatory protein C4BP. Thus, complement proteins and complement regulatory factors are probably coordinately regulated, ensuring that situations that elevate the amount of complement proteins in the host permit a higher level of regulation of complement activity.

Disorders Associated with Defects in Synthesis of Complement Proteins

The primary role of the complement system is the neutralization or destruction of harmful microorganisms. Experiments with complement-deficient strains of mice and clinical observations in human patients with congenital defects in complement proteins have emphasized the critical importance of the complement system to innate defense against microbial infection—observed primarily in patients who have deficiencies in the alternative pathway (e.g., factor B or factor D deficiency) or defects that affect both the classical and alternative pathways (e.g., C3 deficiency). Such individuals are predisposed to bacterial infections (e.g., recurrent streptococcal pneumonia and bacterial meningitis), which usually manifest at a very early age. It is interesting that individuals with genetic defects that permit complement activation but prevent final assembly of the MAC (e.g., defects in components C6 through C9) do not appear to be at an increased risk for most infections, suggesting that defense against infection usually is achieved through other modes of complement action (e.g., opsonization by C3b deposition). When such individuals are found to be susceptible to infection, it is usually to infection by gram-negative bacteria such as *Neisseria* spp. This indicates that disruption of the gram-negative outer membrane by the MAC plays some role in protection of the host. Curiously, complement activation in C9-deficient individuals has been found to be capable of a reduced but measurable level of bacteriolysis. This small amount of bacteriolytic activity is probably attributable to formation of the C5b678 complex, which is capable of disrupting membranes, albeit to a lower degree than a complete MAC.

Individuals with genetic defects that prevent the classical pathway of activation without affecting the alternative pathway (e.g., C4 deficiency or C2 deficiency) have a very different phenotype. They do not suffer from recurrent infections (perhaps indicating that the alternative pathway is more important for immunity to bacterial infections) but from chronic autoimmune conditions such as systemic lupus erythematosus, rheumatoid arthritis, and glomerulonephritis. These conditions are brought about by immune complex-mediated reactions similar to a type III hypersensitivity reaction, underscoring a second important role of the complement system, the removal of immune complexes from the blood. When a soluble antigen with a repetitive structure is presented to the immune system, more than one antibody molecule can bind to it. Furthermore, one antibody molecule can bind to two separate molecules of the antigen. Thus, great lattice-like complexes of antibodies and antigens can form. Since these immune complexes can trigger complement activation, foci of inflammation develop wherever the complexes are deposited, causing diseases such as glomerulonephritis (if deposited in the kidney) and pemphigus (if deposited in the skin). To prevent such inflammation, elaborate systems have evolved for clearing immune complexes before they precipitate in tissues. The system in primates is particularly elegant. Primate erythrocytes express CR1 on their surface.

Circulating immune complexes are coated with C3b as a result of classical pathway complement activation and bind to erythrocytes via CR1. Upon passing through the reticuloendothelial system (spleen and liver macrophages, Kupffer cells; also called the *mononuclear phagocyte system*), C3b is enzymatically cleaved to iC3b and the complexes are released from CR1 on erythrocytes and ligated and ingested by macrophages bearing CR3 and CR4 (Fig. 5.18A). As a result, this material is removed from the erythrocytes on a single pass through the hepatic or splenic circulation and the material is destroyed by the macrophages. Thus, primates use erythrocytes as a packaging mechanism to extract immune complexes from the bloodstream and deliver them to macrophages. The type III immune complex disorders that result from defects in C2, C4, or CR1 are due to the persistence of immune complexes in the circulation, giving them time to become lodged on vascular surfaces and initiate the type III reaction (Fig. 5.18B). In nonprimates, platelets (rather than erythrocytes) expressing CR1 may serve as the packaging mechanism for immune complex clearance.

The last class of complement disorders consists of those that affect complement regulatory proteins. Given its immense destructive potential and its ability to activate and enhance inflammatory reactions, the complement system requires tight regulation. Regulation is partially mediated by proteins that bind to activated complement components and mediate their inactivation. The protein C1 inhibitor (C1inh) binds to component C1 and causes it to dissociate into free C1q and C1r$_2$s$_2$. The regulatory proteins factor H, factor I, CR1, C4BP, and MCP all recognize the C3 convertases and bring about their dissociation and eventual inactivation. As would be predicted, genetic defects in any of these regulatory proteins result in inappropriate or prolonged complement activation and subsequent inflammation. Defects in C1 inhibitor are associated with lupus erythematosus and angioedema that likely result from type III reactions. Defects in factor H result in renal disease brought about by type III reactions in the glomeruli. Factor I defects result in lupus-like autoimmune condition. These examples underscore the important role normally played by the various complement regulatory mechanisms.

Summary

The complement system is the fundamental mechanism by which the body distinguishes uninjured self from

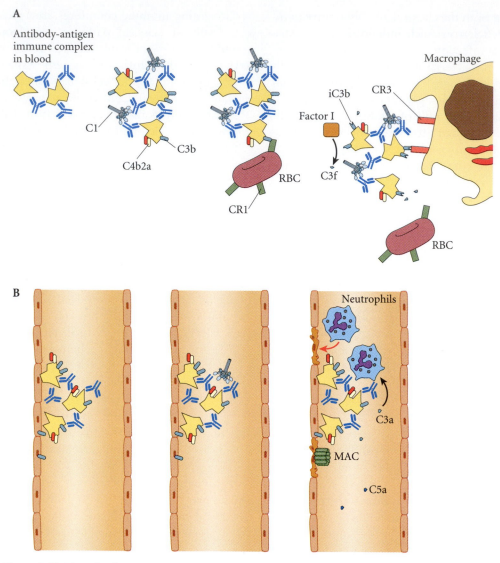

Figure 5.18 The role of complement in clearing immune complexes from the circulation. (**A**) Circulating immune complexes become substrates for activation of the classical complement cascade. Complement fragment C3b attaches to these immune complexes, mediating attachment of the complexes to red blood cells (RBC) via CR1. The RBC circulates to the liver, where CR1 acts as a cofactor for factor I-mediated cleavage of fragment C3b, forming the two products iC3b and C3f. iC3b is not bound by CR1, and so the RBC releases the immune complex, which is immediately bound by macrophages via CR3 or CR4 (not shown). The macrophage ingests the immune complex. (**B**) Genetic defects that impair classical pathway complement activation and genetic defects in CR1 impair this clearance mechanism. The result is persistence of circulating immune complexes, which eventually become embedded on blood vessel walls, triggering complement activation. MAC-mediated injury ensues, and complement split products generated during complement activation (C3a and C5a) attract neutrophils to the site (black arrow). The neutrophils can cause further tissue injury by releasing hydrolytic enzymes and oxidative products such as superoxide (red arrow).

injured self and invading organisms. This system functions in a manner that is both highly specific (based on either antibody specificity or the surface biochemistry of its target) and highly regulated (so as not to occur inappropriately on the surface of normal host cells). Once recognition or activation has begun, complement split products function as inflammatory mediators that elicit vascular and immune cell responses in the host, producing a classic inflammatory response. Immune cells attracted to such sites expose cell surface receptor proteins that recognize particular fragments of C3 and fulfill the biologic function of phagocytosis. Thus, complement constitutes the fundamental proinflammatory response system that can trigger and regulate the remainder of the immune response.

Suggested Reading

Barrington, R., M. Zhang, M. Fischer, and M. C. Carroll. 2001. The role of complement in inflammation and adaptive immunity. *Immunol. Rev.* **180:**5–15.

Fujita, T. 2002. Evolution of the lectin-complement pathway and its role in innate immunity. *Nat. Rev. Immunol.* **2:**346–353.

Law, S. K., and A. W. Dodds. 1997. The internal thioester and the covalent binding properties of the complement proteins C3 and C4. *Protein Sci.* **16:**263–274.

Molina, H. 2002. The murine complement regulator Crry: new insights into the immunobiology of complement regulation. *Cell. Mol. Life Sci.* **59:**220–229.

Nielsen, C. H., and R. G. Leslie. 2002. Complement's participation in acquired immunity. *J. Leukoc. Biol.* **72:**249–261.

Sahu, A., and J. D. Lambris. 2001. Structure and biology of complement protein C3, a connecting link between innate and acquired immunity. *Immunol. Rev.* **180:**35–48.

Smith, G. P., and R. A. Smith. 2001. Membrane-targeted complement inhibitors. *Mol. Immunol.* **38:**249–255.

Spear, G. T., M. Hart, G. G. Olinger, F. B. Hashemi, and M. Saifuddin. 2001. The role of the complement system in virus infections. *Curr. Top. Microbiol. Immunol.* **260:**229–245.

Walport, M. J. 2001. Complement. First of two parts. *N. Engl. J. Med.* **344:**1058–1066.

Walport, M. J. 2001. Complement. Second of two parts. *N. Engl. J. Med.* **344:**1140–1144.

ANTIBODIES

SECTION II

Antibodies

Ronald B. Corley

Antibodies, or immunoglobulins, are multimeric glycoproteins that are expressed in both membrane-bound and soluble forms. As cell surface proteins, antibodies define the B-lymphocyte population and serve as the antigen-specific component of the B-cell receptor complex. The immunoglobulin receptor on B cells plays an important role in the activation of B cells during immune responses and in the internalization of antigen for its presentation to T cells. As soluble molecules, antibodies are found in blood and secretions and serve to recognize and clear foreign antigens from the circulation. Clearance of antigen often involves other serum components and cells such as complement and phagocytes. Antibodies thus represent the primary molecular factor that mediates the antigen-specific activity of the adaptive humoral immune response. Antibodies can be generated against almost any chemical substance and therefore must be capable of great structural diversity. Yet, antibodies also initiate the important biologic effector functions required for the elimination of foreign antigens and thus must maintain significant constancy. To understand how these two disparate features of antibody function—the capacity to recognize vast numbers of antigens and the ability to carry out conserved effector functions—are accomplished by a single molecular structure was one of the great scientific quests of the 20th century. In addition to resolving this dilemma, studies of the nature of antibody structure provided important insights into the cellular basis of immune responses, contributed to our understanding of the relationships between protein structure and function, provided basic information leading to the comprehension of eukaryotic gene structure, and helped elucidate the molecular mechanisms by which tissue-specific gene expression is regulated. In addition, an understanding of how antibodies carry out their effector functions through interactions with other cells and soluble proteins not only has identified key features of the biology of the adaptive immune system but also has provided important and novel insights into the interactions between the innate and adaptive immune systems.

Chemical Structure of Antibodies

Early Studies

The classic studies of Edward Jenner in the 1790s and Louis Pasteur in the 1870s demonstrated experimentally that animals, including humans, could be specifically immunized against infectious agents. By the beginning of the 20th century, a number of studies had already established several important parameters of humoral immunity, i.e., immunity carried out by antibodies. Studies by Emil von Behring and Shibasaburo Kitasato, in 1890, had effectively demonstrated that immune serum obtained from animals resistant to diphtheria could protect naive (nonimmunized) animals from challenge by the same bacterium. Transfer of immune serum to nonimmune recipients is the basis for passive protection. The substance in immune serum was specific in that it neutralized the toxins from diphtheria but did not protect animals from challenge with unrelated pathogens or their products. An important feature of the immune serum, revealed in other studies, was its ability to interact specifically with different antigens, such as different strains of bacteria. This was shown by the ability of immune serum to cause bacteria to clump (agglutinate) and, under certain conditions, to even bring about the destruction, or lysis, of the bacteria. This reaction is now known to require serum substances called complement. Karl Landsteiner, in 1900, coined the name *antikörper* (antibody) for the substance that reacted specifically with the bacteria.

The important contribution that antibodies made to destroying harmful bacteria was suggested by the classic studies of Jules Bordet in the 1890s. Bordet demonstrated that multiple factors were needed to bring about the destruction of the bacteria and that the antibodies could be distinguished from other needed constituents of immune serum. Although freshly isolated immune serum mixed with bacteria such as *Vibrio cholerae*, the causative agent of cholera, destroyed the bacteria, immune serum that had been heat treated at 58°C before incubation with the bacteria could not. Addition of fresh but nonimmune serum to the heated immune serum could reconstitute the lytic activity, suggesting that the immune serum contained two substances, a specific antibody that was induced upon immunization and resistant to destruction at 58°C and a nonspecific activity that was present even in nonimmune serum. This latter activity has been called *complement,* and even today heat inactivation is a common technique used to eliminate the effects of complement. Thus, while antibodies contribute the specific antigen-recognition part of the humoral immune response, biologic activities needed to carry out the protective effects of the antibody (i.e., effector functions) reside in other serum proteins with which the antibodies can interact. Other functions of antibodies were later found to depend on an interaction of antibodies with cell surface receptors present on numerous immune cell types.

Monomer Unit Structure: Heavy and Light Chains

The complexity of antibodies was manifested in their multiple properties of being highly specific and highly diverse but also sufficiently constant in order to activate common effector functions. Elucidation of the chemical structure of antibodies required that they be separated from other serum substances. As with many other scientific problems, questions about the structure of antibodies preceded the capacity to answer them because the necessary technology was lacking. However, several important advances made in the first few decades of the 20th century helped point antibody studies in the right direction. First, antibodies were shown to be proteins. Lloyd Felton and Howard Bailey (1926) purified antibodies and used them to immunoprecipitate polysaccharide antigens. They found that the immunoprecipitates included protein as well as polysaccharide, indicating that antibodies are proteins. Antibodies also were shown to have different solubility in the presence of salts such as ammonium sulfate $[(NH_4)_2SO_4]$ that distinguished them from other serum substances, such as albumin. In serum saturated to 45% with $(NH_4)_2SO_4$, albumin (so called because it became opaque, like egg whites, when heated) remained soluble but antibodies in the serum did not. The precipitate that fell out of serum in the presence of $(NH_4)_2SO_4$ was called the *globulin* fraction. The antibodies in this immune globulin fraction were therefore referred to as *immunoglobulin.*

To further separate antibodies from other serum proteins, Arne Tiselius and Elvin Kabat, in 1939, applied a newly developed technology, an electrophoretic method developed by Tiselius, that permitted additional separation of serum proteins. This procedure not only separated the globulin fractions from albumin but also separated the globulins into three fractions, the so-called alpha, beta, and gamma fractions (Fig. 6.1). In this now classic experiment, Tiselius and Kabat found that the gamma globulin fraction was larger in serum from immune than

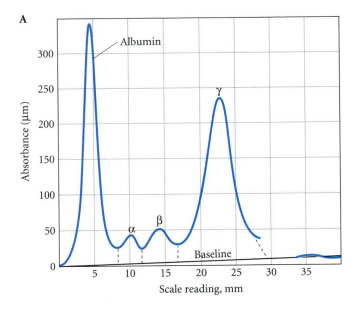

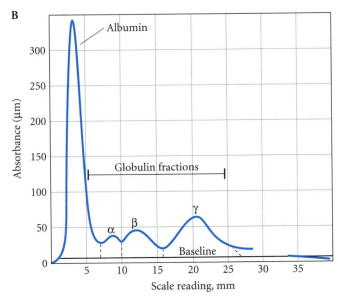

Figure 6.1 Electrophoresis of rabbit antiserum containing anti-egg albumin immunoglobulins before (**A**) and after (**B**) adsorption of the antibody with egg albumin. The demonstration that immunoglobulins were in the gamma globulin fraction is shown by the decreased amount of material in this fraction following removal of antibodies by adsorption. Reproduced from A. Tiselius and E. A. Kabat, *J. Exp. Med.* **69:**119–131, 1939, with permission.

from nonimmune animals. Further, this fraction could be reduced to its nonimmune quantity by first adsorbing the immune serum with the specific antigen (Fig. 6.1). Because the gamma globulin fraction was identified as a major antibody-containing fraction, antibodies came to be referred to as *gamma globulins* and the antibodies purified from these fractions, as *immunoglobulin G*. Other studies revealed that antibodies were complex and

could be separated on the basis of size. This separation was accomplished initially by density-gradient ultracentrifugation of immunoglobulins in sucrose solutions (represented as a sedimentation coefficient, which was a number followed by the letter S), allowing for the calculation of size. The bigger the value of S, the larger the molecule. One of the fractions containing antibody activity was large and had the sedimentation property at 20°C in water ($S_{20,w}$) of molecules of approximately 950,000 daltons ($S_{20,w} = 19S$), whereas the majority of antibodies were smaller, approximately 150,000 daltons ($S_{20,w} = 7S$).

The 7S gamma globulin fraction was used as the starting material in the elegant series of experiments performed by Rodney R. Porter, Gerald M. Edelman, and Alfred Nisonoff between 1959 and 1964, among others, that eventually led to the elucidation of the structure of antibodies and the awarding of the Nobel Prize for medicine or physiology in 1972 to Porter and Edelman. Porter subjected the 7S-immunoglobulin fractions to proteolytic digestion using papain, an enzyme isolated from papaya (used commercially today as a meat tenderizer). The papain-digested material was then fractionated on carboxymethyl cellulose, an anion-exchange resin that allows proteins to be separated according to their charge (Fig. 6.2). Two fractions (I and II) capable of binding antigen were identified, each with a molecular mass of about 50,000 daltons (50 kilodaltons [kDa]). A

Figure 6.2 Fractionation of a papain digest of rabbit gamma globulin by gradient elution (sodium acetate, pH 5.5, 0.01 to 0.9 M) and carboxymethyl cellulose chromatography. Note that fractions 1 and 2 both contain Fab components, while fraction 3 is the Fc component. The different elution profiles of the Fab components reflect charge heterogeneity within the polyclonal antiserum. Adapted from R. R. Porter, *Nature* **182:**670–671, 1958, with permission.

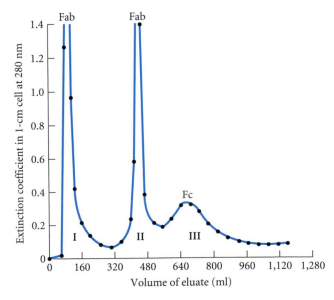

third fraction, also with a mass of 50 kDa, had the interesting property of forming crystals at neutral pH and low ionic strength but was totally devoid of antigen-binding activity. Fractions I and II became known as *Fab* because they were the fractions containing antigen-binding activity. Fraction III was referred to as *Fc,* for its propensity to form crystals. Although fractions I and II were able to bind antigen, they were unable to precipitate or agglutinate antigens, suggesting that they were univalent and thus able to bind to only one antigenic epitope at a time (Table 6.1).

Nisonoff used another proteolytic enzyme, pepsin, to digest gamma globulins. He observed that pepsin digestion resulted in a product approximately two-thirds the size of native gamma globulins. In contrast to the Fab fractions, the product of pepsin digestion precipitated antigen, suggesting that it was at least bivalent. No Fc fraction was obtained. It is now clear that this fraction was absent because pepsin digests the Fc region into small peptides. When the pepsin digest was further treated with reducing agents such as 2-mercaptoethanol, the antibody was reduced to a fraction approximately 55 kDa in size that had the capacity to bind but not to precipitate antigen, suggesting a univalent structure. The pepsin digest with antigen-binding activity was therefore considered to be bivalent and was referred to as $F(ab)'_2$, while the reduced pepsin digest was referred to as *Fab',* to distinguish this larger product from the smaller Fab produced by papain digestion.

To determine if gamma globulins were composed of more than one chain, Edelman and coworkers, and later

Porter, reduced the gamma globulins and alkylated them to prevent re-formation of disulfide bonds that often link protein chains together, and then denatured the antibodies and separated them into different sizes by gel filtration. Two protein bands were revealed, a larger band that fractionated as a 50-kDa protein and a smaller band that appeared to be about 25 kDa in size. These proteins were, respectively, designated as the heavy (H) and light (L) chains. To determine the stoichiometry, Porter and colleagues fractionated gamma globulins that had been reduced, alkylated, and denatured by gel filtration (Fig. 6.3). They found that 70% of the total mass of the gamma globulins was in the H-chain peak, suggesting the presence of two H chains (0.7×150 kDa $= 105$ kDa, or $\sim 2 \times 50$ kDa). Similarly, 30% of the mass was in the L-chain peak, suggesting the presence of two L chains (0.3×150 kDa $= 45$ kDa, or $\sim 2 \times 25$ kDa). Thus, antibodies appeared to be in an H_2L_2 configuration.

The arrangement of the H and L chains was determined by reducing the Fab fragments, which were found to contain one L chain and a component of an H chain, called the *Fd fragment.* Consistent with the presence of L and H chains in the Fab fragments, anti-antibodies to the Fab fragment prepared in another species reacted with both L and H chains. On the other hand, antibodies to the Fc component reacted only with isolated H chains, suggesting that the Fc is composed entirely of the H chain.

From these cumulative results, Porter and colleagues suggested a prototypic structure for the immunoglobulin (antibody) molecule—a substantially correct model that

Table 6.1 Fragments of antibody molecules

Fragment	Definition
Fab	A monomeric antigen-binding fragment of an immunoglobulin molecule created by papain digestion consisting of an intact L chain and the V_H and C_H1 domains of the H chain
Fc	A constant-region fragment resulting from papain digestion consisting of a dimer of the H-chain constant region but lacking the C_H1 domains
$F(ab)'_2$	A dimeric antigen-binding fragment of a immunoglobulin molecule created by pepsin digestion consisting of an intact L chain and the V_H and C_H1 domains; it is dimeric because pepsin cleaves below an interchain disulfide bridge between two H chains
$F(ab)'$	A monomer resulting from the reduction of the disulfide bonds between the two H chains of the $F(ab)'_2$, this fragment includes part of the hinge region of IgG
Fd	The H-chain component obtained by reduction and denaturation of the Fab fragment
Variable region	The N-terminal highly variable domain (~ 110 amino acids) of H and L chains; variable regions are responsible for the antigen-binding specificity
Constant region	The C-proximal domains of H and L chains that are more constant. The constant region of L chains is composed of one domain, whereas those of H chains are three or four domains, depending on the isotype. Constant regions are responsible for the biologic functions of antibodies.
Fv	The $V_H - V_L$ dimer forming the variable region of the Fab fragment

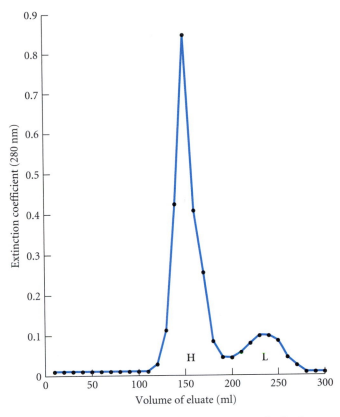

Figure 6.3 Separation of H and L chains from IgG antibodies by fractionation of reduced rabbit gamma globulin on Sephadex G-75 in 1 N acetic acid. Adapted from J. B. Fleischman et al., *Arch. Biochem. Biophys. Suppl.* **1:**174–180, 1962, with permission.

required only minor revision when the complete sequence of an antibody was obtained and all disulfide bond assignments were made (Fig. 6.4). This model suggested that the antigen-binding domains, made up of both H and L chains, were localized at one end of the molecule (the amino, or N, termini of the contributing H and L chains), whereas the Fc domain, composed only of H chain, was oriented at the other end (the carboxyl, or C, termini of each H chain). The Fc domain is now known to be important in initiating the effector functions of antibodies. This model explained the dual properties of antibodies—specific antigen recognition localized to one end of the molecule and biologic effector functions mediated by a different part of the molecule. This model also indicated that the diversity in antigen recognition could be carried out by varying the antigen-recognition part of the antibody, whereas the conserved biologic effector functions could be maintained by keeping the Fc region fairly constant in all antibody molecules with that specific function. But the big question this posed for geneticists and biochemists was, How do you make a

structure with sufficient diversity at one end to mediate antigenic specificity while maintaining conserved biologic effector functions?

Variable and Constant Regions

To understand how antibody specificity is achieved, it was first essential to have access to a homogeneous source of antibodies. It was well appreciated that serum antibodies were too heterogeneous for sequence analysis and that sources of homogeneous antibodies were necessary. Before the advent of hybridoma technology in 1974, only the availability of spontaneously arising tumors composed of plasma cells made this analysis possible. Plasma cells are the B-lineage cells dedicated to the secretion of antibodies. In humans, the primary sources of plasma cell tumors (plasmacytomas) were patients with multiple myeloma, a disease of the bone characterized by the uncontrolled proliferation of plasma cells. Plasmacytomas also were found to develop spontaneously in certain inbred strains of mice. In 1962, Michael Potter discovered that the incidence of tumor formation could be increased by administering certain irritants and carcinogenic substances to these mice, thus increasing the number of unique plasmacytomas available. Recognition that plasmacytomas in humans and experimental animals secreted immunoglobulins and could be used as homogeneous sources of antibodies for large-scale production and purification permitted the initial sequencing and structural studies—impossible tasks otherwise. In addition, the availability of plasmacytomas that could be adapted to grow and secrete antibodies in vitro was essential for the somatic-cell genetic approaches that eventually led to the production of hybridomas by Georges Köhler and Cesar Milstein in 1974.

The availability of plasmacytomas and myelomas was important for a number of reasons. These tumor cells served as homogeneous sources of antibodies of different classes (e.g., IgM or IgG) against which specific antibodies could be raised. This led to the identification of the different L-chain and H-chain isotypes and made identification of the antibody classes possible. Antibodies from these tumors were also crucial for sequence analysis. In this regard, an important characteristic of patients with multiple myeloma was the excretion of free L chains in their urine. These L chains, called *Bence-Jones proteins,* could easily be purified and therefore served as the major source of material for the early sequencing experiments that led to the identification of variable and constant regions in L chains, as well as to hypervariable regions found within the variable region. Moreover, Bence-Jones proteins could be crystallized and served as a source for many of the early studies of three-dimensional

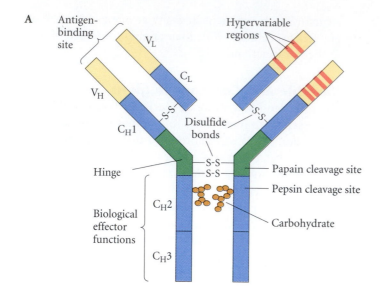

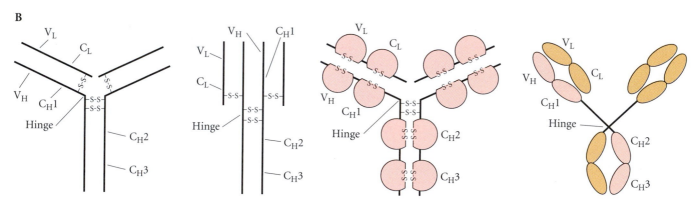

Figure 6.4 (A) Schematic diagram of an intact immunoglobulin antibody showing the variable and constant regions of the H and L chains. The CDRs, also known as the HV regions, are illustrated in the variable-region domains. Also shown are the intradomain disulfide bonds, hinge region, and associated asparagine-linked carbohydrates. Note the positions of the pepsin and papain cleavage sites relative to the interchain disulfide bonds that link the two H chains in the hinge region. (B) Different types of diagrams typically used to represent immunoglobulin molecules. The two diagrams on the left depict each protein chain as a solid line; the two diagrams on the right emphasize the domain structure of the protein chains, representing each domain structure as either a loop or an oval. All the diagrams use the symbol s-s to represent disulfide linkages.

conformation that contributed to our understanding of antibody structure.

Light chains

Comparisons of the sequences of Bence-Jones protein L chains from a number of different patients made clear that L chains could be divided into two roughly equal halves, or domains, each approximately 110 amino acid residues. The N-terminal half was highly variable and termed the V_L (variable light) region, whereas the C-terminal half was highly conserved and termed the C_L (constant light) region. In addition, two major types, or isotypes, of L chains previously identified by anti-antibodies

to myeloma proteins could be distinguished by their C-terminal sequences and were referred to as kappa (κ) and lambda (λ) L chains. L chains were found to contain 214 to 216 amino acid residues, suggesting a molecular mass of 22,900 to 23,112 daltons (assuming an average of 107 daltons per amino acid). This was in good agreement with the predicted size of the L chain based on the estimates from earlier biochemical studies.

Careful examination of a large number of V_L regions revealed that they were not uniformly variable. For example, a number of highly conserved, even invariant, amino acids were found at specific positions within the L chain, such as cysteine residues at positions 23 and 88. The conservation of these residues at particular locations suggested that they played an important role in the overall structure of the L chain, perhaps as a result of the formation of an intradomain disulfide loop, a deduction later confirmed by three-dimensional structural analysis. Of interest was the presence of two cysteine residues in similar relative positions in the C-terminal half of the L chain, suggesting that these different portions of the L chain had an overall similar structure.

Heavy chains

Although the H chains are larger than the L chains, sequence analysis revealed that the structure of H chains was similar to that of L chains. Thus, H chains contained an N-terminal domain of about 110 amino acids that showed significant sequence variability when the sequences of a number of H chains were compared. This region is designated V_H (variable heavy). The rest of the protein was more conserved and designated the C_H (constant heavy) region. As with the V_L region, there are two invariant cysteine residues in the V_H regions in similar positions and with similar spacing. The C_H regions, although larger than the C_L region, exhibited similar characteristics, and the larger size of the C_H region compared with the C_L was accounted for by the use of multiple blocks of amino acids to form the full region. Each block consisted of approximately 110 amino acids and contained two invariant cysteine residues spaced 60 to 70 residues apart. The comparable structures of the V_H regions, the V_L regions, and the C_L and C_H constant regions suggested that they evolved from a common ancestral gene. The regions of about 100 amino acids with conserved cysteines that can form an *intrachain* disulfide bond are referred to as *immunoglobulin domains*. As with the L chain, the sequences of the C_H chains revealed the existence of distinct forms, or *isotypes*, varying considerably from each other in sequence but nonetheless having the same characteristic domain structure. There are now known to be five major isotypes of H chains common to all mammalian species (known as α, γ, μ, δ, and ε, which define the antibody classes described in Table 6.2). It is important that although the amino acid sequences of the five isotype constant regions differ dramatically *from each other*, antibodies *within a given isotype* still display a high level of amino acid conservation within their constant regions. The different H-chain isotypes show approximately 30% sequence homology, suggesting that the genes encoding these proteins diverged early in the evolution of the antibodies.

Myelomas and plasmacytomas, like normal plasma cells, generally secrete antibodies of a single class, defined by H and L chains of a single isotype. Thus, the antibodies secreted by these tumors contain only one antibody L-chain isotype (κ or λ) and one H-chain isotype (e.g., α, γ, μ), which is referred to as "isotype restriction." However, it was known that plasma cells first started out making one kind of antibody, IgM, and then switched over to making antibody of a different isotype but with specificity for the same antigen. It was difficult to understand how antigenic specificity could be maintained while switching of the constant regions occurred until molecular genetic approaches revealed how antibody genes are assembled and expressed. Further, it was difficult to understand how antibody proteins could be so variable at one end and, at least within a single isotype, remain invariant at the other end. Again, this puzzle was solved only after it was possible to use molecular genetic approaches to define the genetic basis for generating the structure of antibody H and L chains.

The immunoglobulin fold

The net result of the analysis of the amino acid sequences of antibodies suggested that they were composed of multiple units of approximately 110 amino acids, each with two conserved cysteine residues, spaced approximately 60 amino acids apart, that could be involved in disulfide bonding—the immunoglobulin domains. As early as 1966, Robert L. Hill and colleagues suggested an evolutionary relationship between these domains: that the antibody L and H chains could have been constructed by stringing together domains that had evolved by duplication and divergence of these domains from a common primordial gene. Analysis of the three-dimensional structure of antibodies by X-ray crystallography has lent strong support to this view, demonstrating that each domain folds into a similar tertiary structure, referred to as the *immunoglobulin fold*. The immunoglobulin domain is now known to be the basic building block used not only by antibodies but also by a wide array of proteins, especially those with some type of recognition or interaction function. These are collectively referred to as members of the *immunoglobulin superfamily*. The evolutionary success of the immunoglobulin domain no doubt results in part from its ability to facilitate noncovalent interactions between domains, allowing it to be a structural subunit for different kinds of proteins that form by oligomerization.

All L chains, whether κ or λ, are composed of two immunoglobulin domains, one at the V_L region and the other comprising the C_L region. In addition to the V_H region at the N terminus of each H chain, the C_H region is composed of multiple domains. There are either three (γ, α, or δ) or four (μ and ε) C_H regions designated as

Table 6.2 Characteristics of antibody classes

Property	IgM	IgG				IgA		IgE	IgD
		IgG1	IgG2	IgG3	IgG4	IgA1	IgA2		
H-chain isotype	μ	γ_1	γ_2	γ_3	γ_4	α_1	α_2	ε	δ
No of constant domains	4	3	3	3	3	3	3	4	3
Usual molecular form(s)	Pentamer, hexamer	Monomer	Monomer	Monomer	Monomer	Monomer dimer, tetramer	Monomer dimer, tetramer	Monomer	Monomer
Molecular weight (kDa)	950, 1,140	150	150	150	150	160, 330, 650	160, 330, 650	190	180
Serum level (mg/ml)	1.5	9	3	1	0.5	3	0.5	0.003	0.03
% of Ig in serum	8	49	16	5	3	16	3	0.02	0.2
Serum half-life days	5	23	23	8	23	6	6	2 (in serum)	3
Carbohydrate content	10	3	3	3	3	7 (average, in serum)	7 (average, in serum)	13	9
Primary functions	Primary antibody responses	Secondary antibody responses; protection of fetus	Secondary antibody responses; protection of fetus	Secondary antibody responses; protection of fetus	Secondary antibody responses; protection of fetus	Secretory immunity; secondary antibody responses	Secretory immunity; secondary antibody responses	Antiparasite responses; allergy	Unknown (marker for mature B cells)
Complement activation: classical pathway	Yes	Yes	No[a]	Yes	No	No	No	No	No
Complement activation: alternative pathway	No	No	No[a]	No	No	Yes	No	No	No
Binds to macrophage Fc receptors	No	Yes	No[a]	Yes	No	No	No	Yes (Fcε)	No
Crosses placenta	No	Yes	Yes	Yes	Yes	No	No	No	No
Present in secretions	Yes	No	No	No	No	Yes	Yes	No	No
Induces mast cell deregulation	No	No	No	No	No	No	No	Yes	No

[a] The ability of IgG2 to activate complement has been controversial, but data now appear to show definitively that it is incapable of activating complement.

C_H1, C_H2, C_H3, and C_H4. The α, δ, or γ H chains with three constant-region domains also contain a flexible *hinge region* that appears to be important for their antigen-binding function.

X-ray crystallographic studies revealed that the variable and constant regions independently fold into the characteristic compact globular structure that typifies the immunoglobulin fold (Fig. 6.5). The immunoglobulin fold consists of two separate β-pleated sheets that are joined and thus stabilized by the intradomain disulfide bond, providing the explanation for the conservation of the two cysteine residues at defined intervals within each immunoglobulin domain. Each β-pleated sheet is composed of three or four antiparallel β-strands, such that each immunoglobulin domain contains one β-pleated sheet with three strands (the three-strand face) and the second with four strands (four-strand face). The β-strands characteristically have alternating hydrophobic and hydrophilic amino acids whose side chains are arranged with the hydrophobic sequences oriented toward the interior of the globular structure and the hydrophilic sequences oriented such that they are exposed to solvent (usually water). This motif is essential for the formation and stability of both the secondary and tertiary structure of the immunoglobulin domain. Not unexpectedly, the positioning of the hydrophobic residues along the β-strands is highly conserved. Each of the β-strands is connected by loops of varying size; in the case of the variable regions, some of these strands contain the hypervariable regions and constitute the antigen-binding domains (Fig. 6.5).

Despite their overall structural similarities, the variable and constant regions have subtle differences in their structure. Both V_H and V_L are somewhat longer than constant regions (approximately 16 amino acid residues). These residues make up an extra pair of β-loops on the three-strand face of the variable-region domain; thus, this face actually contains five strands (Fig. 6.5). That both V_H and V_L contain these extra amino acids suggests that the structure of the variable region was established before evolutionary divergence of the two variable regions.

The structure of the immunoglobulin fold exhibits two important features essential for the function of the antibody molecule. First, the structure of the immunoglobulin domain is highly suited to fostering noncovalent interactions with other protein domains, a feature of particular importance in the overall structure and function of the immunoglobulin molecule. In the case of immunoglobulin chains, the immunoglobulin fold allows for interactions between similar domains as needed, as exemplified by the interactions of the two C_H3 domains within a single IgG molecule. These interactions are crucial for the formation and stability of the immunoglobulin monomeric subunit, composed of two H and two L chains (H_2L_2). In addition, the immunoglobulin fold makes it possible for nonidentical domains to interact, which in the case

Figure 6.5 Ribbon diagram of L chain in three dimensions showing the variable and constant domains. β-strands appear as flattened arrows, and shading illustrates the β-strands forming the four-stranded and three-stranded sides. Numbers show amino acid positions in the variable and constant regions. The intradomain disulfide bonds stabilizing the associated four- and three-stranded sides are represented by black bars. Note the additional β-strands within the variable region. Reprinted from M. Schiffer et al., *Biochemistry* 12:4620–4631, 1973, with permission.

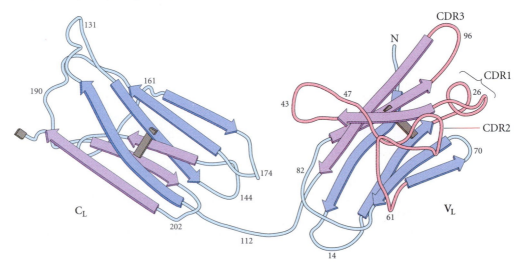

of antibodies includes pairing of C_H1 with C_L and of V_H with V_L. This feature obviously allows for the important interactions essential for the proper association of immunoglobulin H and L chains and thus for the formation of the antigen-binding sites.

The second important feature of the immunoglobulin fold for antibody function is that it permits significant variability in the number of amino acid residues that can be accommodated in the loops that connect the β-strands. Although the β-sheet structure dominates the secondary structure of the immunoglobulin fold, the possibility of variability permits significant flexibility in the evolution of the immunoglobulin domain because loops of varying size and complexity can be incorporated without affecting the overall three-dimensional structure of the immunoglobulin molecule, as long as the hydrophobic core structures are maintained. This feature allows for the incredible binding diversity of antibodies, in that the hypervariable regions of the immunoglobulin V_H and V_L domains that constitute the antigen-binding sites are contained within the loops.

Variable-Region Domains: Structure and Function

Having established that the N-terminal domains of both the H and L chains constitute the variable regions of antibody molecules, it was important to determine the extent of variability within this region. Early comparisons of variable-region amino acid sequences showed that some positions exhibited significant variability while amino acids at other positions were much more conserved or even invariant. To visualize the differences in variability of the different amino acid positions in the variable region, Tai Te Wu and Elvin A. Kabat (1970) developed a method, called the variability index (VI), by which they could assign a numerical value to each position that would reveal the extent of its variability. They defined the VI as the number of different amino acids found at a given position divided by the frequency of the most common amino acid in that position. Thus, the VI could vary from 1 for an invariant position [$VI_{min} = 1/(20/20)$] to 400 for extreme hypervariability ($VI_{max} = 20/(1/20)$). By plotting the VI at each position, it became immediately obvious that the variable region contained stretches of amino acids that were particularly variable, with intervening stretches that were much less variable (Fig. 6.6). The highly variable regions were termed *hypervariable* (HV) regions, and the less variable stretches were called *framework* regions (FR). Three major HV regions could easily be defined within each of the V_H and V_L regions. The most straightforward interpretation was that the antigen-binding specificity of the antibody was determined by

amino acids within the HV regions, a prediction subsequently borne out by experimental data. Indeed, Wu and Kabat referred to the HV regions as *complementarity-determining regions* (CDRs)—predicting that these regions were likely to contribute to the antibody-combining site by forming a structure complementary to an antigenic determinant such that the antigenic epitope could be encompassed by the HV regions. This prediction was experimentally proven by three-dimensional structural studies carried out in the 1980s.

Antigen binding: general features

Antigen-antibody interactions are noncovalent and as such constitute reversible reactions. As with other noncovalent interactions, antibodies bind to antigens only if the release of free energy by the binding reaction is sufficient to be thermodynamically favored. The interactions between antigens and antibodies use forces similar to those associated with other noncovalent interactions, including the formation of hydrogen bonds, van der Waals interactions, and the formation of salt bridges. As such, the binding of antigens to antibodies can be reversed, making antibodies reagents of choice in a process called *affinity purification.* Here an antibody to an antigen is immobilized on a solid surface, and an impure solution containing the antigen of interest is added under conditions that allow the antigen to bind to the antibody. The other components of the solution that do not bind are washed away, then the antigen is dissociated from the antibody and collected in the dissociating solution. Common agents used to dissociate antigens from antibodies include low (or high) pH and the use of high concentrations of chaotropic salts.

The "goodness of fit," or strength of binding between an antibody and its antigen, is reflected in the affinity of the interaction. Like other binding reactions between biomolecules (hormones and their receptors, enzymes and their substrates), the interactions between antibodies and their ligands are described by basic thermodynamic principles. Affinity reflects the ability of the antigen to stably associate with the antibody; this is the association constant of the antigen-antibody interaction. However, once associated, a high-affinity interaction will be characterized by the ability of the complex to be maintained—the dissociation constant. If the association constant, or "on" rate, is high but the dissociation constant, or "off" rate, is also high, then there will not be an overall high affinity of the antigen for the antibody. Alternately, if the association constant is low but the complex is stable with a slow dissociation, a high-affinity interaction of antigen and antibody can nonetheless occur. To quantify the *dissociation constant,* a value is determined that reflects the concen-

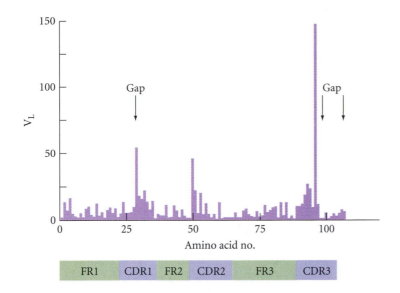

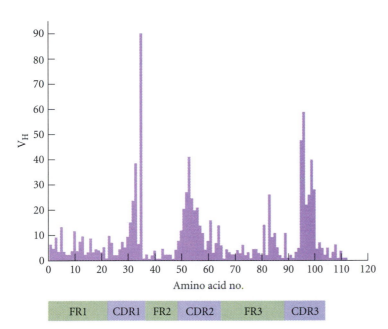

Figure 6.6 Variability plots of the human H and L chain variable regions. Variability plots are based on the comparison of sequences of a number of different L chains (**top**) and H chains (**bottom**). In both cases sequences were aligned for maximum homology. Positions where differences in sequence length exist are identified as gaps. The VI (on the vertical axis) is a calculated value ranging from 1 (no variability at that amino acid position) to 400 (completely random use of all 20 amino acids at that position). The positions of the CDRs and FRs are identified. (**Top**) Adapted from T. T. Wu and E. A. Kabat, *J. Exp. Med.* **132:**211–240, 1970. (**Bottom**) Adapted from E. A. Kabat, *Structural Concepts in Immunology and Immunochemistry,* 2nd ed. (Rinehart and Winston, New York, N.Y., 1976).

tration of antigen (in moles) allowing half of the antibody molecules to be bound. Thus, the smaller the dissociation constant, termed K_d, the higher the affinity. Naturally occurring antibodies do not alter the antigen they bind, and antigen-antibody reactions are essentially always reversible. One exception brought about by modern molecular technologies is the production of so-called catalytic antibodies, which are designed to have a variable region that mimics the transitional state of a catalyst and therefore promotes a chemical change in the target antigen (i.e., the "substrate").

The affinity of an antibody can be measured experimentally by equilibrium dialysis. However, during an immune response populations of antibodies to the target antigen are made. These antibodies differ on the basis of specificity for different epitopes on the antigen and the ability of related, but different, antibodies to bind to the same epitope, usually with different affinities. The affinity of antibodies generated during immune responses varies, with the K_d ranging between 5×10^6 and 5×10^9. In any immune response, the different antibodies produced to the antigen will generally have different affinities. As a result, there is an average affinity of antibodies to a particular antigen that reflects the affinity properties of the diverse antibodies produced.

During immune responses, the average affinity of the antibodies produced in response to antigens generally increases over time, especially during a secondary immune response. This process, termed *affinity matura-tion,* is now known to reflect the accumulation of select-ed mutations that occur in the genes encoding antibody proteins that occur following activation of B cells by spe-cific antigen. The antibodies with increased affinity com-pared with the initial, germ line or nonmutated, counter-parts appear during an immune response because variant B cells producing antibodies with a better ability to bind antigen (i.e., higher affinity) are actively selected to pro-liferate and mature into antibody-secreting plasma cells.

Antibody-combining site: affinity labeling

The first experimental evidence that the HV regions were involved in antigen binding came from affinity-labeling studies pioneered in 1962 by Leon Wofsy, Henry Metzger, and S. J. Singer, who used the same techniques that were successful in identifying the active sites of enzymes. Affinity labeling involves the use of reactive haptens (small antigens that can be bound by antibodies but do not by themselves elicit antibody responses) to both bind and specifically label antigen-binding sites on antibodies. In affinity labeling, a hapten is selected that interacts reversibly with the antibody-combining site in the usual fashion but is also designed to include a highly reactive chemical group capable of binding covalently to the anti-body once the hapten is initially bound in the usual non-covalent manner. In general, the reactive haptens that have been used to bind irreversibly with amino acid residues in the antibody molecule that come in close con-tact with the hapten include those with tyrosines that can form azo groups, or modified lysine residues. Although the amino acid residues that are specifically involved in antibody binding cannot be definitively identified by this method, amino acids that have specific side chains neigh-boring the antibody-combining site are labeled. Such studies therefore localized the antigen-binding sites on the antibody molecules and were the first to confirm that amino acid residues within or around the HV regions were involved in antigen binding. Moreover, amino acids in both the V_H and V_L were labeled, a result suggesting that residues from the variable regions of both of the anti-body chains were able to contact the antigen.

More common approaches to defining the antibody-binding site that are available today involve the crystal-lization of the antigen-binding domains along with the antigen, followed by the elucidation of the structure by X-ray diffraction methods. In the age of recombinant DNA methodology, mutational analysis of defined antigen-binding sites can be accomplished, followed by re-expression of the altered H and L chains in anti-body-secreting cells. The effect of individual mutations

on the binding of antibodies to antigens has been an important adjunct to the crystallographic studies. Together, these studies have demonstrated that the HV regions contain important contact sites for the antibody with its antigen and thus represent the CDRs predicted by Wu and Kabat.

Antibody-combining site: X-ray crystallography

Direct evidence of the involvement of the amino acids within the HV regions in antigen binding came from X-ray crystallographic studies in which the Fab region was crystallized and the three-dimensional structure of the Fab bound to antigen was characterized. In addition to proving a direct relationship between the amino acids within the CDRs and antigen binding, these studies pro-vided insights into the nature of antigen-antibody inter-actions and the tremendous flexibility exhibited by the antigen-binding regions. The CDRs generally fall within the loop structures connecting the β-strands of the vari-able region, with CDR2 falling within the extra loop char-acteristic of the variable regions (Fig. 6.5). The tremen-dous variation in the specificity of antibodies is reflected in the variations in the length and precise amino acid sequence of these loops as well as in the combination of sequences provided by the two variable regions, V_H and V_L. The more conserved FRs around the CDRs make up the β-pleated sheet structure of the V_H and V_L regions, essentially serving as scaffolding supporting the CDRs. It is interesting that the three-dimensional structure of the FRs of most antibody variable regions can be superim-posed, whereas the structure of the loops encompassing the six CDRs exhibit a high degree of structural variation and orientation. Consequently, the structure of the immunoglobulin variable regions provides the constancy by which overall structure of an antibody is maintained but has the flexibility necessary for significant diversity in antigen binding.

X-ray crystallographic studies have shown that the antibody-combining site exhibits extraordinary variabili-ty in several important ways. First, the orientation and size of the combining site vary to bind specifically to cog-nate the antigen. Thus, small antigens might fit within a pocket, or cleft, while the epitopes on larger macromole-cules are generally bound over broader and more planar surfaces. The surface areas of the antigens and antibodies involved in contact vary significantly (Table 6.3). Second, important contact sites generally are found in both the V_H and V_L regions, but variability exists in the degree of importance of these different variable regions in binding, depending on the antigen, and on the number of available

Table 6.3 Contact area between Fab fragments and antigens[a]

Fab	Fab contact area (Å²)[b]	Antigen	Antigen mol mass[c] (kDa)	Antigen contact area (Å²)	Antigen buried contact area (Å²)	% Antigen buried
Small antigens						
McPC603	161	Phosphocholine	169	169	137	81
DB3	286	Progesterone	314	277	246	89
Se155-4	297	Dodecasaccharide	1,416	378	248	66
4-4-20	308	Fluorescein	334	282	266	94
AN02	350	Dinitrophenyl spin-label	392	344	232	67
17/9	468	HA[d] peptide	1,055	742	436	59
BV04	515	D(pT)₃	932	687	454	66
B13/2	560	C-helix peptide	818	701	462	66
131	725	Angiotensin II	1,046	ND[e]	620	ND
Globular protein antigens						
D1.3	690	Lysozyme	14,000	5,564	680	12
HyHEL-10	721	Lysozyme	14,000	5,414	774	14
HyHEL-5	746	Lysozyme	14,000	5,436	750	14
NC41	916	Neuraminidase	50,000	14,638	899	6

[a] Contact area determined by computer analysis of X-ray crystallographic data of Fab fragments bound to their respective antigens. Adapted from I. A. Wilson and R. L. Stanfield, *Curr. Opin. Struct. Biol.* **3:**113–118, 1993, with permission.
[b] 1 Å = 0.1 nm.
[c] mol mass, molecular mass.
[d] HA, hemagglutinin.
[e] ND, not determined.

CDRs actually used (from the maximum of six, three each within each variable region). Finally, in some cases, contacts might be made between the antigen and amino acids within the FRs, which apparently stabilize binding in some cases. Thus, as was predicted from the original solution of the immunoglobulin fold, this structure accommodates significant variation.

Initial crystallographic studies were carried out using small antigens, such as haptens or small carbohydrates, to characterize the binding sites. These studies showed that the antibody-combining site appeared as a pocket, or cleft, into which the antigenic determinant could fit, like a lock and key (Fig. 6.7 and 6.8). These studies confirmed both that small antigens could fit in a binding site and that different CDRs were involved, depending on the antigen. However, it is not possible to fit larger epitopes on macromolecules into a "pocket-like" binding site on antibodies. Such epitopes involve significant contact across large interfaces on the surface of the antigens and antibodies (Fig. 6.9). Due to the diversity of epitopes on an antigen, the overall population of antibodies that bind to that antigen do so in different ways (Fig. 6.9).

Because the affinity of an antibody can change during the course of an immune response, due to changes or mutations in the genes that encode the variable regions, it was important to understand the molecular and biochemical basis for this. Recent studies that compared the binding of a germ line, unmutated antihapten antibody, and its mutated counterpart showed that the mutated antibody had a 30,000 times greater affinity than the unmutated antibody for the antigen. Of interest is the finding that the improvement of binding of unmutated antibody is accompanied by significant structural alterations in the orientation of the antigen-combining site (Fig. 6.10A). This is of interest, since germ line (or so-called natural) antibodies characteristic of the "nonimmune repertoire" are frequently capable of binding more than one structurally unrelated antigen (a feature termed *multireactivity* or *polyreactivity*). The ability of the binding sites of these antibodies to change their structure to accommodate an antigen may help explain multireactivity.

In contrast to the germ line antibody variable region, the antibody-combining site of the mutated antibody underwent little change during antigen binding (Fig. 6.10B). This difference appeared to be due to mutations affecting the orientation of the antibody-combining site and the combining site itself, such that it now assumed the lock-and-key motif characteristic of other high-affinity antibodies. These data emphasized the tremendous variability in the ability of antibodies to bind anti-

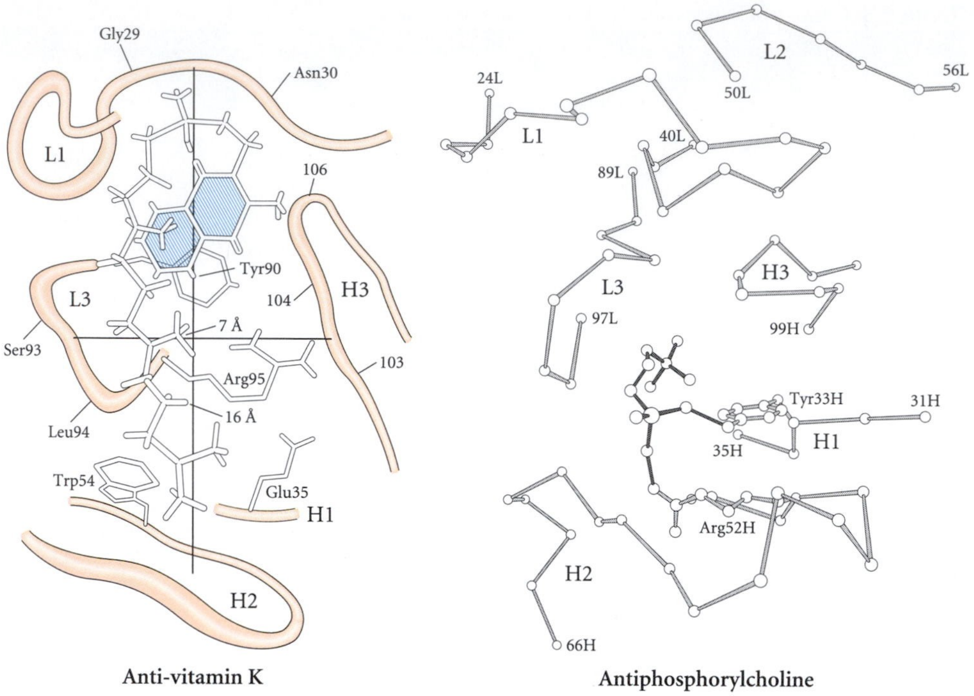

Figure 6.7 Binding sites of human myeloma protein "New" with its target antigen, vitamin K, in the antigen-binding site (**left**) and of mouse myeloma McPC603 with phosphorylcholine (PC) antigen in the site (**right**). The HV regions of the two antibody-binding sites are oriented in the same way, and the identity of the three major HV regions from both L and H chains are identified in the contact sites. Reprinted from D. A. Davies et al., *Annu. Rev. Biochem.* **44**:639–667, 1975, with permission.

Gly29

Asn30

L1

106

Tyr90

L3

104

H3

Ser93

7 Å

103

Arg95

Leu94

16 Å

Trp54

Glu35

H1

H2

Anti-vitamin K

24L

L2

50L

56L

L1

40L

89L

H3

L3

97L

99H

Tyr33H

31H

35H

H1

Arg52H

H2

66H

Antiphosphorylcholine

Figure 6.8 Stereo views of the binding of angiotensin II to the Fab region of a high-affinity monoclonal antibody. (**Top**) Side view (**Bottom**) Front view (looking into the binding site). Only the van der Waals surfaces are shown for the Fab and appear in green. The peptide hormone is shown in red. Reprinted from K. C. Garcia et al., *Science* **257**:502–507, 1992, with permission.

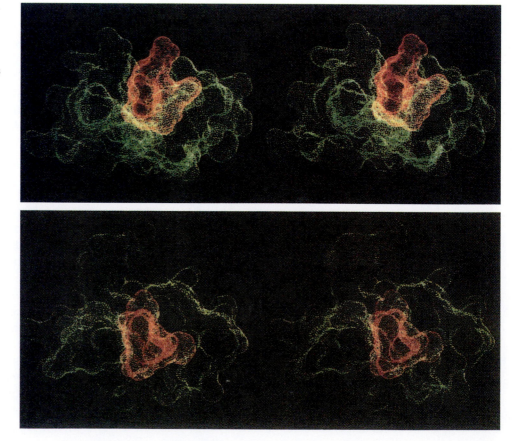

A End-on view

B Side view

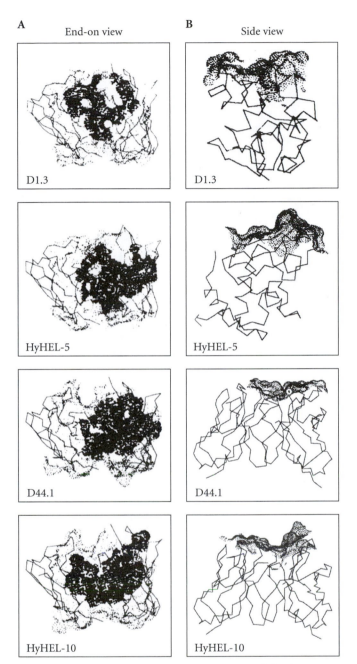

D1.3

HyHEL-5

D44.1

HyHEL-10

D1.3

HyHEL-5

D44.1

HyHEL-10

Figure 6.9 Binding sites of different antibodies to a defined antigen, lysozyme. (**A**) Stereo view of antigen-combining sites of four different antilysozyme antibodies. (**B**) Schematic view of these same antibodies and the epitopes recognized on the antigen. Note the excellent fit between the epitope on the antigen (**top**) and the complementary antigen-binding site in the antibody (**bottom**). For clarity, the epitopes are pulled away from the paratopes (antigen-combining sites). Reprinted from E. A. Padlan, *Adv. Protein Chem.* **49:**57–133, 1996.

gen, provided some perspective into the different natures of natural and antigen-selected antibodies, and provided the first structural insights into the evolution of antibody-combining sites during immune responses.

Constant-Region Domains: Structure and Function

The antibody molecule has two major functions: the first is to recognize and bind the antigen and the second is to initiate one or more biologic effector functions to elicit the removal or elimination of the foreign antigen. Whereas the variable-region domains, V_H and V_L, are responsible for antigen binding, the constant-region domains, specifically those of the H chains, are associated with the various biologic functions of the antibody molecules. In addition, the constant region provides flexibility to the molecule through the hinge region, enabling the molecule to bend, rotate, and flex, features that differ depending on the antibody isotype but that are important in antigen binding and biologic activities. The H chains are glycosylated on defined asparagine (N) residues. These N-linked glycans are important for the biologic functions of antibodies and contribute to other characteristics of the antibody molecule, such as its clearance from the blood or secretions.

The constant-region domain of the L chain

The L chain, whether κ or λ, has only one constant-region domain. The C_L domain has no known biologic functions, but its existence is crucial to the overall structure of the immunoglobulin molecule. The C_L domain interacts with the C_H1 domain of the H chain, and these interactions are stabilized by an interchain disulfide bond via cysteine residues in the C_L and C_H1 domains. As a result of its interactions with C_H1, the C_L domain serves to stabilize the crucial interactions of the Fab region of the immunoglobulin molecule and to extend the antigen-binding domains away from the hinge, serving as a "spacer" between the hinge and the antigen-binding domains. Further, association of the L chain is required for the proper folding of the C_H1 domain of the H chain. Immunoglobulin H chains cannot be secreted without associated L chains, and thus the L chain helps ensure that only functional, antigen-binding molecules are secreted by plasma cells.

The constant regions of the H chains

All mammals have five types of antibody molecules, as defined by their H chains, each of which is responsible for one or more of the diverse biologic activities carried out by antibodies. It is likely that the genes encoding for the constant regions of the H chains (referred to as IGHC) arose by gene duplication from a common ancestor before mammalian speciation. Consistent with this hypothesis is the sequence homology exhibited by the different H chains, which share up to 30% identity at the amino acid level. Note, however, that the presence of antibodies is not restricted to mammals. Antibodies have been found in all

A

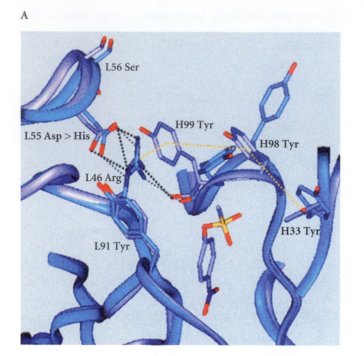

B

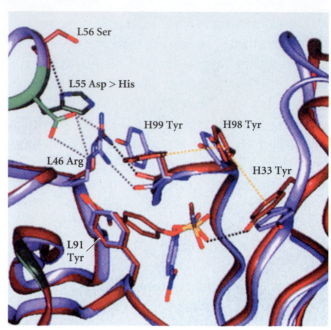

Figure 6.10 Structural changes that occur following binding of an antibody to hapten. The diagrams depict the conformation of the antigen-binding site of the antibody before (**A**) and after (**B**) binding to the antigen. Modified from G. J. Wedemayer et al., *Science* **276:**1665–1669, 1997, with permission.

vertebrates tested and even in the primitive cartilaginous fishes. However, in many nonmammalian species, only one identifiable form of immunoglobulin, namely IgM, is found.

Antibodies exist both as soluble, secreted proteins and as membrane forms. As a membrane protein, the immunoglobulin molecule is anchored via a hydrophobic transmembrane segment in the plasma membrane. Membrane immunoglobulin (mIg) serves as the antigen receptor on B cells and plays an important role in the activation of antigen-specific B cells during immune responses. The sequences that distinguish membrane and secretory antibodies are found at the end of the C terminus of the H chains and arise as the result of differential splicing of a precursor RNA, which gives rise to either the membrane or secretory forms of immunoglobulin. The C terminus of the H chain of secreted antibodies contains hydrophilic amino acid residues of varying lengths, depending on the isotype. The membrane form contains a conventional hydrophobic transmembrane segment of about 26 amino acids and a cytoplasmic tail of variable length that extends into the cytoplasm of the B cell (Fig. 6.11).

Functions of the H-chain domains

All of the known biologic functions of antibody molecules are determined by the nature of the H chain; thus,

considerable attention has been focused on understanding the structure and functions of the individual immunoglobulin H-chain domains. Depending on the isotype of the antibody, the constant region of the H chain contains three or four C_H domains. Those antibodies that have three constant-region domains, namely the γ, α, and δ H chains of IgG, IgA, and IgD, respectively, also contain a flexible hinge region between C_H1 and C_H2, whereas those containing four constant-region domains, μ and ε, lack the flexible hinge. These two H chains have, instead, an additional constant-region domain, the C_H2 domain of these H chains, $C_\mu2$ or $C_\varepsilon2$, that substitutes for the hinge.

The first H-chain constant region, C_H1, lies within the Fab fragment and covalently associates with the C_L domain. This interaction is probably of great importance in allowing a diverse array of V_H and V_L regions to associate to form an antigen-binding site. During the development of B cells from committed progenitors, the variable regions of V_H and V_L are assembled from individual genes (called IGHV, IGHD, and IGHJ genes for H chains, IGKV and IGKJ for κ L chains, and IGLV and IGLJ for λ L chains) by a process of recombination to form complete variable regions. Because this process is random, the resulting V_H and V_L antibody domains produced in a single cell may not interact efficiently with one another, but the stabilizing effect

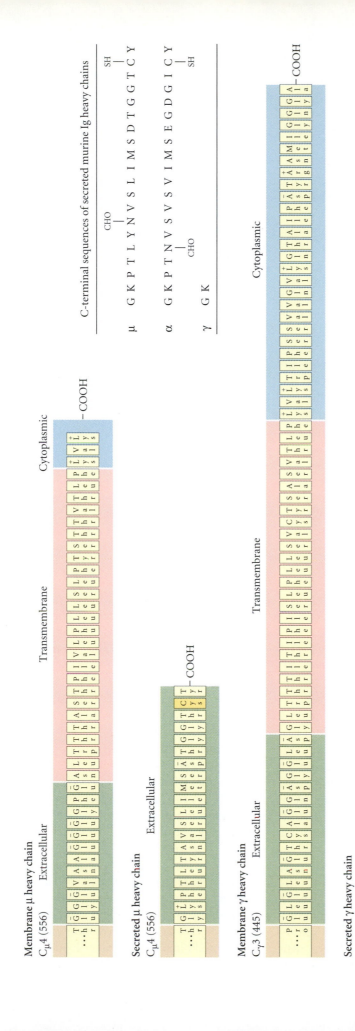

Figure 6.11 Comparison of carboxy termini of the integral membrane and secreted forms of the H chains of IgM and IgG. Amino acid sequences of the transmembrane regions and cytoplasmic tails of membrane μ and γ H chains are compared with the secretory tail pieces of the secreted μ and γ H chains. The different carboxy termini result from differential splicing from a precursor RNA species. A penultimate cysteine in the secreted μ H chain (highlighted) is involved in the interchain disulfide bonding for production of polymeric IgM.

of C_H-C_L interactions can serve to ensure the utilization of a higher number of combinations by B cells in the developing repertoire, thus increasing variability.

The C_H1 domain also plays an important role in the assembly of antibodies. Like other secretory proteins of the constitutive exocytic pathway, immunoglobulin H and L chains are synthesized at the rough endoplasmic reticulum (ER) and translocated into the ER lumen. During this process, molecular chaperones serve to facilitate the proper folding of the immunoglobulin proteins. Chaperone interactions with H chains also serve to prevent H-chain aggregation before their assembly, which occurs by the formation either of H_2 dimers and then H_2L_2 monomeric subunits or HL half-monomers prior to full monomer formation, depending on the isotype. In either case, H chains remain stably associated with the molecular chaperone BiP/GRP78 until HL pairing has occurred. This interaction occurs via sites in the C_H1 domain. Thus, the C_H1 domain serves as a component of the "quality control" mechanisms that ensures that only functional antigen-binding antibodies, comprising both H and L chains, are expressed as receptors on the B-cell surface or are secreted by antibody-secreting cells. Consequently, H chains, unlike L chains, are never secreted alone unless the C_H1 domain is absent. This occurs in certain disease states, in which the C_H1 domain is not properly spliced into the synthesized H chain and naturally occurs in one subclass of IgG antibodies found in camelid species. In the latter case, these single-chain antibodies appear to be used as functional components of the humoral immune system and serve as useful models for the generation of a new class of engineered antibodies.

The major biologic functions of antibody molecules, including transfer across the placenta, complement activation, and Fc-receptor binding, are defined by sequences within the Fc region of the appropriate H-chain isotypes. These sequences are normally encoded within the C_H2 and C_H3 domains or their equivalents, the C_H3 and C_H4 domains, in μ and ε chains. The binding site for the complement component C1q is present in the C_H2 domain (C_H3 for the μ chain) in those antibodies that activate complement (Table 6.2). Activation of the complement cascade leads to the opsonization and clearance of antigens. Other components are released during the activation of complement and serve as mediators of inflammation and enhance the efficiency of the immune response.

The Fc region, especially the hinge and C_H2 domains of IgG (or C_H2 and C_H3 of μ and ε chains), also plays an important role in interacting with Fc receptors. Fc receptors are expressed on a variety of cells, including cells of the innate immune system, such as macrophages, neutrophils, basophils, and natural killer (NK) cells. The binding of antigen-antibody complexes to Fc receptors on phagocytic cells leads to the opsonization of the antigen. Other important effector functions, such as destruction of antibody-bound targets by antibody-dependent cellular cytotoxicity, occur following the interactions with the Fc receptors on NK cells.

IgE also binds Fc receptors on certain cells, including mast cells and basophils, via interaction with binding sites on the ε chain. The interaction of antigen with the IgE on these cells leads to allergic reactions and to various protective responses against parasites. The Fc regions of some H chains also contain sites that are directly recognized and bound by specific bacterial proteins, for example, the protein A of *Staphylococcus aureus*. Whether this interaction represents an innate mechanism that allows an antibody to target bacteria nonspecifically or is a bacterial strategy for hampering its host's defenses can only be speculated.

IgG, IgE, and IgD are secreted as monomers in the conventional H_2L_2 monomeric form. However, IgM and IgA are usually (IgM) or frequently (IgA) secreted as polymers. The secreted form of both the μ and α chains contains an evolutionarily conserved secretory tailpiece that contains a penultimate cysteine residue (Fig. 6.11). Polymerization between monomeric subunits occurs via interchain disulfide bond formation involving these cysteines. J chain, a short polypeptide that is an important component of polymeric antibodies, is also linked to the antibody via this cysteine residue. The polymeric forms of IgM and IgA are crucial for their biologic functions. The secretory tailpiece also contains a second conserved motif, an asparagine-linked glycosylation site. This site is essential for proper polymerization, and recent data suggest that the presence of the carbohydrate is also important for biologic function.

The Hinge Region

The hinge region separates the Fab region from the Fc in γ, α, and δ chains. Hinges have no homology with immunoglobulin domains. The hinge regions contain cysteine residues that are involved in the disulfide bonding of the two H chains that form the H_2 of the immunoglobulin monomer. The hinge regions vary in length and are rich in proline, serine, and threonine residues. This amino acid composition gives hinges their flexibility, which in turn allows the Fab portion of immunoglobulin molecules to bend, flex, and rotate relative to the Fc region (Fig. 6.12A and B). Flexibility allows immunoglobulin molecules to bind epitopes on large antigens bivalently (Fig. 6.12C). The added flexibility afforded by the hinge region also makes it possible for the C_H2 domain in IgG to be exposed to mediators, such as C1q, or Fc receptors at the same time the antibody is bound to the antigen. Evidence for the importance of the hinge region comes from experiments using deletion

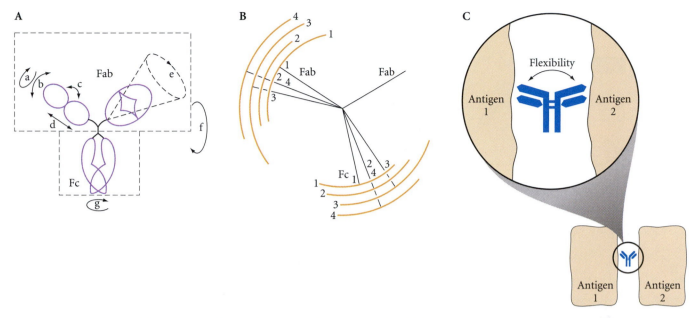

Figure 6.12 Diagrams showing the modes of flexibility of IgG. (**A**) (**a**) Rotation around the long axis; (**b**) bending to the hinge; (**c**) bending between the variable and first constant region; (**d**) compression; (**e**) "wagging"; (**f**) planar folding between Fab and Fc regions; (**g**) rotation of the Fc. (**B**) Comparison of the amount of flexibility around the hinge regions of the four human IgG subclasses (labeled 1, 2, 3, and 4). The straight lines show the angles that can be achieved between the two Fab arms and the Fc region. The partially circular lines indicate the potential distance traversed by the antigen-binding sites of different IgG subclasses. (**C**) Segmental flexibility of immunoglobulins can facilitate antigen binding when the antigen has steric constraints, e.g., large monovalent antigens. An antibody may be capable of binding to two such large antigens simultaneously if there is sufficient flexibility between the two Fab fragments. The bottom diagram shows the antigens and antibody at lower magnification to emphasize the large relative size of the antigen. (**A and B**) Adapted from K. H. Roux et al., *J. Immunol.* **159**:3372–3382, 1997, with permission.

mutants. When the hinge region is missing, important biologic activities, such as complement fixation, are lacking.

The J Chain

The J chain is a 15-kDa glycoprotein that is covalently associated with polymeric IgM and IgA. The association of J chain with these two polymeric antibodies is accomplished by disulfide bond formation between two specific cysteine residues on the J chain, Cys14 and Cys68, and the conserved cysteine residue in the secretory tailpiece of IgM and IgA. Most data are consistent with the presence of one, and only one, J chain per IgM or IgA polymer. Thus, the J chain "bridges" only two μ or two α chains in the secreted IgM or IgA polymer, respectively (Fig. 6.13).

IgM can be secreted as pentamers and hexamers, but the pentamer is the major form found in vivo. J chain is found only in the IgM pentamers and never in hexamers (Fig. 6.13) and is always found in the polymeric immunoglobulin in secretions. Recent studies using J-chain-deficient mice, produced by targeted disruption, have shown that J chain is required for the interaction of IgA, and presumably for IgM as well, with the polymeric immunoglobulin (poly-Ig) receptor that transports these

antibodies from the basal side of the epithelium, where the antibodies are made, through the epithelial cell and out onto the luminal side of the mucosal surface. Because of its important role in this process, J chain is crucial to the normal functioning of the secretory immune system.

At one time, it was believed that J chain was required for the formation of IgM and IgA polymers; it is now clear, however, that both types of polymers can be assembled and secreted by plasma cells in the complete absence of J chain. In IgM-secreting cells, J chain does not initiate the formation of the polymer but rather is added at a terminal step in IgM assembly, before the completed polymer is released from the ER to be transported out of the cell. Recent results suggest that J chain drives the preferential assembly of IgM pentamers, preventing hexamer production, in these cells. Although the reason for this is not clear, it may be that hexameric IgM has deleterious effects, perhaps because of its unusually high capacity for activating complement. J chain has recently been found in invertebrate species that do not have any immunoglobulins. This suggests that J chain is an evolutionarily conserved protein that may have evolved functions before its use as a component of polymeric antibodies.

A

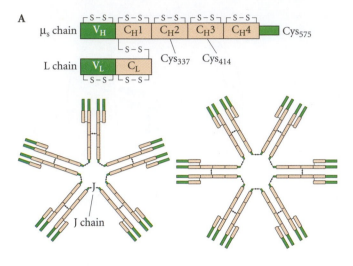

B

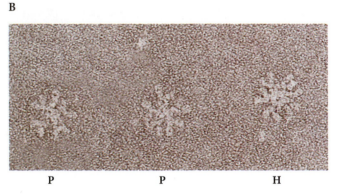

P   P   H

Figure 6.13 Structure of pentameric and hexameric IgM. (**A**) Diagrammatic representations of IgM. The top shows the domain structure of the covalently linked IgM H and L chains, the intradomain S-S bonds, and the free Cys residues used for interchain S-S bonding between monomeric and polymeric structures. The pentamer and hexamer are schematically represented. Note that the J chain is present only in the pentameric form of IgM. (**B**) Electron micrograph of IgM pentamers and hexamers. The average size of an extended IgM pentamer is 30 nanometers (nm). In this electron micrograph, 5 to 10 of the 10 binding sites of pentamers can be observed.

Membrane Forms of Antibodies: the B-Cell Receptor

Because major functions of antibodies are carried out in their secreted form, it is essential that cells capable of producing antibodies of the needed specificities be stimulated effectively during immune responses. The B-cell receptor complex evolved to accomplish this. This complex is composed of mIg and accessory proteins and has at least two functions. First, it serves as the receptor to select cells on the basis of their antigen specificity and thus contains a signaling function resulting in activation of the antigen-specific B cells following the binding of antigen. Second, antigen bound to surface antibodies is internalized efficiently for transport into endosomes, where the antigen is

introduced into the presentation pathway to associate with the major histocompatibility complex (MHC) class II antigen. This allows the B cells to act as antigen-presenting cells to stimulate antigen-specific T cells, helping to ensure specificity of the immune response and facilitating the activation of antigen-specific T and B cells.

mIg of all isotypes is noncovalently associated with two heterodimeric complexes of the Ig-α and Ig-β proteins (Fig. 6.14). Although the mIg lends specificity to the B-cell receptor complex, the Ig-α and Ig-β proteins form its active signaling component by interacting with important kinases (via their cytoplasmic tail regions) that initiate the activation of B cells. Ig-α and Ig-β are also important in the trafficking of newly synthesized mIg from the ER to the plasma membrane.

Glycosylation

Antibodies are glycoproteins and, as such, contain one or more types of carbohydrate modifications. All H chains are glycosylated, whereas L chains are not unless N-linked glycosylation motifs are present in the variable-region sequence. In the variable region, carbohydrate can affect the

Figure 6.14 Diagram of a B-cell receptor that is composed of the Ig molecule and two associated Ig-α/Ig-β complexes. The cytoplasmic tails of the Ig-αβ complexes are involved in recruitment of kinases responsible for the intracellular signal transduction following the binding of antigen to the mIg.

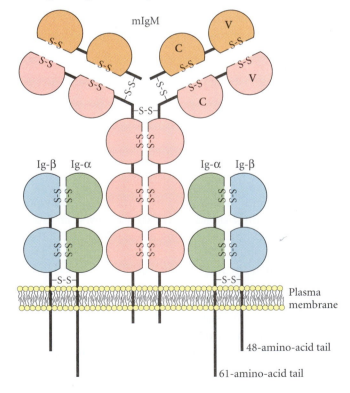

specificity of antigen binding. The role of carbohydrate on H chains is not well understood. As for other glycoproteins, it is possible that the carbohydrate content affects the stability of the molecule and influences the half-life of the protein in serum, although relevant data are conflicting. It is clear, however, that the elimination of the carbohydrate on H chains can affect antibody structure or function. For example, elimination of the N-linked glycosylation site in the C_H2 domain of IgG affects its ability to interact with C1q, suggesting that the carbohydrate plays an important role in sterically maintaining or exposing this site. As already mentioned, elimination of the N-linked glycosylation motif on the secretory tailpiece of IgM results in the incorrect formation of IgM polymers.

One of the IgA subclasses in humans, IgA1, is heavily O-glycosylated on serine residues in the hinge region. The presence of the carbohydrates is believed to protect the accessible hinge region from nonspecific proteases present in secretions lining mucosal surfaces. Interestingly, some pathogenic bacteria have evolved a protease (the IgA protease) that specifically cleaves the IgA1 hinge region, but the IgA2 hinge region is not affected by this protease.

Antigenic Determinants of Immunoglobulins

Immunoglobulins are glycoproteins and, as such, are potent immunogens when introduced into different species, where they are recognized as "foreign." Therefore, antibodies can be used to induce other antibodies by appropriate immunizations. These anti-antibodies proved to be extremely useful for initially characterizing antibody classes and subclasses and for elucidating the genetic relationships between immunoglobulin constant-region genes and variable regions before the genetic organization of immunoglobulin loci was understood. Anti-antibodies are still commonly used, for example, to determine concentrations of antibodies in serum or as experimental tools to gain insights into the regulation of immune responses.

Because antibodies are complex glycoproteins, different types of epitopes (antigenic determinants) can be recognized, depending on the immunization protocol used and the method of screening for anti-antibodies. The epitope types recognized fall into three broad classes, defined as isotypes, allotypes, and idiotypes. Each type is localized in specific ways on the immunoglobulin proteins to form different epitopes.

Antibody isotypes

Isotypic determinants define epitopes on the constant regions of antibody proteins. They distinguish each H-chain class (i.e., μ, δ, γ, α, and ε) and L-chain type (i.e., κ and λ) from one another within an individual species. Each member of the species normally will contain all isotypes within its genome and express them; as such, serum antibodies will always contain representatives of each combination of antibody class (e.g., IgM, κ; IgM, λ; and IgG, κ) unless an underlying genetic defect or an acquired defect caused by disease interferes with normal development or alters antibody expression or secretion.

Because the protein sequences of each class of antibody differ among species, anti-isotypic antibodies are produced by immunizing one species with the antibodies of another. Anti-isotypic antibodies can also recognize antibody subclasses. The five major classes of H chains and the two classes of L chains share only about 30% sequence homology, but subclasses are much more closely related, sharing 60 to 90% sequence identity. Thus, subclasses are believed to represent more recent gene duplication and divergence events in the diversification of the immunoglobulin loci. In support of this is the finding that the same distribution of subclasses is not found in all mammalian species. For example, humans have two functional genes for the α chain, IGHA1 and IGHA2, and thus have two subclasses of IgA, whereas mice have only one locus. Both mice and humans have four known γ-chain isotypes and therefore produce four different IgG subclasses, designated IgG1, IgG2, IgG3, and IgG4 in humans and as IgG1, IgG2a, IgG2b (which is closely related to IgG2a), and IgG3 in mice. Although these subclasses are highly related, they can be distinguished by differences in their biologic effector functions. In some cases, these have been directly attributable to differences in sequences in or near the binding sites for different effector molecules, such as C1q. In other cases, differences in hinge length and flexibility appear to alter the effector activities. L chains may also exhibit subtypes. For example, λ L-chain genes exist in multiple copies in humans and mice; consequently different λ L-chain isotypes exist.

Allotypes

Although each member of a species inherits the same complement of immunoglobulin isotypes, more than one allelic form of each gene may exist, a reflection of subtle genetic differences in the sequences of these genes. These allelic variants are transmitted according to standard Mendelian genetics. Anti-allotypic antibodies can readily be made by injecting one member of a species with an antibody exhibiting an allelic difference from another member of the same species. Anti-allotypic antibodies are commonly elicited in humans following transfusions of whole blood and are sometimes naturally produced during pregnancy.

In general, allotypes reflect differences in the constant-region sequences of individual genes. In some species, however, variable-region allotypes have also been defined. In humans, allotypic variants are known for each of the IgG subclasses, for IgA2 and IgE, and for κ L chains. The standard system for naming human immunoglobulin allotypes uses the designations G1m, G2m, G3m, A2m, and Em to refer to allelic forms of the genes encoding the H chains of IgG1, IgG2, IgG3, IgA2, and IgE, respectively [G1m(f) is a practical example of this nomenclature system, referring to allele "f" of the gene encoding the γ-1 H chain]. The same system uses the designation Km (previously called Inv) to refer to allelic forms of the gene encoding the κ L chain. Numerous studies have been conducted to compare the relative quantities of the different allotypic forms of antibodies present in human serum and to determine whether any of the allelic forms are associated with protective or non-protective immune function. Such studies show that certain allotypic forms of immunoglobulin H chains are present in the serum in higher concentrations than other allotypic forms, owing to a greater percentage of B cells producing those allotypic forms and to a longer in vivo half-life of some allotypic forms.

Idiotypic determinants

Idiotypic determinants are found in the variable regions of antibody molecules. Because of the almost limitless sequence diversity found in the variable regions of antibody H and L chains, it is not surprising that these regions not only form to bind antigen but also can elicit antibody responses themselves. Each antibody V_H-V_L combination may possess many idiotypic determinants (or idiotopes); the combination of the idiotopes is referred to as the *idiotype*. Idiotypic determinants are formed by the folding of the V_H and V_L regions and may be expressed on individual V_H or V_L regions; they may also be formed by combinations of V_H and V_L. Thus, idiotypic determinants may represent sequences integral to the combining site or unique structural features of the Fd region that is not part of the antigen-combining site. As a result, anti-idiotypic antibodies that bind to idiotopes involved in antigen binding can inhibit binding, whereas idiotypic antibodies directed to epitopes outside the antigen-binding site do not inhibit binding.

Because of the clonal nature of the antibody response, both membrane and secreted antibodies derived from a single clone of cells will express identical idiotypes unless the cells have undergone somatic hypermutation and altered their sequence during the humoral response. However, because of the diversity of the variable regions in an animal, few antibodies will share idiotypes. Thus, progeny of individual clones can be followed using anti-idiotypic antibodies, a procedure that has proven invaluable in delineating certain features of B-cell responses to antigens.

Anti-idiotypic antibodies are generally produced experimentally by immunizing different species or genetically different individuals of the same species with a monoclonal antibody and then selecting for the anti-idiotypic specificities by eliminating anti-isotypic or anti-allotypic antibodies or by selecting the appropriate antibodies using hybridoma technology. Under certain circumstances, however, idiotypic determinants can also be immunogenic in the same individual in which they are expressed; for example, if the concentration of the antibody expressing the idiotype reaches a certain minimum threshold value. Most antibody variable regions are expressed at concentrations below those required to elicit a detectable immune response and do not activate the accessory functions necessary to generate a detectable immune response. However, under certain experimental conditions, in which very high antibody responses of restricted specificities have been elicited, animals have been shown to generate anti-idiotypic antibodies to antibodies used early in the response. The frequency with which this occurs is not known, and it is not clear what physiologic consequences, if any, this may have on immune responses to foreign antigens. One possible role for idiotype–anti-idiotype interactions may be in the generation of early immune repertoires.

Classification of Antibodies
Antibody Classes and Their Functions

Antibodies bind antigen; however, only in rare cases, such as the neutralization of a toxin before it poisons a cell, does this binding event per se effectively inactivate a pathogenic process. In all other cases, antibody binding is only the first in a cascade of events that lead to antigen elimination. The elimination of antigens is initiated by the biologic activities of antibodies, which are properties of the H-chain constant regions. These functions are summarized in Table 6.2, and the structures of the different H chains are shown in Fig. 6.15.

IgM

IgM is the first isotype secreted in immune responses and is the isotype expressed on primary B cells that have recently emerged from the fetal liver or the bone marrow. As a cell surface receptor, IgM is expressed in monomeric form, as are all B-cell receptors irrespective of isotype. Following the binding of antigen and stimulation of B cells by mitogens or activated T cells, B cells enlarge, enter the cell cycle, and may differentiate into plasma cells,

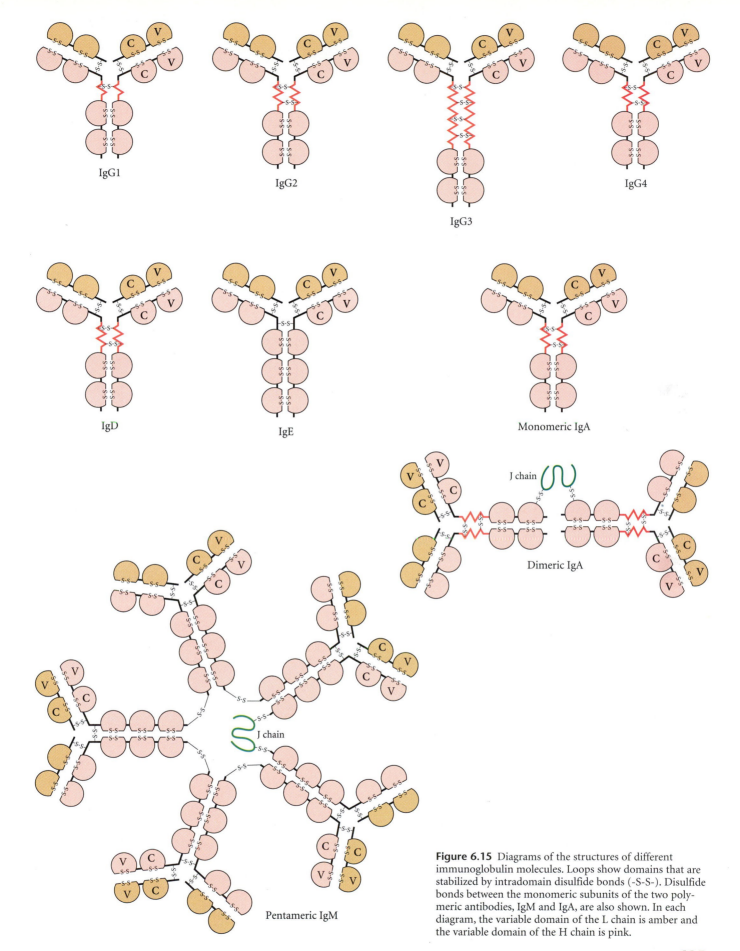

Figure 6.15 Diagrams of the structures of different immunoglobulin molecules. Loops show domains that are stabilized by intradomain disulfide bonds (-S-S-). Disulfide bonds between the monomeric subunits of the two polymeric antibodies, IgM and IgA, are also shown. In each diagram, the variable domain of the L chain is amber and the variable domain of the H chain is pink.

135

which are factories for high-rate synthesis and secretion of antibodies of the appropriate class. At least some of the progeny of the clone derived from primary or naive B cells will secrete IgM, whereas others may undergo the process of isotype switching and secrete antibody with the same antigen-binding site but with different H-chain constant regions: either α, γ, or ε.

IgM accounts for 5 to 10% of the total serum immunoglobulin and is found in concentrations ranging from 0.5 to 1.5 milligrams per milliliter (mg/ml). Serum IgM usually binds its antigen with very low affinity because most is secreted before affinity maturation and selection, which changes the affinity of the variable region for the selecting antigen. As much as one-third of serum IgM also is polyreactive, meaning that these antibodies can bind to and clear a number of antigens even if these are not the antigens that elicited their secretion. Polyreactive antibodies generally have a low affinity for these multiple antigens.

Secreted IgM is almost polymeric in form, and most of the IgM polymers are pentameric, giving it 10 antigen-binding sites per IgM molecule. Therefore, while IgM generally has a low affinity for antigen, its *avidity* is generally higher because of its ability to bind antigen multivalently. This may be the basis for binding of polyreactive IgM antibodies to multiple, unrelated antigens. IgM is very important in primary immune responses because of its high capacity for activating the complement cascade. In contrast to IgG, which requires at least two molecules bound to antigen in sufficiently close proximity to activate complement, IgM requires only one molecule because of its binding to C1q. This can be very important in initiating the clearance of pathogens before higher-affinity antibodies are generated. C1q has low average affinity for its binding site on immunoglobulins (in IgM, this site is found in the C_H3 domain, the homolog of C_H2 in IgG), but the ability to bind multivalently significantly increases the affinity, resulting in the activation of other components of the complement cascade. Whereas IgM itself does not bind Fc receptors on phagocytic cells, the target antigen can nonetheless be opsonized by the interaction of the complement components deposited on the antigen with complement receptors on phagocytes. For example, complement receptor 1 (CR1, CD35) interacts with C3b and C4b, and recent evidence indicates that this receptor also binds C1q. Thus, through the complement system, IgM can be a potent opsonin.

Recent evidence suggests that IgM is also important in the initiation of the adaptive immune response. Antigen-IgM complexes bound to follicular dendritic cells, together with attached complement components, appear to be very important in the activation of B cells. Presumably the IgM antibodies are present due to polyreactivity or perhaps production of IgM antibody induced by environmental exposures that cross-reacts with antigens activating adaptive responses. The antigen components of such IgM immune complexes interact with the B-cell antigen receptor, whereas C3b and C3d fragments in the immune complexes interact with the CD19 and CD21 B-cell coreceptors. Thus, the presence of complement fragments in the immune complexes effectively lowers the threshold of antigen required to stimulate B cells. These interactions may also be crucial for the formation and propagation of germinal centers, environments within the spleen and lymph nodes essential for somatic mutation and expansion.

IgM can be found in secretions at mucosal surfaces and in breast milk, although at much lower concentrations than IgA. This appears to be due to recognition of J chain by the poly-Ig receptor present on the basal side of mucosal epithelial cells that transports the IgM out onto the mucosal surface (see Fig. 6.16), although little direct information concerning the molecular details of this interaction is available.

It has recently been found that IgM can be secreted as hexamers. IgM hexamers lack J chain but contain a sixth monomeric μ_2L_2 subunit. Of interest is the finding that IgM hexamers are at least 10 to 20 times more efficient at activating complement than are IgM pentamers. IgM hexamers are normally found only in extremely small quantities in normal serum; consequently the physiologic function of IgM hexamers remains unclear. However, the recent findings that IgM hexamers may be abundant in some IgM-mediated autoimmune diseases may indicate that hexamers have deleterious effects, perhaps as a consequence of their high capacity for activating complement.

IgG and IgG subclasses

IgG is the most abundant immunoglobulin in serum, accounting for approximately 80% of the total of serum antibodies, with normal serum concentrations being 10 mg/ml or higher. In humans, IgG1 is the most abundant of the subclasses and IgG4 is the least abundant (Table 6.2).

IgG antibodies of high affinity can inactivate viruses directly or neutralize bacterial toxins by their binding. However, most biologic effects of IgG antibodies are elicited through their interaction with complement or Fc receptors on various cell types. A major function of IgG is to activate the classical complement pathway. Although C1q interacts rather weakly with the Fc region of individual IgG molecules—with an affinity of only 100

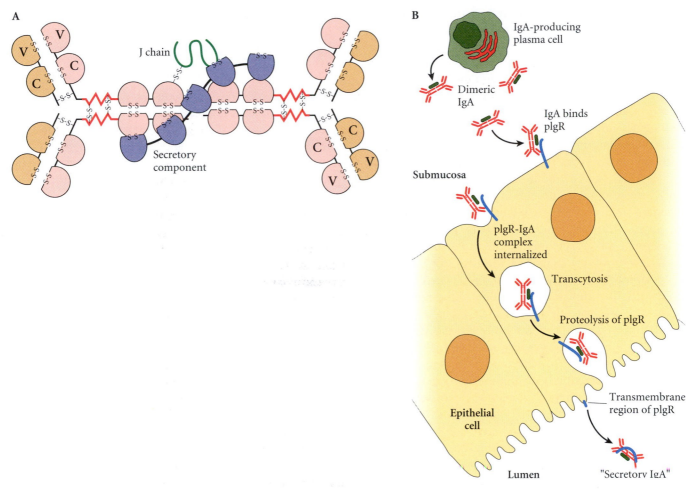

Figure 6.16 Structure and function of secretory IgA. (A) Structure of dimeric IgA as found in the secretions showing the presence of secretory component, which helps protect the polymeric molecule from proteolysis. (B) Schematic diagram showing the formation of secretory IgA by mucosal plasma cells. This dimeric IgA is bound by the poly-Ig receptor owing to the presence of J chain. The poly-Ig receptor–IgA complex is transported from the apical to the basolateral surface of the epithelial cell, where the IgA is released following the cleavage of the poly-Ig receptor. The cleaved portion of the poly-Ig receptor that remains covalently associated with IgA is the secretory component.

μM—the binding affinity is significantly increased if multiple IgG molecules are bound close together to epitopes on the antigenic surface. When such binding occurs, the aggregates of the IgG molecules facilitate the binding of multiple C1q molecules, interacting with a subset of the six C1q heads connected by a collagen-like stem to a central stalk. This increases the affinity of IgG for C1q to as much as 10 nM, initiating the activation of subsequent components of the complement cascade. However, not all subclasses of IgG are equally effective at activating complement. In humans, both IgG1 and IgG3 activate complement very effectively. Although IgG3 binds C1q most avidly, it is not always better than IgG1 at activating complement, perhaps because of a decreased

segmental flexibility around the hinge region or unknown factors that may influence complement activation. In humans, neither IgG2 nor IgG4 binds C1q, and this failure has been directly attributed to sequence differences in the C_H2 domain. Traditionally, human IgG2 has been thought to be able to activate complement from species other than humans, such as rabbits, under experimental conditions. However, IgG2 can activate human complement when bound to some polyvalent antigens, such as bacterial surface polysaccharides where the presence of a highly repetitive basic structure leads to the presence of high-density identical epitopes on the antigens' surface. The activation of complement by IgG1 and IgG3 increases their ability to act as potent opsonins.

In addition to activating complement, IgG also binds to Fc receptors, a property that considerably increases the range of effector functions carried out by several of the IgG subclasses. For example, IgG1 and IgG3 and, to a lesser extent, IgG4, but not IgG2, bind to the high-affinity Fc receptor, FcγR type I (FcγRI, or CD64). This receptor can bind to uncomplexed IgG, is constitutively expressed on monocytes and macrophages, and can be induced on neutrophils by interferon-gamma. IgG also can interact with two other types of Fcγ receptors, FcγRII (CD32) and FcγRIII (CD16), both of which interact effectively only with immune complexes of antigen and IgG. These receptors are broadly expressed on myeloid and other cell types, and thus the interactions with IgG can lead to numerous biologic activities. For example, the interaction of antigen-antibody complexes with FcγR on phagocytic cells can lead to increased opsonization, which can occur even without complement activation (although complement increases the effect). The interaction of IgG with FcγRIIB, an FcγR expressed on B cells, leads to the inhibition of B-cell responsiveness when antigen is cross-linked to both the FcγRIIB and the B-cell receptor. Finally, the interaction of IgG bound to target cells with the FcγRIII receptor on NK cells leads to death of the target cell through a process called *antibody-dependent-cellular cytotoxicity.*

IgG antibodies are also important in protecting the unborn fetus. All IgGs are capable of crossing the placenta (albeit with different efficiencies) and thus can confer immunity to antigens to which the mother has been exposed. Placental transfer of IgG keeps the immune system of the fetus from responding to those antigens to which maternal antibody has been transferred. This nonresponsive state decreases over time as the maternal IgG is catabolized, and by 6 to 12 months of age most of the maternal antibody is gone. Under normal circumstances, transplacental antibody appears to be important for the normal development of the immune system. Similarly, several IgG subclasses can bind to an unusual FcγR found

in the gut (FcRn), which, in experimental animals, has been shown to permit transfer of IgG from maternal milk across the intestinal epithelium. This receptor has recently been implicated as important in the homeostatic regulation of IgG serum levels. FcRn interacts with IgG through the interface of the C_H2 and C_H3 domains.

In the mouse, all of the effector functions mentioned above are also carried out by the various IgG subclasses (Table 6.4). As in the human, all four of the mouse IgG subclasses are capable of being transferred to developing fetuses during pregnancy. There are several minor differences in the effector functions of the mouse subclasses compared to the human subclasses. Whereas human IgG1 and IgG3 are capable of activating the classical complement cascade and of binding to macrophage Fc receptors, in the mouse only IgG2a has these activities. Interestingly, mouse IgG1 has the ability to bind to the high-affinity IgE receptor present on the surface of basophils and macrophages. Thus, in the mouse, mast cell degranulation can be triggered by either IgE or IgG1. This is in marked contrast to the human immune system, where mast cell degranulation is only triggered by IgE. These differences in activity make it difficult to draw analogies between mouse and human IgG subclasses.

IgA and IgA subclasses

IgA represents only 10 to 15% of serum antibodies, but the amount of IgA synthesized and secreted is greater than that of any other immunoglobulin class. Most of the IgA is produced by IgA-secreting plasma cells concentrated below mucous membrane surfaces. IgA is the dominant isotype in secretions (e.g., tears, salivary glands, bile), and most of the IgA synthesized is secreted by the lymphoid tissues located in the submucosal area of mucosal surfaces. Following secretion from plasma cells, the IgA is transported onto the mucosal surface. Like IgM, IgA is secreted in polymeric form, but IgA exists predominantly as dimers, with smaller amounts of trimers or tetramers. The majority of these polymers contain the

Table 6.4 Comparison of the effector functions of IgG subclasses of humans and mice

Effector function	Human				Mouse			
	IgG1	IgG2	IgG3	IgG4	IgG1	IgG2a	IgG2b	IgG3
Complement activation: classical pathway	Yes	No[a]	Yes	No	No	Yes	No	No
Complement activation: alternative pathway	No	No[a]	No	No	No	No	No	No
Binds to macrophage Fc receptors	Yes	No[a]	Yes	No	No	Yes	No	No
Crosses placenta	Yes	Yes	Yes	Yes	Yes	Yes	Yes	Yes
Present in secretions	No	No	No	No	No	No	No	No
Induces mast cell deregulation	No	No	No	No	Yes	No	No	No

[a] The ability of human IgG2 to activate complement has been controversial, but data now appear to show definitively that it is incapable of activating complement.

J-chain protein. However, unlike IgM, IgA also is secreted at significant levels as monomers, and much of the serum IgA is present in this form. In secretions, however, essentially all of the IgA is polymeric.

IgA is transported into secretions as a result of its interaction with the poly-Ig receptor (Fig. 6.16). This receptor is present on the basolateral surface of epithelial cells and binds polymeric antibodies containing J chain. When IgA is bound to the poly-Ig receptor, the complex is internalized by receptor-mediated endocytosis. The receptor, with its intact antibody, is transported in vesicles through the epithelial cell to the apical surface, where the vesicle fuses with the apical membrane. The poly-Ig receptor is cleaved enzymatically, releasing the bound antibody together with a fragment of the receptor called *secretory component*. Secretory component remains associated with the IgA through a covalent attachment with one of the α chains.

Secretory component helps protect the protease-sensitive sites in the IgA hinge region from proteolysis. The high susceptibility of the IgA hinge to proteolysis may contribute to the short serum half-life of IgA monomers. In secretions, protection from proteolysis is of critical importance to the function of IgA, which is constantly exposed to bacterial and host proteases. The hinge of IgA1 is heavily O-glycosylated, a factor that also may protect this subclass from proteolysis. Of interest is the evolution of an "IgA protease" in several bacterial species that cleaves this hinge. Presumably the IgA protease counteracts host defenses on mucosal surfaces, although it has been difficult to obtain direct evidence for this. For example, although *Neisseria gonorrhoeae*, the causative agent of gonorrhea, produces an IgA1 protease, its activity could not be detected in the cervical secretions of women with gonorrhea, and experimental infection of male volunteers with a mutant that did not make IgA1 protease did not reveal any decreased ability of the mutant bacterial strain to cause infection. However, because humans have a second class of IgA, IgA2, which lacks sites sensitive to the bacterial IgA1 protease, many have speculated that the microbial proteases may have been the selective pressure that led to the evolution of the IGHA2 gene in humans that encodes for the α_2 H chain.

IgA likely participates in the first line of defense against pathogens that enter through the mucosal surfaces, since IgA is found in all external secretions of the gastrointestinal tract, the mucosal surfaces of the pulmonary tract, and urogenital tracts. However, lack of production of IgA does not seem to greatly affect the susceptibility of humans to infection. IgA immunodeficiency is common in certain populations (1 in 625 Scandinavians lacks IgA), and the vast majority of these individuals do not manifest any increased susceptibility to infection. Presumably, the IgM and IgG present on mucosal surfaces, although in much lower amounts than IgA, can compensate for its loss. However, when it is present, IgA can be an important component of mucosal immunity. Because IgA is polymeric, secretory IgA can cross-link pathogens with multiple epitopes, thus enhancing the ability of IgA to prevent pathogens from moving to the part of the body they prefer to infect. The binding of IgA to bacterial and viral pathogens can inhibit attachment at mucosal surfaces and thus prevent infection. Complexes of IgA and antigen also are easily entrapped within the mucous lining of the mucosal surface and eliminated by ciliated epithelial cells of the respiratory tract or by peristalsis of the gut. IgA also likely plays an important role in protection of the newborn, since it is actively transported across breast epithelium into milk. It helps protect infants from infections until their own humoral immune system has matured.

IgE

IgE is found at extremely low concentrations in the serum, and most of the secreted IgE is bound by high-affinity IgE receptor (FcεRI) present on tissue-based mast cells and basophils in the serum. Receptor-bound IgE is very stable and survives for extended periods. When engaged by antigen on the surface of these cells, multiple IgE molecules are cross-linked, leading to the release of cytoplasmic granules (degranulation) and their stored contents from the mast cells and basophils. The granules are filled with potent inflammatory agents and vasoactive compounds including histamines, slow-reacting substances of anaphylaxis, and other mediators of strong physiologic reactions. These mediators can lead to anaphylaxis, a potentially lethal response if systemic anaphylaxis is elicited, as well as to allergies and asthma in susceptible individuals; the prevalence of both of these conditions is increasing in Western nations.

The main function for IgE is believed to be in immune responses to certain parasites, such as nematodes, where mast cells and eosinophils are particularly important mediators of immunity. The primary protective effect is probably due to the degranulation of the cells caused by cross-linking of FcεRI upon the binding of antigen to two or more IgE molecules. In these cases, the granule contents are felt to mediate protective immunity, a process that goes awry in IgE-mediated allergic responses. It is also possible that IgE bound to eosinophils in tissues infected with large, multicellular parasites mediates direct destruction of these parasites. Since nematodes and similar parasites are much too large to be phagocytosed or lysed by complement, an alternative means for their destruction is needed.

IgD

Among the immunoglobulin subclasses, IgD is present at the second lowest concentration in serum, and it has no known functions in the serum. Indeed, in some animals such as mice, defects in the δ gene prevent secretion of IgD, yet no defects are known to be associated with a lack of serum IgD. IgD is present as a surface receptor on all mature IgM-positive B cells, and numerous studies attest to a function for IgD in B-cell activation. Like IgM, membrane IgD is associated with Ig-α and Ig-β, and B cells can be activated through surface IgD. It has been postulated that the hinge of IgD permits more flexible binding, since this hinge is lacking in IgM, and thus may increase the ability of the B cell to cross-link antigen with its surface B-cell receptor. However, the precise role for IgD in B-cell function is unknown and is the subject of active controversy.

Nonmammalian Immunoglobulin Isotypes

The study of humoral immunity usually focuses on antibodies of mice and humans, and with good reason. Knowledge of the human immune system is of obvious import to those involved in the fields of medicine or related health sciences, and the mouse immune system has provided the model system that serves as the very foundation of modern immunology. Nevertheless, from a functional standpoint as well as an evolutionary one, it is informative to consider the structure and function of antibody isotypes that are uniquely found in species other than humans and mice.

IgY

One of the most well-studied nonmammalian immunoglobulin isotypes is IgY, which is found in avian, amphibian, and reptilian species. Like the immunoglobulins of mice and humans, IgY consists of two immunoglobulin H chains and two immunoglobulin L chains. However, IgY exists in two structural forms. One form is larger than human and murine IgG and similar in size to IgM, whereas the second form is smaller than mammalian IgG. Although the relationship between these two forms has not been resolved by conventional biochemical approaches, examinations of the gene and its cDNA have shown that the two forms of IgY are generated by alternative splicing of a single IgY upsilon H-chain RNA transcript. Comparisons of the nucleotide sequences of avian upsilon chain with H chains of mouse and human antibodies suggest that avian IgY is more similar to mammalian IgE than to any other

mammalian isotype. In avian and reptilian species, IgY probably functions together with IgM as the primary serum immunoglobulins, in much the same way that IgM and IgG function as the primary serum immunoglobulins in mice and humans.

IgX

Another nonmammalian immunoglobulin isotype that has been identified is the isotype IgX found in amphibians and cartilaginous fish. Structurally, IgX (sometimes called IgR) is similar to IgM, with one variable domain and four constant domains per H chain. (Note: care should be taken in reviewing the literature on IgX, as this name has frequently been used as a temporary designation for various, newly discovered immunoglobulin isotypes and isoforms, most of which are completely unrelated to the isotype formally named IgX.) Like the avian upsilon chain, the H chain of IgX can be found in many forms derived from alternative RNA processing. Plasma cells secreting IgX are typically found lining the various mucosal surfaces, especially those of the gut. It is therefore assumed that IgX plays a protective role in amphibians analogous to the protective role of human and mouse IgA.

IgW, NAR, and IgNARC

Among the species that have been found to possess a humoral acquired immune system, cartilaginous fish are the most ancient. The humoral immunity of these species is therefore likely to represent an evolutionary branch point that gave rise to the more recently evolved humoral immune systems of mammals. The study of humoral immunity in cartilaginous fish has revealed the presence in these species of three classes of immunoglobulin and immunoglobulin-like proteins: IgW, NAR, and IgNARC. These proteins were discovered in 1996 by a number of workers who used the RACE (rapid amplification of cDNA ends) technique to identify immunoglobulin-like gene products.

The structure of IgW is similar to canonical immunoglobulins (two H chains and two L chains). However, the IgW H chain is unusually long, consisting of six C_H domains in addition to the V_H-chain domain. Despite its unusual size, sequence analysis of IgW suggests that the quaternary structure of IgW seems to be maintained by a series of interchain disulfide binds similar to those found in immunoglobulin isotypes of other species. The first constant domain of IgW H chain has a high degree of homology with the IgM C_H1 domain and thus likely participates in H-chain–L-chain pairing, while both the fourth and sixth C_H domains have cysteine residues in positions favorable for inter-H-chain disulfide bond formation.

Among the most exciting findings regarding the evolution of humoral immunity was the discovery and characterization of NAR (which stands for nurse shark antigen receptor or new antigen receptor). NAR can be best described as an immunoglobulin-like protein, as it possesses an immunoglobulin domain structure, including a variable domain responsible for antigen binding. Sequence analysis reveals that NARs are equally divergent from both immunoglobulins and T-cell antigen receptors. This suggests that NARs may be the evolutionary precursors of both of the latter antigen receptors and one of the evolutionarily early members of the immunoglobulin superfamily.

Unlike canonical immunoglobulin, NAR is a single-chain protein (i.e., it is analogous to an immunoglobulin H chain, lacking association with immunoglobulin L chain). It has long been theorized that "classical" immunoglobulins evolved the H-chain–L-chain structure as a means of increasing their diversity of antigen binding, since different combinations of H chains and L chains allow for a smaller number of genes to encode for proteins, with an overall greater diversity in antigen binding. If true, one would expect single-chain antibodies like NARs to be a distinct disadvantage in terms of diversity. However, NARs appear to show extensive diversity, and a single-chain IgG isotype has been found in camelids that appears to participate in adaptive immune responses. That such immunoglobulins exist in nature (and that they are functional in antigen binding) suggests that, for certain species, single-chain antibodies such as NARs are sufficient to mediate protective immunity against infection.

In summary, while much can be learned from the study of mouse and human immunoglobulin isotypes, it is important to bear in mind that mammalian immunoglobulin isotypes are only two current solutions to the age-old problem of the protection of self from microbial invaders. Organisms representing each branch of the phylogenetic tree have been "experimenting" throughout their evolution to find the optimal antigen-binding molecule for their purposes. Evidence for this sort of evolutionary experimentation is clearly visible in sequence homologies that exist among immunoglobulins of different species, indicating that the various isotypes that exist today are the result of the duplication and divergence of ancestral proteins. Similar evolutionary events not only have led to the optimization of antigen-binding characteristics of immunoglobulins but also have served to exploit the structural and functional features of immunoglobulins for purposes other than antigen binding.

The Immunoglobulin Superfamily

Sequence analysis of immunoglobulin variable and constant regions revealed similarities and the conservation of certain amino acid residues at defined locations, which led to the idea that immunoglobulin domains may have evolved from a single primordial gene. Through gene duplication and subsequent diversification, the production of multidomain proteins such as immunoglobulins became feasible. The domain hypothesis was established when X-ray crystallographic studies revealed a common fold among different but related immunoglobulin-like proteins. This fold is formed by two β-pleated sheets stabilized by a conserved disulfide bond and is now known as the immunoglobulin fold. Moreover, the resolution of the genetic organization of the immunoglobulin gene supported the domain hypothesis since it was revealed that each immunoglobulin domain was encoded by a separate exon, supporting the idea that these domains evolved by gene duplication events.

It is now clear that a large number of proteins use the immunoglobulin domain as the basic building block for their structure (Fig. 6.17). The first nonimmunoglobulin protein shown to contain an immunoglobulin domain was β_2-microglobulin, which is a small protein of about 100 amino acids that is a component of MHC class I proteins. The β_2-microglobulin immunoglobulin domain shares amino acid sequence similarities with other proteins possessing immunoglobulin domains, and X-ray crystallography revealed that the three-dimensional structure of the immunoglobulin domain is conserved. A large number of proteins are now known to fall into this category; most are composed of multiple immunoglobulin domains (Fig. 6.16). Together, these proteins make up the immunoglobulin superfamily. Inclusion in this family requires that the proteins not only have sequences similar to immunoglobulin domains but share key structural features of the immunoglobulin fold as well. Obviously, not all of the proteins have been crystallized; thus, computer analysis for predicting structures is used to assign proteins as members of the immunoglobulin superfamily. However, the methods used for inclusion have clearly been validated by the data for those proteins that have been crystallized.

Proteins that are members of the immunoglobulin superfamily may be secreted or membrane bound, and many of them play important roles in recognition functions in the immune system, as exemplified by antibodies,

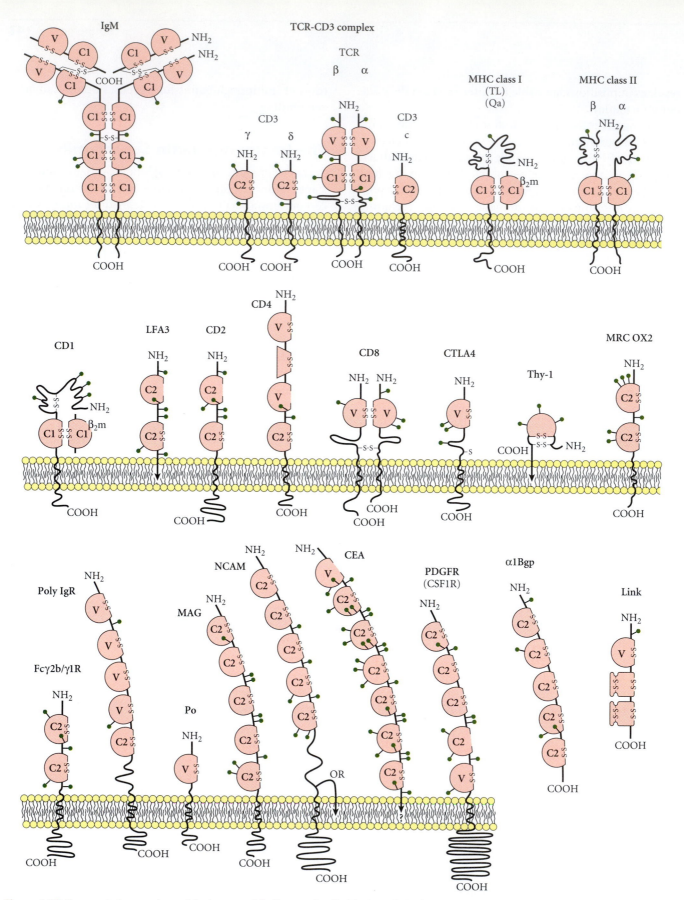

Figure 6.17 Representative members of the immunoglobulin superfamily. The intrachain disulfide bonds are shown, and asparagine (N)-linked glycosylation sites are shown as spikes on the glycoproteins. V and C1 denote domains most homologous to Ig domains, whereas C2 domains are more divergent.

the MHC molecules, and the T-cell receptor. Others, such as adhesion molecules, are involved in cell-cell interactions. Although many are involved in immune function, not all members of this family fall into this category. However, the involvement of most of them in recognition functions of some kind suggests that the immunoglobulin domain has been particularly successful in building molecules for these functions. Indeed, the immunoglobulin superfamily is the largest gene family yet identified and one in which the members possess diverse functions. The identification of members of this family in species from insects to humans suggests that the usefulness of the immunoglobulin domain for protein building was accepted (in evolutionary terms) millions of years ago.

Suggested Reading

Bengten, E., M. Wilson, N. Miller, L. W. Clem, L. Pilstrom, and G. W. Warr. 2000. Immunoglobulin isotypes: structure, function, and genetics. *Curr. Top. Microbiol. Immunol.* **248:**189–219.

Brummendorf, T., and V. Lemmon. 2001. Immunoglobulin superfamily receptors: cis-interactions, intracellular adapters and alternative splicing regulate adhesion. *Curr. Opin. Cell Biol.* **13:**611–618.

Casali, P. E., and W. Schettino. 1996. Structure and function of natural antibodies. *Curr. Top. Microbiol. Immunol.* **210:**167–179.

Crowe, J. E., Jr., R. O. Suara, S. Brock, N. Kallewaard, F. House, and J. H. Weitkamp. 2001. Genetic and structural determinants of virus neutralizing antibodies. *Immunol. Res.* **23:**135–145.

Fearon, D. T., and M. C. Carroll. 2000. Regulation of B lymphocyte responses to foreign and self-antigens by the CD19/CD21 complex. *Annu. Rev. Immunol.* **18:**393–422.

Jefferis, R., and J. Lund. 2002. Interaction sites on human IgG-Fc for Fc gamma receptors: current models. *Immunol. Lett.* **82:**57–65.

Johansen, F. E., R. Braathen, and P. Brandtzaeg. 2000. Role of J chain in secretory immunoglobulin formation. *Scand. J. Immunol.* **52:**240–248.

Padlan, E. A. 1996. X-ray crystallography of antibodies. *Adv. Protein Chem.* **49:**57–133.

Pilstrom, L. 2002. The mysterious immunoglobulin light chain. *Dev. Comp. Immunol.* **26:**207–215.

Preud'homme, J. L., I. Petit, A. Barra, F. Morel, J. C. Lecron, and E. Lelievre. 2000. Structural and functional properties of membrane and secreted IgD. *Mol. Immunol.* **37:**871–887.

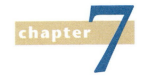

Molecular Genetics of Antibody Diversity

Guillermo E. Taccioli

Observations and Theories Predating Molecular Genetics of Immunoglobulin Genes

One of the most remarkable challenges of the vertebrate immune system is its need to recognize and respond to a virtually unlimited array of antigens. The vast diversity of the antibodies generated by B cells derives largely from the fact that the variable portion of these molecules is assembled differently in each individual lymphocyte using a large number of individual genes. Designation of each of the variable-region genetic components as *genes* is relatively recent, so in much of the immunology literature these are referred to as genetic fragments or gene segments. A similar mechanism is used by T lymphocytes to produce the T-cell antigen receptor (TCR). Despite the functional differences between these two antigen receptors, the molecular processes involved in their generation are almost identical.

Immunoglobulin molecules are homodimers of two identical subunits, with each subunit composed of a heavy (H) chain and a light (L) chain and held together by disulfide bonds. Each of these protein chains has a variable region that forms a part of the antigen-binding site and a constant region that contributes stability to the structure of the antibody and mediates the effector functions of the antibody. In contrast to immunoglobulin molecules, TCR molecules have only been detected anchored to the cell membrane of lymphocytes.

The formation of antibodies was first predicted in 1894 by Paul Ehrlich in his "side-chain hypothesis" (Fig. 7.1A). In a remarkable display of foresight, Ehrlich proposed that B cells possess on their surface a number of different side chains

A

B

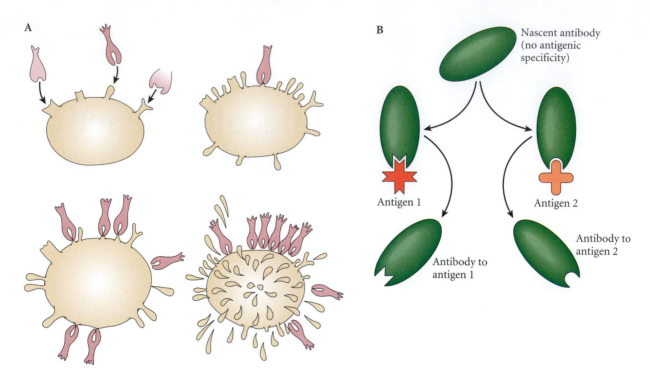

Figure 7.1 Early theories of antibody production. (**A**) Ehrlich's side-chain hypothesis. Ehrlich proposed that B cells possess on their surface a number of different side chains (analogous to antigen receptors) formed by the B cell before its encounter with antigen, each with the ability to bind to a unique antigen. Binding of a foreign body to one side chain would trigger overproduction of and secretion of that particular side chain. (**B**) The instructive hypothesis states that a nascent antibody is a "blank template" with no antigenic specificity at all. Upon its first encounter with antigen, the antibody adopts a conformation permitting specific binding to that particular antigen.

(analogous to antigen receptors) formed by the B cell before it encounters antigen, each side chain having the ability to bind to a unique antigen. Furthermore, he proposed that binding of a foreign body to one side chain would trigger overproduction and secretion of that particular side chain. This idea of antigen-induced selection of side chains is similar to the present view of the clonal selection of antigen-specific B cells proposed in the late 1950s by David Talmage and Frank Macfarlane Burnet.

The seminal studies of Karl Landsteiner in 1936 showed that the immune system has the potential to interact with an almost unlimited array of antigens. The fact that many antigens used by Landsteiner were artificial compounds generated debate among immunologists about the mechanism by which antibodies acquire antigen specificity. The crux of the debate was how a naturally occurring immune mechanism could generate a receptor that could specifically recognize an artificial antigen that had never before existed in nature. To explain this, in 1940 Linus Pauling proposed the "instructive hypothesis" (Fig. 7.1B) that antibodies were highly flexible and upon contact with antigen were molded to form a complemen-

tary binding site. This hypothesis predated the current awareness that the three-dimensional structure of any protein (including an antibody) is defined by its amino acid sequence. According to the present understanding, different antibodies recognize different antigens because they have different amino acid sequences at their antigen-binding site. This realization eventually resulted in the abandonment of the instructive hypothesis.

Another source of contention was the seeming inconsistency between the inheritance of antibody constant regions and the proven variability of antigen binding by antibodies. Genetic studies conducted at the time had determined that genes for antibody constant regions were inherited in a simple Mendelian fashion. However, it was difficult to explain how one individual could inherit a single antibody constant-region allele but also inherit, on the same gene, many different antigen-binding regions. To explain this dilemma, W. J. Dreyer and J. C. Bennett proposed in 1965 that variable regions and constant regions of antibodies must be products of two different genes. The idea of *two genes for one polypeptide chain* in the formation of antibody was revolutionary in that the prevailing dogma stated that each gene in the genome directed the production of one polypeptide. Furthermore, Dreyer and Bennett proposed the existence of several variable-region genes and of a single copy of the gene encoding each constant-region class and subclass (Fig. 7.2). They further predicted that the variable and constant genes would need to come together, or be assembled, to permit the synthesis of a complete single protein chain.

Validation of this theoretical model had to wait until 1976, when Susumu Tonegawa and Nobumichi Hozumi demonstrated that immunoglobulin genes are not inherited in a functional state but rearranged during B-cell differentiation. Using DNA from two different sources—embryonic cells (that did not produce antibody) and myeloma cells (antibody-producing tumor cells derived from a B cell)—they demonstrated that a genetic probe recognizing the antibody κ-chain mRNA detected a different pattern of restriction fragments in the DNA from the myeloma cell than in the DNA from the embryonic cell (Fig. 7.3). They interpreted these results to mean that during the differentiation of a lymphocyte from an

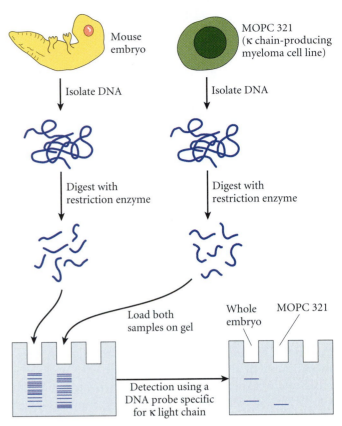

Figure 7.3 Schematic diagram of the experiments of Tonegawa and Hozumi that demonstrated for the first time that production of antibody genes is linked to a physical rearrangement of genomic DNA. DNA from B-cell-like myeloma cells and from non-antibody-producing embryonic cells was digested with restriction endonuclease and the fragments separated by size and then analyzed with a probe that would specifically detect the antibody κ L-chain gene. Tonegawa and Hozumi found that whereas the κ L-chain gene was present on two DNA fragments in non-immunoglobulin-producing cells, the κ-chain gene was present on only one DNA fragment of a unique size in antibody-secreting myeloma cells. This indicates that the antibody-producing cells have DNA rearrangements at or near the antibody genes.

Figure 7.2 Dreyer and Bennett's "two genes, one polypeptide" theory departed from dogma, stating that a single antibody protein chain is produced from two genes. This theory was created to explain the duality of antibody structure (i.e., one portion of an antibody is fairly constant, while another portion is highly variable). According to this theory, during antibody production a gene encoding the highly variable (antigen-binding) portion of the antibody would be joined with the gene encoding the constant region of the antibody. *Eco*RI and *Hin*dIII indicate the positions of the restriction endonuclease recognition sites. Note that the size distribution of restriction fragments after rearrangement differs from that of the same locus before rearrangement. In the example shown, the two *Hin*dIII restriction sites are lost following rearrangement of the DNA to form a functional gene encoding both the variable and constant regions of one antibody chain.

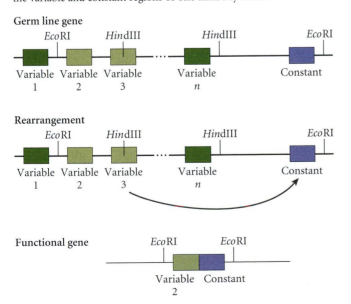

embryonic stage to a fully mature antibody-secreting cell (i.e., myeloma cell) the antibody genes must undergo physical rearrangement at the DNA level. They proposed that the variable and constant regions are separated by a large distance in the germ line configuration in the embryo and that the mechanism that brings these two genes together during differentiation alters the intervening DNA sequence and consequently modifies the distribution of restriction enzyme recognition sites.

Immunoglobulin H-chain genes not only undergo the same type of rearrangement as was initially found for L-chain genes, bringing genes for variable and constant regions together, but also undergo a second, distinct type of DNA recombination event known as *class switch (CS) recombination.* This genetic change allows B cells to express the same variable region encoding antigen-binding specificity with a different constant region, thus switching the antigen recognition property to an antibody of another isotype. This second DNA rearrangement event permits a different effector function of the immunoglobulin molecules that retain the same antigen specificity.

Organization of the Immunoglobulin Genes

Overview

In much of the immunology literature, terms that came into common use after the basic properties of the H- and L-chain loci were known are frequently encountered; however, since 1999 the Human Gene Organization Nomenclature Committee has established specific terminology for designating genes associated with immunoglobulin production. This committee also determined that although multiple gene "segments" were needed to encode a functional immunoglobulin H or L chain, each of the segments would be referred to as a gene. Table 7.1 provides a cross-reference between terminologies. Updated information about the genetic organization of immunoglobulin

genes can be found at http://imgt.cines.fr:8104/textes/IMGTrepertoire/.

In the years since the experiments of Tonegawa and Hozumi, the complete nucleotide sequence and the genetic organization of the loci encoding immunoglobulins have been elucidated. Genes encoding immunoglobulins have a unique organization. The genes for the κ and λ L chains and for the immunoglobulin H-chain locus are each encoded by separate multigene families located on different chromosomes (Table 7.2). Each of these multigene families consists of genes that encode the constant-region domains, preceded by a large number of genes that eventually form the coding region for the antigen-binding variable domain. During the production of a functional and complete antibody gene, these genes are physically rearranged to form a single exon that encodes the variable domain. As it turned out, the genetic information needed to encode a full variable region was also divided into separate genes. Three types of genes known as the V (*variable*), D (*diversity*), and J (*joining*) genes need to be rearranged for the H-chain variable region to be complete, while only two of them, V and J, are used for the L-chain variable region. Preceding each V gene is a small exon encoding a hydrophobic leader sequence (Ls) that is responsible for guiding the nascent H-chain or L-chain protein into the lumen of the endoplasmic reticulum for processing and assembly. A transcriptional promoter is located 5′ from each Ls sequence.

Defining what constitutes an immunoglobulin gene is difficult due to the variety of genes found within the mouse and human genomes. Functional genes are defined as those that are transcribed and translated. However, some of the genes have small changes due to nucleotide changes in conserved promoter sequences, splice sequences, or sequences needed for recombination to occur. These changes will prevent a functional protein from being produced. Other genes appear from sequencing data to be capable of producing a functional mRNA transcript, but no transcript has been

Table 7.1 Correspondence of terminologies used to designate immunoglobulin genes and genetic elements

Region encoded	HUGO[a] designation	Traditional designation
Heavy chains		
V segment	IGHV	V_H
D segment	IGHD[b]	D_H
J segment	IGHJ	J_H
D/J joint	IGHD-J	D-J_H
Entire V(D)J region	IGHV-D-J	$V(D)J$
C region	IGHC	C_H
μ chain	IGHM	C_μ
δ chain	IGHD[b]	C_δ
γ chain	IGHG	C_γ
α chain	IGHA	C_α
ε chain	IGHE	C_ε
Light chains		
κ V chain	IGKV	V_κ
κ J chain	IGKJ	J_κ
Entire VJ region	IGKV-J	VJ_κ
κ C region	IGKC	C_κ
λ V region	IGLV	V_λ
λ J region	IGLJ	J_λ
Entire VJ region	IGLV-J	VJ_λ
λ C region	IGLC	C_λ

[a]HUGO, Human Gene Organization; designation from Nomenclature Committee.

[b]Note that the human immunoglobulin diversity region in the variable portion of the H chain and the human IgD C region are both given the same designation, IGHD. Distinguishing the meaning of these identical terms is done within the context of their use.

Table 7.2 Chromosomal locations of the immunoglobulin H- and L-chain genes known to be used to produce functional immunoglobulin proteins

Gene family	Chromosomal location	
	Human	Mouse
H chain	14[a]	12
L chain		
λ chain	22	16
κ chain	2	6

[a]Although most of the genes for the human H-chain locus are found on chromosome 14, some variable-region elements are also on chromosomes 15 and 16, but it is not yet clear if they can become incorporated into functional genes for antibody H chains.

identified. Some DNA sequences give rise to *pseudogenes,* genes with coding regions containing stop codon(s) and/or frameshift mutation(s). A stop codon or frameshift in the Ls sequence could also make a variable-region gene a pseudogene. Within the DNA loci for the immunoglobulin genes are regions that have some features of an immunoglobulin gene but are otherwise fairly divergent from the known ones, as well as truncated or vestigial genes. Recent information regarding the sequence of variable-region genes indicates that some are found on chromosomes different from the one containing the constant-region gene along with the bulk of the H-chain and L-chain genes. These genetic elements are termed *orphons* but do not contribute to the synthesis of immunoglobulin H- or L-chain polypeptides.

Further complications in determining the number of different genes contributing to production of immunoglobulins arise from differences among individuals in the number of genes they have for producing immunoglobulin polypeptides. Not all of the genes can recombine in a way to produce a functional protein; for this to occur the rearrangement of the genes has to be "productive." Many rearrangements will be "unproductive," meaning that some problem such as the introduction of a stop codon has occurred.

The Immunoglobulin H-Chain (IGH) Locus

The mouse IGH locus

In mice, the IGH locus on chromosome 12 has approximately 185 genes, each of which can function as an individual IGHV gene, but the actual number varies, depending on the strain of mouse. The nucleotides of the IGHV genes encode amino acids 1 through 94 of the immunoglobulin H chain and are located upstream of a cluster of 13 to 14 D genes, designated IGHD (Fig. 7.4). Lying downstream of the IGHD genes, which encode amino acids 95 through 97 of the H chain in a 2-kilobase (kb) cluster, are four genes designated IGHJ, which are approximately 8 kb upstream of the first exon of the IgM constant region (IGHC) and encode amino acids 98 through 113 of the immunoglobulin H-chain variable region.

The sequence of the mouse IGH locus is not complete, so the total number of genetic elements is not yet fully known. The IGHV genes have been divided into 14 to 15 subgroups labeled IGHV1 to IGHV15. Subgroups are formed from closely related IGHV genes, but these related genes are not necessarily grouped together on the chromosome. For example, the IGHV3 subgroup genes map to three locations, and there is one location that is closest to the IGHD region genes that contains interspersed genes for the IGHV2 and IGHV5 subgroups. Murine IGHV families have been categorized into three larger groups, also on the basis

of amino acid sequence homology. The IGHD genes can be divided into four families on the basis of sequence homology. The IGHD cluster is spread over nearly 90 kb, with the 3′-most IGHD gene, D-Q52, located approximately 0.7 kb upstream of the first IGHJ gene designated IGHJ1.

The H-chain constant-region (C_H) locus encompasses nearly 200 kb of DNA and encodes the constant regions of all of the different isotypes of antibody. These constant-region isotypes are arranged sequentially in the IGH-chain locus. In the mouse, this sequence is Cμ-Cδ-Cγ3-Cγ1-Cγ2b-Cγ2a-Cε-Cα or IGHM, IGHD, IGHG3, IGHG1, IGHG2b, IGHE, and IGHA (Fig. 7.4). Each constant-region gene is depicted as a single box for simplicity. In reality, each of these constant-region genes is composed of a number of exons, separated from each other by intronic sequence (Fig. 7.4A, insets). Each exon encodes a separate protein domain, which forms an independently folding unit within the immunoglobulin protein chain. This genetic arrangement has been accepted as support for the hypothesis that the immunoglobulin H-chain and L-chain genes arose as a result of gene duplication during evolution from a primordial gene. This primordial gene probably resembled a single immunoglobulin-like domain and had the ability to bind to foreign proteins. Duplication of this gene resulted in immunoglobulin-like proteins consisting of tandem arrays of immunoglobulin-like domains. Subsequent divergence of these tandem exons permitted the domains that were present on a single protein to carry out different functions (e.g., antigen binding by one domain and effector functions by others).

The human IGH locus

The human IGH locus is on the long arm of chromosome 14 in a region designated 14q32.33 and spans 1,250 kb (Fig. 7.4B), with orphons on chromosomes 15 and 16. There are 123 to 129 IGHV-region genes, depending on the set of genes present on one chromosome. A set of variable-region genes that are found together is referred to as a *haplotype*. The IGHV genes are divided into 6 to 7 subgroups, again depending on the haplotype, but only 38 to 46 of these IGHV-region genes are functional. The IGHD region is composed of 27 genes, arranged into 7 subgroups, of which 23 are known to be functional and 4 are simply acknowledged to be open reading frames. The human IGH locus contains nine IGHJ region genes, of which six are functional. Most humans have nine IGHC-region genes arranged to encode immunoglobulin M (IgM), IgD, IgG3, IgG1, IgA1, IgG2, IgG4, IgE, and IgA2. However, some humans carry haplotypes that have as few as 5 IGHC-region genes due to deletions and as many as 19 due to triplication of part of the locus.

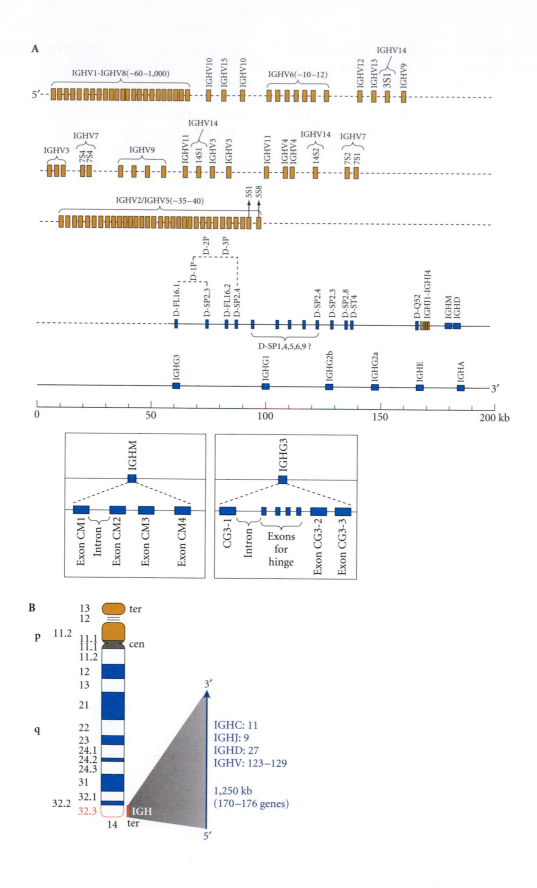

The κ L-Chain (IGK) Locus

The mouse IGK locus

The organization of the murine IGK locus is similar to that of the H-chain locus but less complex. The locus is on mouse chromosome 6 and spans almost 3,200 kb of DNA. The murine IGK locus is composed of 158 IGKV genes that can be grouped into nearly 19 homology-based families; 93 to 99 of the IGKV genes are functional. Downstream of the IGKV cluster are five IGKJ genes, of which four are functional. These J genes are located approximately 2.5 kb upstream of the single IGKC gene, which encodes the κ-chain constant domain (Fig. 7.5). That all mouse immunoglobulin κ chains use this one IGKC gene means that all κ chains have the exact same constant domain.

The human IGK locus

The organization of the IGK locus in humans is similar to that of mice (Fig. 7.6A). It is located on chromosome 2 and spans 1,820 kb of DNA (Fig. 7.6B). In the human IGK cluster there are 76 IGKV-region genes grouped into 7 subgroups, of which 30 to 44 are potentially functional; 5 IGKJ-region genes; and a single IGKC region gene. All five of the IGKJ-region genes are functional. Twenty-eight human IGK orphons have been found on chromosomes 15 and 16. The IGKV-region genes are found in two clusters separated by 800 kb of DNA. Interestingly, human κ L chains, in contrast to those in mice, comprise 60% of the serum immunoglobulin L chains. In mice, κ L chains are found on about 95% of the immunoglobulin proteins.

The λ L-Chain (IGL) Locus

The mouse IGL locus

The murine λ L-chain locus is on chromosome 16 but has an overall arrangement distinct from that of the H chain and the κ L chain. This locus covers 200 kb and is organized into two duplicated units. The first unit contains two functional V genes (IGLV), two J$_\lambda$ genes (IGLJ), and two C$_\lambda$ exons (IGLC) (Fig. 7.7A). However, one of the IGLJ genes (J$_\lambda$4) and one IGLC exon (C$_\lambda$4) are nonfunctional pseudogenes. The second duplicated unit has one IGLV gene, two functional IGLJ genes, and two functional IGLC genes. Rearrangement of the immunoglobulin λ locus involves the joining of a single IGLV gene with one or two of the IGLJ genes that lie within the same duplicated unit as the IGLV gene. Due to the presence of three constant-region genes, mouse IGL chains have three different *isotypes*, which were formerly referred to as *subtypes*.

The human IGL locus

The human IGL locus is on chromosome 22 and extends over 1,050 kb (Fig. 7.7B). There are 70 to 71 IGLV-region genes that span ~900 kb, 7 to 11 IGLJ-region genes, and 7 to 11 IGLC-region genes, depending on the haplotype (Fig. 7.6C). Each of the IGLJ-region genes is followed by an IGLC-region gene to give an IGLJ-IGLC pair. The IGLV genes belong to 11 subgroups. Twenty-nine to 33 of the IGLV-region genes belonging to 10 subgroups are functional. Four to five of the IGLJ-IGLC-region genes are functional. There are six IGL gene orphons.

The Mechanism of Variable-Region Gene Assembly

Overview

During B-cell differentiation, the exon encoding the antigen-binding variable domain is assembled from component V, D, and J genes by a process referred to as *V(D)J recombination*, whereby the DNA of the immunoglobulin locus is physically rearranged. To accomplish this, rearrangements are dependent on conserved DNA sequences called *recombination signal sequences* (RSSs)

Figure 7.4 Genomic organization of the mouse IGH-chain locus. (**A**) The 5′ end of the mouse IGH locus contains genes that are rearranged to form the variable-domain exon. The IGH-chain locus contains three different types of genes to form the complete variable-region gene: IGHV (variable), IGHD (diversity), and IGHJ (joining). In the mouse locus, there are between 100 and 1,000 IGHV genes (the actual number varies among mouse strains and is not fully known at this time). These genes are organized into groups designated IGHV1 to IGHV15, but individual genes are interspersed throughout the IGHV locus. Located upstream of the IGHV region is a cluster of 13 IGHD genes with no ordered nomenclature. The four IGHJ genes lie downstream of the IGHD genes. Each individual IGHV gene is preceded by a leader exon that encodes the hydrophobic leader sequence that guides nascent immunoglobulin proteins into the endoplasmic reticulum; each leader exon has its own promoter. The 3′ end of the IGH-chain locus (starting about 8 kb downstream of the IGHJ genes) contains the genes encoding the constant regions of all of the different isotypes of antibody-IGHC. In the mouse genome, they are arranged sequentially: IGHM, IGHD, IGHG3, IGHG1, IGHG2b, IGHG2a, IGHE, IGHA. It should be noted that each constant-region gene is depicted here as a single box for simplicity. (**Insets**) In reality, each of these constant-region genes is composed of a number of exons separated from each other by intronic sequence. The IGHM-chain gene and the IGHG3 gene are shown as examples. The IGHM chain lacks a hinge region; therefore, its constant gene consists of four exons (CM1 to CM4), each encoding one constant domain. In contrast, the H chain of IGG3 contains a hinge region. Its constant gene contains three exons (CG3-1 to CG3-3) encoding the three constant-region domains and four smaller exons, which together encode the flexible hinge region. (**B**) Chromosomal location and basic organization of the human IGH locus. Located on the long arm of chromosome 14 there are 123 to 129 IGHV, 27 IGHD, 9 IGHJ, and 11 IGHC genes, but not all of the IGHV, IGHD, and IGHJ genes are functional. From IMGT, http://imgt.cines.fr, with permission from M.-P. Lefranc.

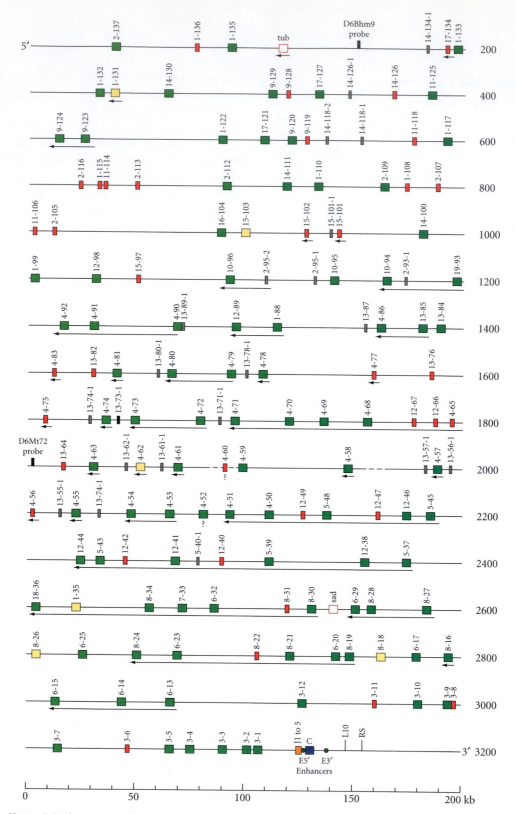

Figure 7.5 The mouse IGK locus on chromosome 6. A total of 158 IGKV genes belonging to 19 subgroups extending over on 3,200 kb of DNA have been identified. Of the IGKV genes, 93 are functional (green), 6 form ORFs that could potentially encode a gene (yellow), and 59 are pseudogenes (red). The known repertoire is 93 established functional IGKV genes belonging to 18 subgroups. ORFs and currently unmapped IGKV genes may change the final number of functional IGKV genes. There are five IGKJ genes (orange) of which one, IGKJ3, is not functional, and one IGKC gene (blue). Genes unrelated to IGK are open boxes. Enhancer elements 5' and 3' (E5' and E3') of the IGKC gene are small circles. From IMGT, http://imgt.cines.fr, with permission from M.-P. Lefranc.

A

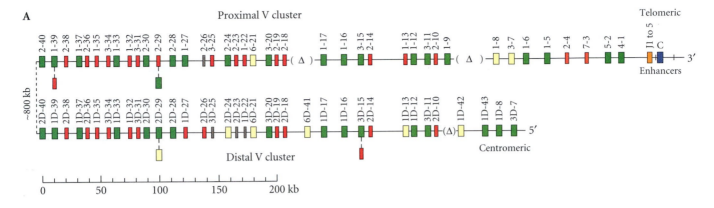

B

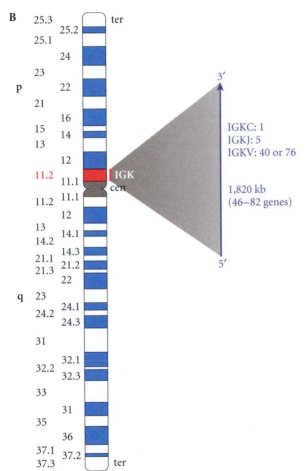

Figure 7.6 Schematic representation of the genomic organization of the human κ L-chain locus on chromosome 2. (**A**) The human IGK locus contains two IGKV-region clusters separated by 800 kb of intervening DNA: the distal cluster containing 36 IGKV genes that is at the 5′ end of the locus and the proximal cluster containing 40 IGKV genes that is at the 3′ end of the locus (shown above the distal cluster). There are five functional human IGKJ genes and a single IGKC gene. The IGKV genes that make up the proximal cluster are designated by a number for the family subgroup of which the gene is a member, followed by a hyphen and a number for where the gene is located in the locus relative to the IGKC-region gene. Smaller numbers are located closer to the IGKC gene. The IGKV genes of the distal cluster have the same numbers as the corresponding genes in the proximal cluster but are further identified with the letter D added. In some cases there are deletions in the clusters; these are indicated by small triangles. Functional genes are shown in green, pseudogenes are red, and open reading frames with the potential to encode a functional gene are yellow. The IGKJ gene cluster is orange, and the IGKC gene is blue. (**B**) Map of the localization of human IGK genes on chromosome 2. From IMGT, http://imgt.cines.fr, with permission from M.-P. Lefranc.

This multistep process is normally restricted to lymphoid cells, so it makes sense for the two crucial protein factors that initiate the process to be lymphoid specific. These protein factors are termed the *recombinase-activating gene products 1 and 2* (RAG-1 and RAG-2). In addition, certain steps of V(D)J recombination are performed by widely expressed factors that are not lymphoid specific. Nevertheless, the restriction of *Rag-1* and *Rag-2* expression to lymphoid cells is normally sufficient to prevent V(D)J recombination from occurring in nonlymphoid cells.

Recombination Signal Sequences

The first step in the V(D)J recombination process is the recognition of the genes to be recombined by the recombinant DNA enzymatic machinery of the B cell. As the immunoglobulin genetic loci of multiple species were being cloned and sequenced, it became apparent that all germ line immunoglobulin genes (V, D, and J genes) were flanked by two closely related conserved sequences, which later were demonstrated to serve as specific target sequences for the RAG-1 and RAG-2 V(D)J recombinases. These RSSs consist of a conserved palindromic heptamer and an adenine, thymidine-rich (AT-rich) nonamer separated from each

that flank each V, D, and J gene. V(D)J recombination is initiated by the generation of precise DNA double-stranded breaks at the end of each gene that is to be joined together. Subsequent processing and ligation lead to the fusion of the two genes to form a *coding joint* that contains the information for the immunoglobulin polypeptide and to fusion of the two RSSs to form a *signal joint*, the byproduct of V(D)J recombination.

A

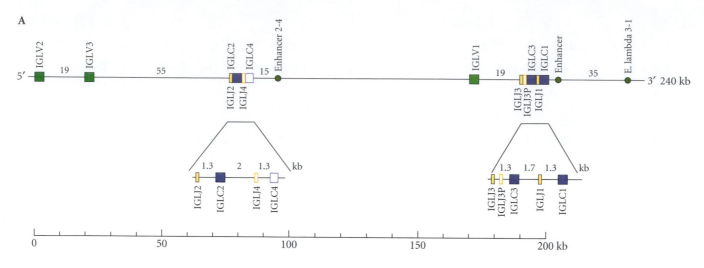

B

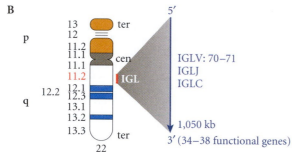

Figure 7.7 The immunoglobulin λ-chain locus. (A) The murine IGL locus on chromosome 16 covers 200 kb and is organized into two duplicated units. The first unit contains two functional IGLV genes (green) and two IGLJ and IGLC genes, of which only one pair is functional (filled yellow and blue; nonfunctional genes in yellow-bordered and open blue box). The second duplicated unit has one IGLV gene, two functional IGLJ genes, two functional IGLC genes, and one IGLJ pseudogene (IGLJ3P). Rearrangement of the mouse immunoglobulin λ locus involves the joining of a single IGLV gene with one or two of the IGLJ genes that lie within the same duplicated unit as the IGLV gene. Thus, only four combinations are possible. For example, IGLV2 and IGLV3 can only recombine with IGLJ2 and IGLC2. Due to the presence of three functional IGLC genes, mouse IGL chains have three different isotypes. (B) The human IGL locus is on chromosome 22 and extends over 1,050 kb. As depicted as a chromosomal representation, there are 70 to 71 IGLV-region genes and 7 to 11 pairs of IGLJ/IGLC genes. Twenty-nine to 33 of the IGLV-region genes belonging to 10 subgroups are functional. Four to five of the IGLJ/IGLC-region genes are functional. From IMGT, http://imgt.cines.fr, with permission from M.-P. Lefranc.

other by a spacer of either 12 or 23 bp (Fig. 7.8). Thus, there are two types of RSSs differentiated by the length of their spacer. Although the sequence of this intervening spacer does not appear to be important for recombination to proceed, the length of the spacer (i.e., the distance between the heptamer and nonamer elements) is crucial. Coincidentally, 12 bp and 23 bp correspond, respectively, to one and two turns of the DNA helix. Thus, in both sequences the heptamer and nonamer are at the same relative positions along the circumference of the DNA helix.

Close examination of the types of RSSs that successfully mediate V(D)J rearrangements led to the additional observation that recombination occurs primarily between genes located on the same chromosome and between genes flanked by RSSs with different spacer lengths. In other words, a gene flanked by a 12-bp RSS can recombine *only* with a gene flanked by a 23-bp RSS and vice versa—a rule that is called the "12/23 rule" or the "one turn/two turn rule." In the immunoglobulin H-chain locus, IGHV genes are flanked 3′ by a 23-bp RSS, and IGHJ genes are flanked

5′ by a 23-bp RSS. IGHD genes are flanked both 3′ and 5′ by a 12-bp RSS (Fig. 7.9A). Therefore, the rearrangement of an IGHD gene is restricted to an IGHV gene or an IGHJ gene; an IGHD gene cannot recombine with another IGHD gene since both genes have the same RSSs flanking the 5′ and 3′ sides. An analogous restriction prevents the joining of IGHV genes directly to IGHJ genes. A similar strategy is employed during rearrangement of immunoglobulin L chains. In the κ-chain locus, the IGKV genes are flanked 3′ by 12-bp RSSs while the IGKJ genes are flanked 5′ by 23-bp RSSs (Fig. 7.9B). Conversely, in the λ-chain locus, the IGLV genes are flanked 3′ by 23-bp RSSs while the IGLJ genes are flanked 5′ by 12-bp RSSs (Fig. 7.9C). In both cases, an IGLV gene can recombine only with an IGLJ gene and never with another IGLV gene. Finally, elegant experiments performed by K. Mizuuchi and M. Gellert and colleagues using extrachromosomal substrates clearly demonstrated that the RSSs are sufficient to target V(D)J recombinase activity and that this site-specific recombination is restricted to lymphocytes.

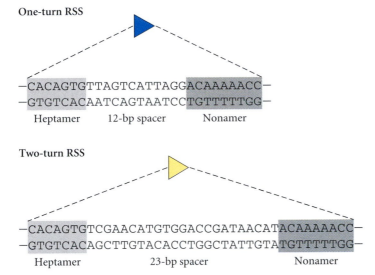

One-turn RSS

CACAGTGTTAGTCATTAGGACAAAAACC
GTGTCACAATCAGTAATCCTGTTTTTGG

Heptamer   12-bp spacer   Nonamer

Two-turn RSS

CACAGTGTCGAACATGTGGACCGATAACATACAAAAACC
GTGTCACAGCTTGTACACCTGGCTATTGTATGTTTTTGG

Heptamer   23-bp spacer   Nonamer

Figure 7.8 V(D)J recombination is precisely targeted to IGV, IGD, and IGJ segments by RSSs that flank each gene in the germ line DNA. An RSS consists of three elements: a palindromic heptamer, an AT-rich nonamer, and a spacer. The nucleotide sequences of the heptamer and nonamer are critical for V(D)J recombination to occur, while the length of the spacer (but not its nucleotide sequence) is important. Depending on the spacer length, RSSs exist in two varieties, called 12-bp and 23-bp. The blue triangle represents the 12-bp RSS, and the yellow triangle represents the 23-bp RSS.

Deletional joining versus inversional joining

Analysis of the genomic DNA of immunoglobulin-producing cell lines has demonstrated that the relative orientation of two genes in the germ line (embryonic) configuration dictates the fate of the intervening sequence that connects the two genes. The molecular basis of this phenomenon is the bringing together of the RSSs that flank the two genes to be joined during recombination in a synapse in which the RSSs lie close together (Fig. 7.10A). Thus, genes lying in the same transcriptional orientation (in the germ line configuration) are connected to each other by a *deletional* mechanism. Synapse formation must involve a looping of the intervening DNA, and when the genes are recombined, the DNA between the two genes will be permanently removed from the genome (Fig. 7.10B). In contrast, genes arranged in opposite transcriptional orientation are rearranged by an *inversional* mechanism. In an inversional recombination event, the sequence intervening between the two genes is not removed from the genome but is flipped in its orientation (Fig. 7.10C).

DNA Rearrangements during V(D)J Recombination

Regardless of whether V(D)J recombination proceeds by a deletional or an inversional mechanism, this process always will involve the formation of two new junctions, the *coding joint* and the *signal joint*. The coding joint is the union between the two genes, whereas the signal joint is the union between the two RSSs that originally flanked the genes. It is noteworthy that although two different types of genetic junctions (coding joint and signal joint) are formed during V(D)J recombination, these two junctions

appear to be generated by distinct pathways. Determination of the nucleotide sequences of several signal joints and coding joints showed that the RSSs in signal joints were, in fact, perfectly ligated to each other such that no nucleotides were ever added to or removed from the RSSs during the formation of the signal joint. In contrast, coding joints frequently were found to contain nucleotide deletions, addi-

Figure 7.9 Arrangement of 12-bp and 23-bp RSSs in genes of immunoglobulin loci. In the IGH locus, IGHV (V) and IGHJ (J) genes are flanked 5′ and 3′, respectively, by a 23-bp spacer RSS, and IGHD (D) genes are flanked by a 12-bp spacer RSS on both sides. The 12/23 rule ensures that an IGHD gene can recombine only with an IGHV gene or an IGHJ gene, not with another IGHD gene. In the IGK locus, the IGKV genes are flanked 3′ by 12-bp spacer RSSs while the IGKJ genes are flanked 5′ by 23-bp spacer RSSs. In the IGL locus, the IGLV genes are flanked 3′ by 23-bp RSSs while the IGLJ genes are flanked 5′ by 12-bp spacer RSSs. In the case of both L chains, the 12/23 rule ensures that a V-region gene can recombine only with a J-region gene, not with another V-region gene.

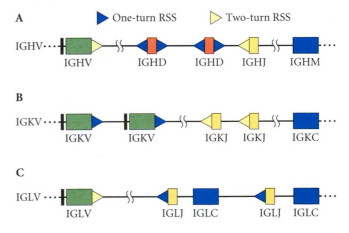

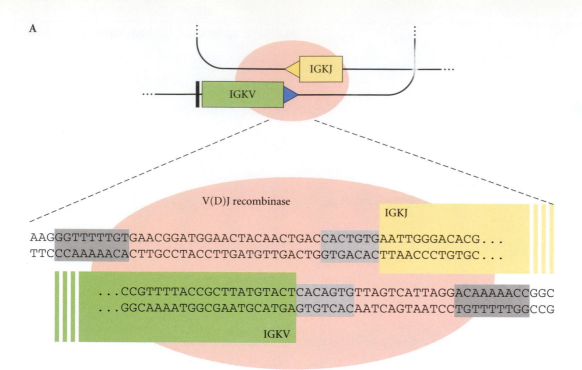
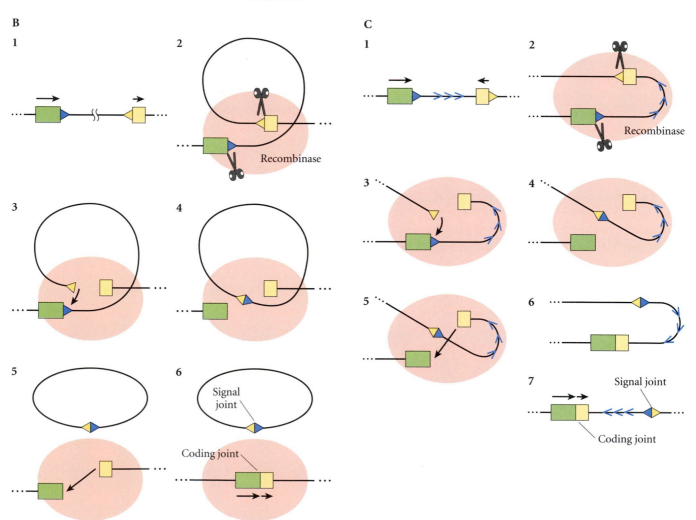

tions, or both when compared with the nucleotide sequences of the genes from which they were derived. Since the joining of the genes for IGH and IGL chains occurs in the nucleotides that will encode the third complementarity-determining region (CDR), incorporation of a lot of potential genetic variation during the DJ and V(D)J recombination steps can provide a much greater degree of antigen-binding diversity. The sequence variations observed in these regions are collectively known as "junctional diversity" and represent an important source for generating much of the antigen-binding repertoire that is engendered in the variable-region sequence.

Protein Factors Involved in V(D)J Recombination

The recombination of variable-region genes involves a number of steps that may be summarized by the following events (Fig. 7.11):

1. Recognition of the RSS by a complex consisting of the proteins RAG-1 and RAG-2, followed by the formation of a synapse, bringing the genes to be recombined into proximity.
2. Generation of a nick by RAG proteins, with the ligation of signal ends to form a signal joint. This occurs concomitantly with a *trans*-esterification reaction at the coding ends that simultaneously produces a *hairpin loop* structure.
3. Opening of the hairpin structure, possibly forming single-stranded DNA overhangs that will serve as templates for addition of random nucleotides to the DNA known as P-nucleotide addition.
4. Nucleotide trimming, presumably by an exonuclease.
5. Optional addition of more nucleotides in a process termed *N-nucleotide addition* that occurs when the enzyme terminal deoxynucleotidyl transferase (TdT) is present.
6. Alignment, polymerization, and ligation of the DNA double-strand break to restore the integrity of the chromosome.

Reporter constructs used to study V(D)J recombination

Since V(D)J recombination of B cells normally occurs in the bone marrow, the scientific study of this process required the development of in vitro methods to artificially produce the recombination of the IG genes and observe them at work. Most of these methods involve the use of immortalized cell lines that are transfected with artificial genetic constructs (called *recombination substrates*) that contain RSSs that flank convenient DNA sequences. The latter sequences are engineered into the DNA constructs such that V(D)J recombination at the RSSs yields a final DNA product that can easily be detected.

Stably introduced recombination substrates

The introduction of recombination substrates, either as retroviral vectors or by stable transfection methods, into transformed B-cell lines has been an important tool for assaying mechanistic and regulatory aspects of V(D)J recombination. Most important, such vectors have provided an invaluable tool for identifying and cloning the genes that encode essential protein components of the V(D)J recombination reaction, defining both *lymphoid-specific components* and *non-lymphoid-specific components* needed for V(D)J recombination.

The most widely used type of artificial substrate includes a constitutive promoter that drives the expression of a selectable marker gene, such as the guanosine phosphoribosyl transferase (*gpt*), which provides resistance to the drug mycophenolic acid. However, the selectable marker is oriented in the reverse orientation in the original vector (Fig. 7.12A). Therefore, the selectable marker is expressed only after inversional joining by a V(D)J recombination process, using RSSs that are engineered to flank the genes that are the targets of the recombination machinery. Cells harboring a stably integrated copy of this vector that has undergone inversional V(D)J rearrangement can therefore be easily identified as being resistant to the drug mycophenolic acid (Fig. 7.12B).

Figure 7.10 The relative orientation of genes in the germ line configuration determines the mechanism by which V(D)J recombination proceeds. (A) During recombination of two genes (in this case, a κ-chain IGKV gene and a κ-chain IGKJ gene), the RSSs that flank the two genes are brought together in a *synapse*, in which the RSSs lie close together and are oriented in the same direction. The 3' end of the IGKV locus is joined to the 5' end of the IGKJ locus. (B) If the two genes lie in the same transcriptional orientation (indicated by black arrows) in the germ line configuration, recombination must involve formation of a loop in the DNA. When the genes are recombined, the DNA sequence intervening between the two genes is permanently removed from the genome by a looping-deletion mechanism. Scissors indicate the action of an endonuclease at the boundary of the heptamer of the RSS. The thin arrow indicates joining of free DNA ends. (C) If the two genes lie in opposite transcriptional orientations (indicated by black arrows), recombination requires only that the DNA bend back on itself to form the RSS synapse. Recombination in this case results not in the deletion of the intervening sequence but rather in its inversion (or "flipping") within the genome. The blue arrowheads are included to emphasize the inversion of the intervening sequence. In this case the coding joint and signal joint remain on the chromosome with no DNA deleted.

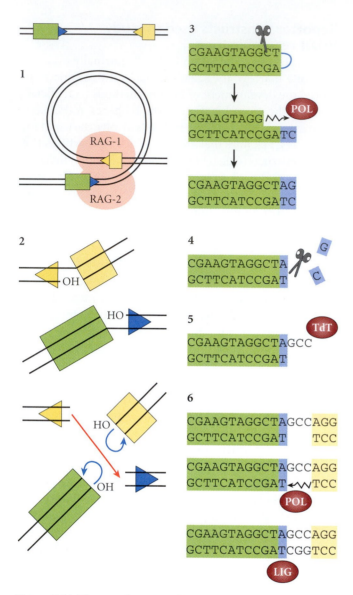

Figure 7.11 The recombination of V-region genes involves a number of steps. (**1**) The first step is recognition of the RSSs by the *Rag* complex, followed by the formation of a synapse. (**2**) A single-stranded nick is introduced by the *Rag* gene products (**top**) followed by the ligation of signal ends to form a signal joint (red arrow), and the *trans*-esterification reaction at the coding joint, which simultaneously produces a hairpin loop structure (blue arrows). (**3**) The hairpin structure is cleaved to form single-stranded DNA overhangs (blue), which will lead to P-nucleotide addition. The overhang is used as a template by a DNA polymerase (POL), which synthesizes the complementary strand. This panel shows the hairpin loop at the end of the V gene as an example. (**4**) The free DNA ends are trimmed, presumably by an exonuclease (represented by a pair of scissors). (**5**) In some cases, during rearrangement of the H-chain, N-nucleotides are added by the enzyme TdT. (**6**) The free DNA ends are then aligned (**top**), polymerized by a DNA POL to fill existing gaps (**middle**), and the DNA double-strand break ligated together (LIG) (**bottom**) to restore the integrity of the chromosome.

Transient recombination substrates

A more versatile substrate involved the development of shuttle vectors that can be transiently transfected into eukaryotic cell lines where V(D)J recombination can take place followed by transformation of the vector DNA into bacteria to amplify the products of V(D)J recombinant (Fig. 7.13). Although the principle of recombination is similar to the one described above, this method permits the recovery and analysis of large amounts of DNA resulting from independent recombination events. This type of vector contains a constitutive marker, such as an ampicillin resistance (Amp^r) gene and a bacterial chloramphenicol acetyltransferase (*cat*) gene, which upon expression confers chloramphenicol resistance to bacteria carrying the vector (Fig. 7.13). For *cat* to be expressed in the bacterium and confer resistance to chloramphenicol, the strong bacterial *lac* promoter must be placed in front of the *cat* gene by removing a transcription terminator (OOP) that lies between the promoter and the *cat* gene. Because the OOP is flanked by RSSs, its removal is mediated by V(D)J recombination when the vector is in the eukaryotic cell.

These types of vectors have proven useful in the identification of both lymphoid- and non-lymphoid-specific components of V(D)J recombination. V(D)J recombination activity can be estimated by the relative amount of rearranged *cat* activity (based on the acquisition of chloramphenicol resistance) compared with the total amount of *amp* activity recovered (based on the constitutive expression of ampicillin resistance). Also, depending on the relative orientation of the RSSs in these vectors, they can be used for the study of coding (Fig. 7.13A) or signal (Fig. 7.13B) joints. The determination of nucleotide sequences of coding joints and signal joints in cloned recombination products permits the study of the mechanistic details of the reaction, such as the occurrence of nucleotide additions and deletions in the coding joint.

Lymphoid-specific components of V(D)J recombination

Recombination-activating genes (RAGs)

A crucial advance in our understanding of the mechanisms involved in V(D)J recombination came from experiments, similar to those depicted in Fig. 7.12, that resulted in the identification of the genes that encode the recombinase enzymes. The pioneering work in this field, conducted by D. G. Schatz, M. A. Oettinger, and David Baltimore in the 1980s, involved the use of rodent fibroblasts that were first stably transfected with a recombination substrate that conferred drug resistance after inversional recombination using a *gpt* marker (Fig. 7.12).

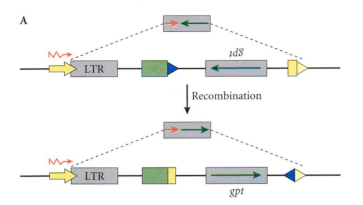

Figure 7.12 Experimental use of an artificial recombination substrate to measure recombination. (**A**) The substrate consists of a strong, constitutive promoter (e.g., one contained in a retroviral long terminal repeat [LTR]) and two genes, one that has a 12-bp RSS and the other that has a 23-bp RSS. The red zigzag arrow indicates the direction of transcription from the LTR promoter. The genes are oriented in the substrate such that they are recombined by inversional joining. Between the two genes is a selectable marker gene (in this example, the gene *gpt*, whose product creates resistance to the drug mycophenolic acid). The selectable marker is placed into the substrate in the wrong orientation to encode a functional protein (**top**). Inversional recombination results in flipping of the *gpt* gene to the proper orientation and in production of the Gpt protein, conferring drug resistance (**bottom**). The red arrows represent the orientation of the promoter, and the light blue arrows represent the orientation of the *gpt* gene. (**B**) This recombination substrate can be used to isolate and identify genes encoding proteins that are essential for V(D)J recombination. (**1**) The recombination substrate is stably transfected into a cell. (**2**) This stable transfectant is then transiently transfected with a cDNA library. (**3**) Transient transfectants that receive a gene encoding a recombinase (red cDNA) will recombine the artificial substrate, thus inverting the *gpt* gene so that it is in the correct orientation to be expressed. (**4**) Addition of mycophenolic acid to the transient transfectants allows selection of cells that received DNA (red) encoding the recombinase. The piece of DNA conferring resistance can be isolated, cloned, sequenced, and analyzed for protein structure and function.

These stably transfected fibroblasts were then further transfected with genomic DNA from a human B-cell line and selected for *gpt* expression. It was expected that fibroblasts receiving genomic DNA that contained the gene(s) encoding the V(D)J recombinase would rearrange the recombination substrate and thus become drug resistant. Indeed, this happened, and so the genes *Rag-1* and *Rag-2* were identified and cloned.

The *Rag* genes encode nuclear phosphoproteins that do not share substantial homology with other known genes but contain motifs found in proteins implicated in transcription and/or recombination. The mechanistic role of RAG-1 and RAG-2 in the recognition of RSSs, the formation of the RSS synapse, and the generation of the single-stranded DNA nick at the RSS has recently been re-created in vitro (steps 1 and 2 in Fig. 7.11). This, in conjunction with the fact that nonlymphoid cells transfected with the *Rag-1* and *Rag-2* genes become capable of V(D)J recombination, demonstrates that these two gene products alone are sufficient for the early

steps of this process. Also, as predicted, given the direct role of RAG-1 and RAG-2 in V(D)J recombination, V(D)J recombination is impaired in transgenic mice with deletions in either of the *Rag* genes, resulting in a complete absence of B cells and T cells (since T cells also use the *Rag* genes to produce their antigen receptor), a condition called *severe combined immunodeficiency*. However, except for this combined immunodeficiency, such transgenic mice appear to be normal (and are healthy if kept in a germ-free environment), suggesting that the *Rag* genes function exclusively in lymphocyte development.

TdT

V(D)J recombination can be accompanied by nontemplated (i.e., noncoded in the DNA) addition of nucleotides at the coding junction of variable-region genes (step 5 of Fig. 7.11). Since these additions occur at junctions where D-J and V-D-J genes are joined together, they can strongly affect the amino acid sequence of the final antibody variable

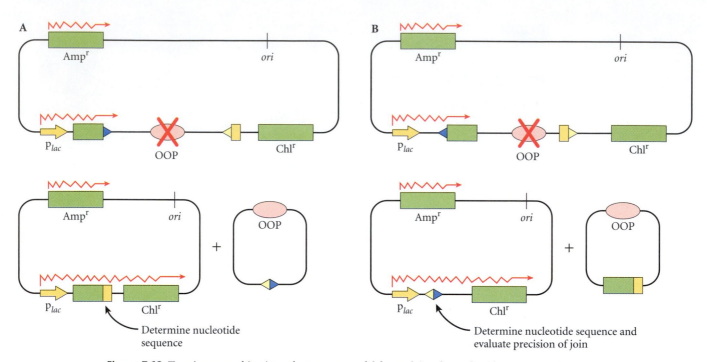

Figure 7.13 Transient recombination substrates are useful for studying the nucleotide sequences of coding (A) and signal (B) joints that are formed during V(D)J recombination and are therefore useful for ascertaining the contribution of P-nucleotide addition, N-nucleotide addition, and junctional flexibility to individual recombination events. The substrate (top of each panel) consists of a bacterial promoter (p_{lac}) that drives expression of a selectable marker (in this example, the Chl^r gene, which confers resistance to the antibiotic chloramphenicol [Chl]). Between the promoter and the selectable marker is a transcriptional terminator (OOP) that is flanked by RSSs. The RSSs are oriented so recombination will result in deletional joining of the RSSs, removing the OOP and allowing expression of the Chl^r resistance marker. Depending on the original orientation of the RSSs in the recombination substrate, the substrate can be used to study the nucleotide sequences of coding joints (A) or signal joints (B). The substrate also contains a bacterial origin of replication (*ori*) and a constitutive marker for selection in bacteria (e.g., one encoding ampicillin resistance; Amp^r) that allows cloning of DNA that has been recombined for analysis of the types of joining reactions that have taken place.

region and thus its antigenic specificity. This addition of nucleotides is mediated by the DNA polymerase TdT, and the process is termed N-nucleotide addition. TdT is present at progenitor stages of lymphocytes in bone marrow and thymus but not in circulating lymphocytes. That TdT is responsible for N-nucleotide addition was initially suggested by the correlation between expression of TdT in lymphocytes and the presence of N-nucleotides in rearranged variable-region genes. This correlation is most dramatic in B-lymphocyte development in mice. Examination of the expression of TdT during mouse B-cell development shows that TdT is expressed transiently during the pro-B-cell stage but ceases to be expressed by the time the B cell reaches the pre-B-cell stage (Fig. 7.14). The pro-B-cell stage is marked by the rearrangement of the immunoglobulin H-chain gene, and examination of the coding joints of a rearranged H chain reveals numerous examples of added N-nucleotides. In contrast, the immunoglobulin L-chain genes

are rearranged during the pre-B-cell stage of development, after expression of TdT has ceased. Thus, N-nucleotides are never found in the coding joints of murine immunoglobulin L-chain genes. Several studies have demonstrated that humans express TdT throughout B-cell development and, accordingly, N-nucleotides appear in both immunoglobulin H-chain and L-chain genes.

The role of TdT in N-nucleotide addition has recently been proven through the generation of mice with a targeted disruption of the gene encoding TdT. Lymphocytes isolated from these animals undergo V(D)J recombination but lack N-nucleotide additions, demonstrating that TdT activity is not essential for this recombination process per se but rather contributes to the diversity of the final antigen-receptor repertoire. Although it is true that N-nucleotide addition may also be found in signal joints, this is rare compared with the occurrence of N-nucleotides at coding joints.

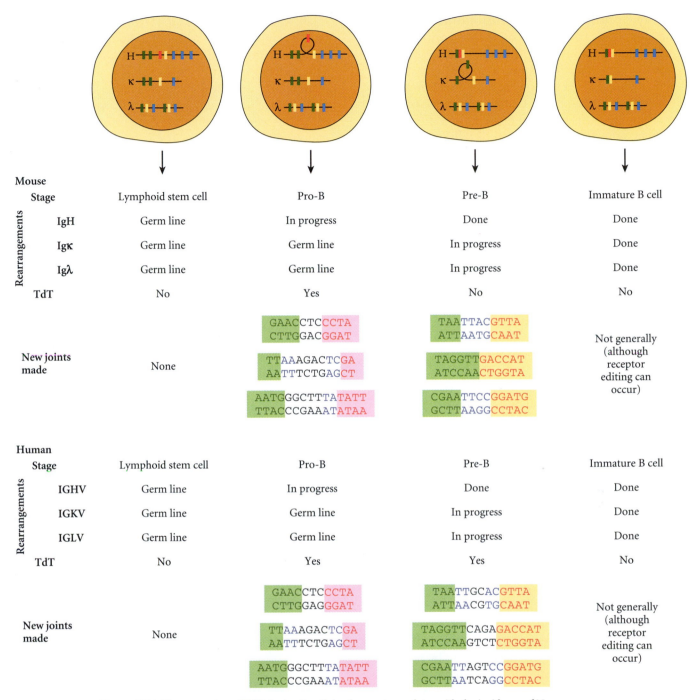

Figure 7.14 The expression of TdT during B-cell development correlates with the incidence of N-nucleotide addition. In the mouse, the enzyme TdT is expressed during the pro-B-cell stage of maturation, when the immunoglobulin H chain is being rearranged. Accordingly, immunoglobulin H-chain coding joints contain N-nucleotides (in black text). By the time the B cell reaches the pre-B-cell stage, when L-chain rearrangement is occurring, TdT expression is shut off. Coding joints of the L-chain genes do not contain N-nucleotides, although they may still contain P-nucleotides (blue text).

Non-lymphoid-specific components

The possibility that non-lymphoid-specific proteins could be involved in V(D)J recombination was first suggested by the characterization of a novel mutation in a murine gene that led to a severe combined immunodeficiency (Scid) phenotype that was distinct from that found in *Rag*-deficient mice. *Rag*-deficient mice demonstrate a complete absence of both B cells and T cells because of a failure of the earliest steps of V(D)J recombination that are required to form these cells and have no DNA breaks at the immunoglobulin loci (Fig. 7.15A). In contrast to *Rag*-deficient mice, the newly identified Scid mice have functional RAG-1 and RAG-2 enzymes and are capable of initiating the V(D)J recombination reaction to produce DNA double-stranded breaks at RSSs. Nevertheless, the Scid mice are deficient in mature B and T cells, presumably because of another defect in the V(D)J recombination process. Upon further investigation, the lymphoid precursor cells in these Scid mice were found to produce signal joints normally but to be unable to form coding joints properly. Therefore, although the early part of the V(D)J recombination process (formation of single-stranded DNA nicks and *trans*-esterification to produce signal joints) occurs normally in these Scid mice, they are not able to generate functional antigen-receptor genes because of their inability to correctly religate the coding joints (Fig. 7.15B). These immunodeficient mice were eventually found to be defective in DNA double-strand break repair (DSBR) in both lymphoid and nonlymphoid cells. This finding demonstrates that at least one enzyme used by many cell lineages for general DNA repair functions also is used by lymphocytes for V(D)J recombination.

Direct evidence for a link between V(D)J recombination and the DSBR enzymes came from the characterization of three radiosensitive Chinese hamster ovary (CHO) cell lines that exhibit defects in DNA repair. These experiments involved rendering these nonlymphoid cells capable of initiating V(D)J recombination by forcing the expression of the *Rag* genes. Similar to DSBR-defective mouse strains, none of the mutant CHO lines appeared to have defects in their ability to initiate the V(D)J recombination reaction when transfected with artificial recombination substrates. However, all of these cell lines failed to repair the DNA double-stranded breaks that were generated. The defects in two of these cell lines appeared to be due to mutations in members of a particular protein complex called *DNA-dependent protein kinase* (DNA-PK), a mammalian protein serine/threonine kinase that must be bound to DNA to be activated. Biochemical analyses have established that this complex contains three subunits, including components designated Ku70 and Ku80, which together form the DNA-binding component of the complex along with a 460-kilodalton (kDa) catalytic subunit, DNA-PKcs (Fig. 7.15C). After DNA-PK is activated in vitro, it phosphorylates a number of substrates, including the Ku subunits and a variety of transcription factors. These properties of the DNA-PK have led to the suggestion that it may be involved in recombination and/or DNA repair. The roles of the three subunits of this complex in V(D)J recombination have been recently confirmed in vivo by the generation of transgenic mice deficient in each of the DNA-PK subunits that have an immunodeficiency phenotype owing to an impairment in coding joint formation.

Complementation analysis of the third CHO mutant permitted localization of its defect to a gene designated *XRCC4*. The protein product of the *XRCC4* gene has recently been shown to interact strongly with DNA ligase IV, suggesting that this gene is involved in regulation of the final step of V(D)J recombination, the ligation of the free coding ends. These results have recently been confirmed by the generation of transgenic mice deficient in both XRCC4 and DNA ligase IV (Fig. 7.15C).

Recently, the gene responsible for a novel human SCID was identified. Fibroblasts isolated from those patients show defective V(D)J recombination and an increased sensitivity to ionizing radiation that resemble those identified in murine Scid. *Artemis* was identified by positional cloning and encodes a 78-kDa protein with homology to metallo-β-lactamases which not only forms a complex in vivo with DNA-PKcs but also is a substrate for the DNA-PK. Recombinant Artemis has an intrinsic 5′-to-3′ exonuclease activity and acquired endonuclease activity after phosphorylation by DNA-PK. Like DNA-PKcs, Artemis is detectable only in vertebrates.

Overall, V(D)J recombination involves both the lymphoid-specific *Rag* gene products as well as proteins that are generally used by many cells for maintaining the integrity of the cell's DNA.

Generation of Antibody Diversity

To generate the enormous receptor diversity required by the immune system, vertebrates have evolved somatic diversification mechanisms that maximize the coding potential that can be generated from the limited number of germ line antibody genes.

Combinatorial Rearrangement of V, D, and J Genes

The foremost mechanism of antibody diversification is the combinatorial rearrangement of immunoglobulin genes. This mechanism alone results in antibody diversi-

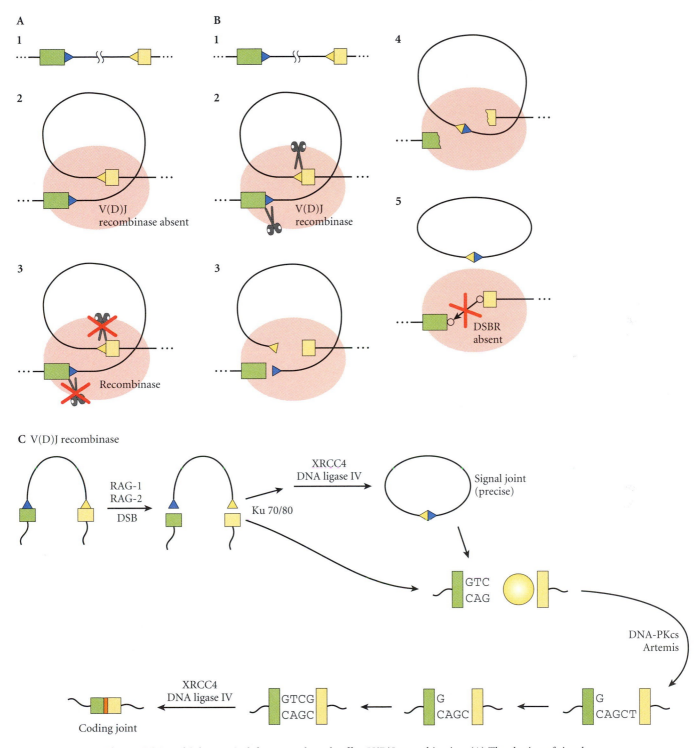

Figure 7.15 Multiple genetic defects can adversely affect V(D)J recombination. **(A)** The cloning of signal joints and coding joints from recombination events occurring in mutant B cells has demonstrated that B cells lacking functional RAG proteins are still capable of forming RSS synapses (2) but fail to initiate V(D)J recombination, since single-stranded DNA nicks are not produced (3). Scissors represent an endonuclease. **(B)** In contrast, B cells deficient in the DNA-PKcs enzyme initiate V(D)J recombination by forming RSS synapses (2) and single-stranded DNA nicks (2) but are impaired in generating joints correctly (**3 to 5**). **(C)** A synopsis of DSBR enzymes that are required for V(D)J recombination. See text for details.

Table 7.3 Numbers of potentially functional V, D, and J genes in mouse and human immunoglobulin loci[a]

Gene	No. of genes					
	Human			Mouse		
	H chain	κ chain	λ chain	H chain	κ chain	λ chain
V	38–46	30–44	29–33	185	93–99	3
D	23–27			14		
J	6	5	4–5	4	4	3
No. of combinations[b]	5,244–7,452	150–220	116–165	10,304	372–396	4[c]

[a]Based on data that can be obtained from IMGT, http://imgt.cines.fr, with permission from M.-P. Lefranc. Numbers are based on known functional genes and potentially functional genes for which a protein product has not been confirmed. Pseudogenes and vestigial genes are not included.
[b]Number of combinations is equal to IGHV × IGHD × IGHJ or IGKV × IGKJ.
[c]In the mouse λ chain, each V gene can only rearrange with some of the J genes.

ty equal to the product of the numbers of V, D (if present), and J genes in a given immunoglobulin locus. Table 7.3 shows the diversity (i.e., the number of different antigenic specificities) generated by combinatorial rearrangement of V, D, and J genes. Note that in both mice and humans, hundreds, or even thousands, of combinations are possible for each immunoglobulin variable region, the notable exception being the mouse λ L chain, which is capable of only three variable-region combinations ($V_\lambda 2$ $J_\lambda 2$, $V_\lambda 1$ $J_\lambda 3$, and $V_\lambda 1$ $J_\lambda 1$) because of the extremely limited number of functional genes. It is important to realize that the calculations in Table 7.3 represent the maximal number of possible combinations, many of which will not actually encode antibodies. However, although the rearrangement process is usually thought to occur in a totally random fashion, in actuality it is not a random event; there is a bias toward preferential formation of some V(D)J combinations and less common production of other combinations.

H-Chain–L-Chain Pairing

Since the actual antigen-binding site of an antibody is determined by an H-chain–L-chain pair, the overall antigenic specificity of the antibody is actually influenced by the final variable regions of both the H and L chains. Mathematically, the amount of antigenic diversity created by such H-chain–L-chain pairing can be expressed as the product of the number of possible H-chain combinations and the number of possible L-chain (κ + λ) combinations. In the human, the amount of potential diversity calculated from available sequence and function data would be as follows.

H-chain diversity: 38 to 46 IGHV genes, 23 to 27 IGHD genes, and 6 IGHJ genes, or 5,244 to 7,452 possible H-chain variable-region combinations

L-chain diversity: 30 to 44 IGKV genes and 5 IGKJ genes, or 150 to 220 possible κ L-chain variable regions

29 to 33 IGLV genes and 4 to 5 IGLJ genes, or 116 to 165 possible λ L-chain variable regions

Total possible diversity: low end, $(5,244 \times 150) + (5,244 \times 116) = 1.39 \times 10^6$ HL combinations; high end, $(7,452 \times 220) + (7,452 \times 165) = 2.87 \times 10^6$ HL combinations

The influence on antigenic specificity of H-chain–L-chain pairing is most simply thought of as a result of the physical contacts the CDRs of both immunoglobulin chains make with the antigen. However, several research groups have conducted experiments that typically involve the introduction of known point mutations into either the H chain or the L chain genes for some part of the variable region, followed by measurement of how this affects the strength of the antigen binding to the antibody, known as the antigen-binding affinity. The results show that the final antigenic specificity of an H-chain–L-chain pair may not be as straightforward as the mere piecing together of the two halves of an antigen-binding site. This finding has been interpreted to mean that the H-chain variable domain and L-chain variable domain influence each other at the antibody-binding site, so that a mutation in one chain can produce slight conformational shifts in both variable domains.

Another important consideration in the antigen diversity created by V_H-L_H pairing is the relative contributions of the H- and L-chain variable regions to antigen binding. The calculation shown above showing that the combination of 7,452 IGHV genes with a total of 385 IGLV genes will result in approximately 2.87 million specificities is actually an overestimation because it is based on the presumption that the V_H and L_H regions make equal contributions to antigen binding. This is not always the case: the contribution of the V_H region to antigen binding is frequently greater than that of the V_L region.

In summary, the mechanisms of combinatorial rearrangement of V, D, and J genes and of H-chain–L-chain pairing are capable of generating fairly great antigen-binding diversity in the antibody repertoire. This diversity, however, is probably not sufficient to deal with the 10^8 to 10^{10} different antigens a host organism is likely to encounter throughout its lifetime. Four other molecular mechanisms exist that increase the antigenic diversity that can be generated. Three such mechanisms, P-nucleotide addition, junctional flexibility, and N-nucleotide addition, act during the process of V(D)J recombination to modify the junctions between V, D, and J genes. The fourth mechanism, somatic hypermutation (SHM), acts long after the process of V(D)J recombination is completed and usually happens during the process of B-cell activation.

Palindromic Nucleotide (P-Nucleotide) Addition

V(D)J recombination involves the cleavage of DNA at the RSSs that flank each gene followed by the spontaneous formation of hairpin loops (step 2 of Fig. 7.11). These nucleotides forming the hairpin loops must be cleaved by an endonuclease before the coding joints can be formed by ligation of the DNA double-stranded ends. Sometimes

a hairpin loop is cleaved open at the point of its formation (Fig. 7.16A) so that the end of the gene is restored to its original state. However, often the hairpin loop is cleaved open asymmetrically (Fig. 7.16B and C). In such cases, the hairpin loop contains an overhang of nucleotides on one strand. These overhangs are usually 2 (Fig. 7.16B) to 4 (Fig. 7.16C) nucleotides in length, depending on where the asymmetric cleavage occurs, and are repaired by a DNA polymerase that fills in the gap. Since these overhangs originate from double-stranded DNA, the nucleotides at the 5′ end of the addition are always complementary to those at the 3′ end of the addition; the base-pair additions are therefore palindromic. Thus, these nucleotide additions are termed palindromic (P)-nucleotide additions.

Addition of P-nucleotides results in a change in the total number of nucleotides in the final, rearranged variable-domain exon. One major repercussion of this event is that the reading frame of the exon may be altered, which can happen any time the total change in nucleotide number is not evenly divisible by three (because of the triplet code of protein translation). If the reading frame is shifted, it is likely that the rearranged variable-domain exon will not be functional, as it will contain many premature termination codons (Fig. 7.17). It should be noted, however, that this total change in nucleotide number is ultimately affected not only by P-nucleotide addi-

Figure 7.16 The opening of hairpin loops at the coding joint can occur at different nucleotide positions. The examples shown depict opening of a hairpin loop at a variable gene (in green text) before its ligation to a diversity gene (in red text). (**A**) If the opening of the loop (by the action of an endonuclease, represented by a pair of scissors) occurs at the same place where the loop formed, the gene remains unchanged from its original state. (**B and C**) If the hairpin loop is opened asymmetrically, single-stranded DNA overhangs will be generated at the end of the gene. When filled in by DNA POL, these overhangs will become palindromic (P-nucleotide) additions (shown in blue text). The single-stranded overhangs can be two nucleotides (**B**) or four nucleotides (**C**), depending on the location of the asymmetric cleavage.

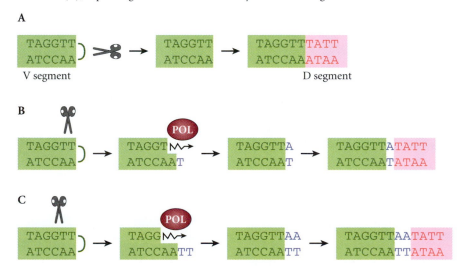

No. of nucleotides added (+) or removed (−)	Nucleotide sequence and amino acid sequence
0	V D AAGGTTAA TATTGATAGAGTA TTCCAATT ATAACTATCTCAT LysValAsnIleAspArgVal →
−1	V D AAGGTTA TATTGATAGAGTA TTCCAAT ATAACTATCTCAT LysValIleLeuIleGlu →
−2	V D AAGGTT TATTGATAGAGTA TTCCAA ATAACTATCTCAT LysValTyr ···
+1	V D AAGGTTAA A TATTGATAGAGTA TTCCAATT T ATAACTATCTCAT LysValLysTyr ···
+3	V D AAGGTTAA ATT TATTGATAGAGTA TTCCAATT TAA ATAACTATCTCAT LysValLysPheIleAspArgVal →

Figure 7.17 The removal or addition of individual nucleotides at the end of a gene (by P-nucleotide addition, junctional flexibility, or N-nucleotide addition) can enhance antibody diversity but also can cause RF shifts that can result in premature chain termination. The example shown depicts a V-D junction when 0 to 3 nucleotides are added or removed from the genes before formation of the coding joint. Blue letters indicate nucleotides added by the enzyme Tdt. The right-pointing arrow after some amino acid sequences indicates that translation continues beyond the point shown.

tion but also by the processes of junctional flexibility and N-nucleotide addition that further contribute to antibody diversity. The reading frame of the final, rearranged exon will depend on the sum total of nucleotide changes contributed by all three of these mechanisms.

If it is assumed that the reading frame is maintained after V(D)J recombination, the amino acid sequence of the variable domain will be greatly influenced by the addition of P-nucleotides. However, since P-nucleotides are added at the junctions of the IGHV, IGHD, and IGHJ genes in H chains and the IGKV/IGKJ and IGLV/IGLJ genes in the L chain, they only influence the amino acid sequence downstream of the junctions made between the appropriate IG genes. Because the first two CDRs of the V

domain are encoded upstream of these junctions entirely within the V gene, they are not affected by P-nucleotide addition; only CDR3 is affected by P-nucleotide addition since it is the only CDR encoded by sequences in the IGHD-J (for H chains) or IGKV-J/IGLV-J (for L chains) genes (Fig. 7.18).

Artemis, a protein responsible for hairpin opening, has been recently identified. It is regulated by phosphorylation by DNA-PK. Interestingly, the lack of DNA-PK activity in murine models defective in either Ku80 or DNA-PKcs is accompanied by an accumulation of hairpin coding ends along with a defect in the endonuclease responsible for their opening.

Junctional Flexibility

After the hairpin loop is opened (possibly resulting in the addition of P-nucleotides), the free DNA ends can be trimmed, usually with the removal of 1 to 10 nucleotides. This loss of nucleotides from the free end of the gene is termed *junctional flexibility.* The mechanism of nucleotide loss has not been clarified, but it is reasonable to speculate that an exonuclease is involved. This exonuclease activity can remove not only P-nucleotides that have already been added to the gene but also nucleotides that were originally part of the immunoglobulin genes. Because junctional flexibility involves the removal of individual nucleotides from the end of an immunoglobulin gene, it can produce tremendous diversity in the rearranged variable-domain exon, but it also has the potential to alter the reading frame of the exon (Fig. 7.17). Similar to P-nucleotide addition, sequence alterations due to junctional flexibility occur only in CDR3 of the immunoglobulin variable region.

Figure 7.18 Diagram of a rearranged variable-domain exon, highlighting the alignment of the V, D, and J genes with the codons encoding the three hypervariable loops (CDRs) of the domain. Note that CDRs 1 and 2 lie entirely within the IGHV gene, upstream of the IGHV-D and IGHD-J junctions. For this reason, these two CDRs are unaffected by junctional diversity. Only CDR3 is encoded by the IGHV-D and IGHD-J genes, and only CDR3 is diversified by the mechanisms of junctional flexibility, N-nucleotide addition, and P-nucleotide addition. P, nucleotides created as palindromic additions; N, nucleotides added by TdT.

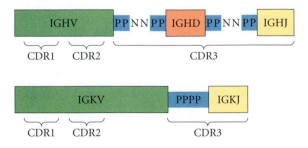

Nontemplated Nucleotide (N-Nucleotide) Addition

After the hairpin DNA loops have been opened and exonuclease trimming has occurred, additional nucleotides can be attached to the free DNA end by the enzyme TdT. TdT adds several (usually 1 to 10) nucleotides to the end of the gene with a G or C preference. Nucleotides added by the action of TdT are termed N-nucleotides since their addition is nontemplated. Like P-nucleotide addition and junctional flexibility, N-nucleotide addition has the potential to alter the reading frame of the variable-domain exon and affects only the sequence of CDR3 of the immunoglobulin chain. In mouse B cells, N-nucleotide addition is restricted to the immunoglobulin IGHV chain, since the enzyme TdT is expressed only by B cells at the pro-B-cell maturational stage when the IGHV-D-J genes are rearranged (Fig. 7.14).

After P-nucleotide addition, junctional flexibility, and N-nucleotide addition are complete, enzymatic activities such as those of the non-lymphoid-specific DNA polymerases and ligases repair the DNA ends and join the two genes together to complete the recombination process and restore the integrity of the chromosome.

Somatic Hypermutation

Combinatorial rearrangement of V, D, and J genes is the primary mechanism by which antibody diversity is generated. Junctional diversity, created by deletion and/or addition of nucleotides from the coding joints, further contributes to the diversity of CDR3. All of these mechanisms have in common their occurrence during the process of V(D)J recombination that occurs in B cells developing in the bone marrow and, thus, before the B cell had contact with antigen. This starting pool of antigenic specificities, called the *primary antigen receptor repertoire,* is therefore very efficient at generating a large and versatile array of immunoglobulin antigen receptors. However, because of the randomness of this process, it is incapable of "intentionally" producing antibodies specific for any one particular antigen and of improving any given antibody so that it binds its antigen more avidly. These two abilities, which are absolutely essential for the production of high-affinity, high-specificity antibody, are mediated by mechanisms that occur after the process of V(D)J recombination has ceased. The first of these abilities (production of antibodies for a particular antigen) is mediated by the process of clonal selection, wherein B cells that have randomly produced a particular antigen receptor are selected for proliferation following contact with the antigen. The second of these abilities (improvement of an existing antibody so that it binds its antigen more avidly) is mediated by the process of SHM, which

involves the introduction of point mutations into the variable regions of the immunoglobulin H and L chains at a relatively high rate (about 1 mutation per 1,000 bp). This mutation process alters individual nucleotides in IGKV-J, IGLV-J, and IGHV-D-J exons.

SHM differs from P-nucleotide addition, junctional flexibility, and N-nucleotide addition in several important respects. First, whereas the other mechanisms proceed via the addition or deletion of individual nucleotides from the junctions of the genes, SHM usually involves point mutations that do not change the total number of nucleotides present. As a result, SHM is not likely to cause frameshift mutations and therefore causes premature chain termination only in the unlikely event that a point mutation creates a stop codon (e.g., GGA → TGA). Second, whereas P-nucleotide addition, junctional flexibility, and N-nucleotide addition influence only CDR3 of the variable domain, SHM affects the entire variable-domain exon and can therefore affect all three CDRs and the entire framework of the variable domain (Fig. 7.19). The occurrence of SHM is influenced by the proximity of the gene to the promoter region for the immunoglobulin protein.

Role of somatic hypermutation in affinity maturation

SHM results in the introduction of point mutations, small deletions and insertions in the variable-domain exons of antibody genes. These mutations can have no effect, a negative effect, or a positive effect on the affinity of the antibody for its antigen. Since the ultimate goal of

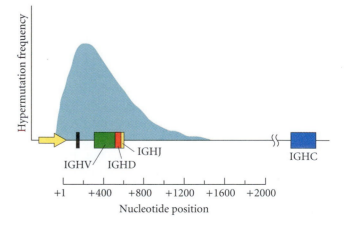

Figure 7.19 The frequency of mutations in SHM is dependent solely on the relative position of the immunoglobulin promoter and is not due to any quality unique to immunoglobulin genes. The nucleotide positions are shown on the horizontal axis in the bottom panel and indicate distance from the promoter.

the humoral immune response is the generation of antibody with high affinity for its antigen, another step is required to distinguish those B cells whose antigen receptor has been improved by the process of SHM from those that have been either unaffected or worsened by hypermutation. This entire process, including SHM and the selection event that follows it, is termed *affinity maturation*. Our present view of the clonal selection of antigen-specific B cells was proposed in the late 1950s by Talmage, Burnet, and Lederberg, who also conceived the notion that a high rate of mutation confined to a few genes in antibody-producing cells was responsible for the different antibody specificities. The existence of affinity maturation explains the early observation that antibodies produced by an animal after a second or third exposure to a given antigen usually have a higher affinity for that antigen than the antibodies produced by the same animal after its first exposure to the antigen.

The SHM process occurs in the germinal center of the secondary lymphoid follicle. The proliferating B-cell blasts (centroblasts) undergoing hypermutation are in a physiologic state that makes them extremely susceptible to programmed cell death (apoptosis). To avoid undergoing apoptosis, the centroblasts must be continuously stimulated by follicular dendritic cells (FDCs) present in the germinal center to receive *survival signals*. The centroblasts must bind to antigen-antibody immune complexes present on the FDC surface (these immune complex-containing bodies are called *iccosomes*) in order to receive the survival signals. Since the antigen present in iccosomes exists in limiting quantities, B cells with higher-affinity receptors are at a competitive advantage for survival (Fig. 7.20).

By comparing a large number of immunoglobulin gene sequences before and after affinity maturation, it is possible to map out the amino acid substitutions resulting from this process (Fig. 7.21). The mutations present in the variable domains of the antibody are not distributed randomly across the entire variable domain but are concentrated in the CDRs. The concentration of mutations in CDRs is a result of the selection event that follows the mutational process and is not due to the mutational process itself. Since the driving force for this selection event is the high-affinity binding of membrane immunoglobulin (mIg), an antibody for antigen, mutations in non-antigen-binding portions of the antibody would confer no competitive advantage on a B cell. Indeed, mutations introduced into the framework regions of an antibody are likely to result in misfolding of the variable domain of the antibody, probably ablating the ability of that antibody to bind antigen.

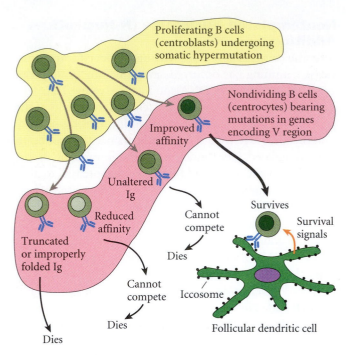

Figure 7.20 Affinity maturation is brought about by the random introduction of point mutations into immunoglobulin variable-domain exons (by SHM) followed by the selection of B cells with immunoglobulin mutations resulting in an increased affinity for antigen. After proliferation and SHM, the B cells become extremely susceptible to apoptosis and can survive only if they receive essential signals from FDCs located in the basal light zone of the germinal center. To receive these signals, the B cell must bind to antigen that is present as immune complexes (called iccosomes) on the membrane of the FDCs. Since the amount of antigen in the iccosomes is present in limiting quantities, the B cells must compete with each other for antigen binding. As a result, only those B cells with the highest affinity for antigen receive survival signals.

Experiments with transgenic animals show that the frequency of mutation directly correlates to the level of transcription and that the role of enhancers as targeting sequences for *cis*-acting factors can be uncoupled from their role in driving transcription. It is also clear that a sequence preference exists and that the surrounding sequences exert a modulating role, but what really targets the mutator machinery remains elusive. In this context, the folding of transcribed mRNA into stem-loop structures might slow the transcriptional machinery and favor kinetically the recruitment of the mutator complex.

A theory of how such mutation might occur was originally proposed in the 1960s by Brenner and Milstein. They envisaged the presence of a specific nuclease that, by an unknown mechanism, generates DNA cleavage in the antibody genes, with error-prone repair fixing the lesion into a mutation. Although the original model predicted the presence of single-strand DNA breaks as a way to explain intermediates for mutagenesis, recent findings by

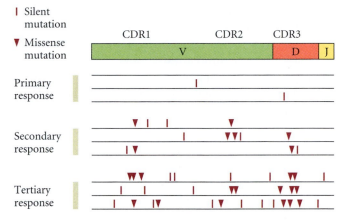

Figure 7.21 Distribution of point mutations that accumulate after affinity maturation. The diagram shows the amino acid map of the variable H and variable L domains after an initial encounter with antigen (primary) and after a second or third (tertiary) encounter with the same antigen. For each encounter, the amino acid sequence is marked with arrowheads to indicate the location of point mutations. Note that the distribution of point mutations is confined largely to the CDRs of the variable domains and differs dramatically from that of mutations introduced by SHM (Fig. 7.19). The reason for this difference is that the mutations shown are the combined result of SHM and affinity maturation. Mutations in the CDRs are selected for since they are most likely to result in an increase in antigen-binding affinity.

Sale and Neuberger and by Papavasiliou and Schatz demonstrate the existence of double-strand breaks (DSBs) restricted to IGHV regions and colocalizing with mutations. Generation of these DSBs is promoter and enhancer dependent.

The process of mutagenesis could be understood as the result of an error-prone processing of DNA breaks or of defective repair. In this context, efforts have been made to link SHM and known DNA repair pathways. Although the results were largely negative, B cells isolated from mice defective in the DNA mismatch repair protein Msh-2 exhibit an abnormal spectrum of mutations with a bias toward G or C nucleotides. However, inactivation of other subunits of the mismatch recognition complex of which Msh-2 is a component does not have an impact on SHM. These results suggest that an alternative role for Msh-2, such as recognition of a variety of DNA structures, might be involved in the recruitment of nucleases that triggers DNA repair.

Vertebrates have evolved two fundamentally different pathways for repairing DSBs: homologous recombination, which requires extensive regions of homology, and mechanisms that require little or no homology. It is not clear how many mechanisms fall into the latter category, but the major pathway in mammalian cells is DNA nonhomologous end joining (NHEJ).

As we have seen, DSBs generated by V(D)J recombina-

tion are repaired by NHEJ pathways and occur almost exclusive in the G_1 phase of the cell cycle. In contrast, DSBs generated by SHM are found in G_2, which helps to explain the lack of success in the effort to link NHEJ pathways with SHM. However, studies by Neuberger and colleagues provide evidence for a link between SHM and homologous recombination. When they disrupted the *XRCC2* or *XRCC3* gene, which is involved in homologous recombination, in chicken DT40 cells, the frequency of untemplated point mutations was much higher than in wild-type controls. It is worth noting that the mechanism of diversification of IGV genes in chickens is primarily gene conversion with few associated mutations (see below), a mechanism that was basically intact in the *XRCC2* and *XRCC3* mutants. These results suggest a potential overlap between gene conversion and SHM.

Recently, an activation-induced cytidine deaminase (AID) activity has been identified as a pivotal player in the generation of antibody diversity and has been linked to three unrelated reactions responsible for immunoglobulin assembly and modification.

Receptor Editing, a Means of Rescuing an Autoreactive B Cell from Negative Selection

Classically, it was thought that V(D)J rearrangements that encode immunoglobulins with undesirable (e.g., autoreactive) specificities lead to their elimination by the process of *negative selection*, which causes potentially autoreactive lymphocytes to undergo programmed cell death at an early stage of their development. More recent data suggest that immunoglobulin gene rearrangement could continue even after assembly of an undesirable functional B-cell mIg receptor. This gives rise to an alternative means of eliminating self-reactive B cells by a mechanism known as *receptor editing*. This process, different from anergy or deletion, serves to eliminate potentially autoreactive B cells by replacing their mIg receptor.

Secondary rearrangements can occur at both H- and L-chain genes, but the mechanism of replacement is different at the two loci. In H chains, cryptic RSSs embedded in IGHV genes upstream of those that initially were used to form the V-region encoding domain can be used so that the upstream IGHV gene can recombine with the initially formed IGHV-D-J gene to eliminate the undesirable V-region gene and produce hybrid genes for the V region. In L chains, the undesirable IGKV/IGKJ rearranged genes can be entirely replaced by secondary rearrangements of IGKV genes that recombine with a surviving downstream IGKJ gene. Thus, κ locus structure permits a replacement reaction, leading to receptor editing.

It now appears most likely that autoreactivity initially prevents B-cell developmental progression and promotes receptor editing that allows some cells to change their antigenic specificity. Although self-reactive B cells that fail to alter their receptors eventually die, death is not immediate and is delayed to a rate similar to the rate of turnover of pre-B cells that fail to generate any receptor at all. Several lines of evidence suggest that receptor editing in immature B cells is focused primarily on the V regions of the immunoglobulin L-chain loci.

Besides providing an elegant mechanism for maintaining self-tolerance, receptor editing may have an additional biologic benefit. It is universally recognized that the V(D)J recombination is far from random and that it results in an overrepresentation of certain recombined genes. Although the absence of D genes in recombined IGKV-J or IGLV-J genes facilitates receptor editing but limits receptor diversity, secondary rearrangements may play a role in diversification; this, in turn, suggests that receptor editing may be an important force in diversification of the antibody repertoire.

Interestingly, even mature B cells that have interacted with antigen can undergo receptor editing during the immune response in germinal centers. This process, known as *receptor revision,* may serve as a means of rescuing a B cell that was originally not self-reactive but then became self-reactive as a result of SHM. Molecular studies have proposed that receptor editing is a highly regulated process involving the reexpression of *Rag* genes in mature B lymphocytes. Many such studies have been carried out in transgenic mice genetically engineered to produce B cells solely expressing self-reactive immunoglobulins. Usually these B cells will be eliminated by negative selection, but in many cases mature B cells are found in these animals. These now non-self-reactive B cells express the original transgenic H chain with a newly rearranged L chain. The newly expressed H-chain–L-chain combination is no longer self-reactive despite continued expression by the B cell of the transgenic (self-reactive) H chain.

Other Mechanisms of Immunoglobulin Diversity in Other Species

The molecular mechanisms that generate a primary antibody repertoire through a combinational joining of V, D, and J genes operate in human and many rodent immune systems. Substantial differences in the timing, tissue site, and mechanism of immunoglobulin diversity exist in different vertebrate species. For example, birds create their repertoire by gene conversion from germ line pseudogenes. In this scenario, V-region genes that cannot be expressed as part of a protein on their own jump or translocate into an expression site that contains the genetic information for a full-length immunoglobulin protein. Sheep rely more heavily on somatic hypermutation, and rabbits use a combination of these mechanisms. The life stage at which the primary repertoire develops varies among species as well. This process is restricted to neonates in some species but occurs throughout life in others.

Productive and Nonproductive Rearrangements: Allelic Exclusion

Junctional diversity represents a very important source of variable-region repertoire, but this diversification also can produce translational reading-frame shifts (Fig. 7.17). These frame-shifted mRNA sequences cannot be translated into a functional protein and are therefore referred to as nonproductive rearrangements.

Since every progenitor cell begins its differentiation with two alleles of each gene, one maternally inherited and one paternally inherited, every pro-B cell has two chances of producing each immunoglobulin chain. If the rearrangement is productive during either the first or second attempt, the B cell will be allowed to proceed to the next maturation step. In contrast, unsuccessful attempts in both alleles at any stage will trigger the B cell to undergo apoptosis, since in this case the B cell will be incapable of producing a functional antigen receptor.

The protein products of V(D)J recombination not only serve to regulate B-cell development, activating subsequent recombination events at the proper times, they also regulate antigen specificity. The strict antigenic specificity of the immune system requires each B lymphocyte to express one kind of immunoglobulin molecule on its surface with only one antigenic specificity. This is true of the variable regions of both immunoglobulin H and L chains and is regulated by a mechanism referred to as *allelic exclusion.* By this mechanism, if a B cell makes a successful rearrangement of an immunoglobulin gene on its first attempt (i.e., the first of its two alleles), the B cell will not attempt to rearrange the second allele of that gene, since the genomic locus of that immunoglobulin chain will become inaccessible to the recombination enzymes. The precise molecular mechanism of allelic exclusion has yet to be elucidated.

In addition, B cells potentially could recombine either their κ or λ immunoglobulin L-chain genes, but not both. A phenomenon known as *isotypic exclusion* operates to achieve this control. This mechanism ensures that a B cell will express only one functional immunoglobulin L chain. In addition, this regulatory process ensures that functional

B cells will express only one unique immunoglobulin on the surface with only antigenic specificity.

B-Cell Differentiation

Antigen-Independent Development

In mammals, B-cell differentiation occurs in the liver during the early stages of fetal development. However, later in fetal development, or shortly after birth (depending on the species), the bone marrow becomes the site of lymphopoiesis and remains so throughout adult life. B-cell differentiation is a tightly regulated process that proceeds through many stages and involves several sequentially ordered rearrangements of immunoglobulin genes and the expression of functional immunoglobulin gene products. The expression of these immunoglobulin protein products from successfully rearranged immunoglobulin genes serves to regulate developmental events during B-cell maturation.

B-cell differentiation starts with the progenitor B-cell (pro-B-cell) stage, when rearrangement of the immunoglobulin H chain occurs (Fig. 7.22). This process occurs in two steps, the first involving rearrangement of an IGHD gene to an IGHJ gene and the second involving rearrangement of an IGHV gene to the rearranged IGHD-J genes. Successful production of an IGHV-D-J gene rearrangement allows transient expression of the single IGHM H chain at the cell surface that occurs in combination with other proteins. One of these is known as the surrogate L chain. Two other proteins, designated Ig-α and Ig-β, are also needed for the μ H chain and surrogate L chain to be present in the plasma membrane. These proteins form a complex known as the pre-B-cell receptor (pre-BCR). Surface expression of this receptor is required for further B-cell development and allows the cell to proceed to the precursor B-cell (pre-B-cell) stage. Presumably, binding of the pre-BCR to a yet-unidentified ligand on the membrane of a bone marrow stromal cell initiates a cytoplasmic signal within the pro-B cell that signals development to the pre-B-cell stage. This signal terminates all further rearrangement of the immunoglobulin H chain, leading to allelic exclusion, and also activates VJ recombination of the immunoglobulin L-chain genes (Fig. 7.22).

The immunoglobulin L-chain loci (κ or λ) are rearranged in a sequential fashion after successful rearrangement of the immunoglobulin H-chain locus (Fig. 7.22). In mice, this process always begins with rearrangement of the immunoglobulin κ locus. Successful rearrangement of the first attempted IGKV/IGKJ genes results in allelic exclusion of the remaining immunoglobulin L-chain genes,

while unsuccessful rearrangements at both κ alleles allow IGLV/IGLJ recombination at the immunoglobulin λ-chain loci to proceed. The fact that the κ-chain IGKV and IGKJ genes are always rearranged before the λ-chain IGKV and IGKJ genes explains the preponderance (95%) of κ-chain-containing immunoglobulin in mice. In humans, the choice to initially rearrange κ chain or λ chain seems to be more random and is reflected in the nearly equal use of the two L-chain types in human immunoglobulin (60% κ, 40% λ). Successful rearrangement and expression of an L-chain protein product result in assembly of a complete IgM molecule anchored in the B-cell membrane along with the Ig-α and Ig-β proteins, and trigger progression of the B cell to the "immature B-cell" stage of development.

At this stage, self-reactive B cells are negatively selected by deletion or anergy. B cells that are initially targeted for elimination by negative selection have a chance to be further modified by the L-chain editing process. If L-chain editing fails to create a functional antigen receptor that is not self-reactive, the B cell will die by apoptosis. B cells that survive this selection process can complete their development, proceeding to the "mature B-cell" stage. This final developmental step is heralded by the appearance of membrane IgD in addition to membrane IgM on the surface of the B cell. Mature lymphocytes with a complete immunoglobulin receptor can migrate to the peripheral lymphoid organs (spleen, lymph node, Peyer's patches) waiting to encounter foreign antigen.

Antigen-Dependent Development

The recognition of cognate antigen by a BCR will trigger a clonal expansion of the B cell bearing the antigen-specific receptor. During this expansion, the process of affinity maturation fine-tunes the specificity and affinity of the B cell's receptor. B lymphocytes of the selected clone can differentiate into short-lived plasma cells surviving for several days, which secrete abundant amounts of soluble immunoglobulin molecules. Some of the B cells that result from antigen-driven expansion become long-lived memory cells. Such memory cells are capable of initiating a quick immune response if and when the host organism is reexposed to the same antigen.

During this differentiation process, activated B cells also may undergo another type of genomic rearrangement known as CS recombination, which results in the production of antibody isotypes IgG, IgA, and IgE. This process maximizes the efficiency of antibody production by creating different isotypes that retain the same antigenic specificity as the original antibody but carry out different effector functions.

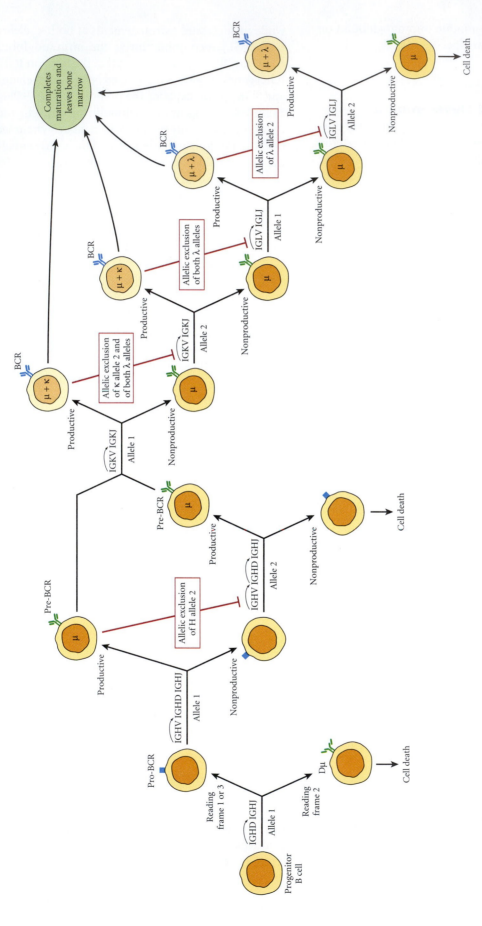

Figure 7.22 Rearrangement of the mouse IGH- and IGL-chain loci occurs in a defined sequence, always beginning with the IGH-chain locus. IGH-chain rearrangement proceeds in two steps, the first being the juxtaposition of one IGHD gene and one IGHJ gene. The IGHD and IGHJ genes can be joined in any of three RFs. If the joining occurs in RF2, a truncated form of the H chain (called D_μ) will be produced, which ultimately signals cell death. If the joining occurs in either RF1 or RF3, however, the IGHDJ gene will be joined to an IGHV gene. This step of maturation is marked by the appearance on the cell membrane of the pro-BCR, consisting of Ig-α, Ig-β, and calnexin. Successful rearrangement of the first IGH allele will inhibit rearrangement of the second IGH allele (allelic exclusion). If the first IGH allele is rearranged nonproductively, rearrangement will occur at the second IGH allele. If neither IGH allele is rearranged productively, the B cell dies by apoptosis. If one of the IGH alleles is rearranged productively, the immunoglobulin κ-chain (IGK) locus will become accessible to the recombination machinery. Note that the λ–chain locus is not rearranged at this time. Successful rearrangement of the first IGK allele will inhibit rearrangement of the second IGK allele (allelic exclusion). If the first IGK allele is rearranged nonproductively, rearrangement will occur at the second IGK allele. If one of the IGK alleles is rearranged productively, the λ-chain (IGL) locus will become accessible to the recombination machinery. Successful rearrangement of the first IGK allele will inhibit rearrangement of the second IGK allele by allelic exclusion. If the first IGL allele is rearranged nonproductively, rearrangement will occur at the second IGL allele. If one of the IGL alleles is rearranged productively, the recombination machinery is shut off and the B cell will produce an IgM/κ antibody. If neither IGK allele is rearranged productively, the λ-chain (IGL) locus will become accessible to the recombination machinery. Successful rearrangement of the first IGL allele will inhibit rearrangement of the second IGL allele by allelic exclusion. If the first IGL allele is rearranged nonproductively, rearrangement will occur at the second IGL allele. If one of the IGL alleles is rearranged productively, the B cell will produce an IgM/λ antibody. If neither IGL allele is rearranged productively, the B cell dies by apoptosis.

Overview of Model Systems for Study of B-Cell Differentiation

Use of cell lines

The availability of tumor cell lines representing different stages of B-cell differentiation has provided an invaluable tool for the molecular dissection of B-cell differentiation. For example, the ability of the Abelson murine leukemia virus (A-MuLV) to transform cells derived from bone marrow or fetal liver permitted the establishment of cell lines representative of these early cell stages. Although these A-MuLV cell lines do not fully differentiate in culture and express abnormal levels of V(D)J recombination activity, they proved useful in elucidating the normal sequences of endogenous immunoglobulin gene rearrangements.

More recently, nontransformed B-cell precursors have been propagated in long-term cultures from bone marrow cells. The use of appropriate stromal cell lines to simulate the hematopoietic bone marrow cells and the addition of specific growth factors and cytokines such as interleukin-7 have allowed re-creation of hematopoietic conditions in the laboratory and have provided a means of characterizing this process more finely and under more realistic conditions than could previously be obtained with transformed B-cell lines.

Finally, normal mature murine B cells can be activated in culture to proliferate and secrete immunoglobulin. This is accomplished by treatment of the B cells with nonspecific activators such as cross-linking antibody specific for a B cell's surface immunoglobulin receptor and bacterial lipopolysaccharide, alone or in combination with cytokines. These systems have proven useful for studying the molecular events involved in B-cell activation and the impact of cytokines on CS recombination.

Use of animal models

The ability to generate transgenic and somatic chimeric mice is another powerful tool for studying in vivo aspects of B-cell differentiation. For example, the generation of mice deficient in one of the key genes involved in V(D)J recombination (e.g., *Rag-2*) not only served to demonstrate that B- and T-cell lines have the same recombination machinery, since both immunoglobulin and TCR rearrangements are defective in such mice, but also provided a murine model for the study of immunodeficiency disorders.

Moreover, complementation of blastocysts isolated from *Rag-2*$^{-/-}$ animals is a powerful alternative system for rapidly assessing the role of particular genes in the development of the immune system and for circumventing some of the problems of the embryonic lethal phenotypes if the activity is required for early developmental events in cells other than lymphocytes (Fig. 7.23).

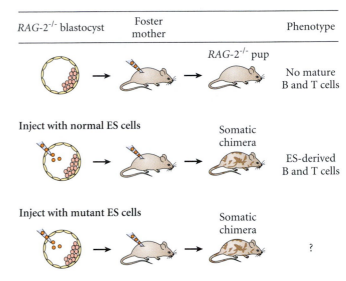

RAG-2$^{-/-}$ blastocyst	Foster mother		Phenotype
		RAG-2$^{-/-}$ pup	No mature B and T cells
Inject with normal ES cells		Somatic chimera	ES-derived B and T cells
Inject with mutant ES cells		Somatic chimera	?

Figure 7.23 *Rag-2*$^{-/-}$ mice have deficiencies of B cells and T cells because of an inability to carry out variable-region gene recombination for either immunoglobulin or T-cell receptor production (**top**). Blastocysts from *Rag-2*$^{-/-}$ mice can be rescued from this immunodeficient state by receiving an injection of *Rag-2*$^{+/+}$ embryonic stem (ES) cells (**middle**). The targeted disruption of various genes in the ES cells prior to their being injected into the *Rag-2*$^{-/-}$ blastocyst is a useful way of assessing the role of the disrupted genes in B-cell or T-cell development (**bottom**). The resultant somatic chimera mice can be tested for the presence of mature B and T cells, and if none is found, the DNA of the mouse can be analyzed to see what gene was disrupted to prevent the ES cells from restoring B- or T-cell development.

Last, introduction of fully rearranged immunoglobulin genes into the germ line of mice has permitted the study of B-cell regulatory events such as allelic exclusion and constitutes a powerful tool for understanding processes such as CS recombination. The introduction of prerearranged immunoglobulin transgenes that recognize self antigens also has allowed such transgenic technology to be applied to the study of self-tolerance.

Surrogate L-Chain Genes

The transition from pro-B cell to pre-B cell in B-cell development relies on the expression on the B-cell surface of the pre-BCR, which consists of a successfully rearranged immunoglobulin H chain complexed with two proteins called *surrogate L chains* (Fig. 7.24A). These two nonrearranging λ-chain-related genes have been determined experimentally to play a crucial role in B-cell maturation in both mice and humans and are termed λ5 (the human counterpart is called *14.1*) and *VpreB*. λ5 and *VpreB* are located on the same chromosome about 5 kb apart but are not linked to the λ immunoglobulin L-chain locus.

The murine λ5 gene is organized in three exons separated by introns of about 1.3 kb. Amino acid sequencing

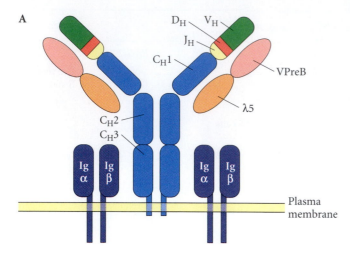

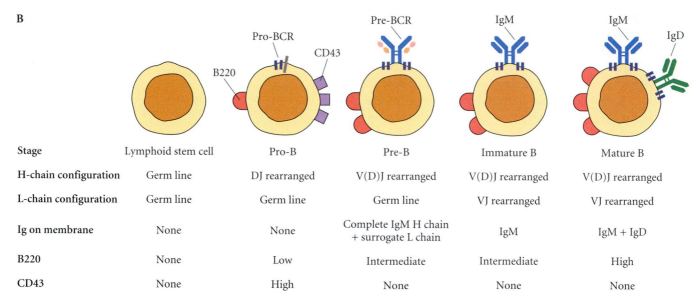

Figure 7.24 B-cell maturation. (**A**) A diagram of the pre-BCR. In this complex, membrane-bound immunoglobulin H chain is associated with the surrogate L chain (comprising the proteins λ5 and VpreB) and the signaling components Ig-α and Ig-β. (**B**) Schematic representation of B-cell development, highlighting status of IGH-chain and IGL-chain rearrangement and membrane expression of immunoglobulin, the B220 phosphatase, and CD43 glycoprotein. During the pro-B-cell stage, the cell can transiently express on its surface the pro-BCR. The pro-BCR consists of the proteins Ig-α, Ig-β, and calnexin and appears on the membrane of the B cell at the developmental stage where the immunoglobulin H chain is incompletely rearranged and has only completed IGHD-J rearrangement (Fig. 7.22).

Stage	Lymphoid stem cell	Pro-B	Pre-B	Immature B	Mature B
H-chain configuration	Germ line	DJ rearranged	V(D)J rearranged	V(D)J rearranged	V(D)J rearranged
L-chain configuration	Germ line	Germ line	Germ line	VJ rearranged	VJ rearranged
Ig on membrane	None	None	Complete IgM H chain + surrogate L chain	IgM	IgM + IgD
B220	None	Low	Intermediate	Intermediate	High
CD43	None	High	None	None	None

has revealed certain areas of homology to conventional IGLV, IGLJ, and IGLC genes, strongly suggesting that the λ5 locus may have arisen by duplication of the conventional immunoglobulin λ locus. In contrast, the *VpreB* gene resembles a conventional IGLV gene, including the presence of a leader sequence as an upstream exon.

The λ5 and VpreB gene products are utilized as the C-like and V-like components, respectively, of the surrogate L chain. In association with the productively rearranged IGHM chain, Ig-α and Ig-β, λ5 and VpreB allow the assembly of the pre-BCR (Fig. 7.24A). In this complex, λ5 is covalently associated with membrane-bound μ H chain, while VpreB is noncovalently associated with this complex. Experiments involving ablation of λ5 in mice by gene targeting demonstrate the requirement of this gene product for efficient differentiation of pro-B cells, suggesting a role in signaling successful immunoglobulin H-chain rearrangement.

Surface Marker Expression during Early B-Cell Stages

B-cell maturation involves rearrangement of functional immunoglobulin H and L chains and occurs in developmental stages that are dependent on these genetic recombination events. These developmental stages also correlate with the expression by B cells of certain cell surface markers (Fig. 7.24B). Chief among the markers used for tracking B-cell differentiation are B220 (a B-cell-specific isoform of the CD45 protein tyrosine phosphatase), CD43 (a sialoprotein estimated to play a role in regulating cell-cell adhesion), and membrane IgM and IgD. H-chain recombination is initiated in B cells that express low levels of B220 (B220[lo]) and CD43 (CD43[+]), but no detectable mIgM or mIgD. The pre-BCR is an important and useful cell surface marker, as it identifies cells that have a rearranged H but not L chain. Also noteworthy is a brief expression by a pro-B cell of the *pro-BCR* (Fig. 7.24B), which is composed of Ig-α, Ig-β, and calnexin. The pro-BCR is expressed after completion of only the first step of V(D)J recombination at the level of IGHD-IGHJ gene rearrangement. However, because of variations in the sites where transcription of the IGHD-IGHJ joints is initiated, a reading frame known as reading frame 2 (RF$_2$) encodes a truncated polypeptide known as D$_\mu$ that, when present on the pre-B-cell surface associated with Ig-α–Ig-β and surrogate L chain, generates a defective receptor that inhibits further variable-region gene rearrangements and halts B-cell differentiation (Fig. 7.22).

Successful assembly and expression of immunoglobulin H chain allow the cell to progress to a pre-B-cell stage, in which the B cells rearrange their immunoglobulin L chain and become B220$^+$, CD43$^-$, mIgM$^+$, and mIgD$^-$ (called *immature B cells*). Last, mature B cells (B220$^+$, CD43$^-$, mIgM$^+$, and mIgD$^+$) can migrate to the peripheral lymphoid organs.

Regulation of Immunoglobulin Expression

As with other eukaryotic genes, control of immunoglobulin H- and L-chain transcription involves *cis*-acting genetic elements, including a promoter located upstream of the variable gene (immediately 5$'$ of the leader exon) and enhancer elements. The locations of these elements in germ line immunoglobulin DNA are shown in Fig. 7.25A.

Transcription of immunoglobulin loci is strongly correlated with V(D)J recombination, in that only a low level of transcription is detectable before gene rearrangement occurs. After V(D)J rearrangement, however, transcriptional activity increases approximately 1,000-fold. It is thought that this is because the transcriptional enhancer elements of the immunoglobulin loci in the unrearranged (germ line) configuration are too far away from the immunoglobulin promoters to affect transcription from them (Fig. 7.25B, top). During V(D)J recombination, the promoter region immediately upstream of the variable gene is brought into closer proximity (Fig. 7.25B, bottom) with the enhancer elements, which lie 5$'$ of the C$_\mu$ (in the immunoglobulin H-chain locus) and 3$'$ of the constant regions (in all immunoglobulin loci). Thus, the DNA rearrangement process involved in the generation of a functional variable region also provides a means to regulate immunoglobulin gene expression by bringing together positive regulatory sequences involved in the transcription of immunoglobulin H- and L-chain loci.

Transcription at the Immunoglobulin Loci
The immunoglobulin H-chain locus
Before the formation of a completely recombined immunoglobulin gene, low-level transcription is initiated at the locus through the use of several cryptic promoters

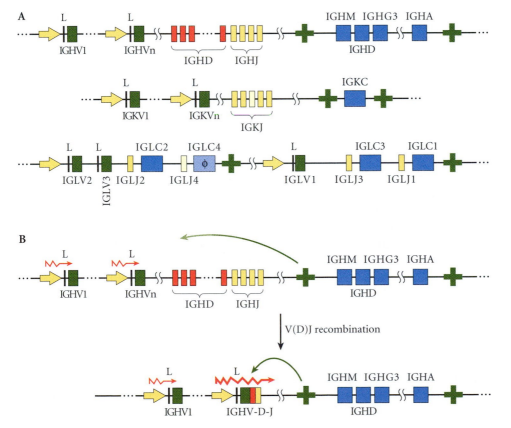

Figure 7.25 (A) Genomic arrangements of the mouse immunoglobulin IGH locus (**top**), IGK locus (**middle**), and IGL locus (**bottom**), highlighting the locations of promoters (yellow arrows) and enhancers (green plus signs). (B) The promoters preceding each V-region gene are all very weak and are unable to direct transcription in the absence of enhancer activity. In the genomic configuration (before IGHV-D-J rearrangement occurs), the promoters are too far away from the enhancers to benefit from the enhancers' activity (top, short red squiggly arrows). IGHV-D-J production brings the promoter close enough to the enhancers such that the latter can amplify transcription (**bottom**, long red squiggly arrow).

located upstream of the various germ line immunoglobulin genes. For example, the murine IGHJ-IGHC region is transcribed before assembly of a complete V(D)J unit. Experiments conducted in pre-B-cell lines isolated from *Rag*-deficient mice show the presence of a transcript that appears to initiate just 5′ to the IGHD genes (encoding the D component of the variable domain). Another germ line μ-specific transcript, known as I_μ, initiates in the IGHJ-IGHC intron just downstream of the enhancer. A mature I_μ transcript consists of a 5′ exon spliced to the IgM constant-region coding exons. However, no polypeptide product of this transcript has been detected, a property of what is known as *sterile transcripts*.

Rearrangement and joining of IGHD-IGHJ genes allow the transcription from a cryptic promoter 5′ of the IGHD gene to be initiated (D_μ). One of the RFs of this transcript allows the translation of a polypeptide containing a truncated IGHD gene. The truncated protein product is responsible for the RF2 counterselection. Last, during the immature B-cell stage, germ line transcription can be detected from promoters 5′ of IGHV genes. These transcripts are generally terminated downstream of the IGHV coding sequences and likely represent part of a transcription-based mechanism that regulates V(D)J recombination.

Sterile transcripts at the immunoglobulin H-chain locus are not limited to the IGHV, IGHD, and IGHJ genes but also are found throughout the portion of the locus encoding the IGHC genes. In these cases, transcription begins at a cryptic promoter located immediately upstream of regulatory elements known as *switch regions*, which lie upstream of each IGHC gene. These sterile transcripts play an important role in CS recombination.

The immunoglobulin L-chain locus

During B-lymphocyte differentiation, germ line IGKJ-IGKC transcription, which initiates 5′ of the IGKJ genes, appears to be specifically induced prior to IGKV-IGKJ rearrangement. Of interest is the finding that these transcripts are induced by the expression of immunoglobulin H chain in the B cell. This finding has led to the notion that expression of the immunoglobulin H-chain protein activates the germ line immunoglobulin L-chain locus. The mechanism by which this signal is delivered is likely to involve the expression of the pre-BCR and is therefore likely to be similar to the signal that mediates allelic exclusion of the H chain.

Sequential rearrangement of κ- and λ-chain genes

After successful rearrangement of an antibody H-chain gene, the B cell needs to rearrange its L-chain genes to produce a complete (H_2L_2) antibody molecule. This process requires strict regulation in several respects. First, L-chain rearrangement needs to be regulated such that this process occurs only after H-chain rearrangement is successfully completed and only one L-chain transcript is produced. The second level at which immunoglobulin L-chain rearrangement is regulated is the determination of which L-chain type (κ or λ) is ultimately produced by the cell. Several mechanisms have been proposed to explain the allelic and isotypic exclusion phenomena. While stochastic (random) rearrangements and feedback mechanisms play a role, directed regulatory processes, such as the kinetics and the efficacy of gene rearrangements, are also responsible. In addition, L-chain loci are subjected to feedback suppression similar to that for H-chain loci. However, the evidence for feedback suppression in L-chain gene rearrangement is less compelling.

Immunoglobulin H-Chain Isotype Expression during B-Cell Differentiation
Differential processing of primary transcripts

Expression of the membrane or secreted form of immunoglobulin

Any antibody can exist in a membrane-bound form on the surface of a B cell where it participates in B-cell activation as a part of the BCR or can be secreted by the B cell to perform immune effector functions. The regulated synthesis of these two forms of a given antibody is achieved through the alternative usage of two exons encoding the hydrophobic stretch or "membrane anchor" amino acids at the carboxy terminus of the immunoglobulin H chain. This is achieved at the RNA level by differential processing of the H-chain primary transcript. As shown in Fig. 7.26, the genetic region encoding an immunoglobulin H chain has two different polyadenylation [poly(A)] addition signals. One of these poly(A) sites (site 1) is located immediately downstream of the last immunoglobulin constant-region exon ($C_\mu4$ in Fig. 7.26), while the other poly(A) site (site 2) is located several kilobases downstream of the constant-region exons, immediately after two small exons called M1 and M2. M1 and M2 encode the amino acids that make up the hydrophobic transmembrane and hydrophilic intracellular domains, respectively, of the membrane-bound form of the immunoglobulin H chain. Utilization of the poly(A) site 3′ of exon $C_\mu4$ will terminate the transcript at this place, removing the M1 and M2 exons from the mature transcript and allowing the incorporation of amino acids that encode the hydrophilic secreted terminus of the immunoglobulin H chain. In contrast, utilization of the poly(A) site 3′ of exon M2 retains the M1 and M2 exons in the mature H-chain transcript, allowing production of the transmembrane form of the immunoglobulin H chain.

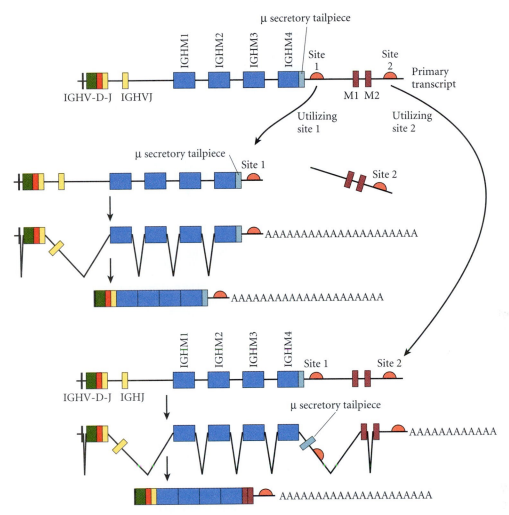

Figure 7.26 Alternative usage of two poly(A) addition sites in the immunoglobulin H-chain constant (IGHC) region, which is accompanied by alternative RNA splicing, determines the selective production of either secreted or membrane-bound immunoglobulin. Use of a poly(A) site involves RNA cleavage at the site by an endonuclease and attachment of a poly(A) tail (AAAAA...) to the transcript. Utilization of the poly(A) site close to 3′ exon IGHM4 (site 1) terminates the transcript at this place, removing the M1 and M2 exons from the mature transcript and allowing incorporation of amino acids that encode the secreted terminus of the IGHC. In contrast, utilization of the poly(A) site 3′ of exon M2 (site 2) retains the M1 and M2 exons in the mature IGHC transcript, allowing production of the transmembrane form of the IGHC. Simultaneously, utilization of site 2 results in an alternative splicing scheme that removes from the transcript the hydrophilic secreted tail of the IGHC and includes in the transcript the M1 and M2 exons, which encode the hydrophobic transmembrane and hydrophilic cytoplasmic domains, respectively, of the membrane-bound form of the IGHC.

Alternative usage of the two poly(A) addition sites of the immunoglobulin H-chain transcript is accompanied by alternative RNA splicing events. Utilization of the poly(A) site 3′ to the M2 exon results in splicing from a splice donor site within the $C_\mu 4$ exon to a splice acceptor site at the 5′ end of the M1 exon (Fig. 7.26). A second splicing event occurs, utilizing a splice donor located at the 3′ end of M1 and a splice acceptor at the 5′ end of M2. This alternative splicing scheme simultaneously removes from the transcript the hydrophilic secreted terminus of the immunoglobulin H chain and includes in the tran-

script the M1 and M2 exons. Since resting B cells produce only membrane-bound immunoglobulin, whereas plasma cells produce only secreted immunoglobulin, it is assumed that stage-specific splicing factors regulate this alternative splicing event.

Antigen-independent expression of IgD

Production of IgD also uses an alternative splicing mechanism (Fig. 7.27) similar to that used to selectively produce membrane and secreted IgM antibody (Fig. 7.26). Because IgM and IgD are produced by alternative splic-

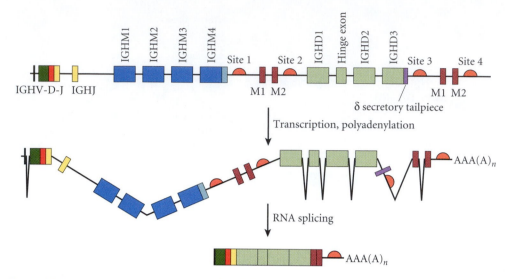

Figure 7.27 A mechanism similar to that used to differentially produce secreted and membrane-bound immunoglobulin (Fig. 7.26) is also responsible for the simultaneous production of IgM and IgD by a single B cell. A primary IGHC transcript contains the coding sequences necessary for the production of secreted IGHM, membrane-bound IgM, secreted IgD, and membrane-bound IgD. In the example shown, the utilization of polyadenylation [$AAA(A)_n$] site 4 allows the production of membrane-bound IgD. Note that this mechanism regulates *only* the production of IgM and IgD, since all other isotypes are produced by class switch recombination, which requires rearrangement of DNA.

ing, it is possible for one B cell to simultaneously produce both IgM and IgD. Coexpression of IgD and IgM antibodies with the same antigenic specificity is a characteristic feature of mature, naive B cells that emerge from bone marrow following hematopoiesis. The mechanism that allows such simultaneous expression involves alternative splicing as well as alternative usage of multiple poly(A) addition sites. This is the only circumstance in both mice and humans that a non-IgM isotype is expressed in the absence of antigenic stimulation. It is also the only example in these two species of simultaneous expression of two antibody isotypes by a single normal B cell. No effector function has been assigned to IgD, and this isotype is normally present in serum in minute quantities (about 30 micrograms per milliliter). However, membrane-bound IgD exists on the B-cell surface as a part of a BCR complex containing Igα and Igβ proteins. Moreover, the acquisition by a maturing B cell of the ability to produce IgD via alternative mRNA splicing strongly correlates with the functional maturity (immune competence) of the B cell. Because of these facts, the role of IgD is thought to be limited to that of membrane-bound IgD on the surface of the resting B cell where it contributes to the regulation of B-cell development or activation.

CS recombination

One of the most perplexing puzzles in the molecular genetics of antibody production was the ability of an ani-

mal to produce different isotype antibodies of identical antigenic specificity. For example, early immunologists knew that one animal could make antibody of one isotype upon initial exposure to an antigen but could produce an antibody of identical specificity, but different isotype, upon a second exposure to the same antigen. We now know that this is made possible through a process known as CS recombination. CS recombination is another mechanism by which DNA is physically rearranged in B cells and is distinct from V(D)J recombination (Table 7.4). In CS recombination, the IGHV-D-J exon encoding the H-chain variable domain is moved from its original position 5′ of the IGHM constant-region exons to a new position immediately 5′ of the constant regions of another antibody isotype. The DNA sequences that originally lay between the original position of the IGHV-D-J exon and its new position are permanently removed from the genome by a looping-deletion mechanism (Fig. 7.28A). The important exception to this rule is the C_δ region, which is expressed not through CS recombination but through the alternative splicing mechanism that gives rise to membrane-bound or secreted immunoglobulin (Fig. 7.27). In contrast to V(D)J recombination, which occurs during B-cell development in the absence of antigen, switch recombination generally occurs in mature B cells and *after* antigen stimulation.

Although the exact mechanism of CS recombination is unclear, the DNA rearrangement involved in this

Table 7.4 A comparison of V(D)J recombination and class switch recombination

Characteristic	V(D)J recombination	Class switch recombination
Immunoglobulin chain affected	Heavy and light	Heavy only
Antigen dependence	Independent	Dependent
Cell types	B cells and T cells	B cells only
Maturational stage	Progenitor and precursor	Mature, activated
Specificity	Site specific	Region specific
Target *cis*-acting sequence	RSS	Switch region
Mechanism of rearrangement	Deletion or inversion	Deletion
Purpose of process	Antigenic diversity	Change of isotype of Ig
Likelihood of nonproductive rearrangement	Likely	Not possible
Reading frame affected?	Possible	Not possible
trans-acting factors	RAG-1, RAG-2, TdT, DSBR enzymes	Activation-induced cytidine deaminase

process is known to be different from the one that operates in V(D)J recombination. As in the site-specific recombination process involved in variable-domain assembly, flanking sequences known as switch regions are necessary to activate CS recombination. These switch regions are located 2 to 3 kb upstream of each IGHC gene (except C$_\delta$) and are composed mainly of a tandem repeat of a pentameric GC-rich motif (Fig. 7.28A). However, because the switch regions lie within introns, not at the junctions or coding regions, the imprecision of CS recombination has no effect on translational RFs. Thus, all rearrangements are productive. Each switch region is preceded by an *I exon* (Fig. 7.28B), which in turn is preceded by a promoter. As with V(D)J recombination, germ line transcription from the I exon promoter precedes the switch to production of a particular IGHC gene.

Transcription begins at the I-region promoter, runs through the switch region and the constant-domain exons, and undergoes termination and polyadenylation at the normal sites downstream of the IGHC exons. The primary transcript thus generated undergoes splicing to join the I exon to the IGHC exons, with the deletion of the intervening introns (Fig. 7.28B). This results in the production of a mature mRNA sterile transcript that does not encode a functional protein. Although the role of this sterile transcript is unknown, induction of these transcripts is necessary but not sufficient to induce CS recombination. The action of RNA polymerase on the switch region is thought to be important for altering chromatin structure and rendering the switch region accessible to the machinery that leads to CS recombination. The particular IGHC region to be affected by CS recombination can be modulated by the presence of specific cytokines. By analogy to the findings on the control of V(D)J recombination, germ

line transcription precedes the recombination of that particular IGHC gene with a rearranged and functional IGHV-D-J gene. Thus, the cytokine climate of a particular immune response, which is influenced in part by the activation of T helper type 1 versus T helper type 2 cells, and in part by localized inflammatory events, can affect the choice of which antibody isotype will predominate after B-cell activation (Fig. 7.28C).

CS recombination appears to be strictly a B-cell specific event and, in addition to being regulated by contact-dependent signals and cytokines from T cells, is induced and regulated by antigen. Interestingly, some antigens cannot be processed and presented by T cells but nonetheless elicit antibodies; these are called T-cell-independent antigens (see chapters 8 and 10) and can also trigger CS recombination. For example, CS recombination can be induced in cultured mouse B cells by a number of different T-independent antigens. In contrast to widely held beliefs among some immunologists, some, but not all, T-independent antigens such as purified bacterial polysaccharide capsules used to immunize humans induce CS recombination. Therefore, it is thought that multiple events can serve as signals triggering CS recombination.

An AID in the Generation of Immunoglobulin Diversity

Several proteins that bind to or cleave S regions in vitro have been identified, but the in vivo relevance in CS recombination remains unclear. However, in a screen for molecules differentially expressed after induction of CS recombination in the B-cell lymphoma CH12F3-2, an enzyme called AID has been identified by T. Honjo and colleagues. With sequence homology to RNA editing deaminases, AID is preferentially localized in secondary

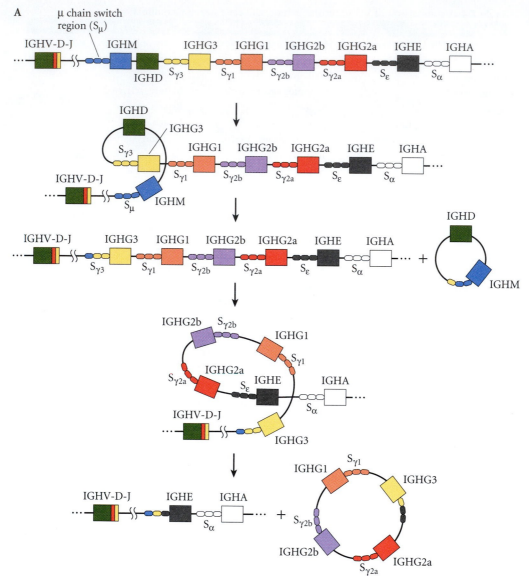

Figure 7.28 CS recombination is the means by which a B cell changes from production of an antibody of one isotype to production of an antibody of a different isotype but the same antigenic specificity. This is accomplished by the physical rearrangement of the IGHC locus that moves the IGHV-D-J gene from an initial location (immediately upstream of the exons encoding the constant region of IGHM) to a location immediately upstream of the exons encoding the constant region of another IGHC isotype. (**A**) Switch regions serve as the *cis*-acting elements that target CS recombination to the appropriate location in the immunoglobulin locus and consist of tandem-repetitive sequences. A switch region is represented as an array of ellipses. During CS recombination, a recombination event causes a crossover of two switch regions belonging to different isotype exons. DNA sequences that lie between the original location of the IGHV-D-J gene and its final location are removed permanently from the genome by a looping deletion mechanism. Since the switch regions are tandem repeats, the synapse formed between the two switch regions can occur in one of several different registers, resulting in an imprecise recombination event. Since this recombination event happens in an intron, the imprecision of recombination has no effect on the translational reading frame. (**B**) CS recombination at a given switch region is thought to be activated by the initiation of sterile transcription from a promoter (yellow arrow) located upstream of the switch region, at the so-called I exon. This sterile transcript (red zigzag arrow) is processed by polyadenylation and splicing (splicing joins the I exon to the constant-region exons), just like a normal productive transcript. This transcription may help make the chromatin structure at the switch region accessible to the recombinase machinery. (**C**) The choice of isotype during CS recombination is governed in part by cytokines. The example shown depicts the action of interleukin-4 (IL-4) in causing preferential class switching to the isotype IgE. IL-4 mediates this effect by inducing sterile transcription at the I exon promoter of the ε-chain switch region (S_ε).

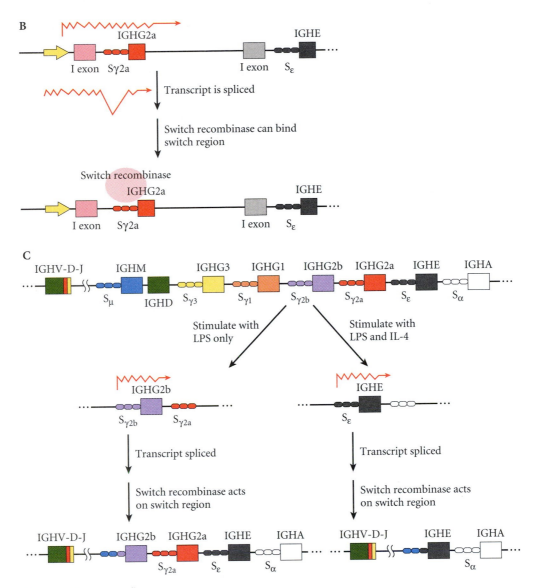

Figure 7.28 *(continued)*

lymphoid organs. More important, mice and humans deficient in this protein are impaired in CS recombination and, surprisingly, in SHM. A recent study using the chicken cell line DT40 implicated AID as essential for diversification of IGV genes by gene conversion.

In fact, several potential parallels between CS recombination and SHM can be drawn: (i) both reactions take place in germinal center B cells in response to antigen stimulation, but they occur independently of each other; (ii) although CS recombination is confined to the vicinity of switch recombination regions and SHM spreads over the IGV gene, DNA cleavage is associated with mutation, and switch recombination regions are often mutated; (iii) both processes are tightly linked to transcription;

(iv) Msh-2 deficiencies generate similar phenotypes in SHM and CS recombination; and (v) there is an AID requirement, i.e., expression of AID is sufficient to activate SHM in B-cell hybridomas and CS recombination in 3T3 fibroblasts.

As discussed above, SHM breaks appear primarily during G_2, consistent with the fact that the NHEJ pathway has no impact on the repair of those lesions. However, studies have implicated NHEJ, Ku70, Ku80, and DNA-PKcs in CS recombination, but junctions of this transaction contain a high frequency of point mutations, an atypical outcome for this type of repair. In the same context, the repair of DSBs generated by CS recombination is proposed to occur in G_1 based on the abundance of repair foci associated with this transaction which contain AID and Nbs1. How many more repair processes are involved in this reaction and how these pathways are orchestrated are unknown.

Early studies showed that when S regions are transcribed in vitro, transcripts remain on the template DNA, forming DNA-RNA hybrids. Recently, Ming and Alt showed that the displaced nontemplate strand remains largely single stranded and that the hybrid adopts an R-loop structure that can be recognized and cleaved by an endonuclease involved in nucleotide excision repair. This model is based entirely on in vitro data, and in vivo validation is not available; however, it provides an attractive model for the generation of secondary structures that might serve as motifs recognized by factors like Msh2.

Although the exact function of AID is speculative and its role may be indirect as an RNA editing enzyme for the mRNA of an endonuclease for the DNA breaks, three gene diversification processes might be initiated by a common type of DNA lesion. Finally, when Neuberger and colleagues forced the expression of AID in *Escherichia coli*, they found that it confers a mutator phenotype and is consistent with a deaminating function of dC residues in DNA. These results led them to propose that the diversification of immunoglobulin, SHM, CS recombination, and gene conversion is triggered by AID-mediated deamination of dC residues and that the outcome depends on how this lesion is resolved by the different DNA repair pathways.

Summary

One of the major mysteries of the generation of diversity in antigen binding among immunoglobulin proteins has been solved in the past 20 years by understanding the mechanism of V(D)J recombination in antibody genes. Two or three genes, encoding V, J, and D portions of the immunoglobulin variable region, can recombine to form a single gene encoding the entire variable region, a process that occurs during B-cell development in the bone marrow. This rearrangement is mediated by specific nucleotide sequences in the IGV, IGJ, and IGD genes, known as recombination signaling sequences, and is involved in both lymphoid-specific factors (RAG-1 and RAG-2) and non-lymphoid-specific factors. Additional mechanisms for the generation of diversity encompass combinatorial binding of the different IGV, IGJ, and IGD genes, pairing of different H and L chains to produce immunoglobulin of different antigenic specificity, and changes introduced into the third CDR by junctional flexibility and P-nucleotide and N-nucleotide addition. Further diversity is generated by the process of somatic hypermutation, where B cells responding to an antigenic stimulus accumulate point mutations in the regions of the genes that code for the CDRs, that leads to antibody with a higher affinity for the antigen. Affecting these processes are control points allowing changes to the immunoglobulin genes, including receptor editing and receptor revision, that contribute to the elimination of potentially self-reactive B cells.

B cells differentiate in the absence of antigen (antigen-independent development) in the bone marrow (or sometimes other organs in other animals), going through a series of defined stages that start with rearrangement of the H-chain IGHD and IGHJ genes. There are numerous regulatory processes that control B-cell development, including transcriptional regulation of the immunoglobulin genes, allelic exclusion, and sequential rearrangement of L-chain variable-region genes. Following a predetermined series of changes in gene expression and synthesis of mIg, a B cell that can leave the bone marrow and seed the secondary lymphoid organs is produced. If stimulated by antigen, the B cell can undergo CS recombination to combine the same genes that form the variable region with a gene for a different constant region, resulting in isotype switching. The overall understanding we now have of the genetics of antibody production has been a major advance in modern molecular biology and medicine, and, so far, the use of a limited number of multiple genes to produce the tremendous number of possible antibody molecules is only replicated with genes encoding the TCR. No other biologic process appears yet to be based on similar molecular genetic mechanisms.

Suggested Reading

Blunt, T., N. J. Finnie, G. E. Taccioli, G. C. M. Smith, J. Demengeot, T. M. Gottlieb, R. Mizuta, A. J. Varghese, F. W. Alt, P. A. Jeggo, and S. P. Jackson. 1995. Defective DNA-dependent protein kinase activity is linked to V(D)J recombination and DNA repair defects associated with the murine *SCID* mutation. *Cell* **80**:813–823.

Fugmann, S. D., A. I. Lee, P. E. Shockett, I. J. Viley, and D. G. Schatz. 2000. The RAG proteins and V(D)J recombination: complexes, ends, and transposition. *Annu. Rev. Immunol.* **18**: 495–527.

Gellert, M. 2002. V(D)J recombination: RAG proteins, repair factors, and regulation. *Annu. Rev. Biochem.* **71**:101–132.

Grawunder, U., and E. Harfst. 2001. How to make ends meet in V(D)J recombination. *Curr. Opin. Immunol.* **13**:186–194.

Honjo, T., K. Kinoshita, and M. Muramatsu. 2002. Molecular

mechanism of class switch recombination: linkage with somatic mutation. *Annu. Rev. Immunol.* **20**:165–196.

Lefranc, M.-P., and G. Lefranc. 2001. *The Immunoglobulin Facts Book.* Academic Press, New York, N.Y.

Ma, Y., U. Pannicke, K. Schwarz, and M. Lieber. 2002. Hairpin opening and overhang processing by an artemis/DNA-dependent protein kinase complex in nonhomologous end joining and V(D)J recombination. *Cell* **108**:781–794.

Meffre, E., R. Casellas, and M. C. Nussenzweig. 2000. Antibody regulation of B cell development. *Nat Immunol.* **1**:379–385.

Nemanzee, D. 2000. Receptor selection in B and T lymphocytes. *Annu. Rev. Immunol.* **18**:19–51.

Neuberger, M. S., M. R. Ehrenstein, C. Rada, J. Sale, F. D. Batista, G. Williams, and C. Milstein. 2000. Memory in the B-cell compartment: antibody affinity maturation. *Philos. Trans. R. Soc. Lond. B* **355**:357–360.

Papavasiliou, F. N., and D. G. Schatz. 2002. Somatic hypermutation of immunoglobulin genes: merging mechanisms for genetic diversity. *Cell* **109**(Suppl.):S35–S44.

Sadofsky, M. J. 2001. The RAG proteins in V(D)J recombination: more than just a nuclease. *Nucleic Acids Res.* **29**:1399–1409.

Sleckman, B. P., J. R. Gorman, and W. Alt. 1996. Accessibility control of antigen-receptor variable-region gene assembly: role of cis-acting elements. *Annu. Rev. Immunol.* **14**:459–481.

Stavnezer, J. 1996. Immunoglobulin class switching. *Curr. Opin. Immunol.* **8**:199–205.

Tonegawa, S. 1983. Somatic generation of antibody diversity. *Nature* **302**:575–581.

Vercelli, D. 2002. Novel insights into class switch recombination. *Curr. Opin. Allergy Clin. Immunol.* **2**:147–151.

chapter 8

Antigens, Antigenicity, and Immunogenicity

Gerald B. Pier

The initiation of an immune response requires the interaction between T cells, B cells, and antigen-presenting cells (APCs), which form central components of almost all immune responses, and antigens, substances recognized as foreign by the immune system. Therefore, antigens initiate an immune response whose goal is to eliminate the antigens from an organism and restore homeostasis. Most antigens possess the property of *foreignness,* although in certain pathologic situations, indigenous or self antigens are able to provoke immune responses. Antigens must have numerous chemical and physical properties in order to initiate an immune response and combine with the immune effectors thus generated. Some antigens are incapable of eliciting an immune response on their own and must be chemically modified or combined with other substances to become immunogenic. Such immune-enhancing factors are termed *adjuvants,* which activate cells of the immune system by using components of the innate immune system, such as the Toll-like receptors (see Table 2.2 and Fig. 2.7 and 2.8). T and B cells may also be activated in a nonspecific manner by certain substances such as superantigens that bypass the normal processing pathways required for immune stimulation.

The immune response is initiated when antigens are internalized and processed by APCs and then antigenic peptides derived from the initial antigen are complexed with major histocompatibility complex (MHC) class II proteins. The peptide-MHC complex then interacts with the T-cell receptor (TCR) on the surface of CD4$^+$ T lymphocytes. Full activation of the T cell requires interactions between additional ligands present on the surface of activated APCs, such as CD80 and CD86 (see Fig. 3.8) and receptors on the surface of T cells, such as

CD28, to form the costimulatory complex. The MHC-peptide-TCR and costimulatory interactions form the basis for the two-signal model of T-cell activation. T-cell activation in turn leads to proliferation and functional differentiation of the T cell into helper and cytotoxic T cells.

For antigens that can provoke an antibody response, B lymphocytes will also interact directly with the antigen to produce antibodies. Only a small portion of the antigen will bind specifically to the recognition molecules of the immune system: antibodies and TCRs. These portions of the antigen are called *epitopes* or *antigenic determinants* (interchangeable terms) (Fig. 8.1). T-cell-stimulatory antigenic peptides must bind to both MHC proteins and TCRs, whereas B-cell epitopes bind to the antigen-binding site on membrane immunoglobulins. Specific chemical properties of antigens and configurations of epitopes determine whether they will be recognized by T cells or B cells. For example, T cells generally recognize linear peptides derived from antigenic proteins that are complexed to MHC molecules. B cells tend to recognize epitopes formed by the three-dimensional conformation taken on by an antigen, which often means that disparate parts of an antigen that are in close physical proximity due to molecular folding form a B-cell epitope. The immune system evolved in a way such that different recognition pathways are pivotal for controlling immune responsiveness. Antigens activate the adaptive immune response and represent the major factors that control the intensity and duration of an immune reaction. Therefore, properties determining the ability of an antigen to initiate an immune response and to interact subsequently with the effector cells and molecules of the immune system, represent the driving force of the adaptive immune response.

Figure 8.1 Demonstration of the locations of epitopes and paratopes in the interactions of antigens with the TCR (**A**) and B-cell receptor (**B**). The epitope is a portion of the antigen that makes physical contact with the receptor. Ab, antibody; Ag, antigen.

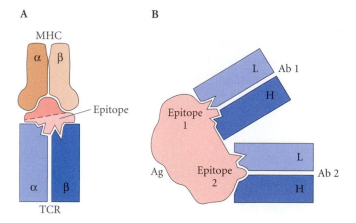

General Properties of Antigens

Most antigens are foreign, or nonself, substances. The concept of foreignness is based on whether the immune system of a specific individual has the potential to respond to the antigen. Most self molecules within one's own body induce tolerance in their immune system, and tolerance prevents responses to self antigens; everything else is potentially foreign or nonself to the immune system. Some antigens differ slightly from self substances but are often still able to provoke an immune reaction. When they do, an autoimmune response can be generated whereby the self substance is recognized and destroyed, often manifesting as a severe pathologic condition.

The ability of an antigen to combine with antibody reflects the property of *antigenicity*. However, not all antigens are capable of provoking an immune response. Antigens that also provoke immune responses are called *immunogens*. The distinction between antigenicity and immunogenicity can be seen by examining antigen-antibody reactions; a substance that is antigenic but not immunogenic would likely bind to a B-cell membrane immunoglobulin receptor but fail to provoke subsequent antibody production by that B cell. When the nonimmunogenic antigen is altered such that it becomes immunogenic, one can obtain antibodies to the antigen that will react with the nonimmunogenic form of the antigen. Immunogenicity ultimately depends on several properties, such as molecular size, epitope density, charge of the antigen, and individual host factors that relate to whether the necessary cells to make an antibody response are present. In other words, immunogens form the subset of antigens that are able to elicit an immune response following a primary interaction with the immune system.

A large number of chemical structures are potentially antigenic, meaning that materials with widely divergent chemical compositions can act as antigens. In reality, however, a hierarchy of immunogenic properties exists, as defined by the antigen's chemical composition, whereby foreign proteins and polysaccharides rank as the best immunogens for mammals. Nucleic acids and phospholipids can be immunogenic under certain conditions, but because of their structural conservation across biologic systems, these substances tend to require special conditions to provoke an immune response. Small molecules, such as hormones, lipids, simple sugars, metabolic by-products, and organic chemicals, can be readily antigenic, although they usually need to be conjugated to a larger macromolecule such as a protein to become immunogenic. In addition to its chemical nature, an antigen must possess certain physical and biologic properties to be immunogenic. The size of the antigen and its toxicity to the host are among the criteria that have the greatest impact on immunogenicity. The adaptive immune response is endowed with the ability to respond to a vast number (perhaps >10^{12}) of chemically unrelated antigens, although this response is also marked by extreme specificity, manifested as the ability to distinguish even slight chemical differences between closely related substances. Thus, most individuals are able to express TCRs and secrete antibodies specific to myriad antigens.

Activation of T Cells and B Cells by Antigen

Nature of B- and T-Cell Epitopes

One of the signals required to initiate an immune response to a protein comes in the form of processed antigenic peptide, derived by proteolysis of a parent protein, complexed to an MHC molecule, and presented on the surface of an APC. This complex will next physically contact the membrane-anchored TCR on a T cell. Thus, only a small portion of the initial protein antigen actually comes into physical contact with the TCR. It has also recently been shown that certain bacterial glycolipids can be presented to T cells when complexed to nonclassical MHC proteins that are members of the cell surface glycoproteins collectively known as the CD1 family. Most other nonprotein antigens cannot be processed and presented to T cells of the mammalian immune system; mammals lack enzymes for breaking down substances such as bacterial polysaccharides into small enough structures for binding to MHC molecules. However, because these antigens often stimulate good antibody responses, they clearly must bind to the B-cell membrane immunoglobulin receptors.

Most antigens express multiple epitopes (i.e., are multivalent), and it is clear that different immune effectors can be produced against different epitopes on the same molecule. However, TCRs and antibodies recognize markedly different types of epitopes. TCRs on CD4+ T cells recognize only segments of protein antigens bound to MHC class II molecules. Each protein antigen is internalized and processed into its component peptide fragments by degradative enzymes in the cytoplasm or cytoplasmic vacuoles of APCs. TCRs on CD8+ T cells recognize portions of protein antigens complexed to MHC class I molecules. There are two recognized pathways for processing proteins into antigenic peptides within an APC; one, the endogenous pathway, involves processing peptides produced within the cell and generally results in binding of the peptide to MHC class I. The other pathway, the exogenous pathway, takes in antigens from outside the APC and processes them for binding to MHC

class II. However, there are important exceptions to these general statements. In theory, any linear portion of a protein antigen capable of being degraded into a peptide fragment of approximately 8 to 20 amino acids has the potential to be a T-cell epitope. In reality, this situation is more complex.

To engage a TCR, peptide fragments must be produced inside an APC; be properly transported to an endosome, where they can noncovalently associate with an MHC class II protein; and from there be transported to the cell surface. In addition, the host must have a TCR capable of recognizing the peptide-MHC protein complex in order to physically contact the presented antigenic epitope, ultimately leading to T-cell activation. B-cell surface immunoglobulin often binds noncontiguous surfaces on the antigen brought together in three-dimensional space by molecular folding events. Such folding gives the antigen a tertiary conformation. These physically close surfaces then bind to the variable region of the immunoglobulin molecule. These types of antigenic determinants are referred to as *conformational epitopes* (Fig. 8.2). A linear epitope, comprising a continuous string of amino acids, less frequently forms an antigenic determinant for a B cell. Such a linear type of epitope is called a *sequential determinant.*

T-Cell Epitopes and Peptide Binding to MHC Molecules

The mechanism of antigen recognition employed by the TCR differs substantially from that used by immunoglobulin molecules on B cells. T cells respond to peptide and glycolipid fragments of larger antigens. Peptides ranging from 7 to 20 amino acids in length can stimulate T-cell responses, although the optimal length is about 8 to 10 amino acids for peptides presented by MHC class I molecules and 13 to 18 amino acids for MHC class II-bound peptides. Because the antigenic peptide must interact with both an MHC protein and a TCR, there must be at least two interaction sites per antigenic peptide: one for the TCR and one for the MHC protein.

Studies by J. L. Strominger, D. C. Wiley, and colleagues, P. J. Bjorkman and colleagues, and P. A. Peterson, I. A. Wilson, and coworkers (1992 to 1994) have determined the three-dimensional structure of MHC class I and class II proteins bound to peptides. This work provided important insights into the nature of T-cell epitopes. Most humans have a limited number of MHC genes (six class I and around eight class II), but the proteins they encode are capable of presenting a large repertoire of peptide antigens to T cells. Clearly, one MHC molecule can bind many different peptides, but it is also clear that there are some structural similarities in the peptides that bind to a

A

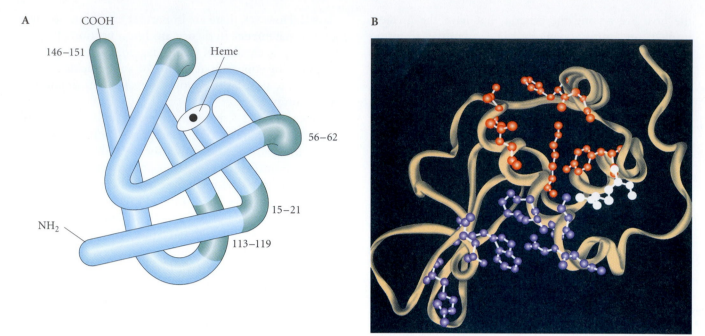

B

Figure 8.2 Illustration of the difference between sequential epitopes and conformational epitopes. (A) Sequential epitopes (blue regions) are composed of amino acids that are contiguous in a primary amino acid sequence of the protein antigen (e.g., amino acids 15 to 21). Adapted from M. Z. Atassi and A. L. Kazim, *Adv. Exp. Med. Biol.* **98:**19–40, 1978, with permission. (B) In contrast, a conformational epitope is composed of amino acids that are separated from each other in the primary structure of the protein antigen but are brought together in the native, folded structure of the antigen. The ball-and-stick portions of the model highlight amino acids in three different regions of the antigen's primary sequence (color coded in blue, red, and white) that together form one conformational epitope. Adapted from W. G. Laver et al., *Cell* **61:**553–556, 1990, with permission.

given allelic variant of an MHC molecule. The peptides bound to MHC proteins do not take on tertiary conformation but rather are bound as an extended helical structure. One important feature of peptide binding to MHC proteins is that the dissociation of the complex is very slow under physiologic conditions. This means that once a peptide is bound to MHC proteins it tends to stay bound. Certain auxiliary proteins, such as calnexin and HLA-DM, aid in the loading of peptide into MHC molecules, likely allowing for the flexibility needed for binding of many different peptides by one MHC molecule.

Peptide binding by MHC class I

MHC class I molecules present antigenic peptides to CD8$^+$ T cells. These peptides are usually, but not always, derived from proteins manufactured within the cytosol of the cell and are subsequently broken down into peptide fragments by proteolytic structures such as the proteasome. Under steady-state conditions, class I proteins bind peptides derived from endogenous or self molecules. However, because of the removal of self-reactive T cells during their maturation in the thymus or due to specific inhibitory mechanisms that prevent potentially self-

reactive T cells that may have made it out of the thymus into the periphery, such presentation of self peptides usually does not elicit any autoimmune or pathologic consequences. Cytosolically produced peptides are moved from the cytoplasm to the interior or lumen of the endoplasmic reticulum (ER) where the class I protein is being made. Here the peptide is complexed to the newly synthesized MHC class I molecule, which forms a stable structure that can be transported to the cell membrane.

Once bound to MHC protein, the peptide sits in a groove at the membrane-distal end of the MHC protein. As peptides lie in the binding groove of the MHC protein, certain peptide residues (called the *agretope*) are directed toward the MHC protein and are actually responsible for maintaining the physical interaction between MHC and antigenic peptide. Other peptide residues (called the epitope) point outward, away from the MHC protein, and are most important for interactions with the T-cell antigen receptor (Fig. 8.3). The peptide-binding groove is formed by α-helical and β-sheet regions of the MHC protein and is structurally different in class I and class II MHC proteins. The peptide-binding groove of the MHC class I protein is closed at both ends, such that the peptide

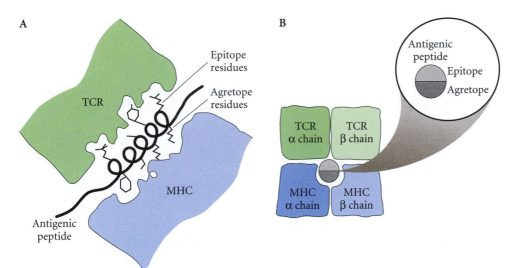

Figure 8.3 Binding of a TCR to its cognate antigenic peptide requires the simultaneous interaction of the peptide with both the TCR (on the T cell) and the MHC (on either a target cell or an APC). The physical region of the peptide that contacts the MHC is termed the agretope, and the region that contacts the TCR is termed the epitope. (A) Side view of peptide. The antigenic peptide is depicted in a helical configuration, with the amino acid side chains making contact with either the MHC or the TCR. (B) End-on view of peptide showing that both chains of TCR and MHC are involved in interaction with antigen.

is contained entirely within the groove. Pockets at the end of the binding groove, which are usually nonpolar, accommodate an amino acid side chain branching off the antigenic peptide. The groove usually contains peptides 8 to 10 amino acids in length, although nonamers predominate as MHC class I ligands. The amino acid residues at positions 2 and 3 on the peptide and at its carboxy terminus (usually position 9 of the peptide) are conserved for the variety of peptides that bind to a particular MHC class I molecule and are referred to as *anchor residues*. Anchoring via these terminal residues appears to confer a certain degree of specificity on the peptide-MHC interaction. Since the peptide-binding groove is made up of different amino acids, depending on the allelic variant of the MHC molecule, different MHC class I alleles prefer different anchor residues at the carboxy terminus of the peptide and, therefore, bind to different antigenic peptides.

The nature of the peptides bound to class I molecules has been elucidated by techniques whereby bound peptides are eluted from class I proteins, separated on chromatography columns, and then analyzed by mass spectrometric methods to determine the peptide's composition. About 100,000 individual class I molecules are found on a cell's surface, and up to 2,000 different peptides are bound to these molecules. It has been estimated that a specific peptide may be found on 100 to 4,000 MHC class I molecules on a cell's surface.

For a single class I molecule to bind thousands of different nonameric peptides, there must be some flexibility in the placement of the peptide in the binding groove. This occurs in the middle portion of the peptide, which can bend or arch away from the floor of the peptide-binding groove. The middle part of the peptide may not come into close contact with the MHC molecule but may

affect interaction with the TCR. Indeed, recent structural determinations of the binding of TCRs to MHC-peptide complexes show there is a strong analogy between TCR-peptide-MHC binding and antigen-antibody binding. The TCR expresses regions analogous to the certain complementarity-determining regions (CDRs) in the variable region of the antibody. In the TCR, certain portions of the variable regions bind to the carboxy terminus of the peptide-MHC complex, other portions bind to the amino terminus, and still others bind to the middle part of the peptide in the MHC-binding groove.

Peptide binding by MHC class II

MHC class II molecules present peptide antigens to CD4+ T cells. Usually these peptides are derived from exogenous proteins taken into the cell by pinocytosis or phagocytosis, although it is clear that some cytosol-produced antigens can also be complexed to MHC class II molecules. Proteolytic peptides derived from such endocytosed antigens are loaded onto MHC class II molecules. This loading process takes place in endosomal vesicles.

Similar to MHC class I, MHC class II has a peptide-binding groove at its membrane-distal end, also formed by α-helical and β-sheet regions of the MHC protein. However, unlike the groove of MHC class I, the peptide-binding groove of the MHC class II protein is open at both ends, allowing peptides with a variety of lengths (13 to 25 amino acids in length) to occupy the groove. Peptides bind to class II molecules via a central core of nine amino acids that twist into a ribbon-like helix. The open-ended nature of the class II binding groove allows for the presence of residues flanking the central core. In cases where extremely long peptides are so bound, several amino acids of the antigenic peptide protrude from each of the open ends of the class II binding groove. The crystal structures of both mouse and human MHC class II-bound peptides have been determined, and there appears to be a high level of conservation in the types of amino acids that anchor the peptides to residues in the class II molecule. The central core of nine amino acids is characterized by the presence of hydrophobic amino acids at the first peptide-binding residue and a lysine or arginine at the ninth position. At peptide-binding position 4, there tends to be a hydrophobic amino acid, and at binding position 6, an asparagine, aspartic acid, or glutamine residue. Interestingly, of the class II molecules whose structures are known, there is a conservation of amino acids in the binding pocket that forces the peptide to take on a twisted-ribbon structure in order to rest in the pocket (Fig. 8.4). This puts more constraint on the type of peptide that can form a class II epitope, and hence there is less variability in peptides bound to class II molecules than in those bound to class I molecules.

Many peptides bound by class II molecules contain proline residues at position 2 from the amino terminus and at the carboxy terminus. These are not involved in binding to the class II molecule but instead hang out over the edge of the binding groove. This conservation in structure is thought to reflect the proteolytic activity of enzymes that generate the peptides for binding to class II molecules.

Host Factors Affecting the Selection of Antigenic Peptides

T-cell epitopes on an antigenic protein are often concealed as a result of the tertiary conformation taken on by the folded protein, indicating that one of the functions of anti-

gen processing is to expose these internal peptides. The part of the protein destined to become a T-cell epitope may be identifiable to some degree from the structure of the intact protein but is determined, in part, by the genetic constitution of the host animal. Most important in this respect is the combination of alleles that the host animal possesses at its MHC genetic locus (collectively termed the host animal's MHC *haplotype*). MHC class I and class II proteins exist within a given species as a large family of alleles, but only a small portion of these alleles will be expressed on the cells of any single individual within the species. The different alleles of MHC class I and class II vary in their affinity for distinct, potentially antigenic peptides. It has recently been proposed that the conserved structural motifs in the anchoring portions of the class II-bound peptides may be related to loading of these peptides into the class II groove at the low pH present in the endosome. A somewhat unexpected finding about MHC class II epitopes is the observation that peptide residues flanking the anchor residues and lying outside the peptide-binding groove also influence TCR binding and that, after initial loading of the peptides onto MHC molecules, the peptides are susceptible to further modification by surface proteases such as aminopeptidase M (CD13). E. E. Sercarz and colleagues have suggested that, at some point, T-cell epitopes are selected on the basis of their ability to bind MHC proteins as the original protein antigen becomes linearized. The MHC-binding portion of the peptide would, therefore, be selected according to its affinity for MHC molecules as the foreign protein unfolds and is processed.

Additional variation in the selection of antigenic peptides is attributable to proteins that are part of the protein-degrading apparatus known as the proteasome, altering the spectrum of antigenic peptides generated for eventual trafficking into the ER and loading onto MHC class I. Different alleles of LMP2, LMP7, and LMP10 have been shown to vary in the way they modify the proteolytic specificity of the proteasome. Also, the two genes encoding the transporter associated with antigen processing (TAP1 and TAP2), which transports peptides generated by the proteasome into the ER, are genetically polymorphic (i.e., exist as a large family of alleles within the population), and these different alleles of TAP1 and TAP2 have varying specificities with regard to their selection of peptides to be transported into the ER. However, while it is true that the MHC haplotype of the host animal influences the selection of antigenic peptides at several levels, it must also be understood that selection of these peptides may vary even among individual mice derived from the same inbred line. This variation has been postulated to be based on each animal's particular inflammatory state, APC population, and other, as yet undefined, possibly

Figure 8.4 Antigenic peptides bound to MHC class I (A) and MHC class II (B) proteins. In both cases, the antigenic peptide lies in a groove that is situated between two α-helical regions of the MHC protein. The MHC class I molecule (white) is shown with a peptide antigen (red) from human immunodeficiency virus reverse transcriptase (amino acids 309 to 317). β₂-Microglobulin is shown in blue. The MHC class II diagram shows a DR molecule with the α chain in white, the β chain in blue, and the embedded red peptide lying in a pocket with open ends. Reprinted with permission from D. A. A. Vignali and J. L. Strominger, *Immunologist* **2:**112–118, 1994.

A
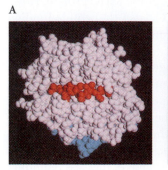

B
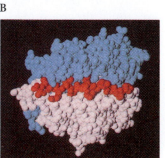

environmental, factors capable of influencing antigen processing. Therefore, although our understanding of antigen processing has become sophisticated, the prediction of the immunogenicity of peptides generated from any given whole antigenic protein will still be influenced by subtle factors.

Recognition of the MHC-Complexed T-Cell Epitope

The TCR must first interact with a combination of peptide and MHC, thus forming a trimolecular complex. Since part of the peptide is contained within the MHC protein groove, the TCR must interact with the remaining peptide portion, exposed for recognition (Fig. 8.3). The side of the peptide that binds to the MHC protein (i.e., the agretope) tends to be hydrophobic, while the opposite side of the peptide, which interacts directly with the TCR (the epitope), is hydrophilic, making the immunogenic peptide amphipathic overall. Computer algorithms have been developed to predict T-cell epitopes within protein antigens, based on a system that relies on assigning a score to each peptide by its degree of amphipathicity, yielding a relatively accurate correlation between the peptide's score and its potential ability to form a T-cell epitope. However, the actual selection of T-cell epitopes may vary considerably among individuals, as detailed above, making it difficult to predict the location and sequence of epitopes from their primary protein structure.

In addition to the binding of peptide-MHC to the TCR, other signals are derived from the APC–T-cell interaction that result in T-cell proliferation and differentiation. Prominent interactions include CD80/CD86 on the APC and CD28, cytotoxic T-lymphocyte antigen 4 (CTLA-4; also called CD152) on the T cell, inducible costimulator and its ligand, and PD-1 and the PD-1 ligand pathway. These interactions are complex, providing both stimulatory (i.e., CD28) and inhibitory (i.e., CTLA-4) signals to the T cell. How these various signals are integrated and interpreted by the T cell is not well understood. However, without some costimulatory signal the MHC-peptide-TCR interaction itself is insufficient to activate a T cell and can put the T cell in a state of anergy where it becomes refractory to responding to the antigenic peptide-MHC complex.

Experimental evidence for the compartmentalization of binding activities within an antigenic peptide comes both from structural determinations of peptide-MHC complexes and from mutational studies in which amino acids of the antigenic peptide are altered. M. M. Davis and colleagues have used this *altered peptide ligand* technique to identify amino acid residues on the peptide that come

into physical contact with the TCR (Fig. 8.5). These are distinct from those affecting peptide binding to MHC proteins. B. D. Evavold and P. M. Allen analyzed these altered peptide ligands for the ability to activate T cells and induce the synthesis of cytokines. Through these studies, they discovered a gradation of signaling events occurring within the T cell related to differences in the T-cell epitopes recognized. The strength of the interaction of the MHC–T-cell epitope with the TCR determines whether a full-fledged T-cell response occurs or whether an inhibitory (antagonistic) response occurs, leading to suppression of T-cell activity. Another facet of T-cell epitopes, described by J. A. Berzofsky, R. N. Germain, and associates, is that the amino acid residues not involved in binding to either MHC proteins or TCRs must nonetheless be permissive for these two binding events to occur and thus for subsequent TCR engagement to be successful. In other words, those amino acids not directly involved in MHC protein binding or TCR engagement still affect the immunogenicity of the epitope. Changes in amino acid residues that do not compromise MHC or TCR engagement would likely have no effect on the epitope's immunologic function, whereas amino acid changes in these nonbinding residues resulting in the loss of the integrity of MHC binding and/or recognition of the MHC-peptide complex by the TCR will ultimately result in a change or loss of immunogenicity. Peptides that activate a T cell expressing a specific TCR are referred to as *agonist* peptides, those that only partially activate the T cell are called *partial agonist peptides,* and peptides that inhibit a T cell from responding are known as *antagonist peptides.*

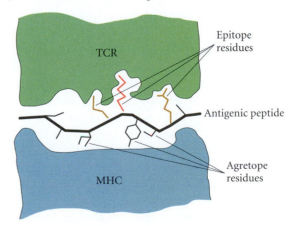

Figure 8.5 Schematic representation of peptide bound to both MHC and TCR, showing amino acids of the peptide that make significant contributions to TCR binding. The amino acid side chain that makes the most extensive interaction with the TCR is colored red, while the side chains of two amino acids that make lesser (although still significant) interactions are colored orange.

B-Cell Epitopes

Studies on the nature of B-cell epitopes date back to the 1950s, when L. Pauling first showed that an antigenic epitope must be in close physical proximity to the antigen-binding site on an antibody molecule for immune complex formation to occur. A paradigm established by E. Kabat around the same time indicated that a dextran polymer about six monosaccharides in length will occupy the antigen-binding site of an antibody. More recent crystallographic analysis of carbohydrate epitopes bound to antibody indicates that four to eight monosaccharide residues will fill an antigen-binding site. Although it is not commonly appreciated, carbohydrate antigens, like protein antigens, bind to antibodies in the context of their tertiary conformation. B-cell antigens can form conformational epitopes based on noncovalent folding of the antigen molecule, bringing into close proximity portions of the antigen that are distant from each other in the antigen's primary monosaccharide or amino acid sequence (Fig. 8.2). Sequential epitopes can also form on protein antigens, usually from portions of protein molecules containing α-helical bends. Regardless of whether they are sequential or conformational, B-cell epitopes must always be exposed on the antigen's surface in order for the whole molecule to bind to antibody. In addition, B-cell epitopes are often hydrophilic because they are usually found exposed in aqueous environments. Internal portions of a molecule cannot bind to membrane immunoglobulin to induce an immune response, so antibodies to these concealed structures would be synthesized only under extremely unusual circumstances.

B-cell epitopes tend to be located on protein antigens at sites where a certain amount of mobility exists in the protein's overall structure, allowing these epitopes to undergo conformational changes to bind immunoglobulin. Thus the amino and carboxy termini of proteins often form B-cell epitopes due to their mobility in three-dimensional space. By changing shape in such a way as to achieve maximal complementarity with respect to the antigen-binding site, the binding of a B-cell epitope to antibody is stabilized. Validation of this concept came from studies of I. A. Wilson and coworkers, who determined the three-dimensional structure of the Fab portion of an antibody to a peptide from the influenza virus hemagglutinin antigen, both with and without the peptide epitope bound to the Fab fragment. They found that the third CDR on the antibody heavy chain underwent a major conformational change when the antigen was bound (Fig. 8.6). This conformational change in the antibody created a pocket capable of binding the peptide epitope. Since antibodies can undergo changes in structure

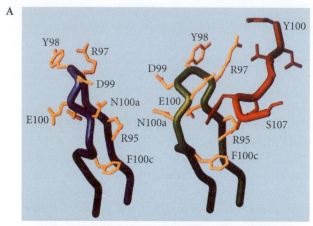

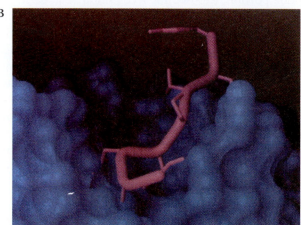

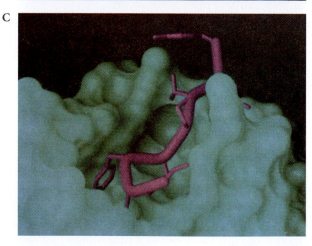

Figure 8.6 Demonstration of how an antigen-binding site on an antibody molecule undergoes conformational changes to accommodate antigen upon binding. (**A**) Comparison of the loop in the third CDR of the heavy chain in the unligated (**left**) and ligated (**right**) state. Note in particular the different positions of amino acids 99 and 100 (aspartic acid and asparagine, respectively). (**B and C**) Shape of the antigen-binding pocket in the unligated (**B**) and ligated (**C**) state. The peptide is positioned in panel B as it is in the ligated state but without the antigen-binding pocket undergoing the conformational change. Reprinted from J. M. Rini et al., *Science* **255:**959–965, 1992, with permission.

when they bind antigens, there is an induced fit between the B-cell epitope and its immunoglobulin *paratope* (the portion of the immunoglobulin that contacts the antigenic epitope). These findings remind us that older, discredited theories about antigen-antibody binding, which had suggested that antigen instructed antibody how to fold around it, contained some truth after all.

B cells that bind to protein antigens can become activated to process and present antigenic peptides to T cells. Thus, B cells are a type of APC. As with other interactions of T-cells with APC, costimulatory interactions also play an important role in B-cell activation, maturation, and differentiation. This principally involves cell surface molecules CD40 and CD40 ligand (originally designated CD40L, but now designated as CD154), but other interactions between B cells and T cells also contribute to the development of an antibody response.

Some B-cell antibody responses can be made in the absence of T-cell help (see Fig. 1.13 and chapter 15 for more detailed discussion). Antigens that elicit antibody in the absence of T-cell help are known as T-independent (TI) antigens. In general, TI antigens are nonprotein antigens that cannot be processed and presented by APCs, including B cells, to T cells. They usually contain multiple repetitive repeats of epitopes that are thought to activate B cells by extensively cross-linking the membrane immunoglobulin, which provides a sufficiently strong signal for the B cells to develop into antibody-secreting cells. Some protein antigens with similar antigenic properties can also function as TI antigens. Antigens that get processed and presented by APCs to T cells and elicit T-cell help are referred to as T-dependent antigens.

Anti-Idiotype Antibodies

Anti-idiotypic antibodies can function to mimic antigens, further inducing anti-anti-idiotypic antibodies, homologous to the original primary antibody, and thus capable of binding the original antigen responsible for inducing formation of the initial primary antibody (Fig. 8.7). Structural studies have now confirmed this concept of antigenic mimicry. For example, when an anti-idiotype antibody is raised to an antibody induced by a peptide hormone, comparative analysis of the structural conformation taken on by the CDR loop on the anti-idiotype has revealed a substantial degree of complementary structure between the initial antihormone antibody and the anti-idiotype antibody. This observation provides structural evidence that the antigen-binding site of the anti-idiotypic antibody takes on the same shape structure as the initial antigen of which the anti-idiotype is a molecular mimic.

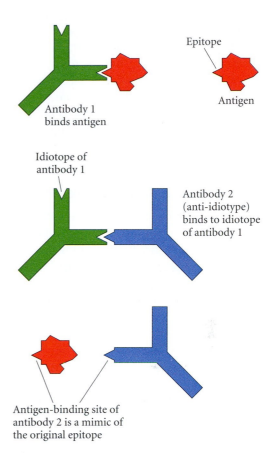

Figure 8.7 The idiotype–anti-idiotype network for generating B-cell responses to related epitopes. An epitope on an antigen stimulates an antibody response (antibody 1) that binds to the antigen. Within the antigen-binding site of antibody 1 are new antigenic determinants, not previously present in the host at a high level, that form the idiotopes. Antibody 2 responds to an idiotope on antibody 1, binding to the antigen-binding site in much the same way as the immunizing antigenic epitope. The result is that the antigen-binding site (or idiotype) of antibody 2 is closely related to the three-dimensional shape of the original immunizing epitope. Antibody 2 can now be used as a surrogate for the original antigen.

Immunodominance of Epitopes

As has been noted for T-cell epitopes, there is a discrepancy between the potential number of B-cell epitopes on an antigen and the actual number of different antibodies induced in an individual animal or person. Certain epitopes tend to be *immunodominant*, meaning they will elicit the strongest immune response, although the identity of these epitopes depends on an individual's immunologic history and genetic constitution. Therefore, even after vaccination, antibodies to a particular antigen may not be directed against the majority of the B-cell epitopes expressed by the antigen. The actual number of epitopes that could be identified on various proteins proved to be much larger than the number identified by analysis of sera from individual animals. Thus, many antigens are able to present multiple potential epitopes, but each individual responds to only a subset of these. Such an immune response, directed at only a subset of antigenic epitopes, can still be totally effective at eliminating the antigen. This points out another important facet of the immune response: an immune response is more likely to be successful if the antigen contains a large number of different epitopes.

Antigenicity and Immunogenicity

The ability of an epitope to bind to either an antibody or a TCR is necessary, but not sufficient, for induction of an immune response. Specifically, for antibody production, membrane immunoglobulin on the surface of B cells must encounter the epitope as part of a much larger molecule, even though antibodies, once produced, will bind only to the smaller epitope. To elucidate the differences between antigenicity and immunogenicity, K. Landsteiner, in the 1920s, synthesized numerous small organic compounds that, by themselves, could not induce antibodies but, after coupling or conjugation to a larger molecule, could induce antibodies capable of binding the free compound. These experiments introduced the concepts of *haptens* and *carriers,* forming one of the major experimental tools used in modern immunology. Haptens are small antigenic epitopes that bind specifically to antibodies, while carriers are structures that, when conjugated to the immunologically inactive hapten, impart the property of immunogenicity to the hapten. Antigens that are immunogenic on their own are sometimes referred to as *complete antigens,* while haptens are sometimes called *incomplete antigens.* Complete antigens usually possess both T- and B-cell epitopes (i.e., are multivalent), whereas haptens, because of their extremely small size, generally comprise only a single epitope. This system has proven extremely useful for studying the properties of antibodies; the hapten-carrier complex can be used to induce antibodies, while the isolated hapten alone, with its much simpler structure, can be used to study how antibodies bind to antigens (Fig. 8.8).

Factors Affecting Immunogenicity

Immunogenicity depends on both host and antigen factors. Even among genetically identical animals, each antigen varies in its immunogenicity, probably reflecting the impact of an individual's immunologic history on the state of its immune system. Nonetheless, certain general factors, or properties, shared by most immunogens have been defined, and as such, a classification system has been devised on the basis of these similarities.

Foreignness

Foreignness is crucial to the induction of an immune response. One of the hallmarks of the immune system is the ability to distinguish between self and nonself antigens and to respond to nonself antigens upon recognition. Foreignness is both relative and contextual, not absolute. Foreignness can be defined as chemical differences between the antigen and components of one's own body, but foreignness is also dependent on the contextual state of the immune system. What is determined by the immune system to be self represents only those self antigens to which the immune system is exposed and to which it becomes unresponsive or tolerant. Not all self components will be exposed to the immune system (i.e., cytoplasmic antigens that are degraded before being exposed to cells of the immune system).

To prevent immune responses to those self antigens that gain access to cells of the immune system, a process occurs during T- and B-cell development to eliminate potentially self-reactive lymphocytes. If neonatal animals are exposed to a nominally foreign antigen, a state of nonresponsiveness to the foreign substance can be induced in some instances that lasts into adulthood, suggesting that the animal's immune system acquires some of the properties of self-nonself discrimination during early development. Phylogenetically related animals are less likely to recognize each other's antigens as foreign and to respond to them immunologically because of evolutionary conservation of genes and associated gene products. Similarly, molecules like collagen that are highly conserved throughout evolution are poorly immunogenic in most animals. However, if a self molecule is somehow sequestered from the immune system, for example, inside a cell, it may be immunogenic when isolated and injected into an appropriate host.

Chemical complexity

In general, the more complex a molecule, the more immunogenic it is. All four of the structural levels giving rise to a protein's native conformation are able to affect immunogenicity (Fig. 8.9). At the primary level, most amino acid substitutions will affect higher structural levels. The secondary structure (involving β-sheets and α-helix formations), tertiary conformation (achieved through further protein folding via the use of hydrophobic exclusion, disulfide linkages, and other chemical interactions), and, where applicable, complexing of multiple polypeptides to yield a quaternary structure are all able to affect antigen structure and thus the ability of the antigen to be recognized by immune cells and subsequently induce a response. Simple polymers of single amino acids

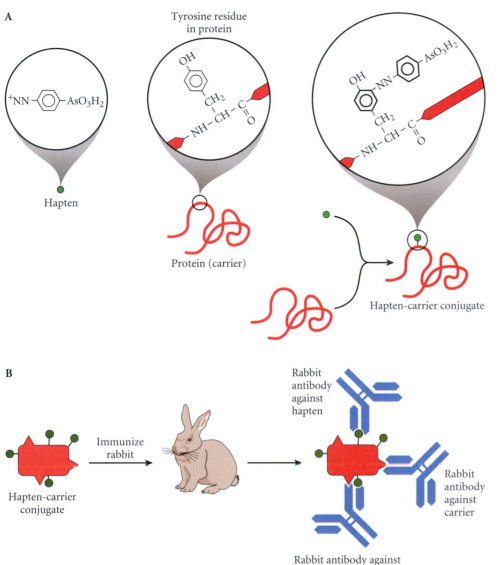

Figure 8.8 Use of hapten-carrier conjugates to study the factors affecting immunogenicity and antigenicity of an antigen. (A) Covalent conjugation of the hapten, diazoarsanilic acid, to the tyrosine-containing carrier protein forms the hapten-carrier conjugate. (B) The hapten-carrier conjugate (immunogen) gives rise to the antibodies of different specificities, which are determined by testing sera against the indicated structure. Some antibodies generated against the conjugate recognize epitopes on the carrier, while other antibodies recognize the hapten portion of the conjugate. Still other antibodies recognize *neoepitopes* that comprise both hapten and carrier structures.

tend to be poorly immunogenic and are unable to take on a defined three-dimensional shape. Copolymers of two or more amino acids can be immunogenic, particularly if they contain complex aromatic amino acids. Chemical complexity is likely important in terms of stimulating an immune response, since an antigen must be able to take on a shape to interact with membrane immunoglobulin on the B-cell surface, yet be amenable to proteolytic degradation in order to be processed into T-cell epitopes.

The contribution of chemical complexity to a polysaccharide's immunogenicity is less clear than its contribution to a protein's immunogenicity. Growing evidence shows that polysaccharides, like proteins, produce conformational epitopes, indicating that polymer complexity correlates with increased immunogenicity. However, some simple polysaccharide polymers, such as the α-2 → 9-linked sialic acid homopolymer of group C *Neisseria meningitidis,* are readily immunogenic in humans, whereas a closely related antigen, the α-2 → 8-linked sialic acid homopolymer of group B *N. meningitidis,* is nonimmunogenic in humans. The eight or so capsular polysaccharides of group B streptococci, which form important etiologic agents for infections contracted by newborns, have the same constituent sugars, although they are arranged in different orders on the basis of variable linkage patterns and sugar conformations. Despite their similarities at the subunit level, these polysaccharides show diverse immunogenicity in humans, with population

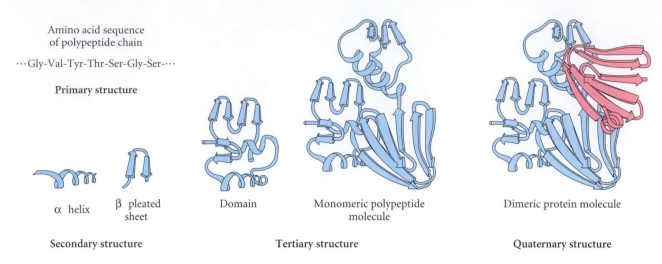

Amino acid sequence
of polypeptide chain

···Gly-Val-Tyr-Thr-Ser-Gly-Ser-···

Primary structure

α helix   β pleated
                 sheet

Domain   Monomeric polypeptide   Dimeric protein molecule
                molecule

Secondary structure   **Tertiary structure**   **Quaternary structure**

Figure 8.9 Aspects of protein structure affecting immunogenicity.

responses to an individual immunogen ranging from 30 to more than 80%. Since polysaccharides are not processed and presented to T cells, chemical factors affecting the immunogenicity of this class of antigens are poorly understood. As such, polysaccharide antigen immunogenicity cannot be estimated from a general set of guidelines and must thus be determined experimentally for each different antigen.

Molecular size

Immunogenicity correlates directly with molecular size. Although proteins as small as 1,000 daltons can, under certain circumstances, be immunogenic, most proteins smaller than 10,000 daltons are poorly immunogenic. In general, the most immunogenic proteins have a mass greater than 10,000 daltons. For polysaccharides, a minimum molecular mass of around 100,000 daltons is associated with potential for generating an immune response. Small molecules can be coupled to protein carriers to enhance their immunogenicity, as has been demonstrated in the hapten-carrier system. Some antigens that are poorly immunogenic can achieve increased immunogenicity by conjugation to protein carriers; this has been done with several poorly immunogenic bacterial polysaccharide antigens, for example, the conjugated capsular polysaccharide of *Haemophilus influenzae* type b, which has already proven to be a highly successful childhood vaccine.

T-cell interactions

For proteins, the ability to stimulate T-cell responses is critical for immunogenicity, since T helper cells are needed to produce immune-stimulating cytokines. This means that the immunogen must be susceptible to processing and presentation by APCs. Processed antigens essentially are degraded fragments of the immunogen. Thus, protein sensitivity to degradation by intracellular proteases is critical for immunogenicity. If a protein cannot be degraded, peptide fragments of it cannot bind to MHC proteins to be presented to the TCR. This phenomenon has been shown experimentally using polymers of D-amino acids, which are mirror images (enantiomers) of the L-amino acids used by most terrestrial organisms in their proteins. Mammalian proteases can degrade only L-amino acid-bearing proteins, while synthetic proteins made up of D-amino acids cannot be degraded and thus are nonimmunogenic. Large aggregates of proteins, as well as immune complexes, tend to be highly immunogenic because of their increased size, and thus their greater ability to be taken up by APCs, processed, and presented to T cells.

Dose and route of administration

Immune responses, like most biologic responses, are maximal when the stimulus is present at an optimal concentration and in an optimal location to interact with responding cells. Most immunogens have a dose range that is optimal for eliciting T- and B-cell responses, although that dose range may not be the same for these two cell types. Suboptimal and supraoptimal doses will not provoke immune responses. For example, the optimal dose of dextran in a mouse is between 0.1 microgram (μg) and 10 μg; at doses lower than 0.1 μg or higher than 10 μg, the intensity of the immune response decreases. In some cases, an incorrect dose of antigen can actually be paralyzing, or *tolerogenic,* to the immune system, driving it into a state of long-lasting nonresponsiveness. When this occurs, even subsequent exposure to optimal doses of immunogens fails to elicit an immune response. Mice immunized with doses of bovine serum albumin (BSA) ranging from 10^{-11} to 1 gram (g) and subsequently boosted with an optimal 10-milligram (mg) dose 14 days later had a bell-shaped curve of secondary responses to the optimal dose. Mice given suboptimal and supraoptimal initial doses had impaired secondary responses compared with controls that received the optimal initial immunizing dose (Fig. 8.10). In addition to the requirement for an optimal dose, multiple doses of antigen often are needed to maximize immunogenicity, as exemplified by the hepatitis B vaccine given to humans, for which three or four doses are routinely needed for the induction of full immunity.

Another factor affecting immunogenicity is the route of antigen administration. Natural immunization usually occurs when an antigen crosses a mucosal surface, be it gastrointestinal, respiratory, or genitourinary. A break in the skin or absorption through it also can serve as a route for natural immunization. If an antigen is encountered on a mucosal surface, it must be able to penetrate that surface and enter the submucosal space, where lymphocytes are found. The site of antigen entry will influence the isotype of antibody produced, in that mucosal immunization promotes formation of both immunoglobulin A (IgA) and IgG antibodies. Experimental vaccination can deliver antigens by intradermal, subcutaneous, intramuscular, intravenous, or intraperitoneal routes, as well as by oral and respiratory routes. Different routes of administration result in quantitatively or qualitatively different immune responses, in part because of the diversity of the populations of APCs that reside at each anatomic site. APCs are responsible for distributing the antigen to the local lymph nodes, and the particular array of T cells and B cells present in the nodes will affect the quality and quantity of T-cell responses and, subsequently, of antibodies secreted. There are some indications that intradermal administration of antigen provokes T-cell responses, whereas systemic distribution via intravenous or intraperitoneal immunization tends to favor antibody production.

Adjuvants

Sometimes it is necessary to boost an immune response generated by a poorly immunogenic antigen. Boosting can often be accomplished by addition of an adjuvant to the immunizing mixture. Adjuvants enhance immunity, usually by provoking a more intense and prolonged immune response. In humans, only one type of adjuvant, derived from aluminum-containing compounds complexed to either phosphates or hydroxides (alum), has been approved for clinical use, but numerous others are currently under investigation. Adjuvants commonly used in animals, such as complete Freund adjuvant, are too toxic for human use.

Enhancing immunogenicity through the use of adjuvants has been attributed to several mechanisms (see Fig. 21.6). Adjuvants are able to alter antigen distribution and to prolong their persistence in the host, allowing for an extended interaction with lymphocytes and thus a greater chance of immune stimulation. The adjuvant effects attributed to alum are believed to be due to delay in release of the antigen produced by its adsorption onto the salt precipitate, resulting in more prolonged exposure to the antigen. Adjuvants increase the number of costimulatory molecules on the surface of APCs, which enhances lymphocyte activation. Many adjuvants nonspecifically stimulate lymphocytes and APCs, probably through the induction of cytokine production.

Figure 8.10 Dose dependency of the immune response of mice to BSA. Mice were given an initial dose of BSA ranging from 10 picograms (10^{-11} g) to 1 g. Fourteen days later they were given the optimal dose of 10 mg of BSA, and antibody titers were measured 7 days later. Animals given suboptimal (10^{-11} to 10^{-5} g) or supraoptimal (1 [or 10^{0}] g) doses had a lower secondary response, indicating that these doses interfered with and suppressed the secondary response to the optimal 10-mg dose. Responses of <100% indicate inhibition of secondary antibody production, whereas responses of >100% indicate that priming has occurred for an increased secondary booster response. Adapted from N. A. Mitchison, *Proc. R. Soc. Ser. B* **161:**275, 1964, with permission.

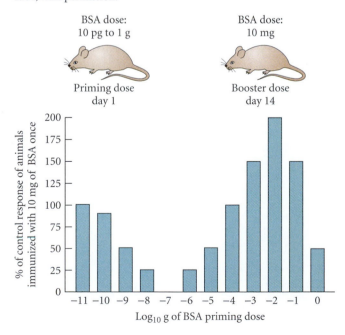

Adjuvants are particularly useful as components of vaccines (see chapter 21 for additional details) and come in a variety of formulations, all toxic to some degree. When an adjuvant is used, its immune-enhancing properties must be weighed against its toxic side effects. Sometimes chemical derivatives of a toxic adjuvant, which retain most of the adjuvant's activity but lack most of its toxic properties, can be used instead of the original adjuvant. For example, a component of the toxic bacterial lipopolysaccharide, termed monophosphoryl lipid A, retains much of the original adjuvant's effects while having a greatly reduced toxicity. Much progress has recently been made in developing and testing newer adjuvants possessing both immune-enhancing properties and acceptable side effects (Table 8.1).

The chemical compositions of adjuvants span a wide range. Many incorporate lipids or lipid-like factors, which may account for their ability to perturb immune cell membranes. Another group of adjuvants derived from microbial components may interact with host receptors for the microbial product and provide a signal alerting the host to activate an inflammatory response. Chemical variants of these microbial products, which retain high levels of adjuvant activity and low levels of toxicity, have been synthesized for vaccine use. Several relatively new adjuvants have shown promise in phase 1 human clinical trials. These results raise hopes that someday these compounds will be important components of vaccines designed to protect against diseases such as human immunodeficiency virus infection and malaria. A better understanding of the ways in which adjuvants operate, coupled with a better knowledge of the plethora of signals activating each different aspect of the immune system, will pave the way to the design of adjuvants capable of augmenting the immune response to a given antigen in a precise manner. For example, an individual adjuvant or specific combination of adjuvants may promote a cell-mediated response or production of a particular IgG isotype, according to which is most effective in eliminating the offending antigen.

Important Antigens from Infectious Agents

The identification of antigens important in provoking immune responses that are protective against infection with microbial pathogens rests on knowledge of how groups of microorganisms cause disease, how the disease can be diagnosed, and how immunity against microbial pathogens is manifested. Clearly, microbial products that directly cause pathology, such as toxins, would be important antigens toward which a neutralizing immune response should be directed. In diseases such as diphtheria, tetanus, botulism, and menstrual toxic shock syndrome, a secreted bacterial toxin is responsible for the disease and immunity is manifested as antibodies specific to each toxin. For many infectious agents, however, the individual microbial antigens responsible for pathology have not been identified. The chemical nature of microbial antigens and the epitopes they express directly influence

Table 8.1 Type of adjuvants currently used or under investigation

Adjuvant	Mode of action[a]	Relative toxicity
Complete Freund's adjuvant	Activates TH1 cells through TLR2 and TLR4	Very high
Alum	Activates TH2 cells	Very low
Immunostimulating complexes	Activate CD4$^+$ cells Induce interferon-gamma Modulate MHC class II	Low
Non-ionic block polymers	Increase antibody responses Activate TH1 cells	Low
Monophosphoryl lipid A	Induces interferon-gamma and TNF Induces TH1 cells Inhibits TH2 cells Activates through TLR4	Moderate
Muramyl dipeptides	Induce humoral responses Augment both antibody and cellular responses when given as oil-in-water emulsion Induce IL-1 secretion Activate through TLR2	Moderate
Cytokines	Activity based on biologic specificity	Moderate

[a]TH cell, helper T cell.

the immune response and ultimately can determine the nature of protective immunity and the types of immune effectors that might be measured and used as a diagnostic tool for a particular infection.

Viral Antigens

Viruses are obligate intracellular organisms generally composed of pieces of either DNA or RNA encased in a protein or lipoprotein coat. Immune responses directed to viral proteins require T-cell involvement and encompass both cell-mediated and humoral effectors. Viral antigens that induce neutralizing antibodies and specific cytotoxic T cells are the most efficient at generating a state of protective immunity (Fig. 8.11). However, it is often difficult to predict which particular viral epitope or even which viral protein will be the target of protective immunity. Viruses often possess the ability to alter their surface protein composition to evade preexisting host immune

effectors. This is one reason why individuals can experience the common cold, influenza, or similar infections year after year: each infection is caused by an immunologically distinct strain of virus, which has "escaped" the host's immune response to previous strains of the virus.

Epitopes most effective at inducing protection are usually found on the viral surface. Proteins expressing these epitopes are needed for binding of virus to cellular receptors used for viral entry into cells or for the early steps in viral infection inside a cell. Obviously, an antibody that either inhibited virus binding to its receptor or prevented its internalization by the host cell could prevent infection. Once inside a cell, most viruses release their internal nucleic acid. Antibodies that bind to the virus before it becomes intracellular that can then block this step will be highly effective at neutralizing viral activity. Some viruses are coated with the plasma membrane derived from the host cell they had previously infected. Complement-fixing antibodies sometimes kill these agents by disrupting the membrane coat. Epitopes capable of promoting opsonization also can be effective at inducing protective immunity to viruses.

Bacterial Antigens

Bacteria generally cause disease by one of two mechanisms: secretion of a toxic product (as in tetanus, diphtheria, toxic shock syndrome, and botulism) or invasion and growth in an inappropriate host tissue (as in pneumococcal pneumonia or spinal meningitis). Immunity to extracellular products, such as toxins, usually involves the production of neutralizing antibodies. Bacterial protein toxins exert a wide variety of effects on host cells (Table 8.2). Vaccines composed of detoxified versions of some of these proteins have been highly successful in reducing the morbidity and mortality from many of these toxin-mediated diseases. In some instances, a toxin is derived from the bacterial surface when the organism either sheds its coat or is disrupted and lysed. In the case of gram-negative bacteria, the outer cell membrane lipopolysaccharide or endotoxin can be toxic to the host, often to the point of lethality. This material is made up of a toxic lipid component, known as lipid A, and an immunogenic, but usually nontoxic, polysaccharide. Antibodies to the polysaccharide portion can be protective. In the case of gram-positive bacteria, the cell wall teichoic acid and peptidoglycan can have pathologic effects by inducing toxic levels of host-derived cytokines such as interleukin-1 (IL-1) and tumor necrosis factor alpha (TNF-α). Toxic effects of bacterial antigens appear to be due to the activation of Toll-like receptors, notably TLR2 and TLR4.

Figure 8.11 Antigens involved in the host response to viruses. (a) Viral-envelope antigens can be the targets of antibodies, which can either block host-cell infection or trigger complement-mediated killing of free virions. Viral infection of a host cell will result in the production of viral proteins within the infected cell. (b) Some of these viral proteins may be processed and presented to cytotoxic T lymphocytes on MHC class I. (c) Alternatively, the infection may induce overproduction of host proteins such as stress-response proteins or may alter the production or peptide loading of MHC class I, resulting in killing of the infected cell by cytotoxic T lymphocytes or natural killer cells. (d) Finally, viral envelope proteins are expressed on the cell membrane of the infected cell and can be the targets of antibody-mediated killing by either cell-mediated or complement-mediated killing.

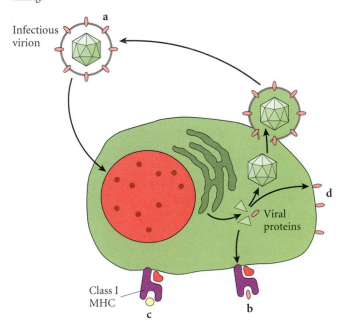

Table 8.2 Toxic proteins of bacteria causing disease

Bacterial strain	Toxin	Biologic effect	Mechanism of immunity
Vibrio cholerae	Cholera toxin	Diarrhea: ADP-ribosyl transferase and activation of adenylate cyclase[a], loosens tight junction	Unclear: subunit B part of vaccines under investigation or in use
	Zona occludens toxin	Diarrhea	Unclear
	Accessory cholera enterotoxin	Diarrhea	Unclear
Escherichia coli	Enterotoxins (2)	Diarrhea: heat-labile toxin similar to cholera toxin; heat-stable toxin activates guanylate cyclase	Unclear
Clostridium botulinum	Botulinus neurotoxin	Neurotoxic: blocks presynaptic release of acetylcholine	Antibodies induced by toxoid
Clostridium tetani	Tetanus toxin	Tetanospasm: spasmodic muscle contractions	Antibodies induced by toxoid
Corynebacterium diphtheriae	Diphtheria toxin	Cellular toxicity: ADP-ribosylates elongation factor 2, inhibits protein chain elongation	Antibodies induced by toxoid
Staphylococcus aureus	Variety of enterotoxins; TSST-1	Superantigens induce cytokine production; enterotoxins cause diarrhea	Not clear for enterotoxins; antibody to TSST-1 protects against infection

[a]ADP, adenosine diphosphate.

When a bacterial pathogen invades host tissues and cells, effective immunity usually entails phagocytic killing of the offending agent before it is able to damage host tissues. Bacterial killing requires the presence of protective antibodies specific for epitopes on the bacterial surface (Fig. 8.12). Many bacteria are coated, or encapsulated, with a polysaccharide antigen. IgM and IgG antibodies to these capsular polysaccharides usually promote phagocytic killing, often in the presence of complement cofactors. In some rare cases, serum IgA also can promote effective opsonic killing, but this process does not involve complement. Rather, specific receptors for the Fc portion of IgA, known as FcαR (CD89), are found on certain phagocytic cells. The polysaccharide portion of the lipopolysaccharide of gram-negative bacteria serves as an effective target for protective antibodies. In the case of gram-positive group A streptococci, which are the major cause of strep throat, surface proteins, called M proteins, are targets for protective antibodies. Some bacterial pathogens avoid host immune responses by coating themselves with polysaccharides that share considerable homology with those found in humans: group B *N. meningitidis* and the K1 group of *Escherichia coli* encase themselves in a sialic acid-based polysaccharide coat that is chemically identical to an antigen present on human cell surfaces. Proteins present in the outer membrane of gram-negative bacteria or embedded into the cell wall of gram-positive bacteria also may serve as targets for immune effectors. Overall, many different epitopes are detected on bacterial surfaces, some of which are targets for protective immunity. However, surface polysaccharide antigens seem to predominate as targets for protective immunity against bacteria that are pathogenic for humans. The success of vaccines composed of purified and/or conjugated polysaccharides is consistent with the importance of these chemical structures as antigens provoking immunity to bacterial infections.

Fungal Antigens

The pathogenic factors with which fungi are endowed and the immune mechanisms that act against them are not well understood. However, the frequent infection of immunocompromised patients with such microbes argues that the acquired immune response plays an important protective role against fungi in normal healthy individuals. Serious fungal infections are generally encountered in immunocompromised hosts (e.g., people with cancer or acquired immunodeficiency syndrome), although some fungi are able to cause disease in otherwise healthy individuals. The type of disease caused by fungal infections is usually dependent on fungal tropism for target organs or tissues, leading to their preferential colonization. For example, lethal bloodstream infections can occur when pathogenic fungi gain access to the circulatory system and are able to successfully grow there, whereas growth in the meninges of the brain can lead to life-threatening meningitis. Non-life-threatening fungal infections, such as athlete's foot, ringworm (which is not caused by a worm at all), and similar skin infections, occur commonly, as do diseases affecting other tissues,

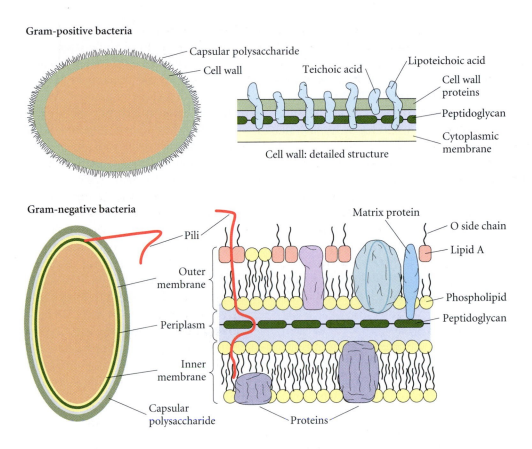

Figure 8.12 Architecture of the gram-positive and gram-negative bacterial cell wall. Prominent structures often involved in provoking immune responses are displayed. All bacteria have an inner cytoplasmic membrane and cell well, composed of peptidoglycan, surrounding the cytoplasmic membrane. Gram-negative bacteria have an additional outer membrane that contains proteins and lipopolysaccharide. Often capsular polysaccharides surround bacterial cells. The antigens most commonly used for immunologic diagnosis and as targets for protective antibodies are found on the outer surface, where they can readily interact with immunologic effectors such as antibody. Reprinted from G. B. Pier, p. 767–774, *in* K. J. Isselbacher et al. (ed)., *Harrison's Principles of Internal Medicine*, 7th ed. (McGraw-Hill, New York, N.Y., 2001), with permission.

such as vaginitis and oral thrush. Most efforts at characterizing fungal antigens have focused on those used for diagnosis of infection. These antigens either are detected directly in infected body fluids or are used indirectly to measure antibody responses in individuals suspected of being infected with the fungus in question. Fungi produce both glycoprotein and polysaccharide antigens, which have been employed in the evaluation of parameters defining both the level of infection caused by a certain fungus and the quality of immunity induced by it.

Polysaccharides such as the glucuronoxylomannan capsular polysaccharide produced by *Cryptococcus neoformans* are important in the infectious process used by this fungus; antibody to this antigen has shown protective effects, and detection of the cryptococcal capsular polysaccharide provides a useful tool for infection diagnosis.

Candida albicans produces mannose polymers (mannan), and *Aspergillus fumigatus* produces a galactomannan (mannan substituted with additional galactose groups), both of which are used in antigen-detecting assays, thus acting as useful diagnostic markers.

Protein and glycoprotein antigens are also used to diagnose fungal infections and may be involved in the pathogenic process employed by these microbes. Impaired cell-mediated immunity is a predisposing factor for fungal infections, indicating that the development of T-cell delayed-type sensitivity responses to fungal protein antigens is important in resisting these infections. Histoplasmosis is a common fungal infection endemic to parts of the midwestern United States. A serologic diagnosis can be made using histoplasmin, a preparation whose two major antigens are glycoproteins. Blastomycosis is another fungal infection that can occur in otherwise healthy individuals. A complex protein extract from this fungus, termed antigen A, has been somewhat useful in the serodiagnosis of this infection. An intriguing finding indicates that one of the targets for protective antibodies to *C. albicans* is a heat shock protein, hsp90. Heat shock proteins are highly conserved and may provide major target antigens for cells of the immune system.

Parasitic Antigens

Protozoan parasites and helminths are very large infectious agents with complicated life cycles. Together, these pathogens infect more than half of the world's population. Most of the important antigens characterized for these parasites are proteins or glycoproteins. In addition, some parasites, like the trematodes (flukes) from the genus *Schistosoma,* can cover themselves with host-derived antigens, including MHC proteins, and escape immune recognition by appearing syngeneic to the host. An additional set of significant antigens has immunosuppressive properties, which serve to blunt the host's immune attack. The most widely studied parasitic antigens are those that undergo antigenic shifts, in which the target epitopes of the immune response change during the course of infection.

The African trypanosomes, which cause sleeping sickness, cover themselves with a surface protein known as the variant-specific surface glycoprotein (Fig. 8.13). More than 1,000 different alleles of the gene encoding this protein have been identified. Antigenic polymorphism in malarial parasites also is thought to contribute to the pathologic

process, principally due to avoidance of acquired host immunity. To acquire some degree of resistance to the effects of malarial infection, human adults in areas where malaria is endemic develop a form of cross-protective immunity after years of infection. Whether this immunity is due to a broad-spectrum antibody response encompassing most of the antigenic variants of malarial parasites or to a more specific response directed at the more conserved, yet less immunogenic, antigens is not clear. The circumsporozoite protein coating the surface of the sporozoite phase of *Plasmodium falciparum,* the form of the malaria agent that is injected into the animal host from an *Anopheles* mosquito bite, has been investigated as a potential vaccine candidate. It has been found that antibodies directed to a four-amino-acid repeat within this protein are able to neutralize the parasite's infectivity. Additional malarial antigens, derived from the blood-stage form, are currently being evaluated as possible vaccines, with preliminary results suggesting that cell-mediated immune effectors are critical to the provision of effective immunity. Enzymes such as proteases and parasite heat shock proteins may be potential targets for immunologic attack and/or serodiagnosis.

Superantigens

Superantigens do not manifest their activity as do normal antigens but rather function as polyclonal stimulators of subsets of T cells. Superantigens bind promiscuously to MHC molecules, forming a bridge with the variable region of the TCR β chains, encoded by the TRBV genes

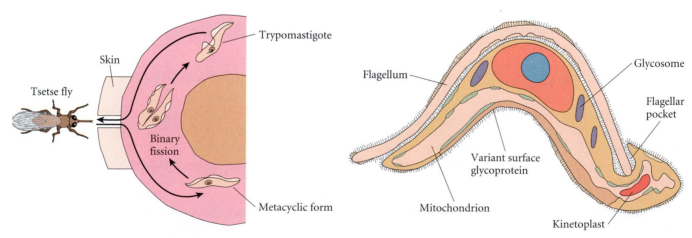

Figure 8.13 (**Left**) Life cycle of *Trypanosoma brucei,* the cause of African sleeping sickness. (**Right**) Cross-section of *T. brucei* showing structural features. The variant surface glycoprotein is a major antigen seen by the immune system. The parasite has more than 10^3 genes for this glycoprotein and changes the antigenic structure to evade host defenses. Reprinted from P. Borst, *Immunol. Today* **12**:A29–A33, 1991, and Anonymous, *Immunol. Today* **12**:A46–A47, 1991, with permission from Elsevier.

and comprising part of the αβ TCR (Fig. 8.14). Most often the superantigen binds to an MHC class II molecule, but evidence for binding to class I molecules and cell adhesion molecules has been found. Instead of activating T cells through specific TCR recognition of a peptide-MHC complex, superantigens activate a subset of T cells expressing a particular TRBV protein by engagement of the TCR outside the antigen-binding cleft, which normally binds to an antigenic peptide in complex with an MHC molecule. In addition, the binding to MHC molecules also takes place outside the peptide-binding cleft, usually involving a conserved region of the MHC protein. These unusual binding properties result in the bridging of MHC on the APCs and all T cells bearing one or more specific TRBV chains, leading to the selective activation of that T-cell subset. Thus, a given superantigen does not activate all T cells but only those with TRBV that act as receptors for the particular superantigen.

Two forms of superantigens have been identified: self and foreign. Self (or *endogenous*) superantigens are exemplified by the minor lymphocyte-stimulating determinants found in mice. These antigens were originally identified by their ability to stimulate polyclonal proliferation of T cells in culture when mice of the same MHC haplotype but of different strains were used as stimulators and responders in T-cell proliferation assays. Since the cells were matched at the major histocompatibility locus, yet still initiated a T-cell response, other, minor, antigenic epitopes had to be present to provoke the proliferation of the responding T cells. The minor lymphocyte-stimulating antigens are now known to be encoded by the genome of the endogenous retrovirus, mouse mammary tumor virus (MMTV). The DNA from this virus is actually integrated into mouse chromosomal DNA and passed on to the offspring via germ line cells. Although the DNA for

minor lymphocyte-stimulating superantigens encodes a transmembrane protein, a soluble form that also functions as a superantigen probably exists. The evolutionary reasons for maintaining the MMTV genome integrated into mouse DNA are purely speculative, although the suggestion that an integrated MMTV genome may prevent additional MMTV infections in mice seems like a reasonable extrapolation, based on selective pressures for increased survival.

Foreign (or *exogenous*) superantigens are usually found in toxins produced by gram-positive bacteria, such as staphylococci and streptococci, by an antigen produced by *Mycoplasma arthritidis,* and by some viruses. Several of the bacterial superantigens cause food poisoning, while one of them, toxic shock syndrome toxin 1 (TSST-1), causes, as its name implies, toxic shock syndrome. TSST-1 is a potent inducer of IL-1 and TNF-α, which could explain, in part, both its T-cell stimulatory capacity and some of the clinical manifestations attributed to this syndrome (e.g., high fever, muscular weakness, and a drop in blood pressure leading to shock).

Both self and foreign superantigens appear to bind similar portions of MHC proteins, although different TRBV proteins are recognized on the T cell by the different superantigens. Binding leads to a selective activation of T cells expressing the appropriate TRBV element. Transgenic mice, in which most T cells express the TRBV26 polypeptide (formerly referred to as the $V_{\beta}3$ polypeptide), undergo vigorous cellular proliferation in response to the superantigen known as staphylococcal enterotoxin A (SEA). In contrast, nontransgenic mice, which express TRBV26 on only about 10% of their T cells, require 1,000-fold higher concentrations of SEA in order to generate vigorous cellular proliferation. Although the involvement of the TRBV protein in T-cell activation by superantigens is well estab-

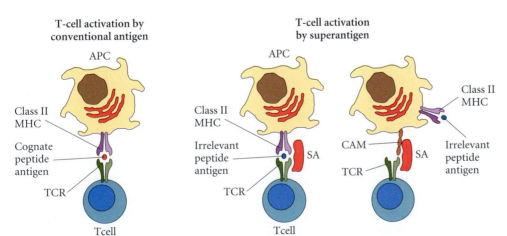

T-cell activation by conventional antigen	T-cell activation by superantigen
APC	APC
Class II MHC	Class II MHC / Class II MHC
Cognate peptide antigen	Irrelevant peptide antigen / CAM / Irrelevant peptide antigen
TCR	TCR / TCR
T cell	T cell

Figure 8.14 Difference between normal antigenic stimulation of T cells (**left**) and stimulation by a superantigen (**right**). Unlike the normal antigen, which must be processed and presented by an APC, a superantigen (SA) remains intact and binds to nonpolymorphic portions of the MHC class II protein and to β chains of the TCR from a particular family of V_{β} chains. Some superantigens bind to cell adhesion molecules (CAM) and β chains of the TCR.

lished, T cells bearing certain TRAV elements in association with TRBV can be stimulated by staphylococcal enterotoxin B. This work demonstrates that, at least in some instances, the TRAV elements of the TCR can influence T-cell activation by superantigen. It appears that the TRAV element of the TCR alters the conformation of the TRBV element to one that is more favorable for superantigen binding.

Mitogens

Study of the cellular events involved in lymphocyte activation is difficult because only a few antigen-specific cells interact with tiny amounts of native or processed antigen in organs such as lymph node or spleen. Much of what we know about lymphocyte responses following activation is derived from in vitro experiments, in which many cells can be activated and their responses subsequently studied under laboratory conditions. The observed responses are thought to reflect those that occur naturally following antigenic stimuli. To mimic lymphocyte functional responses to antigen activation, immunologists often have employed *mitogens* as antigen surrogates. However, mitogens are not usually considered to be true antigens in terms of stimulating T- and B-cell responses specific to the mitogen.

Mitogens represent a broader class of polyclonal activators than do superantigens, in that mitogens tend to activate all cells of a certain type in a totally nonspecific manner (that is, while the superantigen SEA activates all T cells expressing TRBV26, a mitogen may activate *all T cells,* regardless of TRBV usage). Mitogens are used to induce polyclonal cellular activation and proliferation. Some mitogens activate T cells, while others, such as bacterial lipopolysaccharide, activate mouse B cells; still others activate both types of lymphocyte. Many mitogens are lectins, proteins that specifically interact with carbohydrate residues. Common T-cell mitogens include concanavalin A, phytohemagglutinin, and pokeweed mitogen. These mitogens bind surface carbohydrates on cells and may also promote cellular agglutination. Although mitogens are an experimentally useful surrogate for measuring lymphocyte responses to antigens, the results of such experiments must be interpreted with caution since these responses may deviate considerably from the true in vivo situation. Mitogen-like preparations, including monoclonal antibodies that bind to lymphocyte surface antigens and activate these cells, have also been employed to study the cellular events involved in lymphocyte activation.

Mitogens have been useful for studying signal transduction mechanisms, cellular proliferation, and the production of cytokines and their complementary receptors. These are all closely linked events in lymphocyte biology, driving the cell through its cycle and ultimately yielding a mature cell capable of carrying out its specific function. Other systems used in these studies include cloned T-cell lines and T-cell/T-cell hybridomas.

Summary

The term *antigen* refers to any molecule or structure that can bind specifically to the clonotypic receptors of lymphocytes (antibody and the TCR). Antigens can be of any known class of biomolecule: protein, carbohydrate, lipid, or nucleic acid. Binding of an antigen to its specific receptor sometimes, but not always, leads to activation of the lymphocyte bearing the antigen receptor. Antigens that are capable of specifically activating a lymphocyte are termed immunogens. Many factors determine whether a given antigen will be immunogenic. Some of these factors are intrinsic to the antigen: foreignness, chemical complexity, and size. Other factors affecting immunogenicity are dependent not on the antigen itself, but on the conditions under which the host encounters the antigen. Antigen dose is an extremely important factor; moderate doses of antigen stimulate an immune response, whereas doses above and below this optimal range fail to produce a response. The route by which the antigen enters the host also is critical.

Lymphocytes that specifically recognize an antigen usually do not contact the entire antigen; rather, they contact a portion of the antigen termed the epitope. Epitopes that are recognized by B cells usually comprise a portion of the antigen that resides on the antigen's surface, where the epitope is available to interact with an antibody. Epitopes recognized by T cells are very different, comprising short (8 to 20 amino acids) peptides derived from the original protein antigen by proteolysis. To be recognized by a T cell, this peptide must first be bound to an MHC protein on the surface of another host cell, which *presents* the peptide to the T cell. Because of this required process of proteolysis and binding of short peptides to MHC, most T-cell epitopes are proteins. Antigens recognized by B cells do not have these restrictions. Therefore, B cells frequently recognize antigens of all biochemical classes (protein, carbohydrate, etc.).

The epitopes recognized by B cells and T cells have in common that they are bound by antigen receptors in a highly specific manner. However, lymphocytes can also be activated in a less specific fashion by other classes of stimulators. *Superantigens* are proteins encoded by bacteria or retroviruses that bind to MHC proteins and TCRs by a mechanism that relies on only a small portion of the TCR variable region. All TCRs that possess this portion of the

TCR are stimulated by a given superantigen. Therefore, a single superantigen can stimulate about 5 to 20% of the T cells in an individual host (as compared to the 0.001 to 0.01% of T cells stimulated by most conventional antigens). This large amount of T-cell activation can have pathological consequences for the host.

Still other stimulators can activate lymphocytes in a manner even less specific than that of superantigens. These molecules are termed mitogens. Mitogens usually bypass the antigen receptor altogether, causing a nonspecific aggregation of stimulatory receptors on the lymphocyte or directly activating the lymphocyte's signal transduction machinery. Although not an accurate representation of in vivo lymphocyte activation, mitogens can be useful for many experimental approaches where lymphocyte activation is needed.

Suggested Reading

Cox, J. C., and A. R. Coulter. 1997. Adjuvants—a classification and review of their modes of action. *Vaccine* **15**:248–256.

Fremont, D. H., W. A. Hendrickson, P. Marrack, and J. Kappler. 1996. Structures of an MHC class II molecule with covalently bound single peptides. *Science* **272**:1001–1004.

Hudecz, F. 2001. Manipulation of epitope function by modification of peptide structure: a minireview. *Biologicals* **29**:197–207.

Kaisho, T., and S. Akira. 2002. Toll-like receptors as adjuvant receptors. *Biochim. Biophys. Acta* **589**:1–13.

Llewelyn, M., and J. Cohen. 2002. Superantigens: microbial agents that corrupt immunity. *Lancet Infect. Dis.* **2**:156–162.

Marchalonis, J. J., M. K. Adelman, I. F. Robey, S. F. Schluter, and A. B. Edmundson. 2001. Exquisite specificity and peptide epitope recognition promiscuity, properties shared by antibodies from sharks to humans. *J. Mol. Recognit.* **14**:110–121.

Ramsland, P. A., E. Yuriev, and A. B. Edmundson. 2001. Immunoglobulin cross-reactivity examined by library screening, crystallography and docking studies. *Comb. Chem. High Throughput Screen.* **4**:397–408.

Regner, M. 2001. Cross-reactivity in T-cell antigen recognition. *Immunol. Cell Biol.* **79**:91–100.

Rini, J. M., U. Schulze-Gahmen, and I. A. Wilson. 1992. Structural evidence for induced fit as a mechanism for antibody-antigen recognition. *Science* **255**:959–965.

Rubin, B., L. Alibaud, A. Huchenq-Champagne, J. Arnaud, M. L. Toribio, and J. Constans. 2002. Some hints concerning the shape of T-cell receptor structures. *Scand. J. Immunol.* **55**:111–118.

Rudolph, M. G., J. G. Luz, and I. A. Wilson. 2002. Structural and thermodynamic correlates of T cell signaling. *Annu. Rev. Biophys. Biomol. Struct.* **31**:121–149.

Rudolph, M. G., and I. A. Wilson. 2002. The specificity of TCR/pMHC interaction. *Curr. Opin. Immunol.* **14**:52–65.

Thomas, J. W. 2001. Antigen-specific responses in autoimmunity and tolerance. *Immunol. Res.* **23**:235–244.

Van Regenmortel, M. H. 2001. Antigenicity and immunogenicity of synthetic peptides. *Biologicals* **29**:209–213.

chapter 9

Antibody-Antigen Interactions and Measurements of Immunologic Reactions

Johannes Huebner

topics covered

▲ Antigenic specificity

▲ Physical nature of the antibody-antigen interaction

▲ Chemical forces that influence antibody-antigen interactions

▲ Cross-reactivity

▲ Affinity versus avidity

▲ Assays used to measure antibody-antigen interactions

The interaction of antibodies with antigen is one of the fundamental mechanisms of host immunity. The high specificity of this interaction has made it one of the principal paradigms for understanding molecular recognition in biologic systems. This interaction is also the basis of a large number of diagnostic tests for diseases. Many of these tests are widely used by the medical and scientific communities and therefore have applications outside the field of immunology.

Antibody-antigen interactions are in many respects comparable to enzyme-substrate interactions, in that both are highly specific, reversible, and based on noncovalent intermolecular interactions. The major difference between antibody-antigen and enzyme-substrate interactions is that antibody-antigen interactions do not usually change the chemical structure of either partner whereas enzyme-substrate interactions commonly result in a change in the chemical structure of the substrate, resulting in the formation of a "product."

Gaining an understanding of the structural basis of antigen specificity has been a major thrust of immunology research in recent years as the use of antibodies has extended to a growing number of applications in modern medicine and biotechnology, such as the diagnosis of infections and tumors; the detection of chemicals, drugs, and hormones; and the development of vaccines.

The Concept of Specificity

Since many of the antibody-mediated reactions involved in the elimination of invading bacteria and viruses also are potentially dangerous to the host's uninfected tissues, antibody specificity is essential for directing these immune reactions to the foreign material while leaving the host's uninfected cells and tissues unharmed. *Specificity* refers to the usual reactivity of one antibody to only one antigenic determinant. It is probably true that any accessible area on the surface of a molecule can be antigenic. Because there are millions of possible antigenic

structures, the immune system must be able to create an equally diverse population of antibody molecules.

The Molecular Basis of Specificity

The structural basis of the antigen-binding specificity of an antibody lies in complementarity-determining regions (CDRs), which are located in the Fab regions of the antibody at the amino termini of the heavy and light chains. Both the specificity and the affinity of antibody-antigen binding depend on the three-dimensional conformation of both molecules. Over the past several years, two different models have been proposed to explain antigen binding by antibodies (Fig. 9.1), and recently a third model has received experimental support. The first is the *lock-and-key model*, which describes antibody-antigen binding as the perfect fit of two rigid, complementary shapes. This model presumes that antibody-antigen binding events are unlikely because of the stringency of the requirement for complementarity between antibody and antigen (i.e., the two molecules must fit each other perfectly). The second model is the *induced-fit model*, which presumes that the antigen, the antibody, or both can change their conformation to allow for a better fit between the two molecules. Since this model predicts that an antigen-binding site of the antibody can adopt a range of closely related conformations, it follows that antibody-antigen binding is not so unlikely after all, since an antibody that does not fit a given antigen perfectly can change its conformation to permit binding. An important implication of the induced-fit model is a reduction in antibody-antigen specificity, since the ability of an antibody to subtly change the shape of its antigen-binding site might allow the site to bind multiple antigens. This could explain the frequently observed phenomenon of *cross-reactivity*, in which an antibody originally generated to one antigen is

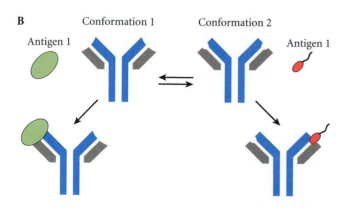

Figure 9.1 The lock-and-key, induced-fit, and equilibrium models help explain the interaction of antibodies with antigen. (**A**) According to the lock-and-key model, the CDRs of the antibody (black and dark blue triangles and rectangles) must be a perfect complement for the antigen's epitope for binding to occur. In contrast, the induced-fit model states that the CDRs of the antibody are able to alter their shape to some degree to adopt a conformation that is complementary to the epitope of the antigen. According to this model, the CDRs do not have to initially match the epitope perfectly for high-affinity binding to occur. (**B**) In the equilibrium model one antibody exists in two isomeric forms that are both always available because they are in equilibrium, with each form able to bind to different and exclusive epitopes. When one isomeric form binds to its cognate antigen, it can no longer switch back to the other form; thus, to maintain the equilibrium, more of the form binding to the antigen is formed. This continues until all of the antigen is bound and the equilibrium can be maintained. Panel B is reprinted with permission from J. Foote, *Science* **299:**1327–1328, 2003.

also capable of binding other, unrelated antigens. The third recently proposed model suggests that the same antibody can exist in two different conformations, each with different antigen-binding sites, and that in liquid solution these conformations are in equilibrium (Fig. 9.1B). For example, one isomer of the antibody may form a shallow surface at the antigen-binding site, whereas another isomer forms a deep pocket. Both forms are available for binding to antigen, as the equilibrium they are in means that rapid interconversion between the two forms occurs. When an antigen that binds to one of the forms is present, it removes some of its specific isomer from the equilibrium, and there is subsequent compensation for the removal with more of the antigen-binding isomer being formed. This continues until all of the antigen is bound and the equilibrium can be maintained. Over the years, the study of a large number of antibody-antigen complexes has led to the conclusion that the lock-and-key and the induced-fit models are correct and that the equilibrium model may also be operative for some antibodies. Overall, the nature of antibody-antigen binding varies from one antibody-antigen pair to another. Some pairs bind in a lock-and-key fashion, while others demonstrate some degree of induced-fit characteristics or bind to different isomers formed from the equilibrium reaction. Comparisons of these binding events indicate that induced-fit-type interactions, although they appear to be more likely than lock-and-key-type interactions, tend to be of lower affinity, probably because an antibody capable of induced-fit binding must have fairly flexible, mobile CDRs. Binding of such an antibody to an antigen would inevitably immobilize the CDRs, thereby reducing the entropy of the binding reaction and making it less favorable from an energetics standpoint.

Crystallographic Evidence of Specificity

The three-dimensional structures of many antibody molecules have been elucidated by X-ray crystallography. Not only have these studies provided us with an idea of how antibodies appear in actual, three-dimensional space, they also have led to a more concrete understanding of the structural basis of antibody-antigen interactions.

The preparation of crystals for X-ray diffraction studies requires a homogeneous population of molecules because the crystals must consist of a regularly repeating subunit, the antibody-antigen complex, in this case. Because of the heterogeneity of the antibodies in whole serum, they are not suitable for the formation of crystals. This problem was solved with the identification of a patient with multiple myeloma, who had a plasmacytoma that was clonal in nature (i.e., all of the tumor cells were derived from the same original parent cell and were therefore genetically identical). All of the antibodies, called myeloma proteins, produced by the tumor cells were identical. About 30 years ago the initial studies on the antibody-antigen interaction were performed on antibodies specific for the antigens vitamin K and phosphorylcholine. These studies provided some information about the antibody-antigen interaction; however, the ability to produce homogeneous antibody to a particular antigen represented an even greater advance. Initially, this was accomplished by the induction of tumors in mice that had been hyperimmunized with the antigen of interest. Later, the field of immunology was revolutionized by the advent of hybridoma technology, which permitted immunologists to produce homogeneous antibodies specific for any antigenic epitope they desired. Further advances in molecular genetic techniques made it possible to isolate and sequence the antibody genes carried by the hybridoma and to systematically introduce mutations into various portions of the gene encoding the antigen-binding part of the antibody. Such studies made it possible to dissect the antibody-antigen interaction at the level of the individual amino acid.

The analysis of one antibody-antigen complex, that between the antigen hen egg lysozyme (HEL) and the HEL-specific (anti-HEL) monoclonal antibody D1.3, has yielded much information about antigen binding and is one of the prototype antibody-antigen pairs studied in immunology. Comparison of the structure of the HEL-D1.3 complex with the structures of each molecule alone led to the conclusion that neither of these molecules underwent significant conformational changes during antibody-antigen binding. This indicated that the binding event was similar to a lock-and-key-type interaction. Also, it was presumed, on the basis of the locations of functional groups such as hydroxyl groups and amino groups, that the intermolecular forces between the antibody and the antigen were mostly van der Waals interactions and hydrogen bonds. Furthermore, it was discovered that this antibody-antigen binding event was mediated by 17 amino acids of the antibody and 16 amino acids of the antigen. Of the 17 antibody amino acids that contributed to binding, 6 belonged to light-chain CDRs, 9 belonged to heavy-chain CDRs, and 2 belonged to framework regions. Equally interesting information was gathered from the identification of the HEL amino acids that made contact with the antibody and formed the antigenic epitope. It was found that the 16 amino acids were not consecutive in the primary amino acid sequence of the antigen and formed a conformational or nonsequential epitope. This structural analysis confirmed that three-dimensional folding (the conformation) of the antigen helped bring these nonsequential amino acids together on the surface of the antigen to form the epitope (see Fig. 8.2).

Further evidence for the existence of conformational epitopes has been obtained in studies of the ability of antibodies raised to a native, intact protein antigen to bind proteolytic fragments of that antigen. In many cases, the antibody cannot recognize the fragments, indicating that the amino acids that make up the epitope are not all contiguous but are brought together in the native protein by the three-dimensional folding of the protein antigen. Not all epitopes are conformational, however. A small portion of antibodies raised to a protein antigen also will recognize proteolytic fragments derived from that antigen. Similarly, antibodies raised to fragments of a protein will sometimes also recognize the intact protein. In these cases, the epitope recognized by the antibody comprises a stretch of amino acids that occur sequentially in the intact protein. Thus, the epitope is preserved whether it exists as a part of the intact protein antigen or as a short isolated peptide. It should be noted that, in all crystallographic studies of antibody interactions with intact protein antigens, the antibody and antigen interact through multiple points of contact involving discontinuous portions of the antigen, even when the epitope had originally been defined as a linear epitope. Therefore, although typically a distinction is made between linear epitopes and conformational epitopes, it is probably more accurate to consider all antibody-antigen interactions as involving conformational epitopes but that, in some cases, a linear region of the protein antigen makes enough contacts with the antibody to be sufficient for antibody binding.

In conceptualizing the antigen-antibody interaction, one must keep in mind that the structures studied in X-ray crystallographic analyses are static, whereas in reality the interaction of an antibody with its antigen is a dynamic process. In addition, the chemical and physical conditions necessary for the formation of crystals, including low temperature, organic solvents, and high salt concentrations, can alter the way the antibody and antigen interact. For all of these reasons, the structure that exists in the crystal may or may not reflect the behavior of antibodies and antigens in solution, and thus, one must be careful when interpreting or considering this type of experimental data.

Deviations from Absolute Specificity
Cross-Reactivity
Although antigenic specificity is one of the central features of the acquired immune system, it has long been acknowledged that the specificity of antibodies is not always absolute, and not uncommonly antibody produced in response to one antigen will also recognize an antigen that is distinct from the original one, a phenomenon termed cross-reactivity. There are several reasons for cross-reactivity (Fig. 9.2).

The first reason for cross-reactivity is the presence of a shared antigen on seemingly different cells, tissues, or microorganisms. For example, although the CD4 plasma membrane molecule is principally found on T cells, some neural cells also express it. If there was a need to distinguish nerve cells from T cells in a biologic sample, use of an antibody to CD4 may not give the needed distinction (Fig. 9.2A). In this case, an antibody raised to the CD4 antigen reacts with T lymphocytes and nerve cells. Many cells and tissues from different species also share antigens that can give rise to cross-reactivity. Another example of this phenomenon involves an antigen known as the Forssman antigen, a sphingolipid that is ubiquitous on the surface of cells from a number of animals (e.g., it is present on most hamster and horse cells but is absent on rabbit and rat cells).

The second type of cross-reactivity occurs when different antigens bear a shared epitope recognized by an antibody. This often occurs when the antigen is from closely related sources (Fig. 9.2B). For example, serum albumins from humans and chimpanzees share many antigenic epitopes and an antibody raised to albumin from one of these sources will readily bind the other. In contrast, albumin from a more distantly related species such as a chicken will have little cross-reactivity because there are few shared epitopes. It is possible to make the antibodies raised to human serum albumin specific for this antigen and not cross-reactive with chimpanzee serum albumin. To do this, the chimpanzee albumin antigen is added to the anti-human albumin antisera to bind to and thus adsorb out the cross-reactive antibodies that recognize albumin from both species. This process leaves behind only antibodies that recognize epitopes found on human serum albumin (Fig. 9.2C).

Third, cross-reactivity can occur if two unrelated antigens bear epitopes that are similar but not identical (Fig. 9.2D). One important consequence of this type of cross-reactivity is that a cross-reacting antibody will recognize each antigen with a different affinity because the two antigens do not bear identical epitopes. Usually, the original antigen (the one to which the antibody was raised) is bound by the antibody with high affinity and the second, cross-reactive antigen is bound with a lower affinity. Many examples of these are found among microbial antigens. For example, many bacteria modify their surfaces by

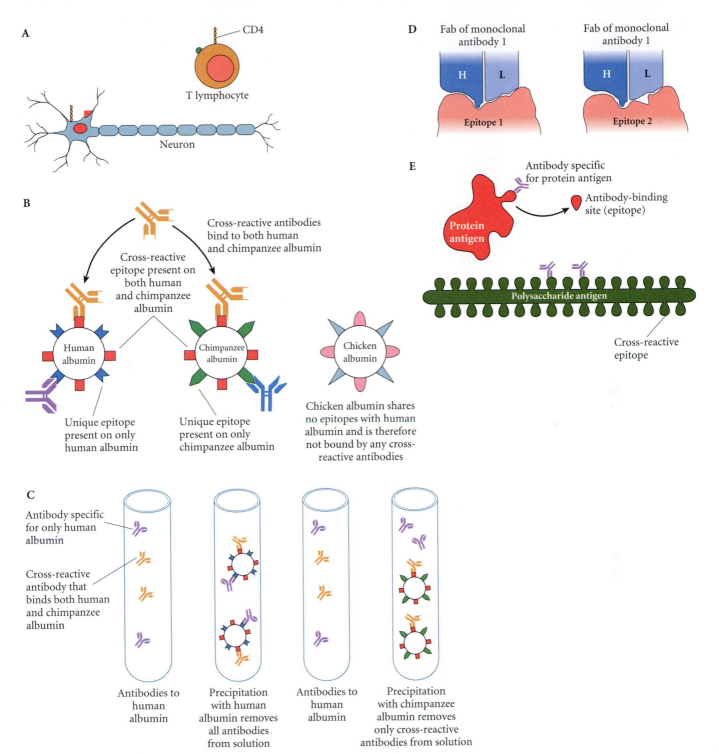

Figure 9.2 The molecular bases of cross-reactivity. **(A)** Cross-reactivity can occur if the same antigen is present on different cell types or in different tissues. In the example shown, an antibody that is meant to bind to T lymphocytes and that recognizes an epitope on the CD4 protein (orange) will cross-react with neurons, since the latter also express the CD4 protein. There are other potential antigens (green circle and red triangle) on T cells and neurons that will not be cross-reactive, since they are expressed on either T lymphocytes or neurons. **(B)** Cross-reactivity can also result from the presence of identical epitopes on the surface of two nonidentical antigens. Serum albumins from chimpanzees and humans are closely related and thus share a large number of epitopes (red rectangles) that elicit antibodies (orange) that bind to this shared epitope on both albumins. Both human and chimpanzee albumins contain a number of unique epitopes that are not cross-reactive. Albumin in chicken blood is much more distantly related and, therefore, there are no shared antigenic epitopes and little or no reactivity of antibodies to human or chimpanzee albumin with chicken albumin. **(C)** When human albumin is added to antibodies generated against human albumin (**left and left center**), all of the anti-albumin antibodies will be bound to and precipitated by the antigen. In contrast, when chimpanzee albumin is added to the antibodies generated against human albumin (**right center and right**), only the antibodies in the antiserum that recognize the cross-reactive epitopes (orange antibodies) are bound to the chimpanzee albumin. If these immune complexes are separated from the unbound antibodies by centrifugation (precipitation), what remains soluble in the supernatant is antibodies specific to human serum albumin epitopes (pink antibodies). **(D)** Cross-reactivity can result when two antigens possess similar (but not identical) epitopes. In the example shown, a monoclonal antibody is intended to be specific for "epitope 1." However, in this case monoclonal antibody 1 cross-reacts with "epitope 2," since epitope 2 is very similar to epitope 1. It is likely that the antibody will bind to epitope 2 more weakly than it binds to epitope 1. **(E)** Two chemically unrelated entities, such as a protein antigen and a carbohydrate antigen, can have similar, cross-reactive epitopes.

adding an acetate molecule to a hydroxyl or amino group. Antibodies that recognize the acetylated form of the antigen will often also recognize the nonacetylated form as well, making it difficult to use antibodies to distinguish between the acetylated and nonacetylated forms of the antigen.

Fourth, cross-reactivity can occur when chemically distinct and seemingly unrelated epitopes nonetheless take on the same overall configuration in three-dimensional space, such that an antibody to one of the structures is also able to bind to the other (Fig. 9.2E). There is a large medical interest in obtaining antibodies to polysaccharide antigens on the surfaces of microbes, particularly bacteria, as these antibodies often mediate protective immunity and can be given passively to infected individuals for antimicrobial therapy. But some polysaccharides are poorly immunogenic, particularly in young children, and one strategy to find immunogens that induce antibody to the polysaccharides is to look for small peptides that mimic the overall three-dimensional structure of the polysaccharide. In this scenario, an investigator can take an antibody to a polysaccharide raised in an animal, screen it against a large library of highly variant peptides, and see which peptides bind the antipolysaccharide antibody strongly. These haptenic peptides can then be coupled to larger carrier molecules and used to induce antibodies to the polysaccharide. Thus the amino-acid-based peptide and the monosaccharide-based polysaccharide form the same antigenic epitope in spite of their very different chemical nature.

Cross-reactivity is sometimes exploited in the development of diagnostic tests. For example, antibodies cross-reactive for cardiolipin, an antigen present on heart tissues of humans and cattle, are formed during infection with *Treponema pallidum*, the causative agent of syphilis. Cardiolipin is used as an antigen to detect the presence of antibodies to *T. pallidum* and help make the diagnosis of syphilis. Another example is the occurrence of antibodies that cross-react with sheep erythrocytes in patients infected with Epstein-Barr virus (EBV), which can cause mononucleosis and other diseases. The presence of antibodies that cause sheep erythrocytes to clump (agglutinate) is a rapid and inexpensive test for detecting EBV infection (Fig. 9.3). In both of these examples it is antibody produced by the host in response to the microbial antigens that is detected, not the microbe itself.

Due to the potential cross-reactivity of antibodies to different antigens, certain pathogens take advantage of the fact that the host usually will not create an immune response to self antigens by coating themselves with molecules that are identical or similar to host molecules. This allows the microbe to avoid host immune responses by appearing to be the same as the host's own cells or tissues, a process known as *molecular mimicry*. An example is the ubiquitous occurrence on human cells of short oligosaccharide structures on glycoproteins containing *N*-acetylneuraminic acid. Some bacteria, such as *Escherichia coli* and *Neisseria meningitidis*, incorporate *N*-acetylneuraminic acid structures identical to the human oligosaccharide into the microbial capsular polysaccharides, making the host's immune system unable to immunologically respond to this protective antigen of the bacterium, which it mistakenly sees as a self antigen.

Molecular mimicry not only can affect the ability of a bacterium to infect a given host, it also can have important repercussions in the host after the bacterial infection has resolved. Such repercussions usually take the form of autoimmune disorders that occur because antibodies produced to a bacterial antigen during infection can cross-react with self antigens. A prototypic example is the M proteins that are on the surface of group A streptococci, the causative agent of strep throat and other, more serious, streptococcal infections. Antibodies produced to M proteins during a throat infection can cross-react with antigens on the plasma membranes of human heart muscle cells. This is the pathophysiologic basis for the disease rheumatic fever. Another example of an autoimmune disease attributable to molecular mimicry is the neurologic damage in Chagas' disease, caused by the protozoan parasite *Trypanosoma cruzi*. Neurologic damage is caused by the production of antibodies to a 12-amino-acid-long region of a *T. cruzi* protein that cross-reacts with human nerve cells, resulting in nerve damage.

Polyfunctional Binding Sites

A number of antibody molecules have been identified that have the ability to bind with low affinity to multiple antigenic epitopes. This polyreactivity is often a property of the so-called *natural antibodies* that exist in animals that have never been immunized or have never encountered a specific foreign antigen. Most of these antibodies probably are produced by a population of B cells that express unmutated germ line immunoglobulin genes. One potential antigen source of the polyreactive antibodies is the microbial organisms that rapidly colonize the skin, gastrointestinal tract, and other mucosal surfaces shortly after birth. Since these natural antibodies are mostly polyvalent immunoglobulin M (IgM) antibodies, their low affinity is compensated for by a high avidity, a property of multivalent antibodies that increases their overall ability to bind to an antigen. Natural antibodies are thought to be important in the host's early defense against a variety of

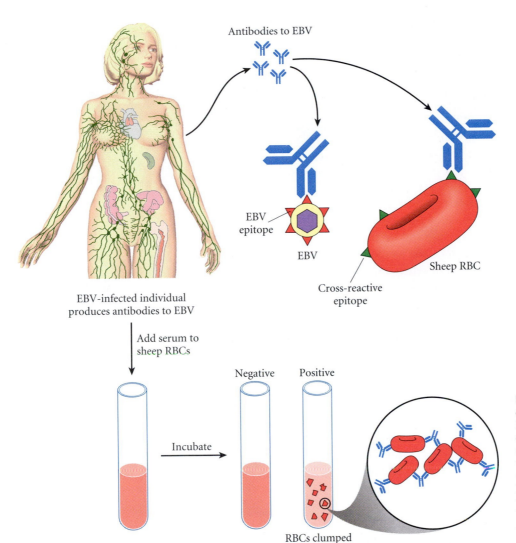

EBV epitope

EBV

Antibodies to EBV

Cross-reactive epitope

Sheep RBC

EBV-infected individual produces antibodies to EBV

Add serum to sheep RBCs

Negative   Positive

Incubate

RBCs clumped

Figure 9.3 The application of cross-reactivity as a diagnostic tool. Individuals infected with EBV produce antibodies to EBV that are cross-reactive with an antigen on the surface of sheep red blood cells (RBCs). Therefore, if serum from an EBV-infected individual is mixed with sheep RBCs (**bottom**), the antibodies to EBV will agglutinate (or clump) the RBCs, giving a positive reaction.

bacterial and viral pathogens and have also been implicated in autoimmune responses.

The Physical Nature of the Antibody-Antigen Interaction

The Concept of Antibody Affinity

Affinity is one of the most important concepts that define the antibody-antigen interaction. This term refers to the overall strength of all of the noncovalent interactions that take place between a single antibody-binding site and a single epitope. This strength is due to two factors: the rate at which the antibody binds to the antigen, known as the forward rate or on rate, and the rate at which the antibody dissociates from the antigen, known as the off rate. High-affinity antibodies bind to their epitope very tightly, and this is usually due to a low rate of dissociation of the antibody from the epitope. Low-affinity antibodies tend to either bind poorly to the antigen, due to a low association rate, or fail to remain tightly bound to the antigen, due to a high dissociation rate. This interaction can be expressed using the law of mass action.

The Law of Mass Action and Its Application to Antigen-Antibody Binding

The reaction between antigen and antibody can be described by the following formula:

$$Ag + Ab \leftrightarrows Ag - Ab$$

The forward rate whereby the antigen-antibody complex is formed represents the association constant (k_{on}), and the reverse or off rate is represented by the dissociation constant (k_{off}). The ratio of the concentration of the immune complexes, [Ag − Ab], to the individual concentrations of free antigen, [Ag], and free antibody, [Ab], is the equilibrium constant of the specific reaction, designated K_a, and represents the affinity of the antibody-antigen interaction:

$$K_a = [Ag - Ab]/[Ag][Ab]$$

The equilibrium dissociation constant, K_d, is defined as the reciprocal of K_a (i.e., $1/K_a$) and is given by the following formula:

$$K_d = [Ag][Ab]/[Ag - Ab]$$

To determine the affinity, the antibody-antigen interaction must take place under equilibrium conditions (i.e., the concentrations of free antigen, antibody, and bound immune complexes become stable). Further, the formula is representative of the affinity constant only when binding is a simple one-step reaction with no conformational changes of either antibody or antigen occurring upon binding. Unless all of these conditions are met, the affinity constants obtained are only approximations of the actual values.

The measurement of affinity is usually done by mixing antibody and antigen in various concentrations and determining the concentrations of free components as well as immune complexes when equilibrium is reached. This can be accomplished by a variety of methods, including filtration, equilibrium dialysis, radioimmunoassay, enzyme-linked immunosorbent assay, and fluorescent measurements. Antibody affinity can also be measured with biosensors, which measure intermolecular binding by tracking minute changes in the refractive index of a surface as molecules bind to and dissociate from that surface. Typically, either the antibody or the antigen is immobilized on the surface and the other (antigen or antibody) is applied as a soluble molecule (Fig. 9.4A). Biosensors are advantageous because they can measure binding events in real time (Fig. 9.4B), allowing determination of not only the equilibrium constants K_a and K_d but also the kinetic rate constants k_{on} and k_{off}, which indicate the actual speed with which the antigen binds to, and is released from, the antibody.

The determination of K_a has traditionally been measured using equilibrium dialysis. This method relies on the use of a dialysis chamber and an antigen that is small enough to pass through the semipermeable membrane; antibody, however, is too large to cross the membrane. When only the antigen is present, it will diffuse equally into both compartments and achieve an identical concentration on both sides of the membrane (Fig. 9.5A). However, when a known amount of antibody is added to only one side of the semipermeable membrane, the binding of the antigen to the antibody will increase the total

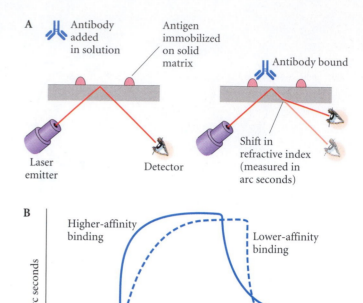

Figure 9.4. The use of a biosensor device for the real-time measurement of antibody-antigen interactions. (**A**) Antigen is covalently conjugated to the surface of a chip, and antibody is added to the solution above the surface of the chip. Meanwhile, a laser beam is bounced off the bottom surface of the chip. Binding or dissociation of the antibody to the surface of the chip results in mass changes near the surface, which alters its refractive index. This changes the angle of the reflected beam, which can be detected by a panel of photomultiplier tubes (right). (**B**) A sample readout from a biosensor device in a hypothetical experiment similar to that depicted in panel A. Antibody is added at the time point marked by the arrow labeled "a," and the binding event is measured over time. The change in the refractive index of the laser light is measured as a shift in the angular distance of the refracted light and is reported in arc seconds (60 arc seconds in an arc minute; 60 arc minutes equal 1 degree on a 360-degree circle; 3,600 arc seconds/degree). After a period of seconds to minutes, the binding event is complete, and the change in the refractive index levels off. If the antibody solution is then removed and the chip is washed using a solution that lacks antibody (time point marked with arrow b), the antibody that is already bound to the chip will dissociate. High-affinity antibodies bind rapidly (fast change in refractive index), lower-affinity antibodies bind more slowly. Similarly, antibodies with a low dissociation constant that stay bound to the antigen are removed slowly and there is a slower change in the refractive index, whereas antibodies with a high dissociation constant that are quickly washed off the antigen have a more rapid decrease in the refractive index.

concentration of antigen inside the chamber due to both antibody-bound antigen and free antigen, with the concentration of the free antigen balanced on both sides of the membrane (Fig. 9.5B).

When the antigen is present in excess, the concentration of free antigenic epitopes, [Ag], can be compared with the total number of antigenic epitopes, [Ag$_{total}$], by the following equation:

$$[Ag] = [Ag_{total}] - [Ag - Ab]$$

with $[Ag - Ab]$ being the concentration of the antibody-antigen complex. Similarly, the concentration of free antibody sites, $[Ab]$, is compared with the total number of the

Figure 9.5 Equilibrium dialysis to measure antibody affinity. **(A)** A small antigen can diffuse freely between the inside and outside of the dialysis tubing made of a semipermeable membrane, and the concentration of the antigen on both sides of the membrane eventually reaches equilibrium. **(B)** If antibody molecules are placed inside the tubing, the large antibodies cannot diffuse through the dialysis membrane. The affinity of the antibody for the antigen corresponds to the amount of antigen that is kept inside the tubing compared with the concentration of free antigen outside. If the antigen is detectable by some tag such as a radioactive label, the amount of free antigen outside the membrane can be measured. It is assumed that the concentration of free antigen inside the membrane equals the concentration of free antigen outside the membrane. Any additional radioactivity inside the membrane represents the amount of bound antigen or the amount of antigen complexed to antibody $(Ag - Ab)$. **(C)** These data can be transformed by the Scatchard equation to estimate the affinity of an antibody for its antigen. If the value $[Ag - Ab]/[Ag_{free}]$ (the concentration of antigen-antibody complexes divided by the concentration of free antigen) is plotted as a function of $[Ag - Ab]$ (the concentration of antigen-antibody complexes), then the slope of the graph corresponds to K_d (the dissociation constant).

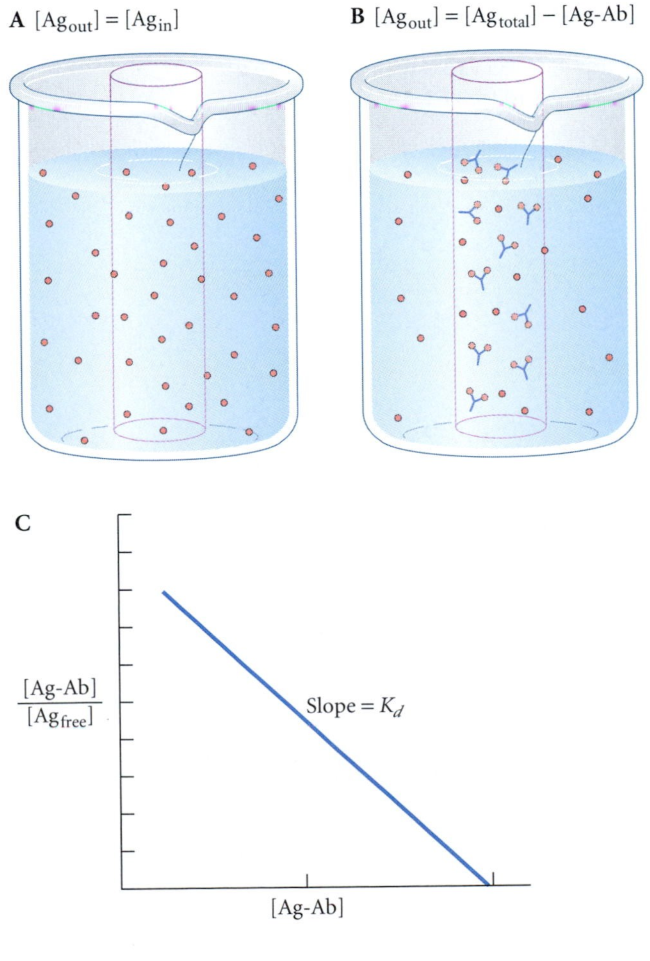

A $[Ag_{out}] = [Ag_{in}]$ **B** $[Ag_{out}] = [Ag_{total}] - [Ag-Ab]$

C

$\frac{[Ag-Ab]}{[Ag_{free}]}$ Slope = K_d

$[Ag-Ab]$

antibody sites, $[Ab_{total}]$, by the following equation:

$$[Ab] = [Ab_{total}] - [Ag - Ab]$$

Thus, the formula

$$K_d = [Ag][Ab]/[Ag - Ab]$$

can then be rewritten as

$$K_d = [Ag]([Ab_{total}] - [Ag - Ab])/[Ag - Ab]$$

or

$$[Ag - Ab]/[Ab_{total}] = [Ag]/([Ag] + K_d)$$

These results can then be plotted using the *Scatchard equation*, a linear plot of this transformation that is derived by varying the antigen concentration while keeping the antibody concentration constant:

$$[Ag - Ab]/[Ag] = ([Ab_{total}] - [Ag - Ab])/K_d$$

To calculate K_d (or K_a, which is equal to $1/K_d$), only the concentration of the antibody-antigen complex, $[Ag - Ab]$, has to be measured, while the other factors are already known. By increasing the amount of antigen that is added, the concentration of antibody-antigen complex is measured and plotted, resulting in a graph (Fig. 9.5C) that allows the determination of K_a (as the slope of the line) as well as $[Ab_{total}]$, representing the valence of the antibody (as the x intercept of the line).

The Concept of Antibody Avidity

The term *avidity* is used to describe the potential antigen-binding ability of an entire antibody molecule. Avidity differs from affinity because all antibodies have more than one antigen-binding site (2 for IgG, IgD, and IgE; 2 or 4 for IgA; and 10 or 12 for IgM). If the antigenic particle has more than one copy of the epitope due to chemical repeats in the antigen, the antibodies will bind the antigen more strongly because the antibody likely will bind simultaneously to more than one site on the antigen. This occurs, for example, when the antigen is a large polysaccharide composed of multiple tandem repeats of a short oligosaccharide structure. Although every antibody has more than one antigen-binding site (and therefore has an avidity for its antigen that is greater than the affinity of each of its antigen-binding sites), the avidity effect is most pronounced in IgM since antibodies of this isotype each have 10 to 12 antigen-binding sites.

Forces between Antigens and Antibodies

The reversibility of antibody-antigen interactions implies that the binding conferred by the noncovalent forces generally is very weak and highly dependent on the distance between the partners. Four molecular interaction forces account for the binding affinity of antigens and antibody (Fig. 9.6).

Hydrogen bonds occur when a hydrogen ion is shared between two electronegative atoms such as oxygen in carboxyl groups and nitrogen in amino groups. The amino groups and carboxyl groups that terminate many amino acid side chains (e.g., the amino group of the arginine side chain or the carboxyl group of the aspartic acid side chain) provide the essential constituents for hydrogen bonds.

Electrostatic forces consist of the attraction between negatively and positively charged groups that form so-called *salt bridges*. These are the strongest of all noncova-lent bonds but are relatively uncommon in naturally occurring antibody-antigen interactions.

Hydrophobic interactions occur when a large region of hydrophobic groups on the antibody interacts with a similar region on the antigen, excluding water from the space between the antibody and antigen to achieve a thermodynamically stable interaction.

van der Waals forces are relatively weak electrical forces that attract neutral molecules to one another. Small, rapid fluctuations in the shape of electron clouds produce instantaneous dipoles around atoms that induce polarization in the electron clouds of nearby atoms. The attractive forces result from the small charge differences between

Figure 9.6 Chemical forces in antigen-antibody interactions. From top to bottom in the figure, hydrogen bonds form when a single hydrogen atom is shared between highly electronegative atoms such as oxygen and nitrogen. The figure depicts a hydrogen bond between a threonine on the antigen and an asparagine on the antibody. Electrostatic interactions represent simple attraction between oppositely charged chemical groups on the two binding molecules. A positively charged amine group on a histidine molecule on the antigen is attracted to a negatively charged carboxyl group on an aspartic acid on the antibody. Hydrophobic interactions represent an energetically favorable juxtaposition of hydrophobic molecules (or hydrophobic regions of molecules), where the hydrophobic chemical groups get close enough to each other that water molecules are excluded from the space between them. The hydrophobic (aliphatic) regions of leucine and threonine amino acids on the antigen come extremely close to alanine and leucine amino acids on the antibody. While water molecules surround the aliphatic groups, all water is excluded from the space between the aliphatic groups. van der Waals forces (enlarged area) are weak electrostatic attractions that occur when two molecules (such as an antibody and antigen) get very near each other. The proximity of the two molecules causes local distortions in the electron clouds (gray) of both molecules, producing regions of higher electron (e⁻) density (darker gray) and regions of lower electron density (lighter gray). The areas of higher electron density have a partial negative charge (δ⁻), while the areas of lower electron density have a partial positive charge (δ⁺). Electrostatic attractions occur between partial positive charges and partial negative charges.

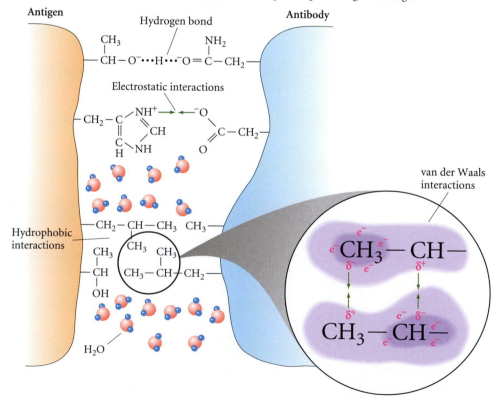

the neighboring atoms. Although van der Waals forces are relatively weak compared with the other types of interactions discussed above, they become quite strong when a large surface area of the antibody comes into close proximity with a large surface area of the antigen. The strength of the van der Waals forces varies in proportion to the distance between the antigenic epitope and antigen-binding site on the antibody. The attractive forces decrease or increase by a factor of the distance raised to the seventh power. Thus the attractive forces decrease rapidly as molecules move apart or increase drastically as they get close together. Such interactions probably explain the observation that the shape of most antibody-combining sites is highly complementary to that of its epitope, since such complementarity allows for close contact of a large surface area of the two molecules.

Types of Assays To Measure Antigen-Antibody Interactions

Tests based on antigen-antibody interactions are used widely in many fields because of their sensitivity, simplicity, and universal application of the concept that antibodies bind tightly and specifically to antigens (Table 9.1). The introduction of radioimmunoassays in the 1960s lowered the sensitivity threshold, allowing detection of substances in the concentration range of picomoles (10^{-12} moles) and making the analysis of small amounts of body fluids possible, and even routine.

One concept that is central to many immunologic reactions is that of *titer*, which indicates the relative amount of antibody present in an antiserum that can bind to a constant amount of antigen. The relative amount is usually determined by making dilutions of an antiserum and testing the dilutions for their ability to react with an antigen. Usually the titer is the reciprocal of the highest dilution (i.e., lowest concentration) that gives a detectable signal in the test being used that is above the background level. Although this measurement is used to indicate the presence of specific antibodies in a sample, it is not necessarily correlated with affinity, because a given titer can be the result of either a high concentration of low-affinity antibodies or a low concentration of high-affinity antibodies. Absolute measurement of the concentration of antibody in a serum is the most precise measure, but this is often difficult to determine as precise standards and standardized test conditions are needed to make the determination of antibody concentration.

Precipitin Reactions

Precipitation reactions are performed with soluble antigens that are mixed with specific antisera. The antibody-antigen interaction results in the buildup of large lattices that precipitate out of solution as seen by the formation of a visible insoluble product within the reaction tube. Now a fairly obsolete test, the precipitin reaction provides important insights into the nature of the antigen-antibody interaction. A number of factors involved in the formation of the aggregates have to be controlled, including pH and ionic strength of the solution. These tests are also dependent on the concentration of antigen and antibody. The precipitin reaction is negative (no precipitation is observed) at both high and low antibody concentrations, and only becomes positive (precipitation is observed) when the antibody and antigen are mixed together in the right proportions. The explanation of this phenomenon (Fig. 9.7A) indicates that at high antibody concentrations there will be far more antibody present

Table 9.1 Tests based on antigen-antibody interactions

Test	Parameter	Sensitivity	Example
Ring test (precipitation)	Antigen	20–200 µg/ml	Serogrouping of streptococci
Single immunodiffusion Mancini test	Antigen	10–50 µg/ml	Detection and measurement of bacterial antigens
Double immunodiffusion Ouchterlony test	Antigen or antibody	20–200 µg/ml	Detection and measurement of candida antigens
Immunoelectrophoresis	Antigen	20–200 µg/ml	Analysis of serum proteins
Rocket immunoelectrophoresis	Antigen	2 µg/ml	Analysis of serum proteins
Direct agglutination	Antigen	0.3 µg/ml	Blood typing
Passive agglutination	Antigen or antibody	0.5–5 ng/ml	Detection and measurement of bacterial antigens
ELISA	Antigen or antibody	0.5 ng/ml	Detection and measurement of viral antigens
RIA	Antigen	0.5 ng/ml	Detection and measurement of viral antigens

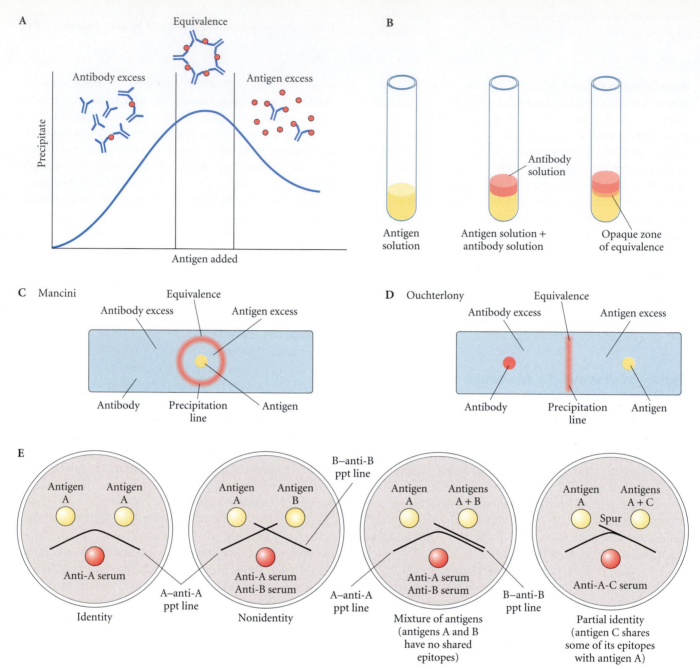

Figure 9.7 Antibody precipitation reactions. (**A**) With increasing amounts of antigen added to a constant amount of antibody, the amount of precipitate will increase until the point of antigen excess, which prevents efficient cross-linking of antibody-antigen complexes. When antibody predominates (antibody excess, low antigen concentration), very few of the antibodies bind antigen, and those that do usually bind it monovalently. As antigen concentrations increase, a high level of cross-linking between the antigen and antibody can occur, giving rise to large, insoluble precipitates. The optimal ratio of antibody to antigen occurs in the zone of equivalence. As the amount of antigen increases further, all of the antibody is saturated and again large complexes cannot form, reducing the size of the precipitates (antigen excess). (**B**) Fluid-phase immunoprecipitation. An antibody solution is overlaid onto a solution that contains antigen. Over time, antibodies and antigens that diffuse across the interface form lattices, which appear as an opaque ring. (**C**) Single radial immunodiffusion, also called the Mancini test, starts with antibodies added to the gel matrix. The antigen is applied into a hole punched into the gel. As the antigen diffuses into the gel, a precipitation ring forms when the optimal ratio between the reactants is achieved. Beyond the outer edge, the reaction is in antibody excess and no precipitate forms. The diameter of the precipitation ring is proportional to the amount of antigen added. (**D**) The Ouchterlony double immunodiffusion test with antigen and antibody applied into different holes diffusing toward each other to form a precipitin line at the zone of equivalence. (**E**) The Ouchterlony test can be used to determine the identities of antigens in an unknown solution. Antigen solutions are placed into wells cut into agar plates. An additional well that is equidistant from all antigen-containing wells is filled with an antibody solution (for example, antiserum). Visible lines of precipitation (ppt) form where diffused antibody and antigen bind to each other and form lattices. If two adjacent wells contain the identical antigen, then a single precipitation line will form (far left panel). If two adjacent wells contain different antigens, each antigen will be precipitated by a different antibody in the antiserum. The result will be two lines of precipitation that cross each other (second panel from left). If one well contains several antigens, then multiple lines of precipitation are possible, some of which may demonstrate identity with antigens in adjacent wells (second panel from right). Last, when more than one antigen is present in a well it is possible that one of the antigens will possess some epitopes that are cross-reactive with epitopes on the other antigen but possess other epitopes that are not cross-reactive. In this case, antibodies that can react with epitopes common to both antigens will form a precipitation line of identity, while other antibodies that bind non-cross-reactive epitopes will diffuse past the line of identity and form a precipitation line with the specific epitope, resulting in a "spur" on the precipitation line (far right panel).

than there are antigenic epitopes available. This will result in the binding of many antibodies to one antigen molecule, making cross-linking of antigen molecules by the antibodies impossible. This is sometimes referred to as the *prozone* effect. Only at the optimal concentration ratios, termed the *equivalence zone*, can cross-linking of antigen molecules occur and measurable lattices and/or large aggregates form. When the antigen concentration exceeds that of the antibody, aggregation again cannot occur due to the excess availability of antigen. Since lattice-network buildup is dependent on the valency of the antibody, IgM antibodies with their 10 to 12 antigen-binding sites are best able to mediate precipitin reactions, whereas other antibodies, such as IgG, can bind to the antigenic determinants but are less able to cross-link and therefore precipitate the antigen molecules.

Fluid-Phase Immunoprecipitation or "Ring Test"

The so-called *ring test* is an easy and rapid way to perform an immunoprecipitation assay (Fig. 9.7B). A solution of the antigen is overlaid with the appropriate antiserum, and a white or opaque ring of precipitate will form at the interface. Allowing the antibody and antigen solutions to diffuse into each other permits the equivalence zone to form on its own. This precipitate eventually will sediment to the bottom of the reaction tube and can be measured. This method is still used today in the serogrouping of bacterial pathogens such as streptococci.

Gel-Based Immunoprecipitation

A number of different procedures have been developed that couple the immunologic properties of the precipitin reaction with the diffusion of antigens and antibodies in gel matrices to establish equivalence zones resulting in the formation of a visible precipitate within the gel matrix. Antibodies and antigens can migrate in gels at a diffusion rate that is correlated with both the size and the concentration of the molecules. Gels can be cast out of liquid agar, agarose, or similar materials that solidify at room temperatures. Once solidified, wells of defined sizes can be punched at specific locations within the gel matrix into which antigen or antibody solutions can be placed. As these two reactants diffuse toward each other through the porous gel, visible precipitates will form as lines in the equivalence zone when an optimal ratio between antibodies and antigen is achieved.

Single immunodiffusion

The single radial immunodiffusion test was introduced in 1957 by Feinberg and modified in 1965 by Mancini to use gel-based immunoprecipitation to measure the concentration of antigen in an unknown solution. A plate or glass slide is covered with liquid agar or agarose that contains antisera that is added to the entire gel at a defined concentration. When it solidifies, the entire gel matrix contains a homogeneous amount of antibody. The antigen solution is placed in wells that are cut out of the gel, and the antigen diffuses out from the well and forms a visible precipitate around the antigen well (Fig. 9.7C). The diameter of the precipitation line around the well is proportional to the concentration of the antigen, and the assay can be standardized with known amounts of antigen to quantify the amount of antigen in an unknown sample.

Double immunodiffusion

The double immunodiffusion test was developed by Örjan Ouchterlony and is also based on the principle of diffusion of antigen and antisera in a gel to form a zone of equivalence. In this instance plain agar or agarose gels are made, wells cut into the gel matrix, and then antisera and antigen placed in different wells so they can diffuse toward each other. At the equivalence zone precipitation lines develop (Fig. 9.7D). The use of specific arrangements of the wells allows for a comparison of the antigenic relatedness of different antigens or antisera. When a central well is surrounded by a ring of outer wells and antiserum is placed in the center well, precipitates form in the gel that indicate the relatedness of different antigens placed in the outer wells (Fig. 9.7E). If the precipitin line that is formed between antigens in adjacent wells is continuous, this indicates these are identical antigens in relation to the test antibody. If the antigens are unrelated but the antiserum solution contains antibodies to both antigens, crossed lines will form. If a spur between the precipitin lines forms, this indicates a partial identity or cross-reactivity of the antibody with the antigen, and is usually attributable to the presence of epitopes on one of the antigens that are not present on the cross-reactive antigen. In this case, antibodies that can react with epitopes on only one of the antigens diffuse past the zone of equivalence with the cross-reactive antigen and then form a precipitin line with the more reactive or specific antigen. The relatedness of different antisera to a single antigen can also be tested in double diffusion by placing antigen in the center wells and antisera in the outer wells.

Immunoelectrophoresis

Electric fields can be used to move antibodies or antigens in gels. Immunoelectrophoresis involves an initial separation of an antigen mixture in an electric field applied to a gel on a slide into which the antigen is loaded, usually in a small well (Fig. 9.8A). After electrical separation, wherein the antigens migrate in the gel on the basis of their charge and size, a trough parallel to the migration of the antigen in the electric field is cut out of the agarose gel. This trough is then filled with the appropriate antiserum, which will passively diffuse toward the separated antigen (Fig. 9.8B). A precipitation line will appear in the equivalence zone between antigen and antiserum (Fig. 9.8C). Because this technique contains an electrophoretic separation step, it allows complex mixtures of antigens to be analyzed because of their different electrophoretic mobility.

Figure 9.8 Immunoelectrophoresis. (A) A mixture of antigens (A⁻ and B⁻ represent negatively charged antigens, while C⁺ represents a positively charged antigen) is added to a hole punched into an agarose or similar gel. (B) An electric field is applied; it separates the different antigens by their charge and size. Although antigens A and B are both negatively charged, antigen A is larger and hence moves more slowly through the gel toward the positive pole. After the electric field is shut off, two troughs (dark blue and orange) are cut into the gel and are filled with antisera to the various antigens. In this example, a mixture of antibodies to antigens A and C is added to the lower trough, and antiserum directed to antigen B is added to the upper trough. (C) After the electrical field is shut off, the migrated antigens diffuse out concentrically from the location to which they electrophoresed. The antibodies in each antiserum also diffuse away from the troughs. An antibody-antigen precipitation reaction occurs in the gel at each equivalence zone, allowing the simultaneous identification of different antigens.

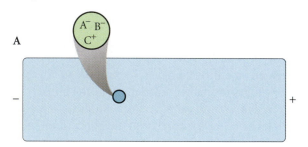

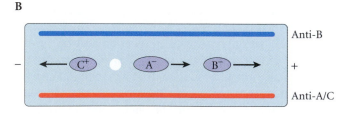

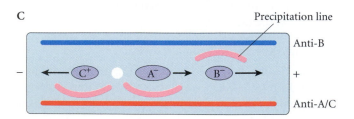

A widely used immunoassay is the *Western blot*, which has increased sensitivity and also uses the principle of separation of antigens in an electric field to analyze different solutions (Fig. 9.9). The antigens are initially separated in an acrylamide or similar thin gel, with the migration of the antigen dependent on its size and charge, the concentration of the acrylamide, the strength of the electric field, and the buffers used to conduct the electricity across the gel. This stage is called polyacrylamide gel electrophoresis and, in and of itself, can be used for analysis of certain molecular constituents of a solution, such as proteins. These can be visualized in the gel with certain stains. For immunologic detection of antigens using the Western blot, the antigens in the gel are transferred or blotted to a membrane, which is then immersed in a solution of antibodies that can bind to the immobilized antigen. If the antigen of interest is present, the binding of specific antibody can be detected. This is most often accomplished by adding a secondary antibody that can actually bind to the first antibody, a so-called anti-antibody. This anti-antibody is labeled with an enzyme or other material that allows its presence to be detected when it is bound to the gel. The use of both a primary antibody specific to the antigen of interest and a secondary antibody amplifies the sensitivity of the test to permit detection of small amounts of antigen.

The *rocket immunoelectrophoresis* technique was introduced by C. B. Laurell in 1966 and represents an immunoprecipitation reaction that can also be used to quantify antigen levels. Antigen solutions are placed into wells that are cut out of an agarose gel containing a homogeneous concentration of specific antiserum. An electric field is applied, causing the antigen to migrate and form precipitation lines at the point of equivalence. The height of the characteristic rocket shape of the precipitation line is proportional to the amount of antigen (Fig. 9.10), and comparison of the heights of the unknown samples with the heights in wells containing known amounts of antigen can be used to standardize the assay.

Agglutination

A number of assays use the aggregation and sedimentation of insoluble particles to detect the formation of immune complexes. Different types of particles have been used for this purpose, but latex beads and erythrocytes are most common. The particles are coupled with the antigen of interest and are then mixed with a test serum. The visible clumping of the beads or erythrocytes is a positive reaction (Fig. 9.11A). This type of assay is rapid, is inexpensive, can be evaluated by eye, and is thus easy to read. The antibodies used in these assays are called *agglutinins*, and IgM anti-

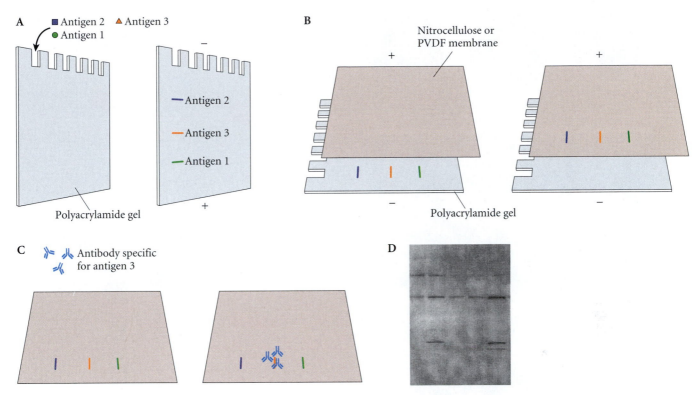

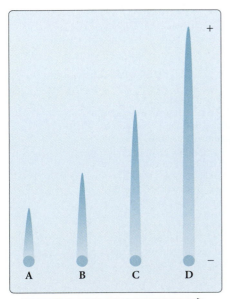

Figure 9.9 Western blot assay. (**A**) A mixture of different antigens is combined with the negatively charged detergent sodium dodecyl sulfate and is applied to the top of a thin polyacrylamide gel. An electric field is applied. Because of the negatively charged sodium dodecyl sulfate, all antigens migrate toward the positive electrode at a rate that is inversely related to their molecular sizes. Large antigens (for example, antigen 2) migrate more slowly, while small antigens (for example, antigen 1) migrate faster. (**B**) The separated antigens are transferred to a flexible membrane made of nitrocellulose or polyvinylidene fluoride (PVDF) by overlaying the membrane on the gel and applying an electric field. (**C**) The membrane is then immersed in a solution containing antibody specific for one or more of the antigens bound to the membrane. The bound antibody can then be detected with an enzyme-linked secondary antibody and an enzyme substrate (not shown). The result is a visible line at the place in the gel to which the antigen had migrated. (**D**) A sample Western blot.

Figure 9.10 Rocket immunoelectrophoresis. This is a combination of single immunodiffusion (Fig. 9.7C) and immunoelectrophoresis (Fig. 9.8). Antiserum is mixed into a gel such as agarose, as is done in single immunodiffusion. Next, an antigen solution is applied to wells and then an electrical field is applied to move the antigen through the gel (as in immunoelectrophoresis). A precipitation line will form at the equivalence point between antigen and antibody concentration. The height of the rocket-shaped precipitation line corresponds to the amount of antigen applied.

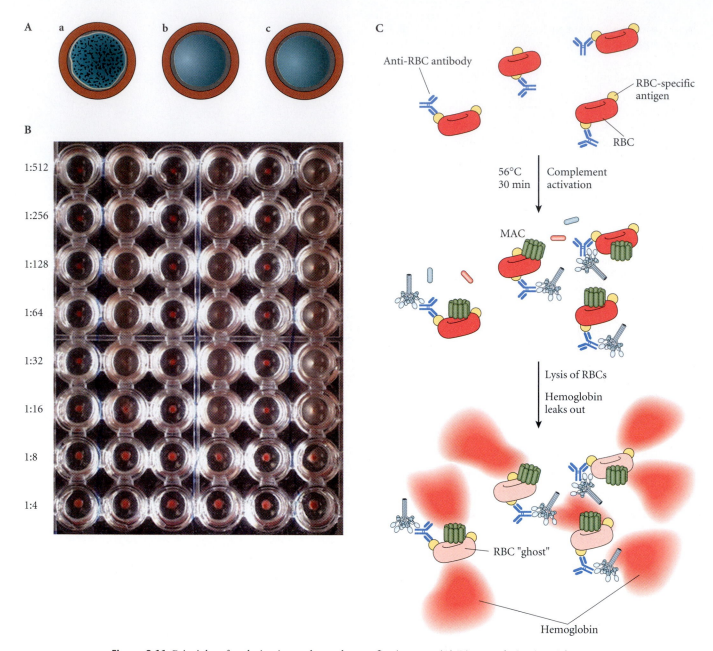

Figure 9.11 Principles of agglutination and complement fixation tests. (**A**) Direct agglutination. A latex bead is coated with an antigen and a test serum is added. Visible agglutination of the latex bead is indicative of a positive reaction well. Negative results are shown in wells b and c. (**B**) The hemagglutination inhibition test can be used to detect and measure antibodies directed against viruses that agglutinate erythrocytes (red blood cells [RBCs]). If antibodies to a virus that can agglutinate erythrocytes are present in a serum sample, they will inhibit hemagglutination induced by the virus. Hemagglutination is detected by the formation of a lattice of RBCs coating the wells. Wells with a pellet of RBCs at the bottom indicate the presence of antibodies, which prevents viral hemagglutination, allowing the RBCs to roll to the bottom of the wells. Serial dilutions of sera give titers that are able to prevent agglutination (i.e., >1:512 in column 1, 1:16 in column 2, etc.). Photo courtesy of A. Angulo, Texas Veterinary Medical Center. (**C**) Complement fixation. After an RBC is coated with an antigen (yellow semicircles) and specific antibody is added, a complement source can also be added. During an incubation step, antibody-coated red cells are lysed by complement activation on or near the cell surface. The hemoglobin released from the lysed cells can be measured spectrophotometrically. The remnants of the lysed RBCs are referred to as "ghosts"; they are transparent because of their lack of hemoglobin.

bodies, because of their larger number of antigen-binding sites per molecule, are about 100 times more effective than IgG antibodies. Like precipitation-based assays, agglutination-based assays depend on an optimal ratio of antibody and antigen and are, therefore, disposed to prozone effects.

It is also possible to conjugate particles such as latex beads to antibodies and use them for the agglutination of antigens in solutions. These latex agglutination tests are the basis of a number of kits for the rapid identification of pathogenic bacteria and fungi such as *N. meningitidis* and *Cryptococcus neoformans*. Another variant, called the coagglutination assay, uses *Staphylococcus aureus* as an antibody-carrying particle. This assay takes advantage of the ability of the protein A on the surface of this bacterium to bind the Fc portion of IgG antibodies from certain animals. In coagglutination assays, the binding of the antigen to the antibody immobilized via protein A to the bacterial surface causes the *S. aureus* cells to agglutinate.

Direct hemagglutination and blood typing

The antigen-carrying particles in direct hemagglutination assays are erythrocytes, and the antigens being measured are present on the surface of the red blood cells. This type of assay is routinely performed before blood transfusions to identify ABO antigens on the donor's and recipient's red blood cells. These antigens define an individual's "blood group." The antigens are composed of glycoproteins on the cell surface. Variation in structures of the carbohydrates substituting the protein accounts for the different blood groups. Blood-group antigens are expressed in a codominant fashion. Persons with two genes for the A factor will have blood group A; these individuals have naturally occurring antibodies to the B antigen. Conversely, persons with two genes for the B factor will have blood group B; these individuals have naturally occurring antibodies to the A antigen. Some people have both antigens present on their erythrocytes (blood group AB) and will therefore have antibodies to neither antigen A nor B as these are self antigens. Individuals who possess neither the A nor the B factor gene, and thus make neither A nor B antigen, have type O blood and natural antibodies to both the A and B antigens. Before the transfusion of blood or blood products, the blood of a patient will be tested with known antisera directed to the A and B antigens. The identification of the blood type according to this test is shown in Table 9.2. From this table it can be ascertained that people with blood type O can be universal blood donors, since the red blood cells will not be seen as foreign by any recipient. Similarly, individuals with the AB blood group are universal recipients of blood, as they have neither antibody to the A or B antigen. Blood transfusion is somewhat

Table 9.2 Identification of blood types by direct hemagglutination assays

Blood group	Antigen	Antibodies
A	A	Anti-B
B	B	Anti-A
AB	AB	None
O	–	Anti-A and anti-B

more complex due to the presence or absence of the Rh antigen, making people either Rh positive or Rh negative. Whereas Rh-positive individuals can get blood from either Rh-positive or -negative donors, Rh-negative individuals can only get blood from other Rh-negative people. Rh-negative humans do not have naturally occurring antibody to the Rh antigen, but they can recognize Rh-positive red cells as foreign, mount an antibody response to this antigen, and destroy the transfused red blood cells.

Passive (indirect) agglutination

Erythrocytes, latex beads, or colored gelatin particles can be treated to carry antigens. The binding of specific antibodies directed to these antigens agglutinates these particles (Fig. 9.11B). To determine whether someone has an ongoing or recent infection, it is often useful to see if he or she has a titer of an antibody to an antigen expressed by the infecting microbe. One commonly used diagnostic assay is the *T. pallidum* particle agglutination test, which is used in the diagnosis of syphilis. Colored gelatin particles are coupled with antigens from *T. pallidum*, and patients' sera are tested for their ability to agglutinate the gelatin particles. A positive result indicates a recent or ongoing syphilis infection.

Complement fixation test

The passive agglutination assay using erythrocytes can be extended to be somewhat more quantitative by adding a source of lytic complement to the reaction. Antibodies bound to antigens on the red cell surface activate complement and release hemoglobin from the red cell (Fig. 9.11C). Spectrophotometric measurement of the amount of hemoglobin can be used to provide a titer or other measure of antibody activity. Once commonly used, this assay is relatively infrequently used now.

Bacterial agglutination

Live or killed bacteria have been used as particles in a number of agglutination assays to detect specific antibodies. In 1896, Max Grüber and Herbert E. Durham, using sera raised in animals to be specific for known bacteria, developed a method to identify unknown bacteria. Georges F. I. Widal used a suspension of inactivated

Salmonella cells as particles to confirm the diagnosis of typhoid by agglutination of patient sera. Most of these older tests have been replaced by latex agglutination assays, which are more sensitive and specific.

Enzyme-Linked Immunoassays

Covalent coupling of enzymes to antibodies allows for a number of easy and versatile tests to be performed and are commonly referred to as *enzyme immunoassays*. These methods do not require the use of radioactivity as do radioimmunoassays, and the detection reaction usually involves having an enzyme convert a colorless substrate to a colored product that can be measured in a spectrophotometer. Both qualitative and quantitative reactions are easy to detect, and the test can be standardized by using samples with a known quantity of antigen and/or antibody. Commonly used enzymes to label antibodies include horseradish peroxidase and alkaline phosphatase. The most common form of the enzyme immunoassay is the enzyme-linked immunosorbent assay (ELISA), which is now the standard immunologic test in many clinical and research laboratories. Several different variants of the ELISA have been created.

An *indirect ELISA* can be used to detect and measure the concentration of specific antibodies to an antigen (Fig. 9.12A). The bottom of the wells of a microtiter plate (usu-ally containing 96 wells arranged in 8 rows and 12 columns in a block of polycarbonate or a similar plastic) is coated with antigen, and after washing away excess, unbound antigen, the test serum is added into the wells of the plate. Antigen-specific antibodies will bind to the surface-attached antigen whereas all the unbound antibodies will be removed in a subsequent washing. The specifically bound antibodies are then detected with isotype- or allotype-specific secondary antibodies, which are chemically conjugated to an enzyme. Again, the unbound secondary antibodies are washed away, and a colorless substrate for the enzyme is added. The change in color of the substrate is directly proportional to the amount of enzyme present, and the color change is monitored and quantified with an appropriate spectrophotometric reader. This is reported as an optical density or some mathematical transformation of the optical density. A large number of tests can be processed simultaneously using 96-well microtiter plates.

The ELISA format can also be used to measure the amount of antigen present in an unknown sample. This is usually done using a *sandwich ELISA* (also called a *capture ELISA*), in which the plates are coated with an antibody specific for the test antigen (Fig. 9.12B). The solution that contains antigen is then applied to the wells, and the immobilized antibody on the surface of the plate will

Figure 9.12 ELISA. (**A**) Indirect ELISA. Wells of microtiter plates are coated with antigen (green circles). A test sample is then applied; it may or may not contain antibody that binds specifically to the immobilized antigen. After unbound primary antibody is washed away, a secondary antibody that is specific for the primary antibody is added. If the primary antibody is specific for the immobilized antigen, and if it binds to the immobilized antigen (left wells), then the primary antibody will still be present after the washing step and can be bound by the secondary antibody. If the primary antibody is not specific for the coated antigen (middle wells) or if no primary antibody is added (right wells), then no secondary antibody will be bound. The secondary antibody is chemically conjugated to an enzyme that leads to a color reaction after the application of an appropriate chromogenic substrate. In the example shown, the secondary antibody is conjugated to the enzyme alkaline phosphatase (blue circles), which catalyzes the conversion of *para*-nitrophenylphosphate (pNPP) to *para*-nitrophenol (pNP). The optical density of the color reaction can be detected quantitatively with a spectrophotometric reader. (**B**) Sandwich ELISAs are used to detect or measure antigen. The wells of a microtiter plate are coated with a capture antibody. The test solution containing the antigen is applied. If antigen reactive with the immobilized capture antibody is present (left wells), it will be bound. If the antigen is not specifically bound by the capture antibody (middle wells), or if no antigen is added (right wells), then no antigen will be bound. A secondary antibody, which recognizes an epitope on the antigen that is different than the epitope recognized by the capture antibody, is then used. This secondary antibody is conjugated with an enzyme that catalyzes a color reaction when the chromogenic substrate is applied. (**C**) ELISPOT test to detect ASC. Wells of a microtiter plate are coated with antigen, and a source of ASC (such as a single cell suspension derived from an immune spleen) is applied. If a given cell is an ASC, the antibody produced by the cell will bind to the antigen surrounding the ASC. After incubation and washing, enzyme-linked secondary antibodies to the secreted antibodies are applied, and after washing a chromogenic substrate that gives rise to an insoluble product is added. The precipitate will form a spot that can be counted as being derived from one ASC. Courtesy of BD Biosciences; original photo © 2003 BD Biosciences. (**D**) RIA. (**Top**) Before the RIA is performed, a radioactive label must be applied to an antigen (for example, a protein antigen might be synthesized in the presence of a radiolabeled amino acid). (**Bottom**) The radiolabeled antigen is then reacted with a test antiserum. If antigen-specific antibodies are present, they bind to the labeled antigen. The antibodies are then precipitated by addition of an antibody-binding protein such as protein A, and the protein A-antibody complex is pelleted by centrifugation. In a positive test (**bottom left**), the radioactive label is detected in the pellet, while in a negative test (**bottom right**), the radioactive label remains in solution.

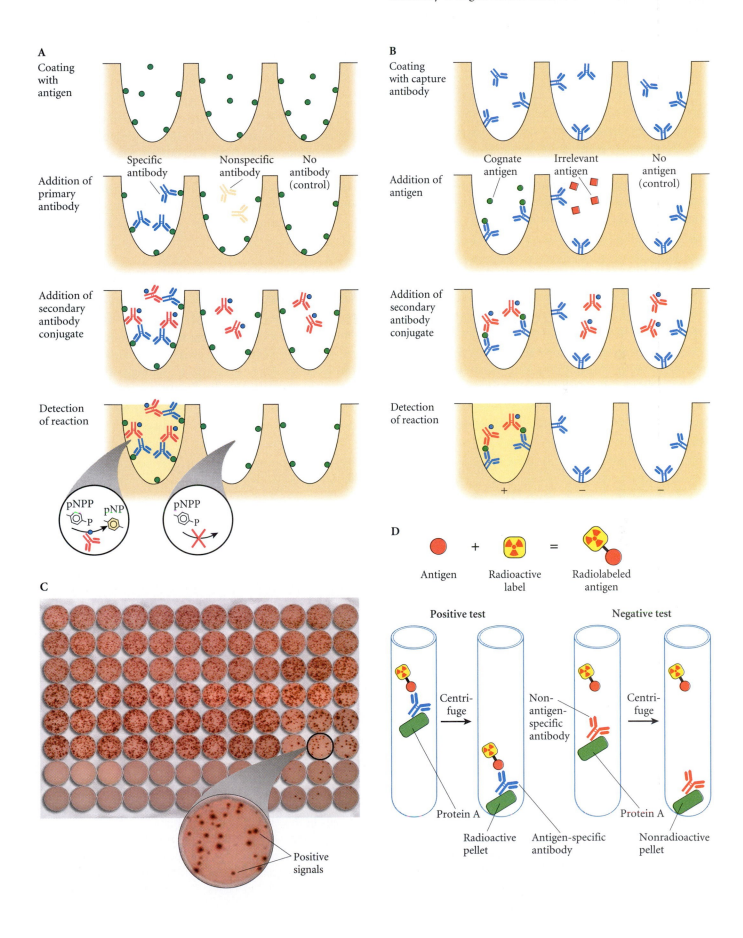

A
Coating with antigen

Addition of primary antibody

Specific antibody   Nonspecific antibody   No antibody (control)

Addition of secondary antibody conjugate

Detection of reaction

pNPP → pNP   pNPP ✗

B
Coating with capture antibody

Addition of antigen

Cognate antigen   Irrelevant antigen   No antigen (control)

Addition of secondary antibody conjugate

Detection of reaction

+   −   −

C

Positive signals

D

Antigen   +   Radioactive label   =   Radiolabeled antigen

Positive test   Negative test

Centrifuge   Centrifuge

Non-antigen-specific antibody

Protein A   Protein A

Radioactive pellet   Antigen-specific antibody   Nonradioactive pellet capture the antigen from the solution. After the unbound antigen is washed away, a secondary antibody conjugated with an enzyme is added. This secondary antibody must be specific for the test antigen but has to recognize a different epitope than the coating antibody. Again, after washing, the chromogenic substrate for the bound enzyme is added and the color change monitored. The secondary antibody does not necessarily have to be coupled to an enzyme. One can use the same principle used in the indirect ELISA by adding an enzyme-linked anti-antibody to the reactions to detect the binding of an unlabeled secondary antibody.

ELISPOT assays

For many years a workhorse assay of immunologists was the hemolytic plaque assay that could be used to detect individual antibody-secreting cells (ASC) in the secondary lymphoid tissue of an animal. In this assay the target antigen was either a red blood cell, usually from a sheep, or a red blood cell to which an antigen had been coupled. The red cells and ASC (from an immunized animal) were mixed in warm, molten agarose, spread on a glass slide, and the ASC allowed to secrete antibody into the gel that could bind to the red cell. After an incubation period some complement was added to diffuse into the gel, and in those places where antibody had bound to the red cell, there was complemented-mediated lysis and the formation of a hole or plaque in the slide. The plaques were counted to quantify the number of ASC.

This assay has been recently replaced by incorporating ELISA technology into the measurement of ASC. This assay, known as an *ELISPOT* assay, utilizes antigen bound to the well of a microtiter plate as the starting step (Fig. 9.12C). The ASC are added to the well, and if they secrete antigen-specific antibody, it will be bound to the antigen surrounding the ASC. After washing away the ASC, enzyme-conjugated secondary antibodies of the appropriate specificity can be added, washed away after incubation, and a substrate for the enzyme added that produces a colored but insoluble product that precipitates around the spot where the ASC were. These can again be counted to quantify the number of ASC in a tissue sample.

Radioimmunoassay

The development of the radioimmunoassay (RIA) in 1960 by Solomon Berson and Rosalyn Yalow introduced a fast and very sensitive method that revolutionized laboratory medicine and was applicable to a variety of substances (Fig. 9.12D). With the use of specific antisera, this method can detect traces in the range of 1 picomole per liter. The RIA relies on the competitive binding of the test antigen and a radioactively labeled antigen that is added together with a specific antibody in a known concentration. Once equilibrium is achieved, the bound and unbound fractions of antigen are separated by differential precipitation, and the radioactivity of the antibody-antigen complex is measured. With the addition of increasing amounts of (unlabeled) test antigen, the fraction of radioactive antigen in the antibody-antigen complex diminishes in a manner that is proportional to the amount of unlabeled antigen that is added. The assay involves the use of radioisotopes; a variety of β- and γ-emitting isotopes have been used to label antigens.

Use of Antibodies To Differentiate Tissues and Cells

Fluorescence Cell Sorting

Flow cytometry is a technique that allows multiple properties of single cells to be analyzed quantitatively by using antibodies or other cell surface binding entities such as lectins that are labeled with fluorescent markers. A related technique (called *fluorescence-activated cell sorting* [*FACS*]) allows cells to be physically separated into subpopulations on the basis of detectable surface properties (Fig. 9.13A). For both of these techniques, cells are suspended in a liquid and reacted with an antibody or other specific detecting reagent labeled with a fluorescent dye. As in other assays, the primary antibody or detecting reagent does not have to be labeled itself, but a secondary, fluorescently labeled antibody can be used to detect the presence of the primary antibody or reagent on the cell surface. The cells are placed into the flow cytometer that directs them single-file past a laser beam and a detector. The laser provides light of a single wavelength that activates the fluorescent molecule. Modern flow cytometers possess a number of channels that allow simultaneous analysis of different fluorophores, using mirrors and bandpass filters to distinguish the different fluorophores. Activation of the fluorophore by light of a specific wavelength causes the molecule to emit a photon of a specific and different wavelength, often in the visible spectrum, that can be detected by photomultiplier tubes tuned to detect the emitted photons. Several detectors read the reflected light, categorizing the light according to both its intensity and scattering pattern. This information may be used to evaluate the size, shape, and optical homogeneity of cells in the sample (Fig. 9.13B).

The FACS technique extends the detection capability of the flow cytometer by incorporating electronics that direct a single cell through a predetermined gate for collection into different tubes. The gate is set to allow pas-

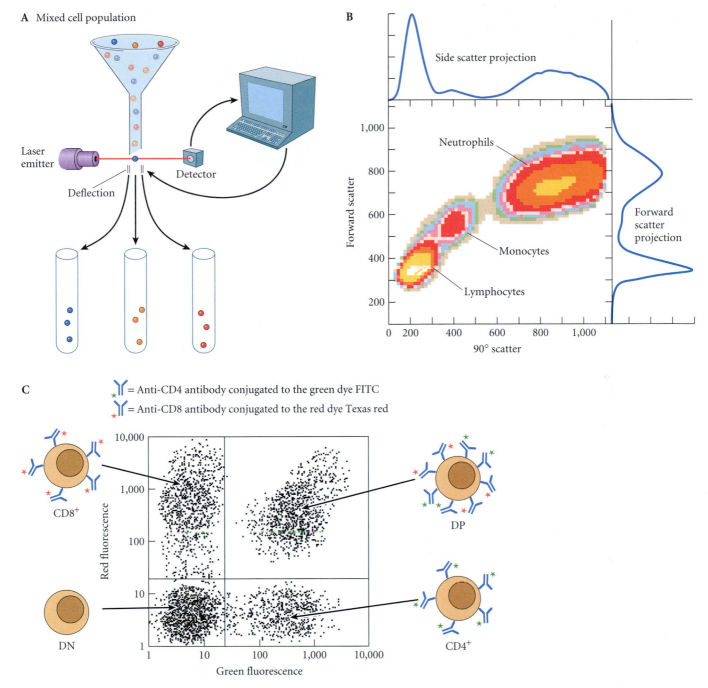

A Mixed cell population

Laser emitter

Deflection

Detector

B

Side scatter projection

Forward scatter

Neutrophils

Monocytes

Lymphocytes

Forward scatter projection

90° scatter

C

$\bar{Y}$ = Anti-CD4 antibody conjugated to the green dye FITC

$\bar{Y}$ = Anti-CD8 antibody conjugated to the red dye Texas red

CD8⁺

DP

Red fluorescence

DN

CD4⁺

Green fluorescence

Figure 9.13 Flow cytometry and FACS can be used to measure subpopulation frequencies of cells in suspension and can separate the subpopulations. (**A**) Cells can be identified in a number of ways, all based on expression or labeling with a fluorescent molecule. Recombinant cells can be made to express fluorescing proteins, and levels of fluorescence are determined under different conditions of cell stimuli. Also, cells can be reacted with fluorescently tagged antibodies that specifically bind to antigens of interest. These methods can identify the cells in the overall population that express that antigen. The cells are then passed through a nozzle that creates a flow of single cells. Separation (or "sorting") of different cell subpopulations is achieved by deflecting the flow of cells into one of several pathways. (**B**) Flow cytometric measurements are then made when the cells pass through a laser beam. Depending on how much of the laser light is adsorbed and scattered, certain characteristics of the single cells can be measured and analyzed by a computer system connected to the apparatus. For larger cells, the light passing through is scattered over a wider angle, producing a high level of "forward scatter." For cells with complex structures in their cytoplasm, such as granules, there is a greater degree of side or 90° scatter. The data can be depicted graphically by using a relative scale of intensities. Thus, neutrophils, which are the largest and most granular of the leukocytes, have high levels of forward and 90° scatter. Monocytes are somewhat smaller and less granular, giving an intermediate level of forward and 90° scatter, and lymphocytes are the smaller leukocytes with the least granular cytoplasm. In addition, the amount of fluorescence given off by each cell is measured. (**C**) A dual-parameter dot plot using two different antibodies (anti-CD4 and anti-CD8) labeled with two different fluorophores (the green dye fluorescein isothiocyanate [FITC] and the red dye Texas red) shows the types of T cells one would find in a thymus. Cells expressing neither CD4 nor CD8 (double negative [DN] cells) would be plotted in the lower left quadrant, CD4⁺ T cells would be plotted in the lower right quadrant, CD8⁺ T cells would be plotted in the upper left quadrant, and double-positive (DP) (CD4⁺ CD8⁺) cells would be plotted in the upper right quadrant.

227

sage of cells with a certain level of fluorescent intensity. This way cells with different surface markers can be sorted into different populations that define not only the presence or absence of a surface marker but the amount of marker present on an individual cell. Sorting of cells in this manner is a key technique in modern biologic investigations.

One application of flow cytometry in immunology is the analysis of subpopulation frequencies of cells possessing specific cell surface markers such as CD4 and CD8. In this case, antibodies specific for these surface markers are added to a sample containing T cells, such as white blood cells. Antibody of each antigenic specificity is labeled with a different fluorophore; for example, the antibody recognizing CD4 might be labeled with a dye that fluoresces green, while the antibody recognizing CD8 might be labeled with a dye that fluoresces red. By simultaneously measuring the amount of red and green light being emitted from each cell in the sample, the device can report the relative levels of expression of CD4 and CD8 by each cell (Fig. 9.13C). Such a technique would be useful for monitoring the number of CD4$^+$ T cells in the blood of an individual with human immunodeficiency virus infection.

Microscopic Detection of Cells and Antigens: Light Microscopy and Electron Microscopy

Microscopes can be used to locate antigens in tissue preparations. The linkage of fluorophores to antibodies can be used in immunofluorescence microscopy to stain and identify various antigens, such as virus particles, bacteria, and tumor antigens in microscopic tissue sections. The tissue sections have to be prepared by gentle methods such as cryosectioning that leave protein antigens intact. The labeled antibodies will usually be applied to the embedded and sectioned sample. Observation of the presence of the fluorophore-labeled antibody requires a fluorescent microscope with a light source, often in the ultraviolet range, capable of emitting the activating wavelength for the fluorophore. The emitted photons, in the visible spectrum, can be seen with the unaided eye using the microscope. This method has the advantage of making it possible to observe the distribution in a tissue of an antigen of interest (Fig. 9.14A). A confocal laser microscope is a sophisticated instrument that not only allows for immunofluorescent detection of antigens in labeled tissue sections but can also focus the laser beam in various planes through tissues or even individual cells to visualize where in the tissue or cell an antigen is actually located.

Antibodies coupled to electron-dense material such as microscopic gold particles are used in immune electron microscopy in place of fluorophores. Gold particles will appear as black dots in electron micrographs, and particles of different sizes can be used to distinguish between different antigens present in the same tissue (Fig. 9.14B). This technique makes it possible to visualize specific features on cells such as bacterial capsules, viral surfaces, or cell organelles.

Measurements of Immunity to Infection

A variety of effector mechanisms are involved in the battle of the immune system with invading microorganisms. The immune system uses several mechanisms, such as the complement cascade and cytotoxic leukocytes, in the destruction of pathogenic microbes. Assays to measure immunity are designed to not only detect the mere interaction of an antigen with an antibody but also the ability of that antigen-antibody complex to recruit various immune effector mechanisms to bring about an end result such as the killing of a microorganism. Thus, the common readout of these assays is the enumeration of viable microorganisms before and after exposure to immunologic effectors.

Neutralization Assays

Neutralization assays test the ability of specific antibodies to neutralize the deleterious effects of viruses, bacteria, bacterial toxins, or other microbial by-products on biologic systems (Fig. 9.15A). The ability of antibodies to neutralize toxins such as tetanus and botulinum can be tested in animal experiments or tissue culture. One group of animals or set of tissue culture wells is given the test material suspected to contain the toxin and a second group of animals or tissue culture wells receives an antiserum to the toxin before being exposed to the toxin. If the antiserum contains antibodies that can bind the toxin and inactivate it, the animals or tissue culture cells that received toxin alone should develop symptoms of toxicity whereas the animals or cells that received the antiserum should be protected and remain healthy.

In viral neutralization assays, a known concentration of infectious viral particles is mixed with diluted antiserum and incubated for a certain period (Fig. 9.15B). The mixture is then injected into animals or is added to appropriate host cells cultured in the laboratory. The presence of neutralizing antibodies in the diluted serum will prevent disease in the animals or inhibit viral growth in a cell culture. As the antibodies become more dilute,

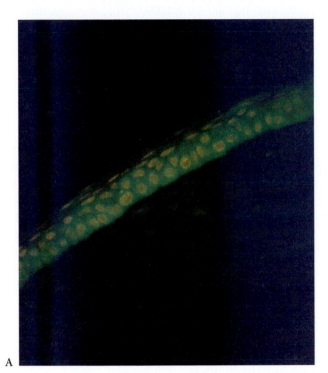 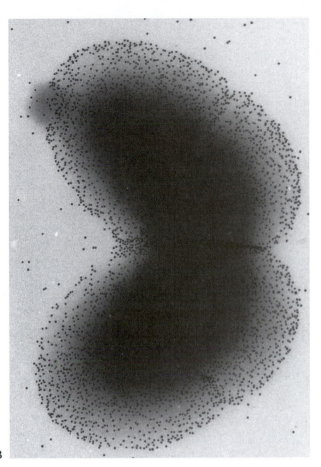

A   B

Figure 9.14 The use of antibodies for the microscopic detection of antigens. (A) Fluorescent immunohisto-chemistry allows for detection of antigens by light microscopy. In this case, the antigen of interest (an ion-channel protein) is detected in epithelium with the use of an antibody that is covalently coupled to the green fluorescent dye fluorescein isothiocyanate. (B) Immunogold electron microscopy is a process whereby antigens are bound by antibodies covalently coupled to gold particles. The primary antibody in this instance is directed against a capsular or surface polysaccharide of a bacterium (*Enterococcus faecalis*) and the binding of this IgG antibody is detected by addition of protein A (an IgG-binding protein) conjugated to 20-nanometer gold particles.

the protective effect will disappear. Neutralizing antibodies are correlated with protection from viral infection because they bind to viral proteins critical in the pathogenesis of disease and disrupt the function of a viral protein that is essential to the binding, entry, or biologic activity of the virus in host cells.

Opsonophagocytic Assay for Extracellular Pathogens

Opsonophagocytosis is the mechanism typically used by the host to fight extracellular bacteria and some pathogenic fungi. A number of congenital and acquired disorders associated with frequent bacterial and fungal infections are caused by deficiencies in phagocytic function, indicating the importance of opsonic killing in immunity

to these infections. Phagocytosis usually involves recognition of a microbe by a phagocyte such as a macrophage or neutrophil and its subsequent attachment to and ingestion of the organism. The immune system recognizes or "targets" an infectious microbe for phagocytosis by tagging it with either opsonic complement proteins such as C3b and/or an IgG molecule (Fig. 9.15C). Binding of either C3b or IgG to the surface of the invading microbe *opsonizes* it for more efficient phagocytosis by polymorphonuclear leukocytes or other phagocytes. These phagocytes possess specific receptors for the complement components (complement receptors) and Fc receptors for the IgG. Opsonophagocytic assays, therefore, involve four components: antibodies, complement, phagocytes, and microorganisms. Viable microbial cells are enumerated

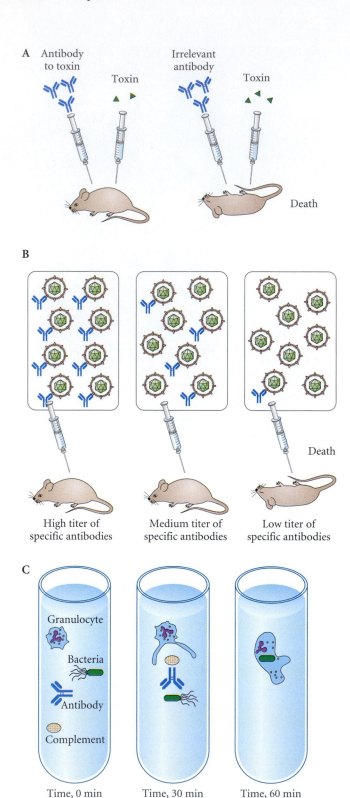

before the components are mixed and at various time points thereafter. The amount of opsonophagocytic killing is defined as the number of bacteria killed during a defined incubation period. A positive result reflects the ability of the phagocytes to kill bacteria, the presence of bacterium-specific antibodies, and the availability of effective complement components. This type of assay can, therefore, be used to study any of these immune system components.

Measurements of Cell-Mediated Immunity

In addition to many tests utilizing antibodies to detect antigens and immunologic effector functions, there are a number of important assays commonly used by immunologists to measure cell-mediated immunity. In general, this refers to T-cell responses to antigen presented on major histocompatibility complex (MHC) class I or class II molecules, but some of these assays can be used to measure natural killer cell function, antibody-dependent cellular cytotoxicity, nonspecific responses to mitogens, or determinations of factors that activate or modify the behavior of lymphocytes. The two central assays are lymphocyte activation and proliferation, wherein an appropriate measure of a T-cell response that results in cellular proliferation or production of cytokines is used, and cytotoxicity, wherein the ability of an activated, often immune, cell to kill a target cell expressing appropriate antigens or cellular markers is measured. Variations on these two assays are commonly used to support a variety of hypotheses being tested to characterize the molecular and cellular basis of immune responses.

Figure 9.15 Biologically relevant immunoassays. (A) Toxin neutralization. In this assay, toxin (green triangles) produced by a microbe is given to an animal that will die from exposure to the toxin. If a specific immune serum is added, the toxin will be neutralized and the animal protected from the toxic effects. (B) Virus neutralization. A suspension of virus particles treated with a control or test serum is given to an animal. If the test serum can neutralize the virus, the animals will be protected, while animals treated only with control serum will die. The reduction in this level of infectivity can be quantified in the virus neutralization assay by varying the amount of neutralizing antibody added to the viral inoculum. (C) Opsonophagocytic killing assay. In the presence of phagocytic cells (granulocytes), antibody, and complement (left), bacteria are opsonized by the antibody and complement split products (middle, after 30 minutes). Receptors on the surface of the phagocyte bind to the immobilized complement and immunoglobulin, which facilitates ingestion and killing of the microbe. By 60 to 90 minutes (right), the majority of the bacteria are opsonized, phagocytosed, and killed in the presence of an immune serum with a large amount of antibody. Almost all antibodies mediating protective immunity to bacterial infections have this property.

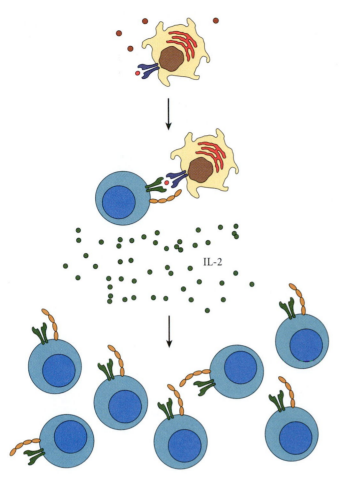

Figure 9.16 Lymphocyte proliferation or activation assay. Antigen-presenting cells (yellow) take up, process, and present antigen (red dots) on MHC class II to antigen-specific CD4+ T cells (blue). The specific T cells proliferate in response to the presentation of the antigen and release IL-2 (T-cell growth factor) (green dots), which can be measured by ELISA. Alternately, [³H]thymidine can be added 12 to 24 hours before the end of the assay, and actively proliferating T cells will incorporate it into their newly synthesized DNA. Increases in nuclear [³H]thymidine can be detected by scintillation counting.

Lymphocyte Proliferation and Response of T Cells to Antigenic Stimulus

This assay is generally used to measure the response of a T cell to antigen presented on an antigen-presenting cell. CD4+ T cells and MHC class II antigen-presenting cells are the basic components (Fig. 9.16). The antigen-presenting cells, T cells (obtained from previously immunized animals), and antigen are mixed together in a cell culture well and the reaction usually proceeds for 3 to 5 days. During this time the antigen is processed, presented, and recognized by an immune T cell, which becomes activated and proliferates in response to this stimulus. The readout can be a number of assays, but the most common ones are direct measures of cellular proliferation. One commonly used measure involves the addition of tritium-labeled [³H]thymidine, which is incorporated into the replicating DNA of the proliferating cells and can easily be measured by collecting the DNA on small pieces of filter paper and determining the incorporated radioactive counts. Another measure of proliferation is the production of interleukin-2 (IL-2) (T-cell growth factor). Other cytokines that may be made in response to stimulation (IL-4, interferon-gamma, etc.) can also be measured. Cytokine determinations usually involve capture-based ELISAs. This test is useful not only for measuring T-cell immune responses but can also be used to analyze the role of MHC in antigen presentation, the response of T cells to mitogens or to generic stimuli like antibody to the CD3 antigen that also activates T cells, or virtually any

Figure 9.17 Cytotoxicity assay. **(A)** An epithelial cell (beige) presents an antigen (red dot) on MHC class I; CD8+ T cells (blue) recognize the antigen as foreign and lyse the epithelial cell in response to the presentation of the antigen on MHC class I molecules. The lysis of the epithelial cells is accompanied by the release of cytoplasmic lactate dehydrogenase (LDH; green triangles) that can be measured to quantify the cytotoxic effect. Alternatively (not shown), the target cell can be labeled with ⁵¹Cr, and this radioactive marker is released when the cell is killed. **(B)** The cytotoxicity assay can be made quantitative by varying the ratio of effector cytotoxic cells to target cells. Populations of cells with more potent cytotoxic activity will kill more targets at lower E:T ratios.

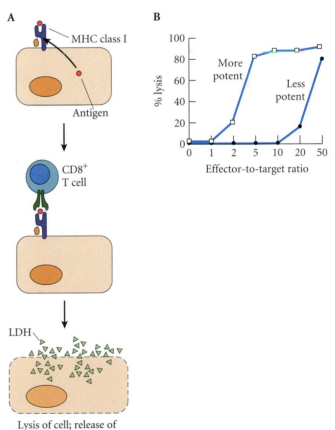

experimental method where the readout is a cellular response defined by activation and proliferation.

Cytotoxic Responses

A second major function of T cells is to kill target cells. This usually involves CD8[+] T-cell responses to antigen presented on MHC class I. In this case, the antigen is not necessarily presented on an antigen-presenting cell but on any cell that can produce the antigenic target in association with MHC class I (i.e., the target cell). In these assays, the target cell is often labeled with a marker that will be released upon the cell's death—often this is radiolabeled chromium sulfate (^{51}Cr label) (Fig. 9.17). Other measures of cellular cytotoxicity, such as release of cytoplasmic lactate dehydrogenase, are also used. The target cell is then exposed to the effector cell, usually a cytotoxic T cell. This is done at different ratios of effector to target cells (E:T ratio). After a period of interaction, usually in the range of 4 to 18 hours, the release of the ^{51}Cr or lactate dehydrogenase is measured. Higher levels of radioactivity or enzyme activity indicate a greater degree of cytotoxicity. A lower ratio of E:T giving a measurable and significant response is indicative of either greater cytotoxic T-cell activity or greater numbers of cytotoxic T cells present. Cytotoxicity assays can also be used to measure the activity of natural killer cells or the occasional cytotoxic CD4[+] cell.

Summary

The basis for the specificity of antigen-antibody reactions is now well understood at many levels. From crystal structures it is now known that the antigenic epitope and antigen-binding site on an antibody take on a complementary shape and need to achieve a close physical proximity in order for the antibody to bind. Cross-reactivity can be a property of certain antibodies, explainable by the presence of the same antigen or antigenic epitope on different target antigens, or the three-dimensional configuration of chemically different antigens that coincidentally achieve the same configuration. The strength of an antigen-antibody reaction can be quantified by a variety of techniques, and the multivalency of antibody molecules confers on them the property of avidity, or an increased strength in the binding to antigens that is above the intrinsic affinity of the antigen-binding site. A large variety of laboratory techniques for determining antigen-antibody reactions and cellular responses to antigens have been developed, and sensitive analyses of single cell responses of immunologic relevance are now routinely made. Understanding the chemical and biophysical basis for the antigen-antibody reaction has been the basis for the development of these critical tools for the study of immunology and immunologic phenomena. Along with assays of cell-mediated immunity, the tools to delve into the most intricate details of cells and molecules of the immune system are now available on a routine basis to many investigators.

Suggested Reading

Bosshard, H. R. 2001. Molecular recognition by induced fit: how fit is the concept? *News Physiol. Sci.* **16**:171–173.

Djavadi-Ohaniance, L., M. E. Goldberg, and B. Friguet. 1996. Measuring antibody affinity in solution, p. 77–97. *In* J. McCafferty, H. R. Hoogenboom, and D. J. Chiswell (ed.), *Antibody Engineering, a Practical Approach.* IRL Press, Oxford, United Kingdom.

Gabdoulline R. R., and R. C. Wade. 2002. Biomolecular diffusional association. *Curr. Opin. Struct. Biol.* **12**:204–213.

Padlan, E. A. 1994. *Antibody-Antigen Complexes.* R. G. Landes, Austin, Tex.

Rose, N. R., R. G. Hamilton, and B. Detrick (ed.). 2002. *Manual of Clinical Laboratory Immunology,* 6th ed. American Society for Microbiology, Washington, D.C.

Zayats, M., O. A. Raitman, V. I. Chegel, A. B. Kharitonov, and I. Willner. 2002. Probing antigen-antibody binding processes by impedance measurements on ion-sensitive field-effect transistor devices and complementary surface plasmon resonance analyses: development of cholera toxin sensors. *Anal. Chem.* **74**:4763–4773.

chapter 10

B-Lymphocyte Activation and Antibody Production

Lee M. Wetzler and Hilde-Kari Guttormsen

Antibodies are essential mediators of immunity to pathogens that survive and multiply in extracellular spaces and utilize the extracellular milieu to spread within host tissues. B lymphocytes are the primary effector cells of the humoral immune response, going through various stages starting with maturing in the bone marrow, circulating in the blood and lymphatics, and, following antigen encounter, maturing into plasma cells (that secrete antibodies) and memory cells. Antibodies also form part of the B-cell antigen-receptor complex.

The maturational process occurs in the bone marrow and involves variable region gene assembly and productive gene rearrangements leading to a large array of antibody diversity. The process also involves B-cell progression through several stages associated with the elimination of autoreactive B cells by negative selection and finally the release to the periphery of mature B cells expressing membrane immunoglobulin M (mIgM) and mIgD. This process occurs in an antigen-independent fashion.

Upon entry into the periphery, the mature B cells are ready to respond to their cognate antigen, which leads to activation of the B cell and antibody production. This process involves a large number of B-cell components, particularly the mIg on the surface and associated structures that form the *B-cell antigen receptor* (BCR), and the *B-cell coreceptor* complex involved in signal transduction and B-cell activation in response to antigenic stimuli. B cells respond to antigens in both a *T-cell-dependent* and *T-cell-independent* fashion, depending on the nature of the antigenic stimulus, and the production of antibody-secreting plasma cells depends heavily on B cells directly interacting with other cells and the production of cytokines to activate and drive the antibody response.

Interaction of Antigen and B Lymphocyte: the BCR

BCR Structure and Expression

The BCR consists in part of membrane-bound immunoglobulin and belongs to a class of receptors that includes the T-cell receptor (TCR) and the Fc receptors for IgE (FcεRI) and IgG (FcγRIII) (Fig. 10.1). All of these receptors contain a complex hetero-oligomeric structure made up of a ligand-binding subunit(s) and signal-transduction subunits. The antigen-binding portion of the BCR is mIg, which is similar in structure to secreted antibody except for the attachment of a membrane-spanning region and a cytoplasmic anchor to the carboxy termini of

Figure 10.1 Structure of the BCR. Schematic representation of the BCR complex, the TCR complex, and the Fc receptors for IgE (FcεR1) and IgG (FcγRIII), emphasizing the areas they have in common. The thicker lines in the cytoplasmic regions of each ligand represent ITAM. Ti, idiotypic TCR (TCR α/β or TCR γ/δ). Based on Fig. 1 of C. M. Pleiman et al., *Immunol. Today* 15:393–399, 1994.

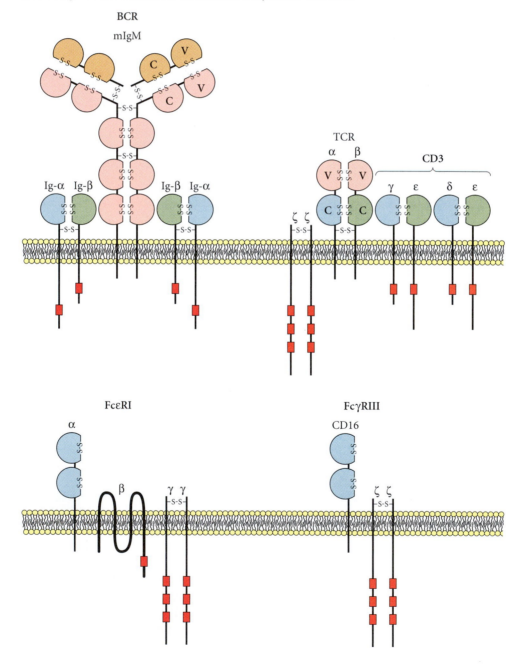

the heavy (H) chains of the mIg (see Fig. 6.14). The isotype of the mIg varies from one B cell to another and depends mostly on the maturational state of the B cell and its immunologic history. Immature B cells that have not yet reached functional competence express only mIgM; mature B cells that have not yet encountered their cognate antigen (i.e., *naive* B cells) express mIgD in addition to mIgM. As class switching occurs following antigenic activation, expression of mIgM is exchanged for expression of immunoglobulins of different isotypes (IgG, IgA, and IgE). Therefore, the membrane of memory B cells that have undergone the process of isotype switching can contain mIgG, mIgA, or mIgE. The cytoplasmic anchor of the mIg, which distinguishes it from soluble immunoglobulin, is usually short, ranging from 3 amino acids for mIgM and mIgD (Lys-Val-Lys) to 28 for mIgG. The intramembranous portion of mIg is usually 25 amino acids long and differs from the transmembranous region of the TCR in that the latter contains several charged amino acids that are needed for interactions with other receptor proteins, whereas the transmembranous region of mIg lacks charged amino acids but instead has many hydroxyl-containing amino acids that can interact with other polypeptides.

In addition to mIg, the BCR contains the proteins Ig-α (CD79a) and Ig-β (CD79b), which function as the signal-transduction portion of the BCR (Fig. 10.1). Ig-α and Ig-β are the products of the *mb-1* and *B29* genes, respectively, and are members of the immunoglobulin superfamily that form a disulfide-linked heterodimer. During antigen recognition by the BCR, Ig-α and Ig-β mediate signal transduction through their interaction with cytoplasmic Src family tyrosine kinases such as Lyn and Fyn. BCR signal transduction is the key event in B-cell activation.

Surface expression of a BCR is a characteristic of any mature B cell that is in a resting (nonactivated) state, whether it is a naive or a memory cell. Two early forms of the BCR, termed the pro-BCR and pre-BCR, appear on the B-cell surface before the completion of V(D)J gene rearrangements and production of a functional mIg (Fig. 10.2). The *pro-BCR* includes Ig-α and Ig-β along with the protein calnexin. During the generation of B lymphocytes, pro-BCR-mediated cell signaling events involving phosphorylation of intracellular proteins and production of intermediates that cause Ca^{2+} levels to increase are required for cell survival and further maturation. Calcium flux triggered by the pro-BCR signals the initiation of the next phase of V(D)J rearrangement: combination of a variable (V) segment with the already rearranged DJ segment. Completion of this step defines the next stage of B-lymphocyte development, the pre-B-II stage. In this stage of development, the H chain is completely rearranged and associates with the *surrogate light (L) chains*, V_{Pre-B} and λ5, as well as with Ig-α and Ig-β to form the *pre-BCR*. Cross-linking of this pre-BCR complex can induce mobilization of both extracellular and intracellular calcium but cannot trigger phospholipase C (PLC) activation. Subsequent rearrangement of the immunoglobulin L chain leads to formation of the BCR, containing intact mIg (μ_2L_2), Ig-α, and Ig-β. At this stage of B-cell development (the immature B-cell stage), the B lymphocyte attains antigen specificity since it has functional immunoglobulin H- and L-chain genes. In addition, both calcium mobilization and PLC activation, with generation of inositol trisphosphate (IP_3), can occur upon cross-linking of the BCR.

In the periphery mature B cells are ready to interact with antigen, become activated, differentiate, expand

Figure 10.2 Development of the mIg on the B cell. As the B cell develops, the surface immunoglobulin is assembled. At first a complex consisting of Ig-α, Ig-β, and the protein calnexin appears on the plasma membrane. This complex is called the pro-BCR. After immunoglobulin H-chain rearrangement is completed, the pre-BCR is formed, consisting of Ig-α, Ig-β, the rearranged Ig H (μ) chain, and the surrogate L chain (made up of the V_{Pre-B} and λ5 proteins). As B-cell development progresses, the L chains are assembled and the mature IgM antibody appears on the cell surface, also in association with the Ig-α and Ig-β proteins. The isotype of the mIg on a mature B cell includes both IgM and IgD.

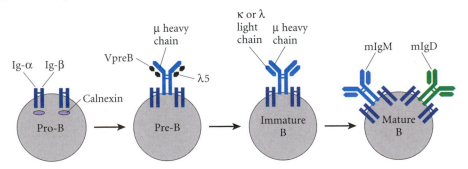

clonally, and mature into antibody-secreting plasma cells. This process is completely antigen driven. In the absence of antigen the B cell has a relatively short half-life, ranging from weeks to no more than a couple of months. However, when a B cell encounters an antigen, a series of signaling events ensues, emanating first from the BCR, then from the BCR coreceptor, followed by interactions with other cells, notably T cells and follicular dendritic cells (FDCs), culminating in antibody secretion and memory cell development. As expected, there are important regulatory checkpoints during B-cell responses to antigen, including effects from T cells, cytokines, the consequences of somatic mutation, and final maturational signals. While still incomplete, there is nonetheless a detailed picture of the molecular and cellular factors that turn resting B cells into potent machines for production of antibody.

Signal-Transduction Events after Engagement of the BCR

When the BCR is cross-linked in vivo or in vitro by direct antigen engagement, a series of intracellular signaling events are set in motion that initiate activation of the B lymphocyte. Treatment with antibody to immunoglobulin in vitro, which causes cross-linking of the BCR, has been used as a model of antigen-mediated B-cell activation. As is the case with many immune activation processes, the signaling events leading to B-cell activation are highly regulated.

The signaling capacity of the BCR resides primarily in the cytoplasmic tails of the Ig-α and Ig-β proteins, although the cytoplasmic tails of some mIg isotypes have also been found to play an important role in signaling.

The regions of Ig-α and Ig-β that are involved with receptor-mediated activation of the B cells are the *immunoreceptor tyrosine-based activation motifs* (ITAMs), which are 26 amino acids long and contain tyrosine phosphorylation sites for regulation of signal transduction. The B-cell ITAMs have also been called the antigen receptor homology 1 motif, the antigen recognition activation motif, and the tyrosine-based activation motif. The overall structure of the ITAM is $D/E-X_7-D/E-X_2-Y-X_2-L/I-X_7-Y-X_2-L/I$ (where D is aspartic acid, Y is tyrosine, L is leucine, I is isoleucine, and X is any amino acid). This region has also been found in the cytoplasmic regions of other proteins with a function homologous to that of Ig-α and Ig-β: TCRζ, TCRη, CD3ε, CD3γ, FcεR1β, FcεR1γ, FcγRIII, and possibly CD22 (Fig. 10.1). The ITAM-containing cytoplasmic tails of these proteins mediate signaling by recruiting signal-transduction molecules to the receptor complex (see Fig. 2.6). ITAM-containing proteins have the ability to transduce intracellular signals such as kinase activity and Ca^{2+} influx, leading to cellular effects typical of cell activation.

Early signaling events

Once the BCRs are specifically bound by antigen (or cross-linked by antibodies to immunoglobulin), various protein tyrosine kinases (PTK) are recruited to the ITAM sequences of Ig-α and Ig-β (Fig. 10.3). Analogous to the situation that occurs during T-cell activation, B-cell activation involves phosphate modifications of tyrosine residues within the Ig-α and Ig-β ITAMs and on associated Src family PTK. The tyrosine phosphorylation of PTK allows further recruitment of additional kinases

Figure 10.3 Signal transduction via the BCR. Once the BCRs are specifically bound by antigen (or cross-linked by antibodies to immunoglobulin), various PTK are recruited to the ITAM sequences of Ig-α and Ig-β. p72^{syk}, a member of the Syk/ZAP-70 family of kinases, appears to be constitutively associated with the cytoplasmic tail of the immunoglobulin μ heavy chain and upon BCR cross-linking may autophosphorylate itself (top left panel, green circle). p72^{syk} autophosphorylation allows Src-family kinases such as p53/56^{lyn}, p59^{fyn}, and p55^{blk} to bind p72^{syk} via their SH2 domains, but prior to the SH2-mediated binding to p72^{syk}, these Src-family kinases need to be tyrosine dephosphorylated by CD45 (B220) (top right panel, arrow 1). Upon association with p72^{syk}, these PTK are activated by phosphorylation by p72^{syk} (arrow 2). The activated kinase molecules in turn phosphorylate Ig-α and Ig-β in their ITAM sequences (top right panel, arrows 3). It is also possible that p72^{syk} tyrosine phosphorylates the ITAMs of Ig-α and Ig-β directly (top right panel, arrows 4); however, the mechanism by which p72^{syk} mediates this process is unknown. The latter mechanism may be due to the creation of a lattice-like network of BCRs upon cross-linkage, allowing *trans*-phosphorylation of the tyrosine residues on p72^{syk} and Ig-α and Ig-β and further recruitment and binding of Src-family kinases and p72^{srk}. It is possible that both of these scenarios occur. Src-family kinases are recruited and reoriented via binding through their SH2 domains to ITAMs (bottom left panel). In addition, an adapter protein with SH2 domains, Shc, also is recruited, undergoing tyrosine phosphorylation and allowing association with Grb2 and Sos1 (other SH2-containing adapter proteins) and activation of the p21^{ras} pathway (bottom right panel). p53/56^{lyn} and p72^{syk} are important for liberation of intracellular Ca^{2+} after antigen binding, but p53/56^{lyn} carries this out via the p21^{ras} system. p72^{syk} mediates Ca^{2+} mobilization through activation of PLCγ2, which cleaves phosphatidylinositol bisphosphate into inositol trisphosphate and diacylglycerol. The result of all these events is the transcription of gene products necessary for B-cell activation, differentiation, proliferation and antibody production. Based on Fig. 1 of C. M. Pleiman et al., *Immunol. Today* 15:393–399, 1994.

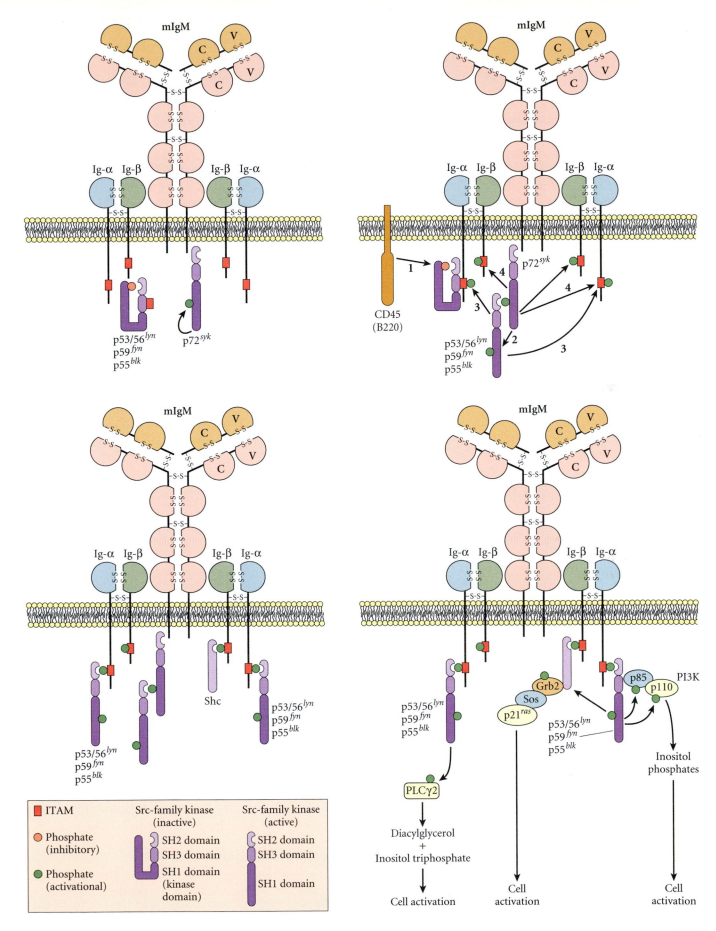

and other enzymes important in the signal transduction. Phosphorylation of other effector molecules (e.g., kinases, phosphatases, and phospholipases) increases the enzymatic activity of these effector molecules to increase the intracellular levels of IP$_3$ and Ca^{2+}, which ultimately affect gene transcription.

The first event after BCR engagement is activation of the Src family kinases, p55^{blk}, p59^{fyn}, p56^{lck}, p53/56^{lyn}, and by a member of the Syk/ZAP-70 family of kinases, distantly related to the Src family kinases, termed p72^{syk} (Fig. 10.3). It is thought that one or some of these kinases need to constitutively associate with the cytoplasmic domains of the BCR to be capable of phosphorylating the BCR ITAMs upon antigen binding. Some studies have revealed that the Src family kinases bind to the ITAM region of the Ig-α component of the BCR in resting B cells. This interaction has been shown to require the 10 amino-terminal amino acids of the kinase and a 4-amino-acid sequence (aspartic acid-cysteine-serine-methionine [DCSM]) within the ITAM region of Ig-α. The equivalent region on Ig-β is QTAT, which cannot bind the Src family kinases.

Src kinases normally exist in the cell in an inactive state maintained by phosphorylation of an "inhibitory tyrosine" located at the carboxy terminus of the kinase; it is probably in this state that the Src kinase exists while it associates with Ig-α in the inactive B cell (see Fig. 2.6B). The initiating event of BCR-mediated signaling could be activation of Ig-α-associated Src kinases by tyrosine dephosphorylation, which allows them to phosphorylate the ITAMs of the BCR complex. Phosphorylated ITAMs have a 20-fold higher avidity than the DCSM residues of Ig-α for binding Src family kinases. The area of the Src family kinases that binds to phosphorylated tyrosine residues in the ITAM region is the Src homology 2 (SH2) domain. Interestingly, binding of an Src family kinase to phosphorylated ITAMs diminishes the ability of the Src kinase to bind the Ig-α DCSM motif, suggesting that SH2-mediated binding of the kinases to the BCR alters the tertiary structure of the Src family kinase. This may be another mechanism of regulating kinase activation.

There is some evidence that the p72^{syk} kinase also plays an important role in early phosphorylation events during B-cell activation. Some investigators have shown that p72^{syk} can bind to the cytoplasmic tail of the immunoglobulin μ H chain. When Ig-α and Ig-β are stripped from the BCR complex (leaving only the mIg), p72^{syk} is still present in the complex. The inability of p72^{syk} knockout mice to signal through the BCR suggests that p72^{syk} is important for this process. p72^{syk} is thought to be important for tyrosine phosphorylation of the ITAMs of Ig-α and Ig-β; however, the mechanism by which p72^{syk} mediates this process is unknown. One possibility is that p72^{syk} autophosphory-

lates itself, allowing other Src family kinases such as p53/56^{lyn}, p59^{fyn}, and p55^{blk} to bind p72^{syk} via their SH2 domains and, in turn, to phosphorylate Ig-α and Ig-β. Another possibility is that cross-linking of the BCR by antigen binding helps forms a lattice-like network of BCRs, allowing *trans*-phosphorylation of the tyrosine residues on p72^{syk} and Ig-α and Ig-β and further recruitment and binding of Src family kinases and p72^{syk}. It is possible that both of these scenarios occur, depending on the mode of BCR activation, with antigens expressing few repetitive epitopes triggering the former mechanism and antigens with a high density of repetitive epitopes triggering the latter. In either case, once the initial tyrosine phosphorylation occurs, Src family kinases are recruited and reoriented via binding through their SH2 domains to ITAMs. In addition, an adapter protein with SH2 domains, Shc, also is recruited, undergoing tyrosine phosphorylation and allowing association with Grb2 and Sos1 (other SH2-containing adapter proteins) and activation of the p21^{ras} pathway (Fig. 10.3), as evidenced by p21^{ras} colocalizing with the BCR during B-cell activation. Two newly defined adapter proteins, Blnk (B-cell linker) and LAB (linker for activation in B cells), may also be involved in downstream signaling associated with engagement of the BCR. They both appear to be tyrosine phosphorylated by p72^{syk}, which has previously been recruited to the BCR membrane complex. LAB is membrane bound and may help to recruit Grb to the membrane (similar to the function of LAT [linker for activation in T cells]). Blnk can bind to Grb and may help recruit PLCγ to the BCR activation complex.

Recent evidence indicates that membrane microdomains, called lipid rafts, have a role in B-cell activation as platforms for BCR signaling and might also act in antigen trafficking. These lipid rafts seem to function by virtue of their ability to segregate proteins laterally in the plane of the plasma membrane. Cross-linking of the BCR and its coreceptor complex by complement-tagged antigens (see Fig. 5.14) will result in translocation of both to the lipid rafts, leading to stable raft association and prolonged signaling. The src kinase Lyn appears to be associated with the lipid rafts, and when the BCR associates with these rafts upon cross-linking, Lyn may initiate signaling by phosphorylating the tails of the BCR and associated Ig-α and Ig-β as another mechanism of initiating B-cell activation.

Later signaling events

Like many biologic signaling cascades, BCR-mediated signal transduction liberates bound intracellular Ca^{2+} stores, utilizing both IP$_3$ and diacylglycerol (DAG)-dependent and -independent triggers. The various BCR-associated protein kinases have different roles in these cellular acti-

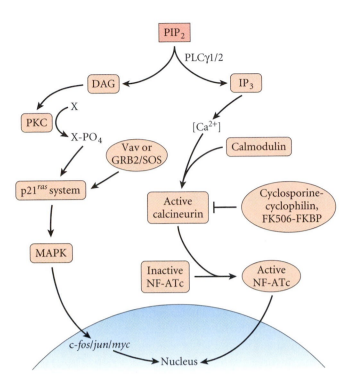

Figure 10.4 PLC breakdown of PIP_2. The cascade of events is initiated by PLC breakdown of PIP_2 into IP_3 and DAG. PKC is then activated by DAG, leading to phosphorylation of a variety of cellular proteins, including MAPK. MAPK activation leads to nuclear translocation of various transcription activators, such as c-Jun, Fos, and Myc. Production of IP_3 leads to release of intracellular Ca^{2+}, which binds to and activates the regulatory protein calmodulin. Activated calmodulin increases the activity of different enzymes, especially the phosphatase calcineurin. Calcineurin, in turn, can dephosphorylate the transcription factor NF-AT, activating it in the process. Calcineurin is the molecular target of the immunosuppressive drugs cyclosporine and FK506.

vation events. For example, both $p53/56^{lyn}$ and $p72^{syk}$ are important for liberation of intracellular Ca^{2+} after antigen binding, but $p53/56^{lyn}$ carries this out through PLC-independent mechanisms. $p72^{syk}$ seems to mediate Ca^{2+} mobilization through activation of PLC, which cleaves phosphatidylinositol disphosphate into IP_3 and DAG. It is likely that $p72^{syk}$ and $p53/56^{lyn}$ act synergistically. Protein kinase C (PKC) is then activated by DAG, leading to phosphorylation of a variety of cellular proteins, including mitogen-activated protein kinase (MAPK) and phosphomyristin C. MAPKs are a family of serine/threonine kinases important for transcriptional and translational regulation and are involved in microtubule function, c-Jun/AP-1 transcriptional activation, and the activation of other serine/threonine kinases. Intracellular Ca^{2+}, whether liberated by PLC-dependent or -independent mechanisms, binds to and activates the regulatory protein calmodulin. Activated calmodulin increases the activity of different enzymes, especially the phosphatase calcineurin. Calcineurin, in turn, can dephosphorylate the transcrip-

tion factor NF-AT, activating it in the process. Calcineurin is the molecular target of the immunosuppressive drugs cyclosporin A and FK506 (Fig. 10.4). Last, signaling by the BCR may be further enhanced through recruitment of phosphoinositide-3-kinase (PI3K) to the receptor complex. PI3K may contribute to signaling by increasing levels of various phosphoinositol molecules (inositol-3-phosphate, inositol-3,4-diphosphate, inositol-3,4,5-triphosphate) with unknown signaling capacities. The end result of all these events is the transcription of gene products necessary for B-cell activation, differentiation, proliferation, and antibody production.

Regulation of BCR Signal Transduction

Antigen binding and signal transduction via the BCR provide only one part of the signaling cascade needed to activate B cells. Other B-cell surface molecules, cytokines, and cellular ligands expressed by T cells and FDCs are also needed for full function of a B cell. Numerous other changes take place during B-cell activation and differentiation, including isotype switching and somatic mutation. To coordinate and control all of the important processes, a variety of factors influence the signals initially emanating from the BCR following antigen ligation.

CD19/CD21/CD81: the B-Cell Coreceptor

The CD19/CD21/CD81 complex is normally expressed on the surface of B lymphocytes, where it plays an important costimulatory role in B-cell activation. CD19 is a 95-kilodalton (kDa) glycoprotein that is expressed early in B-cell development, but not on plasma cells. Expression is restricted to B cells and FDCs. Its extracellular region has two immunoglobulin-like domains (making it a member of the immunoglobulin gene superfamily), while its 240-amino-acid cytoplasmic tail has no known homology with other proteins. When the BCR and CD19 are brought close together, this decreases the threshold needed for the BCR to activate the B cell. Thus, it is thought that the activation level of the B cell is decreased when antigen bridges CD19 and the BCR through mIg.

CD19 knockout mice have been useful for defining some functions of CD19 in B-cell activation and antigen-driven antibody responses. Mice lacking CD19 respond normally to highly repetitive antigens such as polysaccharides that are known as thymus-independent (TI) type 2 antigens. In the absence of CD19, mice do not respond normally to thymus-dependent (TD) antigens such as proteins. However, affinity maturation of immunoglobulins and germinal center formation are defective, processes that are due to B-cell interactions with T cells. Therefore, even though CD19 appears to be important for BCR-mediated B-cell activation, its function seems to be restricted to conditions in which B lymphocytes must interact with T lymphocytes.

CD19 forms a complex on the cell surface with CD21 (also called CR2 for complement receptor 2), a 145-kDa glycoprotein member of the complement-receptor family, and with CD81, a 26-kDa protein. CD21 is expressed exclusively on mature B cells and FDCs. It has an external sequence made up of 15 or 16 repeats of a 60- to 70-amino-acid sequence, termed *short consensus repeats,* and a 37-amino-acid cytoplasmic tail. It is a receptor for the complement split products iC3b, C3dg, and C3d. Since CD21 is expressed later during B-cell development than CD19 or CD81, there must be some variation in the makeup of the CD19/CD21/CD81 complex during B-cell development.

CD81 is expressed on various cell types, including B and T lymphocytes, neuroblastoma cells, melanoma cells, and fibroblasts. B cells express CD81 during their entire lineage development, but it is not expressed on plasma cells. CD81 has four hydrophobic areas that are large enough to transverse the plasma membrane of the B cell, and both the NH_2- and COOH-terminal regions are cytoplasmic. It is, thus, a member of the tetraspan family of transmembrane proteins. The various members of this family have been shown to be involved in regulation of cell growth, motility, and signal transduction.

CD19 engagement increases in a number of B-cell activities, including tyrosine phosphorylation of cytoplasmic and cell surface proteins, PLC activity, inositol phospholipid turnover, Ca^{2+} mobilization, PKC activity, and activation of the transcription factor NF-κB. Various PTK, including p59^{fyn}, p53/56^{lyn}, and p56^{lck}, are associated with the cytoplasmic portion of CD19, and other proteins involved in signal transduction, such as PLCγ1 and the guanidine nucleotide exchange factor p95^{vav}, which activates the p21^{ras} pathway, can recognize phosphotyrosine motifs present in CD19.

Since CD21 is a member of the complement-receptor family, the CD19/CD21/CD81 complex is thought to play a major role in B-cell activation in response to complement-containing antigen complexes. Since many antigens will activate complement, particularly through the alternative pathway, and become covalently tagged with complement split products such as C3b and iC3b, the antigen-complement complexes bind *simultaneously* to both the mIg in the BCR and CD19/CD21/CD81. The mIg portion of the BCR provides the cognate recognition of the antigenic epitope and CD19 recognizes the bound complement fragments. During cross-linking of the CD19/CD21/CD81 complex, CD19-associated PTKs are activated, with subsequent phosphorylation of CD19.

These kinases (such as Src family kinases) will also come into close proximity to the BCR complex, allowing for CD19 engagement to potentiate antigen-driven B-cell activation. This system allows antigens that have been coated with activated complement proteins (such as bacterial surfaces, which are natural activators of the complement system) to activate B cells more readily.

CD22

CD22 is a 135-kDa B-cell lineage-associated surface protein and a member of the immunoglobulin superfamily. CD22 is present in the cytoplasm of B cells at pre- and pro-B-cell stages. Surface expression of CD22 tightly correlates with mIgD expression on mature B cells and has ITAM regions available for phosphorylation. Surface expression of CD22 increases during B-cell activation, then decreases on the surface of the plasma cell during antibody production. There are two isoforms, CD22α and CD22β, the former containing five immunoglobulin-like domains and the latter containing seven. CD22β is the major form expressed on mature B cells. Thus far, the only CD22 mRNA that has been detected in mice is that of the β isoform.

Although only a small percentage (1 to 2%) of CD22 has been found to associate directly with mIg, CD22 engagement, like CD19 engagement, appears to lower the threshold for antigen-initiated signaling through the BCR. PTK activity has been found to occur following CD22 engagement. Surface IgM cross-linking induces phosphorylation of the tyrosine residues in the CD22 cytoplasmic tails in regions with ITAMs. These areas can associate with the SH2 domains of the tyrosine kinases p53/56^{lyn} and p72^{syk}. p72^{syk} recruitment is particularly important, as this kinase can activate PLC and generate IP$_3$. The original PTK that phosphorylates CD22 is unknown, but any of the PTKs mentioned above could be candidates.

CD45

Phosphorylation of tyrosine residues on transmembrane proteins and cytoplasmic proteins by PTK is essential for signal transduction and B-cell activation. It is, therefore, logical that dephosphorylation of such residues would be an important regulatory event in such models. CD45 actually designates a family of related transmembrane glycoproteins, present on T and B lymphocytes, that have protein tyrosine phosphatase (PTP) activity and arise from a single gene by alternative mRNA splicing. Because of its presence on numerous types of white blood cell, CD45 has also been termed *leukocyte common antigen.* The molecular size range of CD45 is 180 to 220 kDa. It has a variable NH_2-terminal region followed by a perimembranous cystine-rich region and two cytoplasmic repeat domains (CDI and CDII) that contain the phosphatase activity. The cytoplasmic domains are the most highly conserved of the entire protein; amino acid homology between the different isoforms is approximately 85% in this region and similar to that of other transmembrane PTPs. Three main isoforms of CD45 have been identified on lymphocytes: CD45RA, CD45RB, and CD45RO. These isoforms differ from each other in their extracellular domains. The mRNA encoding CD45RA contains exon A of the CD45 gene; mRNA encoding CD45RB contains exon B; and mRNA encoding CD45R0 contains neither exon A nor exon B. The highest molecular weight form (CD45RA, also designated B220) is found on B cells and appears early in B-cell differentiation.

It would appear that CD45 PTP activity would abolish or inhibit B-cell activation, since most of the PTKs and membrane proteins (e.g., Ig-α/Ig-β dimers and mIgM/D) require tyrosine phosphorylation for activation. To the contrary, the presence of CD45 is required for B-cell activation after BCR engagement by antigen or specific anti-immunoglobulin monoclonal antibodies (MAbs). For example, in a cell line that expresses mIgM but not CD45, B-cell activation is abnormal upon engagement of the BCR: Ca^{2+} mobilization is not detected, and PLC, MAPK, and p21^{ras} are not activated. When this cell line is transfected with CD45 cDNA, CD45 is expressed and the Ca^{2+} response and p21^{ras} activity return to normal.

The PTP activity of CD45 is directed against a number of different proteins in the B cell, indicating multiple targets for regulation of B-cell responses by CD45. Several phosphotyrosine-containing proteins have been shown to coprecipitate with CD45 in immunoprecipitation assays. These proteins have been identified as the Src family kinases p53/56^{lyn} and Ig-α and Ig-β of the BCR complex. It has been demonstrated in a number of different ways that CD45 has PTP activity toward the Ig-α/Ig-β complex. Tyrosine residues present in the ITAM regions of Ig-α and Ig-β can be phosphorylated and subsequently act as substrate for CD45, rapidly becoming dephosphorylated. When phosphorylated, these regions of Ig-α and Ig-β will bind the SH2 domains of Src family kinases. Dephosphorylation of the tyrosine residues in ITAM of Ig-α and Ig-β prevents Src kinase association. Moreover, when cells are treated with sodium orthovanadate (a PTP inhibitor), Ig-α and Ig-β become hyperphosphorylated. One role for CD45 may be to maintain Ig-α and Ig-β in a dephosphorylated state in resting or naive B cells, thereby preventing aberrant activation.

In addition to acting on the Ig-α/Ig-β complex, CD45 acts on Src family kinases that associate with the BCR complex. The Src family kinases contain a conserved tyro-sine residue near their carboxy terminus, which can be phosphorylated. If this tyrosine residue is substituted with a phenylalanine that cannot be phosphorylated, constitutive PTK activity is induced. Phosphorylation of this carboxy-terminal tyrosine can, therefore, decrease the PTK activity of Src family kinases, indicating that CD45 plays a role in regulating kinase activity (see Fig. 2.6B) and explaining the finding that CD45 PTP activity is necessary for B-cell activation and the signal transduction cascade.

CD19 and CD22 may also be targets for PTP activity by CD45. Tyrosine residues on the proteins can be phosphorylated, and reversal of this process can affect their function. Tyrosine phosphorylation of residues on CD19 can allow binding of Src family kinases via their SH2 domains. Simultaneous cross-linking of CD19 and CD45 can decrease Ca^{2+} mobilization from intracellular stores, where cross-linking of CD19 alone can increase Ca^{2+} mobilization from intracellular stores. The ability of CD45 to dephosphorylate CD19 may prevent the interaction of CD19 with PTK, thus affecting CD19-mediated events after BCR engagement. CD22 interacts with the BCR (see above), and BCR engagement phosphorylates tyrosine residues in the cytoplasmic ITAM regions of CD22. When CD45 is immunoprecipitated from B cells, CD22 coprecipitates with it, suggesting that CD45 can be a part of the BCR/CD22 complex.

In summary, CD45 can have either positive or negative effects on B-cell activation and associated events (e.g., Ca^{2+} mobilization and phosphoinositol hydrolysis). It is likely that CD45 maintains Ig-α, Ig-β, CD19, and CD22 in a dephosphorylated state in resting B cells, thus preventing aberrant activation of the B cells. In addition, CD45 appears to have an integral role in the PTK activity of key Src family kinases, which then could affect the tyrosine phosphorylation of other proteins important in B-cell activation, including PLC, PI3K, p95^{vav}, Shc, and MAPK. These contrasting functions of CD45 can explain the seemingly contradictory findings that CD45 PTP activity can be associated with both B-cell activation and inhibition of B-cell activation through the BCR.

CD20

CD20 is an integral membrane protein found only on B cells. The phosphorylation of CD20 is associated with B-cell activation. CD20 exists as dimer or tetramer and most likely passes through the membrane four times, with both NH$_2$- and COOH-terminal ends located within the cytoplasm, similar to the tetraspan family of proteins. The structure is conserved among species (human, mouse, and rat). There is also distinct homology and similarity in overall structure with the β chain of the high-affinity IgE Fc receptor (FcϵRI). Three forms of CD20 have been found with apparent molecular masses of 33, 35, and 37 kDa, depending on the degree of phosphorylation of the protein. When B cells are activated, expression of the lower-molecular-weight form decreases and expression of the two higher-molecular-weight forms increases.

CD20 is not phosphorylated in resting B cells but is the predominant protein phosphorylated upon activation of B cells and B-cell lines. It has been shown that various kinases can phosphorylate CD20, including PKC, casein kinase II, and calcium/calmodulin protein kinase II. CD20 is involved in B-cell activation, signal transduction, and regulation of cell cycle progression. CD20 phosphorylation increases expression of major histocompatibility complex (MHC) class II, CD18 (integrin β_2 subunit), CD58 (LFA-3), oncogenes (c-*myc* and B-*myb*), and PTK activity and subsequent phosphorylation of myriad cellular proteins. CD20 can act as a Ca^{2+} channel, and it has been hypothesized that changes in intracellular Ca^{2+} concentration are regulated by the opening and closing of CD20. Differential CD20 phosphorylation may affect its Ca^{2+} channel activity.

CD5: a Questionable Role for Expression and Function on B Cells?

CD5 (called Ly-1 in mice) is a monomeric 67-kDa glycoprotein present on most T cells and on a subset of B cells. Although CD5 is not expressed at all by B cells present in the lymph nodes, it is expressed on a substantial fraction of peritoneal and pleural B cells and on a minor population of B cells in the spleen. CD5 is also highly expressed on certain types of B-lymphocyte leukemic cells. The cysteine-rich extracellular domain of CD5 shares homology with the macrophage scavenger receptors. This domain consists of a 100-amino-acid stretch with six conserved cysteines. CD5 also possesses a cytoplasmic tail that may be a target for phosphorylation.

Much of the work regarding CD5 has been done with mice. Murine B lymphocytes expressing CD5 have been called "B-1" cells (differentiating them from "classical" B cells, which have been named "B-2" cells). B-1 cells can be differentiated from other B cells by their ability to replicate outside the bone marrow. A yet unknown feedback mechanism must exist to regulate the number of CD5-positive B-1 cells present in the host. B-1 cells are the main producers of IgM in serum. However, the variable region of the IgM repertoire is oligoclonal. B-1 cells are thought to be the source of natural and autoreactive antibodies. Specific strains of mice that express autoimmune phenotypes have higher numbers of CD5-positive B cells than do outbred mice or other inbred mice not predisposed to autoimmunity (e.g., BALB/c). In addition, a mouse strain, known as "moth-eaten" mice, is prone to

production of autoantibodies and autoimmune disease. Their B-cell population is extremely abnormal, with almost all B cells expressing CD5, which likely contributes to their autoimmune disease.

The function of CD5 on B cells remains elusive. The CD5 cytoplasmic tail contains multiple potential sites for tyrosine and serine/threonine phosphorylation. CD5 can be associated with the BCR, and upon B-cell activation via BCR cross-linking in vitro, CD5 is phosphorylated on tyrosine residues in its cytoplasmic tail. The ligand for CD5 is CD72, a 45-kDa glycoprotein and C-type lectin expressed during all stages of B-cell maturation except on plasma cells. It is believed that the main function of CD72 expression on B cells is to allow B cells to interact with CD5-expressing T cells. Upon B-cell–B-cell interaction through CD72 binding of CD5, signaling events occur in B cells, including increased PTK activity, a slow steady increase in intracellular levels of Ca^{2+} levels, and phosphoinositol diphosphate (PIP_2) hydrolysis. The exact function of CD72, however, is unclear. There is speculation that CD5-CD72 interactions between CD5-positive B cells and CD72-positive B cells are important for B-cell activation in response to thymus-independent antigens. CD5 knockout mice have normal B- and T-cell populations and do not demonstrate any abnormality in their response to antigens. Overall, a major role for CD5 in B-cell activation is not clear, but its presence on a subpopulation of B cells may be an important marker to identify B cells with some specialized functions.

Role of Fc Receptors in B-Cell Activity

It has been known for some time that IgG-containing immune complexes may decrease B-cell activation mediated through BCR cross-linking. The molecular basis for this inhibitory activity was discovered when the structure and function of the IgG Fc receptor, FcγRIIB, were discerned. FcγRIIB is a low-affinity receptor for the IgG Fc region and is the only IgG FcR on B cells. The cytoplasmic portion of this molecule was found to contain an immunoreceptor tyrosine-based inhibitory motif (ITIM) region. The ITIM region is I/V/L/SxYxxL/V (where x is any amino acid) and has been found in the cytoplasmic region of many inhibitory receptors. Phosphorylation of this specific region has been shown to be necessary and sufficient to inhibit BCR-mediated B-cell activation as characterized by calcium mobilization and cellular proliferation.

Phosphorylation of the tyrosine of the ITIM region occurs upon BCR coligation with the FcR, as would normally occur upon binding of immune complexes to the surface of a B cell. In the immune complex, the antigen binds to the mIg in the BCR while the Fc portion of the IgG molecules in the complex bind to the FcR. This coligation allows a close juxtaposition of the ITAM region of the BCR complex, which has bound Lyn kinase, with the ITIM regions of the FcγRIIB. Lyn phosphorylates the ITIM of FcγRIIB. This modification generates an SH2 recognition domain, which becomes the binding site for the inhibitory molecule SH2-containing inositol polyphosphate 5-phosphatase (SHIP).

There are two separate inhibitory activities of FcγRIIB based on recruitment of SHIP (Fig. 10.5A): inhibition of

Figure 10.5 Effect of simultaneous binding of the antibody-antigen complex to the BCR and the Fc receptor (FcγRII) on B-cell activation and signaling events. (**A**) When antigen in an antibody-antigen immune complex binds to the surface immunoglobulin of the BCR and the Fc portion of the antibody binds to the inhibitory FcR present on B cells, FcγRII, these two molecules are brought into close proximity. This allows phosphorylation of the ITIM region of this FcR by p53/56^{lyn} kinase and recruitment of the phosphatase SHIP (SH2-containing inositol polyphosphate 5-phosphatase). There are two separate inhibitory activities of FcγRII based on recruitment of SHIP, inhibition of ITAM-triggered calcium mobilization, and ITAM-triggered cellular proliferation due to the effect of SHIP activity on two different signaling pathways. Inhibition of calcium mobilization requires the phosphatase activity of SHIP to hydrolyze PIP$_3$ bound to PLCγ to PIP$_2$, eliciting dissociation of Btk and PLCγ from the BCR complex like Btk and PLCγ (**1**). Prevention or arrest of proliferation in B cells can also be due to SHIP's activating the adapter protein Dok either directly or by allowing recruitment of Dok to the membrane to allow access to Lyn kinase. Dok activation can lead to subsequent inactivation of MAPK (**2**). Moreover, dephosphorylation by SHIP of PIP$_3$ bound to Akt inactivates PIP$_3$ and enhances susceptibility of the B cell to apoptosis (**3**). (*Figure continues*)

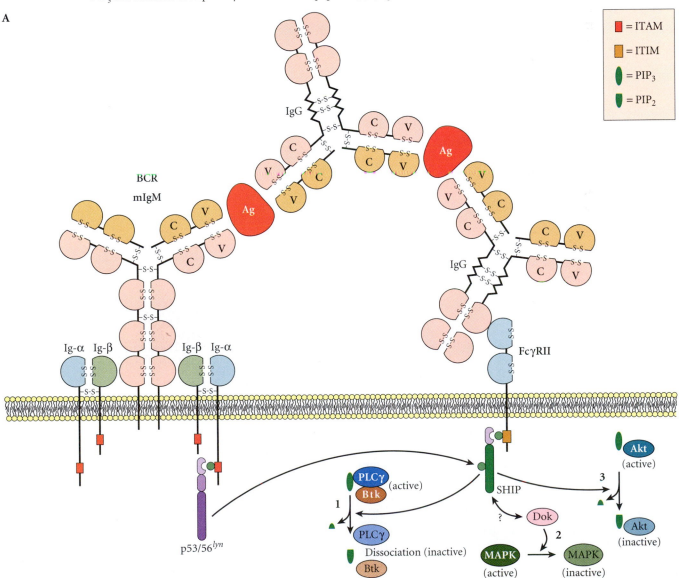

B

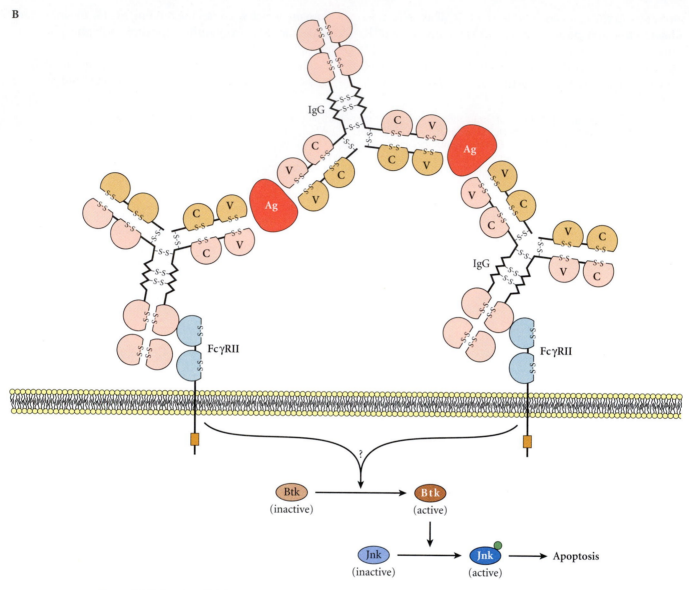

Figure 10.5 *(continued)* (**B**) There is a third B-cell inhibitory activity of FcγRII that is independent of ITIM and SHIP and that requires homoaggregation of the Fc receptor. Clustering of FcγRII, which can occur with immune complexes binding to B cells whose mIg does not recognize the antigen portion of the complex, elicits a proapoptotic signal through its transmembrane sequence. This requires the presence and activation of Btk, which further activates Jnk, allowing for induction of apoptosis. Interestingly, recruitment of SHIP blocks this proapoptotic signal, likely through induction of dissociation of Btk from the BCR cytoplasmic complex. Based on A. L. Defranco and D. A. Law, *Science* **268:**263–264, 1995.

ITAM-triggered calcium mobilization and inhibition of cellular proliferation due to the inhibitory effect of SHIP on two different signaling pathways. Inhibiting calcium mobilization requires the phosphatase activity of SHIP to hydrolyze PIP$_3$ to PIP$_2$. This causes dissociation of adapter and signaling proteins like Btk and PLCγ from the BCR complex (Fig. 10.3). Another pathway leading to the arrest of proliferation in B cells is due to SHIP activating an adapter protein called Dok. Dok activation leads to

inactivation of MAPKs. In Dok-deficient B cells, FcγRIIB-triggered arrest of BCR-induced proliferation does not occur, but these cells retain their ability to inhibit calcium influx.

There is a third B-cell inhibitory activity of FcγRIIB that is independent of ITIMs and SHIP and requires aggregation of the Fc receptor (Fig. 10.5B). Clustering of FcγRIIB, which can occur with immune complexes binding to B cells whose mIg does not recognize any of the antigenic epitopes in the complex, promotes apoptosis. This requires the association of Btk with the BCR, which normally is part of an activating pathway. Recruitment of SHIP blocks this form of apoptosis, likely through induction of the dissociation of Btk from the BCR cytoplasmic complex. This process would prevent inappropriate activation of B cells that cannot recognize an antigen when the B cells bind immune complexes.

Germinal Centers and B-Cell Maturation

The Initial Encounter of B Cell with Antigen

The lymph node and comparable lymphoid tissues, especially the spleen, are the center of activity where B cells proliferate and undergo somatic mutation leading to affinity maturation and isotype switching. The immune response starts out with dendritic cells (DCs) that have migrated into the lymph node and express both intact and processed antigen on their surface. The DCs were initially immature cells present in the tissues where they picked up the antigen. During migration and entry into the lymph node, the DCs mature into antigen-presenting cells (APCs) that can present antigen to the T cells. The DCs are present in the T-cell-rich zone through which naive T cells traffic. This gives the rare T cell that can recognize processed antigen-MHC the opportunity to find its proper antigen and become activated (Fig. 10.6). This interaction is stabilized by coreceptors and other adhesive molecules that bind DCs to T cells. For an antigen-specific B cell to encounter antigen it too must pass through the T-cell area and become trapped in an area where the early immune response is initiated.

The journey of naive antigen-specific B cells begins when the newly formed B cell enters the circulation and then traffics into the lymph node via the high endothelial venules or goes into other lymphoid tissue. Given the rarity of B cells expressing mIg for a specific antigen, and the need to find helper T (TH) cells that can bind to processed and presented peptide fragments of the antigen, it is somewhat remarkable that following entry into the lymphoid tissues a B cell will be able to find the area where antigen activation is taking place. Nonetheless, this does occur, and upon encountering antigen, the migrating B cells stop their migration and are held in place by the activation of cell surface adhesion molecules and the production of chemokine receptors such as CCR7, which binds to both MIP-3β and the secondary lymphoid chemokine. These are the same factors that keep the migrating T cells in the lymphoid tissue once they have encountered peptide-MHC. Following B-cell binding of

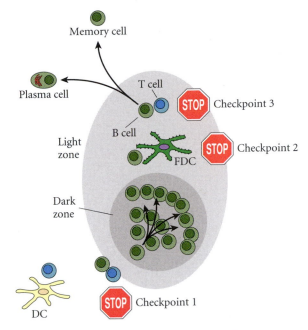

Figure 10.6 Antigen-dependent B-cell maturation in the germinal center is a multistep process involving several regulatory checkpoints. Antigen is first encountered in the T-cell-rich paracortical region of the lymph node, when a DC presents antigen to a T cell on MHC class II. Antigen-specific T cells migrate to the B-cell-rich cortical region where the primary lymphoid follicles reside. Here, antigen-specific B cells present antigen to antigen-specific T cells, and the B cell receives survival signals from the T cells in the form of CD40-CD40-L interactions and T-cell-secreted cytokines (checkpoint 1). B cells activated in this way migrate into the primary follicle and initiate the germinal center reaction. B-cell centroblasts proliferate in the dark zone of the germinal center and during this time undergo the process of somatic hypermutation to diversify their antibody genes. B cells that stop proliferating (centrocytes) then enter the light zone of the germinal center. Here, B cells with mutated antibody genes must compete with each other for binding to antigen on the surface of FDCs. Centrocytes with the highest affinity for antigen receive survival signals from the FDCs (checkpoint 2) and migrate to the apical region of the light zone, where they must interact with antigen-specific T cells (checkpoint 3). B cells that receive help from T cells at checkpoint 3 continue their maturation to become memory or plasma cells and also undergo the process of isotype switching under the regulation of T-cell-derived cytokines.

the antigen via mIg, it can also process and present the antigen to the T cells in the vicinity. Many of the T cells have already been activated by the DCs, making them very responsive to antigen presented by B cells (Fig. 10.6). Once this occurs, the T cells can activate the B cells via CD40-CD40L and MHC-TCR interactions.

During clonal expansion of antigen-specific B cells, a single B cell can expand into a population of cells that contain antibody variants with different affinities for the antigen. This *affinity maturation* is due to somatic hypermutation that provides for the genetic changes leading to the increased antibody affinity. This initial maturation occurs in the dark zone of the primary lymphoid follicle or germinal center (Fig. 10.6). However, during the phase of clonal expansion, these *centroblasts* downregulate the expression of the surface immunoglobulin or BCR and form nonproliferating *centrocytes,* which move into the light zone of the germinal center and associate with FDCs, which can present intact antigen to the B cells. At this point, the B cells now express mutated BCRs, and cells with higher-affinity mIg are selected while cells with lower affinity undergo apoptosis via Fas/FasL interactions. High-affinity binding and cross-linking of the BCR along with CD40-CD40L interactions induce resistance to apoptosis of B cells (Fig. 10.7), while CD40-CD40L interaction alone can upregulate Fas expression on B cells and increase susceptibility to Fas-mediated apoptosis. CD40L can be supplied by T cells or FDCs. Isotype switching also occurs at this point. Earlier, the isotype of the mIg is IgM or IgD; upon somatic hypermutation,

Figure 10.7 Survival signals received by B cells in the germinal center can be mediated at the level of Fas-triggered apoptosis. (**A**) In a proliferating centrocyte, the apoptotic pathway is inhibited since the initiating caspase, caspase-8, is maintained in its inactive precursor form (pro-caspase-8) by the protein FLIP (FLIP, FLICE inhibitory protein; FLICE, FADD-like IL-1β converting enzyme). (**B**) Centrocytes that do not continue to receive survival signals diminish their expression of FLIP, allowing the conversion of pro-caspase-8 to its active form. (**C**) During the germinal center reaction, B cells with a high affinity for antigen can avoid apoptosis because of enhanced FLIP expression. FLIP expression is increased by mIg binding to antigen-antibody complexes on FDCs (checkpoint 2 in Fig. 10.6) or by CD40-CD40L interactions (checkpoints 1 and 3).

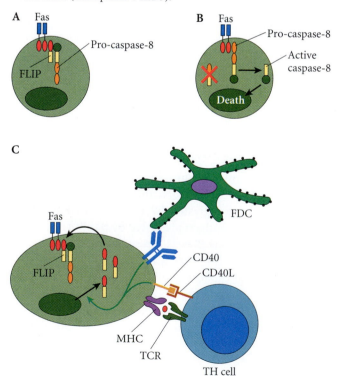

affinity maturation, and selection of higher-affinity antibody-producing B cells (as determined by an interaction of antigen with the mIg), the isotype of the Ig switches to other isotypes, i.e., IgG, IgE, or IgA.

The Secondary Phase of the B-Cell Response

Antibody is initially produced by plasma cells in the germinal center but declines after 2 to 4 weeks. The decline is due to selection of higher-affinity antibody-producing plasma cells and deletion of lower-affinity cells by apoptosis. As the number of plasma cells declines, these higher-affinity cells begin to migrate and accumulate in the bone marrow, where 80 to 90% of the antigen-specific plasma cells now reside. A small number of memory B cells expressing high-affinity mIg as part of the BCR reside in the lymph nodes where these original reactions occur. These B cells can be differentiated from naive B cells by increased surface expression of CD27 and CD148. Upon a secondary encounter with the antigen, antibody responses occur in the lymph node and spleen, as this is where most of the memory B cells are located. These B cells proliferate and some differentiate into antibody-producing plasma cells. After this secondary response subsides, the level of peripheral plasma cells increases, and again, the majority of antibody-specific plasma cells reside in the bone marrow.

Interaction of B Cells with FDCs

The process by which APCs (e.g., macrophages and DCs) present antigen to T cells and the T cells in turn activate B cells is considered the *classic antigen presentation pathway.* It has been shown that an alternative and possibly a more important pathway for antigen interaction with B cells occurs in the lymph node. This *alternative antigen presentation pathway* takes advantage of environments rich in specific antibodies and requires significant involvement of FDCs. FDCs are stellate cells that present antigen to B cells in lymphoid follicles. Despite their name, FDCs are not the same as DCs, as the two cell types have several immunologically important differences. Primarily, FDCs are not classified as APCs, since they do not express MHC class II proteins on their surface, and therefore cannot present antigenic peptides to T cells. However, FDCs have a mechanism for presenting antigens to B cells that does not depend on MHC proteins.

The sequence of events of the alternative pathway is as follows. At first, antigen is transported to the lymph node via the afferent lymph vessels and then to the follicle by cells that are antigen-transport cells. The antigen-transport cells do not process antigen while transporting them to the lymph node and are not well defined but appear to be monocytic and perhaps of the same lineage as FDCs. Once the intact antigen is "transported" to the lymph follicle, an *FDC antigen-retaining reticulum* develops. The antigen interacts with the FDC either directly or as part of immune complexes bound to Fc receptors on the FDC's membrane. It appears that a single antigen-transport site develops into a single antigen-retaining reticulum, which induces the development of a single germinal center. The FDCs then produce plasma membrane-bound structures termed *iccosomes* (immune complex-coated bodies). The iccosomes allow for an enhanced, direct interaction between intact antigen and the B cells. The B cells endocytose the iccosomes, process the antigen, and present the antigen-derived oligopeptides to TH cells. As a result, two phases of the germinal center response are induced: (i) an early phase (3 to 7 days) in which antibody-forming cell precursors are differentiated and migrate to the medulla of the lymph node and to the bone marrow and (ii) a late phase (7 to 12 days) of differentiation of B memory cells.

This late phase involves feedback regulation caused by the changes in the levels of antigen-specific antibody. During the maintenance phase of the immune response free antigen, free antibody, and antigen-antibody complexes are in equilibrium, with various ratios of the three components in the lymphoid organs. Newly produced antibodies cover the antigen in the FDC reticulum, thus terminating the immunogenic stimulus. The cross-linking of the antigen in the dendrites of the FDC forms "ball of yarn"-like structures throughout the germinal center soon after the germinal center reaches its peak size, and this masking of the antigen results in retention of the antigen in the germinal center. When the antibody levels decline, the antigen is revealed, the balls of yarn unravel, and memory B cells are stimulated by the newly unmasked antigen. The persistence of antigen allows for affinity maturation and selection of B cells with high affinity for the antigen, whereas the lower-affinity B cells have much more difficulty interacting with the FDC antigen reticulum and therefore undergo apoptosis.

During the second encounter with the antigen, a similar set of events take place, but the sequence takes place at an accelerated pace in the presence of circulating antibody that recognizes the antigen. The antigen receptors on the B cells compete with specific antibody produced during the primary response. Only B cells with surface immunoglobulin that binds the antigen better than the existing antibodies contribute to the secondary response. This improved binding is achieved through somatic hypermutation of the DNA encoding the immunoglobulin variable domains (the complementarity-determining regions) and results in changes in the antigen-binding site. Through a variation of clonal selection, B cells with higher-affinity antibodies are selected.

Several lines of evidence support the requirement of FDCs for formation of a germinal center. In vitro, B cells have been shown to cluster around FDCs and proliferate as they do in germinal centers if the proportion of T cells, B cells, and FDCs is "correct." When the FDCs are removed from the cocultures, B cells do not proliferate. The interaction of FDCs with B cells is mediated not just by the specific antigen but by other ligands, especially CD54-CD11a/CD18 interactions. Anti-CD54 MAb can block B-cell–FDC clustering in vitro. FDCs can also activate B cells and induce upregulation of B7-1/B7-2 and MHC class II molecules, which allows for much-improved interactions with T cells.

Antibody Production by B Lymphocytes

The activation of B cells to differentiate into antibody-producing plasma cells and memory cells starts with engagement of mIg by antigen. However, as there are many different kinds of antigens, the subsequent steps leading to antibody production and memory can be quite different, depending on the type of antigen to which the B cell is responding. Antigens are placed into two broad classes, depending on the requirement of B cells for T-cell help in producing antibody. T-cell help is based on the ability of APCs, including B cells, to process and present the antigen to T cells. TI antigens, such as bacterial polysaccharides and lipopolysaccharides, cannot be processed and presented by APCs and, therefore, cannot activate TH cells. These antigens stimulate plasma cell maturation and antibody production but generally cannot induce immunologic memory (Table 10.1). Many, but not all, TI antigens only induce IgM responses, failing to induce class switching. This is seen more commonly in mice than in humans, who respond to a number of TI antigens with IgG and IgA. TD antigens, principally proteins, are processed and presented by APCs to T cells and induce antibody production, class switching, and immunologic memory in both mice and humans.

TI Antibody Response
Structure of TI Antigens
TI antigens stimulate antibody production in the absence of MHC class II-restricted T-cell help (Table 10.1) since they cannot be processed into peptides that can be bound to MHC molecules. Therefore, by definition, TI antigens

Table 10.1 Properties of TI and TD antigens[a]

TD antigens		TI antigens
Type 1	**Type 2**	
Bacterial cell wall components	Polysaccharides, can be polypeptides or polynucleotides	Bacterial proteins such as tetanus and diphtheria toxoids
Mitogens or polyclonal B-cell activators	High molecular weight, repeating antigenic determinants	Proteins such as ovalbumin or haptenated derivative
	Slowly metabolized	Sheep erythrocytes, nucleated cells, viruses, parasites
	May be tolerogenic in large doses	May be tolerogenic in low and large doses
Generate few (if any) memory B cells	Generate few (if any) memory B cells	Generate memory B cells
Stimulate responses in nude mice (lacking mature T cells)	Stimulate responses in nude mice (lacking mature T cells)	No response in nude mice (lacking mature T cells)
Activate the alternative complement pathway	Activate the alternative complement pathway (some)	
Stimulate responses in neonates	Fail to stimulate responses in neonates	Stimulate responses in neonates
Stimulate responses in Xid mice	Fail to stimulate responses in Xid mice	Stimulate responses in Xid mice

[a] Based in part on K. E. Stein, *J. Infect. Dis.* **165**(Suppl. 1):S49–S52, 1992 (Tables 1 and 2).

cannot stimulate T cells through TCR-MHC-peptide interactions. TI antigens are often categorized as either type 1 or type 2 (TI-1 or TI-2) on the basis of the ability of the antigen to induce an antibody response in immature or mature B cells. This distinction was made using either nude mice, which lack a thymus, or another strain of mouse known as the Xid mouse. Xid mice have an X-linked immunodeficiency and are only able to generate immature B-cell population. TI-1 antigens can, nonetheless, promote B-cell responses in nude and Xid mice. In contrast, TI-2 antigens can elicit antibody responses in a variety of wild-type mice with mature B-cell populations. This difference in the behavior of TI-1 and TI-2 antigens in Xid mice can be explained by the mechanism by which each class of antigen stimulates B cells.

TI-1 Antigens

Many of the TI-1 antigens are components of bacterial cell walls (Table 10.1). Bacterial lipopolysaccharide (LPS), a major constituent of the outer membrane of gram-negative bacteria, is the best studied TI-1 antigen. LPS has a crucial property of TI-1 antigens: it is a B-cell mitogen in mice (but not humans). Thus, LPS stimulates mouse B cells to divide even in the absence of recognition of the LPS as an antigen by the mIg. At low concentrations, LPS binds to mIg on LPS-antigen-specific B cells and elicits secretion of LPS-specific antibodies. However, at higher concentrations of LPS, all B cells are stimulated to divide,

resulting in a polyclonal B-cell activation. This also leads to production of many antibodies of multiple specificities, but in general the titer and affinity of the antibodies are low.

Most TI-1 antigens are also potent activators of macrophages, which can secrete cytokines and growth factors that can be used by neighboring B cells to differentiate and proliferate. Macrophages ingest bacteria and degrade their cell walls into mitogenic components. The macrophages are thus induced to secrete interleukin-1 (IL-1), IL-6, IL-8, IL-12, and tumor necrosis factor alpha (TNF-α), with resultant lymphocyte activation and increased antibody production from B cells in the local vicinity.

TI-2 Antigens

TI-2 antigens are generally large molecular mass, multivalent (i.e., repetitive antigenic epitopes) antigens that are poorly degraded in vivo. Classic examples are bacterial capsular polysaccharides and flagella. Flagella, which are used by microbes to propel themselves around their environment, are made up of thousands of identical polypeptide subunits, termed flagellin monomers. This makes the large flagellum an antigen with a highly repetitive structure of recurring epitopes. Binding of TI-2 antigens by the B cell through its BCR generates very strong and efficient intracellular activation signals, and the B cell is stimulated to differentiate and proliferate into plasma cells without help from T cells. The efficient cross-linking of the BCR by the repeating antigenic epitopes likely accounts for the TI properties of these antigens. Anti-immunoglobulin is an efficient activator of B cells, due to a similar type of cross-linking of the surface mIg molecules. Anti-immunoglobulin conjugated to dextran molecules is 10,000 times more potent than soluble anti-immunoglobulin in inducing B-cell proliferation and phosphoinositol breakdown, indicative of the potency of highly aggregated BCR complexes in initiating B-cell activation.

TI-2 antigens stimulate mature B cells only and are unable to stimulate responses in Xid mice. Although T-cell help is not required for antibody production in response to TI-2 antigens, responses to these antigens can be enhanced by T cells. There is a reduction in antibody response to TI-2 antigens if TH cells are depleted at the time of immunization with a TI-2 antigen. However, the mechanism by which TI-2 antigens stimulate TH cells is unknown. Immune responses to TI antigens may be influenced by direct T-cell contact with B cells in a TCR-independent fashion or through cytokine networks that become activated when TI-2 antigens interact with B cells and other APCs. Another characteristic of TI-2 antigens is their ability to activate the complement cascade via the alternative pathway. This may participate in B-cell responses to TI-2 antigens by enhancing signaling through the BCR-coreceptor complex, wherein the complement-coated TI-2 antigens bind strongly to the CD21 (CR2) component of the coreceptor.

Kinetics and Characteristics of the Antibody Response to TI Antigens

TI antigens are often thought to elicit primarily IgM responses, without induction of class switching. Although this belief is held firmly by many immunologists, in fact, the situation is more complex. Mice, in general, produce primarily IgM to TI antigens, but there are numerous examples of TI antigens that induce switching to IgG in mice. Most of these are bacterial polysaccharides, which are intensely studied due to their importance in disease and because they are the most commonly used antigen in antibacterial vaccines. Humans tend to be more disposed to producing both IgG and IgA in response to TI antigens. Again, however, there are exceptions. A vaccine to 23 different capsular polysaccharides of *Streptococcus pneumoniae*, the causative agent of classic bacterial pneumonia, generates IgG and IgA responses in immunized adult humans. Other capsular polysaccharides, however, induce only IgM responses in humans. This classification is further confused by the fact that many bacterial polysaccha-

rides do not stimulate any antibody response, including IgM, when injected into children less than 2 years of age. This poor immune response in young children has led to the conclusion that the immature human immune system cannot respond at all to TI antigens. Again, however, there are exceptions, with some TI antigens being immunogenic in infants.

The kinetics of an antibody response to TI antigens is informative with regard to the mechanism by which they stimulate B cells. Whereas the peak antibody levels are seen within 2 to 4 weeks of immunization, much like a protein, high levels of antibody to TI antigens can persist for 5 to 8 years after a single injection. In some instances, the preexisting serum level of antibodies to a TI antigen that are present before an immunization will predict the overall level of antibodies produced in response to the antigen, although this can be modified by other basic immunogenic properties of the antigen. Thus, it seems that some individuals are genetically or otherwise predisposed to make good antibody responses to particular TI antigens. However, what does universally typify an immune response to a TI antigen is the lack of a memory response. Thus, following immunization serum antibody levels peak within a month and slowly decline over a 5 to 8 year period. Repeated injections at short intervals following the initial injection do not result in a booster or anamnestic response. Individuals who are revaccinated after there has been a decline in antibody levels will produce antibodies to the second challenge, but the overall levels will not exceed those achieved with the initial, single dose of TI antigen. Thus, the overall antibody level can be raised back up to the peak level achieved shortly after vaccination, but not beyond it. This contrasts with the response to a TD antigen, where repeated doses lead to increasing levels of antibody following each dose.

TD Antibody Response
Structure of TD Antigens

TD antigens comprise soluble proteins, peptides, whole cells, viruses, parasites and essentially any antigens that are unable to induce antibody production when T cells are not present (e.g., in athymic nude mice) (Table 10.1). APCs are critical components of the response to TD antigens due to their ability to take up aggregated or particulate antigens, process the protein antigens, and present the peptides to T cells. The processed TD antigens associate with MHC molecules at the surface of the APCs, thus allowing the APCs to interact with T cells in part through ligation of their TCR complex, as well as through binding of accessory and adhesion molecules.

Soluble proteins have been used as model antigens for studying the TD antibody response, since such proteins elicit no antibody response in the absence of mature T cells. The requirement for TH cells cannot be replaced merely by cytokines, and there must be a physical, cognate interaction between the TH cell and the B cell for to the latter to become activated and differentiate into an antibody-secreting cell.

T-cell help can also be delivered to a B cell when that B cell presents processed protein antigen to an antigen-specific T cell. To internalize antigens so that they may be processed and presented on MHC class II, a B cell can use its antigen receptor (mIg) for receptor-mediated endocytosis. Fluid-phase pinocytosis is an alternative, but a much less efficient, mode for uptake of antigen. The internalized protein antigen is processed by proteolysis into fragments 13 to 25 amino acids long, and these T-cell epitopes combine with MHC class II molecules in a subcellular compartment in the endocytic pathway of presentation. The MHC class II-peptide complex is then transported to the surface of the B cell, where it can be recognized by antigen-specific CD4 TH cells. The activated T cell then supplies contact-dependent, as well as soluble, activation signals to the B cell to initiate B-cell activation, proliferation, and differentiation.

Kinetics of TD Antibody Response

Upon primary immunization with an antigen, there is a lag phase when no specific antibodies are detectable in serum (Fig. 10.8). During this lag phase the antigen is recognized, processed, and presented to the appropriate TH cells of the immune system, which are themselves activat-ed and proliferate and differentiate into mature TH cells. These TH cells can then assist the full activation of B cells into antibody-producing plasma cells. After this lag phase (usually 7 to 10 days) antibodies specific to the antigen can be detected in serum. Antibodies of the IgM isotype dominate in the early *primary response*, whereas specific IgG appears in the serum days later after isotype switching has had an opportunity to occur. The antibody production decreases rapidly following clearance of the antigenic stimuli; the actual time before levels of circulating antibody return to baseline levels varies for different antigens.

When an individual encounters the same antigen again, the response to the antigen will be faster and more efficient. The *secondary antibody response* is superior to the primary response in several ways. The rate of production of antibody is higher during the secondary exposure, leading to rapid increases in serum antibody levels, and more total antibody is produced in a secondary response. Because of the ongoing process of somatic hypermutation and the accompanying process of affinity maturation, antibodies produced during the secondary response will have a higher affinity for the antigen. Finally, the antibodies produced during the secondary response represent several isotypes (IgG, IgA, and IgE) due to isotype switching that occurs late in the primary response. Antibodies of these isotypes carry out a broad array of effector functions.

T-Cell Dependence and Conjugate Vaccines

Children younger than 2 years of age and immunocompromised patients are especially susceptible to infections with encapsulated bacteria such as group B streptococci, *S. pneumoniae, Haemophilus influenzae* type b (Hib), and *Neisseria meningitidis*. Capsular polysaccharides from several of these bacteria have been purified and used as vaccine antigens and have been shown to induce protective immunity. However, the polysaccharides are TI-2 antigens and have only induced a moderate immune response in humans. Furthermore, booster injections or encounter with the pathogen after immunization with the polysaccharides has only been demonstrated to bring the antibody levels back to the original immunization levels without any augmented (booster) response or switching of the immunoglobulin produced to more efficient isotypes. All of these deficiencies in the antibody response result from the inability of TI-2 antigens to activate TH cells.

The application of the carrier-hapten principle of antigen presentation (see Fig. 8.8) was first described by Karl

Figure 10.8 Primary and secondary antibody response. The number of IgM antibodies in the secondary response varies with different antigens. It can be higher than that of the primary response, lower, or in some instances, not detectable. However, in the secondary response, IgG, and sometimes IgA, predominates and accounts for most of the total specific antibody.

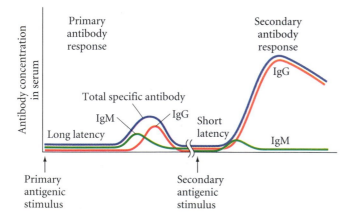

Landsteiner in 1924. The first successful synthesis of a conjugate bacterial vaccine was accomplished by Oswald Avery and Walter Goebel in the 1930s. They conjugated pneumococcal type III capsular polysaccharide to horse serum globulin and demonstrated a booster response to the polysaccharide upon repeated vaccination in rabbits. In the past decade, many research groups have tried to convert the response of TI antigens to that of a TD antigen by covalently coupling the TI polysaccharide antigen to carrier proteins in an attempt to increase the immunogenicity of the polysaccharide.

Such glycoprotein conjugates have been used successfully as vaccine antigens. Hib polysaccharide-protein conjugate vaccines are immunogenic and protective against invasive Hib infection and reduce oropharyngeal carriage of Hib. Infection with Hib has been eradicated in several countries owing to successful vaccination of all infants with Hib conjugate vaccines. The immunoglobulin isotype switch induced after immunization with Hib conjugated to a carrier protein has been demonstrated in rodents but

Figure 10.9 Recruiting T-cell help for polysaccharide (PS) antigens. The membrane immunoglobulin of the BCR-specific for PS can be cross-linked by the repeating epitopes of the PS component of a protein-PS conjugate vaccine. The conjugate is internalized by receptor-mediated endocytosis. The carrier protein is processed, and the oligopeptide T-cell epitopes form complexes with the MHC class II molecules, which are then transported to the cell surface. The peptide-MHC class II complex is presented to T cells specific for the carrier T-cell epitopes. The TH is activated and secretes cytokines that activate the B cells, thus stimulating the B cell to differentiate and giving rise to a clone of anti-polysaccharide-producing cells. Adapted from G. R. Siber, *Science* 265:1385–1387, 1994.

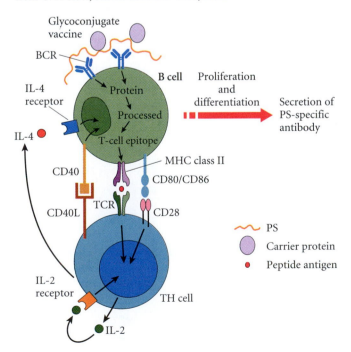

not in humans. Hib conjugate vaccines given to mice induce isotype switching from immunoglobulins of the IgM isotype to a preponderance of those of the IgG isotype. This IgG response consists of specific antibodies of all IgG subclasses, but the majority are IgG1. However, in humans, polyribosylribitol phosphate (PRP) gives rise to antibodies of IgG1 and IgG2 subclasses whether or not the polysaccharide is conjugated. Thus, TH cells are involved in the antipolysaccharide response but by a mechanism that is still not known. A model describing the mechanism of immune induction by glycoconjugate vaccines is displayed in Fig. 10.9; the surface immunoglobulins of polysaccharide-specific B cells are cross-linked by the carbohydrate-protein conjugate, with subsequent internalization of the antigen-receptor complex by receptor-mediated endocytosis. The protein component is subsequently processed by proteolysis. Some of the resultant peptides may form complexes with MHC class II molecules and be transported to the surface to be presented for appropriate peptide-MHC class II-specific TH cells. The activated TH cell begins to divide and secretes cytokines that activate the B cell, stimulating it to differentiate and give rise to a clone of antibody-producing plasma cells specific for the polysaccharide, as these B cells have originally bound the vaccine construct through the polysaccharide component.

B-Lymphocyte Interaction with T Lymphocytes

Contact Interaction between B and T Lymphocytes

Activation of B and T cells involves a reciprocal dialogue between the two cell types, resulting in the activation of both cell types. During this dialogue, the B cell serves as an APC to activate the TH cell, while the TH cell provides the B cell with activation signals essential for full B-cell activation. As with T-cell activation by other APCs, two signals are needed: signal 1 is delivered via the interaction of the MHC on APCs and the TCR on T lymphocytes, and the second, or co-stimulatory, signal (signal 2) is usually delivered by the binding of CD80 and CD86 on B cells to CD28 on T cells. CD80 and CD86 can also bind to CTLA-4 (cytotoxic T lymphocyte antigen 4) on T cells, but this results in an inhibitory signal to the T cell. In addition, there is a recently described set of additional coreceptors that is intimately involved in B-cell–T-cell interactions and important for induction of B-cell immunoglobulin isotype switching: inducible costimulator (ICOS) on T cells and ICOS ligand (also called B7h, B7-related protein, or B7RP-1) on B cells. The interaction of CD40 on B cells and CD40 ligand (CD40L) on T cells

Table 10.2 Coligands involved in B-cell–T-cell interactions

B cell	T cell
MHC class II	TCR/CD3, CD4
CD40	CD40L (gp39)
CD80 (B7-1)	CTLA-4, CD28
CD86 (B7-2)	CD28, CTLA-4
B7h	ICOS
CD19	?
CD21	CD23
CD22	CD45RO, ?
CD54 (ICAM-1)	LFA-1 (CD11c/18)
LFA-1 (CD11c/18)	CD54 (ICAM-1)
LFA-3	CD2
CD58	
CD59	
CD72	CD5
CD5 (subset of B cells)	CD72

is also integral to B-cell activation. Other sets of receptors and counterreceptors (Table 10.2) are involved in T-cell–B-cell interactions, but these other interactions only augment the response of the costimulatory ligands by further stabilizing the T-cell–B-cell interaction and decreasing the threshold of B-cell activation. The combined action of signals 1 and 2 leads to activation of T lymphocytes, which release cytokines that in turn activate the B lymphocytes.

CD80 and CD86

The CD80 and CD86 molecules are part of the B7 family of immune activators, which is a group of structurally and functionally related proteins expressed by B cells and other APCs. These are essential regulators of T-cell activation by antigen-presenting B cells. The family was originally designated as B7 molecules but is more recently identified using the CD nomenclature: CD80 is also referred to as B7-1 or BB1, and CD86 is also referred to as B7-2. The more recently discovered B7h protein has not yet been given a CD designation.

The B7 proteins are members of the immunoglobulin superfamily and consist of a single immunoglobulin V-like region and a single immunoglobulin C2-set domain (Fig. 10.10). CD80 is approximately 50 to 60 kDa after posttranscriptional glycosylation (30 kDa when unmodified). Expression of the B7 proteins on B cells is stimulated by numerous molecules and signals, including LPS, dextran, MHC cross-linking, and CD40 engagement. In fact, CD80 was first identified as a B-cell activation marker, since it is not expressed on resting B cells but can only be detected 24 to 72 hours after B-cell activation.

CD86 is similar to CD80 in overall structure, although the timing of expression of CD86 is different from that of CD80; expression of CD80 is increased much more rapidly after B-cell stimulation and is detectable on B-cell membranes in less than 24 hours. The molecular mass of unglycosylated human CD86 is 34 kDa. The difference between the molecular masses of CD80 and CD86 is attributable to 44 extra amino acids in the cytoplasmic tail of CD86. Unlike CD80, the cytoplasmic tail of CD86 contains three potential sites of phosphorylation by PKC, which may account for some differences in function and expression of these two molecules. Both CD80 and CD86 contain numerous sites for N-linked glycosylation and both are probably heavily glycosylated. For both humans and mice, homology between CD80 and CD86 is approximately 25%. The areas of greatest homology are in the immunoglobulin-like regions and are likely related to their ligand functions (i.e., they are the binding sites for CD28 and/or CTLA-4). In contrast, there is little homology between the cytoplasmic tails of CD80 and CD86.

CD80 and CD86 have different functions that are most likely related to their differing affinities for CD28 and CTLA-4 on T cells. CD80 has a much higher affinity for CTLA-4 than for CD28. CTLA-4 engagement is thought to terminate T-cell activation; therefore, CD80 may primarily initiate this function. Also, costimulation of TH cells by CD80 has been found to influence the TH1/TH2 polarity differently than costimulation by CD86, with CD80 preferentially stimulating a TH1 phenotype and CD86 preferentially stimulating a TH2 phenotype. Given the important role of TH1/TH2 cytokines on both B-cell activation and isotype selection, the relative strength of CD80 and CD86 costimulation may have a profound

Figure 10.10 Schematic representation of B-cell costimulatory ligands CD80 (B7-1) and CD86 (B7-2). P, areas of tyrosine phosphorylation.

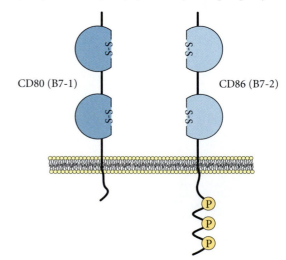

impact on the intensity and quality of the humoral immune response.

CD40 and CD40L

CD40 is an integral membrane protein on the surface of B lymphocytes, DCs, and FDCs. CD40 binds to CD40L (also designated CD154 and gp39) on T lymphocytes. This interaction initiates a host of events that activate B cells, resulting in affinity maturation, isotype switching, and differentiation of proliferating B cells (B-cell blasts) to memory B cells (Fig. 10.11). CD40 interaction with CD40L increases the surface expression of the ligands involved in T cell costimulation (CD80 and CD86 on the B lymphocyte and CD28 and CTLA-4 on the T lymphocyte) and the CD40 receptors/coreceptors may be engaged and activated prior to the B7 proteins and their receptors.

CD40 is a 47- to 50-kDa glycoprotein made up of 277 amino acids with a 193-amino-acid extracellular domain, a 22-amino-acid transmembrane region, and a 62-amino-acid cytoplasmic tail. Human CD40 and murine CD40 share 62% amino acid identity in the extracellular domain and 78% identity in the intracellular regions. CD40 is a member of a new superfamily of cellular proteins designated originally as the p75 low-affinity nerve growth factor receptor family but now more commonly termed the *tumor necrosis factor receptor* family. Members of this family include the receptors for TNF-α and TNF-β, CD27, CD30, OX40, 4-1BB, and Fas (also termed APO-1). The area of greatest amino acid sequence homology in this family is the extracellular region, which reflects the commonality of the binding function of these proteins. The transmembrane and cytoplasmic regions, in contrast, demonstrate greater sequence divergence, thus reflecting the different responses induced by the binding

of the particular ligands to each receptor. CD40 is expressed on all B cells, including mIgD⁺/mIgM⁺ and mIgD⁻/mIgM⁺ B cells, even before the full assembly of mIg genes (Fig. 10.2). Because of this, CD40 was originally thought to be a pan-B-cell marker. However, CD40 is not expressed on plasma cells. CD40 also is found on other APCs, as well as FDCs, T cells, endothelial cells, smooth muscle cells, cardiac myocytes, gastrointestinal mucosa, gallbladder mucosa, bronchus mucosa, and thyroid and parathyroid cells.

Human CD40L consists of 261 amino acids, with 215 in the extracellular domain, 24 in the transmembrane region, and 22 in the cytoplasmic tail. Both murine and human CD40L have an N-linked glycosylation site in their extracellular region. Their amino acid sequence is 78% identical for the whole molecule, 75% for the extracellular region, 96% for the transmembrane region, and 81% for the cytoplasmic tail. CD40L is a member of the TNF superfamily with the typical structure of two packed sheets of eight β-parallel strands in a "β-jellyroll" formation. Other members of this family include TNF-α and TNF-β and ligands for CD27, CD30, and 4-1BB. Their amino acid sequences are not highly similar, but specific regions have conserved amino acids to account for the common tertiary structure. CD40L is expressed primarily on CD4-positive T cells, but it has been demonstrated on CD8-positive T cells and can be detected within 1 to 2 hours after activation on TH0, TH1, and TH2 cell types. Lung mast cells and basophils also express CD40, which is consistent with the ability of basophils to cause B cells to switch isotypes and secrete IgE.

The cytoplasmic domain of CD40 has been shown to be important in signal transduction in B cells. Cross-linking of CD40 results in increased tyrosine phosphorylation of various cellular products, including the Src family kinase p53/56^{lyn} and the p85 subunit of PI3K (increasing its PI3K activity). Most significantly, binding of CD40 by CD40L on T cells increases phosphorylation of PLCγ2, but not PLCγ1. PLCγ2 is essential for B-cell activation, and its activation is consistent with the fact that CD40 ligation increases IP$_3$ levels inside B cells. CD40-CD40L interactions are essential for antigen-driven, T-cell–dependent B-cell activation; they cause resting B cells to enter the cell cycle. Such activation is enhanced by the cytokines IL-4, IL-10, and IL-13.

CD40-dependent B-cell activation is also essential for B-cell maturation and isotype switching, but the specificity of the isotypes is dependent on other cytokines. Evidence of the importance of CD40-CD40L interactions for B-cell maturation and isotype switching is seen in patients with defects in CD40L, which results in a distinct

Figure 10.11 Effect of CD40-CD40L interaction on B cells. Binding of B-cell CD40 to CD40L on T cells elicits a set of events that are essential for efficient B-cell function and antibody production, including isotype switching to IgG and induction of memory B cells. Based on F. H. Durie et al., *Immunol. Today* **15:**406–411, 1994.

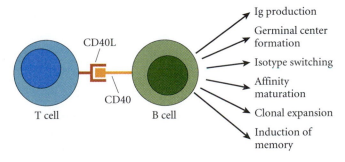

immunodeficiency, X-linked hyper-IgM syndrome. This disease is characterized by increased levels of IgM in serum and reduced levels of IgG, IgA, and IgE. These patients are susceptible to infections by microorganisms against which protection is usually mediated by humoral responses, e.g., encapsulated bacteria. Finally, CD40 activation of B cells seems to be involved in generation of memory B cells.

On T cells, CD40-CD40L interactions can be mediated by a variety of APCs that work in concert with MHC-TCR interactions to further increase the expression of CD40L. When B cells are acting as APCs, CD40 ligation by CD40L also increases the expression of various other cell surface proteins, including CD80, CD86, MHC class II, CD19, CD20, and even more CD40. Thus, it may be that T cells are activated by non-B-cell APCs, such as DCs, resulting in activation of the T cell and further increases in both CD40L and CD28 expression. This activated T cell then can interact with B cells via both MHC class II-TCR and CD40-CD40L. Interaction between CD40 on B cells and CD40L on T cells first increases CD86 expression, thereby increasing the engagement of CD28 on the T cells and resulting in further T-cell activation, which in turn causes increased secretion of different cytokines (e.g., IL-2, IL-4, IL-5, IL-10) that may affect B-cell activity and antibody secretion (Fig. 10.12). CD80 expression, which occurs later in the process (24 to 72 hours), may preferentially bind CTLA-4, inducing a negative response, which decreases T-cell activation and thereby allows the T cell to differentiate into memory T cells.

ICAM-1 and LFA-1

Despite the fact that MHC-TCR, CD40-CD40L, and B7-CD28 appear to be the main pairs of ligands that interact and are involved with B-cell activation, it is clear that they are not the only means by which T and B cells communicate with each other. The CD11a/CD18 (LFA-1)–CD54 (ICAM-1) interaction is also extremely important in controlling B-cell activation. Several lines of evidence support this hypothesis: (i) an active form of CD11a/CD18 is rapidly induced on T cells upon cross-linking of the TCR; (ii) antigen-specific T-cell activation induces a signal to the antigen-presenting B-cell that is dependent on the interaction of CD11a/CD18 with B-cell CD54; and (iii) cross-linking of CD40 on B cells can promote T-cell proliferation that is dependent on the interaction of CD11a/CD18 with B-cell CD54. In addition, patients who have defects in leukocyte adhesion who do not express CD11a/CD18 produce antigen-specific IgM and IgG, but at much lower levels, implying that this complex, interacting with CD54, is important in augmenting antigen-specific immunoglobulin production and induction of B-cell memory. The

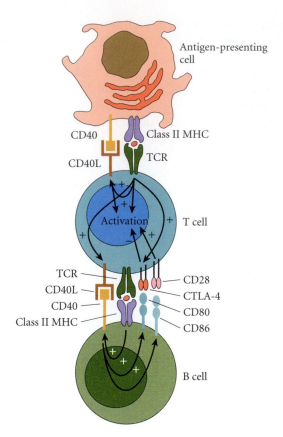

Figure 10.12 Involvement of costimulatory ligands and CD40-CD40L in B- and T-cell activation. A schematic representation of the positive and, possibly, negative effects of the engagement of CD40 on expression of CD40L, B7-1, B7-2, CD28, and CTLA-4 on B cells and T cells. Lymphocyte activation requires two signals. For TD antigens, one signal is transmitted via antigen presentation by MHC class II to the TCR. For TI antigens, the separation of the two signals into distinct entities is less clear, as it appears that the antigen binding to the B cell provides both signals for B-cell activation.

mechanism by which ICAM-1 regulates B-cell activation is not known with certainty. For years, many immunologists believed that the role of ICAM-1 and LFA-1 was simply to tether the B cell to the T cell to maximize the opportunities for other receptors to bind their coreceptors. However, more recent experimental data demonstrate that ICAM-1 engagement induces intracellular signaling, including Ca^{2+} flux and tyrosine phosphorylation. Therefore, ICAM-1 may contribute to B-cell activation by initiating signal-transduction cascades in addition to its important role in B-cell–T-cell adhesion.

Effect of Cytokines on B-Cell Activation and Antibody Production

One of the main regulatory mechanisms for isotype switching and induction of antibody production is the secretion of cytokines by the T lymphocytes. Although it is true that CD40/CD40L interactions initiate isotype switching, cytokines determine which immunoglobulin isotype(s) is produced after the switching occurs. Activated TH1 cells secrete primarily cytokines involved with cell-mediated responses, e.g., IL-2, interferon-gamma (IFN-γ), and IL-12, whereas TH2 cells secrete primarily cytokines involved with the humoral immune response and antibody production, e.g., IL-4, IL-5, IL-6, and IL-10 (Fig. 10.13). The distinction is not absolute, since one mouse Ig isotype, IgG2a, is produced under the influence of the TH1 cytokines. The cytokines with the greatest effect on IgA and IgE antibody production (IL-2, IL-4, and IL-5) are expressed primarily by the TH2 subset. Much of the research ascribing a role for a particular mix of cytokines in antibody production has been performed in murine models, but the same results appear to hold true for antibody production from human B lymphocytes.

Incubation of activated murine B cells with supernatants from activated TH2 clones, primarily containing IL-4 and IL-5, results in significant production of IgE, IgG1, and IgA. When the cytokines present in the supernatant were used individually, purified IL-4 had a great capacity to induce IgE isotype switching and antibody production, along with IgG1 and IgM, but had no effect on IgA production. Total inhibition of IgE production by the addition of anti-IL-4 MAb demonstrated the dependence of IgE production on IL-4. Antibodies of other isotypes (IgG1 and IgM) were only partially inhibited by the addition of anti-IL4 MAb. IL-5 alone induced IgA production and positively affected IgM production but did not affect either IgE or IgG1 production. IL-4 and IL-5 act synergistically. IL-5 can augment the IgE, IgM, and IgG1 production induced by suboptimal levels of IL-4. Similarly, IL-4 can augment the response to IL-5-induced IgA production. IgM production is induced by LPS-acti-

Figure 10.13 Effect of cytokines on B-lymphocyte antibody production. Various cytokines can affect the B cells by priming them for activation and by directing the isotypes of the antibodies they produce. IL-2 can induce production of IgG2a (in mice) and IgG3 (in humans). IFN-γ has a negative effect on antibody production. IL-4 stimulates immunoglobulin production of isotypes IgG, IgG1, and IgE, whereas IL-5 induces IgM and IgG1 with no effect on IgE production. Based on Fig. 2 and 3 of R. F. Coffman et al., *Immunol. Rev.* **102:**5–28, 1988.

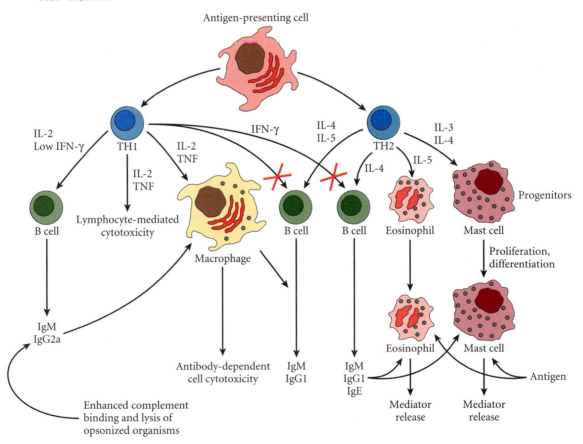

vated B cells whether these cytokines are present or not, but the cytokines are necessary to increase IgM production when B cells are activated by TD antigens.

Many TH1 clones stimulate immunoglobulin production rather poorly compared with that stimulated by TH2 clones. Even though TH1 clones can stimulate B cells to an extent similar to TH2 clones, the level of immunoglobulin production is only 5% of that induced by TH2 clones. This finding suggests that the TH1 clones produce molecules that inhibit immunoglobulin production or that they do not produce enough cytokines necessary for antibody production. IFN-γ and IL-2 are the two main cytokines produced by TH1-type cells. The potent effect on antibody production by IL-4 can be inhibited by IFN-γ but is minimally affected by IL-2. The addition of IFN-γ to B cells cotreated with IL-4 can result in inhibition of the normal IL-4 induction of IgE, IgG1, and IgM antibodies. This is likely due to downregulation of CD40L expression on T cells. The production of IgE is inhibited to a much greater extent by IFN-γ than is production of IgG1 or IgM. When B cells are stimulated to produce antibodies by TH1 cells (which normally results in low levels of antibody production), antibody production can be enhanced by treatment with anti-IFN-γ MAb treatment. Since in this case the B cells are being stimulated by T cells that do not produce IL-4, these data imply that the IFN-γ inhibitory effect on immunoglobulin production is not just specific for IL-4. Indeed, IL-2 (which is also produced by TH1 clones) can induce significant immunoglobulin production, and this positive influence of IL-2 can, in many circumstances, be inhibited by IFN-γ.

A summary of the effect of cytokines on antibody production is displayed in Fig. 10.13 and Table 10.3. APCs present antigen to TH cells—both or either TH1- and TH2-type cells—and various cytokines are released. The TH2 cytokines will affect B cells by inducing IgM, IgG1, and IgE production; this effect can be inhibited by IFN-γ production by stimulated TH1 cells. In addition, TH1 cytokines in the right proportions (relatively high IL-2 levels with relatively low IFN-γ levels) can induce immunoglobulin production, most significantly IgG2a in

mice or IgG1 in humans. Murine IgG2a and human IgG1 bind complement (C1q) and bind to their respective Fc receptors to a much greater extent than do the other IgG subtypes or other isotypes. This finding suggests that although most B-cell antibody production and isotype switching appears to be controlled by TH2-type cytokines, the subtypes likely associated with some protective ability against microorganisms (murine IgG2a or human IgG1) can be induced only by TH1–B-cell interactions.

Isotype Switching

After antigen stimulation, B-cell activation and proliferation occur followed by the production of antibody of isotypes other than IgM. This mechanism of isotype switching enables antibodies of a given antigenic specificity to change their biologic effector function by switching H chains encoded by constant region genes. Isotype switching involves genetic rearrangements (see Fig. 7.28) that bring rearranged V(D)J regions encoding antigenic specificity into close proximity of the different constant region genes, splicing out of intervening DNA and leading to production of mRNA for a different immunoglobulin isotype. The cytokines involved in isotype switching are thought to function by making the switch recombination sites accessible to switch recombinases, which results in the genetic rearrangements that lead to the isotype switching. Along with the observation that the molecular defect in patients with hyper-IgM syndrome is a defective CD40L gene, recent data from transgenic mice also indicate that CD40 on B cells is essential for T-cell-dependent immunoglobulin class switching and germinal center formation, but not for in vivo T-cell-dependent IgM responses and T-cell-independent antibody responses. CD40-deficient mice mounted IgM responses but no IgG, IgA, and IgE response to a TD antigen. However, the mutant mice showed normal IgG and IgM responses to both TI-1 and TI-2 antigens. More recent data indicate that the presence of B7h on B cells, which participates in T-cell activation and costimulation via an interaction with ICOS on the T cells, is also important for induction

Table 10.3 Different cytokines and prostaglandin E_2 induce switching of specific immunoglobulin to different isotypes

Immunomodulator	IgM	IgG3	IgG1	IgG2b	IgG2a	IgA	IgE
IL-4	−	−	+		−		+
IL-5						↑↑ Production	
IFN-γ	−	+	−		+		−
TGF-β[a]	−	−		+		+	
Prostaglandin E_2	−	−					+

[a] TGF, transforming growth factor.

of B-cell immunoglobulin isotype switching. Critical signals for T-cell-independent class switching are unknown. One possible mechanism is that signals elicited by cross-linking of the immunoglobulin receptors of the B cells by multivalent antigens, such as TI antigens, or by polyclonal B-cell activation, such as occurs with LPS, may be sufficient for induction of all the maturation events of B cells, including class switching.

The studies of these CD40-deficient mice suggest that the failure of class switching and secondary immune response are events inseparable from their failure to form germinal centers, since differentiation of memory B cells, affinity maturation, and immunoglobulin class switching of B cells are believed to take place in the germinal centers.

Apoptosis: the Flip Side of B-Cell Activation

To control B-cell activation and prevent overproduction of antibody and possible induction of autoimmune responses, B cells must be killed when their continued activation becomes undesirable. Examples of such circumstances include the acquisition of self-reactivity during somatic hypermutation and the end of a normal immune response after clearance of the stimulating antigen from the host's body. The early development of the immune response is also a critical point for control of B-

cell activation during which autoimmune B cells can be induced. The induction of apoptosis of B cells is therefore extremely important in the regulation of the humoral immune response.

Engagement of B cells by antigen does not necessarily induce B-cell activation. One example has already been given in this chapter: when preformed antigen-antibody complexes simultaneously bind to the BCR and the Fc receptor FcγRIIB1. This results in the dephosphorylation of the cytoplasmic tails of the BCR, causing B-cell tolerance. The lack of this mechanism for inhibition of B-cell activation in moth-eaten mice allows for the overwhelming autoimmune reactions in these animals.

B-cell apoptosis can be initiated when the MHC class II of an already activated B cell is cross-linked. The function of this regulatory mechanism may be to dampen B-cell-mediated T-cell activation once the immune response is activated. Apoptosis can also be induced when CD40L on B cells is engaged in the absence of antigen binding to the BCR. If CD40-CD40L interactions occur in the presence of specific antigen or anti-IgM cross-linking antibody (which will bind to the BCR), Fas-dependent cell death does not occur. This regulatory mechanism may help terminate the immune response once the antigen has been cleared. In addition, this mechanism of B-cell apoptosis may constitute a fail-safe mechanism to eliminate *bystander* (antigen-nonspecific) B cells activated via CD40-CD40L interactions with activated

Figure 10.14 Summary of the outcome of B-cell interaction with antigen and B-cell activation.

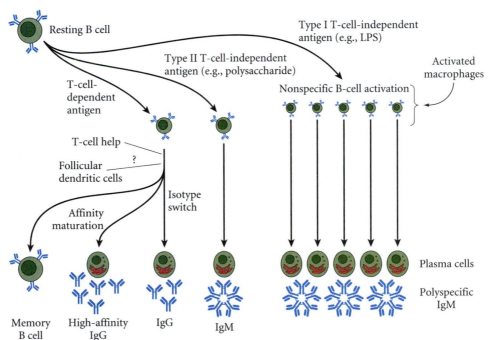

TH cells. Similar to what is observed with most types of leukocytes, the Fas and FasL interaction is essential in mediating B-cell death.

Summary

B lymphocytes are essential for protection from diseases in which antibodies and antibody-mediated protective mechanisms are essential. Antigen binding to mIg of the BCR complex can activate the B cell if the antigen can cross-link the BCR, as typically seen with TI antigens (e.g., carbohydrates), or if antigen-specific T cells can interact with the B cell, as typically seen with TD antigens (e.g., proteins). These events set off a cascade of signal-transduction events. The antigen can be presented to the B cell by FDCs in the germinal center lymph node, the primary area of B-cell maturation. Stimulated B cells produce immunoglobulin. In the case of TD antigens, B cells obtain T-cell help by cell-cell contact and/or cytokine release. The proper cytokines or involvement of interactions between T- and B-cell ligands (CD40-CD40L and B7-2-CD28) can cause B cells to undergo isotype switching and affinity maturation. B cells can also act as APCs and present processed peptides to T cells. Therefore, B cells are activated by TD antigens via two mechanisms: (i) when the antigen is intact, by directly binding the antigen on the BCR, and (ii) after the specific antigen is processed, by binding the processed antigen peptide to the MHC class II protein, presenting the peptide in the context of specific MHC to T cells, and if other B-cell–T-cell ligands interact, eliciting T-cell help to further activate the antigen-specific B cell. This does not occur for TI antigens, such as polysaccharides, as they cannot recruit T cells to augment the B-cell response to them, which is the reason for making protein conjugates: to improve the immune response to polysaccharide-based vaccines. The outcome of B-cell activation and the effect of all the various modulators of B-cell responses are summarized in Fig. 10.14.

Suggested Reading

Berland, R., and H. H. Wortis. 2002. Origins and functions of B-1 cells with notes on the role of CD5. *Annu. Rev. Immunol.* **20:**253–300.

Billadeau, D. D., and P. J. Leibson. 2002. ITAMs versus ITIMs: striking a balance during cell regulation. *J. Clin. Investig.* **109:**161–168.

Bishop, G. A., and B. S. Hostager. 2001. Signaling by CD40 and its mimics in B cell activation. *Immunol. Res.* **24:**97–109.

Frauwirth, K. A., and C. B. Thompson. 2002. Activation and inhibition of lymphocytes by costimulation. *J. Clin. Investig.* **109:**295–299.

Justement, L. B. 2001. The role of the protein tyrosine phosphatase CD45 in regulation of B lymphocyte activation. *Int. Rev. Immunol.* **20:**713–738.

Kurosaki, T. 2002. Regulation of B-cell signal transduction by adaptor proteins. *Nat. Rev. Immunol.* **2:**354–363.

Martin, F., and J. F. Kearney. 2002. Marginal-zone B cells. *Nat. Rev. Immunol.* **2:**323–335.

Poe, J. C., M. Hasegawa, and T. F. Tedder. 2001. CD19, CD21, and CD22: multifaceted response regulators of B lymphocyte signal transduction. *Int. Rev. Immunol.* **20:**739–762.

Sharpe, A. H., and G. J. Freeman. 2002. The B7-CD28 superfamily. *Nat. Rev. Immunol.* **202:**116–126.

van Eijk, M., T. Defrance, A. Hennino, and C. de Groot. 2001. Death-receptor contribution to the germinal-center reaction. *Trends Immunol.* **22:**677–682.

Veillette, A., S. Latour, and D. Davidson. 2002. Negative regulation of immunoreceptor signaling. *Annu. Rev. Immunol.* **20:**669–707.

Wienands, J., and N. Engels. 2001. Multitasking of Ig-alpha and Ig-beta to regulate B cell antigen receptor function. *Int. Rev. Immunol.* **20:**679–696.

Zubler, R. H. 2001. Naive and memory B cells in T-cell-dependent and T-independent responses. *Springer Semin. Immunopathol.* **23:**405–419.

CELLULAR IMMUNITY

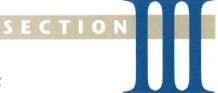

SECTION III

chapter 11

The Major Histocompatibility Complex

Jeffrey B. Lyczak

Recognition of antigen by T cells does not occur through a direct interaction between the T-cell antigen receptor (TCR) and the free, native antigen. Instead, this recognition event requires the processing of antigenic proteins into short peptides and the subsequent binding of these peptides to transmembrane proteins known as the *major histocompatibility complex* (MHC) proteins. The MHC proteins display peptides on the surface of an antigen-presenting cell (APC). Since T lymphocytes recognize antigen only when the antigen is bound to MHC proteins, the latter play a central role in the acquired immune response.

Discovery of the MHC Gene Complex

The first experimental data suggesting the importance of the MHC were obtained in the 1930s by Peter Gorer, who was studying blood group antigens in mice. Gorer had identified four independently segregating genetic regions that encode blood group antigens and named them groups I, II, III, and IV. Later experiments demonstrated that the antigens in group II were crucial for determining the acceptance or rejection of solid tissue grafts. Since this group of antigens regulated the compatibility of the engrafted tissue with its recipient, these antigens were referred to as *histocompatibility antigens* and, more specifically, as *histocompatibility-2 (or H-2) antigens*. The term H-2 is now used specifically to denote the MHC of mice (Fig. 11.1), whereas the term *human leukocyte antigen* (*HLA*) refers to the MHC in humans. The primary function of the MHC gene products is the presentation of antigenic peptides to T lymphocytes, a function discovered in the 1970s that resulted in the award of the 1996 Nobel Prize in physiology and medicine to Peter Doherty and Rolf Zinkernagel.

261

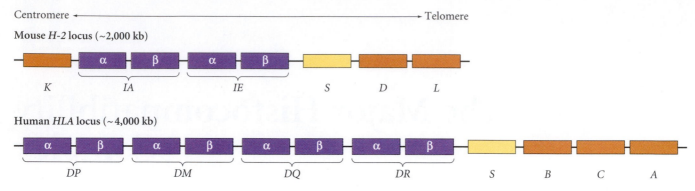

Figure 11.1 General organization of the mouse and human MHC gene clusters. MHC class I genes (orange), which encode proteins that present antigen to CD8$^+$ T cells, are called K, D, and L in mice and A, B, and C in humans. The genes encoding the class II proteins (blue), whose products present antigens to CD4$^+$ T cells, are called IA and IE in mice and DP, DQ, and DR in humans. The class II proteins are the product of two genes (one encoding an MHC α chain and one encoding an MHC β chain). The MHC class III proteins, encoded by genes that lie within the S region, do not function in presentation of antigenic peptides to T lymphocytes. The location of the genes encoding the class III proteins is shown in yellow.

General Arrangement of the MHC Gene Complex

In both mice and humans, all the genes that encode the MHC proteins are present at one genetic region. In the mouse genome, the MHC is a region of chromosome 17 approximately 2,000 kilobases (kb) long (Fig. 11.1). The genes in the MHC are categorized into three classes on the basis of the structure and function of the proteins they encode. Genes encoding the MHC class I products are located at both ends of the MHC, whereas the genes encoding the MHC class II and class III proteins are located between the two class I regions. The MHC class I proteins serve to present antigenic peptides to CD8$^+$ T lymphocytes. MHC class II proteins function in the presentation of antigenic peptides to CD4$^+$ T lymphocytes. Many MHC class III proteins have immune functions unrelated to antigen processing. The class III region of the MHC is also termed the *S region*.

The arrangement of the human MHC genes on chromosome 6 is similar to that of the mouse (Fig. 11.1) except that the human complex is larger (~4,000 kb). The most striking difference in the general arrangement of the mouse and human MHC is the positioning of the entire human MHC class I region at the telomeric end of the complex, with the class II region at the centromeric end. The human MHC class I and class II proteins serve the same functions in antigen presentation as do their mouse counterparts. Like the mouse gene complex, the human class III genes are located telomeric to the class II region and similarly serve several immune-related functions not directly relevant to antigen presentation.

Basic Nomenclature of MHC Genes and Proteins

One of the more perplexing aspects of the MHC is the nomenclature used to denote the genes within this complex. Because the MHC of the mouse is referred to as the H-2 and the gene complex in humans is called the HLA, any reference to these genetic regions or to genes within them is conventionally preceded by either H-2 or HLA, depending on the species. Other names used to denote MHC include the RT1 complex of the rat, the RLA complex of the rabbit, the GPL-A complex of the guinea pig, and the RhLA complex of the rhesus monkey.

Each Class of MHC Proteins Is Made Up of Functionally Related but Distinct Proteins

Mice produce three different types of MHC class I proteins called K, D, and L that are encoded by genes more properly referred to as the H-2K, H-2D, and H-2L genes, respectively, to denote their location within the mouse MHC. The K gene is located at the centromeric end of the H-2 complex, whereas D and L are at the telomeric end (Fig. 11.1). These three genes are expressed codominantly in virtually all nucleated cells of the body, although levels of expression can vary dramatically depending on the cell or tissue. Thus, each mouse cell actually expresses three different MHC class I proteins, each of which is capable of presenting antigenic peptides to CD8$^+$ lymphocytes (Fig. 11.2). The protein product of each MHC class I gene can display hundreds of different antigenic peptides for interaction with CD8$^+$ T lymphocytes. Therefore, a large number of different antigenic peptides,

Target cell

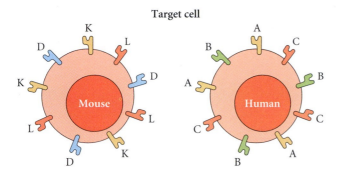

Antigen-presenting cell

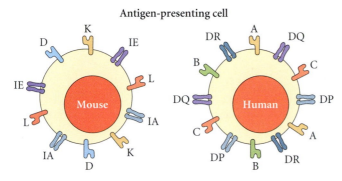

Figure 11.2 (Top) Virtually all cells in the body express MHC class I proteins. Both mice and humans possess three different genes that encode MHC class I proteins. In mice, the MHC class I genes (K, D, and L) are expressed codominantly. Nucleated cells in a mouse express K, D, and L MHC proteins, and nucleated cells in humans express A, B, and C MHC proteins. **(Bottom)** MHC class II proteins are expressed not by every cell but only by a subset of cells known as APCs. The genes encoding MHC class II proteins IA and IE also are expressed codominantly; therefore, every APC of a mouse expresses both IA and IE proteins. APCs express MHC class I proteins as well as MHC class II proteins.

likely thousands, can be bound to the three MHC class I proteins on the surface of each cell. Similar to the mouse gene complex, the human complex has three types of class I genes whose products participate in antigen presentation; these are properly referred to as HLA-A, HLA-B, and HLA-C. Although the arrangement of these genes is different from that of their mouse counterparts, the proteins they encode are similar to those encoded by the mouse K, D, and L genes and have similar functions. Like the mouse class I proteins, the HLA-A, HLA-B, and HLA-C proteins are all simultaneously expressed on virtually all nucleated cells of the body, similarly presenting a wide variety of antigenic peptides to CD8+ T lymphocytes.

MHC class II proteins differ significantly from class I proteins, in that expression of class II proteins is usually restricted to APCs. Cell types typically considered to be APCs are monocytes, macrophages, dendritic cells, and B lymphocytes. MHC class II proteins present antigenic peptides to CD4+ T cells. The mouse genome encodes

two different antigen-presenting MHC class II proteins, called IA and IE (Fig. 11.1), properly referred to as H-2IA and H-2IE. The genes encoding these proteins are clustered together and are located just telomeric to the H-2K gene region. Like MHC class I, cells that express MHC class II simultaneously express both types of class II proteins on a single APC along with MHC class I (Fig. 11.2). MHC class II proteins present a large number of antigenic peptides, such that each APC presents thousands of peptides to a T cell. Unlike the mouse MHC, the human MHC has three regions, called DP, DQ, and DR, giving rise to the HLA-DP, HLA-DQ, and HLA-DR class II proteins. Human MHC class II proteins function like their mouse counterparts, with human APCs expressing HLA-DP, HLA-DQ, and HLA-DR proteins on their surface (Fig. 11.2).

Each MHC class II protein consists of two transmembrane protein subunits (called the α and β chains). Therefore, each MHC class II protein is the product of two genes in the MHC. For purposes of differentiating the α and β chains of the different class II proteins, they are named according to both the MHC protein type and their chain type. However, since there can be more than one nonallelic gene for a particular chain located within a haplotype, the different nonallelic proteins are given a number. The β chain of the HLA-DR protein comes in different nonallelic forms designated as HLA-DRB1, HLA-DRB2, etc. However, there is only one gene per haplotype of the HLA-DR α chain, so it is designated HLA-DRA.

Polymorphism of Genes for Antigen-Presenting MHC Proteins

The genes of the MHC, like many genes, exist throughout the species in a number of allelic forms. Any gene that is maintained in the population in at least two allelic forms is said to be *polymorphic*. The genes of the MHC are unusual, however, in the large number of different alleles that exist at each locus, making the MHC loci highly polymorphic. For the human MHC class I proteins, there are at least 237 different alleles of the HLA-A gene, 472 different alleles of the HLA-B gene, and 113 different alleles of the HLA-C gene (for updated information, see http://www3.ebi.ac.uk/Services/imgt/hla/cgi-bin/statistics.cgi). The high level of MHC polymorphism is a critical factor in immune responses since different allelic forms of an MHC protein are capable of binding to different sets of antigenic peptides. The precedents used for naming the allelic forms of the MHC genes vary depending on the species. For the mouse, it is conventional to indicate the allele name for any given MHC gene with an italicized superscript immediate-

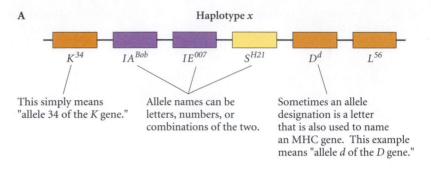

A   Haplotype *x*

K^{34} IA^{Bob} IE^{007} S^{H21} D^d L^{56}

This simply means "allele 34 of the *K* gene."

Allele names can be letters, numbers, or combinations of the two.

Sometimes an allele designation is a letter that is also used to name an MHC gene. This example means "allele *d* of the *D* gene."

B   Haplotype *b*

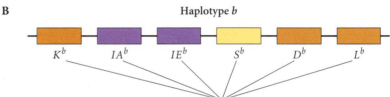

K^b IA^b IE^b S^b D^b L^b

Figure 11.3 Examples of the system used to name alleles of mouse MHC genes. Allele names, given after the name of the MHC protein, are in italicized superscript. (**A**) A hypothetical example. (**B**) The names used for an actual mouse haplotype (for the inbred mouse strain C57BL/6). The allele name *b* was taken from the name of the *b* haplotype.

For simplicity, most of the MHC alleles of inbred mouse strains were given the same names as the haplotype in which they were originally identified. The MHC alleles of haplotype *b* were also named the *b* alleles.

ly following the name of the MHC gene (e.g., *H-2K^d* designates the *d* allele of the mouse class I *K* gene) (Fig. 11.3A). In contrast, human MHC alleles are usually designated with numbers immediately following the name of the MHC gene (Table 11.1; see also http://www.anthonynolan.com/HIG/lists/nomenlist.html). The first designation would be for the gene. For example, HLA-B is a particular locus. For class II genes, wherein a class II protein is made up of two chains, the designation is further extended to include the specific chain. HLA-DRB1 refers to the beta 1 chain of HLA-DR; HLA-DRA refers to the alpha chain. There is only one alpha chain for the human DR class II protein, but multiple beta chains; hence, the beta chains are differentiated by a number. Next comes a designation for a group of related alleles preceded by an asterisk, i.e., HLA-B*08 or HLA-DR*13. The alleles within each group are designated with a second two-digit number, i.e., HLA-B*0801 or HLA-DRB1*1301. Further designations for genetic variations are given in Table 11.1. Official

designations are determined by the World Health Organization Nomenclature Committee for Factors of the HLA System.

Use of Inbred Mouse Strains in Experimental Immunology

Because of the central role of MHC proteins in the host immune response, it is critical to control for this variable in investigations dependent on MHC–T-cell interactions. For this reason, immunology experiments are usually conducted with inbred mouse strains. One of the basic principles of Mendelian genetics is that the alleles in a population will eventually become homogeneous if the population is inbred for a sufficient number of generations. If a mouse strain is inbred for a sufficient number of consecutive generations (usually more than 20 generations), all of the mice of that strain will have identical alleles of all of their genes. This is invaluable from an exper-

Table 11.1 Nomenclature of HLA alleles[a]

Nomenclature	Indicates
HLA	HLA gene complex and a prefix for an HLA gene
HLA-DRB1	Particular HLA locus, i.e., DRB1
HLA-DRB1*13	Group of alleles that encode the DRB1 chain
HLA-DRB1*1301	Specific allele of the DRB1 chain
HLA-DRB1*1301N	Null allele
HLA-DRB1*13012	Allele that differs by a synonymous mutation
HLA-DRB1*1301102	Allele that contains a mutation outside the coding region
HLA-DRB1*1301102N	Null allele that contains a mutation outside the coding region

[a] Reproduced with the permission of Steven G. E. Marsh, http://www.anthonynolan.org.uk/HIG.

imental standpoint, since it permits experiments in which the MHC alleles are identical among all of the individuals of an inbred mouse strain and the MHC no longer represents a source of unwanted experimental variability. In other cases, the MHC alleles can be varied in a controlled manner by selective breeding to allow systematic evaluation of the contributions of different MHC alleles to a given immune response. Such experimental control could never be obtained in a natural (outbred) population, in which virtually every individual animal has a different combination of MHC alleles.

With the establishment of inbred mouse strains starting in the 1940s and 1950s, researchers began assigning a "shorthand" name to the MHC alleles in each strain because they did not yet know the number and locations of the actual MHC genes. Thus, rather than listing the alleles of each MHC gene present in each mouse strain, early researchers referred to the entire MHC genetic region of each inbred mouse strain with a single letter. The term *haplotype* refers to the entire haploid set of MHC alleles contained within the MHC on one chromosome. Thus, the haplotype designation of a lowercase "k" in the mouse was originally defined as an arbitrary designation for a particular set of MHC alleles possessed by the mouse strain CBA. As years passed and other inbred mouse strains were generated, some were found to have the same set of MHC alleles as CBA and were said to be of the *H-2^k* haplotype (pronounced "H two of k" to distinguish it from the class I *H-2K* gene and protein that is simply pronounced "H-two-K" and written using a capital "K"). The MHC haplotypes of other strains that were established were found to be different from those of CBA and were assigned different one-letter designations.

Since each haplotype is a shorthand designation for an entire set of MHC alleles, it is also necessary to have a system for naming the allelic forms of the individual genes that lie within the MHC gene complex. The alleles of each MHC gene in inbred mouse strains are given the same designation as the haplotype in which they were originally defined. The *k* allele of the *H-2K* gene was derived from the *k* haplotype (written *H-2K^k* and pronounced "H-two-K of k"), and the *b* allele of the *H-2K* gene was derived from the *b* haplotype (i.e., *H-2K^b* pronounced "H-two-K of b") (Fig. 11.3B). Figure 11.4A shows the allelic designations of several commonly used inbred mouse strains. Note that some inbred mouse strains have all of the class I, II, and III genes assigned the same haplotype designation. Others, such as the A strain, have a mixed set of haplotype alleles based on the original haplotype designations, and this mixed set is given its own haplotype designation (strain A mice have the *H-2^a* haplotype). This occurs because, after designation

of the initial haplotypes, other inbred strains were found to have allelic variants from more than one haplotype. With many inbred mouse strains now available, there is a large range of mouse MHC haplotypes.

Since by strict definition the term haplotype refers to only one arbitrarily defined set (a haploid set) of MHC genes, each diploid animal bears two different haplotypes of MHC genes (one maternally inherited and one paternally inherited). This can be ignored with inbred mouse strains because the maternal and paternal haplotypes are identical. If mice from two different inbred strains are crossed, however, the F_1 progeny will possess two different MHC haplotypes as long as the two parental mouse strains have different MHC haplotypes. The haplotype of these F_1 progeny is designated by putting both MHC haplotypes in the italicized superscript separated by a slash (Fig. 11.4B and C).

MHC-Congenic Mouse Strains and Their Use in the Study of MHC Function

The establishment of inbred mouse strains with different MHC haplotypes was a major advance in immunologic research because it permitted the examination of immune responses in animals possessing known alleles of the MHC genes. However, comparisons between two different inbred mouse strains still suffer from one great disadvantage: two inbred mouse strains are likely to have allelic differences at many genetic loci in addition to the MHC. Thus, it is difficult to conclude that observed differences between two different mouse strains were due, in fact, to their different MHC haplotypes and not to some other, completely unrelated, allelic difference. For this reason, researchers have developed mouse strains known as MHC-congenic strains. Two mouse strains are said to be congenic if they are genetically identical at all genetic loci except one and are considered MHC-congenic if they are identical at all genetic loci except for a region of the MHC. The convention for naming MHC-congenic strains is to use the name of the strain that represents the majority of the genome, followed by a decimal point and the name of the strain from which the MHC is derived. An MHC-congenic strain with a genetic background from strain "A" at all of its genetic loci except the MHC, which is from strain "B," would be referred to as strain "A.B." If the immune responses of strains A and A.B are found to be different, the difference is likely to be due to the difference between the MHC alleles in the two strains since the MHC alleles represent the only genetic difference between the two strains.

MHC-congenic mouse strains are produced through selective-breeding protocols (Fig. 11.5A). The rationale

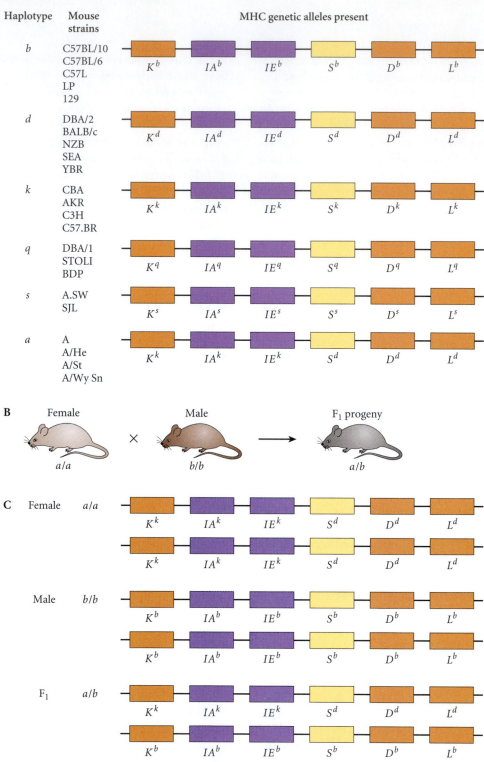

Figure 11.4 (A)The MHC haplotypes of some commonly used inbred mouse strains. The first five haplotypes, b, d, k, q, and s, have each of the corresponding genes in the MHC designated with the same letter as the overall haplotype. Strain A has the same alleles of the K, IA, and IE genes as strain C3H/HeJ (k), but for the S, D, and L regions, strain A mice have the same alleles as does the BALB/c mouse strain (d). (B) If two inbred mouse strains (e.g., strain A expressing the *a* H-2 haplotype and strain C57BL/6 expressing the *b* H-2 haplotype) are crossed, the F₁ progeny will be heterozygous at the MHC region. The MHC haplotype of the progeny is referred to as *H-2ᵃ/ᵇ*. (C) The MHC regions of both chromosomes in each of the mice depicted in panel B. The two parental mice are homozygous, whereas the F₁ is heterozygous and bears one MHC haplotype from each parent.

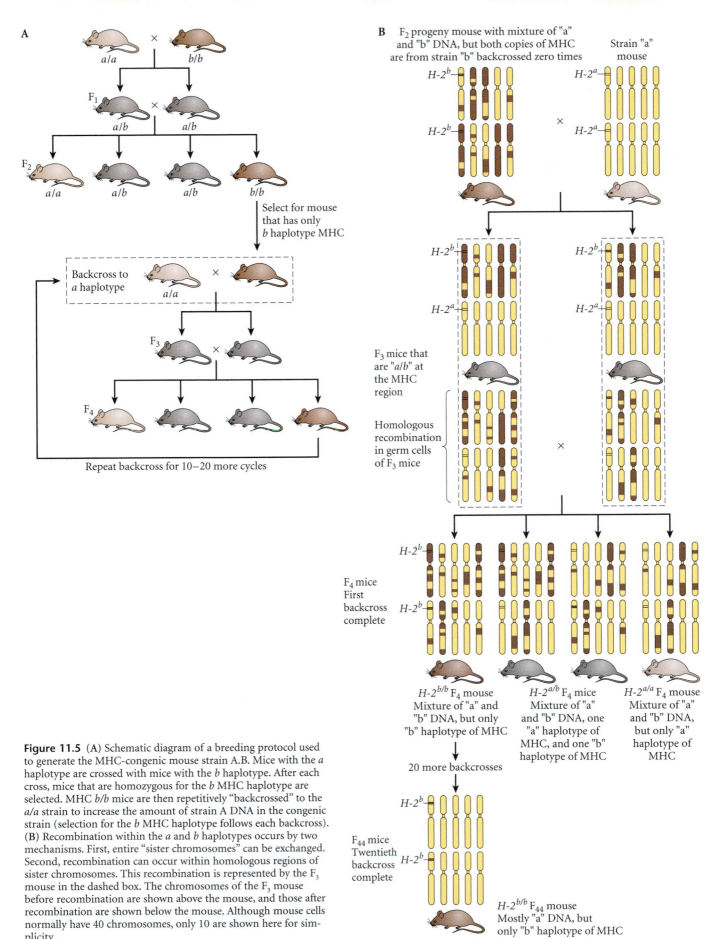

Figure 11.5 (A) Schematic diagram of a breeding protocol used to generate the MHC-congenic mouse strain A.B. Mice with the *a* haplotype are crossed with mice with the *b* haplotype. After each cross, mice that are homozygous for the *b* MHC haplotype are selected. MHC *b/b* mice are then repetitively "backcrossed" to the *a/a* strain to increase the amount of strain A DNA in the congenic strain (selection for the *b* MHC haplotype follows each backcross). (B) Recombination within the *a* and *b* haplotypes occurs by two mechanisms. First, entire "sister chromosomes" can be exchanged. Second, recombination can occur within homologous regions of sister chromosomes. This recombination is represented by the F₃ mouse in the dashed box. The chromosomes of the F₃ mouse before recombination are shown above the mouse, and those after recombination are shown below the mouse. Although mouse cells normally have 40 chromosomes, only 10 are shown here for simplicity.

behind the breeding protocol is to first combine the genetic backgrounds of strains A and B and then repeatedly "backcross" the progeny of the matings to a strain A mouse. Since each subsequent backcross introduces more DNA from strain A into the mice, the progeny of each successive backcross will contain a larger proportion of strain A DNA and less of strain B DNA. To integrate the strain B MHC into a strain A chromosome and replace the strain A MHC genes, breeders rely on intermixing due to genetic exchange between sister chromosomes that occurs by homologous recombination between identical regions of maternal and paternal chromosomes (Fig. 11.5B). The presence of the entire strain B MHC haplotype is detected at each backcross by screening the mice for strain B MHC alleles using a test that can differentiate strain A MHC responses from strain B MHC responses. One way this is accomplished is by engrafting a small piece of strain A skin onto each mouse. Mice that have MHC haplotype *a/a* or *a/b* will not reject the graft since their T cells will recognize the *a* haplotype MHC proteins of the graft as self tissue. However, mice that have the MHC haplotype *b/b* will regard the strain A graft as foreign and reject it. The mice that reject the skin graft are used for subsequent backcrosses.

Recombinant Congenic Mouse Strains

In breeding protocols such as the one depicted in Fig. 11.5, each mouse inherits one MHC haplotype from each parent. Although homologous recombination serves to intermix the DNA of both parents at each generation, such recombinational events within the MHC complex itself occur only rarely because of the relatively small size of the MHC complex ($\sim$2,000 kb in mice). Therefore, the MHC haplotype of each parent is usually inherited as a unit. However, recombination within the MHC complex is not impossible and occurs in about 1% of progeny. Moreover, recombination can encompass the entire MHC complex or only a small part of it, down to individual genes or even portions of genes. Thus, to produce mouse strains congenic at only part of the MHC complex, screening tests need to be used that differentiate responses due to allelic variation at a single gene. For example, a peptide that can be presented to *H-2IA*^{b} but not *H-2IA*^{d} can be used to identify recombinant mice from an *H-2IA*^{d} background that have acquired the *H-2IA*^{b} allele. Once the desired homologous recombination event within the MHC is found, these mice can be backcrossed into the strain with the original non-MHC background to produce *recombinant congenic* animals. These strains are given the same designation as the intended congenic strain except for the addition of the suffix "(R1)," "(R2)," etc., to denote these homologous recombinations within the MHC. Two examples of recombinant congenic haplotypes are shown in Fig. 11.6, where recombination occurs between haplotypes *H-2*^{s} and *H-2*^{d}. The homologous recombination events that give rise to the recombinant congenic haplotype can result in any combination of *s* and *d* alleles. The last example in Fig. 11.6 [strain SJL.D(R2)] shows the result of two homologous recombination events, the first one involving the entire MHC region and the second one limited to the MHC class II genes. The first crossover event introduced the entire *H-2*^{d} MHC region from the DBA/2 strain into the SJL strain (*H-2*^{s}). The second crossover event reintroduced the class

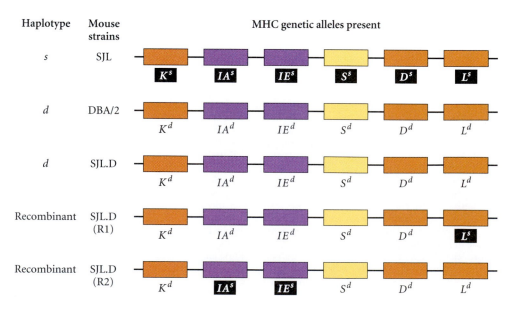

Figure 11.6 The MHC haplotypes of strains SJL (*H-2*^{s}) and DBA/2 (*H-2*^{d}), MHC-congenic strain SJL.D (*H-2*^{d}), and two recombinant congenic strains, SJL.D.(R1) and SJL.D(R2). Strain SJL.D has all of its alleles other than the MHC alleles identical to strain SJL alleles. Strain SJL.D(R1) was generated when a crossover event exchanging the D and L genes on sister chromosomes in heterozygous animals took place, whereas strain SJL.D(R2) is the result of a double crossover event, the first one introducing the entire *H-2*^{d} haplotype into the chromosome of an SJL mouse, and the second event reintroducing the *H-2*^{s} class II genes into the chromosome.

Haplotype	Mouse strains	MHC genetic alleles present					
s	SJL	K^s	IA^s	IE^s	S^s	D^s	L^s
d	DBA/2	K^d	IA^d	IE^d	S^d	D^d	L^d
d	SJL.D	K^d	IA^d	IE^d	S^d	D^d	L^d
Recombinant	SJL.D (R1)	K^d	IA^d	IE^d	S^d	D^d	L^s
Recombinant	SJL.D (R2)	K^d	IA^s	IE^s	S^d	D^d	L^d

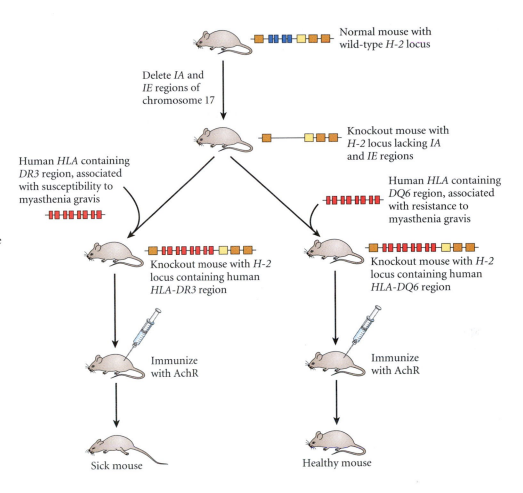

Figure 11.7 Production of MHC-transgenic mice and use in the study of disease. Recombinant DNA encoding different human HLA class II genes (DR3 or DQ6) is inserted into the genome of a starter or founder transgenic mouse lacking the mouse MHC class II genes within the *H-2* gene complex on chromosome 17. This results in transgenic mice expressing either human DR3 or DQ6, which will then serve to direct MHC-restricted T-cell selection. Mice expressing the human class II proteins are immunized with the acetylcholine receptor (AchR) to break tolerance and induce antibodies to AchR. Mice carrying human DR3 genes develop disease, whereas mice with DQ6 genes do not. In humans, HLA-DR3 is found more frequently among individuals with MG than is found in the general population, whereas HLA-DQ6 is found less frequently in individuals with MG than in the general population. Increased and decreased frequencies of allelic variants of genes in individuals with a disease such as MG suggest enhanced susceptibility or resistance to the disease, respectively.

II *IA*^{s} and *IE*^{s} from strain SJL back into the chromosome, but left the MHC genes from strain DBA/2 on both sides of the class II region. Recombinant congenic mice are important tools in immunologic research because they make it possible to dissect the immunologic roles of individual MHC genes. For example, a comparison of an immune response generated using the recombinant congenic animal SJL.D(R1) (Fig. 11.6) with strain SJL.D would allow the role of the class I L gene to be examined independently of that of the other MHC genes.

MHC-Transgenic Mouse Strains

Transgenic mouse technology now allows for the genes that encode MHC proteins to be introduced into a mouse strain as transgenes, obviating the need to develop MHC-congenic mouse strains or recombinant-congenic strains. Another advantage of MHC transgenes is that the MHC genes of one species can be inserted into the genome of a different species. Thus, immune responses to human tumor antigens or antigens derived from human pathogens can be studied in mice that bear human MHC genes. Since the MHC proteins in such mice include

human MHC, it is likely that some of the responding T cells will be specific for antigens that are relevant to the human form of the disease. In one recent study, this experimental system allowed a tumor-specific human cytotoxic T-lymphocyte clone to be studied in a tumor-bearing mouse that possessed a human MHC transgene. In this study, the antigenic peptide bound to the human MHC proteins and the TCR that recognized the antigen were similar to the peptides and TCR that might work during actual tumor rejection in a human patient.

The initiation of many autoimmune diseases is also affected by the alleles of MHC genes that are expressed by an individual animal, with some MHC alleles more likely than others to present self-antigenic peptides to autoreactive T cells. Transgenic mice expressing human MHC proteins but no mouse MHC proteins allow human autoimmune disease to be studied in a mouse model (Fig. 11.7). This was recently done to study the autoimmune disease myasthenia gravis (MG), a disease caused by an antibody response against an individual's own acetylcholine receptor. This antibody blocks nerve transmission across synapses, leading to muscle weakness and other symptoms. Transgenic mice carrying an allele of the human HLA class II complex associated with increased occurrences of MG were more likely to develop clinically significant disease when immunized with acetylcholine receptor molecules compared with transgenic mice that express a human HLA class II molecule that appears to confer resistance to MG. Thus, the APC in the mouse carrying the high-susceptibility human gene processed and presented the acetylcholine receptor antigen in a way that resulted in T-cell help for B cells producing antibody to this antigen, whereas the APC of the mouse with the MG-resistance HLA gene did not. Understanding how different MHC proteins process and present antigens such as autoantigens, and the importance of this for autoimmune diseases, will be a key component of better prevention and treatment strategies for these disorders.

MHC Genes and Linkage Disequilibrium

The large number of allelic variants giving rise to the high level of polymorphism within the MHC could potentially mean that almost every human has his or her own unique MHC genotype. If one multiplies together the number of known alleles for each HLA gene, thus indicating the potential number of HLA haplotypes, then over 10^{17} different haplotypes are possible. In reality, many fewer exist because of the phenomenon of *linkage disequilibrium.* This reflects the observation that the occurrence together on one chromosome of the same allelic variants is much higher than one would predict if allelic variation was randomly assorted over the entire MHC gene complex. This may be due to insufficient time for the different alleles to reach equilibrium in the human population. Since recent estimates indicate that modern humans were derived from a small ancestral population less than 200,000 years ago, the HLA haplotypes available for expansion would be limited. Alternately, certain combinations of HLA-A, -B and -C alleles along with HLA-DR, -DQ, and -DP may have advantageous properties operative under natural selection.

Diversity in MHC allelic variation is further constricted within certain population groups that may have arisen from a small founding population or that have undergone bottlenecks during human expansion and migration. Therefore, in different populations of humans different frequencies for HLA alleles are observed, and there are different patterns of linkage disequilibrium. In some haplotypes, referred to as *extended haplotypes,* the maintenance of the same allelic variants within a haplotype can extend for over 3 million bases. One notable haplotype found among Caucasians is the coinheritance of the HLA-A*010-B*0801-C*0701-DRB1*0301-DQA1*-0501-DQB1*0201-DPA1*0201-DPB1*0101. The maintenance of such strong

linkage disequilibrium has the fortuitous result of making tissue matches (required for successful tissue transplantation) more common than would be expected under conditions of totally random assortment of genetic alleles.

Structure of MHC Class I and Class II Proteins

The primary role of both MHC class I and class II proteins is the presentation of antigenic peptides to T lymphocytes. To accomplish this, both MHC class I and class II proteins must be able to bind antigenic peptides and to subsequently interact with the TCR (Fig. 11.8A). To do this, the peptide-presenting domains of the different MHC alleles must be variable. The MHC proteins must also be able to interact with the conserved CD8 (for MHC class I) or CD4 (for MHC class II) coreceptor molecules. This entails having a conserved part of the MHC molecule that can be recognized by the coreceptors. Because of these similar functions, class I and class II proteins share certain structural features. Both must have protein domains with a surface topology favorable for interaction with antigenic peptides and with the TCR, and both must have domains capable of binding to monomorphic CD4 or CD8.

Subunit Composition of MHC Class I and Class II Proteins

Both MHC class I and class II are heterodimeric proteins (Fig. 11.8B). The two protein chains making up the MHC class II molecule are similar in size and domain configuration. The α chain has a molecular mass of 33 kilodaltons (kDa); the β chain is only slightly smaller (28 kDa). Both the α and the β chains are transmembrane proteins and associate with each other by noncovalent interactions to form the heterodimer. Each MHC class II chain is composed of a membrane-proximal domain (called the α_2 or β_2 domain) that is a member of the immunoglobulin superfamily and a nonimmunoglobulin superfamily membrane-distal domain (called α_1 or β_1). The membrane-distal domains serve the function of binding to antigenic peptides and are also the region of the MHC protein that binds to the TCR during T-cell activation (Fig. 11.8A).

MHC class I proteins comprise one large, transmembrane protein (called the *α chain* or *heavy chain*) paired with a small (12 kDa) conserved protein called β_2-*microglobulin* (β_2m). β_2m does not participate in antigen presentation. The α chain of MHC class I is composed of a membrane-proximal domain (called α_3) that belongs to the immunoglobulin superfamily and two membrane-

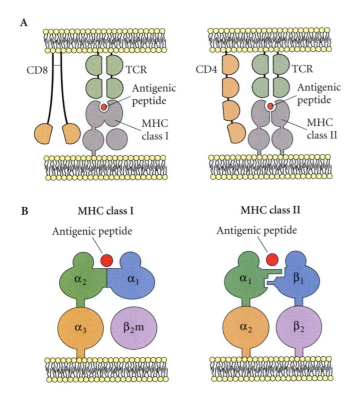

Figure 11.8 Interaction of MHC class I or class II with antigenic peptide, the TCR, and the CD4 or CD8 coreceptors. **(A)** The MHC proteins on an APC present bound peptide to the TCR that recognizes the complex of the peptide and the MHC. The coreceptors CD4 and CD8 facilitate and stabilize the binding of the APC to the T cell. Despite their differences in structure, the two MHC classes must have sufficient similarities to both to be capable of interacting with peptide-MHC complexes. **(B)** Schematic diagrams of MHC class I and class II proteins showing the arrangement of protein domains and the location of the antigen-binding cleft. Domains of MHC class I that are functionally comparable to those in MHC class II share the same colors. MHC class I consists of one transmembrane heavy chain (or α chain) comprising three domains (α_1, α_2, and α_3) and is noncovalently associated with a smaller protein called β_2m. The peptide-binding cleft of MHC class I is formed by the α_1 and α_2 domains. MHC class II consists of two transmembrane protein chains, α and β. The extracellular region of each protein chain contains two domains (α_1 and α_2 or β_1 and β_2). The peptide-binding cleft comprises protein sequences derived from both protein chains (the α_1 domain and the β_1 domain).

erodimer, β_2m occupies the physical space analogous to that occupied by the β_2 domain in MHC class II (Fig. 11.8B). β_2m is a member of the immunoglobulin superfamily of proteins and is encoded by a gene that is not located in the MHC gene complex. Although β_2m plays no direct role in binding to antigenic peptide or in TCR binding, it is a critical component of MHC class I proteins, being necessary for proper folding and stability of MHC class I. Cells that lack a functional β_2m gene are still able to produce MHC class I α chains that can be found in the rough endoplasmic reticulum, but these α chains are not trafficked efficiently to the plasma membrane. Surface expression of MHC class I can be "rescued" in such cells by transfection with a wild-type copy of the gene encoding β_2m.

β_2m also is found complexed with other proteins that are structurally similar to MHC class I, some of which do not function in antigen presentation. These proteins are termed *nonclassical MHC class I proteins*. One example is an iron-transporting protein encoded by the nonclassical MHC gene HFE (originally called HLA-H). Defects in expression of HFE result in the disease hemachromatosis, which is due to iron overload and causes myriad clinical symptoms, including heart defects and pancreatic dysfunction. Similar to classical MHC class I proteins, HFE requires association with β_2m for stability. In the absence of β_2m, cell surface expression of HFE decreases. Although β_2m-deficient mice are typically used as a model system in studies of immune deficiency (because of their inability to present antigenic peptides on MHC class I), these mutant mice will eventually develop symptoms similar to those of human hemachromatosis because of their decreased expression of the mouse ortholog of HFE protein.

Peptide Binding by MHC Class I and Class II Proteins

The regions of MHC class I and class II that physically contact antigenic peptide (the *peptide-binding clefts*) are similar (Fig. 11.9). Both are elongated depressions in the surface of the MHC protein. The floor of the depression is formed by a β-pleated-sheet structure composed of peptide strands of both membrane-distal domains of the MHC protein. The walls of the depression are formed by two long, slightly curved α-helices. Each α-helix is a part of a different membrane-distal domain. An antigenic peptide that binds in the cleft makes contacts with amino acids on the floor and the α-helical walls of the cleft. The portion of the peptide that physically contacts the MHC protein is termed the *agretope*, and each amino acid of the

distal domains (called α_1 and α_2) that are not members of the immunoglobulin superfamily. The two membrane-distal domains of MHC class I form the binding cleft for antigenic peptide and are also the regions of the MHC protein that interact with the TCR. Thus, the peptide-binding domain of MHC class I is formed from the single α chain polypeptide in contrast to the peptide-binding domains of MHC class II proteins, which are formed from both the class II α and β chains.

When expressed on the surface of a cell, the α chain of MHC class I protein is always associated with β_2m, which primarily contacts the α_3 domain of the class I α chain. In the three-dimensional structure of the class I het-

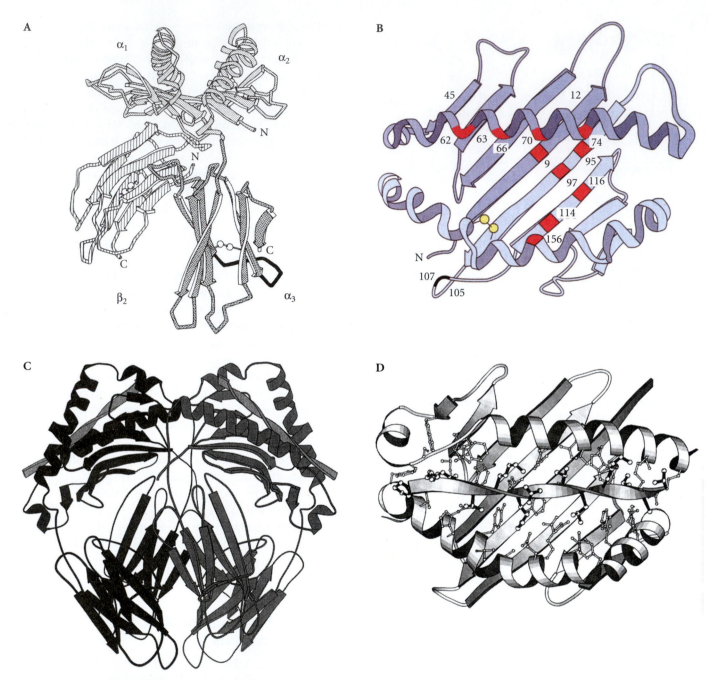

Figure 11.9 The molecular structures of MHC class I (**A and B**) and MHC class II (**C and D**) as seen from a side view (**A and C**) or from the top down into the peptide-binding grooves (**B and D**). The peptide-binding cleft is constructed such that the bottom consists of a β-pleated-sheet lined on both sides by α-helices. In each case the membrane-proximal domains (α_3 and β_2m for MHC class I and α_2 and β_2 for MHC class II) have a structure similar to typical immunoglobulin domains. In panel D, an antigenic peptide is shown bound in the antigen-binding cleft. Amino acid side chains that participate in contacts between the peptide and the MHC are shown (those of the peptide are in black and those of the MHC are in white). (**C**) Two MHC class II proteins. One is shown in black, and the other is shown in gray. The antigenic peptides bound to each MHC class II protein are depicted as light gray ribbons and are located at the top of each class II protein. (**A**) Modified with permission from P. J. Bjorkman et al., *Nature* **329**:506–512, 1987. (**B**) Modified with permission from P. Parham, *Scand. J. Rheumatol.* (Suppl.) **87**:11–20, 1990. (**C**) Modified with permission from P. H. Shafer et al., *Semin. Immunol.* **7**:389–398, 1995. (**D**) Reprinted with permission from L. J. Stern et al., *Nature* **368**:215–221, 1994.

A

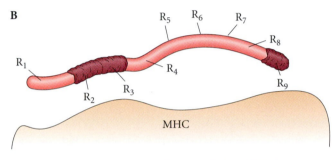

	Amino acid number									
	1	2	3	4	5	6	7	8	9	
H–$2D^d$	NH_2– V	**G**	**P**	Q	K	N	E	N	**L**	–COOH
	NH_2– S	**G**	**P**	R	K	A	I	A	**L**	–COOH
	NH_2– A	**G**	**P**	D	R	T	E	K	**L**	–COOH
	NH_2– I	**G**	**P**	E	R	G	H	N	**L**	–COOH
	NH_2– K	**G**	**P**	E	R	A	N	G	**L**	–COOH
	NH_2– F	**G**	**P**	Y	K	L	N	R	**L**	–COOH
	NH_2– F	**G**	**P**	I	K	F	N	V	**L**	–COOH
	NH_2– F	**G**	**P**	Y	R	F	Y	V	**L**	–COOH
H–$2L^d$	NH_2– Y	**P**	N	V	N	I	H	N	**F**	–COOH
	NH_2– Q	**P**	Q	R	G	R	E	N	**F**	–COOH
	NH_2– A	**P**	Q	P	G	M	E	N	**F**	K –COOH

B

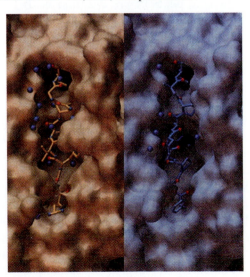

Figure 11.10 (**A**) Antigenic peptides that bind to MHC class I interact with the MHC via anchor residues (in bold type) located at or near both ends of the peptide. The figure shows eight different antigenic peptides that can bind to the H-2D^d MHC class I protein and three different peptides that can bind to the H-2L^d MHC class I protein. Although the nonanchor residues of the peptides differ considerably, the anchor residues of all the peptides that bind a given MHC protein are identical or in some cases closely related. Note also that the anchor residues that confer binding to H-2D^d are different from those that confer binding to H-2L^d. (**B**) Diagram of the interaction of one antigenic peptide with an MHC protein. The physical contact of the anchor residues (residues 2, 3, and 9) with the MHC protein explains the conservation of these residues among peptides that bind the MHC protein. Panel A is modified with permission from V. H. Engelhard, *Curr. Opin. Immunol.* **6:**13–23, 1994.

peptide that binds directly to the MHC is termed an *anchor residue*.

The molecular genetic mechanisms that generate diversity of the TCR have been estimated to be capable of generating TCRs that recognize 10^{13} different antigenic peptides. However, any individual possesses far fewer MHC proteins. For a large number of antigenic peptides to be presented by such a small number of MHC proteins, each MHC protein must have the capacity to bind and present multiple antigenic peptides. MHC binding to antigenic peptides is said to be *promiscuous* as opposed to the high specificity of MHC-peptide-TCR interactions. Several factors are involved in the ability of MHC proteins to bind multiple antigenic peptides. First, only a small subset of the amino acids on the peptide actually come into close

contact with the peptide-binding groove (Fig. 11.10). Since only a few amino acids in the peptide are relevant to MHC binding, most peptides that possess the appropriate anchor residues can bind to a particular MHC protein. Another factor permitting promiscuous binding of antigenic peptides is the conformational shifts on the part of both the peptide and the MHC molecule that frequently accompany peptide binding. These shifts are analogous to the "induced-fit" antigenic conformational epitopes binding to antibody. They contribute to promiscuous binding by allowing the MHC to assume a conformation that efficiently binds a peptide that might otherwise be impossible if the MHC maintained a rigid conformation. A dramatic example of conformational shifts in peptide-MHC binding is illustrated in Fig. 11.11. In this example, the MHC class I protein H-2K^b assumes two different conformations upon binding to two different antigenic peptides.

Differences between Peptides Bound by MHC Class I Proteins and Those Bound by Class II Proteins

The binding of antigenic peptides to MHC class I has several features that distinguish it from peptide binding to MHC class II (Table 11.2). First, the origin of antigenic peptides that bind to MHC class I is different from that of peptides that bind to MHC class II. MHC class I-bound peptides are generally derived from proteins synthesized within the cell (endogenous peptides) and then

Figure 11.11 A model of the van der Waals surface of H-2K^b MHC molecule bound by two different antigenic peptides. The left side shows the vesicular stomatitis virus peptide VSV-8 bound to H-2K^b; the right side shows the same MHC molecule binding the Sendai virus nucleoprotein peptide SEV-9. Note the conformational differences in the MHC protein surface. Reprinted from M. Matsumura et al., *Science* **257:**927–934, 1992, with permission.

Table 11.2 Characteristics of the binding of antigenic peptides to MHC class I and class II proteins

Characteristic	MHC class I	MHC class II
Origin of peptides	Endogenous	Exogenous
Proteolytic enzymes that generate peptides	Proteasome complex	Lysosomal proteases
MHC domains participating in binding	α_1 and α_2	α_1 and β_1
Shape of binding cleft	Closed at both ends	Open at both ends
Peptide length (amino acids)	8–10 (strict limit)	13–18 (can be >18)
Position of anchor residues	Ends of peptide	Spaced along entire length of peptide
Position of ends of peptide	Buried in floor of binding cleft	Protruding from ends of binding cleft
Elevation of peptide from floor of binding cleft	Arched from floor of cleft	Constant elevation from floor of cleft

proteolytically cleaved into short peptides that are transported into the endoplasmic reticulum for loading onto MHC class I. In contrast, peptides that bind to MHC class II are usually derived from "exogenous" proteins that are brought into the cell by endocytosis or phagocytosis, cleaved proteolytically, and then loaded onto MHC class II proteins in specialized endosomal compartments. However, there are numerous exceptions: endogenous peptides binding to class II and exogenous peptides binding to class I.

Most of the other features that distinguish class I-binding peptides from class II-binding peptides are a direct result of subtle differences in the shapes of the antigen-binding clefts of the two classes of MHC (Table 11.2). The peptide-binding cleft of MHC class I has the shape of a groove closed at both ends. As a result, there is a strict limitation on the length of the peptides that are able to bind to MHC class I proteins. The majority of class I-bound antigenic peptides are 9 amino acids long, but these peptides range in length from 8 to 10 amino acids, and it is rare for the length of a class I-bound peptide to be outside this range. An antigenic peptide bound to MHC class I interacts with the MHC protein at both ends of the peptide, while the middle region of the peptide arches away from the MHC. Therefore, the anchor residues of a class I-bound peptide usually reside at or near the ends of the peptides (Fig. 11.10). In some cases, the ends of a class I-bound peptide are actually buried in small depressions in the floor of the peptide-binding cleft of the MHC. Since both ends of the class I-bound peptide are anchored to the binding cleft, the length of the peptide will ultimately determine the degree to which the peptide arches (Fig. 11.12): shorter (8 amino acids) peptides are less arched, and longer (10 amino acids) peptides are more arched. The degree of arching is probably

important to the antigenic epitope that is accessible to the TCR and plays an important role in forming the three-dimensional structure that binds to the TCR.

The interaction of antigenic peptides with MHC class II is different because the peptide-binding cleft of MHC class II is open, rather than closed, at both ends. Therefore, the ends of a class II-bound peptide are free to protrude from the ends of the binding cleft. Thus, the length limitations on peptides that bind to MHC class II are not as stringent as those on peptides that bind to MHC class I. Accordingly, the range in length of class II-bound peptides is much wider (13 to 18 amino acids) than the range of class I-bound peptides. Another consequence of the open-ended nature of the class II peptide-binding cleft is that the peptides bound in this cleft are positioned at a fairly constant elevation across the cleft. Since the ends of a class II-bound peptide are not anchored to the binding cleft, differences in peptide length do not result in "bulging" of the peptide from the cleft. Thus, the anchor residues that form contacts between an antigenic peptide and MHC class II can be spread out along the entire length of the antigenic peptide rather than being limited to the ends of the peptide. It has also been proposed that the portions of the peptide that hang out over the edge of the binding cleft contribute to the formation of the three-dimensional structure of the peptide-MHC complex that interacts with TCR.

Variation in Classical MHC Class I and Class II Proteins and Effect on Peptide Binding

Ideally, the MHC proteins would bind all possible foreign epitopes in the antigenic universe and present them to T cells. Realistically, however, this goal is hindered by limi-

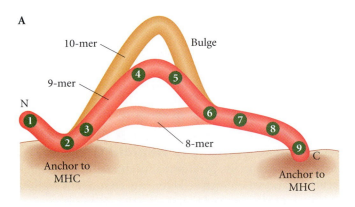

A

10-mer   Bulge

9-mer

N

1 2 3 4 5 6 7 8 9

8-mer

Anchor to
MHC

Anchor to
MHC

C

B

P4

P1

VSV–8

P8

P5

P4

P1

SEV–9

P9

Figure 11.12 Antigenic peptides that bind MHC class I are anchored to the MHC at both ends and bulge away from the MHC at the middle. The degree to which the peptide bulges from the floor of the binding cleft depends on the length of the peptide, with longer peptides bulging further from the floor of the cleft. (A) Representation of the differences in conformation observed for peptides of 8 amino acids, 9 amino acids, and 10 amino acids bound to an MHC class I protein. (B) The conformations of the bound VSV-8 (8 amino acids) and SEV-9 (9 amino acids) peptides shown in Fig. 11.11. The bottom of panel B shows the two peptides superimposed to emphasize the "bulge" of the 9-mer bound to MHC. Panel A is modified with permission from P. Parham, *Nature* **360**:300–301, 1992. Panel B is reprinted with permission from D. Fremont et al., *Science* **257**:919–927, 1992.

tations in the number of MHC proteins possessed by any host organism, with each MHC protein capable of presenting a large but finite number of antigenic peptides to T lymphocytes. Therefore, in all likelihood, the number of antigenic peptides that any host organism is capable of presenting to its T lymphocytes falls far short of the number of antigenic peptides that may be encountered. To maximize the number of peptides that can be presented, MHC molecules have evolved mechanisms to add diversity to their antigen-presentation capacity.

MHC Class I and Class II Polymorphism Allows Binding of Diverse Antigenic Peptides

Although it is not uncommon for genes to exist in several different allelic forms within a population, MHC genes are characterized by the large multiplicity of their allelic forms. The importance of this *polymorphism* can be considered advantageous to both the individual host organism and the entire host population. Since the number of antigenic peptides that can be presented is limited, antigens may exist that cannot be presented on an individual host's MHC proteins. This would occur if a protein antigen contained no internal amino acid sequences that could serve as anchor residues for MHC binding. In this case, a given host organism would be incapable of mounting a specific immune response to that antigen because no T lymphocytes could be activated. The existence of a pathogenic microbe possessing such antigens could be disastrous if all members of the host species had the exact same MHC proteins and an immune response to the antigen was critical in order to resist the infectious microbe. A microbe that possessed such antigens might be able to infect every member of the host species, and thus have the potential to eradicate the entire host species. MHC polymorphism prevents such scenarios for two reasons. First, unlike the inbred mouse strains, organisms in a natural population are outbred and are often heterozygous at most MHC loci (Fig. 11.13). That many individuals possess two different alleles of each MHC gene increases the number of antigenic peptides its APCs can present. This is especially true of the MHC class II proteins: whereas MHC class I proteins are dimers of one polymorphic protein (the MHC heavy chain) and one nonpolymorphic chain (β_2m), MHC class II proteins are heterodimers comprising two polymorphic protein chains. An MHC-heterozygous host bears not only the MHC class II proteins encoded by genes inherited in the MHC of each parent but also "hybrid" MHC class II proteins comprising an α chain from one parental haplotype paired with the β chain of the other parental haplotype. Furthermore, in

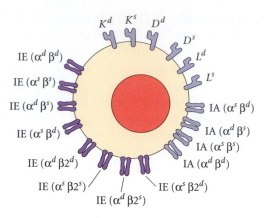

Figure 11.13 Heterozygosity of MHC genes increases the number of different MHC proteins that exist on the surface of a cell. The cell is an APC with the MHC haplotype *d/s*. The *d* and *s* MHC alleles are codominantly expressed, meaning that the APC expresses MHC class I of each haplotype on its surface. The variety of MHC class II molecules expressed on the surface is even greater, since the cell expresses not only the parental MHC types ($\alpha^d\beta^d$ and $\alpha^s\beta^s$) but also "hybrid" class II proteins ($\alpha^d\beta^s$ and $\alpha^s\beta^d$). While the IE α chain of one haplotype can pair with the IE β chain of either haplotype (IE$\alpha^d\beta^d$ or IE$\alpha^d\beta^s$), the α chain of IE can pair *only* with IE β chains (*not* with IA β chains). There is more than one gene encoding the mouse IE β chain, and each of two alleles of the mouse class II IE α chain can produce a protein that pairs up with proteins encoded by either allele of the IE β chain or the IE β2 chain, resulting in eight possible IE proteins on the cell surface.

many instances there is more than one gene for a class II protein chain: in the case of the mouse class II IE protein, there are two genes for β chains, IEβ and IEβ2. MHC polymorphism can protect the host species by a second mechanism: any protein antigen that evades presentation by the MHC of one host organism will almost certainly be presented on the MHC of another host organism of the same species. Thus, it is almost impossible for an antigenic protein to evade presentation by all of the alleles of MHC across the entire host species.

The degree to which MHC alleles differ can be substantial. Some allelic variants of MHC proteins differ by about 5 to 10% in their amino acid sequences. This percentage, however, does not accurately portray the differences in peptide-binding capacity of different MHC alleles because the amino acid variation between MHC alleles is not evenly distributed across the entire MHC coding sequence. Rather, the sequence variation between allelic forms is concentrated at the regions of the MHC protein that contact antigenic peptides. This is obvious when the variability in amino acid sequence is graphed as a function of amino acid position on the MHC protein (Fig. 11.14A). The plot clearly shows that the extent of amino acid variation at the membrane-distal α_1 and α_2 domains, which form the peptide-binding cleft, is

far greater than that in the membrane-proximal domains. Far more dramatic, however, is the distribution of amino acid variability within the membrane-distal domains. Most of the variability within the membrane-distal domains (Fig. 11.14B) occurs among amino acids directed into the actual binding cleft.

Some MHC Class I and Class II Genes Exist in Multiple Copies per Haploid Genome

In many host species, the number of different MHC molecules expressed on each cell is enhanced not only by heterozygosity at many loci but also by the existence of multiple genes encoding for each of the two different chains of the MHC class II molecule. Figure 11.15 depicts detailed maps of the human and mouse MHC gene clusters. Multiple nonallelic genes exist for several MHC proteins. For example, there are two genes in the *H-2* region that encode H-2K proteins.

The genomic organization of MHC genes and their expression can be complex. For example, not all strains of mice can make both β chains of the class II IE protein; some mice lack one of the genes, others carry functional genes. Similarly in humans nine different potential genes for the HLA-DRβ chain have been found in some MHC haplotypes, but five of these are unexpressed pseudogenes. A listing of human HLA genes and other relevant information can be found at http://www.ebi.ac.uk/imgt/hla/index.html.

Serologic and Sequence-Based Identification of MHC Proteins and Relationship to MHC Polymorphism

Since the MHC proteins have been identified as important in transplant rejection, there is a great impetus to find tissue donors whose MHC proteins are closely related to those of the intended recipient of the tissue or organ. Such "matching" of tissues is known to enhance the success of transplantation; the closer the match in MHC proteins, the less likely the donor tissue will be attacked and rejected by the recipient. To classify different alleles and make this information useful to transplant surgeons, a series of immunologic and genetic tools have been developed to enhance the identification of the relatedness of different MHC alleles.

Serologic Identification of MHC Class I Antigens

The earliest means of classifying MHC proteins as more or less related relied on the identification of individuals with specific antibodies that could distinguish proteins

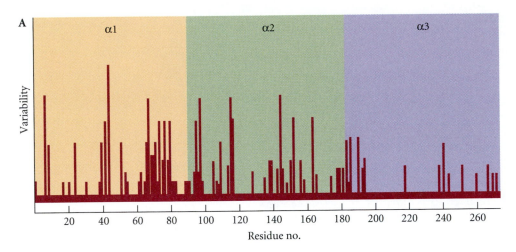

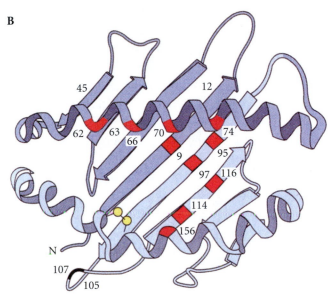

Figure 11.14 Polymorphism of MHC proteins is concentrated in regions of the MHC protein that interact with antigenic peptide. (**A**) Variability is plotted as a function of amino acid position among human MHC class I alleles. Most of the variability among alleles is in the α_1 and α_2 domains; the α_3 domain (which does not bind antigenic peptide) shows little variability. (**B**) Amino acids that are highly variable among different MHC alleles (the amino acids in red) are oriented toward the peptide-binding groove. Panel A is reprinted with permission from R. Sodoyer et al., *EMBO J.* **3**:879–885, 1984. Panel B is reprinted with permission from P. Parham, *Scand. J. Rheumatol.* (Suppl.) **87**:11–20, 1990.

Figure 11.15 Detailed genomic maps of the human and mouse MHC gene clusters. Class I genes are in red, class II genes are in blue, and class III genes are in yellow. Genes whose names appear below each diagram are nonclassical MHC genes. The functions of many nonclassical MHC genes are not yet known.

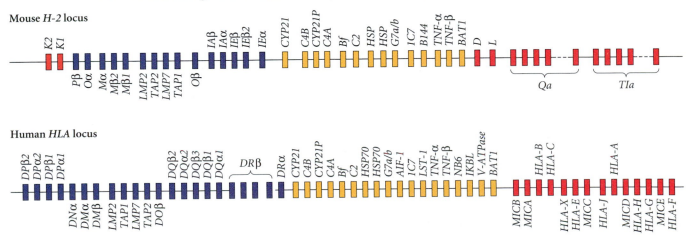

on the basis of epitope expression. These individuals were often multiparous women who made antibody responses to paternal HLA antigens or individuals who received multiple transfusions. The advent of monoclonal antibody technology helped move this field along since large amounts of purified antibody to single epitopes could be produced. The problem, of course, was that MHC proteins, like other proteins, express multiple epitopes. Some of these would be shared among one set of different MHC proteins, others would be shared among a different set of MHC proteins, and other epitopes could be unique to one MHC protein. Shared epitopes are referred to as *public* or *supertypic* determinants, whereas unique epitopes are defined as *private* determinants. Sorting out the complexity of the mixture of public and private epitopes among the class I proteins was no mean feat, but it did lead to the classification of human HLA class I proteins into serologically related types. The different types were designated by the particular HLA class I protein followed by a number, given out in nonsequential order (see http://www.anthonynolan.org. uk/HIG/lists/specs.html). Thus, serologically distinct HLA-A alleles could be classified as HLA-A1, -A2, -A3, -A9, etc. However, as more antibody reagents were developed, it became clear that some of the HLA specificities could be further subdivided into a related set. For example, the antibody that defined the human HLA-A10 protein was found to identify a public epitope; additional reagents further subdivided HLA-A10 into HLA-A25 and HLA-A26. To indicate the relatedness, these are designated HLA-A25(10) and HLA-A26(10), and the original HLA-A10 designation is dropped. Although imperfect, serologic classification of MHC class I alleles has provided a good basis for tissue matching at these loci. Correlations of serologic and genetic types of HLA proteins can be found at http://www.worldmarrow.org/Dictionary/Dict2001Table2.html.

Serologic Identification of MHC Class II Antigens

Initially, the human MHC class II region was designated HLA-D. As a class II protein, it was known to stimulate lymphocyte proliferation in a one-way mixed lymphocyte reaction, a reaction that can take from 3 to 8 days to complete (Fig. 11.16). However, although this assay was useful in the laboratory for classification purposes, it was completely impractical for use in a clinical setting where transplanted tissue had to be matched within hours of removal from a donor. This led to the use of serologic means to classify MHC class II proteins and the designation of human class II proteins as either HLA-DP, -DQ, or -DR. The same problems encountered with serologic

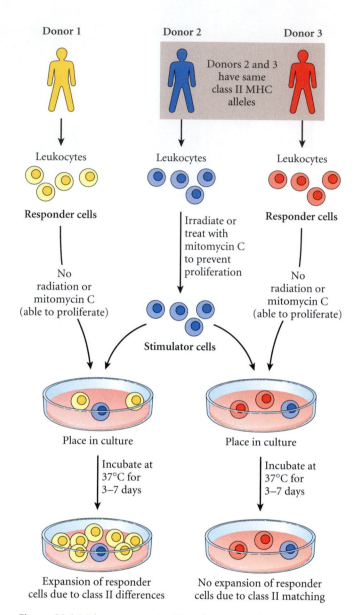

Figure 11.16 The one-way mixed lymphocyte reaction. Three donors of peripheral blood leukocytes are shown; donors 1 and 2 have different MHC class II proteins whereas donors 2 and 3 have the same ones. Leukocytes from donor 2 are irradiated to prevent their proliferating in cell culture and are mixed with leukocytes from donor 1 or donor 3. These are the responder cells. After 3 to 7 days in culture the amount of proliferation of the responder cells is measured. Due to differences in MHC class II between donor 1 and 2, donor 1's lymphocytes recognize the allogeneic class II antigens as foreign and mount a T-cell proliferative response. This can be measured by adding radioactive thymidine to the culture 18 to 24 hours before the end, then harvesting the cells and measuring the amount of radioactivity incorporated into the responding cells' DNA. In contrast, donors 2 and 3 share the same MHC class II haplotype and donor 3 does not recognize donor 2's cells as foreign.

typing of MHC class I are also relevant here: combinations of shared (public) and unique (private) epitopes, based on the use of available reagents, limit the diversity of serologic classification. Also, since the number of genes for a given chain of the human HLA-DR β chain can vary by individual, the actual identity of the HLA-DR type can be tricky. The most important matching for purposes of transplantation in the HLA class II region is at the DRB1 allele. Matching at this allele is used in bone marrow donor registries for identifying potential matches (with more high-resolution mapping including the DQB1 chain for final matching) and for solid organ transplantation, where a fast and reliable typing method is needed.

DNA-Based HLA Typing

With the advent of modern DNA technology in the 1980s, it became possible to classify MHC proteins by allelic variation in the DNA sequences. Because of its obvious implications for clinical transplant medicine, this was principally applied to the identification of allelic variants of genes encoding the human HLA MHC proteins. DNA typing showed there was much more variability in the class I and II genes than could be appreciated by serologic classification. For example, there are about 5 to 10 times as many alleles as there are serotypes of the human HLA class I proteins and 15 to 20 times as many alleles for the HLA-DRB1 chain as there are serotypes. A variety of

DNA typing techniques were thus developed to detect HLA polymorphisms. The polymerase chain reaction (PCR) is currently used to classify human MHC alleles along with a variety of detection techniques for analysis of the products of the PCR. Most commonly used are primers that amplify all of the alleles at a locus (i.e., primers for conserved regions of DNA sequence), leading to amplification of the polymorphic sequences located between the primers. One example of a detection method is shown in Fig. 11.17.

MHC Proteins with Ancillary Roles in Antigen Presentation

Many of the genes present within the MHC do not encode proteins that serve directly in the presentation of antigenic peptides to T lymphocytes. However, some of these nonpresenting proteins play important roles in preparing antigens for eventual presentation to T cells (Table 11.3). Examples are the *LMP-2* and *LMP-7* genes, whose protein products assist in the proteolytic cleavage of protein antigens to form small peptides suitable for MHC binding. Other examples are the *TAP1* and *TAP2* genes, whose protein products transport some antigenic peptides to the appropriate subcellular compartment where the peptides can encounter MHC proteins. Last, the *HLA-DM* and *HLA-DO* genes (*H-2M* and *H-2O* in the mouse) are nonpolymorphic genes that encode pro-

Figure 11.17 Determination of HLA-A type by use of sequence-specific oligonucleotide probes. Arrayed along the strip are lines of oligonucleotides known to represent and differentiate each different HLA-A allele. DNA from test samples is amplified by PCR using primers that are labeled with biotin, thus incorporating the biotin into the test probe. After hybridization, the presence of bound biotin is detected by adding streptavidin coupled to horseradish peroxidase enzyme, followed by a substrate for the enzyme. Those lines with bound probe are then visualized, and computer programs match the pattern to known HLA types. In each lane, there are a reference control and two PCR amplification controls (HLA-A exon 2 and exon 3, which are conserved). Strips 1, 2, 5, 6, and 7 indicate a homozygous genotype, with strips 2, 5, and 6 displaying the pattern for HLA-A*0101. Strips 3 and 4 display the HLA-A genotype of a heterozygous individual. The banding pattern serves as a type of fingerprint to genetically identify different HLA alleles. Reprinted from H. A. Erlich et al., *Immunity* 14:347–356, 2001, with permission.

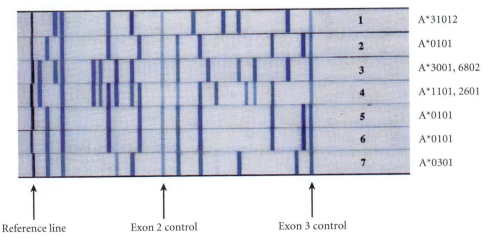

Table 11.3 Non-antigen-presenting MHC class I or II proteins and MHC class III proteins

Protein	Function
Nonclassical class I	
Qa/Tla	Regulation of NK cell activation, T-cell allorecognition
MICA, -B, -C, -D, -E	Antigen-independent stimulation of TCR; regulation and/or activation of T cells
HLA-X	Pseudogene
HLA-E	Regulation of NK cell activation
HLA-J	Pseudogene
HFE (HLA-H)	Iron transport
HLA-G	Regulation of NK cell activation
Nonclassical class II	
DM (M in mice)	Loading of peptides onto classical MHC class II
LMP-2, LMP-7	Regulation of proteolysis of endogenous protein antigens for eventual loading onto classical MHC class I
TAP1, TAP2	Transport of endogenous antigenic peptides into rough endoplasmic reticulum for loading onto classical MHC class I
DO (O in mice)	Regulation of peptide loading onto classical MHC class II
Class III	
CYP21/CYP21P	Steroid 21-hydroxylases
C2, C4A, C4B, Bf	Complement proteins C2, C4, and factor B
HSP70 (HSP in mice)	Heat shock protein
G7a/b	Valyl-tRNA synthetase
AIF-1	Regulator of inflammation, cell adhesion (pseudogene in mouse)
1C7	Regulator of inflammation, cell adhesion?
LST-1 (B144 in mice)	Inhibitor of lymphocyte proliferation
TNF-α, TNF-β	Cytokines
IKBL	Transcriptional regulation
V-ATPase	Proton pump
BAT1	Translational initiation factor

teins that assist in loading antigenic peptides onto MHC class II proteins for subsequent presentation to T cells. Therefore, the MHC gene complex contains genes necessary for several different steps of antigen processing in addition to those that actually serve as presentation platforms for peptides.

MHC Class III: MHC Proteins with No Role in Antigen Presentation

The MHC class III genes (Fig. 11.1 and 11.15) are remarkable in that none of their products play roles in antigen presentation. These genes are not very polymorphic. Some of the class III proteins are immunologically relevant although unrelated to antigen presentation, such as the C2 and C4 complement components and the cytokine tumor necrosis factor (TNF). In contrast, other proteins encoded by genes in this region are completely unrelated to immune function, such as the valyl-tRNA synthetase encoded by the *G7a/b* gene and the heat shock protein HSP70. It is notable, however, that a growing number of MHC class III gene products are being implicated in the innate immune response, for example, the inflammatory response.

Roles of Some Nonclassical MHC Gene Products in Activation of T Cells in Response to Novel Stimuli

Many genes in the MHC gene complex encode proteins that are homologous to classical MHC class I and class II proteins but do not serve in antigen presentation. Only now are the functions of some of these *nonclassical MHC proteins* being deciphered. Although these nonclassical MHC proteins do not present antigens to T cells, many are capable of interacting with the TCR in an antigen-independent manner. Therefore, these nonclassical MHC proteins may provide a way for T lymphocytes to respond to stimuli other than antigenic peptides. An example is MHC class I α-chain-related protein A (MICA). Like classical MHC class I, MICA demonstrates allelic polymorphism, but unlike classical MHC class I, it is expressed on the cell surface in a β_2m-independent manner. Recently, Veronika Groh and coworkers showed that binding of MICA by the $\gamma\delta$ TCR results in activation and acquisition of cytotoxic activity by the T cell, leading to killing of the MICA-expressing target cell by the T cell. These same workers had shown that expression of MICA is greatly increased following a heat shock to the target cell. Therefore, MICA may provide a way for T cells to recognize a target cell that has recently undergone some physical or environmental stress (e.g., cellular injury or viral infection) and to kill that target cell in response. Negative regulatory roles have also been ascribed to nonclassical MHC proteins. The human protein HLA-G, for example, has been postulated to be involved in the downregulation of natural killer (NK) cell responses at the fetal-maternal interface and may therefore help keep the maternal immune system from rejecting genetically different fetal tissue. An additional example of negative regulation of the immune response by nonclassical MHC proteins has been suggested for the class I-like proteins T22 and T10. Expression of these proteins has been found to increase during an immune response, and it is postulated that the TCRs of regulatory T cells recognize T22 and/or T10 proteins when expression of T22 and T10 reaches a certain threshold.

MHC-Like Antigen-Presenting Molecules Encoded by Genes Located outside the MHC and Roles in Presentation of Unusual Antigens

The mechanism of antigen presentation to T lymphocytes was assumed for a while to involve protein antigens exclusively. However, in 1994 Michael Brenner found that non-protein antigens can be presented to T cells to trigger antigen-specific activation of those T cells. The molecules that present these nonprotein antigens are a family of MHC class I-like proteins that make up the *CD1 family*. Thus far, five genes belonging to the CD1 family have been identified in humans (called CD1a, CD1b, CD1c, CD1d, and CD1e). In the mouse, only two CD1 genes have been discovered, both homologous to human CD1d. CD1 proteins are nonpolymorphic proteins similar in structure to MHC class I (Fig. 11.18). Although they normally associate with β_2m, their stable expression on the cell surface does not seem to require β_2m. CD1 proteins differ from classical MHC class I proteins in that the antigen-binding grooves of CD1 proteins are predominantly hydrophobic. CD1 proteins have been found to present various lipid and glycolipid antigens to T cells, with each member of the CD1 family demonstrating a preference for binding a different subset of lipid antigens (Table 11.4). The discovery of the CD1 family and the nonprotein antigens they present has broadened our appreciation of the reactivity of T cells with antigens and has shed new light on the immune response to some diseases, such as mycobacterial infection, where CD1-mediated presentation may be a prominent pathway of immune recognition.

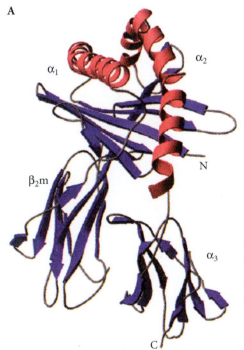

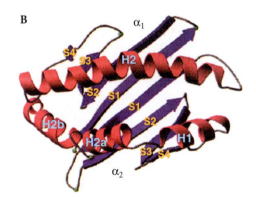

Figure 11.18 Ribbon structure of CD1 molecule illustrating its similarity with classical MHC class I (compare with Fig. 11.9A and B). Like MHC class I, CD1 consists of a transmembrane heavy chain that associates with β_2m. The α_1 and α_2 domains of CD1 form an antigen-binding cleft that has the same overall shape as an MHC class I antigen-binding cleft. However, the interior of the CD1 cleft, unlike that of the classical MHC class I cleft, is hydrophobic, allowing binding and presentation of lipid antigens, which are also hydrophobic. The positions of alpha-helices 1, 2, 2a, and 2b are indicated (H1, H2, H2a, and H2b), as are the positions of beta-strands 1, 2, 3, and 4 (S1, S2, S3, and S4) in the α_1 and α_2 domains. (**A**) Side view of CD1. (**B**) Top view of CD1. Reprinted from Z. Zeng et al., *Science* 277:339–345, 1997, with permission.

Table 11.4 Antigen-binding characteristics of human CD1 proteins

CD1 protein	Antigen	Source of antigen
CD1a	Unknown	Mycobacteria
CD1b	Mycolic acid	Mycobacteria
	Phosphatidylinositol mannosides	Mycobacteria
	Ganglioside GM1	Self cells
CD1c	Isoprenoids	Mycobacteria
CD1d	Glycosylphosphatidylinositols	Self/bacterial
CD1e	Unknown[a]	Unknown[a]

[a] Thus far, CD1e has only been detected intracellularly, in the Golgi apparatus.

Summary

The MHC contains numerous genes whose products function in the presentation of peptide antigens to T lymphocytes. Antigen-presenting MHC proteins fall into two categories: class I and class II. These two classes of MHC protein specialize in the presentation of peptide antigens to different subpopulations of T cells, with MHC class I proteins presenting antigens to CD8[+] T cells and MHC class II proteins presenting antigens to CD4[+] T cells. The structures of both classes of MHC proteins are well suited to their antigen-presenting function. The membrane-distal domains of each MHC protein form a groove-shaped peptide-binding cleft. MHC proteins demonstrate a high degree of polymorphism, meaning that they exist as a large number of allelic forms in most species. The various allelic forms of each MHC protein differ in their antigen-presenting abilities; thus, the presence of such a large number of MHC alleles broadens the spectrum of antigenic peptides that can be presented to T cells for recognition. Some proteins encoded within the MHC do not present antigens to T lymphocytes but have other functions that help regulate the immune response. The nonclassical MHC class I and class II proteins help regulate the loading of antigens onto classical MHC proteins, whereas the MHC class III proteins serve completely unrelated functions in the immune response. The MHC-related family of proteins called CD1 serve a direct role in antigen presentation, although these proteins seem to be most important in the presentation of nonprotein antigens to T cells. The MHC-like protein MICA usually does not present any antigen at all but is expressed only on target cells that have been physically injured, where it serves as a "danger signal" instructing a T cell to kill the damaged target cell. Thus, the MHC proteins serve many roles related to T-cell recognition of target cells and antigens.

Suggested Reading

Alfonso, C., and L. Karlsson. 2000. Nonclassical MHC class II molecules. *Annu. Rev. Immunol.* **18:**113–142.

Hiltbold, E. M., and P. A. Roche. 2002. Trafficking of MHC class II molecules in the late secretory pathway. *Curr. Opin. Immunol.* **14:**30–35.

Maenaka, K., and E. Y. Jones. 1999. MHC superfamily structure and the immune system. *Curr. Opin. Struct. Biol.* **9:**745–753.

Robinson, J. H., and A. A. Delvig. 2002. Diversity in MHC class II antigen presentation. *Immunology* **105:**252–262.

Rouas-Freiss, N., R. M. Goncalves, C. Menier, J. Dausset, and E. D. Carosella. 1997. Direct evidence to support the role of HLA-G in protecting the fetus from maternal uterine natural killer cytolysis. *Proc. Natl. Acad. Sci. USA* **94:**11520–11525.

Yeager, M., M. Carrington, and A. L. Hughes. 2000. Class I and class II MHC bind self peptide sets that are strikingly different in their evolutionary characteristics. *Immunogenetics* **51:**8–15.

chapter 12

Antigen Processing and Presentation

Lee M. Wetzler

The major type of antigen provoking an immune response is a protein or glycoprotein. Other types of antigens, such as polysaccharides and glycolipids, are also important as targets of immunity protecting against infection, but for the most part, it is protein antigens that stimulate the greatest array of immune responses. When an intact foreign protein antigen is recognized as foreign, it must be degraded intracellularly into short peptides by various proteases and placed on the surface groove of either major histocompatibility complex (MHC) class I or class II molecules. Degradation of proteins into antigenic peptides is referred to as *antigen processing,* and expression of the peptide on a cell's surface in association with MHC molecules is referred to as *antigen presentation.* Processed and presented antigens are available to interact with T lymphocytes, which specifically recognize these peptide-MHC complexes via their T-cell receptor (TCR). T lymphocytes are principally divided into two major subpopulations, CD4 and CD8, on the basis of surface expression of one of these coreceptors. However, the particular coreceptor expressed determines the interaction of the T cell with a particular class of MHC protein: CD4$^+$ T cells interact with MHC class II expressed on antigen-presenting cells (APCs) and CD8$^+$ T cells interact with MHC class I presented peptides. The importance of this "class restriction" in the immune response was demonstrated by a number of investigators over the past 30 years, but there is still intense investigation into the finer points of this phenomenon. Even after the basic concept of MHC class restriction in the response of CD4$^+$ and CD8$^+$ T cells to antigenic peptides was defined, the mechanisms whereby the processed peptides were produced and placed onto the antigen-binding groove of the proper MHC protein took considerably more time to elucidate. Over the past 15 years or so the complexity of these mechanisms has been intensively investigated, yet today there still is controversy about various aspects of the pathways involved in antigen processing and presentation.

APCs

The ability to process and present antigens on MHC molecules is a property of virtually all mammalian cells. This property is tied to the presence of MHC class I molecules on most cells. However, this ability to process and present antigen via MHC class I does not initiate an immune response in and of itself. Rather, foreign antigens presented on MHC class I target a cell for destruction by $CD8^+$ cytotoxic T lymphocytes (CTL). Thus, in this context, the cells presenting foreign antigen are, by convention, referred to as target cells. In contrast, professional APCs are those that can process and present antigen associated with MHC class II. This is the initial critical step in the induction of an immune response. A variety of APCs have been identified: dendritic cells, macrophages, and B cells are the major ones. Each of these differs in important ways and in their properties, and one of the most important is the endogenous and inducible level of costimulatory signals that affect the relative potency of the different types of APCs. A detailed discussion of these cells and their function is presented in chapter 3.

Dendritic cells are now known to be the most potent APCs and appear to arise from several precursor populations. They are found throughout the body where they have been classified by a variety of names. Dendritic cells in tissues are in an immature state, where their main function appears to be to ingest foreign antigen. They then move toward local lymph nodes and mature into functional APCs. Dendritic cells constitutively express the CD80 and CD86 costimulatory proteins, which provide the primary signals to naive T cells. These cells are less sensitive to stimulation than are memory T cells.

Macrophages are usually resident within a tissue and do not constitutively produce MHC class II or costimulatory activity. When they encounter a foreign antigen and phagocytose it, they enter a phase of activation that will culminate in their ability to function as APCs. But because macrophages do not express MHC class II constitutively and require antigen-induced activation, their potency as APCs is considerably less than that of dendritic cells. Once activated, macrophages efficiently present antigen via the MHC class II but also need to be stimulated to express the costimulatory ligands CD80 and CD86 in order to inter-

act with helper T cells. Therefore, macrophages are generally considered to be the least potent type of APC. Blood monocytes are believed to be precursors of tissue-fixed macrophages, and for many years immunologists studied these blood cells for antigen-presenting properties because of their ready availability.

B cells constitutively express MHC class II molecules but not costimulatory molecules. B cells recognize antigen via membrane immunoglobulin, so they are specific in regard to the type of antigen that can be processed and presented. Interaction of antigen via the B-cell receptor and coreceptor can lead to B-cell activation of $CD4^+$ T helper cells. B cells are therefore not as effective as dendritic cells as APCs since activation of T cells by B cells includes a lag time necessary for the expression of costimulatory molecules, i.e., CD80 (B7-1) and CD86 (B7-2).

Antigen-Processing Pathways

There are two obvious sources of antigenic peptides: those produced inside a cell and those acquired from outside the cell by endocytosis, pinocytosis, and phagocytosis. As a rule of thumb, antigenic peptides derived from proteins synthesized within a cell are processed and presented on MHC class I proteins via the endogenous or cytosolic processing pathway. In contrast, antigens obtained from outside a cell are processed by the exogenous or endocytic pathway and presented on MHC class II (Fig. 12.1A and B). However, there is a growing number of examples of "cross-presentation" of antigens by the other pathway, so the line between the division of pathways into those that process and present endogenous or exogenous proteins is being blurred (Fig. 12.1C).

The basic division of pathways holds up in a number of instances and can be experimentally demonstrated by use of selective variants of a given antigen. If one immunizes a mouse with an infectious virus, both class I- and class II-restricted T-cell responses will be generated. The class I response comes from the viral proteins being processed by the endogenous pathway, and the class II response from free viral particles released from infected cells that are phagocytosed by professional APCs. If a noninfectious form of the virus is used, only class II-restricted responses are elicited, as only exogenous processing of the free viral particles can occur. In some instances it appears that exogenously acquired proteins can be shunted to the cytosolic pathway for class I presentation and vice versa. However, proteins being processed and presented by these two different pathways go though different stages and cellular compartments and end up associated with either MHC class I or class II proteins.

An intriguing mechanism for cross-priming has been

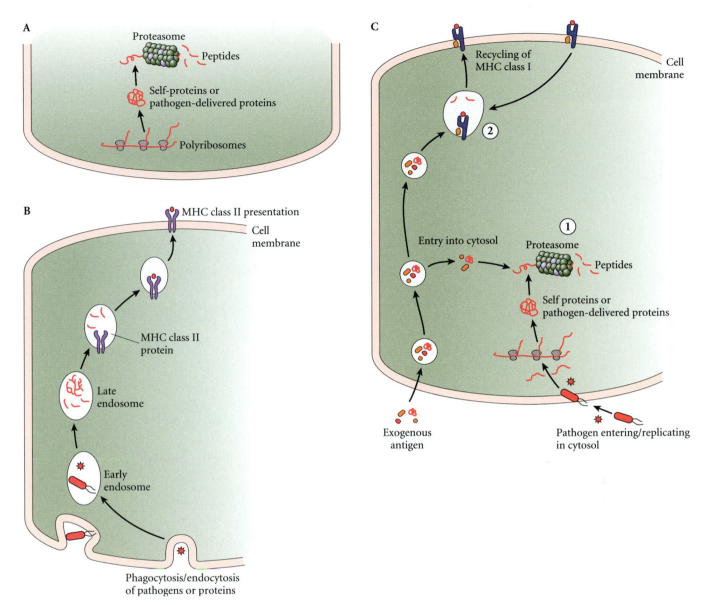

Figure 12.1 Antigen-processing pathways. (**A**) The endogenous pathway utilized by most cells. Proteins are produced within the cellular cytosol on polyribosomes. These are then shunted to the immunoproteasome for degradation. The source of proteins can either be those tagged for degradation or defective ribosomal products. Peptides generated by the immunoproteasome are then made available to the MHC class I peptides for presentation. (**B**) The exogenous pathway utilized by APC. Antigens are taken up by phagocytosis/endocytosis or pinocytosis and shunted into early endosomes. These mature into late endosomes that will fuse with vesicles containing MHC class II proteins, where the two will be brought together and be transported to the surface of the APC. (**C**) Mechanisms of cross-presentation. Exogenous antigens can enter a cell by endocytosis or pinocytosis or by invading the cell and replicating in the cytosol. Exogenous antigens can be shunted to the cytosol for processing via the immunoproteasome. Alternately, peptide fragments of the exogenous antigen can be fused with vesicles containing recycled MHC class I proteins and placed within the antigen-binding groove. Reprinted from M. Larsson et al., *Trends Immunol.* **22**:141–148, 2001, with permission.

proposed by N. Bhardwaj and her colleagues. They have shown that apoptotic or necrotic cells can be engulfed by APCs and the antigens inside these cells processed and presented for activation of both CD4[+] and CD8[+] cells. This could be of particular importance in activating CD8[+] T-cell responses to viral antigens, since it is unlikely that many human viral pathogens infect APCs and produce antigenic peptides via the cytosolic pathway. Apoptosis and necrosis are common responses of cells to infection, and these dying and dead cells are known to be phagocytosed by APCs, providing an opportunity for an exogenously acquired antigen to be presented by MHC class I. Priming of APCs with lysates from infected or tumor cells has been shown to enhance the immunogenicity of the microbial or tumor antigens and may provide a useful strategy for increasing the potency of vaccines.

Antigen Presentation by MHC Class I

One of the major functions of CD8$^+$ T cells responding to antigenic peptides presented by MHC class I molecules is to kill via a cytotoxic activity the cell that is presenting the antigen. This is useful when the cell is infected with an intracellular pathogen or has become transformed into a tumor cell that needs to be eliminated from the body. Viruses are classic examples of intracellular pathogens that provoke a CD8$^+$ CTL response, as the viruses are obligated to use the protein-synthesis machinery of the cells they infect to replicate and grow. By killing the infected cell, the immune response limits further viral growth and allows other immune effectors, such as antibodies, to opsonize the viral particles for clearance via phagocytosis. Bacterial pathogens such as listeriae and mycobacteria can grow inside macrophages and antigens from these pathogens can elicit a protective immune response mediated by CD8$^+$ CTL. Although the bacterium's own protein-synthesis machinery produces its antigens, release of bacterial antigens into the host cell's cytoplasm can shunt them into the processing and presentation pathway. Curiously, it was not clear how a CTL response to an intracellular bacterium would be beneficial for the host, as lysing the infected target cell could release the bacterial cells that could then spread to other cells and extend the infection. Recently R. Modlin and coworkers have found a CTL factor located in acid cytoplasmic granules, named granulysin, that can kill bacteria by increasing their membrane permeability. Thus, it may be that T cells possess inherent antimicrobial factors that directly kill intracellular organisms following the killing of the cell in which they are growing.

Proteasomes and Immunoproteasomes: Antigen Processing for MHC Class I Presentation

Antigens that are destined to be presented on MHC class I proteins are generally synthesized inside the same cell that presents the antigen to T cells; as such, these are termed *endogenous antigens*. Before they can be complexed with an MHC class I protein, endogenous antigens must be cleaved into small (8 to10 amino acids) peptides. Proteolysis within a cell is carried out by a large multicatalytic complex called the *proteasome*, also spelled proteosome (Fig. 12.2). The central structure of the proteasome,

termed the 20S proteasome, has a molecular mass of approximately 700 kilodaltons (kDa). Four portions of the 20S proteasome have been identified, consisting of two seven-membered outer rings of α subunits (α1 to α7), which are on the outside of the structure, and two seven-membered rings of β subunits (β1 to β7), located in the middle of the structure (Fig. 12.2A). Thus, there are 28 total polypeptides, ranging in molecular size from 21 to 31 kDa in the 20S proteasome. The α subunits appear to function as a type of gate through which proteins destined for degradation move, whereas the β subunits contain the proteolytic active portion of the proteasome. A fully functional proteasome consists of a 20S unit complexed to two 19S regulatory subunits, which together make up the 26S proteasome. The 19S subunit has a base containing adenosinetriphosphatase (ATPase) activity and chaperone activity to guide proteins to the gates of the proteasome, along with a "lid" whose function is not known.

The proteolytic activity of proteasomes acts on many cytosolic proteins. The involvement of this activity in antigen processing is only one of its functions, as the proteasome plays a critical role in the continuous turnover of many short-lived regulatory proteins, including transcription factors and cyclins. In the latter of these roles, the 26S proteasome mediates adenosine 5'-triphosphate (ATP)-dependent proteolysis of proteins that have been targeted for degradation by conjugation to the protein ubiquitin. Ubiquitin is a small 76-residue polypeptide that is added in various numbers to cytosolic proteins. It seems that four copies of ubiquitin in a chain (Ub4) may be required to target proteins to the 26S proteasome, as these Ub4 chains exhibit certain structural characteristics that may be recognized by the proteasome, especially by the 19S regulatory subunit of the 26S proteasome. However, this particular proteasome structure does not seem to produce many of the peptides that bind to MHC class I.

Instead, a different type of proteasome, termed the *immunoproteasome*, appears to produce many of the peptides destined to be bound to MHC proteins. Production of the immunoproteasome is dependent on synthesis of subunits regulated by the level of interferon-gamma (IFN-γ). Exposure of a cell to IFN-γ induces synthesis of new 20S proteasomes containing two MHC-encoded proteins, LMP-2 and LMP-7, and a non-MHC-encoded protein, LMP-10 or MECL1. LMP-2, LMP-7, and LMP-10 are also referred to as the β_{1i}, β_{5i}, and β_{2i} proteins, respectively. In the immunoproteasome, these three proteins replace the β_1 or δ, β_5 or ζ, and β_5 (MB1) polypeptide of the regular proteasome. LMP-2 replaces 100% of the β_1 subunits, and LMP-7 replaces 70% of β_2 subunits. Formation of the core 20S structure of the immunopro-

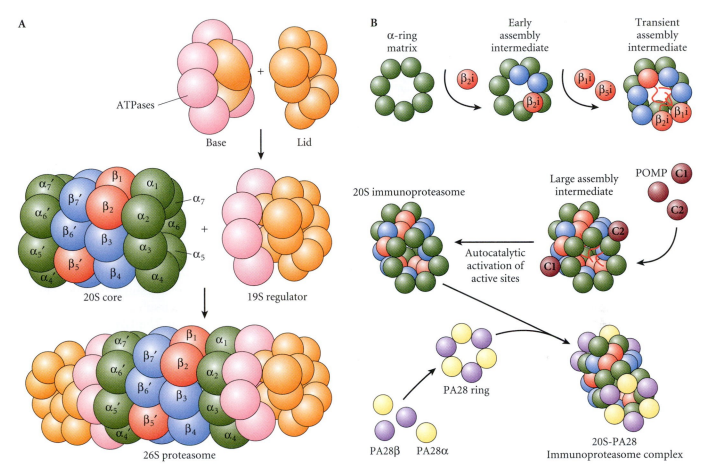

Figure 12.2 Structure of the proteasome. (**A**) The 26S proteasome is thought to provide peptides for the majority of antigen presentation functions. It consists of the 20S core (red, blue, and green) and a 19S regulatory subunit (pink and orange). The 20S proteasome is a tube-shaped complex consisting of two rings of "a" subunits (green) and two rings of "b" subunits (blue and red). The 19S regulatory subunit binds to the 20S proteasome and influences the substrate specificity of the proteasome (e.g., by binding to proteins that have been conjugated to the protein ubiquitin). (**B**) Assembly of the immunoproteasome. An immunoproteasome is formed by an initial seven-membered α ring that provides places for the 7-membered β ring to bind. In the immunoproteasome, the subunits β_{1i} (LMP-2), β_{2i} (LMP-7), and β_{5i} (LMP-10) replace three of the normally occurring β subunits (β_{1i}, β_{2i}, and β_{5i} are shown in red). LMP-2 and LMP-7 are thought to modulate the fine specificity of the proteasome to preferentially produce peptides that can bind to the MHC class I-binding groove. A proteasome maturation protein (POMP) along with chaperones (C) facilitates polymerization into a large assembly, followed by autocatalytic activation of the 20S subunit. Two copies of the PA28 activator, which is thought to alter the specificity of the proteasome by assisting in the unfolding of particularly large substrate proteins, are attached to form the final 20S-PA28 immunoproteasome complex.

teasome also requires chaperone proteins and the proteasome maturation protein, and production of the fully functional immunoproteasome involves generation of active sites via autocatalysis (Fig. 12.2B). Another component of the immunoproteasome is the proteasome activator PA28, also known as the 11S regulator, that is induced by IFN-γ and substitutes for one of the two 19S regulator complexes found in the regular proteasome.

The role of the immunoproteasome in antigen processing, presentation, and T-cell development has been demonstrated by the use of biochemical inhibitors of pro-

teasome catalytic function and in transgenic knockout mice. In vitro, the use of proteasome-specific peptide aldehyde inhibitors prevented both the surface expression of MHC class I and the presentation of MHC class I-restricted antigenic peptides. LMP-2 knockout mice have no decrease in surface expression of MHC class I but have a 60 to 90% decrease in the number of CD8$^+$ T cells. LMP-7 knockout mice have normal numbers of CD8$^+$ T cells but have a decrease in the surface expression of MHC class I. It is possible that the LMP-2 and LMP-7 subunits affect the cleavage preferences of the 26S immunoproteasome, with preferred cleavage following hydrophobic or basic residues. It is hypothesized that these subtle alterations in proteolytic activity have the effect of generating a larger population of peptides capable of binding MHC class I. Thus, in the LMP-2 knockout mice there may be a more restricted set of peptides presented by MHC class I (i.e., a reduction in the quality or diversity of peptides), leading to a reduction in CD8$^+$ T cells, while in the LMP-7 knockout mice there are fewer antigenic peptides produced to bind to MHC class I proteins (i.e., a lowered quantity of peptides). The PA28 regulator consists of six subunits that form a ring that can attach as a cap to both ends of the 20S proteasome (Fig. 12.2B). This regulator enhances the efficiency with which the proteasome processes antigen, possibly by altering the peptide substrate conformation to allow improved proteolysis of larger proteins by the proteasome.

To obtain antigenic peptide fragments for MHC class I presentation, the proteasome must have access to both native and foreign proteins, since peptides from both of these sources are found on surface class I molecules. Although it is generally regarded that these derive from proteins tagged for degradation, many proteins produced in a cell end up in a compartment sequestered from the proteasome or quite stable. Therefore, another source of proteins for producing fragments for MHC class I binding is needed. Recent evidence suggests that these are derived from proteins that are defectively translated on the ribosome, so-called defective ribosomal products. When a problem occurs with synthesizing a protein, it becomes ubiquitinylated and targeted for digestion in the proteasome. This may be due to the close proximity of the proteasome to the polyribosomes producing the cellular proteins. If there is a link between protein translation and production of peptide fragments for MHC presentation, then the immune system would have access to a large array of antigenic peptides.

Peptide Trafficking to MHC Class I and the Transporter Associated with Antigen Processing

When host proteins or foreign antigens are degraded into oligopeptides for presentation by MHC class I, the resulting peptides are located in the cytosol. However, assembly of MHC class I and the loading of antigenic peptides onto MHC class I occur in the endoplasmic reticulum (ER). Therefore, a mechanism for trafficking the peptides into the ER exists. The main effector of this transport is the heterodimeric transporter associated with antigen processing (TAP). TAP is inserted in the ER membrane and, through an ATPase-dependent process, allows transloca-

tion of antigenic peptides into the ER and thus the association of these peptides with MHC class I (Fig. 12.3 and 12.4A). Mice that lack TAP can still present some peptides via class I MHC because many proteins contain signal sequences that direct them into the ER. Exopeptidases that exist in the ER can clip signal sequences from nascent proteins; these signal-sequence peptides have been shown to be able to bind to the MHC class I groove and to be presented on the cell's surface.

TAP consists of two subunits, TAP1 and TAP2, encoded by genes in the MHC and closely linked to LMP-2 and LMP-7. Similarly, TAP1 and TAP2 are IFN-γ-induced proteins. The N terminus of each subunit is largely hydrophobic with multiple predicted transmembrane regions, allowing for insertion in the ER membrane. The C terminus of each subunit has an ATP-binding domain (Fig. 12.3). In addition, there is a single peptide-binding site made up of domains of each subunit at the C-terminal end of the hydrophobic region. The TAP peptide-binding site discriminates between different peptides on the basis of the primary amino acid sequence of each peptide and in this way influences which peptides can enter the ER. Most immunologists believe that the peptide specificity of human TAP is greater than that of mouse or rat TAP. In vitro, human TAP preferentially binds and transports nonameric peptides. Human TAP has a lesser affinity for peptides with acidic amino acids in the C terminus and in

Figure 12.3 Diagram of TAP. TAP is a heterodimer of two polypeptides called TAP1 and TAP2. Both of the polypeptides are members of the ATP-binding cassette family of transporter proteins. The cytosolic nucleotide-binding domains (NBD) bind and hydrolyze ATP to provide energy to drive the transporter function of TAP.

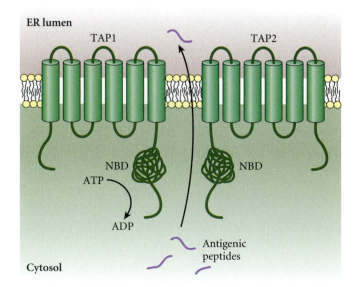

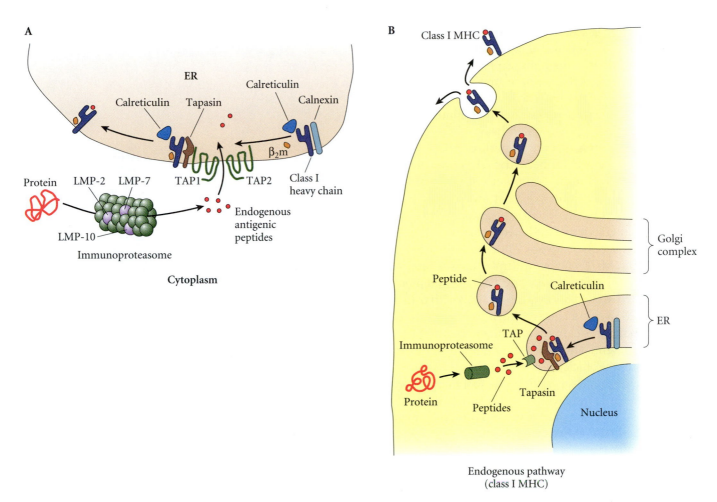

Figure 12.4 (A) Schematic diagram of the assembly of MHC class I peptide cleavage by the proteasome, and peptide transport by TAP. The diagram also shows the loading of endogenous peptide antigens onto MHC class I within the ER and highlights the role in this process of the chaperone proteins calnexin, calreticulin, and tapasin. (B) Export of MHC class I-peptide complexes to the cell surface allows these complexes to be presented to CD8+ T cells.

the first or third position, and the presence of neutral or basic amino acids at these positions increases affinity of TAP for these peptides, increasing their probability of transport into the ER. Murine TAP and rat TAP have slightly different preferences; murine TAP and the rat TAP1/2-B variant preferentially translocate peptides with aromatic or aliphatic C-terminal residues.

Of interest is the finding that peptides that are longer than 10 residues are transported by TAP into the ER. Since MHC class I only binds peptides 8 to 10 amino acids in length, some mechanism must exist to trim these down to fit into the antigen-binding groove. It has been proposed that these longer peptides associate with TAP by means of an internal nonameric sequence that binds with high affinity. The longer peptide then becomes trimmed by exopeptidases in the ER to allow binding to the enclosed MHC class I antigen-binding groove.

Assembly of MHC Class I-Peptide Complex

The MHC class I heterodimer consisting of an α heavy chain and a β_2-microglobulin (β_2m) molecule is assembled in the ER with the aid of a number of chaperones and is brought into close proximity with the TAP complex and the peptides it transports during this assembly process (Fig. 12.4A). Calnexin (p88) is the first chaperone the MHC class I heavy chain encounters. Calnexin aids in the folding and disulfide-bridge formation of the nascent heavy chain and allows the MHC class I dimer to be assembled by facilitating the interaction of the MHC class I with the essential β_2m subunit. Calnexin likely stabilizes the heavy chain-β_2m heterodimer before the peptide is loaded into the MHC groove and helps prevent the MHC class I from leaving the ER prematurely before peptide loading. Another chaperone in the ER, calreticulin, has significant homology with calnexin and can substitute for calnexin during assembly of the heavy chain-β_2m heterodimer. Mutant human cell lines that lack calnexin can still assemble MHC class I and express the MHC class I normally on their surface, demonstrating redundancy in the chaperone system of MHC class I assembly.

Early experiments demonstrated that immunoprecipitation of TAP also precipitated heavy chain-β_2m heterodimers, indicating that the ER portion of TAP must associate with the newly formed MHC class I dimer. It was later demonstrated, using a mutant cell line that lacked MHC class I surface expression, that another chaperone is necessary for full assembly and expression of MHC class I and for the interaction of the heterodimer with TAP. This chaperone was termed *tapasin*. The tapasin gene is tightly linked to the MHC locus. Multiple tapasin molecules (probably four) interact with one TAP heterodimer and bridge TAP to MHC class I via interactions with β_2m. The number of MHC class I heterodimers associated with one TAP heterodimer is equivalent to the number of tapasin molecules present. The presence of tapasin in this complex increases the efficiency of peptide loading onto MHC class I, but it is not clear if this is due to a direct effect on the peptides or simply to the ability of tapasin to place MHC class I in close proximity to TAP. After peptide loading, the MHC class I heterodimer dissociates from tapasin and TAP and is transported to the surface from the ER via the Golgi apparatus (Fig. 12.4B).

MHC class I dimers that do not bind peptide are eventually transferred to the cytosol and degraded by proteasomes. In this case, the class I molecule is transported by the Sec61p complex, the same pore used for the signal-sequence-dependent translocation of soluble and transmembrane proteins into the ER during synthesis on membrane-associated ribosomes. From this information, it appears that the quantity of available peptide may be the limiting factor in MHC class I assembly. This may be important, since a cell that becomes infected by a virus or other intracellular pathogen would need rapid access to available class I molecules to present foreign peptides to T cells.

Viral Evasion of MHC Class I Antigen Presentation

Cell-mediated immunity to intracellular pathogens, especially viruses, is mediated primarily by the presentation of antigen by MHC class I to CD8$^+$ cytotoxic T cells. Many viruses have evolved elegant mechanisms to modulate this host defense mechanism by reducing antigen presentation by MHC class I molecules (Fig. 12.5). Epstein-Barr virus (EBV) is a ubiquitous virus that causes infectious mononucleosis in many parts of the world, but can also cause

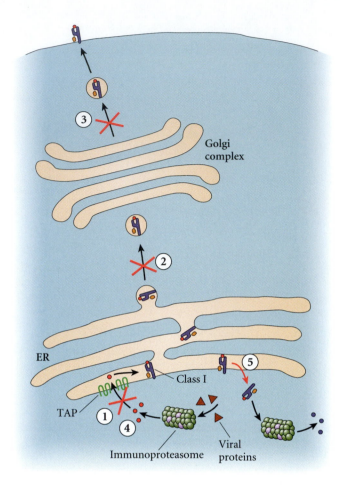

Figure 12.5 Synopsis of immune evasion mechanisms employed by viruses to avoid presentation by MHC class I. (1) The EBV EBNA-1 protein and the HSV ICP47 protein can both interfere with the normal function of TAP. CMV interferes with MHC class I surface expression through (2) the US3 protein, which retains MHC class I in the ER; (3) the gp40 protein, which retains MHC class I in the Golgi complex; (4) the US6 protein, which prevents peptide translocation by TAP; and (5) the US2 and US11 proteins, which induce translocation of MHC class I molecules from the ER into the cytosol.

Burkitt's lymphoma and nasopharyngeal carcinoma. EBV produces the EBNA-1 protein in virus-infected cells. It appears that EBNA-1 can interfere with the normal function of TAP. In addition, an internal repeat region within EBNA-1 can prevent antigen processing of internal EBNA-1-derived peptides, allowing EBNA-1 to persist in the host cell's cytoplasm. Herpes simplex virus (HSV) also avoids class I presentation by affecting TAP function. ICP47, a gene produced early in infection by HSV, coprecipitates with TAP in immunoprecipitation experiments and is a potent inhibitor of TAP function. Hours after HSV infection, MHC class I is found to be retained in the ER rather than exported to the cell's surface.

Cytomegalovirus (CMV) has a number of mechanisms for evading cell-mediated immunity. CMV produces a protein, US3, that can bind MHC class I and cause it to be retained in the ER, preventing its surface expression. The CMV protein gp40 also prevents MHC class I surface expression but causes the MHC to be retained in the Golgi apparatus rather than the ER. Another CMV protein, US6, prevents peptide translocation by TAP. Two other proteins, US2 and US11, independently induce translocation of newly synthesized MHC class I molecules from the ER into the cytosol by an unknown mechanism. It has also been suggested that some viruses may interfere with the function of the proteasome or with production of the immunoproteasome. As proteasome function is critical for cell viability, viral mechanisms for affecting its function cannot result in a shutdown of the proteasome. Nonetheless, if viral products reduce production of antigenic peptides, then there is likely a concomitant reduction in immune responses to the infected cell. It should also be mentioned that many tumor cells are defective in presenting antigen via the MHC class I pathway, due to specific defects in the antigen-processing machinery, including defects in TAP function and decreased surface expression of MHC class I.

Antigen Presentation by MHC Class II

The MHC class II antigen-processing pathway, unlike that of MHC class I, is generally intended to present antigens obtained by endocytosis from the extracellular milieu, although some cytosolic proteins are shunted into this processing pathway. Since these antigens are mostly derived from outside the presenting cell (mainly from organisms that cause extracellular infection), they are termed *exogenous antigens*. The role of the professional APCs—dendritic cells, macrophages, and B cells—in presentation of MHC class II-restricted antigens directs the acquired immune response toward production of protective effectors of immunity—antibody and activated CD4$^+$ helper and effector cells.

Antigen Uptake and Entrance into the Lysosomal/Endosomal Pathway

Exogenous antigens can be taken up by APCs by various pathways. The route of uptake that predominates in any circumstance is dependent on a number of factors, including the type of APC and the presence or absence of preformed antibodies specific for the exogenous antigen. Four mechanisms are used by APCs to internalize exogenous antigen: phagocytosis, receptor-mediated endocytosis, pinocytosis, and macropinocytosis. Macrophages and immature dendritic cells in tissues are very active phagocytes capable of internalizing large, particulate antigens such as whole bacteria. Indeed, phagocytosis is the chief mechanism by which macrophages and immature dendritic cells internalize antigens. Once the dendritic cells move into the lymphoid tissue and mature, they lose their phagocytic capacity. In addition, dendritic cells and macrophages have receptors for complement fragments and antibody Fc regions on their surface. Therefore, exogenous antigens that are coated with antibodies and/or complement split products are more readily ingested than are uncoated antigens. B cells are less efficient than dendritic cells and macrophages at taking up antigens. They are, however, still very potent APCs because of their expression of membrane immunoglobulin, which makes up part of the B-cell antigen receptor.

After the antigen has been internalized by the APC, the endosome (or phagosome) fuses with a specialized vesicle called a *lysosome*, which contains various proteases and other hydrolytic enzymes. The fusion of the phagosome with the lysosome forms a vesicle called a *phagolysosome*, which then enters the endosomal processing pathway. During formation of phagolysosomes, the pH of the vesicles decreases. This decrease in pH is essential for antigen processing since many of the hydrolytic enzymes in the lysosome function optimally at low pH. Protein antigens inside the phagolysosome are degraded into peptides that can eventually be presented by MHC class II molecules. Phagolysosomes encounter MHC molecules by traveling through the endosomal pathway, eventually encountering MHC class II-containing vesicles.

Synthesis of MHC Class II and Trafficking to the Endocytic/Lysosomal Pathway

MHC class II is translated and assembled in the rough ER. During translation, the nascent MHC class II molecules associate with a molecule termed the *invariant chain* (Ii) (Fig. 12.6). One Ii molecule associates with one MHC class II α and β chain heterodimer, and three such complexes form a stable nonamer made up of three Ii molecules and three class II heterodimers. Ii has three distinct functions: (i) it guides the folding of MHC molecules; (ii) it prevents the association of MHC class II heterodimers with antigenic peptides that are present in the ER (these peptides are intended for presentation on MHC class I) by interacting with the peptide-binding groove of the MHC class II; and (iii) it provides a trafficking signal to guide MHC class II to the endosomal/lysosomal pathway. This last function is mediated by dual dileucine-based motifs on the Ii cytoplasmic tail. In its first two functions, Ii acts as a molecular chaperone by assisting both in the folding and assembly of MHC class II and in the formation of proper MHC-peptide complexes. In this respect, Ii serves functions that are roughly analo-

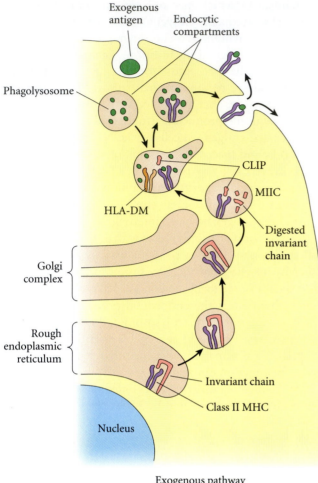

Figure 12.6 Schematic diagram showing the route by which exogenous antigens are processed and presented and MHC class II proteins produced. MHC class II proteins are synthesized in the ER, processed through the Golgi complex, and then membrane vesicles bud off to produce the compartments (MIICs) where the invariant chain is bound to MHC class II and digested to leave only the CLIP peptides behind. The Ii serves a chaperone function, aiding in the assembly of MHC class II in the ER and simultaneously preventing the premature association of endogenous peptides with MHC class II while the latter resides in the ER. Ii also provides targeting signals, ensuring the trafficking of MHC class II to the MIIC. Following fusion of the MHC transport vesicles with phagolysosomes, the CLIP peptide is removed from the MHC class II and exogenous antigenic peptides loaded into the antigen-binding grooves. This complex then moves to the cell surface for interacting with CD4$^+$ T cells.

gous to those served by calnexin and calreticulin in the class I processing pathway.

Once the nonameric complex $(\alpha\beta Ii)_3$ transverses the trans-Golgi network, the transport vesicles containing these complexes can fuse with phagolysosomes (Fig. 12.6). At this point, the lysosomal proteases will cleave Ii into short peptides, leaving only a small peptide called *class II-associated invariant peptide* (CLIP), which remains

in the MHC class II peptide-binding groove. These vesicles, now containing free (i.e., *not* Ii-bound) MHC class II, are called either *MHC class II compartments* (MIIC) or *class II-containing vesicles*. These vesicles are considered to be distinct organelles, are multilamellar, and are acidic. MIICs then fuse with phagolysosomes and permit the newly formed MHC to associate with processed antigenic peptide (Fig. 12.6). Finally, peptide-class II complexes are routed to the plasma membrane to be presented to T cells.

In addition to MHC class II, MIICs contain other proteins called HLA-DM (H-2M in mice), HLA-DO (H-2O in mice), and HLA-DN. These proteins are structurally related to MHC class II and serve chaperone-like functions in that they help remove CLIP from the MHC class II-binding groove to make the latter available for binding to antigenic peptides. It has been demonstrated that HLA-DM stimulates exchange of CLIP for antigenic peptides in the MHC class II-binding groove (Fig. 12.7A). This was

Figure 12.7 The MHC class II-like proteins HLA-DM and HLA-DO modulate the interaction of MHC class II with antigenic peptide. (**A**) HLA-DM helps MHC class II bind antigenic peptides by triggering the removal of CLIP from MHC class II. Whether this occurs by the direct removal of CLIP by HLA-DM (**left**) or indirectly by conformational shifts induced in MHC class II by HLA-DM (**right**) is not yet known. (**B**) HLA-DO negatively regulates HLA-DM-mediated peptide exchange. HLA-DO associates with HLA-DM, and HLA-DM–HLA-DO complexes demonstrate a lower ability to mediate peptide exchange than HLA-DM alone.

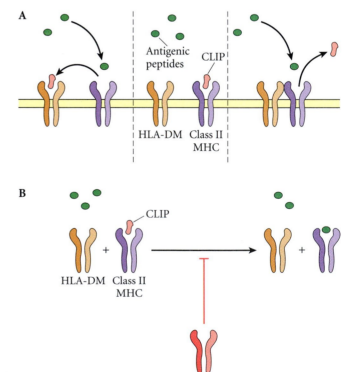

first shown using mutant cell lines lacking HLA-DM; these cells could no longer present antigen via MHC class II, and the majority of the MHC class II on the cell surface contained CLIP in their binding groove. However, the actual mechanism by which HLA-DM mediates this exchange is controversial. One hypothesis is that HLA-DM binds to CLIP very strongly, actively removing CLIP from the class II-binding cleft. Another theory states that HLA-DM binds to MHC class II, thus altering the conformation of the latter so that MHC class II is no longer capable of retaining CLIP in its binding cleft. Another chaperone that exists in the MIIC, HLA-DO, acts to regulate the activity level of HLA-DM (Fig. 12.7B). HLA-DO associates with HLA-DM, and DM-DO complexes demonstrate a lower ability than HLA-DM alone to mediate peptide exchange. Therefore, it is thought that HLA-DO is a negative regulator of HLA-DM activity. The purpose of HLA-DO can only be speculated. The currently available data suggest that the activity of HLA-DM and HLA-DO influences which peptides bind to the class II peptide-binding cleft. When HLA-DM is fully active, the only peptides that are found in the class II-binding cleft are those that fit the cleft perfectly, whereas when HLA-DM activity is limited, a greater variety of peptides (some with a poorer fit for the binding cleft) are found in the cleft. It has been postulated that during positive and negative selection of T lymphocytes, HLA-DO functions to ensure that thymocytes are selected against the widest possible spectrum of self peptides (not just those that bind very well to the binding cleft).

Bacterial Evasion of MHC Class II Immunity

The virulence of some bacterial pathogens requires the inhibition of antigen processing and presentation (Fig. 12.8). For example, shigellae and listeriae are able to escape from an endosome before acidification and lysosomal fusion. These organisms then live in the cytoplasm of their host cell. Employing a different survival strategy, *Legionella* species and mycobacteria alter the phagosomes they inhabit by inhibiting endosome acidification and/or preventing endosome-lysosome fusion. In contrast, leishmanias permit normal acidification and endosome-lysosome fusion but prevent antigen presentation by possibly sequestering MHC class II molecules in these vesicles.

Presentation of Nonclassical, Nonprotein Antigens to T Cells

In recent years it has become apparent that T cells can be stimulated by foreign antigens that are not proteins but are lipid components of bacterial cell walls. Mycolic acid

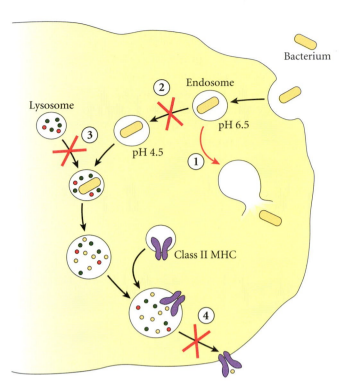

Figure 12.8 Synopsis of immune evasion strategies employed by bacteria to prevent presentation of bacterial antigens on MHC class II. (1) Shigellae and listeriae have the ability to escape from an endosome before acidification and lysosome fusion. *Legionella* species and mycobacteria alter the phagosomes in which they reside (2) by inhibiting endosome acidification and/or (3) preventing endosome-lysosome fusion. (4) Leishmanias permit normal endosome acidification and endosome-lysosome fusion but prevent antigen presentation by trapping MHC class II molecules in these vesicles.

of the cell wall of *Mycobacterium tuberculosis* (the causative agent of tuberculosis) and lipoarabinomannan of the cell wall of *Mycobacterium leprae* (the cause of leprosy) are two examples of lipid antigens that are presented to T cells. Similar to protein antigens presented to T cells, these lipid antigens are usually not recognized directly by the TCR. These antigens are complexed to members of a family of presenting molecules called CD1, which is similar in structure to MHC class I (see Fig. 11.18 and Table 11.4). The two most notable differences between MHC class I and CD1 are that CD1 is nonpolymorphic and that the antigen-binding groove of CD1 is extremely hydrophobic, thus allowing CD1 to bind and present hydrophobic lipid antigens. Each member of the CD1 family has been found to have slightly different preferences for the lipids it presents.

Although the CD1 protein is most similar in structure to MHC class I, the processing pathway that prepares antigens for binding to CD1 more closely resembles the processing pathway used by classical MHC class II in that the glycolipid antigens that eventually bind to CD1 are initially brought into the presenting cell as an exogenous antigen (Fig. 12.9). Such glycolipid antigens have been found to traffic through a series of endocytic compartments. Moreover, some members of the CD1 family have been found to possess cytoplasmic tails that contain trafficking signals that target them to the late endosomal compartments. Thus, CD1 molecules probably bind their antigens in late endosomes after the antigens have been degraded by lysosomal hydrolytic enzymes. It should be emphasized that not all CD1 molecules contain targeting signals for the late endosomes. It is likely that such CD1 molecules (e.g., CD1a) bind to their antigens in other, as yet undefined, subcellular compartments.

Figure 12.9 Diagram showing the route by which microbial lipid antigens (orange) are internalized, processed in phagolysosomes, and presented on CD1 molecules (red) to T cells. The diagram also shows the trafficking of CD1 starting from its point of synthesis in the ER, proceeding to the late endosomal compartment where CD1 encounters processed lipid antigen. The dotted arrows labeled with question marks indicate that some members of the CD1 family (e.g., CD1a) likely do not traffic to the late endosomes and therefore bind antigenic lipids in another, unknown subcellular compartment.

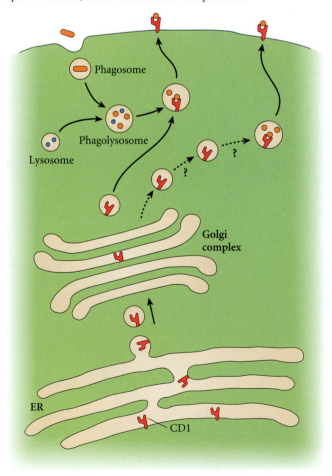

Summary

To activate T-cell recognition of antigenic peptides, protein antigens and some glycolipid antigens need to be processed and presented. Antigen processing can occur in most cells via the endogenous pathway generally leading to presentation of peptides on MHC class I molecules. In professional APCs, antigen processing occurs via the exogenous pathway and leads to presentation of peptides on MHC class II molecules. To produce antigenic fragments for class I binding, cells use the basic function of the proteasome, a cytosolic structure that is modified under the influence of IFN-γ production to become an immunoproteasome. The peptides produced by the immunoproteasome are trafficked to the ER by the TAP proteins, where they can then be placed into the antigen-binding groove of the class I molecule. To produce antigenic fragments for class II binding, the specialized subset of class II-expressing cells, APCs, take up foreign antigens into specialized cytoplasmic vacuoles, degrade the antigens, and complex them to MHC class II. MHC class II is stabilized following synthesis by the invariant chain, and a fragment of this chain, termed CLIP, is left behind in the antigen-binding groove until the MHC class II protein encounters antigenic fragments for loading into the groove. Loading is assisted by MHC class II-like molecules DM and DO (and possible DN). Recently it has been shown that glycolipid antigens can be processed and presented to T cells via the CD1 family of MHC-like molecules. Overall, the processing and presentation of antigenic fragments are essential for TCR recognition and responses to foreign antigens that underlie the initiation of the acquired immune response.

Suggested Reading

Ben-Neriah, Y. 2002. Regulatory functions of ubiquitination in the immune system. *Nat. Immunol.* **3:**20–26.

Bhardwaj, N. 2001. Processing and presentation of antigens by dendritic cells: implications for vaccines. *Trends Mol. Med.* **7:**388–394.

Brocke, P., N. Garbi, F. Momburg, and G. J. Hammerling. 2002. HLA-DM, HLA-DO and tapasin: functional similarities and differences. *Curr. Opin. Immunol.* **14:**22–29.

Hiltbold, E. M., and P. A. Roche. 2002. Trafficking of MHC class II molecules in the late secretory pathway. *Curr. Opin. Immunol.* **14:**30–35.

Kloetzel, P. M. 2001. Antigen processing by the proteasome. *Nat. Rev. Mol. Cell Biol.* **2:**179–187.

Lankat-Buttgereit, B., and R. Tampe. 2002. The transporter associated with antigen processing: function and implications in human diseases. *Physiol. Rev.* **82:**187–204.

Lennon-Dumenil, A. M., A. H. Bakker, P. Wolf-Bryant, H. L. Ploegh, and C. Lagaudriere-Gesbert. 2002. A closer look at proteolysis and MHC-class-II-restricted antigen presentation. *Curr. Opin. Immunol.* 14:15–21.

Mellman, I., and R. M. Steinman. 2001. Dendritic cells: specialized and regulated antigen processing machines. *Cell* 106:255–258.

Niedermann, G. 2002. Immunological functions of the proteasome. *Curr. Top. Microbiol. Immunol.* 268:91–136.

Rivett, A. J., S. Bose, P. Brooks, and K. I. Broadfoot. 2001. Regulation of proteasome complexes by gamma-interferon and phosphorylation. *Biochimie* 83:363–366.

Van den Eynde, B. J., and S. Morel. 2001. Differential processing of class-I-restricted epitopes by the standard proteasome and the immunoproteasome. *Curr. Opin. Immunol.* 13:147–153.

The T-Cell Receptor

Howard Ceri and Chris Mody

In the immune system, specificity is defined through antigen recognition carried out by receptors found on the surface of B and T lymphocytes. On B cells this attribute is mediated by surface immunoglobulin. On T cells, specificity is mediated by the T-cell receptor (TCR) for antigen. Although the TCR bears many similarities to immunoglobulins, key differences between the B-cell receptor (BCR) and the TCR have made the study of the TCR much more difficult. The first major difference is that the TCR is found only as a cell surface molecule, whereas immunoglobulin can be both membrane bound and secreted at high concentrations by B cells. This latter property of B cells provides high concentrations of antibody in a soluble form and ensures the production of high levels of immunoglobulin messenger RNA (mRNA) as a useful tool to study immunoglobulin genetics. The second major difference between antibody and the TCR is the inability of the TCR to recognize antigen directly in its native state. Therefore, direct binding of antigen by TCRs was not detectable and could not be used for the identification and purification of TCRs specific for given antigens. Moreover, the level of expression of TCR mRNA is far lower than that of antibody mRNA. These differences complicated the identification and purification of the TCR.

Isolation and Characterization of the TCR

Functional Assays: the Demonstration of T-Cell Specificity and Self MHC Restriction

The first indications that T cells recognized antigen through a TCR were derived from functional assays using specific target-cell interactions. These experiments, done by Rolf M. Zinkernagel and Peter C. Doherty, not only demonstrated the presence of an antigen-specific TCR but identified a role for self major histocompatibility complex (MHC) in antigen recognition by T cells. Zinkernagel and Doherty used mice infected with lymphocyte choriomeningitis virus (LCMV) to derive target-specific T cells, which could kill LCMV-infected cells from the same strain of mice but not LCMV-infected cells from other strains of mice (Fig. 13.1). This classic experiment showed both antigenic specificity of T-cell killing and MHC restriction of T cells. This surprising finding led to the next obvious question: How does the TCR recognize both the specific antigen and the appropriate MHC molecule? Two explanatory models were proposed. The "dual-receptor" model proposed that that the T cell bears independent receptors, one for antigen and a second for MHC. An alternative "altered-self" model proposed that a single receptor exists that binds a combination of the antigen and MHC molecules, altering the structure of the otherwise self MHC molecule. This question was resolved by the studies of J. W. Kappler and his colleagues in 1981. Kappler started with two independent T-cell hybridomas that expressed TCRs that recognized different antigens in the context of different MHC molecules; the fusion of these hybridomas would yield a single T-cell line express-

Figure 13.1 Killing of virus-infected target cells by T cells is specific for a given virus. Virus-specific T cells are generated by infecting a mouse (strain A) with LCMV and then isolating T lymphocytes from the mouse 2 weeks later. These T cells are then tested for their ability to kill target cells derived from the same mouse strain and infected with either LCMV or a different virus, the mouse mammary tumor virus (MMTV). The T cells from the previously LCMV-infected mouse kill target cells infected with LCMV but do not kill target cells infected with MMTV. Additionally, the immune T cells from strain A mice do not kill strain B cells infected with LCMV, due to production of different MHC proteins by these two different mouse strains.

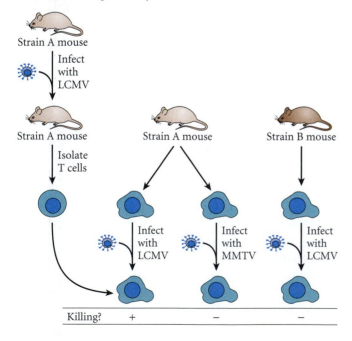

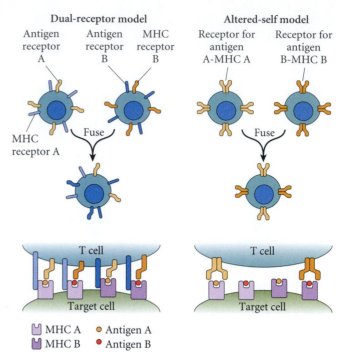

Figure 13.2 Illustration of the proposed dual-receptor and altered-self models of T-cell recognition of antigen-MHC. According to the dual-receptor model (**left**), antigen and MHC are each recognized by a separate receptor molecule on the T cell. Kappler et al. reasoned that if this model is correct, these two receptors should sort independently on the T-cell surface, such that fusion of two T cells (one recognizing antigen A complexed with MHC A and the other recognizing antigen B complexed with MHC B) would produce a hybrid T cell capable of recognizing any combination of antigen A, antigen B, MHC A, and MHC B. In contrast, the altered-self model holds that one TCR recognizes both antigen and MHC (existing as a complex on the target-cell surface). Kappler et al. reasoned that if this model is correct, the same hybrid T cell would recognize antigen A only in the context of MHC A and would recognize antigen B in the context of MHC B. These studies proved conclusively that the altered-self model is the more accurate model.

ing both TCRs. Therefore, if the dual-receptor hypothesis were correct, this fused cell line should recognize either antigen expressed with either MHC molecule; but if the altered-self model were correct, the fused T-cell hybridoma would respond to either antigen but only when expressed in a target cell with the appropriate MHC molecule. The results of this elegant experiment established that the altered-self hypothesis for the recognition of antigen in context of self MHC was the correct model (Fig. 13.2).

The mixed lymphocyte reaction is another type of functional assay that measures the activity of T cells. In these assays the response between lymphocytes from different individuals (allogeneic lymphocytes) can be monitored by measuring (i) the growth of activated lymphocytes responding to the allogeneic cells through the incorporation of [³H]thymidine into replicating DNA, (ii) the activation of responder lymphocytes through the production of specific cytokines, or (iii) the activation of cytotoxic T cells as determined by the killing of specific target cells whose cytoplasm was loaded with ^{51}Cr. These assays demonstrate that foreign, allogeneic MHC molecules can be recognized by T cells from a separate individual because the allogeneic MHC molecules appear to the responding lymphocytes to be the same as a self MHC altered by foreign peptide. Hence, the altered-self model of TCR interactions has been verified by a number of different approaches.

Monoclonal Antibodies and TCR Identification

The initial identification and isolation of the TCR awaited the development of a panel of monoclonal antibodies (MAbs) that could be used to bind specifically to the TCR. These panels were prepared by raising MAbs to T-cell clones and then eliminating those MAbs with reactivity common to all T cells. This resulted in MAbs to T-cell clones that reacted only with one clone, hence identifying an antigen specific to that clone. These "clonotypic" antibodies were, therefore, directed to a T-cell structure antigen believed to be the TCR and was likely analogous to an idiotope determinant on an antibody molecule. The development of clonotypic antibodies permitted the first isolation and study of TCR molecules. The major advancement in this field, however, still had to wait for the development of the techniques for the cloning and sequencing of the TCR genes.

Cloning and Sequencing of the TCR Gene

The isolation and sequencing of the genetic loci encoding the TCR lagged far behind the sequencing of antibody genes. The delay was due in part to the limited amounts of TCR mRNA found in T cells as compared with the high quantity of mRNA for antibody found in B cells. The TCR is found only in a membrane-bound form, with about 30,000 receptors per cell, and therefore a very limited amount of mRNA is needed to maintain TCR protein levels. Human and mouse TCR genes were cloned independently by subtractive hybridization in the same year. This process involved the forming of ^{32}P-labeled complementary DNA (cDNA) from mRNA isolated from T cells (the tester population) and then allowing these cDNAs to hybridize with excess RNA from B cells (the driver population). Genes common to both T cells and B cells would hybridize and could be removed by a chromatography process that separated single-stranded cDNA from double-stranded cDNA-mRNA hybrids, leaving the cDNA specific to T cells as single-stranded, ^{32}P-labeled cDNAs. These cDNAs would include genes for TCR and genes for other T-cell-specific proteins. To find the genes presumed to be specific for the TCR, and hence rearranged from the germ line configuration as are the genes for immunoglobulin molecules, Southern blots were used to find those cDNA molecules that hybridized to a different pattern of restriction-digested DNA when comparing germ line DNA with DNA in the T-cell clones. If no gene rearrangement had occurred, as would be seen with cDNAs derived from non-TCR genes, then the restriction digest pattern would be the same in germ line DNA and T-cell clone DNA (Fig. 13.3). The cDNAs that showed different hybridization patterns in germ line and T-cell DNA were cloned and yielded the predicted genes for TCRs. The subsequent sequencing of these genes allowed for the comparisons of large numbers of TCRs and established their obvious relationship to antibody genes and also provided a means for expressing a large number of recombinant TCRs for protein structural studies.

Structure of the TCR

Structure of the αβ Receptor

Two forms of the TCR exist: the αβ TCR, found on the majority of T cells maturing in the thymus, and the γδ TCR, found on an important but minor subset of the T-cell population. The αβ TCR is composed of one α chain and one β chain linked together by disulfide bonds to produce a structure that resembles a membrane-bound Fab fragment of immunoglobulin (Fig. 13.4). This resemblance results from the presence of two immunoglobulin-fold domains (see Fig. 6.5) in each of the TCR chains, consisting of approximately 100 amino acids organized to form a loop of 60 to 75 amino acids bridged by conserved cysteine residues that form disulfide bonds (Fig. 13.5). As is seen in immunoglobulins, the sequence of the N-terminal domain of the TCR yields a highly variable region when comparing one T cell to the next, while that of the C-terminal domain is constant among T cells. The αβ chains also contain a region similar to the hinge region of immunoglobulins that permits cross-linking of the two chains through disulfide bonds. A transmembrane region, which is characterized by a high level of positively charged amino acids, allows the TCR to be inserted and maintained in the T-cell membrane. This charged property of the transmembrane region allows for the interaction between the TCR and the other members of the TCR complex. Both the α and β chains contain short cytoplasmic tails, which, like the cytoplasmic domains of immunoglobulin, are far too short to play a role in signal

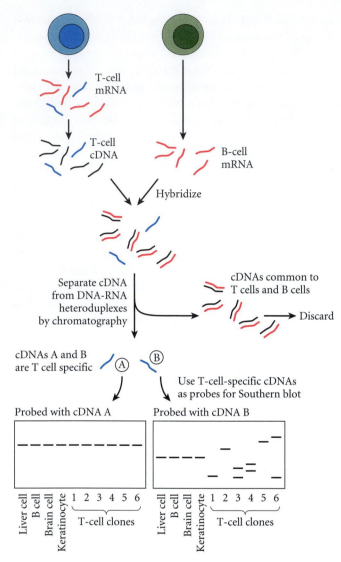

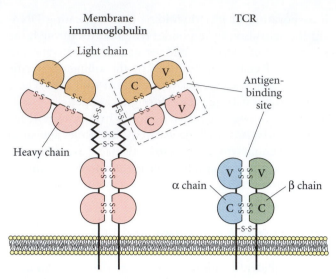

Figure 13.4 The structure of the TCR is similar to that of immunoglobulin (stippled box around one immunoglobulin Fab fragment highlights the region of strongest structural similarity). Like an immunoglobulin, the TCR is composed of two types of protein chains (α and β chains), each consisting of a tandem array of immunoglobulin-like domains. Each protein chain is a different color, and each immunoglobulin-like domain is represented by a shaded circle. In addition, the arrangement of disulfide bonds (-s-s-) is similar in TCR and immunoglobulin, with each immunoglobulin-like domain containing one intradomain disulfide bond and each protein chain attached to the others by interchain disulfide bonds. In each case, the antigen-binding site exists at the interface of two protein chains and is located at the most membrane-distal end of the protein.

Figure 13.3 Strategy used to clone the gene encoding the TCR, which is based on two assumptions: (i) the gene for the TCR is expressed only in T cells, so mRNA for the TCR can be enriched by subtracting the cDNA prepared by reverse transcription from T-cell mRNA with mRNA isolated from a closely related cell type (in this case, a B cell); and (ii) the gene for the TCR should be randomly rearranged in T-cell clones (to generate unique antigenic specificities) but not in B cells or nonlymphoid cells. After non-T-cell-specific cDNAs are removed by hybridization to B-cell RNA followed by chromatography, the T-cell-specific cDNAs are individually cloned and each used as probes in Southern blots of DNA from liver cells, brain cells, keratinocytes, B cells, and various T-cell clones. cDNA A contains a T-cell-specific transcript that is not rearranged and hence does not represent a TCR cDNA. The same banding pattern is attained for all samples on the blot. However, cDNA B contains a TCR gene, as this DNA is rearranged differently in each T-cell clone examined, giving a unique banding pattern for each T-cell clone. Hybridization of one cDNA clone with DNA from multiple T-cell clones is based on the annealing of the constant region genes that are conserved within each different class of TCR chain.

transduction. This quality necessitates the existence of a complex of molecules to carry out the signaling role of the TCR; these molecules are part of the CD3 complex that specifically identifies T cells. The detailed studies of the interaction between the tripartite complex (TCR-MHC antigen-peptide) have been facilitated by the production of soluble TCR and MHC molecules from their gene products by the elimination or substitution of the transmembrane regions. Such experiments have shown the TCR-MHC-peptide interaction is relatively weak. The availability of soluble TCR and MHC has also made it possible to crystallize the TCR-MHC-antigen complexes, permitting the determination of the fine structure of this complex by X-ray diffraction.

Crystallographic data, although limited, have further supported the similarity of TCR to Fab fragments (Fig. 13.5). An obvious similarity between these molecules is the structure or function of the V_α and V_β domains of the TCR, which, like the V_H and V_L domains of immunoglobulin, are composed of both framework regions and hypervariable complementarity-determining regions (CDRs) involved in MHC-antigen recognition. The CDR1 and CDR2 regions, which associate primarily with the MHC component of the MHC-antigen complex,

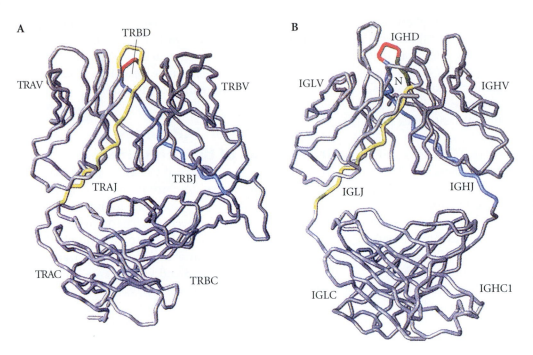

A

TRBD
TRAV
TRBV
TRAJ
TRBJ
TRAC
TRBC

B

IGHD
IGLV
N
IGHV
IGLJ
IGHJ
IGLC
IGHC1

Figure 13.5 A side-by-side comparison of backbone carbon tracings of the TCR (**A**) and an antibody Fab fragment (**B**). TRAJ (J_α) and IGLJ (J_L) are depicted in yellow, TRBJ (J_β) and IGHJ (J_H) are depicted in cyan, and TRBD (D_β) and IGHD (D_H) are shown in red. Green regions indicate areas where nontemplated nucleotides (N-nucleotides) were inserted during V(D)J recombination. Modified from I. A. Wilson and K. C. Garcia, *Curr. Opin. Struct. Biol.* 7:839–848, 1997, with permission.

show less variability, as might be expected, than the CDR3 region, which seems largely responsible for the recognition of a vast potential array of antigenic peptides displayed in the MHC-antigen complex. The TCR is situated diagonally over the MHC-antigen complex, such that the V_α is found at the N-terminal region of the MHC-bound peptide, the V_β is found at the C-terminal region, and the CDR3α and CDR3β lie directly over the peptide (Fig. 13.6). In the variable region of the TCR, a fourth hypervariable loop exists that has no homolog in antibody variable regions.

Structure of the γδ Receptor

The γδ TCR is structurally homologous to the αβ receptor but composed of γ and δ chains in place of the α and β chains that are also linked by disulfide bonds. γδ T cells represent fewer than 5% of the T cells in peripheral lymphoid tissues but account for up to 15% of lymphocytes found among the epithelial cells of the small intestine and as many as 40% of the lymphocytes found among the epithelial cells in the large bowel. These are referred to as intraepithelial lymphocytes. γδ T cells do not mature in the thymus and hence do not undergo the same thymic selection processes as αβ T cells. The functions played by γδ T cells are not well understood, but on the basis of their anatomic distribution, it has been suggested that they mediate an important role in the protection of mucosal surfaces. At mucosal surfaces, γδ T cells are known to respond to intracellular pathogens, including bacteria (listeriae), viruses (human immunodeficiency virus), and

Figure 13.6 Backbone carbon tracings of two TCRs complexed with peptide-MHC. CDRs of the TCRs are color coded as follows: CDR1α (blue), CDR2α (purple), CDR3α (green), CDR1β (cyan), CDR2β (pink), CDR3β (yellow), and HV4 (orange). Reprinted from I. A. Wilson and K. C. Garcia, *Curr. Opin. Struct. Biol.* 7:839–848, 1997, with permission.

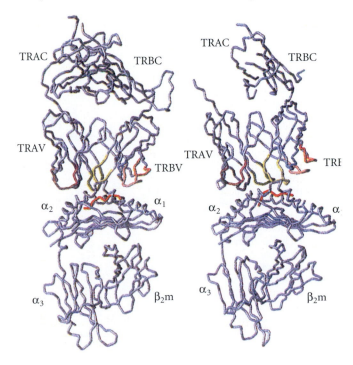

TRAC
TRBC
TRAC
TRBC
TRAV
TRAV
TRBV
TRB
α_2
α_1
α_2
α
α_3
β_2m
α_3
β_2m

parasites (leishmanias), and have also been implicated in the immune response to highly conserved heat shock proteins. This observation has been interpreted to mean that γδ T cells are an immune effector targeted at eliminating aberrant host cells that have undergone physiologic stress, which can be caused by physical damage to a cell or by infection and results in the production of heat shock proteins.

The germ line gene segments of γδ TCRs are significantly less variable than those involved in the αβ TCR gene rearrangement. Evidence indicates that this difference may be due to the interaction of γδ T cells with nonclassical MHC molecules, which possess less polymorphism than the MHC class I and class II molecules. The variability of the γδ TCR changes with aging. The TCR repertoire goes from being broad and diverse in young individuals to being more restricted, approaching oligoclonality, in older individuals. The reason for this reduction in diversity is not known; however, since the reduction is not always observed, it may be the result of an antigen-driven selective process in some individuals. This change in the diversity of

the population may indicate a change in function of these cells. For example, whereas γδ T cells may play an important role in mucosal protection in the young, this role may diminish with age as the immune system matures and acquires significantly more memory function.

Organization of TCR Genes

Organization of the Germ Line

The TCR genes encoding for the α, β, γ, and δ chains of mice have been mapped to chromosomes 14, 6, 13, and 14, respectively. Those in humans are found on chromosomes 14, 7, 7, and 14, respectively. The germ line configurations of TCR genes, like that of immunoglobulin genes, contain multiple variable (V), joining (J), and constant (C) segments for the α and γ TCR genes, and for the β and δ TCR genes they consist of V, J, and C segments along with a diversity (D) segment (Fig. 13.7 and Table 13.1). Therefore, the α and γ chains are analogous to immunoglobulin light chains and the β and δ chains are analogous to immunoglobulin heavy chains. An interest-

Figure 13.7 Germ line organization of the human TCRα (TRA) and TCR δ (TRD) gene families. Functional V genes for both the TRAV and TRDV polypeptides are shown in green, and pseudogenes are shown in red. Variable-region genes with single numbers are not part of a subgroup. Variable-region genes with a hyphenated number (i.e., 13-1) indicate the subgroup (first number) and gene within that subgroup (second number). Genes with a composite designation including a forward slash (/) and a DV number can be incorporated into variable regions of either TCR α or TCR δ chains. Variable-region genes exclusively used in TCR δ chains are designated TRDV. Note TRDV3 is 3′ of the TRDC gene and transcribed in the opposite direction (arrow). Solid yellow bars represent functional joining-region genes, red bars are pseudogenes, and pink bars indicate potential open reading frames for which no protein has yet been found. TCR δ-chain diversity-region genes are in dark blue (TRDD1 to 3). Constant-region genes are in light blue (TRDC and TRAC). Enhancers (cyan) refer to regulatory genetic elements that promote transcription of the genes in this region. From IMGT (http//imgt.cines.fr) with permission from M.-P. Lefranc.

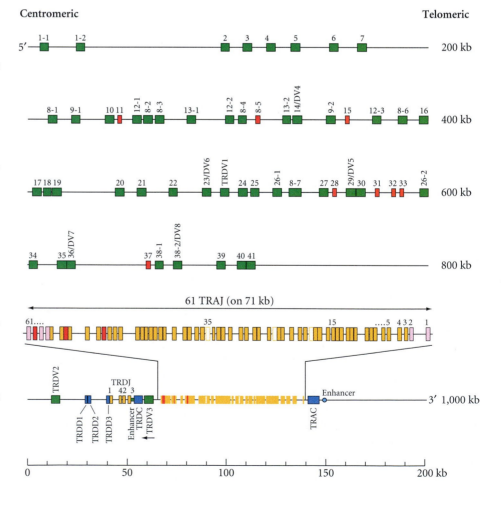

Table 13.1 Comparison of the number of V, D, and J genes in the germ line of human immunoglobulin (Ig) and TCR genes

	V segments		D segments		J segments	
Human gene	Total	Functional	Total	Functional	Total	Functional
IGGH (Ig heavy chain)	51		27		6	
IGLL (Ig light λ chain)	30		0		6	
IGLK (Ig light κ chain)	40		0		5	
TRA (TCR α chain)	54	42–44[a]	0		61	50
TRC (TCR γ chain)	12–15[a]	4–6	0		5	
TRB (TCR β chain)	64–67[a]	40–42	2	2	13	13
TRD (TCR δ chain)	8[b]	8	3	3	4	4

[a] Ranges indicate haplotype variations.
[b] Five of the eight TRDV genes can also be used to produce the TRAV polypeptide.

ing aspect to the arrangement of the TCR genes is the placement of the genes encoding the δ chain between the V and J segments of the α chain. This ensures that one T cell does not simultaneously express both αβ and γδ TCRs, since the rearrangement of the α chain eliminates the genes encoding the δ chain.

Rearrangement of TCR Genes and Analogies to Immunoglobulin Genes

Rearrangement of the TCR genes occurs only in T cells and follows mechanisms analogous to those used in the rearrangement of immunoglobulin genes. Both T cells and B cells express the recombination-activating genes known as *Rag-1* and *Rag-2* that are responsible for rearrangement of these genes. In T cells, however, the *Rag-1* and *Rag-2* gene products (RAG-1 and RAG-2) do not rearrange the immunoglobulin genes because a T-cell-specific protein binds to the 3′ enhancer of the immunoglobulin κ chains and blocks the rearrangement of the immunoglobulin genes. Just as in B cells, RAG-1 and RAG-2 recognize recombination signal sequences (RSSs) that are associated with each of the V, D, and J gene segments of the TCR. In T cells, the RSS regions exist as heptamer and nonamer sequences separated by one-turn spacers of 12 base pairs (bp) or two-turn spacers of 23 bp, as in immunoglobulin genes. Recombination of both immunoglobulin and TCR can occur only between sets of 13-bp and 23-bp spacers, referred to as the 12/23 rule, to ensure the proper alignment of segments (see Fig. 7.8 and 7.9). Also important in the recombination processes are components of the double-strand break-repair mechanism. SCID mice, for example, have defective genes for proteins involved in double-strand break repair and therefore are unable to rearrange either their TCR or immunoglobulin genes. The general process of VJ and V(D)J joining of gene segments to yield functional TCR genes follows a mechanism that is virtually the same as for immunoglobulin genes (see Fig. 7.18).

Generation of Diversity in the TCR

Genetic Basis for the Generation of TCR Variable Regions

In both TCRs and BCRs, antigenic diversity is achieved through a process of rearrangement of the germ line gene sequences. In both cases, a complex set of mechanisms, including multiple germ line segments, combinatorial joining of gene segments, junctional flexibility, P- and N-nucleotide addition, and combinatorial association between the two antigen receptor chains, acts to enhance the level of diversity. However, subtle differences exist in the application of these mechanisms in T cells compared with B cells, accounting for the unique properties of antigen recognition seen in T cells.

An obvious difference in the generation of diversity between immunoglobulin and TCR is the difference in the number of V-gene segments in the germ line of each receptor. The absolute numbers of V segments in the TCR and immunoglobulin germ line vary between haplotypes. Current information about the human and mouse TCR gene loci can be found at http://imgt.cines.fr:8104. The nomenclature for the designation of the genes of the TCR loci has been standardized since 1999 and accepted by the Human Gene Organization Nomenclature Committee. Many genes for a given TCR region are closely related and thus placed into subgroups. Usually, when there are multiple genes present for a single function (i.e., the variable region), the different genes are distinguished from each other by a composite number, the first of which represents the subgroup and the second, preceded by a hyphen (-), the gene within the subgroup. For example, there are two TCR α-chain V segments (TRAV) in subgroup 1 designated TRAV1-1 and TRAV1-2. Some subgroups have only one member, i.e., human TRAV subgroup 2 has only one member, designated TRAV2.

Based on sequencing of the human genome, the number of TRAV segments is 54, of which 42 to 44 are functional (expressed protein), 8 are pseudogenes (no expressed protein), and 2 are not yet characterized. The human TRAV genes are grouped into 32 to 34 subgroups. The TRAV genes are linked to 61 TCR α-chain J gene segments (TRAJ1 to TRAJ61), of which 11 are functional, but the TRAJ genes cluster in a region that is 3′ to both the TRAV genes and all of the TCR δ-chain segments, including the variable (TRDV), diversity (TRDD), joining (TRDJ), and constant (TRDC) region segments (Fig. 13.7). The TRAJ genes are found 5′ to the single TCR α-chain C segment (TRAC).

Among the human TCR β-chain V segments (TRBV) there are 64 to 67 genes belonging to 30 subgroups, of which 40 to 42 in 21 to 23 subgroups are known to be functional (Fig. 13.8). As for the TRAV genes, the TRBV genes would be designated by TRBV followed by a composite number reflecting the subgroup and the gene within the subgroup (i.e., in TRBV subgroup 3 there are two genes, TRBV3-1 and TRBV3-2). All except one of the TRBV genes are located 5′ of the TCR β-chain diversity, joining, and constant region genes; TRBV30 is located 3′ of the DJC cluster and is transcribed in the opposite orientation to the other TRB genes. The genes for the diversity (TRBD), joining (TRBJ), and constant regions (TRBC) for the human TCR β chain are arranged in two,

likely duplicated, clusters. The first cluster has one TRBD gene (TRBD1), six TRBJ genes (J1-1 to J1-6), and one TRBC gene (TRBC1). The second cluster has one TRDB gene (TRBD2), seven TRBJ genes (TRBJ2-1 to 2-7), and one TRBC gene (TRBC2). Each of the two TRBC genes has two known alleles. The alleles are distinguished by an asterisk (*) after the gene designation; hence, the two allelic versions of TRBC1 are written TRBC1*01 and TRBC1*02. The presence of two separate TRBC genes in most humans gives rise to two different β-chain constant region isotypes.

The human TCR γ-chain locus, located on chromosome 7, has 12 to 15 V gene segments (TRGV), of which 4 to 6 are functional (Fig. 13.9). Five of the six are in subgroup 1, the other one in subgroup 2. However, unlike the TRAV genes, the TRGV genes each have their own designation (TRGV1 to TRGV11) and not a designation that includes a subgroup number, a hyphen, and a number for the variant in the subgroup. The TRGV locus is 5′ to two related clusters encoding the TCR γ-chain J genes (TRGJ) and C genes (TRGC). The first cluster has three TRGJ genes and one TRGC gene, and the second cluster two TRGJ genes and one TRGC gene. There are two known allelic variants of the TRGC1 (TRGC1*01 and TRGC1*02)

Figure 13.8 Germ line organization of the human TCRβ (TRB) gene locus. Boxes are not to scale and exons are not indicated. Functional V genes for the TRBV polypeptides are shown in green, pseudogenes are in red, and yellow boxes indicate potential open reading frames for which no protein has yet been found. Variable-region genes with single numbers are not part of a subgroup. Variable-region genes with a hyphenated number (i.e., 3-1) indicate the subgroup (first number) and gene within that subgroup (second number). Darker yellow bars represent two joining-region gene clusters with six or seven genes (J1-1 to J1-6 and J2-1 to J2-7). TCR β-chain diversity-region genes are in light purple (TRBD1 and TRBD2). Constant-region genes are in blue (TRBC1 and C2). Enhancer (cyan) refers to regulatory genetic elements that promote transcription of the genes in this region. Purple boxes (filled, functional; empty, pseudogenes) represent genes not related to TCR production. From IMGT (http://imgt.cines.fr) with permission from M.-P. Lefranc.

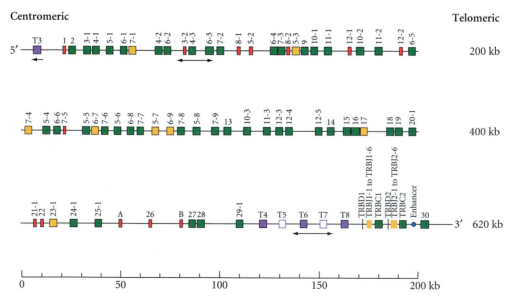

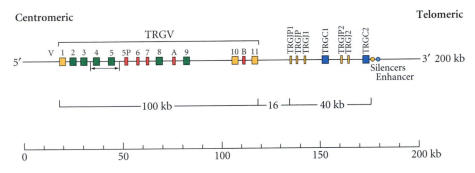

Figure 13.9 Germ line organization of the human TCRγ (TRG) gene locus. Boxes are not to scale and exons are not indicated. A double arrow indicates an insertion or deletion polymorphism. Functional V genes for the TRGV polypeptides are shown in green, pseudogenes are in red, and yellow boxes indicate potential open reading frames for which no protein has yet been found. All TRGV genes that are not pseudogenes are designated by a number. Two clusters represent the TRGJ (orange-yellow) and TRGC (blue) regions. Enhancer (cyan) refers to regulatory genetic elements that promote transcription of the genes in this region. Silencer (yellow circle) refers to a regulatory genetic element that inhibits transcription from the region. From IMGT (http://imgt.cines.fr) with permission from M.-P. Lefranc.

locus and four allelic variants of the TRGC2 locus. The TRGC locus is encoded by four or five exons because of duplication or triplication of exon 2. If an allelic variant of TRGC2 has a duplication of exon 2, it is officially designated as TRGC2(2X). Within the TRGC2(2X) locus there are four known allelic variants, designated TRGC2(2X)*01 to TRGC2(2X)*04. The variant with three replications of exon 2 has only one allelic variant and is designated to TRGC2(3X)*01. The complexity of all of these designations reflects the evolutionary development of the genetic loci for TCR that has occurred in humans and demonstrates the role of duplications within both clusters and even exons in generating polymorphism within the human genome.

With the TCR δ locus located between the TRAV and TRAJ genes, a complicated use of variable region genes from both the α-chain locus and δ-chain locus is seen (Fig. 13.7). There are three separate TRDV genes in three subgroups that are found only in TCR δ chains. One of the TRDV genes, TRDV1, is located among the TRAV genes. There are five V genes designated TRAV/DV, belonging to five subgroups, which can be found rearranged with either D and J segments of the TCR δ locus or with the J segment of the TCR α-locus. Thus, these five genes are found in either TCR α or TCR δ chains. There are three separate TCR δ-locus D genes (TRDD1 to TRDD3), four separate TCR δ-locus J genes (TRDJ1 to TRDJ4), and one TCR δ-locus C gene (TRDC). As was found for the TCR β locus, there is one variable-region gene, TRDV3, located 3′ of the DJC cluster and transcribed in the opposite direction. This suggests there was a single locus ancestral to both the TCR β and TCR δ loci. The use of some of the same vari-

able region genes in either TCR α or TCR δ chains provides another means for generating diversity among TCRs.

In mice, the arrangement of the TCR genes is analogous to that of humans but reflects the differences in the genomes of these two species. For the murine TCR α locus there are 96 TRAV genes, of which 68 are functional and grouped into 23 subgroups (Fig. 13.10). Like the human genome, there are a large number (61) of TRAJ genes in the mouse, 38 of which are functional. There is one mouse TRAC gene with two alleles (TRAC*01 and TRAC*02). For the murine TCR β locus, there are 35 TRBV genes grouped into 31 subgroups, of which 21 are known to be functional (Fig. 13.11). As was also seen for the human TCR β locus, the diversity, joining, and constant region genes are represented by two duplicated clusters, each of which contains one TRBD gene, seven TRBJ genes, and a TRBC gene. There is a TRBV gene, TRBV31, 3′ of the TRBC gene and transcribed in the opposite direction.

TRGV genes in mice fall into five subgroups with seven individual genes (Fig. 13.12). There are four J/C elements (J1 to J4 and C1 to C4). The J3 and C3 genes are not functional and are 3′ to a nonfunctional TRGV gene, TRGV3. For the TRGJ1/TRGC1 and the TRGJ4/TRGC4 regions the J gene is 5′ to the C gene. For the TRGJ2/TRGC2 region, the joining region is 3′ to the constant region. Four of the TRGV genes are 5′ to TRGJ1 and TRGC1, TRJ3 and TRGC3, and TRGC2 and TRGJ2. Two of the TRGV genes lie in between the 3′ end of the TRGJ2 gene and the 5′ end of the TRGJ4 gene. The limited amount of genetic information encoding the mouse TCR γ locus underlies the

Figure 13.10 Germ line organization of the mouse TCRα (TRA) and TCRδ (TRD) gene families. The boxes representing the genes are not to scale. Exons are not shown. Variable-region genes for TRAV and TRDV are designated by a number for the subgroup followed, whenever there are several genes belonging to the same subgroup, by a hyphen and a number for their relative localization. Numbers increase from 5′ to 3′ in the locus. Functional V genes for the TRAV polypeptides are shown in green, pseudogenes are in red, and solid yellow boxes indicate potential open reading frames for which no protein has yet been found. The solid blue line and the dashed blue line below the map represent two parts of the locus that are duplicated. The TRAV genes of the proximal V cluster (closer to the telomere) are designated by a number for the subgroup, followed by a hyphen and a number for the localization from 3′ to 5′ in the locus. The TRAV genes of the distal duplicated V cluster (closer to the centromere) are designated by the same numbers as the corresponding genes in the proximal V cluster, with the letter D added. Single arrows show two genes, TRAV7-2 and TRDV5, whose transcriptional polarity is opposite to that of the TRA JC cluster and the TRD DJC cluster. TRDD-region genes are in dark blue, functional joining-region genes in orange-yellow, pseudogenes in red; and joining-region pink boxes indicate potential open reading frames for which no protein has yet been found. Constant-region genes are in lighter blue. From IMGT (http://imgt.cines.fr) with permission from M.-P. Lefranc.

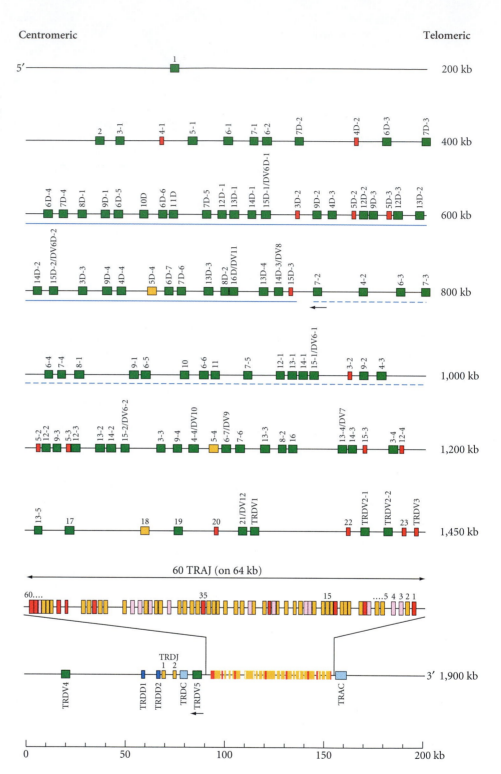

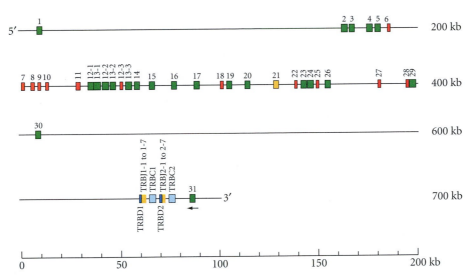

Figure 13.11 Germ line organization of the mouse TCRβ (TRB) gene locus. Boxes are not to scale and exons are not indicated. A single arrow shows the most 3′ TRBV gene whose transcriptional polarity is opposite to that of the DJC cluster. Functional V genes for the TRBV polypeptides are shown in green, pseudogenes are in red, and yellow boxes indicate potential open reading frames for which no protein has yet been found. Variable-region genes with single numbers are not part of a subgroup. Variable-region genes with a hyphenated number (i.e., 3-1) indicate the subgroup (first number) and gene within that subgroup (second number). Orange-yellow bars represent two joining-region gene clusters with six or seven genes (J1-1 to J1-6 and J2-1 to J2-7). TCR β-chain diversity-region genes are in dark blue (TRBD1 and TRBD2). Constant-region genes are in a lighter blue (TRBC1 and C2). From IMGT (http://imgt.cines.fr) with permission from M.-P. Lefranc.

low amount of diversity in recognition of antigen-MHC complexes by this TCR. TRDV gene use in mice is complicated, as it is in humans, by the presence of TRAV genes that can not only rearrange with the TCR α-chain J segments (TRAJ) to give the expected VJ rearrangement but can also rearrange with the TCR δ-chain DJ segments to produce the TCR δ-chain V(D)J segment. Of the 96 mouse TRAV genes, there are 8 TRAV/DV genes that can also join with δ-chain DJ segments (Fig. 13.10). There are 11 additional TCR δ-locus-specific TRDV genes, of which 7 are known to be functional and unknown. Mice have two TRDD genes (TRDD1 and TRDD2), two TRDJ genes (TRDJ1 and TRDJ2), and one TRDC gene. One of the

TRDV genes, TRDV5, lies 3′ to the TRDC gene and is transcribed in the opposite direction, a situation that is orthologous to the human TCR β and TCR δ loci. Until the completion of the sequencing of the mouse genome, the actual complexity and functionality of all of the TRDV genes will not be known.

Generation of TCR Diversity and Interaction with Peptide-MHC

The absence of somatic hypermutation mechanisms in the TCR restricts the level of diversity that can be generated in the CDR1 and CDR2 regions of the TCR, encoded by the V segment. This reduction in the variability of

Figure 13.12 Germ line organization of the mouse TCRγ (TRG) gene locus. Boxes are not to scale and exons are not indicated. Horizontal arrows show genes whose polarity is opposite to that of the locus. Functional V genes for the TRGV polypeptides are shown in green and yellow boxes indicate potential open reading frames for which no protein has yet been found. All mouse TRGV genes are designated by a number. Four clusters represent the TRGJ (orange-yellow) and TRGC (blue) regions. The mouse TRGJ3/C3 cluster is not expressed. Enhancer (cyan) refers to regulatory genetic elements that promote transcription of the genes in this region. From IMGT (http://imgt.cines.fr) with permission from M.-P. Lefranc.

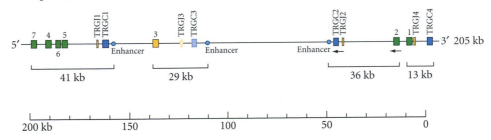

CDR1 and CDR2 in the TCR is, however, consistent with our current model of complex formation between TCR-antigen-MHC. It is believed that CDR1 and CDR2 of the TCR are responsible for the association with the MHC component of the complex, whereas CDR3 is responsible for binding to the antigenic peptide. The variability in the structure of MHC is very much less than that for antigenic peptides bound to the MHC, and hence the level of variability required in the CDR1 and CDR2 regions of the TCR would be significantly less than that required in the CDR3 region. The importance of this specific recognition of MHC by the TCR in the function of the immune system may have applied an evolutionary selective pressure to prevent the use of somatic hypermutation as a mechanism for generating diversity in T cells. Mutations resulting in a change in TCR-MHC interaction could result either in a loss of T-cell function (not recognizing appropriate MHC) or in the induction of autoimmunity (inappropriate interaction with self MHC). This is an especially important consideration, as hypermutation would have the capacity to alter T-cell activity after negative selection has occurred in the thymus.

To compensate for the lack of diversity resulting from limited numbers of V segments and to create greater diversity in the desired CDR3 domain, the germ line of the TCR contains greater numbers of J segments than does the immunoglobulin germ line. This increase in J segments alone can account for significant diversity through combinatorial joining. For example, in a human, the TCAV and TCAJ genes can potentially give rise to 2,200 TCR α chains; in the κ immunoglobulin light chains there might be 200 such combinations possible. The potential diversity of the CDR3 region in the TCR is further increased in several ways. The distribution of the 12/23-bp spacers in the TCR germ line differs from that in the immunoglobulin germ line and contributes to diversity in the TCR in a way not seen in immunoglobulin rearrangement. In immunoglobulin genes, the 12/23 rule allows a D segment to recombine with only a V segment or a J segment, never with another D segment (see chapter 7). In the TCR germ line, a 23-bp spacer is also found 3′ to the V segments and a 12-bp spacer is found 5′ to the J segments, which would allow for VJ joining. To accommodate D joining, a 12-bp spacer is found 5′ of each D region segment and a 23-bp spacer is found 3′ of the D segments (Fig. 13.13). This arrangement could further increase diversity of the CDR3 region by allowing multiple D segments to be inserted between V and J, making it possible to have VDDJ or VDDDJ joining. This usually occurs in the TCR δ chain, as the TCR β chain has only two duplicated TRBD regions. Diversity in the CDR3 domain is ex-

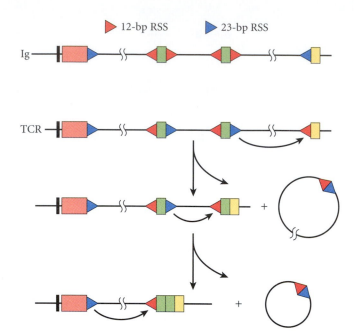

Figure 13.13 Comparison of RSS arrangement in immunoglobulin (Ig) versus that in TCR. Similar to Ig, V, D, and J segments of the TCR chain loci are flanked by 12-bp and 23-bp RSSs. However, the arrangement of these RSSs differs between TCR and Ig. Most notable is the difference in RSS arrangement flanking the D segments. In the Ig heavy-chain locus, the same type of RSS is found upstream and downstream of each D segment, which prevents D segments from joining to each other. In the TCR β- and δ-chain loci, each D segment is flanked upstream by a 12-bp RSS and downstream by a 23-bp RSS. (**Bottom**) The arrangement of RSSs in the TCR β- and δ-chain loci allows joining of multiple D segments in one rearranged variable-domain exon, while still obeying the 12/23 rule.

panded equally in immunoglobulin and TCR by junctional flexibility and P-nucleotide addition (Fig. 13.14); however, N-region nucleotide addition contributes more to CDR3 diversity in the TCR than it does in immunoglobulin, as this mechanism is active on all TCR chains but only on the heavy chain during immunoglobulin-gene rearrangement. These factors maximize the diversity of TCRs where it is necessary (CDR3) but limit diversity where it is not (CDR1 and CDR2).

Production of a Functional Receptor

Since the TCR is found only as a membrane-associated molecule, the final structure of the TCR is much simpler than that of immunoglobulins, being closely related only to the (Fab′)₂ structure (Fig. 13.14). Thus, the three-dimensional structures of the αβ TCR, the γδ TCR, and the (Fab′)₂ show close similarities. Some notable differences include the smaller angle between the variable and constant domains of the γδ TCR and the larger gap be-

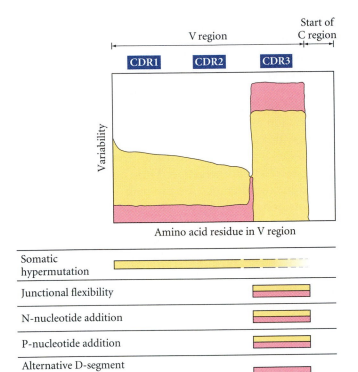

Figure 13.14 Schematic diagram comparing variability within a TCR variable domain versus that within an immunoglobulin domain. For clarity, the TCR curve (pink) is in the foreground on the left side, while the immunoglobulin curve (yellow) is in the foreground on the right side. Bars at the top indicate the extent of the CDRs. The chart below the graph indicates the extent to which various molecular mechanisms contribute to variability in each CDR of the V region.

tween the constant regions of the γ and δ polypeptides when compared to αβ and heavy- and light-chain constant regions. The lack of a soluble form of the TCR obviates the need for the elaborate alternative splicing mechanisms that B cells use to produce membrane-bound or secreted immunoglobulin. T cells also have no need for the class switching seen in the production of immunoglobulin.

For the TCR to produce a functional receptor, it must be assembled into the plasma membrane such that it can recognize an appropriate antigen-MHC complex displayed to the T cell and must also be able to signal this event to the T cell. Signal sequences, preceding the variable domain of each chain, ensure the transport of the protein into the lumen of the endoplasmic reticulum (ER). The TCR is anchored in the ER membrane by its membrane-spanning C terminus. The two immunoglobulin-like domains of each chain are present in the lumen of the ER, where they are glycosylated as part of secondary processing. The TCR is then stabilized by the formation of disulfide bonds between the αβ heterodimer within the hinge-like regions.

Interaction with CD3

Structure of CD3

Production of a stable, transmembrane TCR cannot occur in the absence of another marker of T cells, a multiprotein complex designated as CD3. In addition, the TCR α, β, γ, and δ chains lack large intracellular signaling domains, so expression of TCR on the T-cell surface in association with CD3 provides the biophysical means for transmitting the signal for T-cell activation following binding of the TCR to the MHC-antigen complex. The CD3 complex is made up of five polypeptide chains, named γ, δ, ε, ζ, and η (Fig. 13.15). One of each of the γ, δ, and ε chains is present in the complex, along with a dimer of ζ and η chains; 90% of CD3 complexes possess a ζζ homodimer, and 10% possess a ζη heterodimer. The γ, δ, and ε chains are members of the immunoglobulin superfamily and are required for the association of CD3 with the TCR, whereas the ζ and η chains have a short external region and long cyto-

Figure 13.15 Overall structure of a γδ TCR, αβ TCR, and Fabs. (**A**) γδ TCR (red); (**B**) αβ TCR (green); (**C to E**) three Fabs (blue) showing the angle between the V and C domains. The V domains are at the top of each depiction. The γδ TCR V regions have a smaller angle between them when compared with the other antigen-binding molecules, and the γδ C regions are more separated from each other than the αβ TCR C regions or HL Fab C regions. The δ, β, and H chains are the lighter shades, and the γ, α, and L chains are the darker shades. Reprinted from T. J. Allison et al., *Nature* **411**:820–824, 2001, with permission from D. Garboczi and *Nature* (Macmillan Publishers Ltd.).

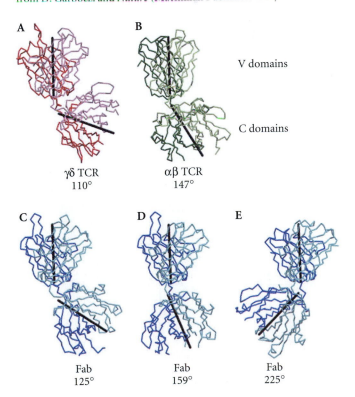

plasmic regions that are responsible for signaling. The negative charge of the transmembrane region of CD3 is due to the presence of many aspartic acid residues that interact with positively charged residues on the transmembrane region of the TCR chains. This ensures that the two are in close proximity and increases the likelihood that each CD3 molecule associates with two or more TCR molecules.

Function of CD3 polypeptides

The CD3 molecule is responsible for transmitting the signal from the membrane-based TCR to cytoplasmic molecules involved in signal transduction within the T cell (Fig. 13.16). The cytoplasmic domains of the CD3 chains have binding domains that interact with tyrosine kinases that are critical for cellular signaling. These binding domains are called *immunoreceptor tyrosine-based activation motifs* (ITAMs). The γ, δ, and ε chains each have a single ITAM, whereas ζ and η each have three copies. The ζ, η, and γ chains associate with the Fyn tyrosine kinase, and the ζ chain associates with the Src homology domain 2 of tyrosine kinase ZAP-70 (Fig. 13.17). These tyrosine kinases are responsible for transmitting activation signals in the T cell after antigen recognition and have also been implicated in positive and negative selection during T-cell maturation in the thymus.

Role of CD4 and CD8 Polypeptides in TCR Function

The affinity of the TCR for MHC-antigen complexes is not particularly high when compared with the affinity of

Figure 13.16 The CD3 complex consists of six polypeptide chains in association with two (or more) TCRs. The CD3 complex depicted contains a homodimer of ζ chains; however, some CD3 complexes contain a ζη heterodimer instead of a ζζ homodimer (not shown). The ζ and η chains have three ITAMs per chain, while the γ, δ, and ε chains have a single ITAM per chain. The ITAMs interact with the Fyn and ZAP-70 protein tyrosine kinase.

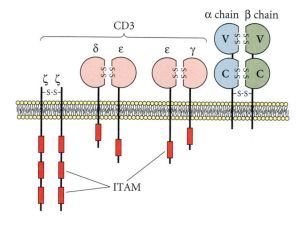

other immune-binding interactions, such as that of immunoglobulin to antigen. There are approximately 8,000 TCRs on the surface of each T cell that need to be engaged to signal the T cell. Signaling can be initiated by as few as 8 to 10 MHC-antigen complexes. Thus, the low affinity of binding and the requirement for rapid association and dissociation of a limited number of MHC-antigen complexes with a large number of TCRs mandate the binding of additional pairs of molecules to strengthen the avidity of the MHC-TCR interaction. These additional receptor-ligand interactions increase the magnitude of the signal transduction events that are responsible for activating T-cell and antigen-presenting cell (APC) responses, heightening the cellular response to antigen presentation and inducing cytokine production by the T cell and the APC. This coordinated spatial arrangement of receptors that bind to their receptive ligands is called the immunologic synapse, which forms the junction between the APC and the responding T cell that is necessary for signaling the T cell.

The subset of T lymphocytes expressing the accessory molecule CD4 on their surface makes up the CD4$^+$ subset of T cells, mostly T helper cells and T cells that mediate delayed-type hypersensitivity (Fig. 13.18A). CD4 is a monomeric 55-kilodalton (kDa) protein that has four immunoglobulin-like domains. Of these immunoglobulin-like domains, the one most distal to the membrane binds to the β2 domain of the MHC class II molecule. The cytoplasmic domain of CD4 contains serine residues that are phosphorylated upon T-cell activation. Ligation of CD4 to the TCR-MHC-antigen complex markedly enhances signal transduction. This ligation is enhanced by the interaction between CD4 and the tyrosine kinase Lck and is an important component of T-cell signal transduction (discussed in chapter 14). Although the interaction of CD4 with MHC class II has classically been thought also to increase the adhesion of the T cell to the APC, recent evidence suggests that adhesion due to CD4 enhances the initial interaction between the TCR and MHC and has a distinctive spatial distribution within the immunologic synapse—a focal cluster of TCRs and accessory molecules that form the junction between the APC and the responding T cell.

Another subpopulation of mature T lymphocytes does not express CD4 but instead expresses the CD8 accessory molecule. These are the CD8$^+$ subset of T cells that often, but not always, mediate cytotoxicity against target cells or have regulatory properties in the immune response (Fig. 13.18B and C). The CD8 molecule usually consists of a typical αβ heterodimer of two different proteins, each approximately 40 kDa in size; however, on some T cells,

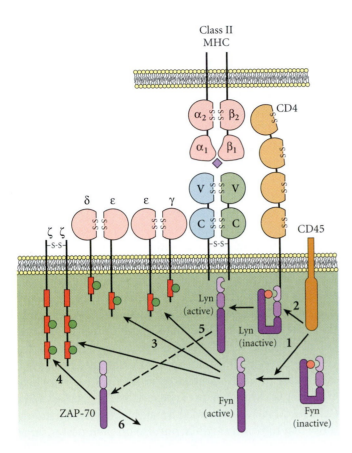

distal domain of CD4 then binds to the β_2 domain of MHC class II, or in the case of CD8$^+$ cells, the CD8 immunoglobulin domains bind to the α_2 and α_3 domains of MHC class I (Fig. 13.18). CD4 undergoes a conformational change that enables membrane-proximal CD4 domains to interact with other CD4 molecules, forming a

Figure 13.18 The CD4 and CD8 accessory molecules. (**A**) The CD4 molecule binds to the β_2 domain of MHC class II. (**B**) The CD8 accessory molecule binds to the α_2 and α_3 domains of MHC class I. (**C**) The stereo view of the structure of a CD8 $\alpha\alpha$ homodimer with HLA-A2 MHC and cognate peptide showing the interaction surfaces of the complex. The HLA-A2 heavy chain (green), β_2 microglobulin (gold), CD8α subunit 1 (red), and CD8α subunit 2 (blue) are depicted schematically, and the peptide bound to the MHC is shown in white as a ball-and-stick representation. The CD8 α chain contains two immunoglobulin-like folds (red and blue), and the loops (thin part of ribbon structure) of the domains, analogous to the CDR loops of variable regions, come in contact with the MHC molecule. The two subunits do not have an equal contribution to the binding to MHC class I. Both subunits make interactions through all of their CDR-like loops with the $\alpha 3$ domain. However, the first subunit domain contacts both the $\alpha 2$ and $\alpha 3$ portions of MHC class I. Reprinted from G. F. Gao et al., *Nature* **387**:630–634, 1997, with permission from E. Y. Jones and *Nature* (Macmillan Publishers Ltd.).

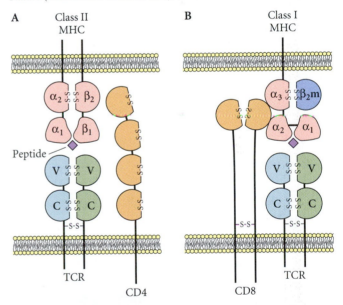

Figure 13.17 Association of the protein kinases Lck, Fyn, and ZAP-70 with components of CD3 results in tyrosine phosphorylation that transmits the signal for cellular activation. The following are the steps of signal transduction: (**1**) the tyrosine phosphatase CD45 removes an inhibitory phosphate group from the Src family kinase Fyn, thus activating Fyn; (**2**) CD45 likewise removes an inhibitory phosphate group from the Lck kinase, activating Lck; (**3**) active Fyn phosphorylates multiple ITAMs on the cytoplasmic tails of the proteins of the CD3 complex; (**4**) phosphorylated ITAMs of CD3 ζ chain form a docking site that recruits the ZAP-70 kinase to CD3; (**5**) (hatched arrow) active Lck phosphorylates and thus activates CD3-bound ZAP-70; (**6**) (not shown) active ZAP-70 phosphorylates and activates phospholipase Cγ1 (PLCγ1). Active PLCγ1 can then mediate downstream signaling events. Dots indicate phosphorylation. Adapted from M. Izquierdo and D. A. Cantrell, *Trends Cell Biol.* **2**:268–271, 1992.

such as $\gamma\delta$ T cells, the two α chains can form an $\alpha\alpha$ homodimer. Each protein chain of CD8 possesses a single immunoglobulin-like domain and a cytoplasmic domain that contains serine residues that are substrates for protein kinases. Like CD4, the cytoplasmic domain of CD8 interacts with Lck for signal transduction, although with an affinity somewhat lower than that of CD4, and also is important in T-cell adhesion to target cells.

The interactions of T cells with either APCs or target cells result in a complex that increases the affinity of the binding of the cells to each other. The TCR binds first to a dimer of the MHC class II molecule. The membrane-

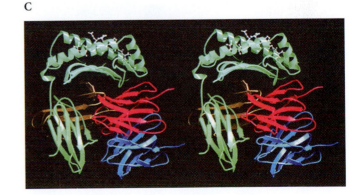

complex. This results in the formation of tetrameric or oligomeric lattice-like receptor aggregates on the surface of the T cell that stabilize cell-cell interactions and initiate signal transduction. Somewhat in contrast to this is the finding that CD8 αα homodimers have almost the same structure in solution that they have when bound to MHC class I.

Role of Other Accessory Molecules in TCR-Based Antigen Recognition

In addition to the accessory function of CD4 and CD8, other receptor-ligand pairs of molecules increase the binding affinity of T cells and APCs and/or signaling of T cells and APCs (Fig. 13.19). These include CD28 and CTLA-4 (CD152) on T cells, which bind to CD80 (B7-71) and CD86 (B7-2) receptors on APCs; inducible costimulator (ICOS) on T cells, which binds to ICOS ligand on APCs; LFA-1 (CD11a/CD18), which binds to ICAM-1 (CD54); CD2, which binds to LFA-3 (CD58); CD45R, which binds to CD22; and CD5, which binds to CD72.

CD80 and CD86 are expressed at low levels on immature dendritic cells and resting monocytes, macrophages, and B cells. Surface expression of both of these molecules is increased following an antigen encounter, with CD86 expression usually preceding CD80 expression by 12 to 24 hours. Both CD80 and CD86 are important in signaling T cells via binding to CD28, which is expressed on about half of the CD8$^+$ T cells and on almost all of the CD4$^+$ T

Figure 13.19 Accessory molecules involved in T-cell binding to an APC. In addition to the MHC-antigen binding to the TCR, other receptor-ligand pairs increase the affinity of binding between a T cell and an APC and can also contribute to signal transduction in T-cell activation. Although CD80 and CD86 both interact with CD28 and CTLA-4, CD80 tends to interact preferentially with CTLA-4 and CD86 tends to interact with CD28.

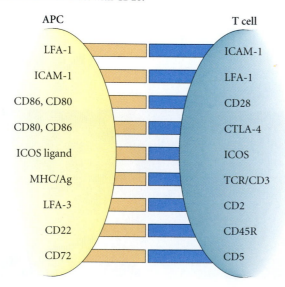

cells. The interaction with CD28 increases the cell-cell adherence, which potentiates overall TCR signaling and is also important in the production of interleukin-2 (IL-2). Failure to ligate CD28 on T cells during antigen recognition sends a negative signal that results in induction of a nonresponsive state (called "anergy") in T cells. Stimulation of CD28 lowers the threshold for TCR engagement, and ligation of CD28 and CD3 is sufficient to stimulate T cells to produce IL-2 and enter the cell cycle. For these reasons, CD28 is considered the dominant costimulatory molecule.

CD2 is expressed on all thymocytes, all T lymphocytes, and large granular lymphocytes. The CD2 ligand, LFA-3, is widely distributed on endothelial cells and epithelial cells and, importantly for antigen presentation, on the surface of APCs. Antibodies to CD2 can stimulate T cells to enter the cell cycle and to proliferate; CD2 is therefore considered an alternate receptor mediating T-cell activation. The interaction between CD2 and LFA-3 also stimulates T cells and APCs to secrete cytokines.

LFA-1 is part of the integrin superfamily of proteins. Like all the proteins in the integrin family, LFA-1 is a heterodimer consisting of an α chain (CD11a) and a β chain (CD18). LFA-1 is expressed on all leukocytes, including those that function as APCs, but also on thymocytes, large granular lymphocytes, activated macrophages, and 50% of bone marrow cells. Its ligand, ICAM-1, is expressed on activated T cells, vascular endothelial cells, tissue macrophages, germinal center dendritic cells, and thymic and mucosal epithelial cells. This interaction is also important for cell-cell adhesion. This adhesion event is an essential structural and function feature of TCR engagement. During the interaction of a T cell with an APC (or target cell), the TCR, MHC, and adhesion molecules undergo a spatial reassortment at the interface of the T cell and APC, producing a dense packing of TCR-MHC-antigen complexes at a relatively small focal point in the area of cell-cell contact that is crucial for T-cell activation. In CD4$^+$ T cells, this involves microdomains (lipid rafts) of the phospholipid membrane bilayer.

In addition to the accessory molecules that function as surface receptors, another group of accessory molecules, cytokines, have a major influence on the T-cell response. A number of cytokines that are released from both the T cell and the APC are important for this response. Chief among them is IL-1, which acts on T lymphocytes to provoke IL-2 production and induces the release of interferon-gamma and granulocyte-macrophage colony-stimulating factor. IL-6 and IL-12 are also important accessory cell cytokines; they are produced by monocytes and macrophages and costimulate T-cell activation.

More recently, another T-cell growth factor, named IL-15, was described. Despite the similarity of its structure to IL-2, IL-15 bears no sequence homology to IL-2 and is produced by monocytes, but not by T cells, and therefore functions in an accessory cell-dependent fashion. It stimulates proliferation of T cells and enhances the cytotoxic activity of T cells and natural killer cells.

Summary

In the immune system, specificity is defined through antigen recognition carried out by unique, but related, receptors found on the surface of B and T lymphocytes. On B cells this attribute is mediated by surface immunoglobulin. On T cells, specificity is mediated by the TCR for antigen. Although the TCR bears many similarities to immunoglobulins, key differences between the BCR and the TCR have made the study of the TCR much more difficult. Nonetheless, the molecular genetic basis for the generation of diversity in antigen recognition is similar. The TCR genes produce proteins that form two heterodimers, $\alpha\beta$ TCR and $\gamma\delta$ TCR, composed of N-terminal variable regions and C-terminal constant regions. $\gamma\delta$ TCRs show a limited diversity in antigen recognition variable regions, and $\gamma\delta$ TCR$^+$ cells have a distribution that tends to be restricted to epithelial and skin surfaces. TCR variable regions are formed on α and γ chains from V and J genes, just like for light chains on antibody. Variable regions for β and δ chains are formed from V, D, and J genes, like immunoglobulin heavy chains. The δ genes are located between the V and J genes for the α chain so that a VJ rearrangement eliminates the possibility that the cell could produce a $\gamma\delta$ TCR. To compensate for the lack of somatic hypermutation in generating TCRs, there are more genes for joining regions in the TRAJ locus, and the recombination signal sequences flanking the diversity-region genes allow for multiple D gene segments to be present on β or δ chains. Junctional flexibility and P- and N-nucleotide additions further contribute to the generation of diversity in TCR. The use of multiple gene segments to produce a functional antigen receptor is so far unique to antibody and TCR molecules. This genetic mechanism is notable for its utility in using a limited amount of genetic information to produce a very large number of proteins that have both a variable and conserved region.

The structure of the TCR is analogous to that of the $(Fab')_2$ fragment of immunoglobulins. The two variable regions complex together to form a site for binding MHC-peptide complexes. The constant regions are close to the membrane. The TCR is associated with the CD3 molecule in the cell membrane of the T cell. Engagement of MHC-peptide on an APC by TCR activates a variety of signals through the ITAMs on the CD3 components. This activation will lead to T-cell growth and differentiation. Supporting the T-cell–APC interaction are a number of other molecular components, including CD4 (for MHC class II), CD8 (for MHC class I), and a variety of others. Overall, the TCR plays a central role in antigen recognition, and the structural diversity in this molecule represents another example of the use of multiple gene segments to produce a functional molecule with the capacity for recognizing an enormous number of MHC-peptide complexes.

Suggested Reading

Allison, T. J., and D. N. Garboczi. 2002. Structure of gamma/delta T cell receptors and their recognition of non-peptide antigens. *Mol. Immunol.* **38:**1051–1061.

Carding, S. R., and P. J. Egan. 2002. Gamma/delta T cells: functional plasticity and heterogeneity. *Nat. Rev. Immunol.* **2:**336–345.

Davis, M. M., J. J. Boniface, Z. Reich, D. L. Lyons, J. Hampl, B. Arden, and Y.-H. Chien. 1998. Ligand recognition by T cell receptors. *Annu. Rev. Immunol.* **16:**523–544.

Khor, B., and B. P. Sleckman. 2002. Allelic exclusion at the TCRbeta locus. *Curr. Opin. Immunol.* **14:**230–234.

LeFranc, M. P., and G. LeFranc. 2001. *The T Cell Receptor Facts Book.* Academic Press, New York, N.Y.

Lord, G. M., R. I. Lechler, and A. J. T. George. 1999. A kinetic differentiation model for the action of altered TCR ligands. *Immunol. Today* **20:**33–39.

Rudolph, M. G., and I. A. Wilson. 2002. The specificity of TCR/pMHC interaction. *Curr. Opin. Immunol.* **14:**52–65.

Rubin, B., L. Alibaud, A. Huchenq-Champagne, J. Arnaud, M. L. Toribio, and J. Constans. 2002. Some hints concerning the shape of T-cell receptor structures. *Scand. J. Immunol.* **55:**111–118.

Wang, J. H., and E. L. Reinherz. 2002. Structural basis of T cell recognition of peptides bound to MHC molecules. *Mol. Immunol.* **38:**1039–1049.

chapter 14

T-Cell Maturation and Activation

Gerald B. Pier, Howard Ceri, Chris Mody, and Michael Preston

topics covered

▲ The maturation and development of T cells in the thymus

▲ Cell surface markers on developing T cells

▲ T-cell commitment to CD4 or CD8 lineage

▲ The role of MHC restriction in T-cell development

▲ How positive selection generates self-restricted T cells

▲ How negative selection eliminates self-reactive T cells

▲ Other mechanisms to maintain proper T-cell function

▲ Cellular and molecular factors regulating T-cell function

▲ How T cells communicate they have engaged an antigen

▲ Signal transduction specific to T-cell activation

▲ T-cell activation by superantigens and mitogens

The concept that there are two major populations of lymphocytes that participate in the immune response—T cells and B cells—was first elucidated in the mid-1960s by Henry Claman and colleagues. Before that time the role and function of the thymus were not known. Incredibly, starting around 1905 and continuing into the 1940s and early 1950s, it was thought that irradiating the "enlarged" thymus of newborns increased their growth rate, and this was done in some instances. The importance of the thymus was revealed in studies that showed that there were lymphocytes derived from the bone marrow whose full function was not realized until they spent time maturing in the thymus. Hence, the term thymus-derived cell or T cell was applied to these cells. T cells were found to be critical for full-fledged immune responses to proteins and to foreign cellular antigens, and were initially characterized as cells that provided help to B cells to produce antibody. Thus, the helper function of T cells (TH cells) was their first appreciated property. Now T cells are known to have multiple other functions; they can be cytotoxic cells, they can interact with phagocytic cells to mediate delayed-type hypersensitivity, and they have regulatory functions that affect the activity of other T cells. The structure of the thymus (see Fig. 4.3) provides an environment where immature thymocytes can interact with a variety of cells, including thymic epithelial cells and dendritic cells, to acquire their final functional properties—expression of a major histocompatibility complex (MHC)-restricted T-cell receptor (TCR), presence of either CD4 or

315

CD8 in the plasma membrane, and ability to interact with antigen-presenting cells (APCs) or nucleated target cells to respond to foreign antigens.

During development of the thymocyte some key events must occur to produce a mature T cell. The genes for the TCR must be rearranged with a particular timing and co-ordinated with expression of the RAG-1 and RAG-2 proteins. The TCR that is produced has to be capable of interacting with presented antigens in an MHC-restricted fashion; this occurs under a process called *positive selection*. T cells expressing self-reactive TCR have to be eliminated; this occurs under a process called *negative selection* and leads to self tolerance. Finally, the TCR restriction to an MHC class I- or MHC class II-bound antigen has to be coordinated with expression of either the CD8 or CD4 coreceptor.

T-Cell Maturation and Development in the Thymus

Early T-Cell Development

Hematopoietic stem cells can give rise to all of the cells found in the blood, and one of the immediate derivatives of the hematopoietic stem cells is the common lymphoid precursor (CLP). The CLP cells will give rise to T cells, B cells, natural killer (NK) cells, and potentially some types of dendritic cells and appear to be mostly committed to these lineages. The CLP cells that enter the thymus become immature thymocytes with germ line configurations for the TCR genes, and they also lack expression of most of the other surface markers that are present on mature T cells such as CD3, CD4, or CD8. The lack of CD3, CD4, and CD8 markers is indicative of *triple-negative* (TN) cells, and the TN cells go through four stages before becoming an immature T cell. These cells are also referred to in the literature as *double-negative* (DN) cells to indicate just the lack of CD4 and CD8. Immature mouse thymocytes entering the thymus express an antigen referred to as Thy-1, but there is no known human equivalent of this marker.

Once in the thymus, the CLP cells start to undergo development into the various T-cell subpopulations. One of the earliest membrane-expressed factors on the CLP cells is the c-kit ligand (CD117) needed to respond to a critical growth factor termed stem cell factor. Activation of c-kit leads to tyrosine kinase activity that is crucial to continued T-cell development (Fig. 14.1). Recently it has been determined that another critical factor for T-cell development is expression of interleukin-7 (IL-7) and the IL-7 receptor (IL-7R) on the TN cells. The IL-7R is composed of two transmembrane proteins; one of these is used by a variety

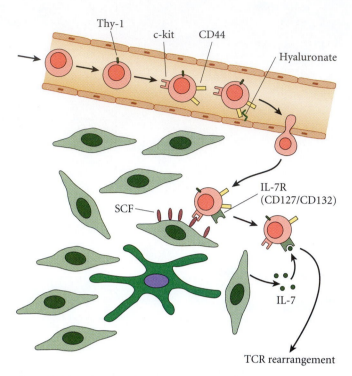

Figure 14.1 Early events in T-cell maturation in the thymus. Precursor thymocytes bearing surface markers (Thy-1, a mouse-specific marker, and c-kit and CD44) enter the thymus, facilitated by CD44 binding to cell surface receptors expressing hyaluronate. c-kit engages its receptor, stem cell factor (SCF), which leads to the production of IL-7R on the cell surface. When IL-7 is made, the IL-7R leads to changes in the chromatin structure and the accessibility of the DNA encoding the γ chain of the TCR to initiate TCR recombination events.

of cytokine receptors and is referred to as the common γ chain (CD132) whereas the other confers a specificity for IL-7 on the receptor and is referred to as the IL-7R α chain (CD127). IL-7 directly affects the rearrangement and transcription of TCR genes. Intracellular signals generated by binding of IL-7 to IL-7R result in changes in the chromatin structure and chemistry that make the TCRγ genes accessible for rearrangement and transcription. In the absence of IL-7 signaling, the TCRγ-chain genes do not rearrange and no γδ T cells develop. Interestingly, in the absence of IL-7 or IL-7R, there is some rearrangement of the TCR δ, α, and β genes but no production of the γδ T cells due to lack of production of γ chains. There is, however, limited production of αβ T cells.

Cellular Markers and T-Cell Development

The stages of T-cell development in the thymus can be analyzed by labeling cell surface markers with specific antibodies and subsequently undertaking flow cytometric analysis (Fig. 14.2). Cells enter and initially reside in the corticomedullary junction of the thymus, and the first identifiable T-cell phenotype arising from the CLP cells expresses CD44 but not CD25 (CD25$^-$ CD44$^+$). CD25 is the α subunit of the IL-2R. CD25$^-$ CD44$^+$ cells retain the potential to become either a B cell or NK cell, but both of these cell types mature in the bone marrow, not in the thymus. The CD25$^-$ CD44$^+$ cells may also give rise to thymic dendritic cells, but this is a controversial notion. In the thymus the CD25$^-$ CD44$^+$ cells are at the TN1 stage and are called thymic lymphoid precursors.

Progression through the next several phases of T-cell development (Fig. 14.3) involves production and function of a number of transcription factors that bind to DNA and modulate gene expression leading to changes in cell surface markers. To go from the TN1 to the TN2 stage, where the cells are now CD25$^+$ CD44$^+$, cellular production of E2A and other similar transcription factors is needed. These transcription factors are members of the basic helix-turn-helix family of activators. In transgenic mice lacking E2A there is a 5- to 10-fold reduction in $\alpha\beta$ T cells and a 10- to 40-fold reduction in $\gamma\delta$ T cells, indicating that this is an essential factor for progressing to the TN2 stage. The TN2 cells are also known as pro-T cells.

Between the TN2 and TN3 stages the pro-T cell becomes committed to expression of either the $\alpha\beta$ or $\gamma\delta$ TCR (Fig. 14.4A). At this point it is not clear if the commitment to production of one or the other is based on an

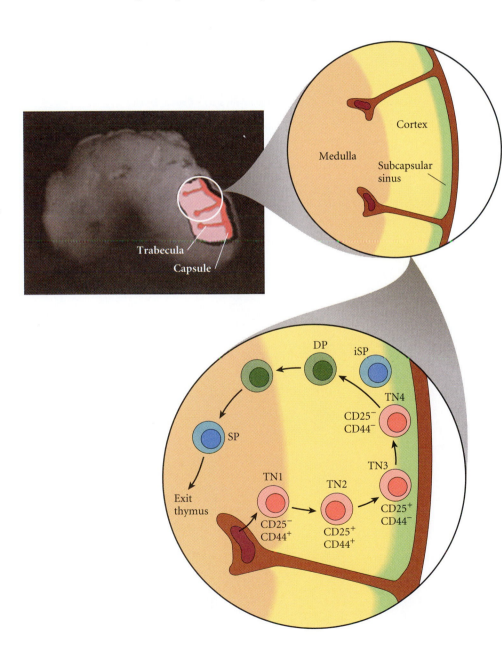

Figure 14.2 Identification of T-cell development in the thymus and correlation with the migration of the cells. The precursor T cells are initially found in the outer cortex and are identified as TN cells because they lack production of CD3, CD4, and CD8. The cells then produce CD3 but still do not express CD4 or CD8 and are called DN. The cells pass through more mature TN stages, then into the DP state, indicating that they express both CD4 and CD8, and finally in the SP state they migrate out of the thymus.

instructive model or a selective model. In the instructive model, a cell with the potential to be either an αβ or γδ T cell will randomly produce either of these TCRs that, once produced, provide critical signals for the further development of the T cell. Thus, the type of TCR made, and not other factors, determines the cell's phenotype. In the selective model, the type of TCR that is made is determined by expression of other factors, potentially produced even before the cell has started to rearrange the αβ or γδ TCR genes. For example, some evidence indicates that the level of expression of CD127 may determine which TCR is made; cells with low-level expression (CD127^{lo}) are likely to become αβ T cells, whereas cells with higher-level expression of CD127 (CD127^{hi}) preferentially become γδ T cells. Overall, the data are incomplete in regard to which of these models is operative in TCR production and what

factors may participate in the selective model, if this is the operative model.

If the cell is going to develop into a γδ T cell, then the genes for TRDV-D-J and TRGV-J (see chapter 13 for a discussion of this nomenclature) will rearrange to form a final gene including the TRDC and TRGC genes that can be transcribed and translated into functional receptor proteins. The T-cell-specific marker, CD3, will be produced along with the γδ TCR. This appears to complete the development of γδ T cells. The γδ T cells are the predominant T-cell population during early fetal development in mice, but start declining relative to αβ T cells just before birth and by adulthood make up only approximately 10% of the T cells.

If the T cell is going to develop into an αβ TCR-expressing T cell, then the next stage of development involves

Figure 14.3 Changes in T cells as they go through development stages in the thymus. The thymic T-cell maturational stage correlates with changes in cell surface markers. The clonogenic lymphoid precursor can give rise to T cells, B cells, or NK cells. The first identifiable T-cell maturation stage, TN1, is characterized by the presence of the CD44 marker (CD44$^+$) and lack of CD25 marker (CD25$^-$). As the cells progress through various TN stages, there are changes associated with the cell surface markers and the generation of TCR. Correlated with these developmental steps are changes in gene expression, notably transcription factors. Most T cells will produce an αβ TCR. Just before production of the TCR α chain at the DP stage, either CD4 or CD8 genes are transcribed, leading to an initial single-positive (iSP) stage. Following full production of the TCR along with CD4 and CD8 the cells become SP, producing only CD4 or CD8 in association with a specific MHC-restricted TCR.

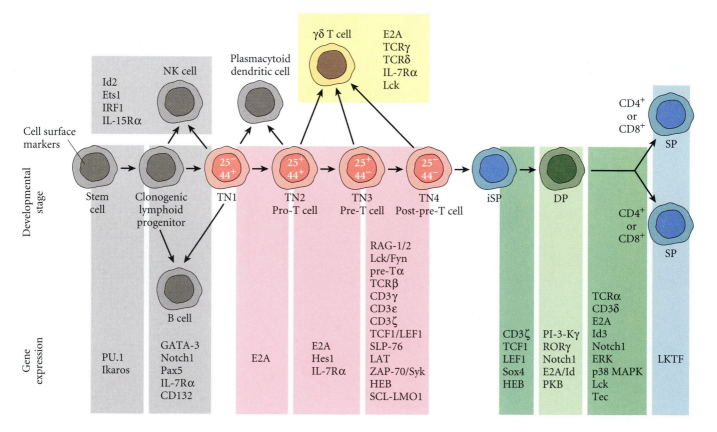

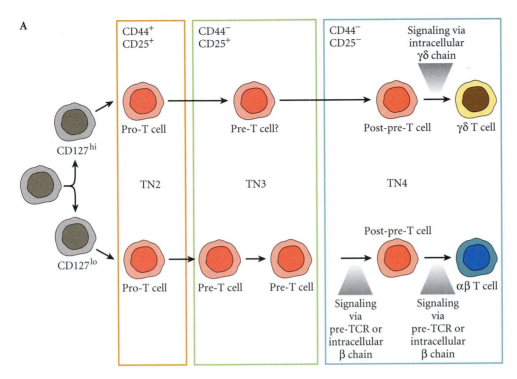

A

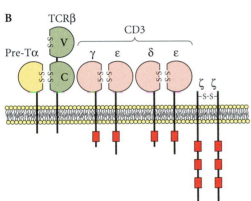

B

Figure 14.4 Commitment to αβ or γδ lineage and formation of the pre-TCR. (**A**) Changes in levels of the IL-7R α chain (CD127) are associated with development of either αβ or γδ T cells. Both development lines appear to involve a CD44⁺ CD25⁺ stage, followed by a CD44⁻ CD25⁺ stage associated with the pre-T-cell stage for αβ T cells. The ultimate fate of the T cell depends on signaling via the type of TCR produced. (**B**) Formation of the pre-TCR complex on a developing αβ T cell. Expression of the TCR β chain requires the presence of an invariant chain termed pre-T alpha (pre-Tα). This receptor is associated with the production of the CD3. Pre-TCR formation signals the cells to expand and differentiate further into mature αβ T cells, a process designated β selection.

progression from the TN2 to the TN3 stage. This is determined by transcription factors and results in a cell that is CD25⁺ and CD44⁻ and is referred to as a pre-T cell. Although it is not fully appreciated what signals this transition, it appears that the maturing T cells usually pass through specific compartments of the thymus as they progress in their development (Fig. 14.4A). Thus, the thymic microenvironment may be critical for signaling the cells to proceed through specific maturation pathways.

At this stage the T cell is likely committed to the αβ lineage, and a number of changes in the cells have been defined as they go from the TN3 pre-T-cell stage to the TN4 post-pre-T-cell stage. At the TN4 stage, the cells are CD25⁻ and CD44⁻. Principal among the changes that oc-

cur going from pre-T-cell to post-pre-T-cell stage is the expression of the pre-Tα surface protein, expression of the RAG-1 and RAG-2 genes, rearrangement of the TRBV-D-J genes to produce a TCR β chain, and expression of CD3 polypeptides (Fig. 14.4B). The TCR β chain is expressed on the developing T-cell plasma membrane in a complex with pre-Tα and CD3, forming the pre-TCR. Although there is pre-TCR on the surface, neither CD4 nor CD8 is expressed, so at this point the cell becomes a truly DN (CD3⁺ CD4⁻/CD8⁻) T cell. Expression of a pre-TCR indicates that the cell has undergone a productive rearrangement of the TRBV-D-J genes, and this also inhibits RAG-2 production, allowing for allelic exclusion to occur in a particular cell.

Expression of the post-pre-TCR at the TN4 stage confers on the developing T cell the capacity to interact with a currently unknown ligand, which transmits signals using the CD3 proteins. Members of the mitogen-activated protein kinase (MAPK) family of serine/threonine kinases that were initially known for their role in signaling for responses to growth and stress factors are critical for further T-cell development as are other signaling pathways (Fig. 14.5). Pre-TCR-mediated signaling may be critical to the decrease in RAG-2 gene expression and also appears to initiate and enhance rearrangements of the TRAV-J genes. During this time the cells migrate back toward the inner cortex of the thymus, where they can be identified using cell surface markers to the CD3 and pre-TCR antigens. It should be noted that the importance of this migration event is not entirely confirmed, since it has been shown that maturation can occasionally proceed to completion in the absence of migration through the thymus.

The cells next begin to increase expression of CD8 or CD4, leading to an immature *single-positive* (SP) cell in the second part of the TN4 stage (Fig. 14.3). Further differentiation, under the influence of transcription factors and possibly the thymic microenvironment, results in the next

identifiable stage, where both CD4 and CD8 are expressed on *double-positive* (DP) cells. These DP cells then become CD44$^-$ CD25$^-$ CD69$^-$ RAG-2^{hi} TCRβ^{lo} and attempt to rearrange their TCR α locus. Several different rearrangements of the α locus can be attempted, and because the α locus does not undergo allelic exclusion, single T cells expressing two different α chains have been described. If an αβ TCR is successfully expressed, the developing T cell will go on to become either a CD4 or CD8 SP cell.

Lineage Commitment

The exact mechanism whereby an αβ T cell becomes an SP cell expressing either the CD4 or CD8 coreceptor is not yet fully elucidated. Recent models suggest that it is not just the ability of the TCR to recognize either a class I- or class II-presenting self antigen that determines lineage commitment but the strength or duration of survival signals provided to the T cell as a result of expression of CD4 or CD8. There are several models that describe the mechanism of lineage commitment, each of which has supportive data (Fig. 14.6). In the instructional model, engagement of MHC class I or MHC class II by a TCR provides the signal that a cell needs to make the changes needed to become CD4$^+$ or CD8$^+$. Thus, a class I-restricted TCR that engages self peptide on MHC class I is instructed to stop making CD4, leaving CD8 as the coreceptor. A similar process would result in production of the CD4 coreceptor on a T cell with a class II-restricted TCR by inhibition of production of CD8. A related model, termed stochastic production, indicates that either the CD4 or CD8 coreceptor emerges under the control of as yet undefined factors following TCR gene rearrangements and production of the membrane TCR. Support for this model comes from observations that maturing T cells in the thymus can express either a high level of CD4 and a mid-level of CD8 (CD4^{hi} CD8^{mid}) or the other configuration (CD4^{mid} CD8^{hi}). If the cell expressed a TCR that was class I restricted but also was a CD4^{hi} cell, it would not receive additional signals needed to survive. DP cells with the same TCR that were CD8^{hi} cells would receive a rescue signal from interacting with MHC class I and survive and mature further, as would cells with a class II-restricted TCR that were CD4^{hi}. Whether a cell that made the "wrong" choice in coreceptor would be given a second chance to produce the correct receptor, analogous perhaps to the receptor editing seen in production of immunoglobulin light chain variable regions, is controversial. One caveat for all of the data generated in support of the instructional or stochastic models is that they have been derived in transgenic mice expressing only one TCR or overexpressing a coreceptor. Documentation that a

Figure 14.5 T-cell development and pre-TCR signaling. Once the pre-TCR complex is formed, signals are sent to the cell via a variety of pathways to promote various activities critical for T-cell development. Much of the signaling occurs through the protein kinases Lck and Fyn. Survival signals involve activation of the p53 transcription factor and inhibition of the Fas-activated death domain (FADD). Proliferation and differentiation signals involve the Ras pathway as well as PLCγ1 and PKC factors. Activation of PKC is also involved in allelic exclusion. ERK is a transcription factor that is needed for survival, proliferation, and differentiation.

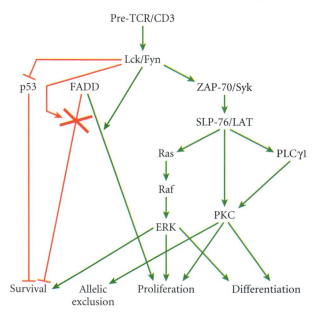

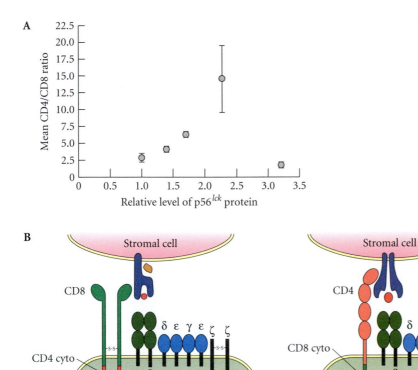

Figure 14.6 Models of lineage commitment to CD4 or CD8. (A) In transgenic mice, increases in the relative levels of p56^{lck} increase the ratio of CD4$^+$ cells to CD8$^+$ cells up to a point. Relative expression over threefold of normal returns the ratio of CD4$^+$ to CD8$^+$ cells to normal. Reprinted from S. J. Sohn et al., *J. Immunol.* **166:**2209–2217, 2001, with permission. (B) Development of an SP cell depends on the strength of the signal from the cytoplasmic domain of the CD4 or CD8 coreceptor. A CD8 extracellular domain binding to MHC class I engineered to express a CD4 cytoplasmic tail (cyt.) will produce a strong Lck signal and develop into a CD4$^+$ T cell in spite of binding to the MHC class I molecule. Similarly, a cell engineered to express a CD4 extracellular domain that binds to MHC class II fused with a CD8 cytoplasmic tail will become a CD8$^+$ T cell.

comparable process occurs in a wild-type situation has not yet been made.

For lineage commitment to proceed, the maturing T cell must decrease production of the inappropriate coreceptor. This appears to be carried out by the strength of coreceptor signaling involving the p56^{lck} (Lck) kinase. This kinase helps determine the CD4 or CD8 fate by influencing the strength or duration of signaling through the TCR complex (Fig. 14.6). CD4 is much more active than CD8 at recruiting Lck to the TCR complex. When the TCR on DP cells engages the MHC-antigen receptor on thymic dendritic cells for a short period, Lck signaling is low and CD8$^+$ cells principally emerge. Longer engagements and thus longer signaling through the receptor complex result in a CD4$^+$ cell. The stronger survival signal from the CD4 coreceptor has been invoked to explain why CD4$^+$ cells outnumber CD8$^+$ cells by a ratio of 2:1. Secondary influences for other regulatory cellular factors can decrease the intensity of Lck signaling, and the cell will then produce a CD8 coreceptor. Conversely, even if a cell has an MHC class I-restricted TCR, if other cellular fac-

tors are present that enhance the strength of the Lck signal, then the cell will become CD4$^+$. For example, in DP cells engineered to express an extracellular domain of CD8 attached to a cytoplasmic tail of CD4, which binds Lck better, even when the TCR on the DP cell engages MHC class I-presented peptide, it still develops into a CD4$^+$ cell (Fig. 14.6B). Similarly, CD8$^+$ cells develop from engineered cells expressing an extracellular CD4 to engage MHC class II and cytoplasmic CD8 domains. Removal of cells expressing incompatible MHC-restricted TCR and the CD4 or CD8 coreceptor will presumably come at a later point in T-cell maturation.

Acquisition of MHC Restriction and Generation of the Mature T-Cell Repertoire

The next process involves selecting T lymphocytes that will form the repertoire necessary for host responses to foreign antigens complexed to self MHC. The predominant conceptions for this process have been designated as "neglect, select, and eliminate" models wherein T cells

Figure 14.7 Schematic diagram showing the thymic cell types that are important in the induction of central tolerance. In the outer cortex of the thymus much of the positive selection takes place. Here the maturing thymocyte interacts with thymic epithelial cells. Those that receive sufficient survival signals due to appropriate interactions with self MHC-peptide can move on to the next stage, negative selection. Those that do not receive sufficient survival signals die by apoptosis. In the medullary area, the thymocytes interact with interdigitating dendritic cells, which arise extrathymically. Here much of the negative selection takes place, where thymocytes that interact too strongly with self MHC-self peptide receive a strong signal due to a high-affinity interaction from the TCR engagement and die by apoptosis.

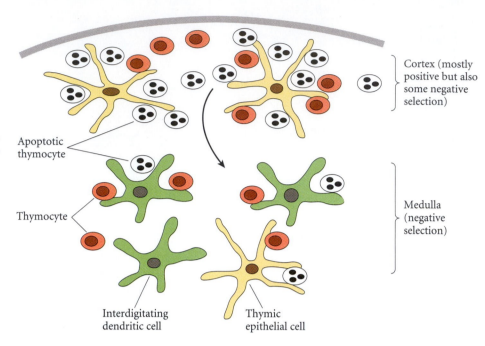

Apoptotic thymocyte

Thymocyte

Interdigitating dendritic cell

Thymic epithelial cell

Cortex (mostly positive but also some negative selection)

Medulla (negative selection)

that cannot interact with peptide-self MHC die from neglect, T cells that react with the proper combination of peptide and MHC are selected for further maturation, and those T cells that react too strongly with self peptide and MHC are eliminated to prevent unwanted autoimmune reactions. At the DP stage, the maturing T cells are still in the thymus, although there is some regional localization in regard to where the next maturational stages occur (Fig. 14.7). In addition, the cellular and molecular mechanisms mediating this selective process have been difficult to unravel. This is because the large array of possible foreign antigens complexed to self MHC that can be recognized by T cells is not available in the thymus for informing the maturing T cells that they have made a self-MHC-restricted TCR recognizing foreign antigen. Furthermore, T cells that make a TCR that cannot recognize foreign antigens complexed to self MHC must be eliminated, apparently through the process of "neglect" where they fail to receive signals needed to proceed further through the maturational stages. The next process that occurs is called positive selection and establishes MHC restriction, the ability to recognize antigenic peptides in the context of self MHC. Interestingly, the acquisition of self-MHC-restricted recognition of foreign antigens is not an intrinsic or genetic property of the T cell, but it is a property learned during maturation in the thymus. Rolf Zinkernagel and coworkers surgically removed the thymus from young mice and then placed a transplanted thymus graft into the thymectomized animal (Fig. 14.8). The T cells

that emerged following maturation in the thymus graft of the recipient were "educated" to react with antigens presented by the MHC of the donor of the thymus graft. Thus, these T cells would only produce an effective immune response if they interacted with APC or target cells expressing the MHC of the thymic donor. They did not respond to antigen presented by the endogenous MHC of the recipient.

Positive Selection

The predominant model that has emerged over the past several years to explain the molecular and cellular bases for positive selection has focused on the affinity or avidity of the interactions of T cells with self peptide presented by self-MHC antigens expressed on epithelial cells in the cortex of the thymus. Other signals provided in this microenvironment of the thymus also play a role in positive selection. For positive selection to occur, the expressed TCR must have a basic binding capacity for self peptide complexed to self MHC class I or class II, but not too strong a binding capacity (Fig. 14.9). If the rearranged TCR has minimal to no capacity to bind to self MHC, then it will not receive survival signals through the receptor complex and will die by apoptosis due to "neglect." This appears to be the fate of 95% or more of the T cells maturing in the thymus. Survival signaling is determined by the kinetics and strength of the TCR-self-MHC interaction. Strength of binding determines the type of signal received through the TCR complex, and strength is deter-

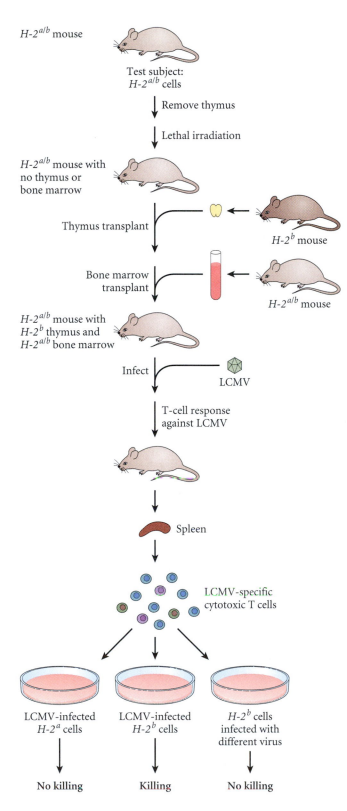

Figure 14.8 T cells are positively selected by the MHC phenotype of the thymus. An F$_1$ heterozygous mouse (*H-2$^{a/b}$*) is thymectomized and lethally irradiated to destroy all of its hematopoietic capacity. This results in an *H-2$^{a/b}$* mouse with no thymus or bone marrow. This mouse then receives a thymus transplant from a mouse with only one of the parental *H-2* haplotypes, *H-2^b*, and a bone marrow transplant from an isogenic *H-2$^{a/b}$* sibling. This leaves a mouse with an endogenous *H-2$^{a/b}$* overall background, an *H-2^b* thymus and *H-2$^{a/b}$* bone marrow. After recovery, the mouse is immunized with lymphocytic choriomeningitis virus (LCMV) to generate cytolytic CD8$^+$ T cells. After an immune response is made, the T cells in the spleen are tested for their ability to kill LCMV-infected *H-2^a* or *H-2^b* cells. The immune T cells efficiently kill the virus infecting *H-2^b* targets, but not *H-2^a* targets, indicating the T cells were positively selected in the thymus to recognize *H-2^b* targets. As a control, H-2^b cells infected with a different virus were not killed, demonstrating the immunologic specificity of the experiment.

mined, in part, by variations in the amino acid sequences in the peptides presented by the MHC. Variant peptides can either initiate or inhibit a mature T-cell response (Fig. 14.10). Those peptides that provide a strong signal and activate mature T cells are referred to as agonist peptides; peptides that provide a weaker signal are termed partial agonist peptides, whereas those that provide a weak signal and inhibit mature T-cell activation are referred to as antagonist peptides.

Many studies indicate that it is the thymic cortical cells that express the peptide-MHC ligands for positive selection. Unlike hematopoietic cells, these cells are relatively

Figure 14.9 Signaling for positive selection of T cells. TCRs that cannot engage self MHC-self peptide die via apoptosis due to neglect because they fail to receive survival signals. Those T cells that produce a TCR able to bind to self MHC-self peptides will receive signals through the TCR complex that affect cell survival. If too strong a binding occurs and a high signal intensity is generated through the TCR, then the cell will not survive. If the binding of TCR to MHC-peptide is of modest affinity, then a pattern of survival signals is generated.

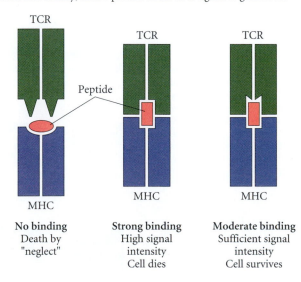

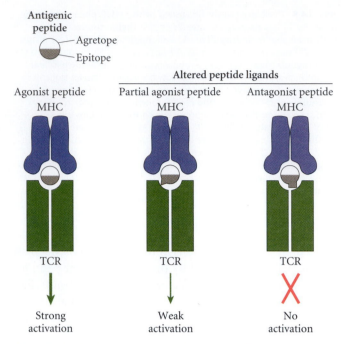

Antigenic peptide
— Agretope
— Epitope

Altered peptide ligands

Agonist peptide	Partial agonist peptide	Antagonist peptide
MHC	MHC	MHC

TCR	TCR	TCR
Strong activation	Weak activation	No activation

Figure 14.10 Peptide influences on the strength of T-cell activation. Alternate forms of peptides that bind to the same MHC and engage the same TCR have an effect on cellular activation delivered through the TCR. Agonist peptides bind to the TCR strongly and give a strong activation or survival signal. Partial agonist peptides weakly activate T cells, whereas antagonist peptides prevent TCR-mediated signaling and lead to no activation.

Although the cellular players involved in positive selection remain unresolved, it may be that both thymic cortical cells and dendritic cells participate in this process, possibly at different stages of positive selection or by mediating different signaling events that overall determine the fate of a DP T cell following positive selection.

Maturation of the DP cells in the thymus appears to be based, in part, on the type of peptide presented by MHC during positive selection—agonist, partial agonist, or antagonist. But there are conflicting data regarding whether agonist or antagonist self peptides complexed to self MHC provide the needed low but sufficient signal to promote further maturation of T cells undergoing positive selection. It is likely that a complex process involving TCR interaction with a number of self-peptide-MHC complexes during positive selection provides a signal that the maturing T cell can "integrate." The overall signal determines the T cell's fate during positive selection (Fig. 14.11). Kinetics plays a key role here, as binding to self MHC with a low affinity due to a high dissociation constant of the TCR with the self MHC can actually transmit survival signals to the DP thymocyte. Although this interaction suggests a threshold level of signaling must occur to promote T-cell survival, it appears that reaching the threshold once is not enough, but it must be sustained for a sufficient time to accumulate survival signals in the DP thymocyte. To accomplish this, there would need to be a lot of association and rapid dissociation events taking place between the TCR and selecting self MHC-peptides. These events would generate signals that are different from those generated from high affinity-interactions of the TCR on mature T cells with MHC-peptide. In this interaction the dissociation rate is slow and hence stable binding of the TCR to MHC-peptide takes place. Stable binding leads to cel-

resistant to irradiation, and this tool has been used to eliminate hematopoietic cells in the thymus to study positive selection. Irradiated thymi repopulated with thymocytes are still capable of undergoing positive selection. However, other investigators have produced data indicating that hematopoietic cells such as dendritic cells present the peptide-MHC complex needed for positive selection.

Figure 14.11 Integrated model of T-cell survival during positive selection. (**Top**) When a TCR that has a moderate association constant for self peptide-MHC and a high dissociation constant is produced, a series of signals are delivered, resulting in a sustained level of the transcription factor ERK, which is needed for T-cell survival. (**Middle**) When there is a high association and low dissociation between the TCR and self peptide-MHC, the T-cell signaling is intense and short-lived and the cell does not receive survival signals to get it through the stage of positive selection. (**Bottom**) If there is no ability of the TCR to bind self peptide-MHC, the cell dies via apoptosis.

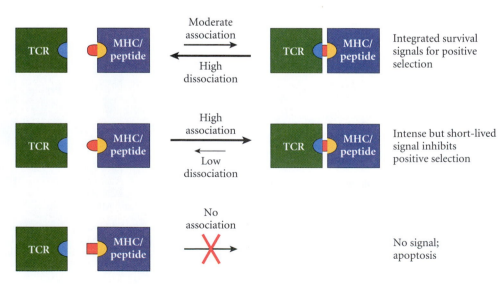

TCR — MHC/peptide	Moderate association → ← High dissociation	TCR — MHC/peptide → Integrated survival signals for positive selection
TCR — MHC/peptide	High association → ← Low dissociation	TCR — MHC/peptide → Intense but short-lived signal inhibits positive selection
TCR — MHC/peptide	No association ✗	No signal; apoptosis

lular internalization of the TCR, which seems to inhibit positive selection. The lower-affinity interactions would provide a lower-intensity, sustained signal. This sustained signal could be integrated into the process of positive selection. In this scenario, the TCR on the maturing T cell's surface would remain on the cell surface and thus continue to provide signals to the cell. This would allow the T cell to proceed and survive the positive selection stage. Those results suggesting that a strong agonist peptide can participate in positive selection would need to be coupled to models wherein the maturational state of the DP T cell undergoing positive selection is at a stage where the agonist peptide-MHC complex does not provide too strong a signal. Indeed, low-affinity binding of TCR to MHC and antigen in the periphery appears to be necessary for survival of T cells.

A key molecular component of positive selection appears to be production of the transcription factor known as extracellular regulated kinase (ERK) that has a strong influence on gene transcription. However, it is not yet clear if it is the sustained production of ERK following low-affinity TCR-self-MHC interactions that accounts for cell survival signals leading to positive selection. Other signals from the thymic cortical cells are known to be involved in positive selection. One possibility is that the thymic cortical cells produce anti-apoptotic factors that promote survival of those T cells with TCRs capable of recognizing self-MHC-bound self peptides.

Tolerance

During the process of T-cell maturation and positive selection, TCRs are generated with a tremendous potential diversity in their ability to bind antigenic peptides. This is critical in order to endow lymphocytes with the ability to recognize and respond to a broad range of harmful pathogens and foreign antigens. However, following positive selection there is still a large likelihood that TCRs that recognize self peptides or even CD1-restricted lipid antigens from the host's own cells will survive. If the cells are strongly reactive with self antigens complexed to self MHC, they could react against the host's own tissues, setting the stage for *autoimmunity*. To prevent such events, the immune system has evolved to be unresponsive to self antigens while maintaining its capacity to react appropriately to foreign antigens. This functional unresponsiveness to self antigens is known as *tolerance*.

One of the earliest ideas to describe immunologic tolerance was the process of clonal deletion wherein lymphocytes reactive to self antigens are killed during their development and therefore never reach functional maturity. Numerous early observations suggested that tolerance was principally acquired during fetal or neonatal development. Exposure of a fetus or very young animal to a self antigen would render it tolerant to that antigen. Some well-known, classic experiments of R. E. Billingham, L. Brent, and P. B. Medawar carried out in 1953 demonstrated that the immune system of a mouse could be made tolerant to otherwise foreign tissues if exposure to foreign tissues occurred sufficiently early in the mouse's development. Frank Macfarlane Burnet in 1959 postulated that immune cells specific for a particular self antigen would be eliminated if that antigen was present during an individual's early development. In the same year, Joshua Lederberg theorized that the lymphocyte's maturational state was the primary factor in determining whether tolerance to self antigens would develop. By extrapolation, these hypotheses predicted that an animal exposed to a foreign antigen before full maturation of the immune system would regard that antigen as self, failing to immunologically respond to it upon reexposure.

As more information about the immune system was gathered, there were important challenges to these observations and the resultant hypotheses regarding the mechanism for self-tolerance. Establishment of self-tolerance only during early development did not account for the continual generation of mature lymphocytes throughout an animal's life. If the immune repertoire were set by birth or shortly thereafter, then neonatal exposure to antigen could form the basis of self-tolerance. However, not only are mature T and B cells being generated throughout an animal's life, many new antigens are expressed along with tissue and organ changes that occur during developmental events such as puberty. Clearly a more active mechanism to prevent production of self-reactive lymphocytes is needed. One of these mechanisms that continues to operate throughout an animal's lifetime is the deletion of self-reactive T cells in the thymus during a process called negative selection. Following positive selection, T cells that are still capable of becoming fully activated by complexes of self MHC and self antigen are deleted in the thymus. Negative selection that occurs in the thymus forms the basis for *central tolerance* or the process whereby the large pool of emerging mature lymphocytes is screened for self-reactivity and eliminated if improperly reactive. Central tolerance also occurs in the bone marrow during B-cell development for the same purpose.

Negative Selection

Generating central tolerance via negative selection involves apoptosis of immature T cells in the thymus following receipt of strong intracellular signals through the

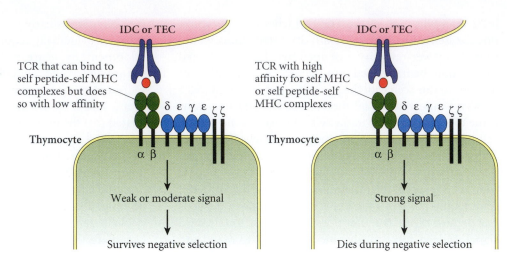

Figure 14.12 Negative selection eliminates self-reactive T cells. T cells that survive positive selection may still be capable of binding to self-peptide-MHC complexes inappropriately. During negative selection, self antigens presented by IDCs or thymic epithelial cells (TEC) that bind to TCR with low affinity give rise to survival signals. The resultant cell can now recognize foreign peptide complexed to self MHC, but not self peptide complexed to self MHC. A high-affinity interaction leads to either more intense or qualitatively different signaling, leading to apoptosis and elimination of self-reactive T cells.

TCR (Fig. 14.12). Although a facet of positive selection includes removal of cells with too high an affinity for self MHC-self peptide, there is still a subsequent step of negative selection that works via a similar overall mechanism. Negative and positive selections have been differentiated into clearly distinct stages in experimental systems, and the apparent redundancy in removal of potentially self-reactive T cells at two distinct steps of thymocyte maturation may reflect the importance of ensuring their elimination. Also, it is likely that some different mechanisms are operative in negative selection that do not involve internalization of TCR bound strongly to self-MHC-peptide complexes. The identification of all of the cellular and molecular factors that mediate negative selection is not yet completed, likely because of complexity and redundancy in the factors that promote negative selection. This makes it difficult to observe overall changes in negative selection following manipulation of a single factor. As with positive selection, controversy particularly exists over which cells in the thymus mediate negative selection and whether it takes place in the cortex or the medulla of the thymus. Recent evidence, however, points to the thymic medulla as a major site for negative selection (Fig. 14.7). There are abundant bone marrow-derived interdigitating dendritic cells (IDCs) that are rich in MHC class II molecules in the medulla, and these cells would be well positioned to eliminate self-reactive CD4$^+$ cells. Also, circulating self antigens enter the thymus from the blood more readily in the thymic medulla, where they can be processed and presented as part of negative selection. However, IDCs may not perform this function universally, since thymocytes have been observed to occasionally complete their maturation (including, presumably, negative selection) without ever entering the thymic medulla. This indicates that cell types other than medullary IDCs

are capable of inducing negative selection, and these cells may be particularly important for eliminating CD8$^+$ T cells. Experiments using thymuses treated with deoxyguanosine, a chemical that destroys all bone marrow-derived cells in the thymus but leaves the thymic epithelium intact, suggested that the thymic cortical epithelium, which is distinct from the cells in the thymic medulla, can provide strong tolerogenic signals to developing thymocytes (Fig. 14.13). Interestingly, the importance of medullary IDCs as sources for signals leading to self-tolerance seems to be dependent on whether the developing T cell is of CD4$^+$ or CD8$^+$ lineage, with the former being more strongly influenced than the latter in the thymic medulla. Effects on CD8$^+$ cells may be mediated by interaction with thymic epithelial cells (Fig. 14.7).

One confounding aspect of attributing the occurrence of self-tolerance in the thymic medulla is that most of the cells in this location are not DP T cells but rather SP CD4$^+$8$^-$ or CD4$^-$8$^+$ cells. Many studies suggest that it is the DP T cell that is the target of negative selection because the DP cells are very susceptible to apoptosis mediated by binding of agonist self peptides on MHC. This is in contrast to the opposite effect when mature T cells that have left the thymus bind foreign antigen on self MHC. Strong binding of TCR on mature T cells to foreign antigen on self MHC elicits survival and proliferation signals, particularly in concert with binding of a costimulatory molecule such as CD28. However, it may be that negative selection occurs with cells that have matured to a certain level but are still immature T cells. Immature T cells express a marker known as heat-stable antigen (HSA), and the majority of SP T cells in the thymic medulla express high levels of HSA (HSA^{hi}), indicating their immature status. These cells appear to retain their sensitivity to apoptosis induced by strong binding of TCR to agonist self peptides presented by self MHC, resulting in negative selection.

Additional elements involved in negative selection have been intensively studied, and it appears that there are contributions from multiple factors with redundancy in their activity. Although it was initially thought that costimulation during negative selection involving CD28 was another means to eliminate self-reactive T cells, this hypothesis was disproven when it was shown that self-reac-

tive cells were readily eliminated in CD28$^{-/-}$ mice. Screening of a panel of potential receptors identified not only CD28, but CD5, CD43, and other T-cell surface molecules that could be engaged during negative selection and promote apoptosis of the cells expressing both HSA and CD4. Another factor thought to play a role in the apoptotic phase of negative selection is CD95 or Fas. Binding of CD95 to its ligand, CD95L (Fas ligand), initiates apoptosis in the CD95-expressing cell. However,

Figure 14.13 The role of thymic epithelial cells in negative selection of CD4$^+$ T cells. In a thymic culture system, intrathymic dendritic cells and other cells arising in the bone marrow were destroyed by incubation in deoxyguanosine, leaving only thymic cells of nonhematopoietic origin. If this thymus is then seeded with fresh thymocytes, mature CD4$^+$ thymocytes are subjected to negative selection, even in the absence of thymic interdigitating dendritic cells. Survival of autoreactive CD8$^+$ T cells indicates a role for bone marrow-derived cells in negative selection of these T cells.

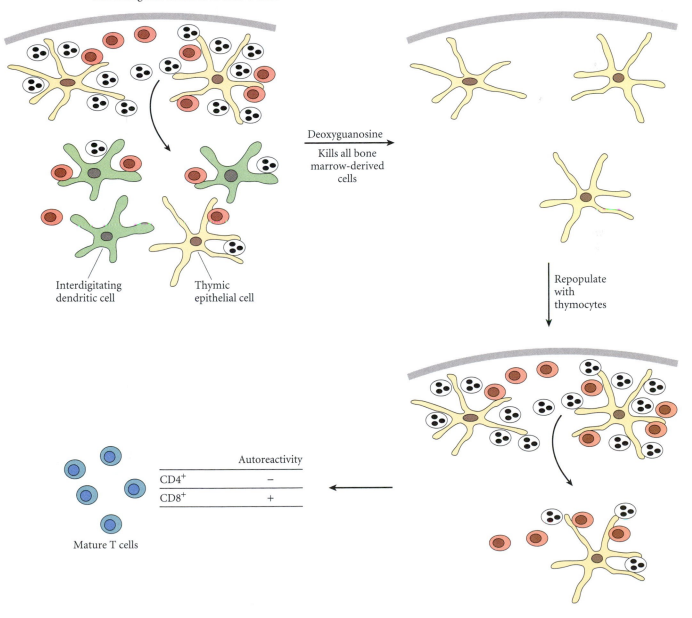

CD95 does not appear to play a role in negative selection except in circumstances wherein there is a very strong signal generated through the TCR, likely due to very high affinity binding to MHC-self peptide. Thus both CD95-independent and CD95-dependent molecular mechanisms influence the generation of apoptosis during negative selection. Cytokines also appear to influence negative selection. Both IL-4 and IL-7 inhibit the CD95-independent apoptosis of the HSA^{hi} CD4^{+} CD8^{-} medullary immature thymocytes but have no effect under conditions of strong stimulus due to CD95-dependent apoptosis. It has been proposed by J. Sprent and coworkers that the CD95-dependent apoptosis functions as a backup pathway in case the CD95-independent pathway fails.

In summary, negative selection is critical for eliminating potentially self-reactive T cells from the set of mature T cells that might have otherwise populated the periphery. However, since there is some indication that closely related molecular mechanisms mediate seemingly contradictory outcomes—positive or negative selection—by binding of TCR to cells presenting strong agonist peptides complexed to self MHC, a full understanding of the processes of positive and negative selection has not yet been generated.

Alloreactivity

Following positive and negative selection the mature T cells theoretically represent a population of cells that are self MHC restricted but not autoreactive. But one component of this model that is not fully understood is the concept of *alloreactivity*, which forms the basis for rejection of foreign tissue transplants as well as for graft-versus-host disease (GVHD). In GVHD transplanted immunologically competent lymphocytes from a donor react against the recipient's tissue antigens, creating a pathologic state due to cell and organ dysfunction induced in the recipient by activation of the donor lymphocytes that see the recipient's tissues as foreign. When T cells from one individual in a species are exposed to cells expressing nonself MHC from another individual in the species, instead of being refractory to stimulus, as one would predict since the stimulating *allogeneic* cell and responder T cells are mismatched at the MHC, the responding T cells are strongly stimulated. Thus, the responding T cells are activated by recognizing antigenic peptides presented on a *nonself* MHC. This response across MHC barriers is referred to as alloreactivity and represents another aspect of immunology wherein two seemingly opposite phenomena are both found to occur and thus must be adequately explained.

The molecular basis for alloreactivity involves the recognition of peptides that are presented by the allogeneic MHC molecules in a way that is similar to the recognition of self MHC complexed with foreign peptide (Fig.14.14). Of course, the peptide that is usually present in the peptide-binding groove of the allogeneic MHC is a self peptide for that cell. This allogeneic MHC and antigen

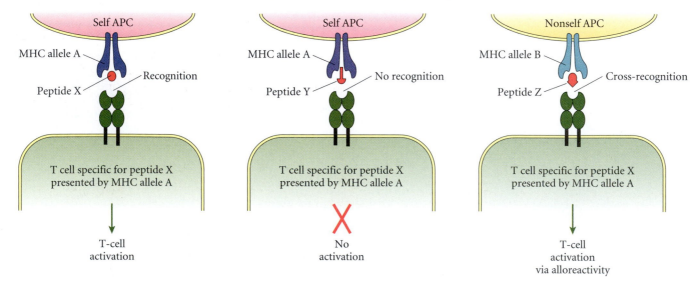

Figure 14.14 Potential basis for alloreactivity. In all cases, a T cell (green) specific for peptide X presented by MHC allele A interacts with different APCs. Self APC (pink) could present peptide X, leading to T-cell activation, or peptide Y, which will not activate the T cell. In some instances when a nonself APC (yellow) presents a peptide (Z) (which can be a self peptide for the nonself APC), the T cell recognizes this complex and is activated. Alloreactivity is actually quite common, with up to 10% of T cells able to respond to a large population of cells expressing nonself MHC but presenting their own cells' peptide antigens.

combination can cross-react with the TCR on the responder or recipient T cells and activate them. Alloreactivity therefore appears to follow the paradigm of agonist and antagonist peptides and stimulation of T cells: foreign MHC with its own self peptide is an agonist for the responding T cells. These mechanisms raise the exciting possibility that antagonist peptides could be placed in the peptide-binding groove of the foreign MHC and inhibit instead of activate T cells of tissue graft recipients or T cells that cause GVHD.

Central Tolerance Does Not Eliminate All Autoreactive Lymphocytes

Even in a healthy individual showing no overt signs of autoimmunity, mature lymphocytes that bear receptors capable of recognizing self antigens can be identified in the circulation. Since central tolerance does not delete all potentially autoreactive T lymphocytes, additional means of tolerance induction are needed to prevent autoimmune

Figure 14.15 Different mechanisms leading to nonresponsiveness of T cells. (**1**) In the thymus, clonal deletion via negative selection eliminates potentially self-reactive T cells. (**2**) Also in the thymus, clonal anergy can put potentially self-reactive T cells into a state of anergy, rendering them nonharmful when they encounter self antigens. (**3**) In the periphery, self-reactive T cells can be eliminated by clonal deletion if they encounter self antigen but do not receive activation signals but instead signals to undergo apoptosis. (**4**) Self-reactive T cells that encounter self antigen in the absence of costimulation can enter an anergic state and remain unresponsive to antigenic stimulus. (**5**) Regulatory or suppressor cells can keep potentially self-reactive T cells in check. (**6**) Immune privilege sites represent places in the body where resident cells constitutively express Fas ligand (CD95L), and when Fas (CD95)-bearing T cells enter the tissue, they undergo apoptosis subsequent to engaging the FasL.

disease. Although apoptosis leading to deletion of self-reactive clones is a major mechanism for negative selection, it also appears that contact of self-reactive T cells with thymic epithelial cells can lead to another type of nonresponsiveness termed central *clonal anergy* (Fig. 14.15). Instead of dying via apoptosis, these self-reactive T cells are rendered unresponsive or anergic to MHC-antigen stimuli, allowing them to live, albeit functionally incapacitated. Again, it is probably the affinity of the TCR for self-MHC-peptide complexes, based on whether the presented peptide is an agonist or antagonist peptide, that determines the fate of the still-maturing T cell. Anergy can potentially be reversible when the functionally inactivated CD4$^+$ cells move out of the thymus into a lymph node. For these reasons, other mechanisms of tolerance that function in the peripheral tissues are necessary to maintain self-tolerance.

Peripheral Tolerance

Peripheral tolerance refers to all of the tolerogenic mechanisms acting on mature lymphocytes that have already proceeded through all of the B- and T-cell maturation stages, have left the primary lymphoid organs, and have entered the periphery (Fig. 14.15). Such mechanisms are needed primarily because the bone marrow and thymus, where central tolerance takes place, do not express every gene product encoded in the genome. For mature T cells leaving the thymus, they are bound to encounter self antigens that were not available during the process of negative selection.

Mechanisms of peripheral tolerance: clonal anergy

The most common mechanism of peripheral tolerance is clonal anergy, the process whereby lymphocytes that recognize a self antigen are kept alive but are placed into a nonresponsive state. The main mechanism of anergy induction in the periphery acts through the delivery of an incomplete activation signal to a resting T cell (Fig. 14.16). T-cell activation requires a main signal, delivered via the TCR during ligation with peptide-MHC and a costimulatory signal, usually provided by CD80 or CD86 on the APC when they bind to CD28 on the T cell. In some cases, other T-cell surface proteins such as CD2, CD5, CD9, or CD44 can substitute for CD28 to deliver the costimulatory signal. However, if a T cell receives the main activation signal in the absence of sufficient costimulation, the T cell enters a state of anergy. Delivery of a costimulatory signal (e.g., CD28) results in reorganization of the T-cell plasma membrane, recruiting the TCR to a complex known as "membrane rafts." Rafts are domains within the plasma membrane that are rich in several protein tyrosine kinases and

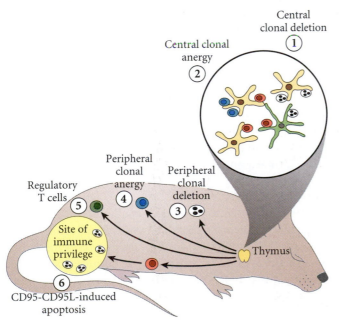

Central clonal deletion
①

Central clonal anergy
②

Peripheral clonal anergy

Peripheral clonal deletion
③

Regulatory T cells

④

⑤

Site of immune privilege

Thymus

⑥

CD95-CD95L-induced apoptosis

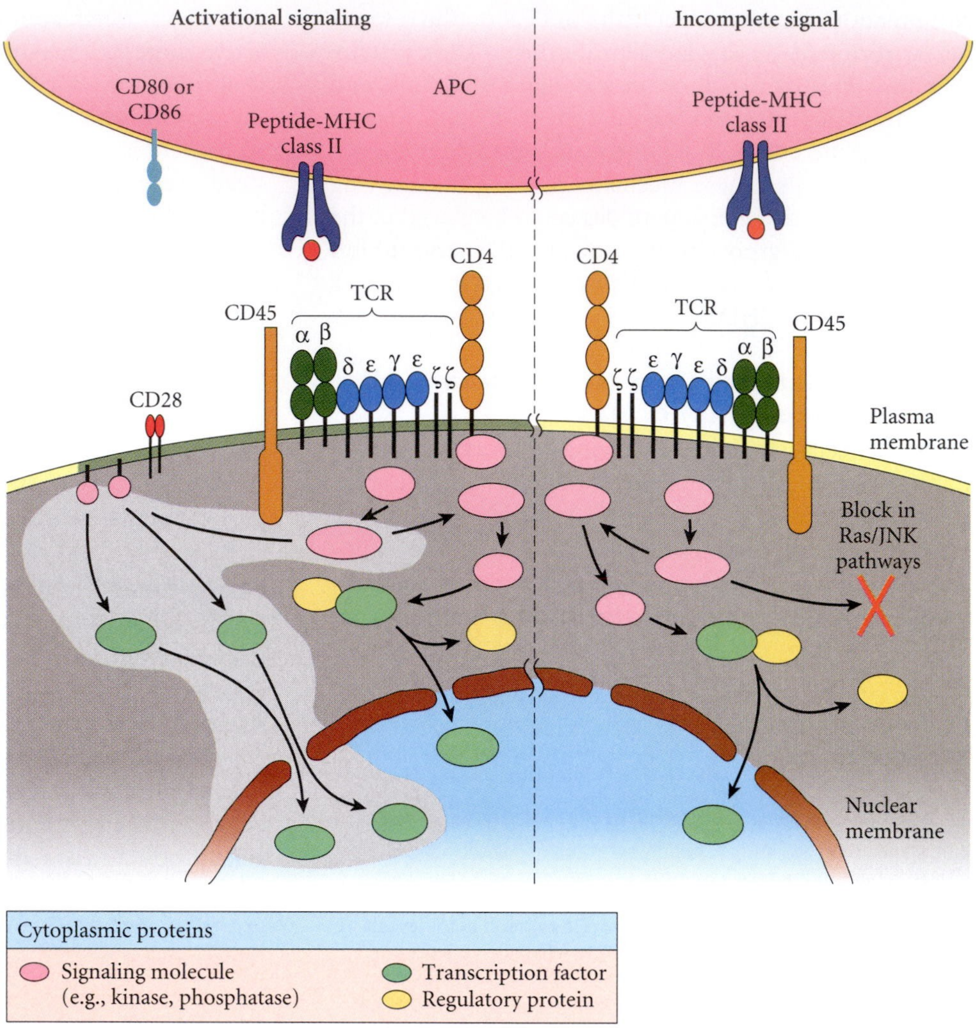

Figure 14.16 T-cell tolerance can be induced by "incomplete" signaling through the TCR. On the left, the T cell receives an activation signal consisting of antigen-MHC binding to TCR/CD3/CD4 as well as costimulatory signals such as the interaction of CD80 or CD86 on the APC with T-cell costimulatory receptor CD28. Engagement of CD28 on the T cell helps mobilize the TCR into membrane rafts (green area of membrane) containing key signaling molecules. Further events downstream of these initial interactions lead ultimately to entry of multiple transcription factors into the nucleus (light gray area) and cellular activation. In contrast, on the right, the T cell receives an incomplete signal consisting of TCR/CD3/CD4 engagement, but no CD28 engagement (tolerogenic signal). The resulting signal cascade fails to activate the T cell because an insufficient level or number of transcription factors enter the nucleus. This incomplete signal instead induces a state of anergy.

certain glycolipids and contain signaling molecules such as the Rac and Ras G proteins. The recruitment of the TCR complex to the rafts results in signal transduction to the nucleus and in cytoskeletal rearrangements necessary for T-cell activation, whereas the absence of costimulation results in incomplete activation. How this incomplete signal initiates entry into the anergic state is still under investigation, but it presumably involves interference with important signaling pathways within the T cell that prevent the T cell from becoming activated.

Anergy is also a state induced in a mature T cell following exposure to antagonistic or partially agonistic peptides on self-MHC molecules. The altered peptides within the MHC bind to T cells in a manner that is qualitatively different from binding of stimulatory foreign peptides. This indicates that the outcome of TCR engagement is not simply an "all-or-none" phenomenon but may vary depending on distinct, and possibly subtle, changes in the spatial orientation of the TCR complex during antigen

binding. Further, the strength of the signals delivered to the T cell from the external interactions of TCR with MHC-peptide and the interactions of costimulatory molecules with their receptors on T cells may influence the outcome of TCR engagement. Since many variant proteins are produced in the body due to splice variations, posttranslational modifications, binding of receptors to ligands, etc., a mechanism of recognition of these as antagonists leading to anergy would be useful to prevent self-T-cell responses.

Lack of danger signal

Another proposed, but controversial, mechanism of peripheral tolerance suggests that mature T cells that are reactive to self antigen and MHC do not respond to self antigens expressed by normal cells because the proper costimulatory signals are only generated when something like a viral infection, oncogenic change, or elaboration of stress signals such as heat shock proteins occurs. P.

Matzinger and colleagues have proposed this idea that a concurrent "danger" signal must be provided along with an antigenic stimulus to activate a T cell. In their view, when a healthy APC expressing only self antigens, or possibly also a target cell for CD8$^+$ cytotoxic T cells, encounters a self-reactive T cell nothing happens, since the presenting cell is not expressing or responding to any danger signals. Although this hypothesis simplifies the issue of self-tolerance in some ways, it ignores other clear data that negative selection and central clonal anergy are important mechanisms for generating tolerance.

Regulatory or suppressor T cells

Peripheral tolerance may also be due to a type of regulatory T cell that inhibits or suppresses immune responses. The existence of so-called T suppressor cells has been hypothesized since the mid-1970s, but there was no clear consensus on what characterized these cells, in regard to either phenotypic markers or activity. One conceptual problem is that the lack of help is functionally equivalent to active suppression, so that it was difficult to distinguish an anergic T cell from a responsive one being kept in check by another T cell. Recently a significant amount of evidence has accrued to document that the thymus produces T cells that are functionally dominant over self-reactive T cells that might escape negative selection. These T cells have recently been relabeled "regulatory" T cells when they are CD4$^+$ cells and "suppressor" T cells when they are CD8$^+$ cells. It is not clear if these cells constitute a unique and stable subpopulation of T cells or are just part of the normal T-cell pool that attains regulatory functions. CD4$^+$ regulatory T cells have been characterized as having a surface marker profile that is CD5^{hi}, CD45RC^{low}, RT6.1$^+$ (a rat T-cell marker), or CD25$^+$. The CD25$^+$ CD4$^+$ subset has been the most studied of the regulatory T cells. None of these markers appears to be associated with the regulatory function of these cells, and these markers are typically found on activated T cells. CD4$^+$ CD25$^+$ regulatory T cells have a variety of functions (Fig. 14.17A), with an important one being control of autoimmune responses. When T-cell-deficient mice such as nude mice are reconstituted with intact T-cell suspensions, no autoimmunity is observed in the recipients (Fig. 14.17B). However, if they are given T cells from which the cells with the regulatory profile have been eliminated (all CD25$^+$ cells or CD4$^+$ CD25$^+$ cells), then almost all of the mice develop autoimmune disease. Transfer of CD8$^+$ CD25$^-$ cells does not induce autoimmunity in recipient mice. If CD25$^+$ cells are added back to the transferred T-cell suspension initially depleted of CD25$^+$ cells, then development of autoimmune disease is prevented.

Regulatory or suppressor cells seem to manifest their activity through several mechanisms. One is similar to the anti-idiotypic network mechanism theorized to explain the maintenance of B-cell homeostasis. Put simply, since each lymphocyte bears a clonotypic antigen receptor (i.e., either membrane immunoglobulin or TCR), the magnitude of the representation of any given antigen receptor in the body is dependent on the number of cells of the lymphocyte clone that express the clonotypic receptor. When a lymphocyte is activated and then proliferates, a much higher number of cells expressing the clonotypic receptor are achieved (i.e., going from 10 to 5,000 cells with the same TCR). At a sufficiently high cell number, the antigen receptor on the clonally expanded cells will become great enough to become immunogenic and stimulate an immune response to this particular antigen receptor (Fig. 14.18). Since this is a T-cell-mediated response, the responding T cell is recognizing the peptide fragments of the variable region of the clonotypic TCR being presented by MHC molecules on the surface of the T cell. An important role for regulatory T cells that produce secondary anti-TCR responses is supported by the finding that autoimmunity is intensified when the secondary anti-TCR T cells are neutralized or killed. Another mechanism may relate to the pattern of cytokines secreted by the regulatory T cells. In addition to the TH1 and TH2 subpopulations of CD4$^+$ cells, there are other subpopulations that secrete transforming growth factor β (designated TH3 cells) or IL-10 (designated Tr1 cells), and these cells have regulatory properties that prevent autoimmune and inflammatory diseases in mice. The secretion of cytokines that suppress T-cell activation or effector function represents another means of regulatory T-cell control in the periphery, although it is not clear if the cytokines themselves are the suppressive factors or are needed more for the proper development of regulatory T cells.

Immune-privileged sites

Another localized mechanism of peripheral tolerance is the existence of "immune-privileged sites," places in the body where lymphocytes are generally excluded. Sites of immune privilege usually are exceptionally delicate or intricate tissues, whose function may be permanently compromised by the collateral damage ("innocent bystander damage") that accompanies an intense immune response. Sites of immune privilege have several mechanisms available for preventing or dampening immune responses. Examples of immune-privileged sites are the eye, the testes, and the developing fetus in the uterus.

Several mechanisms have been proposed or demonstrated to account for immune privilege. In the testes,

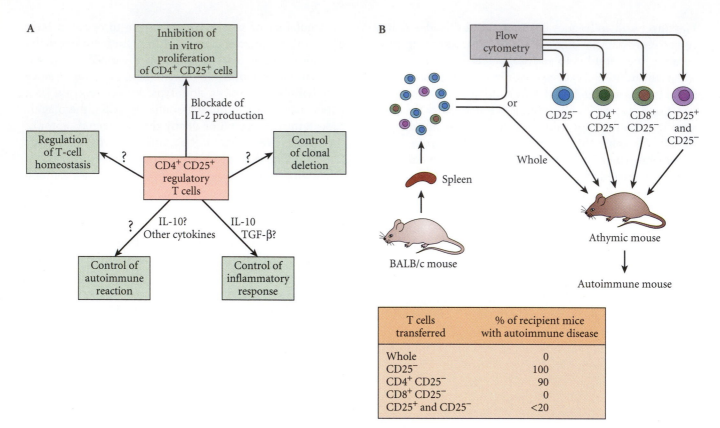

Figure 14.17 (A) Function of regulatory T cells. At the core of this mechanism of T-cell regulation are CD4$^+$ CD25$^+$ T cells that can mediate a variety of functions by secreting soluble factors or possibly via direct cell contact. A blockade of IL-2 production will remove a critical factor T cells need for growth and differentiation. IL-10 and transforming growth factor β (TGF-β) are well-known factors that inhibit lymphocyte function and responses. Regulating T-cell homeostasis and controlling clonal deletion also have been proposed as mechanisms of action of regulatory T cells. (B) Experimental evidence for the existence and function of regulatory T cells. Isolated T cells from the spleen of a normal BALB/c mouse can be separated by flow cytometry on the basis of expression of surface markers. The separated cells can then be transferred in various combinations to an athymic mouse lacking an endogenous immune system. The mice are then monitored for the development of autoimmune disease. Athymic mice that get unfractionated or a whole population of T cells develop no significant autoimmune disease whereas mice that get those T cells lacking CD25 (CD25$^-$) go on to develop autoimmune disease. If CD4$^+$ but CD25$^-$ cells are transferred, then autoimmune disease also frequently develops. In contrast, CD8$^+$ cells that are CD25$^-$ do not promote autoimmune disease, indicating a regulatory role for these T cells. If the population of autoimmune-promoting CD25$^-$ cells are mixed with the autoimmune-inhibiting CD25$^+$ cells, then the latter cells can prevent the development of autoimmune disease.

CD95L is expressed constitutively throughout the tissue on stromal cells. Normally, CD95L is expressed on cytotoxic T lymphocytes (CTLs) and is used by CTLs to trigger apoptosis of target cells expressing CD95. Activated T cells also express CD95 but somehow resist destruction by other CD95L-expressing CTL. In response to this constitutive expression of CD95L by the stromal cells, any immune cells that enter the tissue are immediately induced to undergo apoptosis themselves (Fig. 14.19A).

The existence of other mechanisms of immune privilege has been proposed on the basis of findings from studies that used the placenta as a model system (Fig. 14.19B). The placenta is an interesting tissue because it is a site where maternal and fetal immune systems come in contact with each other in a tissue called the trophoblast. However, during a successful pregnancy, fetal and maternal immune systems ignore each other's existence. Fetal tissues express paternal antigens, which are usually seen as foreign by the mother, and since the fetus only inherits one maternal MHC haplotype, fetal lymphocytes likely could react to maternal self peptides displayed on MHC proteins encoded by the noninherited haplotype. Thus there is a strong potential basis for maternal responses to fetal tissues and vice versa. Mechanisms being investigated to explain the immune privilege at the fetomaternal interface include the absence of expression of antigenic

HLA antigens, the presence of alternate HLA surface molecules that may be tolerogenic instead of immunogenic, production of cytokines and other inhibitory factors that initiate a nonspecific reduction of immunoreactivity, production of "blocking antibodies" that interfere with the activity of cytotoxic cells, and changes in the expression of complement regulatory proteins that prevent the appearance of an inflammatory-like state in the trophoblast. For example, inactivation of the mouse complement regulator protein Crry (a mouse homolog of human complement receptor 1) resulted in the rejection of em-

bryos during pregnancy (Fig. 14.19B); histologic examination of the placenta demonstrated strong complement activation and infiltration by maternal neutrophils. Another mechanism of fetal tolerance might be the result of the amino acid starvation of infiltrating maternal immune cells. The trophoblast expresses the enzyme indoleamine 2,3-dioxygenase (IDO), a tryptophan-catabolizing enzyme that could inhibit lymphocyte proliferation if expressed in the placenta. Support for this hypothesis comes from results showing that treatment of fetuses with an IDO inhibitor led to leukocyte infiltration of the concep-

Figure 14.18 (A) Evidence for the existence of regulatory T cells in an experimental model of multiple sclerosis (experimental autoimmune encephalomyelitis). When injected with myelin basic protein (MBP), MBP-specific CD4$^+$ and CD8$^+$ T cells become activated and expand. The CD4$^+$ cells provide help to the CD8$^+$ cells that mediate the pathologic disease process. These MBP-reactive T cells express TRBV13-2, then attack nerve cells coated with MBP and destroy them, leading to autoimmune encephalomyelitis. (B) If mice are immunized with CD8$^+$ CTL expressing TRBV13-2 or soluble TRBV13-2 molecules, they will develop CD8$^+$ CTL that recognize peptide fragments of TRBV13-2 presented by MHC antigens of TRBV13-2$^+$ T cells. Mature T cells can express both MHC class I and class II. The CTL that can now recognize the TRBV13-2$^+$ cells usually express TRBV31 and are cytolytic to the TRBV13-2$^+$ cells.

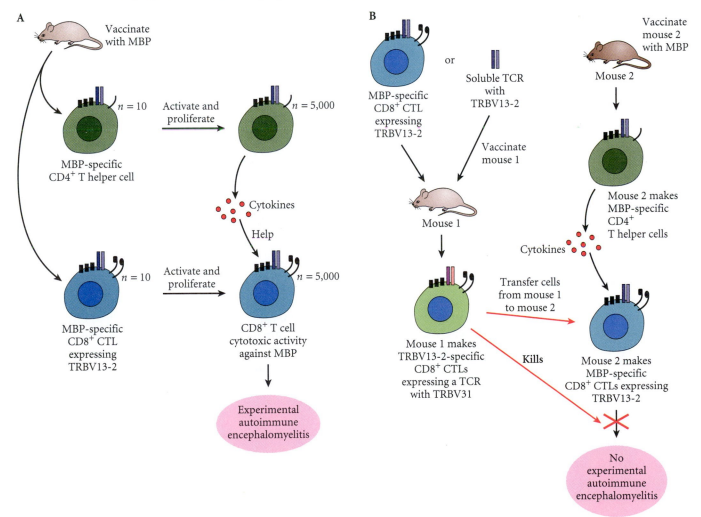

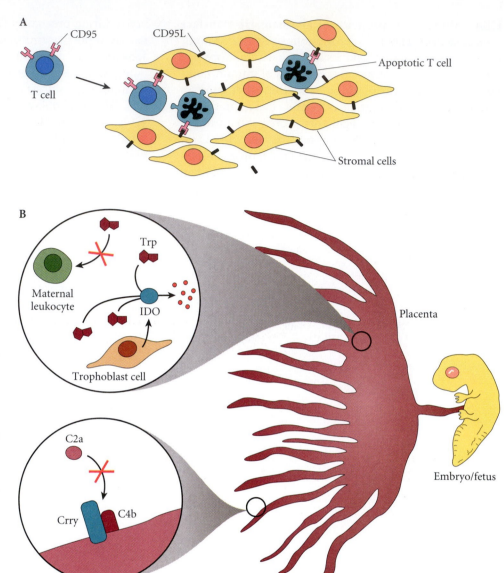

Figure 14.19 Regulation of T-cell and complement activation at sites of immune privilege. (**A**) In the testes, stromal cells constitutively express CD95L (Fas ligand). Binding of CD95L to CD95 (Fas) on T cells triggers apoptosis of the latter, thus preventing immune responses within the testes. (**B**) In the placenta, privilege has been shown to be maintained by two mechanisms. First, IDO secreted by trophoblast cells consumes all available tryptophan (Trp), thus killing immune cells by amino acid starvation. Second, the placenta controls complement activation by constitutive expression of the complement regulatory protein Crry, which binds C4b and prevents the formation of the C4b2a "C3 convertase."

tus and to an immunologically based fetal rejection. Clearly some potent and multifactorial mechanisms mediate immunologic tolerance during pregnancy, and when these mechanisms fail and allow maternal immune responses to the fetus, there is a potential immunologic basis for infertility in some women.

T-Cell Activation and Antigen Recognition

Events in T-Cell Signal Transduction

Antigen-MHC recognition by the TCR

Although considerable information has been gained about the mechanisms of signal transduction in response to MHC-antigen-TCR ligation, these systems remain incom-

pletely defined. Nonetheless, many of the basic events are well understood. APCs constitutively cluster MHC molecules with associated peptides into lipid rafts to concentrate them for presentation to T cells. When a T cell engages MHC-peptide, an *immunological synapse* is formed—an area of cell-cell contact where the MHC-peptide-TCR complex is found in the center with accessory molecules such as ICAM-1 and LFA-1 forming a ring around the synapse (Fig. 14.20A). However, it may be that TCR signaling occurs before the formation of the mature synapse, when the TCR is not concentrated in the center of the synapse but mostly around the periphery (Fig. 14.20B). Regardless of whether signaling takes place at the periphery or center of the synapse, the TCR engages an important protein kinase, Lck. The TCR-CD3-CD4 or TCR-CD3-

CD8 complex transmits the signal indicating a binding event has occurred via a series of protein kinases including Lck, Fyn, and ZAP-70. Lck is a member of the Src family of protein tyrosine kinases, thus expressing Src homology domain 2 (SH2). To the degree to which the signaling steps and factors involved in activating a T cell are understood, there is a hierarchy of steps that transmit the information that the TCR has engaged the proper MHC-peptide combination (an extracellular binding event) to the T-cell nucleus in an orderly fashion. In a CD4$^+$ cell, Lck is concen-

trated on the cytoplasmic side of the lipid raft and is also associated noncovalently with the cytoplasmic tail of the CD4 molecule. Until TCR engagement of MHC-peptide, Lck is maintained in a closed, inactive form due to the presence of phosphate molecules at its C terminus (Fig. 14.21A). When TCR and CD4 are ligated on the surface of T cells, the protein tyrosine phosphatase CD45 dephosphorylates Lck, opening it to produce the form that can be phosphorylated in its activation loop. Phosphorylation activates the kinase activity of Lck. CD45 also dephosphory-

A

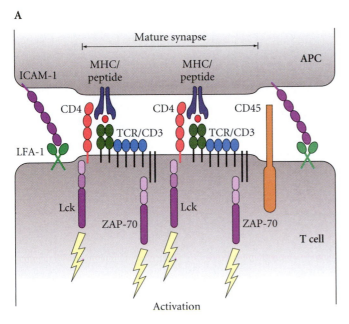

Figure 14.20 The immunologic synapse. (**A**). In one model, binding of TCR to MHC-peptide facilitates movement of this complex into lipid rafts. These molecules are then concentrated in the middle of the synapse. A ring of accessory molecules is formed, involving ICAM-1 and LFA-1 among others to exclude unnecessary factors. (**B**) In another model, most of the TCR engages Lck at the periphery of the synapse before formation of the mature synapse, and TCR-based signaling is mostly over by the time the mature synapse forms. The TCR may be internalized from the synapse by endocytosis for either further intracellular signaling or attenuation of signaling due to removal of the TCR from the cell surface.

B

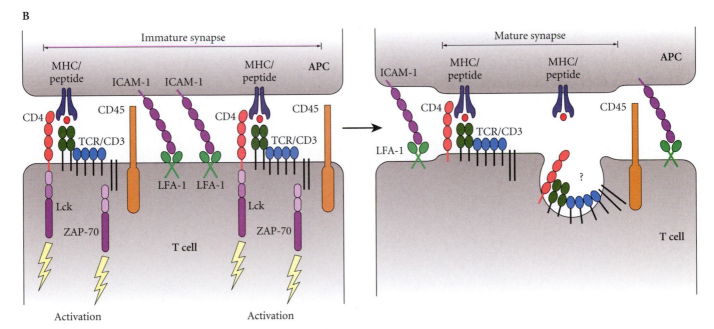

Figure 14.21 Initial events in T-cell activation. (**A**) Following ligation of TCR and CD4 to MHC-peptide, the activity of the CD45 protein tyrosine phosphatase dephosphorylates the terminal phosphate (orange) on p59*fyn* and p56*lck*. (**B**) The activated Fyn and Lck are themselves phosphorylated (green circles) by protein tyrosine kinases, and they then phosphorylate tyrosine molecules located in the cytoplasmic ITAMs (red).

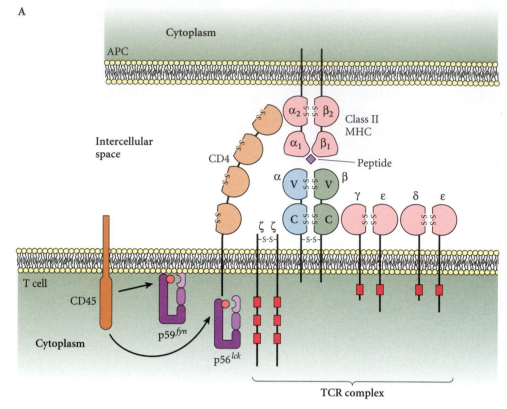

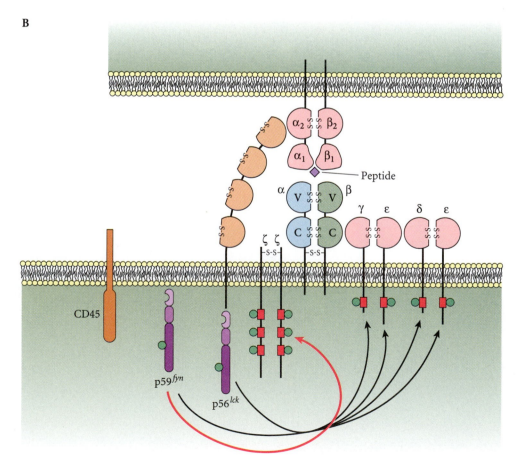

lates another membrane-anchored molecule, Fyn, which is also a Src family kinase. Lck is the principal molecule responsible for the inducible phosphorylation of the immunoreceptor tyrosine-based activation motif (ITAM) activation sites on the γ, δ, and ε chains of CD3 as well as the ζ chains of CD3 (Fig. 14.21B). The protein tyrosine kinase Fyn also interacts with the γ, δ, ε, and ζ chains of CD3. This interaction initiates signaling due to increases in the kinase activity of Fyn on the CD3 subunits.

The newly phosphorylated ITAMs of the ζ chain homodimer of the CD3 molecule provide docking sites for another kinase, ZAP-70, that has tandem SH2 domains (Fig. 14.22A). These SH2 domains are spaced apart in a specific manner that allows them to interact with phosphorylated ITAMs. A splice variant of the ζ chain, known as the η chain, can also form a heterodimeric complex with a ζ chain. After binding to the ITAMs, ZAP-70 is phosphorylated in its activation loops by Lck and Fyn. Activated ZAP-70 then phosphorylates another substrate, LAT (linker of activation in T cells), along with a protein called SLP-76. These become linker or adapter proteins to further amplify T-cell signaling. LAT is a cytoplasmic protein that has a 14-carbon-long fatty acid (palmitic acid) bound to cysteine residues, allowing LAT to be concentrated within the lipid rafts. LAT also has many tyrosines that can be phosphorylated and serve as docking sites for enzymatic signaling molecules that bind via SH2 domains and therefore further promote the signaling process. The complex of activated ZAP-70, LAT, and SLP-76 is then able to activate a number of other targets, prominent among which is *phospholipase Cγ* (PLCγ), which is activated upon phosphorylation.

The kinetics of T-cell activation and its site of occurrence in the membrane or lipid raft are not well established. It was initially proposed that to sustain signal transduction, the lipid rafts are used to amplify TCR-derived signaling within the immunologic synapse. This could occur by binding of the accessory molecule CD28 to CD80 or CD86, which in turn recruits more rafts to the synapse. This process could result in the exclusion of phosphatases that would otherwise interfere with kinase-mediated signaling. But other data indicate that TCR-based signaling is mostly over by the time the mature immunologic synapse forms. Since the rafts also promote cytoskeletal changes, it may be that the function of the immunologic synapse is to direct polarized secretion of cytokines or to modulate TCR-based signaling by promoting endocytosis of the TCR into the T cell. Some receptors, such as the epidermal growth factor receptor, are internalized by cells to promote signaling. Alternately, removal of the TCR from the cell surface by endocytosis out of the synapse may attenuate

signaling. Although the timing of TCR signaling in relation to formation of the immunologic synapse has only recently been studied and is therefore not fully determined, it is clear that formation of the synapse occurs in conjunction with TCR-mediated cell signaling, and this signaling event includes numerous other additional components.

Phosphorylation of PLCγ results in activation of second messengers in the *phosphatidylinositol* pathway (Fig. 14.22B). The critical first step is the hydrolysis of *phosphatidylinositol bisphosphate* (PIP$_2$), which results in formation of *inositol trisphosphate* (IP$_3$) and *diacylglycerol* (DAG). IP$_3$ binds to receptors in the endoplasmic reticulum and is responsible for release of calcium from stores within cellular vacuoles to the cytoplasm. The result of this release is the opening of calcium channels in the plasma membrane and an influx of calcium into the cell. Increased levels of intracellular calcium activate a protein called *calmodulin,* which, through other cellular intermediaries, leads to production of transcription factors that enter the cell nucleus and affect gene transcription. DAG remains associated with the plasma membrane of the T cell and is responsible for phosphorylation of *protein kinase C* (PKC). The resultant activation of PKC leads to its ability to function as a protein kinase, and, along with changes in calcium levels, activates downstream signaling events, including activation of calcineurin and the small GTP-binding protein (*small G protein*) known as Ras.

Small G proteins such as p21^{ras} and CDC42/*rac* represent another type of signaling molecule involved in T-cell activation (Fig. 14.23A). When the costimulatory molecule CD28 is engaged by CD80 or CD86, the small G proteins Rac and Ras are recruited to the cell membrane. Ras is a potent controller of cellular growth. Their activation state is determined by whether they are bound to guanosine diphosphate (GDP) or guanosine triphosphate (GTP) (Fig. 14.23B). When bound to GTP, Ras is active and becomes inactive when a particular enzyme removes a phosphate group from the GTP. To return Ras and other small G proteins to their active, GTP-bound forms, regulatory enzymes known as *guanine-nucleotide exchange factors* act on GDP-bound small G proteins to exchange GDP for GTP. The activated small G proteins initiate other signaling cascades, particularly those that comprise the *MAPK cascade*.

The enzymatic and signaling cascades produced from the interactions initiated by TCR engagement of MHC-peptide are the forces that generate many of the activated transcription factors that participate in regulation of T-cell activity (Fig. 14.24). The major transcription factor is NF-κB, generated from a cytoplasmic precursor held in check by binding to its inhibitor, IκB (inhibitor of κB).

Figure 14.22 Full T-cell activation. (A) ZAP-70, a Src family kinase, binds to phosphorylated ITAMs of the ζ chain homodimer via SH2 domains. ZAP-70 is phosphorylated by Lck and Fyn, and the activated ZAP-70 phosphorylates the linker of activation in T cells (LAT) and SLP-76. LAT is concentrated within the lipid rafts and can be phosphorylated to provide docking sites for enzymatic signaling molecules that bind via SH2 domains. The complex of activated ZAP-70, LAT, and SLP-76 is then able to activate a number of other targets, prominent among which is PLCγ1, which is activated upon phosphorylation. The substrate for PLCγ1 is PIP_2, which results in formation of IP_3 and DAG. (B) Production of IP_3 and DAG results in additional effects that are part of T-cell activation. A major consequence is the activation of second messengers such as calcineurin and PKC. These then act on inactivated forms of transcription factors held in the cytoplasm. Both dephosphorylation (i.e., of NF-AT) and phosphorylation (i.e., of IκB) events produce activated transcription factors that then translocate from the cytoplasm to the nucleus. The transcription factors bind to regulatory regions in chromosomal DNA to activate transcription of genes that characterize an activated T cell.

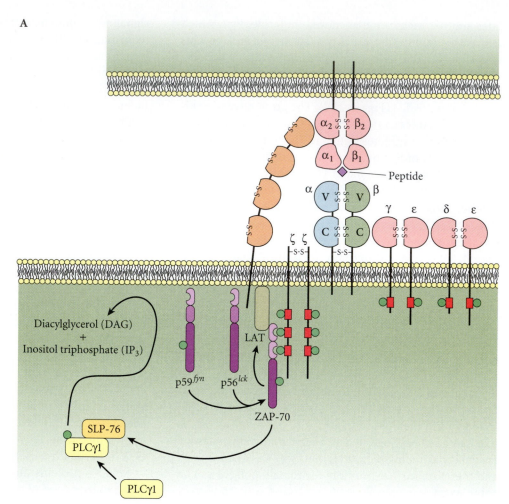

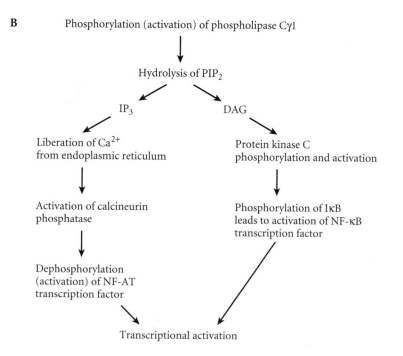

A

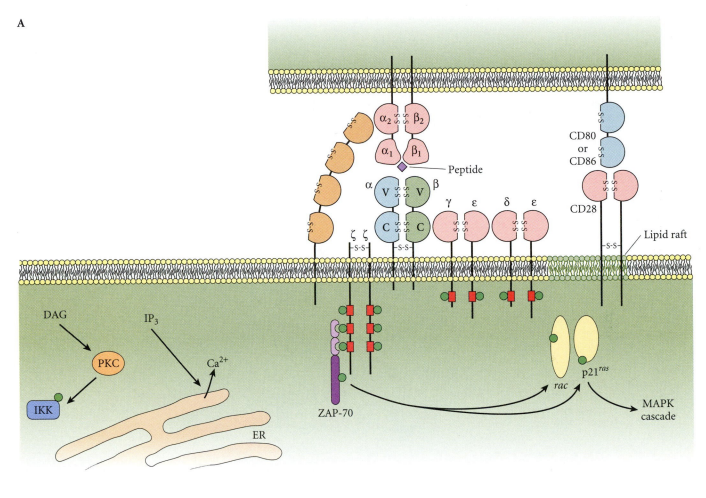

B

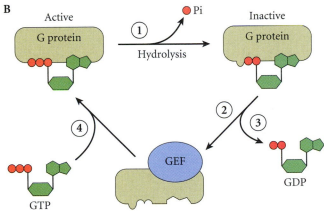

Figure 14.23 G proteins involved in T-cell activation. (**A**) G proteins are potent activators and controllers of cellular growth. Activated ZAP-70 phosphorylates (green circles) p21^{ras} and CDC42/*rac* (yellow ovals) after recruitment of these molecules to the cell membrane when the costimulatory molecule CD28 is engaged by CD80 or CD86. (**B**) The activation state of G proteins is determined by whether they are bound to GDP or GTP. An active G protein is bound to GTP, and becomes inactive when dephosphorylated to produce GDP. Guanine-nucleotide exchange factors (GEF) act on GDP-bound small G proteins to exchange GDP for GTP and reproduce the active form of the G protein. The activated small G proteins initiate other signaling cascades, particularly those that comprise the MAPK cascade.

Activation of an upstream factor, I-κ kinase (IKK), leads to phosphorylation of IκB, which dissociates from NF-κB, is degraded, and frees NF-κB to enter the nucleus to activate gene transcription. Nuclear factor of activated T cells (NF-AT) is generated by dephosphorylation of its inactive precursor by activated calcineurin. The small G protein factors lead to production of the Jun kinase (JNK), which enters the nucleus and phosphorylates its target, Jun. Phosphorylated Jun pairs with another transcription factor, Fos, that together form the AP-1 transcription factor. Other currently unidentified transcription factors are also involved. The net result is that transcription factors that regulate gene expression are induced to enter the nucleus, where they bind to specific sites in promoters or other regions of DNA that regulate gene transcription.

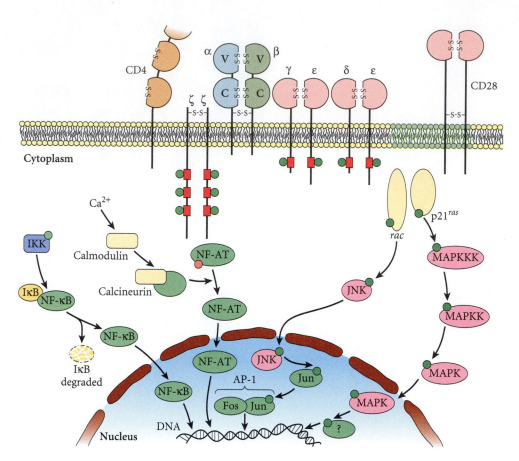

Figure 14.24 Final stages of T-cell activation. Entry of transcription factors into the nucleus with subsequent transcription of genes needed for activation and proliferation mediate the final stages of T-cell activation. NF-κB is derived from an inactive precursor in the cytoplasm. Phosphorylation of the inhibitor of κB (IκB) by IKK releases the active form for nuclear translocation. Calcineurin dephosphorylates NF-AT for its nuclear translocation. Phosphorylated Ras and Rac activate members of the MAPK family—JNK and the MAPK kinase kinase (MAPKKK). Phosphorylated JNK translocates into the nucleus where it acts on a transcription factor, Jun, allowing it to pair with another factor, Fos. This combination forms the AP-1 transcription factor. MAPKKK acts on another kinase, MAPKK, which acts on another kinase, MAPK, that translocates into the nucleus and activates additional transcription factors.

Signaling by accessory molecules

Another effect of CD28 signaling following binding to CD80 or CD86 is enhancement of IL-2 production via activation of the MAPK cascade and production of the cJun transcription factor and formation of the AP-1 heterodimeric DNA-binding element. Binding of CD80 or CD86 to CD28 also results in other changes in the T cell. Ligation recruits phosphatidylinositol 3-kinase to the plasma membrane. The cytoplasmic part of CD28 binds to the adapter proteins of the Grb-2–SOS complex that can signal via the Ras pathway of T-cell activation. CD28 also enhances activation of PLCγ1, Lck, and RAF-1 kinase, stimulates cyclic AMP turnover, and induces the influx of calcium and the generation of phosphoinositides following TCR-mediated signaling. The manner in which all of these activities are controlled and integrated is not well understood, but it is clear that CD28 ligation has multiple effects on T-cell activation.

Signals needed by T-cell activation and consequences of insufficient signaling

T cells that receive signals from CD2, CD28, LFA-1, and a high-affinity interaction with the TCR will enter the cell cycle. Those that receive a stimulus from the TCR alone

receive a negative signal that induces anergy and T-cell unresponsiveness (Fig. 14.16). It was recently determined that a block in the Ras/Jnk signaling pathway is responsible for anergy in T cells. Since CD28 ligation is critical for inducing this particular signaling pathway, then failure to bind to CD28 during antigen presentation can result in anergy. Once the anergic state has been induced, the T cell is refractory to further activation, even when the additional signals needed for T-cell activation are subsequently delivered. The need for costimulation probably arose as part of the regulatory process for preventing inappropriate immune responses. For example, if a TCR is produced but not eliminated in the thymus that can engage a non-APC due to presentation of a self peptide on self MHC, the lack of costimulation prevents inappropriate activation of the T cell.

For T cells to proliferate, they must produce both IL-2 and the IL-2R. IL-2 was named T-cell growth factor following its initial discovery. IL-2 is produced by TH0 cells and TH1 cells and, to a lesser extent, by cytotoxic T cells. IL-2 stimulates proliferation of T cells and the long-term growth of T-cell clones by binding to IL-2R and preventing apoptosis, as well as enhancing the activity of cytotoxic T and NK cells.

Alternate Mechanisms of T-Cell Activation

Alternate mechanisms of T-cell activation other than stimulation of MHC-restricted, antigen-specific activation include the signals provided by superantigens, mitogenic lectins, and antibodies that cross-link receptors on the surface of the T cell. Superantigens include bacterial exoproducts (primarily the staphylococcal and streptococcal enterotoxins that cause toxic shock syndrome, food poisoning, and scalded skin syndrome). These molecules bind to MHC and the TCR, cross-linking the two proteins and bringing them in proximity that facilitates signaling, the primary differences being that superantigen binds to both MHC and the TCR outside of the normal antigen-binding groove and that the affinity of the interaction is much higher than the interaction of TCR with MHC and antigen (Fig. 14.25). Therefore, superantigen does not interact with the MHC-TCR regions that are tailor-made to bind specifically with a given antigenic peptide. Superantigen instead interacts with more highly conserved regions of these proteins and can thus bind to a higher percentage of MHC and TCR molecules than can any conventional antigen. The region of interaction of the TCR with most su-

perantigens is the lateral side wall of the TRBV (V$_\beta$) chain of the TCR. Superantigens usually activate a subset of T cells expressing a particular type of TRBV. For example, staphylococcal enterotoxin B, one of the causes of staphylococcal food poisoning, binds to TCR containing any of the TRBV3, -12, -14, -15, -17, and -20 gene products regardless of the rearrangement and configuration of the CDR3. Other bacterial superantigens bind to different combinations of TRBV. Although these responses are MHC dependent, as they require MHC class II, there is no requirement for processing and presentation by an MHC molecule and the MHC and TCR do not have to be syngeneic, and therefore, the response is not MHC restricted.

Another class of superantigens for mouse T cells are those encoded by certain viral DNAs, such as the mouse mammary tumor virus (MTV). The genes for these *endogenous* superantigens integrate into the host's DNA and the gene product is expressed as a surface molecule. The virus-encoded superantigens stimulate an oligoclonal repertoire of TRBV-bearing T cells. Because the endogenous superantigens are expressed during T-cell development, T cells expressing a TRBV gene product that reacts with an endogenous superantigen are deleted by negative selection. These virally encoded proteins are also termed *minor lymphocyte stimulation* (Mls) antigens because of the role they play, secondary to that of the MHC, in tissue rejection following transplantation. For example, a strain of mouse that contains the *mls2* allele due to infection with MTV-13 will not have any T cells expressing mouse TRBV3, because the Mls2 protein is a superantigen for TCR expressing the TRBV3 protein.

In the laboratory, mitogenic lectins often are used to stimulate T cells. These molecules usually are derived from plants and stimulate (on average) 10 to 20% of the lymphocytes in any given population. Although the mechanism of activation has not been completely delineated, these molecules bind to carbohydrates, usually on surface glycoproteins, and cross-link some of the surface molecules on T cells. Stimulation requires accessory cell function but does not require MHC (MHC independent).

Another laboratory method for activating T cells is to cross-link surface receptors with an antibody or other type of cross-linking agent. Antibodies to both TCR and CD3 cause T cells to undergo activation in a manner analogous to that of cognate engagement of MHC-peptide. Antibodies to CD28 also mimic aspects of T-cell activation and can be used to understand how signaling through the CD28 receptor affects T cells. While obviously not physiologically relevant to T-cell activation, these methods represent important tools for studying the complexity of T-cell responses.

Figure 14.25 Mode of binding of superantigens to MHC-TCR. Normally, the TCR recognizes the MHC-peptide complex on an APC (**left**). Superantigens bind to the variable region of the TCR β chain outside of the antigen-recognition area as well as to the MHC class II on the APC. This mimics cognate recognition by the TCR of peptide-MHC, leading to T-cell activation.

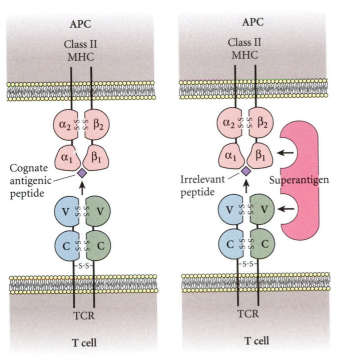

Summary

T cells are an essential component of the cognate, antigen-specific, mechanism of host defense. T cells, like B cells, can identify even very subtle differences in antigens, resulting in a highly specific response. However, T cells differ from B cells in a few fundamental respects. In contrast to B cells, which respond to the conformational epitopes of soluble antigens, T cells respond to the primary amino acid sequence of peptides only when they are presented by an MHC molecule on the surface of an APC that also supplies accessory signals. The TCR recognizes components of both the antigen and the MHC molecule, which have been "learned" during the ontogeny of each individual T cell. In the thymus, each T cell survives only if it responds to self MHC molecules and self antigens with low avidity or signal strength. Strong signals result in deletion of the T cells. The two main functions of T cells are to produce helper and regulatory cytokines and to generate cellular cytotoxicity; unlike B cells, T cells do not secrete their receptors to accomplish their immunologic function. Once the TCR is ligated by MHC and antigen and accessory signals have been provided, the T cell utilizes a signaling pathway that involves a highly complex multicomponent series of tyrosine and serine kinases and adapter proteins that influence transcription, cytokine production, cellular differentiation, effector function, and clonal expansion that provide host defense to a variety of microbial pathogens and tumors.

Suggested Reading

Berg, L. J., and J. Kang. 2001. Molecular determinants of TCR expression and selection. *Curr. Opin. Immunol.* **13:**232–241.

Dykstra, M., A. Cherukuri, and S. K. Pierce. 2001. Rafts and synapses in the spatial organization of immune cell signaling receptors. *J. Leukoc. Biol.* **70:**699–707.

Hermiston, M. L., Z. Xu, R. Majeti, and A. Weiss. 2002. Reciprocal regulation of lymphocyte activation by tyrosine kinases and phosphatases. *J. Clin. Invest.* **109:**9–14.

Maryanski, J. L., V. Attuil, A. Hamrouni, M. Mutin, M. Rossi, A. Aublin, and P. Bucher. 2001. Individuality of Ag-selected and preimmune TCR repertoires. *Immunol. Res.* **23:**75–84.

Nel, A. E. 2002. T-cell activation through the antigen receptor. Part 1: signaling components, signaling pathways, and signal integration at the T-cell antigen receptor synapse. *J. Allergy Clin. Immunol.* **109:**758–770.

Nel, A. E., and N. Slaughter. 2002. T-cell activation through the antigen receptor. Part 2: role of signaling cascades in T-cell differentiation, anergy, immune senescence, and development of immunotherapy. *J. Allergy Clin. Immunol.* **109:**901–915.

Plum, J., M. De Smedt, B. Verhasselt, T. Kerre, D. Vanhecke, B. Vandekerckhove, and G. Leclercq. 2000. T lymphopoiesis. In vitro and in vivo study models. *Ann. N. Y. Acad. Sci.* **917:**724–731.

Rotrosen, D., J. B. Matthews, and J. A. Bluestone. 2002. The immune tolerance network: a new paradigm for developing tolerance-inducing therapies. *J. Allergy Clin. Immunol.* **110:**17–23.

Sen, J. 2001. Signal transduction in thymus development. *Cell Mol. Biol.* **47:**197–215.

Shevach, E. M. 2002. CD4+ CD25+ suppressor T cells: more questions than answers. *Nat. Rev. Immunol.* **2:**389–400.

Singer, A. L., and G. A. Koretzky. 2002. Control of T cell function by positive and negative regulators. *Science* **296:**1639–1640.

Sprent J., and H. Kishimoto. 2001. The thymus and central tolerance. *Philos. Trans. R. Soc. Lond. B. Biol. Sci.* **356:**609–616.

van der Merwe, P. A. 2002. Formation and function of the immunological synapse. *Curr. Opin. Immunol.* **14:**293–298.

Yasutomo, K. 2002. The cellular and molecular mechanism of CD4/CD8 lineage commitment. *J. Med. Invest.* **49:**1–6.

chapter 15

Cellular Communication

Arthur O. Tzianabos and Lee M. Wetzler

Interaction of Cells of the Immune System

Many immune mechanisms depend on the interactions among the cellular components comprising the immune system. These interactions rely on two specific mechanisms: direct contact between cells and soluble intermediary molecules released by these cells that bind to specific receptors on responding cells (Fig. 15.1). Cellular growth and differentiation ensue, leading to a specific immunologic response. The basic components of the immune system that interact, and therefore must communicate with each other, include antigen-presenting cells (APCs), T cells, and B cells. B cells also function as APCs for certain types of T cells. In addition, the activity of other participatory cells, principally leukocytes including monocytes/ macrophages and the granulocytes, is also influenced by cellular communication. In fact, many cells of the body respond to signals and specific interactions from immune cells, making these cells primary mediators of tissue physiology during the course of an immune response. For example, display of antigenic peptides by major histocompatibility complex (MHC) class I turns a tissue cell into a target cell for destruction by cytotoxic T lymphocytes (CTLs).

APCs display peptide fragments of protein antigen on their cell surface MHC class II molecules to facilitate antigen recognition by helper T (TH) lymphocytes (CD4$^+$ cells) via the surface T-cell receptors (TCR). This *cognate interaction* initiates T-cell activation, which is amplified by further interactions among costimulatory molecules present on both the T-cell and APC surfaces. Once T cells are activated by this interaction, they communicate with other cells by production and secretion of a variety of soluble mediators, known as *cytokines*. Cy-

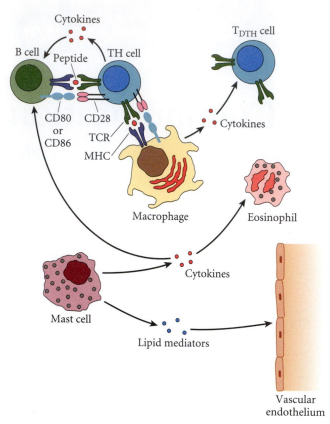

Figure 15.1 Communication between various cells of the immune system relies on both cell contact-dependent signals such as TCR and MHC and CD80 or CD86 and CD28 as well as soluble signals mediated by factors such as cytokines and lipid mediators.

Whereas the MHC-peptide-TCR complex is a critical early step in T-cell activation, APCs must also provide a variety of costimulatory signals to T cells. These costimulatory molecules provide critical signals to the cells as part of their cognate interaction with specific receptors. T-cell activation following engagement of the TCR with antigen-MHC follows a path dictated, in part, by the spectrum of cytokines and costimulatory molecules produced by the APC for the T cell. In some cases the T cells will develop into either a TH1 or TH2 subtype, secreting a specific spectrum of cytokines that either activate other T cells for a cell-mediated or cytotoxic response or help B cells to differentiate into dedicated antibody-secreting plasma cells. Overall, both membrane molecules and soluble cytokines that bind to receptors mediate the cell-to-cell communication critical for initiating and maintaining an immune response.

Mechanisms of Communication

Cell-to-cell contact

One of the major mechanisms by which cells of the immune system communicate with one another is through direct contact with other cells. This can result in the activation of the appropriate cell types, precipitating an immune response directed toward the insulting antigen. Myriad cell surface adhesion molecules and ligands are involved in controlling these cell-cell interactions. These accessory molecules, usually present on the surface of APCs, T cells, and B cells, function together to promote and stabilize cell-cell interactions that then augment the activation of the target cell. Among the cell surface accessory molecules that have been well described for T-cell activation are CD3, CD4, and CD8 present on mature TH cells and CTLs; CD40, which is often found on B cells and dendritic cells, and its ligand CD40L, found on T cells;

tokines have wide-ranging biologic functions, particularly on the immune response. Among the most critical of the T-cell activation events is the production of interleukin-2 (IL-2), a T-cell growth factor that stimulates proliferation of T cells that produce receptors for this cytokine (Fig. 15.2).

Figure 15.2 The cytokine IL-2 provides a crucial soluble signal during the activation of a T cell. (**A**) A naive T cell is presented with cognate antigen peptide complexed to self MHC and also receives sufficient costimulation via CD80 (or CD86)-CD28 interactions. This is sufficient to begin the process of T-cell activation but is not sufficient to cause the T cell to enter the cell cycle. (**B**) The partially activated T cell produces both IL-2 and a high-affinity receptor for IL-2. (**C**) Binding of IL-2 by the same cell that synthesized it (termed autocrine activity) provides the T cell with the final signal it needs to begin proliferating.

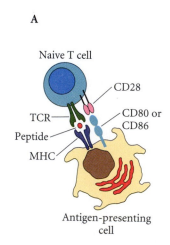

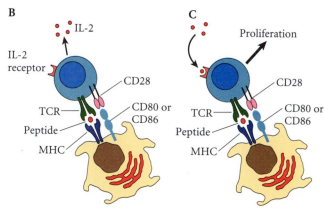

and B7-1 (CD80) and B7-2 (CD86) on APCs that bind to CD28 and CTL antigen 4 (CTLA-4, or CD152) on TH cells. CD28 transduces a stimulatory signal to T cells that is required for costimulation of T cells upon interaction of MHC with the TCR. Conversely, CTLA-4 transduces an inhibitory signal that is necessary for control of T-cell responses. Mice that lack CTLA-4 have hyperactive immune systems and usually die within 4 to 6 weeks as a result of overwhelming lymphocyte infiltration into major organs.

Additional cell surface structures potentiate binding of APCs to T cells and stabilize the interaction, including LFA-1 (lymphocyte function-associated antigen 1, or CD11a/CD18) and CD2 on the surface of T cells and their respective ligands on APCs, ICAM-1 (intercellular adhesion molecule 1, or CD54), and LFA-3 (CD58). The area of interaction between the APC and the T cell, where ligands and antigen-loaded MHC interact, is termed the *immune synapse* (see Fig. 14.20). Cell-cell contact in the synapse includes interactions by adhesion molecules and their receptors such as ICAM-1 and LFA-1, MHC-TCR and CD4 or CD8, CD40-CD40L, and CD28-CD80 and CD86. Many of these interactions, such as ICAM-1–LFA-1, stabilize the cell-cell interaction. The geography of the synapse is not fully defined; although initial studies suggested that the TCR-MHC pairing occurred in the center and the other adhesion and costimulatory molecules were found in the surrounding periphery (see Fig. 14.20), some recent studies question this model and suggest that the initial interaction in the periphery is between MHC and TCR and that, by the time the full immune synapse forms, this interaction is replaced by the binding of the costimulatory molecules to their cognate receptor. Cell-to-cell interactions also are involved in other cell adhesion-dependent host responses, including leukocyte and lymphocyte trafficking toward sites of tissue damage during their extravasation from endothelial venules.

T-cell signaling events initiated by cell-cell contact

The early events in signal transduction leading to T-cell activation and cytokine production can be categorized into two major activation pathways: (i) hydrolysis of plasma membrane inositol phospholipids and (ii) phosphorylation of membrane and cytoplasmic proteins. Following binding of the TCR, phospholipase C catalyzes the hydrolysis of phosphatidylinositol 4,5-bisphosphate, a membrane phospholipid (see Fig. 14.22A), creating a rapid rise in intracellular calcium levels, which in turn activates protein kinase C (see Fig. 14.22B). Phosphorylation of different membrane-bound and cytoplasmic DNA-binding proteins is thought to allow their release from a complex

and allow for transcriptional activation of genes necessary for T-cell activation and cytokine secretion.

B-cell signaling events initiated by cell-cell contact

Binding of antigen to membrane-bound immunoglobulin (usually IgM or IgD) on B cells activates a cascade of biochemical events within the cell. Paramount in this response are the increased levels of expression of membrane molecules that can mediate cell-to-cell contact with T cells. This contact with TH cells provides signals needed for B-cell activation. The major molecules involved in forming the T-cell–B-cell cognate interactions include antigen-bearing MHC class II molecules on the B cell and the TCR on the T cell, ICAM-1 on the B cell and LFA-1 on the T cell, CD40 on the B cell and CD40L on the T cell, and CD80-CD86 (B7-1 and B7-2) on the B cell and CD28–CTLA-4 on the T cell. A new set of costimulatory molecules, inducible costimulator (ICOS) on T cells and ICOS ligand on B cells, have been found to be important for immunoglobulin isotype switching. Mice that lack ICOS are no longer able to switch immunoglobulin isotypes from IgM upon antigen stimulation. Similarly, CD40-CD40L interactions are also important for isotype switching. The expression of many of these cell surface molecules on both the T cell and B cell is increased following engagement of the TCR by antigen plus MHC. A model for the sequential expression of these cell surface molecules is shown in Fig. 15-3.

Structure and Function of Mediators of Cell-to-Cell Contact

Accessory molecules that mediate cell-to-cell adhesion

The accessory molecules LFA-1 (CD11a/CD18), which binds to ICAM-1, and CD2 (LFA-2), which binds to LFA-3, promote cell-to-cell adhesion and are involved in both lymphocyte trafficking and signal transduction (Fig. 15.4). The mechanism of CD2-mediated signaling is not clear but has been postulated to be due to CD2-induced aggregation of lipid rafts on the T-cell membrane. Both CD2 and LFA-3 are members of the immunoglobulin superfamily of molecules, having two immunoglobulin-like extracellular constant-region domains. LFA-1 is an adhesion molecule that is a member of the integrin family, expressed primarily on leukocytes, and when bound to its specific ligand, ICAM-1, stabilizes antigen-specific T-cell activation. Recent experiments have demonstrated that ligation of LFA-1 causes an increase in the transcription of the IL-2 gene. This interaction has also been implicated in T- and B-cell responses, antibody-dependent cytotoxicity,

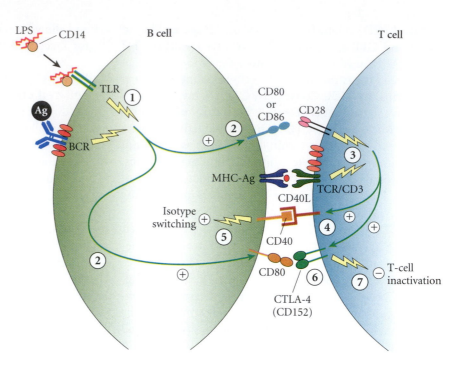

Figure 15.3 T-cell–B-cell interactions involve the increased expression of many counterreceptors by both cells. (1) Activation of B cell begins with either binding of antigen (Ag) by the B-cell antigen receptor (BCR) or binding of a ligand such as bacterial LPS by a pattern-recognition receptor such as a TLR and CD14. (2) These early activation events result in increased expression of CD80 and CD86 by the B cell. (3) Initial activation of the T cell requires both antigen-MHC recognition by the TCR and costimulation such as CD28 binding to CD86. (4) Early T-cell activation results in increased expression of CD40L. (5) CD40L binding to CD40 is an essential signal to stimulate isotype switching in the B cell. (6) Later in T-cell activation, the T cell increases its production of CTLA-4. (7) CTLA-4 binds to CD80 on the B cell, inactivating the T cell and returning the immune system to a quiescent state.

and leukocyte binding of endothelial cells. ICAM-1 is also a member of the immunoglobulin superfamily, has a molecular mass of 80 to 114 kilodaltons (kDa), and is found on a number of cell types. It has recently been shown that expression of LFA-1–ICAM-1 is potentiated by cytokines such as interferon-gamma (IFN-γ), IL-1, tumor necrosis factor (TNF), and IL-8 and is important in regulating inflammatory responses. The binding of LFA-1 on leukocytes to ICAM-1 on endothelial cells lining blood vessels also facilitates rapid extravasation of leukocytes toward inflammatory sites.

Another important member of the integrin family is the VLA-4 (very late activation 4 or CD49d) molecule, which is expressed on a broad spectrum of trafficking immune cells, including T cells, monocytes, and dendritic cells, and acts as a potent cell adhesion structure. VLA-4 expression is increased in response to T-cell activation and is induced by inflammatory mediators. The ligand for this structure is termed VCAM-1 (vascular cell adhesion molecule 1 or CD106) and is a member of the immunoglobulin superfamily. The VLA-4–VCAM-1 interaction has many functions similar to those of the LFA-1–ICAM-1 interaction involved in T-cell activation, T-cell-mediated killing, and lymphocyte extravasation during inflammation. A number of other VLA molecules have also been identified and include VLA-1 through VLA-6 (CD49a through CD49f), due to variations in the VLA α chain.

Figure 15.4 Cell-cell interactions are promoted by several families of cell-adhesion molecules (CAMs). Glycoprotein CAMs called *mucins* are recognized by carbohydrate-binding CAMs that belong to the selectin family. CAMs of the *integrin* family possess a high-affinity binding site for CAMs of the *immunoglobulin superfamily*.

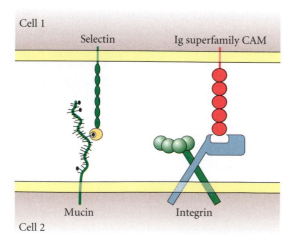

The T-cell coreceptors

The CD4 and CD4 T-cell coreceptors (see Fig. 13.18) stabilize MHC-TCR interactions occurring on the extracellular face of the plasma membrane and are signaling molecules that act on the intracellular face of the plasma membrane. CD4 and CD8 interact with phosphorylating enzymes that control cell growth and function (see Fig. 14.21). Knockout mice that do not express CD4 or CD8 nonetheless develop normal numbers of T cells, and the TCRs can still be restricted to recognizing antigen in the context of MHC class I or II even in the absence of CD4 or CD8 coreceptors. The major role for these coreceptors appears to be to increase the strength of the binding of T cells to antigens presented by MHC molecules.

CD4 is a transmembrane glycoprotein composed of a single polypeptide chain with a molecular mass of about 55 kDa and four extracellular immunoglobulin-like domains, making it a member of the immunoglobulin superfamily of molecules. The cytoplasmic tail contains three serine residues that can be phosphorylated by protein kinases, indicating the site for signal transduction in this molecule. CD4 binds to the β_2 domain of the MHC class II molecule on the APC, and on the T cell, is closely associated with the TCR, although not covalently linked to it. Likely, a complex containing two or more molecules of the TCR, CD3, and CD4 or CD8 is needed for efficient activation of a T cell by an APC.

CD8 is a disulfide-linked molecule composed of two polypeptides, termed CD8-α and CD8-β. The $\alpha\beta$ heterodimer is found on T cells originating in the thymus and seeding the major secondary lymphoid organs such as the spleen and lymph nodes. However, T cells found within the epithelium of the intestinal tract, known as intraepithelial lymphocytes (IELs), are mostly CD8$^+$ cells, wherein the CD8 molecule is composed of two α chains (an α/α homodimer). Each of the CD8 chains is composed of a singular extracellular immunoglobulin-like domain, a transmembrane region, and a modest-sized cytoplasmic tail with potential phosphorylation sites. Mice in which the α chain of CD8 is disrupted by homologous recombination have defective maturation of cytotoxic cells in the thymus but a normal number of IELs. However, these IELs express neither CD4 nor CD8 but express TCRs. In normal animals the CD8 α^+/α^+ cells may mature not in the thymus but in other tissues, such as the intestinal epithelium.

Selectins in cell-cell interactions

Signaling involving cell-cell contact does not function just in the context of lymphocyte activation but also in the context of lymphocyte interactions with the vascular endothelium that brings cells to sites of inflammation. Much of this lymphocyte-endothelial interaction is mediated by the selectin family of adhesion molecules (Fig. 15.4). This family of proteins was identified relatively recently with monoclonal antibodies generated to cytokine-activated endothelial cells. At present, this family comprises three proteins, termed *E-selectin*, *P-selectin*, and *L-selectin*. All three molecules have been determined to regulate leukocyte binding to endothelium at sites of inflammation. Each is composed of a single chain of amino acids with an N-

terminal lectin-like binding domain, followed by a series of short consensus repeat motifs, each of 62 amino acids. Each selectin has specific carbohydrate ligands to which it binds. E-selectin (also known as ELAM-1 or CD62E) is expressed by activated endothelial cells shortly after activation of these cells by inflammatory cytokines such as IL-1 and TNF. Maximal expression occurs 4 to 6 hours after activation and declines 24 to 48 hours later. Therefore, this cell adhesion molecule appears to be critical in initial stages of the inflammatory response and mediates binding to neutrophils, monocytes, and some T cells.

P-selectin (termed CD62P) is a 140-kDa protein that is stored in resting platelets and endothelial cells. This molecule is expressed in response to mediators of the clotting cascade and functions to regulate adhesion of neutrophils and monocytes. L-selectin (CD62L) was the first selectin to be identified and is found on circulating lymphocytes, monocytes, and neutrophils. This cell adhesion molecule also is involved in extravasation of neutrophils and lymphocytes from blood vessels into the surrounding tissue during an inflammatory response. However, L-selectin is constitutively expressed on cell surfaces and is shed shortly after cellular activation. This process is thought to regulate detachment of immune cells from endothelial tissue.

Soluble Mediators of Communication: Cytokines and Chemokines

Biologic Properties of Cytokines

The initial interactions between APCs, T cells, and B cells result in the production of different soluble molecules known as cytokines. These molecules regulate communication between different cells of the immune system. Cytokines are secreted from activated immune cells and have a number of different biologic functions in both humoral and cell-mediated immune responses. During their initial characterization many cytokines were referred to as *lymphokines* if they were produced by lymphocytes or as *monokines* if they were produced by monocytes. However, further work showed that production of most cytokines is not limited to a specific cell type. The terms lymphokine and monokine have therefore fallen out of usage. Many of the cytokines are designated as *interleukins*, a term used to indicate an interaction among leukocytes. The IL designation has been conserved to classify some of the cytokines. Other types of cytokines are in a class known as *chemokines*, generally small molecules that provide signals for cell migration and chemotaxis. The evolving nature of this classification system is shown by the initial designation of one chemokine as IL-8 even though IL-8 does not have properties typical of other interleukins. Naming of new interleukins is under the auspices of an international committee that establishes criteria for certification of a molecule as an interleukin and assigns official designations.

Cytokines are small-molecular-weight molecules possessing some common properties.

1. They have a brief and limited half-life and are not stored in a preformed state but are synthesized and released upon cellular activation.
2. They are produced by a variety of immune cells and have different biologic activities when bound to different cell types (Fig. 15.5A), a phenomenon known as *pleiotropism.*
3. Their biologic functions can be *redundant*, meaning that two different cytokines have comparable effects on target cells (Fig. 15.5B).
4. Many cytokines induce or inhibit the production of other cytokines (Fig. 15.5C), leading to complex *regulatory networks* that modulate the biologic effects of cytokines.
5. They can act to influence the activities of other cytokines, exerting either *antagonistic* or *synergistic* effects.
6. They exert their effects by binding to specific *receptors* on the cellular surface. They may act on the same cell from which they were secreted (*autocrine* activity) or on a proximal cell type (*paracrine* activity). Generally, cytokines work only in the vicinity in which they are secreted, although some, such as IL-1 and TNF-α, will circulate in the blood and exert a systemic or *endocrine* effect (Fig. 15.6).
7. The cellular response of cells to cytokines usually occurs over a period of hours, requiring de novo production of mRNA and protein.

The roles played by these molecules in cellular communication are essential to the immune response.

Cytokines display myriad biologic properties, ultimately coordinating the innate and acquired arms of the immune response. Almost every aspect of cellular communication and interaction in the immune system is modulated in some way by these molecules. A critical aspect of cytokines is their ability to regulate different aspects of host defense. These compounds mediate both nonspecific inflammatory and specific adaptive immune responses. Cytokines are produced by a number of different cell types including monocytes, macrophages, dendritic cells, B cells, and T cells. In some cases these cells produce a panel of cytokines that is characteristic of a particular type of cell, but many cells often can produce the same cytokine. Cytokines amplify or inhibit already existing biologic functions.

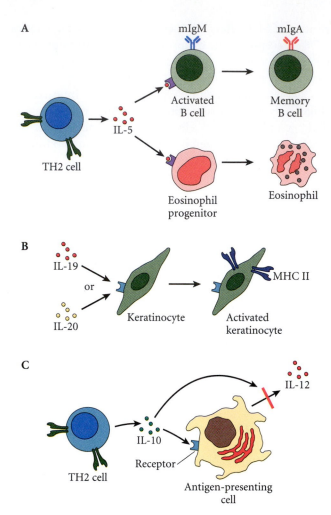

Figure 15.5 Cytokine action is characterized by several qualities. **(A)** Pleiotropism is the ability of one cytokine (for example, IL-5) to affect different target cells, causing different effects in each target cell type. **(B)** Redundancy is the ability of two different cytokines to cause the same effect on the same target cell. In the example shown, IL-19 and IL-20 can cause the same inflammatory responses in keratinocytes because the two cytokines bind to the identical receptor. **(C)** Antagonism is the ability of one cytokine to inhibit the action of another. In the example shown, IL-10 inhibits the action of IL-12 by preventing IL-12 from being synthesized.

The study of cytokines is complicated by the properties noted above: pleiotropism, redundancy, regulation of production of other cytokines, synergy, and antagonism. For example, IL-1 is involved in T-cell activation, hepatocyte production of innate immune mediators such as the acute-phase proteins, and elevation of body temperature due to binding to receptors in the hippocampus, which houses the body's thermostat. IL-4 can affect the growth of T cells, B cells, and mast cells. Redundancy is another complicating property of cytokines; like IL-1, tumor TNF-α can also elevate body temperature through actions in the hippocampus, and IL-6 can stimulate production of

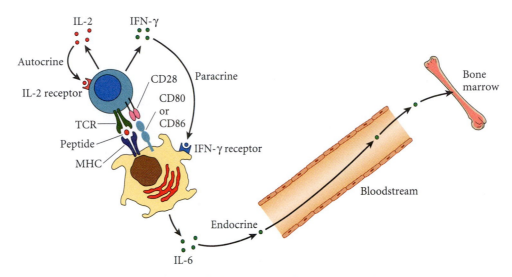

Figure 15.6 Cytokines can act on target cells that are proximal or distant from their point of synthesis. Some cytokines exhibit autocrine activity, meaning that the cytokine exerts an effect on the same cell that synthesizes it. The example shown is IL-2, which is an autocrine growth factor on T cells because the same T cell synthesizes both the cytokine and the cytokine receptor. Cytokines can also act on target cells that are different from the cell that synthesized the cytokine but are still near the cytokine-producing cell. This is termed paracrine activity. Last, cytokines can act on target cells that are distant from their site of synthesis. In the example shown, IL-6 produced by macrophages at the site of a localized infection can enter the bloodstream and act on hematopoietic stem cells in the bone marrow, triggering increased generation of some white blood cell types.

acute-phase proteins. B cells proliferate in response to IL-2, IL-4, and IL-5. Many cytokines initiate very similar responses in cells: IL-2 and IL-15 both promote T-cell proliferation; IL-4, IL-10, and IL-13 all inhibit release of inflammatory cytokines; and IL-12 and IL-18 are both promoters of IFN-γ production.

The fact that most cytokines are neither produced nor act in isolation but function as part of a complex network in which they are both regulators of the production of other cytokines and effectors of biologic activity makes their study enormously challenging. IL-7 increases expression of IL-2 and the IL-2 receptor; transforming growth factor beta increases IL-1 expression. Examination of what is actually occurring in a tissue during cytokine production will be dependent on the activity and function of the regulatory network as much as it will be dependent on the function of specific cytokines. Thus, a change in a tissue or cellular reaction due to elimination or inhibition of a cytokine may not reflect a specific activity of the cytokine but rather the loss of its participation in the normal regulatory network that coordinates and calibrates the overall cytokine expression pattern.

Acting in synergy is another property commonly found among cytokines. To switch to production of IgE, B cells need to be exposed to both IL-4 and IL-5. IL-2 and IL-12 act together to produce CTL responses. Acting antagonistically is another key feature of cytokines used to regulate immune responses. IL-10 production by TH2 cells suppresses the activation of TH1 cells; this is also done in concert with IL-4. IL-10 also counteracts the activity of IL-17, a cytokine that maintains inflammation. The balance of cytokine activities obviously underlies the initiation, maintenance, and ultimately resolution of immune and inflammatory responses. Studying their activities in an in vivo setting can be daunting, since the progression of an immune response through its various stages results not in a production of cytokines one at a time in an orderly fashion but as complex mixtures that may be mediating their effects on different cells at various stages of activation within an inflammatory lesion.

Identification of Cytokines

Almost all cytokines are initially identified on the basis of a biologic activity such as effects on lymphocytes, inflammation, and so forth. Some of these cytokines, such as TNF-α, retain their original designations referring to the initial biologic activity discovered. Although TNF-α can mediate necrosis of tumors, it also interferes with lipid metabolism, resulting in weight loss, which led another group to identify this molecule under a different set of conditions and name it cachectin (*cachexia* is the term used to denote weight loss that typically accompanies certain viral infections). IL-2 was originally called T-cell growth factor.

A

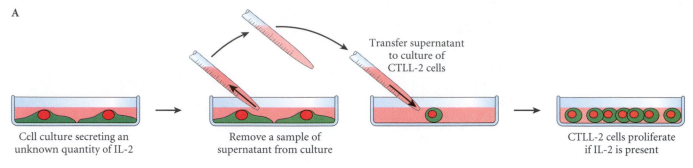

Cell culture secreting an
unknown quantity of IL-2

Remove a sample of
supernatant from culture

Transfer supernatant
to culture of
CTLL-2 cells

CTLL-2 cells proliferate
if IL-2 is present

B

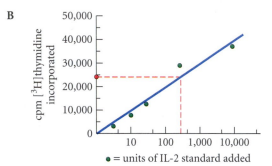

● = units of IL-2 standard added

Figure 15.7 Cytokines can be detected through bioassays that utilize cytokine-responsive indicator cells. CTLL-2 is a cell line that proliferates in response to IL-2. (**A**) If cell culture supernatant containing an unknown quantity of IL-2 is added to a vessel containing CTLL-2 cells, the CTLL-2 cells will proliferate according to how much IL-2 is present in the unknown supernatant. CTLL-2 cell proliferation can be quantitated by carrying out the experiment in the presence of radiolabeled nucleotides (typically [³H]thymidine); in this case, the amount of CTLL-2 cell proliferation will be directly proportional to the amount of radioactivity incorporated into their DNA. (**B**) A sample experiment. A standard curve is generated by culturing CTLL-2 cells in [³H]thymidine as well as known quantities of IL-2 (green data points). The amount of IL-2 in the unknown sample (red data point) is then compared to the standard curve. In the sample experiment, the unknown sample caused CTLL-2 proliferation consistent with approximately 300 units of IL-2. Quantities of some cytokines such as IL-2 are routinely expressed in *units*, since they are so unstable that expressions of mass (such as nanograms) are impractical or misleading.

The rapidly expanding understanding of the roles played by cytokines in inflammatory and other immune responses has required the development of new techniques to identify and characterize these molecules. A number of techniques have been used to detect cytokines, both in vitro and in vivo, and have been helpful in ascribing biologic properties to these peptides. The most widely used technology in identifying cytokines has been the enzyme-linked immunosorbent assay, a technique that uses a specific antibody (in most cases, a monoclonal antibody) that recognizes the cytokine in question (see Fig. 9.12). This type of assay yields information about the type and quantity of cytokine present. Similar assays based on antibody technology, such as the radioimmunoassay, have also been developed to detect cytokines.

Further characterization of cytokines usually requires the use of a biologic assay specific for the cytokine in question. These bioassays are commonly used to identify cytokines and often serve to confirm results obtained from enzyme-linked immunosorbent assays performed in a preliminary identification step. Bioassays take advantage of particular biologic properties associated with the cytokine in question. As an example, the standard bioassay for IL-2 involves the use of the eukaryotic cell line CTLL-2, which proliferates in the presence of IL-2. This line was originally derived from murine spleen cells that had been stimulated by allogeneic cells, followed by propagation with crude T-cell supernatants, making the cell line dependent on exogenous growth factors. A dose-response curve, using recombinant IL-2, was then generated, plotting cell growth (usually measured by the uptake of tritiated thymidine) versus quantity of recombinant IL-2 present. With this bioassay, unknown samples can then be tested and compared with the standard curve to ascertain the presence and quantity of IL-2 in the unknown sample (Fig. 15.7). This type of bioassay is currently available for many of the cytokines identified thus far.

A novel technique has recently been developed that applies molecular biologic techniques to identify and quantitate cytokines. This technique relies on the polymerase chain reaction (PCR) and in situ hybridization technology to identify and quantitate the presence of known cytokines. In addition, PCR has been used to identify novel cytokines. This technique involves the isolation of mRNA from cells that have been activated in some manner to produce the cytokine in question. Once the mRNA has been obtained in pure form, complementary DNA (cDNA) can be derived from the mRNA transcript, using the enzyme reverse transcriptase. The cDNA is then amplified using DNA primers specific for a particular sequence of the cDNA known to encode for the cytokine (Fig. 15.8). Amplified cDNA prepared in this way can also be used for hybridization studies in which these PCR products are used as probes for putative cytokine genes. This technology can also be used to identify novel cytokines, as has been done with the recently discovered IL-13.

Chemokines

Chemokines are a large family of structurally related chemoattractant proteins 8 to 10 kDa in size. They serve as soluble mediators of inflammation and cellular communication and are derived from a variety of cells, with platelets, lymphocytes, activated monocytes/macrophages, and granulocytes being among the prime producers of chemokines. One of the most important functions of chemokines is to induce and regulate leukocyte movements during inflammation as well as during normal trafficking of cells into and out of lymphoid tissues. Chemokines work by affecting the movement of cells along chemotactic gradients, the production of adhesion molecules, and the activation of cellular functions. Chemokines may also have important functions outside the immune system, such as in tissue development.

Chemokines can be divided into four groups based on the arrangement of cysteine residues comprising each chemokine: the C family, the CC family, the CXC family, and the CX_3C family (Fig. 15.9). These molecules are very potent and fast-acting. They change the shape of cells quickly, initiate movement of adhesion molecules to plasma membranes, and induce the production of antimicrobial factors such as toxic oxygen intermediates in phagocytic cells. Since chemokines control inflammatory responses, they also initiate release of granule contents from granulocytes, including proteases, histamine, and toxic proteins.

Chemokine Receptors

There are a large number of chemokines (50 or more). To facilitate cellular changes they must bind to receptors, which are also classified according to the sequence of cysteines in the chemokines. Hence there are C-C and C-X-C chemokine receptors. All chemokine receptors discovered to date are from a family of molecules having a heptahelical structure due to seven domains that span the membrane. On the cytoplasmic side of the receptor are heterotrimeric G proteins, composed of α, β, and γ subunits that are also referred to as large G proteins to distinguish them from small G proteins such as Ras and Rac (see Fig. 14.23). Thus, chemokine receptors are part of the *G-protein-coupled receptor* family, a huge family of cell surface molecules that mediate signal transmission. It has been estimated that over 1% of the entire human genome encodes G-protein-coupled receptors. When the receptor engages the chemokines, the α subunit of the heterotrimeric G protein exchanges GDP for GTP, which results in the dissociation of the G protein into the α and βγ subunits that will lead to signal transmission (Fig. 15.10). A large range of signals are transmitted to the cell, including activation of adenyl and guanyl cyclases and activation of phospholipases and phosphoinositide 3-kinases. These then affect the production of a range of second messengers such as cyclic nucleotides (cAMP and cGMP), phospholipid breakdown products [diacylglycerol, inositol (1,4,5)-trisphosphate, and phosphatidyl inositol (3,4,5)-trisphosphate], arachidonic acid, and phosphatidic acid and also affect intracellular calcium levels.

Most chemokine receptors bind to a number of different chemokines (Table 15.1). Thus, as with cytokines, there is a large degree of complexity associated with chemokine production and regulation of cellular responses due to redundancy, synergism, antagonism, etc. Part of the ability of a cell to respond to a given chemokine lies in the pattern of receptors expressed by the cell. The division of $CD4^+$ T cells into the TH1 and TH2 populations is based on the profile of cytokines produced by the cell. They can also be distinguished on the basis of expression of chemokine receptors. Granulocytes are major participants in inflammation, and different types of these cells express specific patterns of chemokine receptors to mediate the appropriate response during inflammation. Chemokine receptors are now known to play a major role in the pathogenesis of human immunodeficiency virus (HIV) infection leading to AIDS. CXCR4 serves as a coreceptor for viral entry into T cells, and CCR5 serves as a coreceptor for entry into macrophages. Since most HIV infections are initiated by macrophage-tropic strains of virus, people who are genetically deficient in CCR5 are resistant to HIV infection.

Cytokine Receptors and Receptor Signaling

As for the chemokines, the biologic activity of most cytokines is mediated through binding to high-affinity cell surface receptors on target cells. Much of the control of cytokine activity within a certain cell population is achieved by expression of different cytokine receptors on different cells. Three structural domains are necessary for full biologic activity of a cytokine receptor. These functional domains consist of (i) a recognition domain that protrudes from the cell surface and is involved in specific binding of the cytokine, (ii) a hydrophobic transmembrane domain that anchors the receptor to the cell, and (iii) an intracellular signaling domain that uses an enzyme involved in the phosphorylation or dephosphorylation of intracellular proteins. These domains are all required for functional activity of the receptor and may be contained within a single protein or may require the formation of a complex comprising several proteins. Cytokine receptors share structural homologies and can

A

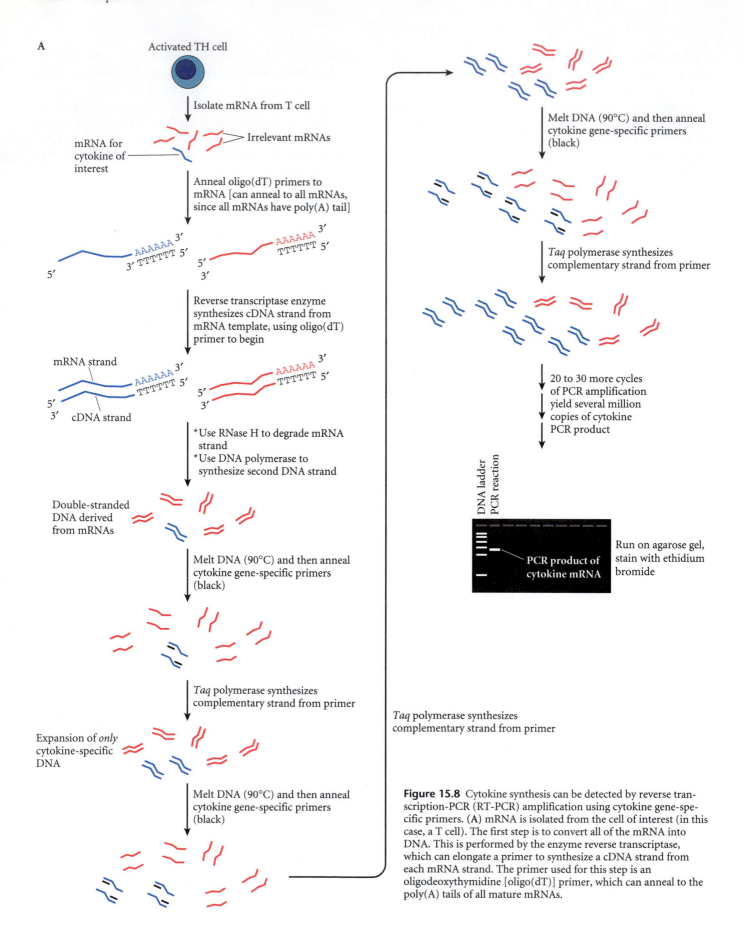

Activated TH cell

Isolate mRNA from T cell

mRNA for cytokine of interest

Irrelevant mRNAs

Anneal oligo(dT) primers to mRNA [can anneal to all mRNAs, since all mRNAs have poly(A) tail]

Reverse transcriptase enzyme synthesizes cDNA strand from mRNA template, using oligo(dT) primer to begin

mRNA strand

cDNA strand

*Use RNase H to degrade mRNA strand
*Use DNA polymerase to synthesize second DNA strand

Double-stranded DNA derived from mRNAs

Melt DNA (90°C) and then anneal cytokine gene-specific primers (black)

Taq polymerase synthesizes complementary strand from primer

Expansion of *only* cytokine-specific DNA

Melt DNA (90°C) and then anneal cytokine gene-specific primers (black)

Melt DNA (90°C) and then anneal cytokine gene-specific primers (black)

Taq polymerase synthesizes complementary strand from primer

20 to 30 more cycles of PCR amplification yield several million copies of cytokine PCR product

DNA ladder
PCR reaction

PCR product of cytokine mRNA

Run on agarose gel, stain with ethidium bromide

Taq polymerase synthesizes complementary strand from primer

Figure 15.8 Cytokine synthesis can be detected by reverse transcription-PCR (RT-PCR) amplification using cytokine gene-specific primers. (**A**) mRNA is isolated from the cell of interest (in this case, a T cell). The first step is to convert all of the mRNA into DNA. This is performed by the enzyme reverse transcriptase, which can elongate a primer to synthesize a cDNA strand from each mRNA strand. The primer used for this step is an oligodeoxythymidine [oligo(dT)] primer, which can anneal to the poly(A) tails of all mature mRNAs.

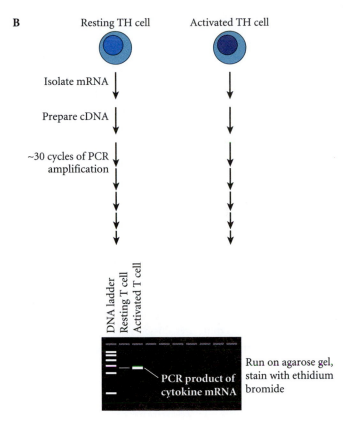

B

Resting TH cell   Activated TH cell

Isolate mRNA

Prepare cDNA

~30 cycles of PCR amplification

DNA ladder
Resting T cell
Activated T cell

PCR product of cytokine mRNA

Run on agarose gel, stain with ethidium bromide

Figure 15.8 *(continued)* These steps are depicted at a higher magnification to emphasize annealing of the oligo(dT) to the poly(A) tails. Reverse transcription yields an RNA-DNA heteroduplex. The RNA strand of this heteroduplex is then degraded by the enzyme RNase H and is replaced with a second DNA strand using a DNA polymerase. Cytokine gene mRNA (blue) is then selectively amplified by PCR using primers (short black lines) that specifically anneal to cytokine gene sequences. Each cycle of PCR amplification consists of "melting" the DNA duplexes, allowing the cytokine gene-specific primers to anneal, and then using *Taq* polymerase to synthesize a complementary DNA strand from the cytokine-specific primer. This results in an exponential amplification of only the cDNA derived from cytokine mRNA. After 20 to 30 cycles of amplification, there is a sufficient amount of cytokine PCR product to detect on an ethidium bromide-stained agarose gel. (**B**) This type of experiment can be used to measure changes in cytokine gene expression. In the example shown, the RT-PCR experiment is performed on mRNA isolated from resting or activated T cells. Analysis of the RT-PCR products from these two samples shows that the activated T cells contain more cytokine mRNA than the resting cells.

Figure 15.9 Structural motifs of the four families of chemokines. The C family, CC family, and CXC family are soluble proteins with conserved cysteine residues (C) at the indicated locations. X indicates the presence of any other amino acid that intervenes between the conserved cysteines. The CX_3C family thus far contains only one member: fractalkine. Fractalkine is a transmembrane protein comprising a membrane-distal domain that contains a structural motif similar to that of chemokines of other families. This domain is followed by a stalk region, and then the transmembrane (TM) and cytoplasmic regions. Modified from S. G. Ward and J. Westwick, *Biochem. J.* **333**(Part 3):457–470, 1998, with permission.

Family	Example(s)	Structural motif
CC family	MIP, MCP, I309, ELC, TECK	C C C C
CXC family	IL-8, Gro, SDF-1, NAP-2, γIP-10	CXC C C
C family	Lymphotactin	C C
CX_3C family	Fractalkine	CXXXC C C Extracellular stalk TM Cytoplasmic

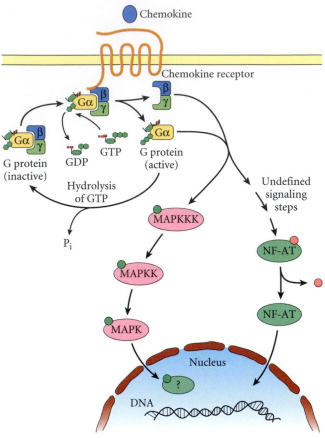

Figure 15.10 Signaling through chemokine receptors utilizes heterotrimeric G proteins. The G protein exists in an inactive state in the cytoplasm, bound to GDP. Chemokine binding allows the chemokine receptor to bind the G protein and function as a guanosine exchange factor, causing the G protein to release the GDP and bind GTP. This activates the G protein. The active subunits of the G protein (Gα-GTP and G$\beta\gamma$) initiate multiple signaling pathways that are still undefined but are known to include the mitogen-activated protein kinase (MAPK) pathway and the transcriptional activator NF-AT (nuclear factor of activated T cells). After signal transduction is complete, the Gα subunit cleaves its bound GTP to GDP, allowing the Gα subunit to reassociate with the G$\beta\gamma$ subunit and inactivate the G protein.

bind different cytokines, usually with different affinities, which accounts for much of the redundant function for these molecules.

Cytokine receptor families

Cytokine receptors are characterized as families of receptors generally on the basis of their structural composition and are usually designated by placing the letter R for receptor after the name of the cytokine to which the receptor binds (i.e., the IL-2 receptor is referred to as IL-2R). The type I cytokine receptor family recognizes a large number of cytokines, including IL-2, IL-3, IL-4, IL-5, IL-6, IL-7, IL-9, IL-11, IL-15, and granulocyte-macrophage

colony-stimulating factor (GM-CSF). These receptors have four conserved cysteine residues in the membrane-distal extracellular domain region, as well as a tryptophan-serine-X-tryptophan-serine (WSXWS) motif within the first 50 amino acids of the membrane proximal domain. This is referred to as the cytokine receptor homology (CRH) domain. The ligands of type I receptors all have a conserved structure consisting of four α-helices. On the intracellular side of these receptors there is more divergence. Since the type I cytokine receptors bind the class of cytokines known as hematopoietin, they are known as the hematopoietin receptors.

Type I cytokine receptors are generally composed of two or three polypeptides. One or two of these contribute to specificity of cytokine binding, while the other one functions as the signal transduction unit. Since many of the type I cytokine receptors share the same signal transduction unit, they will elicit similar cellular responses upon binding of their cognate cytokine. This is likely the basis for the redundant function of some cytokines; their receptors share a common signal-transducing unit. Sometimes the recognition portion of the receptor participates in cellular signaling, and the extracellular domains of the signal-transducing subunit can contribute to cytokine binding. All of the hematopoietin receptors become phosphorylated upon binding of their specific cytokines, but they do not themselves have any kinase activity. This is mediated by other cytoplasmic protein kinases.

Table 15.1 Chemokine receptors and their ligand specificity[a]

Receptor	Ligand(s)
C family	
XCR1	Lymphotactin
CC family	
CCR1	MIP-1α, MIP-5, MCP-2, RANTES
CCR2	MCP-1, MCP-2, MCP-3
CCR3	I-309, MIP-5, MCP-2, MCP-3, MCP-4, eotaxin, eotaxin-2, TARC
CCR4	I-309, RANTES, TARC
CCR5	MCP-2, MIP-1α, MIP-1β, RANTES
CCR6	LARC
CCR7	ELC
CCR8	I-309
CCR9	TECK/CCL25
CCR10	MCP-1, MCP-2, MCP-3, RANTES
CXC family	
CXCR1	IL-8, GCP-2
CXCR2	IL-8, Gro-α, Gro-β, Gro-γ, NAP-2, ENA-78
CXCR3	γIP-10, I-TAC
CXCR4	PBSF
CXCR5	BCA-1
CX$_3$C family	
CX3CR1	Fractalkine

[a]Some data taken from R. Thorpe, *J. Immunol. Methods* **262:**1–3, 2002, with permission from Elsevier Science.

Type II receptors are structurally related to type I receptors and recognize IL-10 family members and interferons. Their extracellular domains contain the same conserved CCCC motif as found in type I receptors but lack the WSXWS membrane-proximal motifs of the class I cytokine receptor subfamilies. The type II receptors are usually heterodimers consisting of a cytokine-recognizing α chain and signal-transducing β chain which do not associate together until the cytokine ligand is present.

Subfamilies of the type I cytokine receptors

Among the class I cytokine receptors there are three major signal transduction subunits shared by different receptors: the β subunit, the gp130 subunit, and the common γ-chain (γc) subunit. This has allowed classification of the type I receptors into subfamilies based on the use of shared signal-transducing subunits.

GM-CSF receptor subfamily

Receptors for GM-CSF, IL-3, and IL-5 are in the GM-CSFR subfamily. They share a common signal-transducing unit designated the β subunit (Fig. 15.11). The other chain of each receptor consists of a polypeptide that confers low-affinity binding of the cognate cytokine to the receptor and is often designated the α subunit. When the cytokine-specific α subunit associates noncovalently with the β subunit, the affinity of the receptor for the cytokine is increased. As might be expected, the biologic functions of GM-CSF, IL-3, and IL-5 can overlap and include release of histamine from mast-cell granules and stimulation of eosinophils. This conclusion correlates with the observation that binding of GM-CSF, IL-3, or IL-5 to a receptor induces a comparable pattern of protein changes, including phosphorylation, in cells expressing the receptors.

The sharing of signal transduction units is also responsible for antagonistic effects of cytokines. Since GM-CSF, IL-3, and IL-5 receptors use the same signal-transducing β subunit, any limited availability of this portion of the receptor will limit the ability of a specific cytokine in this group to activate a target cell. Thus, GM-CSF and IL-3 are antagonistic of each other's function due to competition for the β subunit between the two receptors.

IL-6 receptor subfamily

The IL-6R subfamily is characterized by the presence of a signal-transducing subunit referred to as gp130, which can associate with either one or two other proteins to form a receptor for IL-6, IL-11, oncostatin M, leukemia inhibitory factor, ciliary neurotrophic factor, and cardiotrophin-1. All of these cytokines are structurally related, and many have comparable biologic effects. Oncostatin M, leukemia inhibitory factor, ciliary neurotrophic factor, and cardiotrophin-1 all use a low-affinity binding component referred to as gp190, which is characterized by

Figure 15.11 The GM-CSFR subfamily and IL-2R subfamily of the type I cytokine receptor family. Each receptor is a heterodimer or heterotrimer. The gray ovals represent the bound cytokine. Receptor names are listed above each receptor, and subunit names are listed below each subunit. Subunits with signal transduction capacity are indicated by a lightning bolt icon on their cytoplasmic tail. Within each subfamily, all receptors share a common signaling subunit (the β subunit in the GM-CSFR subfamily and the γc subunit in the IL-2R subfamily) but also contain other subunits that are unique to each receptor and confer cytokine specificity on the receptor. In the GM-CSFR subfamily, the receptor-specific subunit (the α subunit) is able to bind the cytokine alone, without the β subunit. However, the α subunit alone only binds the cytokine with low affinity and fails to transduce a signal upon binding. The β subunits of the IL-2R and the IL-15R are identical.

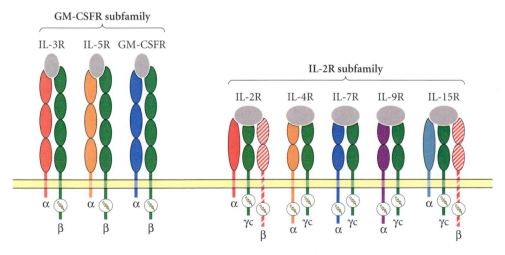

having two of the CRH domains separated by an immunoglobulin-like domain. Between the most membrane-proximal CRH domain and the plasma membrane are three type III fibronectin repeat units, which are found in both the gp130 and gp190 proteins. As with the GM-CSF receptor subfamily, competition for the common gp130 signaling unit underlies antagonistic effects of these cytokines for each other, while the comparable signal transduction emanating from the activated gp130 accounts for the redundancy of the biologic effects of these cytokines. In addition to having effects on immunologic functions such as induction of acute-phase proteins, these cytokines also affect development of cells of the central nervous system and cells of the hematopoietic system.

IL-2 receptor subfamily

The IL-2 subfamily of receptors are bound together by use of a common signal-transducing unit known as the γc. Receptors for IL-2 and IL-15 are made up of three subunits, one of which, the IL-2Rβ subunit, is shared between these two receptors (Fig. 15.11). Again, this similarity likely accounts for the overlapping function of IL-2 and IL-15 in the immune system. The other members of the IL-2R subfamily, IL-7R, IL-9R, and IL-4R, also use the γc for signal transduction but only have a single α-chain protein for recognition of the cytokine. In addition, for some cytokines, another level of complexity arises due to the existence of multiple forms of a receptor. For example, one type of IL-4 receptor consists of IL-4Rα associated with the γc and a second receptor that is composed of IL-4Rα combined with the IL-13Rα, thus explaining the redundancy of function often seen with these two cytokines. The importance of the γc in immune system function was delineated by the finding that mutations in the X-linked gene for this protein result in congenital *X-linked severe combined immunodeficiency*. Similarly, severe immune defects are seen in γc knockout mice, which have significant defects in B, T, and natural killer (NK) cell development. Since IL-7 is so critical for lymphocyte development, the inability to form a functional receptor for IL-7 results in the inability to produce mature lymphocytes.

The IL-2R has been the focus of intense study, and new information on its structure and function continues to accrue. IL-2Rs are found on T cells, B cells, and NK cells. The receptor is a multisubunit molecule, consisting of at least three distinct subunits: the α chain, β chain, and γc. This receptor system is specific to IL-2 and, like other receptors, can be saturated by its ligand. It is clear that both the α subunit and the β subunit participate in cytokine binding and that the β subunit is critical for cellular acti-

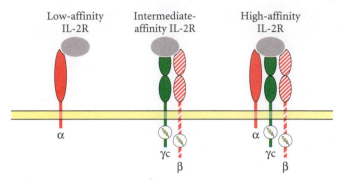

Figure 15.12 The IL-2 receptor exists in three forms, depending on which receptor subunits are expressed by the cell. The α chain alone is a low-affinity receptor. A complex of the β and γc subunits comprises the intermediate-affinity receptor. A complex of all three subunits comprises the high-affinity receptor. Only the intermediate- and high-affinity receptors can transduce signals. The α subunit is not expressed on resting T cells but is expressed on T cells following activation. Therefore, resting T cells express only the intermediate-affinity receptor, whereas activated T cells express the high-affinity and (due to overexpression of the α subunit) low-affinity receptors.

vation by receptor-mediated signaling. Different combinations of the three receptor chains comprise three distinct classes of IL-2Rs. Low-affinity receptors consist of the α subunit alone; intermediate-affinity receptors contain the β and γ subunits; and high-affinity receptors contain all three chains (Fig. 15.12).

Cytokine receptor signaling

Signaling via the type I and II receptors is mediated by binding of the cytokines to the receptor, causing dimerization of the receptor, resulting in the activation of the *Janus kinase* (JAK) family of receptor-associated tyrosine kinases that phosphorylate the *signal transducers and activators of transcription* (STATs) (Fig. 15.13). The JAKs were named after the two-headed Roman god Janus, due to the presence of two symmetrical kinase domains. They associate with the cytoplasmic tails of the cytokine receptors. Activated JAKs phosphorylate tyrosine residues in the cytoplasmic domains of the cytokine receptor molecules, creating Src homology domain 2 docking sites for the STAT proteins that have these domains. Phosphorylated STATs form multimeric complexes, some involving the same proteins (homodimers) and others involving two different proteins (heterodimers). STAT1 is activated via the IFN-γ receptor, and dimers of STAT1 can be further phosphorylated on serine residues to become fully active. The activated STATS are themselves transcription factors that translocate to the nucleus to activate gene transcription. One of the reasons that chemokines exert a very rapid effect on their target cells is the swiftness of the JAK-STAT activation pathway.

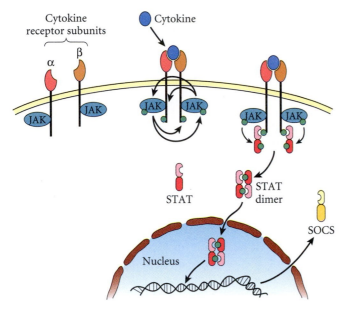

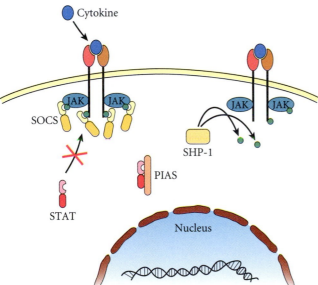

Figure 15.13 Receptors of the hematopoietin family and interferon family signal via the JAKs and STAT family of proteins. (**Top**) Upon binding of the cytokine to the receptor, receptor chains dimerize. JAKs associated with the receptor tails phosphorylate each other and also phosphorylate the cytoplasmic tails of the receptor chains (phosphates are represented as small green circles). The latter event creates docking sites for STAT proteins. STAT proteins docked with the receptor chains are phosphorylated by the JAKs. Phosphorylated STATs are released from the receptor chains and form STAT dimers, which translocate to the nucleus to mediate transcription of activation genes. One gene activated by the STATs is a member of the negative regulator family of proteins SOCS. (**Bottom**) Signaling by these receptors is negatively regulated by several mechanisms. One mechanism is binding of SOCS proteins to phosphorylated JAKs and cytokine receptors, which blocks STAT proteins from associating with the receptors. Secondly, the phosphatase SHP-1 (Src homology domain 2-containing phosphatase) can dephosphorylate the cytokine receptors and JAKs, inactivating the receptor complex. Third, the protein inhibitor of activated STATs (PIAS) can bind and inactivate STAT proteins.

TH1-type cytokine receptors bind and activate STAT4 (i.e., the IL-12R) whereas TH2-type cytokine receptors bind and activate STAT6 (i.e., the IL-4R). STAT4-knockout mice are unable to produce TH1-type T cells, whereas STAT6-knockout mice are unable to produce TH2-type T cells and are defective in IgE production and induction of allergic diseases. Interestingly, STAT4/6-double-knockout mice develop default TH1-type responses. Even though STAT4 and STAT6 are important in developing TH1- versus TH2-type T-cell responses, other transcription factors, such as GATA-3, c-Maf, IRF-1, and T-bet, also are important. There is a family of inhibitors named SOCS (suppressors of cytokine signaling) that can be induced by STATs that will bind to JAK and the cytokine receptors and block cytokine signaling at this point. This is an important mechanism of feedback regulation; SOCS-knockout mice can have severe immune dysfunction and often die from major organ failure due to leukocyte infiltration.

Immunoglobulin superfamily and TNF receptors

The receptor and receptor signaling pathway for IL-1 and IL-18 (type IV receptors) are different from those of the type I and II cytokine receptors, as these receptors are members of the immunoglobulin superfamily. There are two types of IL-1R. Type I IL-1R (IL-1R1) is expressed on almost all cell types and is associated with the IL-1R accessory protein (IL-1RAcP) (Fig. 15.14). IL-1RAcP does not bind IL-1 directly, and therefore the expression of IL-1R1 determines the IL-1 responsiveness of a given cell. The type II IL-1R (IL-1R2) is expressed mainly on B cells, and its main function is to act as a decoy receptor. The IL-18R complex is made up of a heterodimer, IL-18α and IL-18β. The cytoplasmic portions of IL-1R and IL-18R are homologous to the *Drosophila* cell protein Toll and mammalian Toll-like receptors (TLR), pattern-recognition receptors essential for innate immunity (see Fig. 2.8). Signaling through all of these receptors is, therefore, similar. Ligand interaction induces receptor dimerization, which allows binding of the adapter protein MyD88 to the TLR/IL-1R homology domain (TIR on the cytoplasmic portions of these receptors). MyD88 then activates the IL-1R-associated kinase (IRAK), which in turn activates TRAF (TNF receptor-associated factor). TRAF activates nuclear factor κB (NF-κB)-inducing kinase, which then activates inhibitor of κB (IκB) kinase, allowing phosphorylation of IκB, freeing NF-κB, which translocates to the nucleus and induces transcription of a set of genes needed for cell activation.

The TNF family of receptors (TNF-Rs) comprises a large number of receptors with specificity for over 20

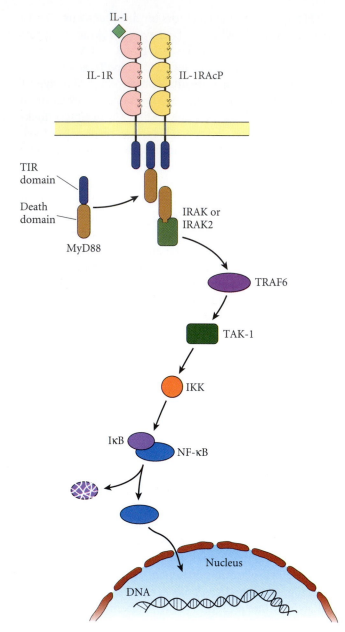

Figure 15.14 The IL-1R belongs to the immunoglobulin superfamily of receptors and transduces signal via a mechanism similar to that used by the TLRs. IL-1RAcP participates in signal transduction but does not participate in ligand binding. Binding of IL-1 to IL-1R and IL-1RAcP causes recruitment of the adapter protein MyD88, which allows IRAK to bind to the receptor complex. This initiates a protein phosphorylation cascade culminating in the phosphorylation of the protein IκB. Phosphorylated IκB is degraded, liberating the transcriptional activator NF-κB, which can then translocate to the nucleus to activate transcription. IKK, IκB kinase; TAK-1, TGF-β-activated kinase 1.

ligands. Official designations for TNF-Rs can be found at http://www.gene.ucl.ac.uk/nomenclature/genefamily/tn-ftop.html. The ones most relevant to the immune system are receptors for TNF-α, lymphotoxin (LT), LIGHT, Fas ligand (FasL), and CD40L and include TNF-R1 (CD120a), TNF-R2 (CD120b), LT-βR, herpes virus entry mediator, Fas (CD95), and CD40. The TNF-R family contains one to four cysteine-rich domains, generally encompassing six cysteines that form three disulfide bonds. Many of these receptors bind to membrane-bound forms of their ligand, although soluble molecules such as TNF-α also can bind to their receptor. Binding of ligand to receptor involves an interaction of a homotrimeric ligand and a homotrimeric receptor. Binding of the TNF-Rs to their cognate ligand can often result in activation of apoptotic death due to the presence of a so-called *death domain* in the cytoplasmic, signaling portion of the receptor. The death domain is found on TNF-R1 and Fas, and engagement of these receptors is important in limiting lymphocyte proliferation to keep overexpansion of these cells in check. Absence of Fas or FasL results in a lymphoproliferative disease in humans and mice and many features of autoimmune disease.

TNF-R1 and TNF-R2 are the two receptors that can bind TNF-α as well as LT. The receptors have molecular masses of 50 to 60 kDa and 75 to 80 kDa, respectively. These receptors have been found on a variety of cell types. For some of the TNF-Rs, such as TNF-R1 and TNF-R2, soluble forms have been found and are hypothesized to effect decreases in TNF responsiveness by binding to soluble or membrane-bound TNF or LT and interfering with binding to signal-transducing membrane-bound forms of the receptor.

Cytokine Families

As the number of known cytokines is large and growing, it becomes difficult to describe all of the individual ones and their importance. Yet the properties of the individual cytokines are very telling in terms of the molecular and cellular interactions among immune cells. Grouping cytokines into families of molecules with broadly related functions is one means to present the important overriding principles and demonstrate the types of interactions and relatedness among cytokines in terms of the biologic effects they have.

Proinflammatory and Inflammatory Cytokines

Proinflammatory and inflammatory cytokines are induced by a variety of cells upon interaction with microbial pathogens or by trauma or damage to host cells. These cytokines initiate a cascade of events essential for innate immunity and "prime" many immune cells to better respond with an acquired immune response. This latter ability is mainly due to increased expression of antigen-presenting MHC on APC cell surfaces along with costimulatory ligands such as CD80 or CD86. The main effect of these cytokines is initiation of the inflammatory cascades and induction of acute-phase responses.

Macrophages are one of the major mediators of inflammation and can be activated through their interaction with a number of different inflammatory and proinflammatory cytokines. The primary effectors of macrophage activation are IFN-γ, TNF-α, and IL-1. These cytokines are also produced by macrophages and therefore serve as autocrine factors for this cell. IFN-γ augments the secretion of TNF-α by macrophages. These cytokines then serve to activate macrophages into producing greater quantities of TNF-α, IL-1, and IL-6, thus acting to increase the inflammatory response. Together, these cytokines are responsible for induction of the acute-phase response (see Fig. 2.14), which is made to microbial pathogens or initiated by noninfectious injury due to burns or trauma. Members of the chemokine family of proteins, MIP-1 and MIP-2, act as macrophage chemoattractant molecules. Another member of the chemokine family, IL-8, is produced by mononuclear phagocytes and is a potent activator and chemoattractant for neutrophils and, to a lesser extent, for eosinophils and basophils.

Although production of these cytokines and chemokines is critical to initiating effective innate immunity, overproduction can have severe consequences for a mammalian host. Endotoxic shock that can occur as part of infection with gram-negative bacteria is a specific disease process characterized by massive release of inflammatory cytokines. This results in vascular collapse and hypotension, together resulting in shock, and occasionally death, and is the paradigm for the adverse effects of inflammatory cytokines. Lipopolysaccharide (LPS; also called endotoxin) is the component of the gram-negative cell membrane that is the major stimulus for cytokine release in response to gram-negative infection. TNF-α released by macrophages in response to LPS has been identified as the cytokine primarily responsible for the symptoms associated with endotoxic shock. Using an in vivo experimental model of LPS-mediated pathology, investigators have shown that high doses of LPS cause disseminated intravascular coagulation, tissue injury, shock, and death. TNF-α is a critical molecular mediator of endotoxic shock and has been shown to elicit similar responses in animals when administered in the absence of LPS. These studies have also shown that TNF-α acts in both autocrine and paracrine fashions on mononuclear phagocytes and lymphocytes, causing the subsequent release of IL-1 and IL-6. These cytokines function to amplify the response, since they share many of the biologic properties of TNF-α. Together, these cytokines activate the coagulation cascade by increasing procoagulant activities in serum.

Long-term TNF-α exposure causes prolonged fever and cachexia (muscle and fat wasting). Elegant studies in animals have shown that administration of antibodies specific for TNF-α reduces many of the biologic manifestations of this cytokine (including death) if these animals are subsequently injected with lethal doses of LPS. It has recently been suggested that therapeutic intervention for TNF-α-associated disease could include the use of monoclonal antibodies to neutralize TNF-α or administration of compounds that impede its synthesis or binding to its receptor. Interestingly, in the setting of microbial infection, such interventions not only were unhelpful in ameliorating the consequences of infection, but, in some studies, interfering with TNF-α activity actually led to more death from infection. This is due to the fact that one needs some TNF-α to fight the infection whereas too much is pathologic. However, in the setting of a local inflammatory response such as arthritis, neutralizing antibodies to TNF-α show a high degree of efficacy in reducing tissue damage and are being studied for similar effects in other localized inflammatory diseases.

The acute-phase response is perhaps the best example of the importance of cytokine modulation of host responses to trauma or bacterial infection. The acute-phase response refers to rapid changes in plasma protein concentrations following burns, pathogenic infections, and other types of trauma. Levels of C-reactive protein, fibrinogen, and amyloid A protein in serum escalate, whereas levels of albumin and transferrin fall. Hepatocytes are the major source of these proteins, and studies have shown that IL-6, in association with IL-1 and TNF-α, is largely responsible for this response. The acute-phase response allows for release of these substances (C-reactive protein and mannose-binding protein), which enhance innate immunity to pathogens, for example, by increasing opsonization of organisms.

Members of the chemokine family, particularly IL-8, are also important mediators of a coordinated inflammatory response. Studies have shown that chemotactic processes associated with the inflammatory response are modulated by early signals, such as release of TNF-α and IL-1. These cytokines increase IL-8 secretion from various cell types, which in turn signals leukocyte recruitment to the sites of tissue damage.

Specific proinflammatory and inflammatory cytokines

IL-1

IL-1 was originally discovered as a costimulator of T cells produced by mononuclear phagocytes. However, IL-1 is currently recognized as a major mediator of the host inflammatory response associated with innate immune mechanisms. A number of stimuli can lead to secretion of IL-1 by monocytes and other APCs, and some populations of dendritic cells may be constitutive producers of IL-1. IL-1 synthesis is induced primarily by the secretion of APC-derived cytokines, such as TNF-α, IFN-γ, or, in an autocrine fashion, even IL-1 itself. Binding of APCs to CD4$^+$ T cells also will induce the APCs to secrete IL-1. IL-1 secretion often follows the exposure of monocyte/macrophages to bacterial products, such as LPS. This explains the increased IL-1 levels in the circulation of animals and humans during gram-negative bacterial sepsis. Along with TNF-α, IL-1 is considered a classic mediator of the acute-phase response. Additional functions of IL-1 include stimulation of secretion of IL-6; induction of expression of IL-2R; and enhancement of the expression of cell-adhesion molecules, which promote cell-cell interactions and inflammatory cell extravasation. IL-1 is also produced by endothelial and epithelial cells and can act on macrophages to produce IL-8, which recruits neutrophils to sites of inflammation.

Two forms of IL-1 have been described: IL-1α and IL-1β. These have been isolated from both mice and humans. Each has a molecular mass of about 17 kDa. One of the characteristics distinguishing the two molecules is the difference in their isoelectric points (pI) (the pI of IL-1α is 5.0 and the pI of IL-1β is 7.0). Each form of IL-1 is the product of two distinct genes, and each is produced as a precursor molecule with a molecular mass of 32 kDa.

IL-1Rs are commonly found on a number of different cell types. Two distinct receptors for both forms of IL-1, known as type I and type II, have been described (see below). A naturally occurring IL-1 inhibitor, known as IL-1 receptor agonist, which binds the IL-1R with the same affinity as IL-1, has been described. Interestingly, this molecule does not have IL-1 activity, instead acting as an IL-1 competitive inhibitor, thus possibly serving to regulate the action of this cytokine.

IL-6

IL-6 is a highly pleiotropic molecule that functions as an autocrine, paracrine, and endocrine activator of inflammation. It is synthesized by monocytes, endothelial cells, and fibroblasts in response to IL-1 and TNF-α. As mentioned earlier, IL-6 is a major mediator of the acute-phase response inducing hepatocytes (liver cells) to secrete a number of plasma proteins that contribute to this host response during bacterial infection. As well as being induced by IL-1 and TNF, IL-6 activities are further complemented by these cytokines. IL-6 also activates B-cell growth and differentiation and may be involved in the induction of B-cell malignancies. IL-6 also stimulates the proliferation of thymocytes and peripheral T cells and can augment NK-cell activity.

IL-6 is a 26-kDa glycoprotein containing two disulfide bonds critical to its biologic activity. Unlike some of the other cytokines, variable glycosylation of IL-6 isolated from different species seems to be important for biologic function. In addition, phosphorylation of this compound at various sites also may be important in regulating its activity. IL-6 binds to a receptor that is susceptible to saturation and composed of two chains, a ligand-binding 80-kDa molecule and a non-ligand-binding signal transducer molecule known as gp130.

Interferons

Interferons were first identified for their ability to confer upon cells in culture resistance to viral infection. Later on it was found that they they could also activate inflammatory cells. There are two forms of interferons, type I and type II. Type I interferons are induced during viral infection and include IFN-α (produced by leukocytes), IFN-β (produced by fibroblasts), and IFN-κ (produced by keratinocytes) (see Fig. 2.10). Type II interferon, better known as IFN-γ, is produced by activated T cells and NK cells and shares many of the antiviral activities of type I interferons. However, IFN-γ is structurally unrelated to IFN-α and IFN-β, binds to a distinct cell surface receptor, and has many immunoregulatory properties not associated with type I interferons.

IFN-γ activates mononuclear phagocytes, allowing these cells to perform many of the functions required to kill ingested microorganisms. This cytokine belongs to a class of molecules that induce the differentiation of monocytes into activated macrophages that also are known as macrophage-activating factors. IFN-γ functions to increase expression of MHC class I and class II on the surface of APCs, increasing their ability to be recognized by T cells when presenting antigen. Many other important biologic properties are associated with IFN-γ. It directly promotes T- and B-cell differentiation and can activate neutrophils and NK cells. It also is a potent stimulus for increased expression of cell-adhesion molecules on immune cells and functions to increase their extravasation from vascular sites to inflammation areas.

Human IFN-γ is a polypeptide of approximately 20 kDa that is variably glycosylated. The receptor for IFN-γ is susceptible to saturation and belongs to a single class of high-affinity receptors. This receptor is found on a variety of lymphoid, monocytic, mast, and endothelial cells and has a molecular mass of approximately 90 kDa.

TNF

Two forms of TNF, TNF-α and TNF-β, are known, but TNF-β is now referred to as LT. These two cytokines share some biologic properties, both in vitro and in vivo, but LT is not generally regarded as an inflammatory cytokine and its primary function is in control of the architecture of secondary lymphoid organs. TNF-α is made up of a basic 17-kDa protein that associates into three subunits. A membrane-bound version of this molecule also exists in both humans and mice. The membrane-bound form can exist as either a 17-kDa or 26-kDa protein. TNF is so named because it was originally identified as a serum factor in LPS-treated animals that could reduce the size of specific tumors. TNF-α secretion by activated macrophages was later found to be a response factor to LPS. At very low concentrations, LPS stimulates TNF-α release from macrophages and also acts as a polyclonal B-cell activator. Although macrophages are the major source of TNF-α, activated T cells, NK cells, and mast cells also can secrete this cytokine. Studies have shown that IFN-α can augment TNF-α production by activated macrophages. At low concentrations, TNF-α has diverse biologic properties. These include the ability to increase the expression of many cell adhesion molecules, such as ICAM-1, which are important in causing leukocyte extravasation, leading to their migration to sites of tissue damage. TNF-α also stimulates the release of the IL-8 family of chemokines, as well as IL-1 and IL-6, from macrophages. TNF-α-knockout mice are also impaired in primary B-cell responses, notably being unable to form primary follicles in lymph nodes and in marginal zones in tissues like the spleen. These mice are more susceptible to intracellular microbes, likely related to the interaction of TNF-α and IFN-γ, both important in activating macrophages for control of intracellular parasites.

At higher concentrations, TNF-α enters the bloodstream and becomes a potent mediator of inflammatory responses to bacteria. In this regard, TNF-α shares many of the biologic functions exhibited by IL-1. Like IL-1, TNF acts as a pyrogen, inducing fever and increasing synthesis of serum proteins from hepatocytes to initiate the acute-phase response to inflammatory stimuli. Since TNF-α causes secretion of IL-1 and IL-6, serum proteins released in response to TNF-α complement those released in response to IL-1 and IL-6, resulting in a coordinated response to augment the efficiency of the inflammatory response. However, very high concentrations of TNF-α can cause severe pathology, and thus a balance must be maintained between producing the proper amount of TNF-α for fighting infection but not too much to make the inflammatory response itself the cause of unwanted responses. High concentrations of TNF-α cause disseminated intravascular coagulation, shock, and tissue damage that can lead to death.

Cytokines and Differentiation of T-Cell Function

The differentiation of CD4⁺ T-cell populations into two distinct groups, TH1 and TH2 cells, is predicated on the patterns of cytokine secreted by the T cells. These distinct T-cell subpopulations determine which type of immune response will be mounted in response to an antigen (Fig. 15.15). However, it is important to point out that the cytokine production pattern has been determined mostly with cloned cells in laboratory settings, and controversy exists as to whether this paradigm of a split into two TH populations occurs in vivo. TH1 clones secrete IFN-γ, TNF, and IL-2 whereas TH2 clones secrete IL-4, IL-5, and IL-10. In vivo studies have demonstrated that different types of pathogens can elicit discrete responses by either of these TH types. A third CD4⁺ population, TH0 cells, has been identified that has a cytokine secretion pattern that lies somewhere between those of TH1 and TH2 clones. However, TH0 cells appear to exert their effects only early in the immune response. These responses were identified originally in the mouse but there is now considerable evidence that these T-cell subsets likely can be found among human T-cell clones. Interestingly, in both humans and mice, most CD8⁺ T-cell clones exhibit a TH1 cytokine pattern.

Cytokines produced by TH1 cells (IFN-γ, TNF, and IL-2) lead to macrophage activation, enhanced antigen presentation, and increased Fc receptor expression and superoxide production. These biologic activities result in effective killing of intracellular and extracellular pathogens and in the development of long-term immunity to these microorganisms. TH1 cells also seem to be important in mediating delayed-type hypersensitivity reactions, including granuloma formation. IL-12 is important in enhancing the expansion of human TH1 cells in vitro and is believed to be a major effector in cell-mediated immunity while inhibiting TH2 cell development (Fig. 15.16). TH2 cells are important in modulating humoral responses to antigens, and cytokines that are typically produced by these cells include IL-4, IL-10, IL-13, and in some TH2 cells, IL-3 and IL-5. These cells also are

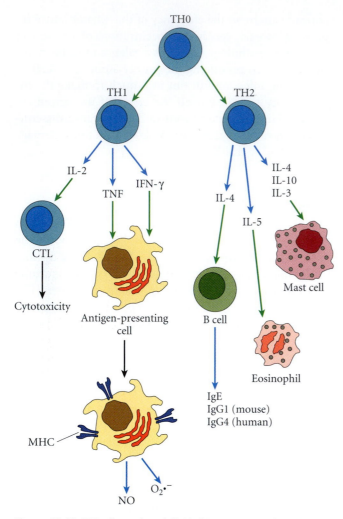

Figure 15.15 TH cells can be subdivided into two main functional categories: TH1 and TH2. TH1 cells secrete primarily IFN-γ, TNF, and IL-2, promoting cell-mediated immunity, whereas TH2 cells secrete primarily IL-4, IL-5, and IL-10, activating humoral immunity as well as granulocytes such as eosinophils and mast cells. Blue arrows indicate synthesis of soluble mediators.

important in coordinating allergic responses to antigens. IL-4 and IL-5 derived from TH2 cells initiate IgE production in B cells and activate eosinophils, respectively, whereas IL-3, IL-4, and IL-10 are responsible for mast-cell activation (Fig. 15.15). These TH2 responses are of vital importance in the immune response to infections with metazoan parasites.

TH1 and TH2 cells regulate each other's activity (Fig. 15.16). The activity of each cell type inhibits the activity of the other, which can skew a given immune response to have either TH1 or TH2 characteristics. This finding presented a puzzle to immunologists: if the action of each TH cell subset inhibits the action of the other, what prevents the TH cell population in a given animal from becoming *permanently* polarized to one phenotype or the other after

a single immune response? The answer lies in a second form of cross-regulation that serves to balance the TH1 and TH2 populations over time. TH1 cells and TH2 cells require different subsets of dendritic cells for their maturation from their common TH0 precursor. Thus, TH1 cells require type 1 dendritic cells (DC1) while TH2 cells require type 2 dendritic cells (DC2) (see Fig. 3.9A). Therefore, a potential means to regulate the balance of TH1 and TH2 cells is by production of the TH2 cytokine IL-4 (see Fig. 3.9B). After being made by activated TH2 cells, IL-4 then inhibits the development of DC2 cells (thus preventing further development of TH2 cells) and also promotes the development of DC1 cells (thus encouraging development of new TH1 cells). A reciprocal form of regulation that promotes TH2 development following a TH1 response has been postulated but has not yet been formally demonstrated. Thus, TH subpopulations seem to have a built-in correction mechanism that prevents either cell type from permanently dominating the T-cell compartment of the host.

The derivation of these T-cell subsets is still unclear. The prevailing hypothesis holds that TH1 and TH2 cells arise from a common precursor cell. Experimental data have shown that exposure to IL-4 during early stages of T-cell activation drives TH2 clonal development such that

Figure 15.16 The two subpopulations of TH cells cross-regulate each other, with TH2 cells negatively regulating TH1-cell development and vice versa. Blue arrows indicate synthesis, green arrows indicate a positive effect, and red lines indicate negative regulation.

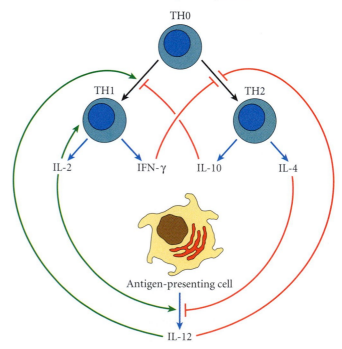

these then go on to secrete high levels of IL-4 upon restimulation. Similarly, the development of TH1 cells can be induced upon exposure to IFN-γ. As mentioned earlier, IL-12 also seems to play an important role in the development of TH1 cells. Furthermore, cytokines produced by either clonal type are able to decrease the activities of the other clonal type, e.g., IFN-γ inhibits TH2 cellular proliferation and the synthesis of many of the cytokines produced by these clones. Meanwhile, cytokines produced by TH2 cells, such as IL-4 and IL-10, inhibit TH1 cell activation and cytokine secretion. It is clear from these studies that a very complex immunomodulatory circuit controls cytokine synthesis by these cells and their respective effector functions.

Cytokines That Control Cell-Mediated Immunity: TH1-Type Cytokines

IL-2

IL-2 was first identified for its ability to stimulate T-cell growth and subsequently was termed T-cell growth factor. CD4$^+$ T cells account for the majority of IL-2 production, but studies have shown that CD8$^+$ cells also produce IL-2. The primary function of IL-2 appears to be autocrine stimulation of CD4$^+$ cell growth. IL-2 also stimulates proliferation of nearby CD4$^+$ and CD8$^+$ T cells in a paracrine fashion. It acts primarily on lymphocytes, and its effects are directly related to the quantity synthesized by activated CD4$^+$ cells. There is evidence suggesting that the amount of IL-2 secreted by activated T cells increases proportionally to the amount of IL-2 to which these T cells are exposed. In addition, IL-2 induces the synthesis of other T-cell-derived cytokines such as IFN-γ. The amount of IL-2 produced by T cells is an important factor in determining the kinetics of the immune response. IL-2 exhibits its effects through binding a specific receptor (Fig. 15.12). This binding brings about increased expression of additional receptor molecules on the cell surface that have an increased affinity for binding IL-2.

IL-2 also stimulates growth of NK cells and allows these cells to exhibit increased cytotoxic activities. This type of cell is important in mediating cell-mediated immune responses and functions as a nonspecific killer of altered or infected target cells. IL-2 participates in converting resting NK cells into lymphokine-activated killer cells, enhancing their ability to perform critical functions during the immune response. This cytokine also functions to augment B-cell growth and antibody production. Although this feature of IL-2 activity is less well understood, IL-2 does not, to any large extent, appear to be involved in antibody isotype switching. Other activities ascribed to IL-2 include

induction of IL-6 production by monocytes and histamine release by mast cells.

Biochemical analysis of IL-2 has demonstrated that it is 14 to 22 kDa, depending on the type of analytic procedure used. There are discrepancies between the apparent molecular weight of human and mouse IL-2, although this appears to be due to the amount of O glycosylation present on each type of molecule. Glycosylation is not required for IL-2 function, whereas reduction of a single disulfide bond between residues 58 and 105 results in a loss of biologic function.

IL-12 and IL-23

IL-12 is a heterodimer composed of a 40-kDa subunit disulfide linked to a 35-kDa subunit. This cytokine mediates a number of cell-mediated immune functions. IL-12 was originally termed NK-cell stimulatory factor since it initially was found to stimulate NK cells. However, more recent studies have demonstrated a broader activity spectrum for IL-12, implicating it as an important mediator for TH1 cell differentiation. IL-12 is produced by dendritic cells, macrophages, and B lymphocytes and stimulates IFN-γ production by NK cells and TH1 clones. A high-affinity receptor for IL-12 has been identified on TH1 cells, confirming its importance as a growth factor for this T-cell subset. IL-12 is extremely important in the control of the development of T cells into TH1 type cells and inhibition of development into TH2 type cells as discussed above. The essential nature of IL-12 signaling and cell activation in protection from pathogens where cell-mediated immunity is needed has been well demonstrated in humans who lack one of the monomers of IL-12R (IL-12Rβ). They are much more susceptible to infection with both mycobacteria and salmonella, two pathogens that have an extensive intracellular lifestyle, and for which TH1-type T-cell responses are required for immunity.

A recently discovered cytokine, IL-23, which is related to IL-12 in form and function, has been described. IL-23 is a heterodimer made up of the p40 subunit that is also found in IL-12 and a unique subunit, p19. Many assays previously performed to measure IL-12 levels were based on measuring the amount of the p40 subunit made, but now it appears that many of these assays may have also been measuring some IL-23 as well. The receptor for IL-23 consists of the β-chain subunit of the IL-12 receptor, IL-2Rβ1, along with a unique signaling chain, IL-23R. IL-23 is secreted by activated dendritic cells and its function is differentiated from that of IL-12 by its ability to induce proliferation of memory T cells (but not naive T cells), while IL-12 has no effect on memory T cells.

IL-15

IL-15 is produced by a wide variety of tissues, including placenta, skeletal muscle, kidney, and activated monocytes and macrophages, although adherent peripheral blood monocytes and macrophages are the primary producers of this cytokine. It is capable of using the β and γ chains of IL-2R for signal transduction and shares many properties with IL-2 despite their lack of any sequence homology. IL-15 has stimulatory activities for NK cells, B cells, and some T cells. Recent evidence suggests that IL-15 has stimulatory activity for γδ T cells. Recently, it has been shown that TNF-α-stimulated fibroblasts express a membrane-bound form of IL-15 during inflammation. Prolonged activation of T cells at the site of inflammation depends on IL-15, since it was prevented by IL-15-neutralizing antibodies. The mechanism of IL-15-mediated activation is thought to involve antiapoptotic effects caused by enhanced synthesis of the antiapoptotic protein Bcl-xL.

IL-16

IL-16, also known as lymphocyte chemoattractant factor, is a T-cell-derived cytokine that induces chemotaxis of CD4$^+$ T cells and CD4$^+$ monocytes and eosinophils. IL-16 also induces expression of IL-2R and MHC class II molecules on CD4$^+$ T cells. The biologic activities of IL-16 are totally dependent on the presence of CD4 receptors on responsive cells. This cytokine is the only lymphocyte chemoattractant that is secreted following serotonin stimulation and may play a role in serotonin-mediated T-cell inflammatory processes. Because of its activity as a chemoattractant, IL-16 has recently been investigated as a key element of pathologic inflammatory states such as inflammatory bowel disease and allergic inflammation.

IL-17

IL-17 has been cloned from a CD4$^+$ T-cell library and is produced in large quantities from primary peripheral blood CD4$^+$ T cells upon stimulation. It induces production of IL-6 and IL-8 and enhances surface expression of ICAM-1 on human fibroblasts. The biologic and immunologic functions attributed to IL-17 are numerous. Intratracheal administration of IL-17 increases neutrophil counts in bronchoalveolar lavage fluids and increases the amount of neutrophil elastase in the bronchoalveolar lavage fluid. IL-17 also regulates expression of several complement components. The receptor for IL-17 binds this cytokine with low affinity and transduces signals via the JAK/STAT pathway, utilizing JAKs 1, 2, and 3, as well as STATs 1, 2, 3, and 4.

Two new cytokines with high homology to IL-17 have recently been identified and cloned. On the basis of the high degree of structural similarity of these cytokines, they were termed IL-17B and IL-17C. However, despite their similarity to IL-17, IL-17B and IL-17C exhibit activities that are different from those of IL-17 and have a different tissue distribution (significantly, IL-17B and IL-17C are not expressed by activated T cells). Yet another member of the growing IL-17 family is IL-17E, a proinflammatory cytokine that stimulates synthesis of IL-8. IL-17E binds to a novel receptor, termed the IL-17 receptor homolog 1.

IL-18

IL-18 is produced by numerous cell types, including T cells, B cells, monocytes, dendritic cells, and nonimmune cell types such as keratinocytes and osteoblasts. IL-18 was identified as a cytokine present in liver extracts that was capable of inducing IFN-γ synthesis, T-cell proliferation, and NK-cell activity. Therefore, the cytokine was originally named IFN-γ-inducing factor. IL-18 is an 18-kDa protein that is structurally related to IL-1. Its receptor (IL-18R) consists of two protein chains originally known as IL-1 receptor-related protein (IL-1Rrp) and accessory protein-like (AcPL). The first of these subunits has IL-18-binding activity, while the second subunit is required for signal transduction. Signaling has been found to proceed via IRAK, TRAF6, and NF-κB.

Early functional studies of IL-18 demonstrated that it activates TH1 cells and represses IgE synthesis. IL-18 was therefore originally considered to be a classic TH1 cytokine, inducing cytotoxic reactions while repressing humoral responses. However, a more recent study showed that IL-18 also can recruit eosinophils into airways, an effect typically observed in TH2-driven responses. The ability of IL-18 to induce eosinophilia was found to depend on its induction of TNF-α synthesis. Therefore, while it is appropriate to consider IL-18 a proinflammatory cytokine, classifying it as either a TH1 or a TH2 cytokine is difficult. Indeed, it is likely that the type of inflammatory response mediated by IL-18 is governed in part by which other cytokines are present during an immune response.

Cytokines That Control B-Cell Function: TH2-Type Cytokines

IL-4

IL-4, a T-cell-derived compound with an apparent molecular mass of approximately 20 kDa, has a wide range of biologic activities and is currently thought to be an important activator of B lymphocytes. IL-4 is also necessary for B-cell differentiation and antibody production and is an important factor in mediating B-cell switching to IgE production. Therefore, our current understanding of IL-4 bioactivity greatly emphasizes the role played by this cytokine in controlling the humoral immune response to antigen. IL-4 also functions to increase expression of MHC class II on B cells and also can act as an autocrine growth factor for $CD4^+$ cells that secrete IL-4, IL-5, and IL-6. Interestingly, IL-4 acts synergistically with IL-3 to activate mast-cell proliferation and can act synergistically with IL-1 to increase antigen presentation and phagocytosis by macrophages.

Production of IL-4 by T cells is now recognized as a major marker for identifying the TH2 subset of $CD4^+$ cells and is also thought to play an important role in decreasing cell-mediated responses via suppression of TH1 clones. IL-4 is believed to act in concert with IL-10 to regulate many immune functions, and it binds to a high-affinity receptor on T cells, B cells, and macrophages.

IL-5

IL-5 is a disulfide-linked dimer with a molecular mass of about 45 kDa under nonreducing conditions. It is produced by activated $CD4^+$ TH2 cells and mast cells and exerts its biologic activities on eosinophils, B cells, and thymocytes. It can stimulate the growth of eosinophils and control their differentiation, enhancing their ability to kill helminths. This ability was demonstrated both in vitro and in vivo by using monoclonal antibodies directed to IL-5, which inhibited the characteristic eosinophilia observed in response to infection with helminth parasites. IL-5 also acts as a costimulator for B-cell growth and differentiation, reportedly acting synergistically with IL-2 and IL-4 to regulate this activity. In addition, IL-5 seems to be important in modulating IgA and IgE production by antibody-producing plasma cells. IL-5 interacts with a multisubunit receptor on target cells composed of two chains: a low-affinity, ligand-binding α chain and a cytoplasmic, signal-transducing β chain.

IL-7

IL-7 is secreted by marrow and thymic stromal cells and is involved in B-cell hematopoiesis. This cytokine is involved in the growth and differentiation of precursor B lymphocytes during the very early stages of maturation and acts on $CD4^-$ $CD8^-$ T-cell precursors in the thymus to potentiate their differentiation. It also acts as a costimulus with concanavalin A to induce murine T-cell proliferation and also can act on $CD8^+$ cells to induce CTL maturation.

At the structural level, the molecular mass of both murine and human IL-7 is approximately 25 kDa. This glycoprotein binds to low- and high-affinity receptors ex-

pressed on B and T cells, respectively. Binding of IL-7 to its complementary receptor results in tyrosine phosphorylation of at least five major cytoplasmic proteins, leading to proto-oncogene transcriptional activation.

IL-9

IL-9 potentiates the growth of human and mouse T-cell lines as well as murine thymic lymphomas in vitro. T cells are believed to be the source of IL-9. It functions to support IL-4-dependent immunoglobulin production and enhance IL-6 synthesis by mast cells. IL-9 has recently been shown to promote the local accumulation of eosinophils during allergic inflammation. This effect probably is due to the ability of IL-9 to promote eosinophil maturation at the site of inflammation. Murine IL-9 has an apparent molecular mass of 32 to 39 kDa, whereas human IL-9 has a molecular mass of 20 to 30 kDa. These discrepancies are most likely due to variations in the amount of glycosylation of the respective proteins. Human and mouse IL-9 exhibit 67% homology at the nucleotide level. This cytokine binds to a 64-kDa protein receptor found on both TH1 and TH2 cells, but so far a single class of high-affinity receptors has been described. The receptor is thought to transduce activating signals through the transcription factor STAT5, since expression of a dominant-negative form of STAT5 ablates IL-9-dependent cells.

IL-10 and IL-10 family members

IL-10 exhibits a number of regulatory activities. This cytokine originally was thought to be produced by TH2 cells, inhibiting production of IFN-γ and IL-2 by TH1 cells. However, other activities have recently been attributed to this cytokine, including the ability to enhance murine T-cell proliferation and to prevent antigen-specific T-cell responses through decreases in MHC class II expression. IL-10 suppresses TNF-α release by macrophages and enhances mast-cell growth in a synergistic interaction with IL-3 and IL-4. It is also an important growth factor for human B cells, increasing their expression of MHC class II. Studies with murine and human IL-10 cDNA have demonstrated that this protein has a molecular mass of 17 to 21 kDa. IL-10R consists of a 110-kDa ligand-binding subunit that associates with a second receptor chain responsible for signal transduction. Signal transduction through the IL-10R requires the participation of the signaling components JAK1 and STAT3.

IL-19, IL-20, IL-21, and IL-22 are recently described members of the newly defined family of IL-10 homology, most of which seem to function primarily in the regulation of inflammation. IL-19 is secreted by monocytes upon stimulation with LPS. Although its function remains unknown, the receptor for IL-19 has recently been shown to be identical to the type I receptor for IL-20. IL-20 is secreted by keratinocytes and binds to a receptor on these same cells. It is therefore thought to play an important autocrine role in skin inflammation. Signaling by the IL-20 receptor has been found to use the STAT3 pathway. IL-21, also called IL-10-related T-cell-inducible factor, is secreted by T cells and mast cells upon stimulation with IL-9. IL-21 binds to a receptor expressed on the surface of hepatocytes and triggers synthesis of several acute-phase proteins via the STAT1 and STAT3 pathways. IL-22 is a distant homolog of IL-10 that is secreted by activated T cells. IL-22 binds to a family of receptors that includes CRF2-4 (cytokine receptor family 2-4) and the newly defined IL-22R. Binding of IL-22 to its receptor(s) signals through a pathway that includes STATs 1, 3, and 5 and has been shown to regulate the production of the TH2 cytokine IL-4. Activity of IL-22 is thought to be regulated by several antagonists called IL-22 receptor antagonists 1 and 2 and IL-22 binding protein, which are encoded by separate genes that lie on the same chromosome and adjacent to the gene that encodes IL-22R.

IL-11

IL-11 is a 20-kDa protein synthesized by bone marrow stromal cells that has pleiotropic effects on both hematopoietic and nonhematopoietic cells. It can stimulate the secretion of immunoglobulin by activated B cells and is involved in the generation of acute-phase proteins (as has been shown with IL-6). IL-11 synergizes with IL-3 to stimulate megakaryopoiesis, and some evidence suggests that IL-11 may potentiate platelet production and regulate bone marrow synthesis. In recent years, IL-11 has come to be appreciated as a regulator of the TH1-TH2 cytokine axis. Early evidence for this came from studies examining the effect of IL-11 on macrophage activation; IL-11 was found to inhibit the production of nitric oxide and TNF-α. Further investigation of this phenomenon revealed that IL-11 inhibits the production of IFN-γ and increases the production of IL-4. Recently, this was demonstrated directly with recombinant IL-11. IL-11R appears to comprise a single peptide with a molecular mass of 151 kDa.

IL-13

IL-13 is a T-cell-derived cytokine with a molecular mass of approximately 10 kDa and properties similar to those of IL-4. It promotes B-cell proliferation but, unlike IL-4, lacks the capacity to stimulate T cells. It does, however, induce immunoglobulin isotype class switching, favoring both IgE and IgG4. IL-13 was recently shown to regulate IFN-γ synthesis and to decrease IL-6 secretion by blood monocytes. Because of its role in inducing IgE synthesis, IL-13 has been studied as part of the immune response to eukaryotic parasites, such as schistosomes and helminths. Synthesis of IL-13 (as well as IL-4) is increased during schistosomiasis, and the IgE synthesis that occurs during the immune response to schistosomes is dependent on production of IL-13. IL-13 also enhances extravasation of eosinophils, which also are thought to be important in the immune response to parasites. However, many of the immune effectors important for the immune response to parasites are also essential components of the allergic response (type I hypersensitivity). Indeed, it has been suggested that IL-13 plays a key role in allergic inflammation in several tissues.

IL-13 mediates its activities via a complex receptor system. IL-13Rα1 binds IL-13 with low affinity but does not signal. However, when IL-13Rα1 combines with IL-4Rα, a signaling high-affinity receptor complex for IL-13 is generated. In contrast, IL-13Rα2 alone binds IL-13 with high affinity but does not signal. IL-13Rα2 is largely an intracellular molecule, whose surface expression is rapidly increased by IFN-γ and results in decreased IL-13 signaling.

IL-14

First identified as a growth factor present in rapidly proliferating B-cell lymphomas, IL-14 is now known to be a T-cell-derived cytokine that stimulates proliferation of activated B lymphocytes but not the proliferation of resting B cells. This molecule also inhibits the secretion of immunoglobulin from stimulated B cells.

Cytokines That Control Cellular and Tissue Development

IL-3

IL-3, first known as multilineage colony-stimulating factor, was originally found as a product of activated CD4$^+$ cells. Further study has shown that activated T lymphocytes are the major source of this cytokine but that NK cells, mast cells, and epidermal cells also produce IL-3. This molecule appears to have diverse biologic roles. One primary function of IL-3 is to promote expansion of a number of bone marrow progenitor cells so that they can differentiate into mature cell types. It also is involved in the stimulation of mast-cell lines, neutrophils, macrophages, basophils, and eosinophils, especially in synergy with IL-4. Two different forms of mouse IL-3 have been identified, each with an apparent molecular mass of 30 to 40 kDa. The two forms have similar biologic properties. Human IL-3 was identified via cDNA cloning from concanavalin A-stimulated TH cells some time after the identification of mouse IL-3. At the DNA level, there is homology of approximately 45% between the human and murine forms of IL-3. IL-3 binds to a multisubunit complex consisting of an α subunit and a β subunit. As seen with IL-2R, the α subunit appears to be important for signal transduction, whereas the β subunit is capable of low-affinity binding.

LT

LT has a molecular mass between 20 kDa and 25 kDa, and there are two protein chains, LT-α and LT-β. Like other members of the TNF family, LT forms a heterotrimer. Some of these are made from three molecules of LT-α while others are made from one LT-α and two LT-β chains (LT-α1β2). The LT-α homotrimer binds to TNF-R1, TNF-R2, and herpesvirus entry mediator receptors, whereas LT-α1β2 binds to the LT-βR. LT is primarily produced by TH1 cells and cytotoxic T cells. Its major effect, however, appears to be in promoting the development of secondary lymphoid tissues. LT-α- and LT-βR-knockout mice lack lymph nodes, and the tissue in the spleen and other secondary lymphoid organs is highly disorganized. Mice lacking only LT-β develop some lymph nodes. In addition to maintaining proper tissue architecture, LT can kill T cells, fibroblasts, and some tumor cells (hence the original designation as TNF-β), inhibit B-cell activity, and activate phagocytic cells such as macrophages and neutrophils.

Colony-stimulating factors

Another class of cytokines responsible for the growth and differentiation of bone marrow progenitor cells has been described. These molecules are responsible for the maturation of new cells and for the replenishing of leukocyte populations depleted during immune and inflammatory reactions. Development of these cells involves the growth and differentiation of precursor cells into mature immune cells that become committed to a particular lineage. Once committed, these cells lose the ability to differentiate into other cell types. The cytokines involved in stimulating this expansion are termed *colony-stimulating factors* (CSFs). There are many different types of CSFs, each acting at different stages of differentiation and on different cell lineages. IL-3, already discussed, is a CSF also known as multilineage CSF. It acts on bone marrow progenitor cells to promote their differentiation into a number of mature cell types.

GM-CSF

GM-CSF is synthesized by activated T cells, macrophages, endothelial cells, and fibroblasts and acts on marrow cultures of granulocytes, macrophages, and eosinophils in vitro. It is capable of stimulating antibody-dependent cytolysis of tumor cells by neutrophils and is presumed to act in both autocrine and paracrine fashions, although it does not enter the circulation, thus precluding any endocrine activity. Human GM-CSF has a molecular mass of 18 to 22 kDa and exerts its effects through binding a high-affinity receptor.

Granulocyte colony-stimulating factor (G-CSF)

G-CSF is produced by the same cells that produce GM-CSF and acts on bone marrow progenitors committed to the granulocyte cell lineage, stimulating neutrophil maturation in particular. G-CSF appears to act downstream from GM-CSF, meaning that it acts later than GM-CSF in the maturation process. G-CSF does not act in an endocrine fashion, since it is unable to enter the general circulation. This cytokine has a molecular mass of 20 kDa and binds to a receptor that is susceptible to saturation.

Monocyte-macrophage colony-stimulating factor (M-CSF)

M-CSF is produced by macrophages, endothelial cells, and fibroblasts and acts locally to stimulate progenitor cells to develop into monocytes. M-CSF has a molecular mass of approximately 40 kDa and binds specifically to a receptor found predominantly on mononuclear phagocytes.

Transforming growth factors

Transforming growth factors (TGFs) were identified when it was found that certain tumors produced factors that would allow normal cells to survive and grow. These activities were ascribed to two compounds, termed TGF-α and TGF-β. TGF-α is a polypeptide factor that stimulates epithelial and mesenchymal cell growth. TGF-β exhibits pleiotropic activities and is secreted by a variety of cell types, including activated monocytes and T cells. This compound exhibits both inhibitory and stimulatory activities, although it is generally considered to be a negative modulator of many other cytokines, especially the proinflammatory ones. TGF-β inhibits T-cell mitogenesis, CTL activation, and macrophage activation. TGF-β is a dimeric protein with a molecular mass of approximately 28 kDa.

Chemokines and IL-8

IL-8 is a member of a large family of structurally related chemoattractant proteins 8 to 10 kDa in size. Also known as the chemokine family, these proteins can be further subdivided into two groups based on the arrangement of cysteine residues comprising each chemokine: the CC family and the CXC family. As a group, these molecules are synthesized by three types of cells: antigen-activated T cells, activated mononuclear cells, and platelets. IL-8 is the best-described member of this family. This peptide is in the CXC family and is usually synthesized by mononuclear phagocytes that have been stimulated with LPS or exogenous IL-1 or TNF. The major function of IL-8 is neutrophil activation and recruitment. Eosinophils, basophils, and lymphocytes also respond to IL-8 but to a lesser degree. IL-8 also augments production of lysosomal enzymes by neutrophils and increases a variety of cell-adhesion molecules. Recent evidence suggests that IL-8 is a dimeric molecule bearing considerable homology to the human MHC class I molecule. This dimer binds two high-affinity receptors known as type I and type II receptors. The type I receptor binds IL-8 only, whereas the type II receptor binds members of the chemokine family in addition to IL-8. Signal transduction through these receptors involves receptor internalization and activation via protein kinase C.

Although IL-8 was the first member of the chemokine family to be identified, other chemotactic peptides have since been described. MCP-1 (monocyte chemoattractant protein 1); RANTES (regulated upon activation, normal T expressed and secreted); and MIP-1α, MIP-1β, and MIP-2 (monocyte inflammatory proteins) are all recently described members of this family. MCP-1 is a member of the CC family and, at nanomolar concentrations, has specific chemoattractant activity for monocytes. In addition, MCP-1 can induce the release of superoxide anion, calcium, and lysosomal enzymes from monocytes. This compound is 76 amino acids long and has one glycosylation site. RANTES is an 8-kDa nonglycosylated protein expressed by T cells. However, its expression by T cells is decreased as a result of T-cell activation. Initially, RANTES was shown to be chemotactic for blood monocytes and for a subset of CD4$^+$ T lymphocytes although recent studies suggest that it also possesses chemotactic activity for basophils and eosinophils. MIP-1 and MIP-2 were originally identified as low-molecular-weight heparin-binding proteins with pleiotropic properties. MIP-1α and MIP-1β are both members of the CC family, whereas MIP-2 is a member of the CXC family of chemokines. MIP-1 and MIP-2 have been characterized as monocyte and T-cell chemoattractants following macrophage activation induced by LPS.

Role of Cytokines in Other Diseases

Recent developments in the understanding of cytokine biology and the singular importance of these compounds in regulating inflammatory and other immune responses have led to a wave of studies examining the role of these mediators in disease processes. In vitro and in vivo models of disease have been successfully used to illustrate the importance of cytokines in modulating host responses to these diseases. These studies have made use of newly developed technologies (including recombinant DNA and monoclonal antibody-based assays) to determine the relative contribution of these various cytokines and their ability to coordinate an effective host response. Major strides have been made toward understanding the involvement of cytokines in infectious disease, cancer, and autoimmune disease. Here, we will focus briefly on the increasing body of work devoted to infectious disease research.

The importance of cytokines in mounting a host response to bacterial, protozoan, or viral pathogens is becoming increasingly clear in light of intensified research efforts during the past few years. With the use of detection technologies discussed in this chapter, as well as animal models of disease and in vitro methodology, specific cytokines have been found to have a major impact on the control of immunologic responses to these pathogens. Murine models of disease pathogenesis have commonly been used for this purpose, showing cytokine responses to accompany a majority of experimentally induced infectious diseases. Perhaps the best understood disease-mediated cytokine response is that mounted during gram-negative bacterial sepsis, as previously described. However, work with bacterial pathogens such as *Mycobacterium tuberculosis*, *Listeria monocytogenes*, group B streptococci, *Campylobacter jejuni*, and *Legionella pneumophila* has shown that cytokines such as TNF, IL-1, and IL-6 also are involved in the host response to these organisms. Furthermore, a number of studies also have centered on the importance of TH1 and TH2 cells in regulating the host response to some of these bacteria. Experimental infection with protozoan pathogens, such as *Schistosoma mansoni*, *Leishmania* spp., and *Plasmodium falciparum*, has been found to elicit a potent cytokine response, efficiently modulating the outcome of these infections.

Summary

Cellular communication is a critical aspect of any coordinated immune or inflammatory response and generally involves cell-to-cell contact and/or cell stimulation by soluble mediators. Cell-to-cell contact results in the release of cytokines that direct cellular function or elicit the recruitment of cells. Numerous cytokines have been identified and their biologic functions characterized. However, it is certain that new compounds belonging to this family of molecules will continue to be discovered. These molecules have wide-ranging activities but exhibit an amazing degree of redundancy in these functions. It is now clear that almost every type of host response, including immune and inflammatory responses, is mediated to some degree by cytokines. Two different subsets of CD4[+] cells (TH1 and TH2 cells) have recently been described that were characterized on the basis of their cytokine profiles. The regulatory activities displayed by the cytokines produced by TH1 and TH2 cells play a major role in controlling the immune response to a variety of infectious diseases. Cell-adhesion molecules, such as LFA-1 and ICAM-1, as well as VLA-4 and VCAM-1, found on lymphocytes and leukocytes, have been found to participate in antigen-dependent and antigen-independent T-cell responses. These and other cell-adhesion molecules are also important in cell-to-cell interactions that control binding of lymphocytes and leukocytes to endothelial cells lining blood vessels and potentiate extravasation of these cells out of blood vessels and into surrounding tissues during inflammatory processes. The selectins, another family of cell-adhesion molecules, have also been found to promote extravasation of these cell types.

Suggested Reading

Alexander, W. S. 2002. Suppressors of cytokine signalling (SOCS) in the immune system. *Nat. Rev. Immunol.* 2:410–416.

Bodmer, J. L., P. Schneider, and J. Tschopp. 2002. The molecular architecture of the TNF superfamily. *Trends Biochem. Sci.* 27:19–26.

Bromley, S. K., W. R. Burack, K. G. Johnson, K. Somersalo, T. N. Sims, C. Sumen, M. M. Davis, A. S. Shaw, P. M. Allen, and M. L. Dustin. 2001. The immunological synapse. *Annu. Rev. Immunol.* 19:375–396.

Colonna, M., A. Krug, and M. Cella. 2002. Interferon-producing cells: on the front line in immune responses against pathogens. *Curr. Opin. Immunol.* 14:373–379.

Dinarello, C. A. 2000. Proinflammatory cytokines. *Chest* 118:503–508.

Ellery, J. M., and P. J. Nicholls. 2002. Alternate signalling pathways from the interleukin-2 receptor. *Cytokine Growth Factor Rev.* 13:27–40.

Kisseleva, T., S. Bhattacharya, J. Braunstein, and C. W. Schindler. 2002. Signaling through the JAK/STAT pathway, recent advances and future challenges. *Gene* 285:1–24.

Liew, F. Y., and I. B. McInnes. 2002. The role of innate mediators in inflammatory responses. *Mol. Immunol.* 38:887–890.

Moore, K. W., R. de Waal Malefyt, R. L. Coffman, and A. O'Garra. 2001. Interleukin-10 and the interleukin-10 receptor. *Annu. Rev. Immunol.* 19:683–765.

Proudfoot, A. E. 2002. Chemokine receptors: multifaceted therapeutic targets. *Nat. Rev. Immunol.* 2:106–115.

Pulendran, B., K. Palucka, and J. Banchereau. 2001. Sensing pathogens and tuning immune responses. *Science* 293:253–256.

Robertson, M. J. 2002. Role of chemokines in the biology of natural killer cells. *J. Leukoc. Biol.* 71:173–183.

IMMUNOLOGIC EFFECTOR SYSTEMS AND IMMUNITY TO INFECTION

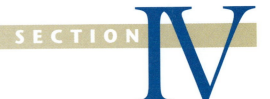

SECTION IV

Cell-Mediated Immunity

William R. Green

Fundamental Aspects of Cell-Mediated Immunity

Cell-mediated immunity (CMI), also known as *cellular immunity*, is a historical definition that now serves to distinguish immune responses that are mediated by cells at the effector phase from those mediated by antibodies in the humoral arm of the immune response. The cells classically associated with CMI are T cells and phagocytic cells, particularly the macrophage (Fig. 16.1). Macrophages and other professional antigen-presenting cells (APCs), including dendritic cells (DCs), are also involved in the generation of CMI responses, as they are involved in generation of antibody responses. Therefore, CMI most meaningfully refers to an effector phase where the T cells provide the specificity for the immune recognition reactions while the phagocytes act on the antigen to kill or inactivate it.

In many settings, CMI responses are needed to kill an intracellular infectious microbe that is often referred to as a facultative intracellular parasite to distinguish it from an obligate intracellular parasite such as a virus. Facultative parasites can live either inside or outside eukaryotic cells. Most facultative intracellular parasites normally infect and grow in a tissue-fixed macrophage or mobile APC in the absence of sufficient CMI. When a CMI response is made, antigen-specific T cells become activated, proliferate, and differentiate to recognize antigenic fragments derived from products made by the intracellular organism presented on major histocompatibility complex (MHC) molecules. What the phagocytes do is become activated by factors secreted by the immune T cells, principally cytokines and chemokines, to become more efficient at killing the intracellular parasite that had

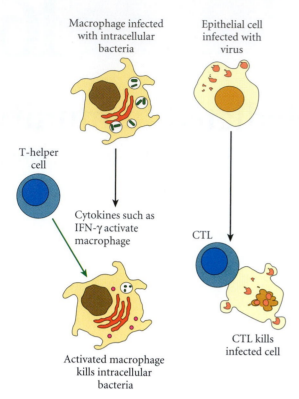

Macrophage infected with intracellular bacteria

Epithelial cell infected with virus

T-helper cell

Cytokines such as IFN-γ activate macrophage

CTL

Activated macrophage kills intracellular bacteria

CTL kills infected cell

Figure 16.1 A synopsis of the elements of CMI. (**Left**) TH cells can provide cytokines to assist in the activation of macrophages. (**Right**) CTLs can kill altered self cells such as tumor cells or virally infected cells.

been successfully surviving within the infected cell. Both T helper (TH) cells, typically CD4$^+$ T cells, and cytotoxic T lymphocytes (CTLs), usually CD8$^+$ T cells, are involved in CMI effector reactions. Of the TH cells, CMI is normally associated with the TH1 subpopulation of T cells, although TH2-type cells, normally associated with the generation of antibody responses, can be involved in CMI in some settings. Because immune responses to microbes that produce many different kinds of antigens and antigenic epitopes generally lead to both antibody- and cell-mediated effector mechanisms, CMI is also typically used to refer to a response in which antibody plays a secondary role in immunity or the actual protective component of the response is mediated by activated cells

The specific CMI reaction known as delayed-type hypersensitivity (DTH) refers to the immune response wherein antigen-specific, CD4$^+$ T cells secrete factors that activate phagocytes. In DTH, microbial antigens presented on the MHC molecules of infected cells are recognized by antigen-specific T cells via their T-cell receptor (TCR) and this causes the T cell to produce soluble factors. Receptors on macrophages and other phagocytic cells bind the factors, leading to activation of the phagocyte. DTH reactions can also be directed at nonliving

antigenic stimuli. Tuberculin tests administered into the dermis of the arm to detect the presence of active tuberculosis are positive when an infected individual's T cells react with MHC-presented fragments of the test antigen, secrete soluble factors, activate local skin phagocytes, and elicit a DTH reaction at the site of injection. This is seen as a red (erythemous), raised area. Poison oak and poison ivy skin sensitivities are also due to DTH reactions.

Another form of CMI involves CTLs, which can kill infected cells and sometimes microbes growing inside the cells. CTLs are able to lyse the infected cell and either directly kill the infecting organism or limit microbial growth via target-cell destruction. For some important intracellular pathogens the CTL releases a factor known as granulysin, which directly kills the infecting organism. CTLs are also able to destroy cells infected with viruses, which are obligate intracellular parasites. This prevents their further growth and spread. For viral infections, antibodies mediate immunity to the establishment of infection whereas CMI mediates resolution of infection. This situation demonstrates how the two major arms of the immune response are complementary via different functional mechanisms.

History

Many of the early experimental systems that served to define the principles of CMI were derived for the study of microbial infections, especially those caused by intracellular bacteria such as *Mycobacterium tuberculosis*. The concept of CMI arose in the 1890s with the work of Elie Metchnikoff, who studied the nature of the cellular response of the host to foreign invasion. He coined the term *microphages*, now known to correspond to polymorphonuclear leukocytes (PMNs or neutrophils), as well as the term *macrophages*. In the early 1900s, H. Zinsser defined the term *bacterial allergy*, which corresponded to his observations that infiltration of mononuclear cells (monocytes and lymphocytes) could lead to the development of local tissue necrosis. In the 1930s and 1940s, K. Landsteiner, F. Jacobs, and M. Chase described reactions involving cellular infiltration invoked by painting skin with chemicals and demonstrated that such reactivity could be transferred from an immune to a naive animal by splenic cells but not by serum containing antibody. G. Mackaness showed in the 1950s that resistance to the intracellular bacterium *Listeria monocytogenes* also was transferred to nonimmune animals only by cells. Eventually it came to be appreciated that T lymphocytes were the key cells in these adoptive transfer experiments. In 1960, A. Govaerts, using a transplantation model in which tissues were transferred between genetically different dogs, demonstrated the properties of CTLs, i.e., lysis of target cells that bear antigens against which the CTLs are directed. Not just with respect to CTLs, but in general, transplantation reactions have been shown to be mediated primarily by T cells and CMI. One exception is the antibody-mediated hyperacute form of tissue rejection. Because transplantation was recognized as a nonphysiologic situation, it was first envisioned that the real function of cells involved in transplantation reactions was immune surveillance against tumors. It is now generally accepted that protection against acute microbial infections, rather than against developing neoplasia, represents the major function of CMI. The recent increase in the incidence of certain infectious diseases due to the emergence of new microbes and the prevalence of human immunodeficiency virus (HIV)-caused immunodeficiency have led to a renewed emphasis on cellular immunity. Many of the pathogens that cause infections in patients with acquired immunodeficiency syndrome (AIDS) are those normally controlled by CMI.

Overlap of Cell-Mediated and Humoral Immunity

A hallmark of CMI reactions is that the critical immune effector reactions are mediated by cells, not by antibodies. However, for some CMI reactions, the antigenic specificity is provided by antibody, which then functions as a bridge between the effector cell and the target antigen. Enhancement of phagocytosis via opsonization (see Fig. 1.17) involves both antibody and phagocytes. Fc receptors (FcR) on cells, including certain nonphagocytic lymphocytes, provide additional connections between CMI and humoral immunity via *antibody-dependent cell-mediated cytotoxicity* (ADCC) (Fig. 16.2). In this reaction, FcR-bearing cells collectively called *K cells* bind antibodies and are then able to engage a target antigen and initiate an appropriate immune reaction that destroys and eliminates the antigen. In addition, antigen-antibody complexes may activate the complement cascade and thereby affect a variety of cells, through both the chemotactic and activation properties of complement fragments and the direct effects on phagocyte binding (via complement receptors) and phagocytosis. Regulation of immunity also uses a number of common mechanistic approaches involving molecular and cellular players that can function in both the humoral and cell-mediated immune systems.

Specific versus Nonspecific Cell-Mediated Immunity

Within the scope of CMI there are both *specific (adaptive)* and *innate* types of cellular immune reactions (Fig. 16.3). Innate CMI responses generally encompass the initial lo-

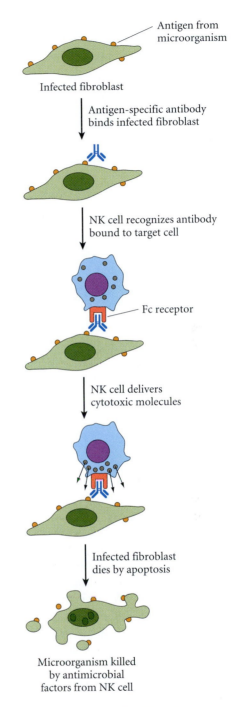

Figure 16.2 FcRs (in particular, FcγRIII or CD16) expressed on the surface of NK cells allow the NK cell to recognize antibody-coated target cells. Target cells recognized by this mechanism will be killed by the NK cell by ADCC.

cal inflammatory response following the introduction of a foreign substance. This response is mediated primarily by phagocytic PMNs, monocytes, and tissue macrophages and by other, nonphagocytic, cells. Another important component of nonspecific cellular immunity involves the

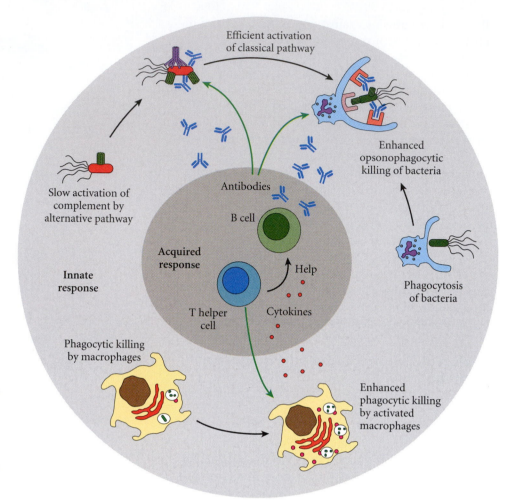

Figure 16.3 Although phagocytosis and complement activation are considered part of the innate (or nonspecific) immune response, products of the specific immune response can enhance the efficiency of these innate immune mechanisms. Antibodies produced by B lymphocytes can mediate classical pathway complement activation and opsonize targets for enhanced phagocytosis. T lymphocytes, particularly TH1 cells, can enhance phagocytic killing by macrophages through their elaboration of cytokines such as IFN-γ, which activates the macrophage.

reticuloendothelial system. In addition to including blood monocytes and macrophages recently extravasated from the blood into tissues, this system consists of connective tissue macrophages, also known as histiocytes, and resident (fixed) macrophages located in a number of organs, including the liver (known as Kupffer cells), alveolar macrophages of the lungs, and other tissues. The phagocytic and endocytic properties of these cells enable them to remove various microbial invaders and foreign substances from the blood and other tissue fluids.

Although some of these same nonspecific cells are subsequently involved in specific CMI, the responses differ qualitatively and quantitatively. Many intracellular pathogens survive and cause disease because shortly following infection they are ingested by sentinel macrophages and grow within them. These pathogens can effectively be eliminated when the same type of cell becomes activated following the emergence of antigen-specific T lymphocytes. For example, *L. monocytogenes* enters the body, infects macrophages, and grows and causes disease from

within the macrophages. But when T cells that recognize listeria antigens emerge, they secrete cytokines that activate the macrophages initiating the specific phase of CMI. The activated macrophages are able to restrict the intracellular multiplication of the bacteria (Fig. 16.4) and also to kill the infecting microbes. Thus, the antigen-specific phase of CMI is particularly effective against intracellular parasites. Interferon-gamma (IFN-γ) is a prominent T-cell factor that activates infected phagocytic cells. The macrophages must also receive a "priming" signal to make them optimally receptive to the activating effect of IFN-γ. This activating signal usually is provided either by certain microbial products, such as lipopolysaccharide (LPS) or lipopeptides, often acting through the Toll-like receptor signal transduction pathway (see Fig. 2.7), or by interaction of the CD40 ligand (CD154) on the T-cell surface with CD40 displayed by the macrophage (Fig. 16.5). T lymphocytes and other cells involved in CMI also produce *chemotactic factors*, which serve to guide phagocytic cells to sites of infection and inflammation.

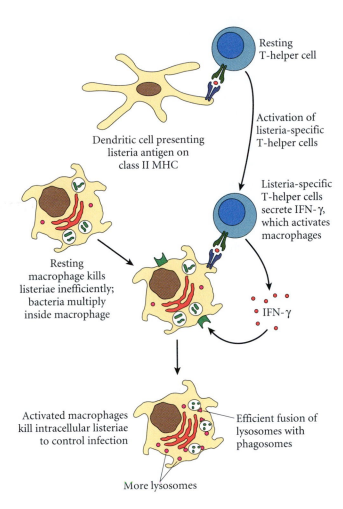

Figure 16.4 Activation of a macrophage not only enhances killing of newly phagocytosed bacteria but also can help a macrophage previously infected with intracellular pathogens (such as listeriae) destroy the pathogen. Upon activation, the macrophage fuses its lysosomes with bacteria-laden vesicles.

Resting T-helper cell

Activation of listeria-specific T-helper cells

Dendritic cell presenting listeria antigen on class II MHC

Listeria-specific T-helper cells secrete IFN-γ, which activates macrophages

Resting macrophage kills listeriae inefficiently; bacteria multiply inside macrophage

IFN-γ

Activated macrophages kill intracellular listeriae to control infection

Efficient fusion of lysosomes with phagosomes

More lysosomes

When foreign antigens are presented by MHC class I molecules, CTLs are the only lytic cells associated with specific CMI per se. Although most CTLs are CD8$^+$, up to 10% or so of CD4$^+$ can be cytotoxic to target cells. Cytotoxicity is mediated by TCR recognition of MHC-peptide on the target cell. Other cytolytic cells, such as natural killer (NK) cells and K cells mediating ADCC, may be involved in some effector aspects of CMI but are considered nonspecific due to their lack of intracellular production of antigen-recognition molecules like TCR (Fig. 16.6). Of course, acquisition of soluble antibody by binding to FcR on these cells gives a type of specificity for cytotoxic activity. NK cells also mediate antibody-independent "natural killing" of virus-infected cells and certain tumor cells due to the interaction of killer-cell activating and inhibitory receptors, which represent another aspect of CMI leading to lysis of cells by recognition of surface molecules expressed on the effector and target.

Other cells of the immune system similarly straddle the border of specific and nonspecific recognition and may have important roles in CMI. One class of these is NKT cells, a subpopulation of T cells that share some characteristics with NK cells. One characteristic is the expression on both cell types of the NK 1.1 marker (mouse) or NKR-P1 (human). NKT cells express CD3 and TCR, but they have a very limited diversity in their TCR usage. Many NKT cells

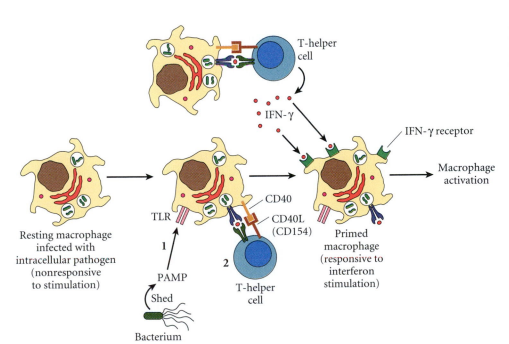

Figure 16.5 Activation of the macrophage by a TH1 cell involves an initial priming step and a subsequent cytokine-mediated step. Priming is essential for making the macrophage responsive to the cytokine IFN-γ and can occur either by binding of pathogen-associated molecular pattern (PAMP) to a Toll-like receptor (TLR) (1) or by engagement of macrophage CD40 protein by CD154 on TH cells (2).

T-helper cell

IFN-γ

IFN-γ receptor

Macrophage activation

CD40

CD40L (CD154)

TLR

1

2

PAMP

Shed

Bacterium

T-helper cell

Resting macrophage infected with intracellular pathogen (nonresponsive to stimulation)

Primed macrophage (responsive to interferon stimulation)

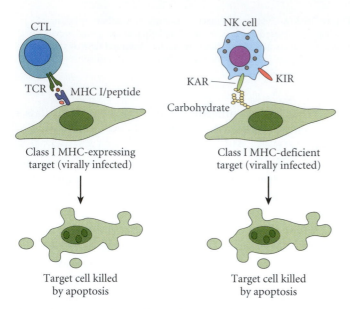

Figure 16.6 Both CTLs and NK cells are capable of cell-mediated cytotoxicity. However, of these two cell types, only the CTL can carry out cytotoxicity in an antigen-specific manner. NK cells have a much more general mechanism of target-cell recognition. NK cells usually engage their target cell by the killer activational receptor (KAR), which binds carbohydrates on the target cell surface. Killing is inhibited if the killer inhibitory receptor (KIR) binds MHC class I protein on the target cell. Thus, by this mechanism NK cells kill targets with abnormal expression of MHC class I.

lack both CD4 and CD8 (double-negative cells), but some do express CD4. They are found in different tissues and in high numbers in the liver. NKT cells recognize antigenic glycopeptides presented by CD1d MHC class I-like molecules of both humans and mice. However, it is not clear exactly how they mediate their effects. Because NKT cells produce high levels of interleukin-4 (IL-4), IFN-γ, and tumor necrosis factor (TNF) following antigenic stimuli, they may be involved both in regulation of other T cells and as effectors of CMI. Skewing of TH cell responses toward a TH2 phenotype is one reported regulatory function of NKT cells. As for effector functions, NKT cells can prevent autoimmune diabetes in diabetes-prone mice, promote resistance to a number of infectious agents, and mediate cytotoxicity against tumor cells growing in the lab. However, many of the determinants of NKT cell function, such as the need for costimulation, the types of signal transduction mechanisms, and the nature of the ligands that activate these cells are not yet known.

Initiating Cell-Mediated Immunity

Eliciting the different types of effector CMI responses depends on the response to foreign antigen that occurs in the inductive and regulatory phases of the immune response. The nature and dose of the antigen, route of antigen entry, and the type of APC presenting the antigen are important in determining the kind of CMI responses produced. The impact of APCs on the generation of different CMI responses is mediated by the effects of APC factors involved in T-cell activation, notably cytokines and cell surface ligands such as CD80 and CD86 for the CD28 receptor on T cells. APC–T-cell interactions can be very influential in determining if a TH1 or TH2 immune response develops, often based on the profile of cytokines produced. The classic TH1 cytokines—IFN-γ, IL-2, and TNF-β or lymphotoxin (LT)—favor CMI, including inflammation and DTH reactions (Fig. 16.7). Production of IFN-γ is especially important because it both promotes (via augmentation of IL-12 production) the differentiation of uncommitted CD4$^+$ TH0 cells to the TH1 pathway and inhibits differentiation to the TH2 subset. As noted earlier, IFN-γ also activates macrophages to become microbicidal to intracellular microbes that have undergone phagocytosis. Production of IL-2 by CD4$^+$ TH1 cells serves to promote both the expansion of this T-cell subset and the growth and differentiation of CD8$^+$ CTLs. Production of cytokines such as IL-12 by macrophages and DCs also strongly favors CMI. Secretion of IL-12 by macrophages can occur early in the immune response via direct stimulation by microbial products or indirectly via stimulation by IFN-γ produced by NK cells. A number of activities of IL-12 enhance CMI, including the augmentation of the differentiation of CD4$^+$ TH0 cells down the TH1 pathway, promotion of cytolytic function of CTLs and NK cells, and stimulation of additional production of IFN-γ.

IFN-γ production by APCs appears to initiate the development of TH1 cells from the uncommitted TH0 cells by stimulating production of a transcription factor known as T-bet (Fig. 16.8). T-bet activation in TH cells promotes the transcription of IFN-γ and IL-12 receptor genes. This allows the IL-12 produced by the APC to function as both a cell survival and growth signal for the T cell. The T-bet factor also prolongs IFN-γ production by the T cell, which mediates, in part, the function of the TH1 subset. T-bet counteracts the development of TH2 cells, which require another transcription factor known as GATA-3 for their activity. IL-12 also promotes the production of IL-18 and IL-18 receptors, which contribute to the development of a TH1 response. Another transcription factor involved in TH1 development is STAT4 (signal transducer and activator of transcription 4). Thus, numerous cytokines and their receptors contribute to the development of CMI effectors.

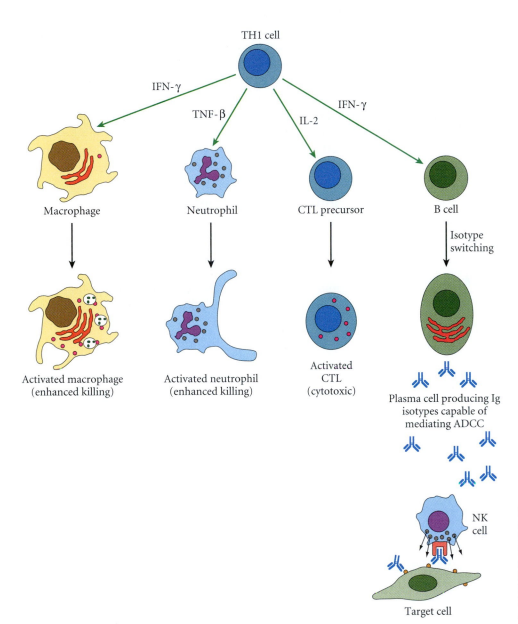

TH1 cell

IFN-γ

TNF-β

IL-2

IFN-γ

Macrophage

Neutrophil

CTL precursor

B cell

Isotype switching

Activated macrophage (enhanced killing)

Activated neutrophil (enhanced killing)

Activated CTL (cytotoxic)

Plasma cell producing Ig isotypes capable of mediating ADCC

NK cell

Target cell

Figure 16.7 Through the secretion of cytokines such as IFN-γ, TNF-β/LT, and IL-2, TH1 cells orchestrate CMI by enhancing the activity of macrophages, neutrophils, and CTLs. Further, TH1 cells can enhance CMI by causing B cells to produce antibody isotypes capable of mediating ADCC.

DTH Reactions

The original definition of DTH was based on immunologic reactions that showed responses peaking at 24 to 48 (sometimes 72) hours after administration of antigen. The use of the term hypersensitivity was predicated on these reactions occurring in immune or hypersensitive individuals. DTH reactions contrast with immediate hypersensitivity reactions, such as those mediating allergies, and manifest themselves within minutes of contact with antigen. As it turned out, DTH reactions are due to specific T-cell responses to antigen, whereas immediate hypersensitivity is due to antibody-mediated reactions. The DTH reaction underlies the tuberculin skin test used to detect tuberculo-

sis: intradermal injection of a purified protein derivative from *M. tuberculosis* stimulates accumulation of memory T cells and activation of local macrophages in infected or previously exposed individuals. The T cells give rise to the red and indurated skin area in about 48 hours, indicative of a positive reaction. A chest X-ray is then needed to distinguish those with active tuberculosis from those merely exposed or previously vaccinated but without active disease.

Characteristics of the DTH Reaction

It is clear that antigen-specific T cells orchestrate the DTH reaction even though they are typically a very small percentage of the total cells present in a lesion. Most of the

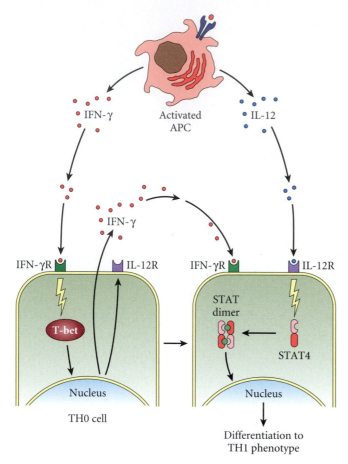

Figure 16.8 Differentiation to the TH1 phenotype begins when a noncommitted TH cell (TH0) binds IFN-γ, triggering a signal transduction cascade that depends on the transcription factor T-bet. This event leads to some TH1 functions (the secretion of IFN-γ) and to acquisition of responsiveness to IL-12 by expression of the IL-12 receptor (IL-12R) on the T cell. Subsequent binding of IL-12 (also produced by APCs) completes the differentiation process by a mechanism that requires the signal transducer protein STAT4. Upon IL-12 binding, STAT4 is phosphorylated, causing dimerization of STAT4 and its translocation to the T cell's nucleus.

cellular infiltrate (>90%) consists of nonspecific effector cells. The specific T cells recruit and activate large numbers of other cells, especially normal macrophages, via chemotaxins and cytokines such as INF-γ. It is convenient to divide DTH into several sequential but overlapping phases: (i) an *induction phase* in which naive (initial or priming response) or memory (actual DTH reaction) T cells recognize their cognate MHC-plus-peptide complex as presented by an APC and are activated; (ii) an *inflammatory phase* during which leukocytes extravasate and accumulate in the affected tissue; (iii) an *effector phase* in which activated macrophages kill the intracellular microbe; and (sometimes) (iv) a *chronic DTH reaction* to certain persistent sources of antigen, such as mycobacterial infections, which are classically characterized by *granu-*

loma formation. Granulomas represent walled-off portions of a tissue within which microbes are trapped in an attempt to keep them from spreading but can also form in response to antigens that the body cannot readily eliminate. Tissue pathology resulting from a DTH response is often due to collateral damage to the surrounding tissues, whether there is a full resolution of infection due to the DTH reaction or infection is contained but not eliminated due to formation of granulomas (Fig. 16.9).

Induction and manifestation of DTH

In primary responses that sensitize for DTH reactions, microbe-derived foreign peptides or possibly glycopeptides are presented by MHC class II to naive antigen-specific CD4$^+$ T cells. Along with attendant costimulation and proper cytokine and cytokine-receptor production, such antigen presentation leads to activation of the responding T cells (Fig. 16.10). These T cells proliferate and differentiate, some becoming helper cells, some becoming memory cells, and some becoming effector T cells such as T$_{DTH}$ cells and CTL. The overall physiology of antigen processing and presentation is fairly well understood, and what is now emerging is the molecular and cellular basis for development of effector TH1 cells, such as production of IL-1, IL-18, their attendant receptors, and activation of specific transcription factors. It is still not entirely clear how a particular microbial antigen can influence these processes. One major factor is likely the way in which microbial antigens are encountered by an APC; those produced within an infected macrophage or similar APC likely promote the production of the cytokines needed for a TH1-based CMI response. In contrast, antigens encountered from outside the APC, such as those made by extracellular bacterial pathogens, provide signals for development of TH2 antibody-mediated responses. Obviously, for the APCs to present MHC class II-restricted endogenous antigens they must have some way to traffic these antigens into the endosomal presentation pathway. Alternately, microbial antigens acquired endocytically or phagocytically by an APC from an infected cell that dies and lyses or undergoes apoptosis in response to infection could be the initiator of CMI.

The DTH reaction in an immune host is also initiated by antigen presentation, but because of the presence of memory T cells, either resident or quickly recruited into the site of infection, the DTH reaction can be activated to eliminate antigens before they can be too harmful. Memory T cells have a much less stringent need for costimulation, so merely engaging their TCR without any other costimulatory factors is often sufficient to cause the T cells to secrete activating cytokines. In addition, a recall DTH response to antigen can occur rapidly in nonlymphatic, peripheral tissues, not just in the lymph nodes. This indicates that APC presentation of antigen and activation of memory T cells already present in a tissue can initiate the early part of CMI, as opposed to needing effector cells to migrate into the area of infection. Tissue macrophages and microvascular endothelial cells lining capillaries and postcapillary venules are likely to be key APCs in the memory DTH response and can additionally be activated by microbial products to be particularly potent phagocytes. Once the DTH response is initiated, cellular infiltration from outside the infected site can occur to sustain the protective inflammatory reaction. Microvascular endothelial cells in the blood vessels of the infected tissue directly interface with circulating memory T cells and other inflammatory cells, leading to their extravasation to enhance the immune response occurring in response to the antigenic challenge.

Inflammation in DTH

Inflammation is a characteristic of both the initial encounter with an antigen, which can prime or initiate the CMI response, and the CMI recall response itself, involving antigen-specific immune reactions. Priming can occur with an inapparent (or subclinical) infection, without any awareness of inflammation. During a recall response to antigen, however, the presence of memory and expanded numbers of effector T cells results in quantitative and qualitative changes leading to a more extensive inflamma-

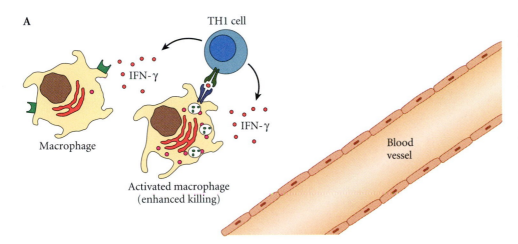

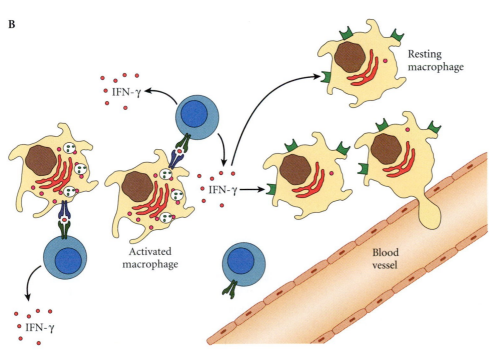

Figure 16.9 The DTH reaction is initiated when macrophages phagocytose antigen and present it to TH1 cells (**A**), the latter of which then secrete cytokines that recruit more macrophages and TH1 cells to the area. The cytokines also activate local macrophages (**B**). If there is a chronic source of antigen, this may ultimately lead to a large mass of activated macrophages and TH1 cells, called a granuloma.

C

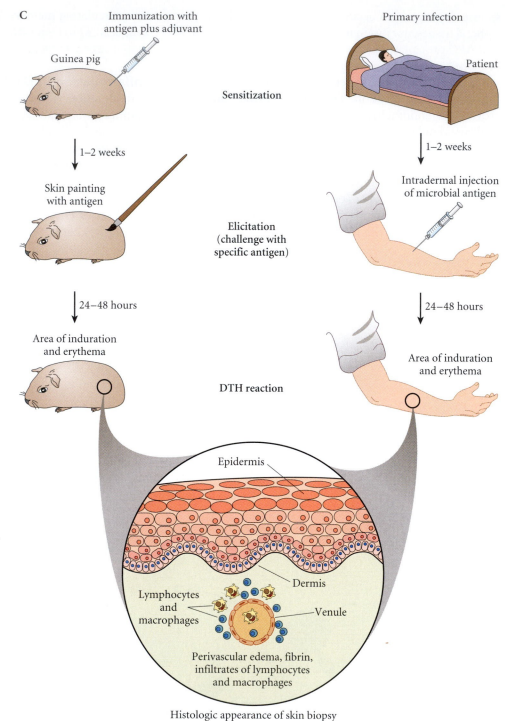

Immunization with antigen plus adjuvant

Guinea pig

Primary infection

Patient

Sensitization

1–2 weeks

1–2 weeks

Skin painting with antigen

Elicitation (challenge with specific antigen)

Intradermal injection of microbial antigen

24–48 hours

24–48 hours

Area of induration and erythema

DTH reaction

Area of induration and erythema

Epidermis

Dermis

Lymphocytes and macrophages

Venule

Perivascular edema, fibrin, infiltrates of lymphocytes and macrophages

Histologic appearance of skin biopsy

Figure 16.9 *(continued)* (C) In live animals, a DTH reaction is observed only after induction of T-cell memory by prior exposure (sensitization) to the antigen. In animals (**left**) this can be accomplished by injection of the antigen, whereas in humans (**right**) this usually occurs by infection with a microorganism such as a mycobacterium. Secondary exposure of the skin to the antigen results in a detectable, red, inflamed, and indurated area. Intentional introduction of the antigen on the skin can be used as an easy and inexpensive test for primary exposure and is the basis of one currently used test for tuberculosis.

tory process than occurs following an initial encounter with antigen. In a primary response the cytokine production necessary to initiate inflammation and infiltration of the site first by PMNs (and eosinophils) and then by mononuclear (monocyte and lymphocyte) cells is triggered primarily by microbial products such as LPS. In contrast, in a recall response, the ability of memory T cells to recognize antigen presented by APCs allows these T cells to accumulate rapidly at the vascular area of the antigenic challenge. Activation of these memory T cells results both in their efficient signaling of endothelial cells through cell surface receptors and production of cytokines that enhance the recruitment and extravasation of PMNs and mononuclear cells. Among the cell surface in-

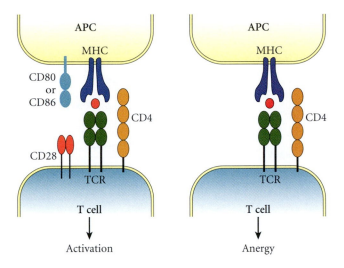

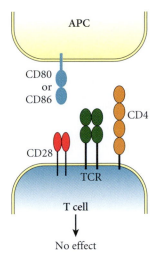

Figure 16.10 For a naive T cell to be activated it must receive two signals from an APC. Signal 1 is the binding of the TCR to MHC-peptide complexes, while signal 2 is the costimulatory signal, which is usually delivered by binding of the CD28 protein of the T cell by the CD80 or CD86 protein of the APC. Delivery of signal 2 alone has no effect on the T cell, whereas delivery of signal 1 alone causes the T cell to enter a state of antigen-specific inactivity called *anergy*.

teractions, the activation molecule CD40 ligand (CD154) of CD4$^+$ T cells plays a major role in that microvascular endothelial cells, as well as professional APCs, express the complementary CD40 receptor. Together with cytokines produced by memory T cells, including TNF-α, TNF-β (LT), and to a lesser extent, IFN-γ, this cell surface signaling causes endothelial cells to initiate several functions that contribute to the accumulation of cells that are critical for eliciting the inflammation associated with DTH.

First, activated endothelial cells enhance local blood flow by their expression of nitric oxide (NO), prostacyclin, and other agents that function as vasodilators. The supply of blood, and hence of inflammatory leukocytes, is thus increased to maximize the potential for extravasation of these cells. Second, the density of cell surface molecules is augmented in activated endothelial cells, resulting in the adherence, first of PMNs and later of monocytes and lymphocytes, to the vascular wall. Endothelial cells on the venule side of the capillaries, analogous to the cells of the high endothelial venules of lymph nodes, are particularly effective in tethering emigrating cells via increased expression of adhesion molecules (Fig. 16.11). Endothelial cells display different adhesion molecules in a sequential manner corresponding to the different waves of extravasating cells. Early PMN recruitment is due to production of endothelial-leukocyte adhesion molecule 1 (ELAM-1, E-selectin, or CD62E), P-selectin, and intracellular adhesion molecule 1 (ICAM-1, CD54). Recruitment of lymphocytes and monocytes is promoted by production of vascular cell adhesion molecule 1 (VCAM-1, CD106) along with an increased level of ICAM-1 (Fig. 16.12). The corresponding ligands on the circulating cells are the integrins VLA-4 (CD49d/CD29) for VCAM-1 and MAC-1 (CD11b/CD18) for ICAM-1. Because one of the ligands of MAC-1, ICAM-

1, is present constitutively on endothelial cells, monocytes adhere and their emigration begins shortly after that of PMNs. Subsequently, binding of monocytes to endothelial cells is sustained and enhanced by the increased levels of ICAM-1. Like monocytes/macrophages, memory CD4$^+$ TH1 cells also express VLA-4 and also LFA-1 (CD11a/CD18), another β$_2$-integrin capable of binding ICAM-1. T-cell infiltration thus can begin early but increases rapidly during the 6- to 12-hour time span and peaks at about 24 to 36 hours. In addition, the constitutive expression by endothelial cells of ICAM-2, which is bound by LFA-1 but not by MAC-1, provides a complementary mechanism that may help T cells bind to the affected microvasculature. Finally, other adhesion-molecule pairs may be involved in PMN, monocyte, and/or T-cell adherence to endothelial cells. For example, PMNs and monocytes/macrophages also express L-selectin (CD62L), which is central to the binding of T lymphocytes to the high endothelial venules of lymph nodes; and activated endothelial cells express P-selectin (CD62P), which also binds sialyl Lewis^x groups. In addition, both PMNs and monocytes/macrophages display LFA-1 on their surfaces and thus can bind to the ICAMs (-1, -2, and -3) (Fig. 16.13).

Activated endothelial cells produce and secrete soluble factors, notably chemokines, that attract additional blood cells to the affected tissue. IL-8 and other members of the CXC chemokine family mediate PMN attraction and activation, and some CC chemokines, such as monocyte chemotactic protein 1, attract primarily monocytes, T cells, and eosinophils but not PMNs. In addition, CXC- and CC-type chemokines synthesized by other cell types (e.g., the CC chemokines are produced especially by activated T cells) can be bound by endothelial cell surface proteoglycans such that the chemokines can interact with

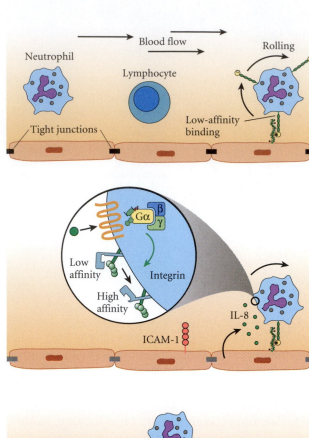

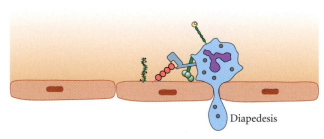

Figure 16.11 Inflammation requires the extravasation of leukocytes from the blood to the interstitial tissue. Extravasation proceeds in several steps, beginning with "rolling adhesion" (**top**) of the leukocyte by selectin-carbohydrate interactions. Most of these early interactions between the leukocyte and endothelial cell are low affinity. During inflammation, interendothelial cell tight junctions dissociate, inflammatory signals lead to the expression of additional adhesion molecules (such as ICAM-1) on the endothelium, and endothelial cells produce chemokines such as IL-8 (green circles) that act on the leukocyte to activate integrin proteins to their high-affinity form (**inset**). This activation event is initiated when the chemokine binds its receptor (orange) on the leukocyte membrane and triggers a G-protein-dependent signaling cascade. Following high-affinity binding, the leukocyte arrests on the endothelial cell surface and leaves the vasculature by *diapedesis*.

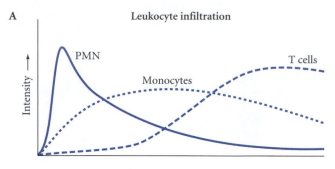

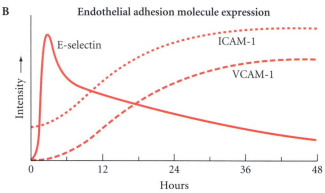

Figure 16.12 (**A**) Neutrophils (PMNs) are the first cells to extravasate to the interstitial tissue. (**B**) This correlates with the early expression of E-selectin on vascular endothelium, which binds to sialyl Lewis^x carbohydrate moieties on the surface of the PMN.

attached migrating cells. Similarly, other activated T-cell-secreted products and CD40L-mediated, contact-dependent signaling induce endothelial cells to alter their morphology and relationship to the basement membrane to facilitate extravasation. These changes are coupled with reorganization of the distribution of endothelial cell-adhesion molecules. Together, these processes facilitate the extravasation of migrating cells and the leakage of plasma molecules into the tissue. Conversion of plasma fibrinogen to fibrin in the affected tissue and fibronectin produce a physical framework that both assists cell emigration and traps cells and fluid, leading to the classic induration characteristic of DTH reactions.

Once in the tissues, other processes help retain the newly emigrated leukocytes at the extravascular site. Retention is cell type specific. PMNs are the first cells to extravasculate in large numbers but are short-lived cells, and their numbers decline relatively early in the CMI inflammatory response with replacement by larger numbers of macrophages and by some T cells. After the accumulation phase, both macrophages and lymphocytes persist in the tissues for many hours before their numbers start to decline gradually, due to death or exit from the tissues via the afferent lymphatics, starting at about 36 to 48 hours after antigen introduction. Retention of macrophages in

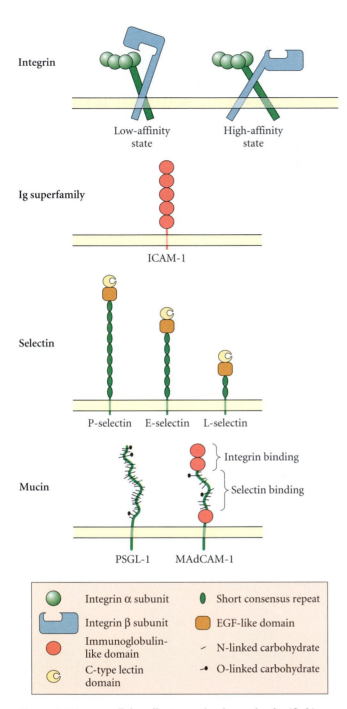

Integrin

Low-affinity
state

High-affinity
state

Ig superfamily

ICAM-1

Selectin

P-selectin   E-selectin   L-selectin

Mucin

Integrin binding

Selectin binding

PSGL-1   MAdCAM-1

	Integrin α subunit		Short consensus repeat
	Integrin β subunit		EGF-like domain
	Immunoglobulin-like domain		N-linked carbohydrate
	C-type lectin domain		O-linked carbohydrate

Figure 16.13 Intercellular adhesion molecules can be classified into several categories on the basis of their structure and function. Molecules of the integrin family bind to Ig superfamily receptors with either low or high affinity, depending on the integrin's activation state. Selectin molecules bind to carbohydrate moieties of mucins via the calcium-dependent (C-type) lectin domain. The mucin MAdCAM (mucosal addressin cell adhesion molecule) is unusual in that it can bind to both integrins (via its Ig-like domains) and selectins (via its carbohydrate moieties).

the tissues is the result of, to some extent, intrinsic characteristics related to their differentiation from blood monocytes to macrophages concomitant with extravasation and the subsequent activation during the DTH effector phase. In addition, macrophage retention is affected by the products of other cells, including activated T-cell-secreted *macrophage inhibitory factor,* one of the earliest described cytokines. Similarly, T-cell activation by antigen leads to an increase in the affinity of the adhesion molecule LFA-1 and to the expression of other adhesion molecules, including those with specificity for extracellular matrix molecules (e.g., collagen, fibronectin, and laminin). Specific T-cell retention works together with antigen-driven clonal expansion to dramatically increase the frequency of antigen-specific T cells in the DTH lesion. Despite this enrichment, the vast majority of the T cells in the affected tissue are not specific for the inciting antigens.

The effector phase

The key cells of the effector phase of the DTH reaction are antigen-specific T cells and macrophages. The T cells provide the antigen recognition and soluble factors needed to activate the effector macrophages and similar phagocytes, the end result of which is greatly enhanced killing of intracellular microbes or containment of other antigens. In some cases there is both a DTH component of immunity and a CTL component. For example, CMI responses to viral infections can lead to direct cytolysis of infected cells by $CD8^+$ CTLs as well as a cell-activating effector phase that inhibits viral growth inside infected cells.

Macrophage activation is primarily mediated by cytokines, particularly IFN-γ, although other cytokines, principally granulocyte-macrophage colony-stimulating factor (GM-CSF), IL-1, TNF-α, and TNF-β/LT, have activating properties. Also, the macrophage must be able to respond to IFN-γ and other cytokines by having the proper receptor. Contact-dependent mechanisms involving the ligation of T-cell surface CD40L (CD154) with CD40 on the macrophage membrane can also promote the effector phase of CMI. Moreover, IFN-γ-activated macrophages have increased levels of Fcγ receptors that promote phagocytosis of opsonized particles and enhanced antigen presentation capacities. Activated macrophages have increased levels of MHC class II, augmentation of class I expression, increased costimulatory ligand display, and other factors. The net result is a positive loop whereby $CD4^+$ TH1 cells that efficiently recognize their cognate foreign peptide-MHC class II complex on the macrophage surface optimally express CD40L and produce IFN-γ to maintain macrophage activation. Microbial products that are active at extremely dilute concentrations can also contribute to enhanced macrophage effector function, and recent evidence has identified CD1-restricted T-cell responses to microbial glycolipids as mediators of macrophage activation in DTH. In addition, certain cytokines, such as TNF-α and IL-1, can synergize with IFN-γ to promote at least some heightened functions characteristic of activated macrophages. Extracellular matrix proteins can be bound by various macrophage cell surface receptors and also prime macrophages to respond to IFN-γ.

Activated macrophages are defined by their enhanced ability to perform one or more functions correlated with removal of foreign antigenic insults and successful resolution of the DTH reaction (Fig. 16.14). Enhanced endocytosis of microbial antigens and phagocytosis of opsonized bacteria via increased FcγR expression are a well-known effector function of activated macrophages. There is also increased fusion of lysosomes to phagosomes within these cells, exposing living microbes to degradative lysosomal enzymes, antimicrobial peptides, and other toxic macrophage products. The activated macrophages are more efficient at killing microbes due to enhanced production of reactive oxygen intermediates (e.g., superoxide anion, hydrogen peroxide, hydroxyl radical) and reactive nitrogen intermediates such as NO. The activated macrophages are able to enhance the production of short-lived mediators of inflammation and also have an increased capacity to enzy-

matically act on other inflammatory molecules such as prostaglandins, leukotrienes, platelet-activating factor, and thrombin and tissue factors, which activate the clotting mechanism.

Because of the breadth of functions encompassed by the activation of macrophages, it is not surprising that some enhanced capabilities transcend the DTH reaction and apply to protective immunity in other contexts. For example, killing of tumor cells by activated macrophages is more efficient owing to several factors: increased FcγR expression and thus enhanced phagocytosis and ADCC; production of TNF-α, which both restricts the blood flow to solid tumors and has direct and indirect toxic effects on some tumor cells; and the production of NO. There is also evidence that NO can inhibit the replication of certain viruses. Production of IL-12 by activated macrophages enhances the activity of NK cells and CTLs against tumors and virus-infected cells. Similarly, IFN-α, produced mainly by mononuclear phagocytes, has a variety of both direct antiviral antiproliferative and indirect negative effects on tumor cells and virus-infected cells.

Beneficial effects of DTH reactions

CMI mediated via the DTH reaction is crucial for resistance to a variety of pathogenic microbes: facultative intracellular bacteria such as *L. monocytogenes*, *M. tuberculosis*, and others; fungi, such as *Candida* species, *Histoplasma capsulatum*, and *Cryptococcus neoformans*; certain protozoan parasites, including *Leishmania major* and *Toxoplasma gondii*; and some helminthic parasites such as *Schistosoma mansoni*. In some instances CMI is an effective mediator of immunity to viral infection. Like many situations regarding immunity to infection, DTH is not the only mediator of resistance: most viral infections are prevented by neutralizing antibodies, but CMI may be needed for recovery from infection; organisms such as *C. neoformans* can be opsonized by antibody to a surface polysaccharide for phagocytic killing, and there are even some examples in animal systems of antibody-mediated resistance to *M. tuberculosis*, the organism and infectious process that provide the strongest examples for the importance of CMI and DTH as immunologic effectors. Yet, there are numerous experimental and clinical observations that emphasize the importance of DTH in resistance and resolution of infection to many different types of pathogens.

Experimental data obtained with mice

Much of the experimental data implicating the importance of DTH come from adoptive transfer experiments in mice. In these situations, nonimmune mice or mice whose immune system is depleted by either genetic ma-

Figure 16.14 Some of the products of activated macrophages. The effects of each product are indicated with green arrows. $O_2 \cdot$, superoxide; H_2O_2, hydrogen peroxide; HOCl, hydrogen hypochlorite.

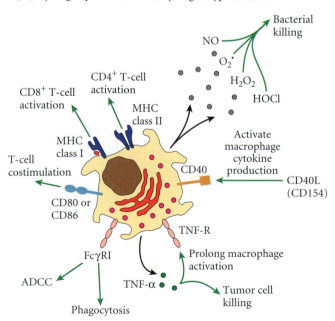

nipulation, antibody treatment to eliminate specific immune cell populations, or irradiation are injected with isogenic T cells, or subpopulations of T cells, then challenged with virulent pathogens. In these systems it is possible to clearly demonstrate the essential role of the CD4$^+$ TH cell compartment, and often cells are polarized to secrete either the TH1 or TH2 cytokine profile. When a specific subset of cells involved in DTH are depleted and there is increased susceptibility to infection, and when the provision of cells from an intact or immune animal reverses this increased susceptibility, there is strong evidence for a role for DTH in immunity to a particular pathogen. Similarly, since DTH relies heavily on production of cytokines, mice whose cytokine production has been disrupted by targeted gene deletions or by treatment with "blocking" antibodies to cytokines become very susceptible to certain infections. For example, IFN-γ gene knockout mice are unable to control a mycobacterial infection and die much more rapidly than mice able to produce IFN-γ in response to the infection (Fig. 16.15).

In some situations it has been possible to show that different inbred strains of mice characteristically mount dominating CMI-based TH1 or antibody-based TH2 responses to a pathogen, and this difference determines their resistance or susceptibility to infection with an intracellular microbe. The most studied and best documented dichotomous response is to the obligate intracellular protozoan parasite, *L. major*, whereby mice that can mount a TH1-dominated DTH response survive infection whereas those that mount a TH2-dominated antibody response are susceptible to infection. As *L. major* lives inside macrophages, it is likely at this stage that the differential factors leading to a TH1 (i.e., IL-12 and IFN-γ) or TH2 (IL-4, IL-5, and IL-10) response are elicited. In humans, where a range of *Leishmania* species cause an array of infections from mild cutaneous lesions to a fatal disease in heavily parasitized patients known as kala-azar (Hindi for "black fever," indicative of the gray color of skin), it is not clear if there is an underlying genetic basis giving rise to a TH1/TH2 dichotomy that influences the severity of infection and disease. Nonetheless, healing and resistance to reinfection in humans are correlated with mounting a strong TH1 response associated with production of IFN-γ and activation of macrophages.

DTH and human disease

There are numerous examples in human medicine of the importance of DTH in the clinical manifestations of infection. Comparative analyses of ill patients with healthy ones who have similarly been exposed to the same pathogen have substantiated that the presence or absence of DTH immune responses (including type 1 versus type 2 cytokine expression in the lesions) is correlated with relative resolution of the infection and formation of protective immunity. Another means to determine the importance of CMI in human immunity to infection is to compare patients who respond differently to infection with the same microbe and determine what the healthier ones have that the sicker ones lack. Leprosy is caused by a member of the mycobacterial genus, *Mycobacterium leprae,* and the disease manifestations come in a broad spectrum characterized by two polar forms, lepromatous and tuberculoid leprosy (Fig. 16.16). In lepromatous leprosy the proliferation of *M. leprae* within infected macrophages is relatively unchecked, so that these cells become literally stuffed with leprosy bacilli, resulting in disseminated and progressive disease. Because *M. leprae* thrives in the cooler areas of the body, there is much initial damage to the skin, but lepromatous patients generally also have cartilage and bone damage and eventually have multiorgan involvement. They also experience diffuse nerve damage. An immune response is not absent here: high titers of specific antibodies are present but are ineffective. Similarly, macrophage activation is inefficient due to poor TH1-based immunity, as shown by the inability of lepromatous patients to mount a positive DTH response to lepromin antigen when it is injected into the skin.

In contrast, patients who have the tuberculoid form of leprosy have lower antibody titers but mount positive lep-

Figure 16.15 The importance of CMI in protection against intracellular pathogens is illustrated by infection of IFN-γ-deficient mice with *Mycobacterium bovis* (attenuated strain BCG). Normal mice (blue line) are able to kill BCG following infection due to an effective TH1-mediated DTH response. However, IFN-γ-deficient mice (red line) are unable to kill the microorganisms and die of overwhelming infection within weeks. Reproduced from D. K. Dalton et al., *Science* 259:1739–1742, 1993, with permission.

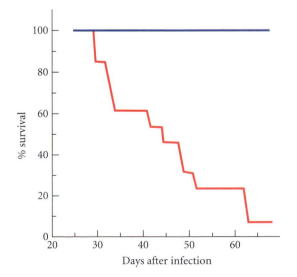

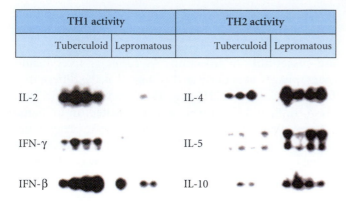

TH1 activity			TH2 activity	
Tuberculoid	Lepromatous		Tuberculoid	Lepromatous

Figure 16.16 The occurrence of two different forms of leprosy correlates with the TH cell (TH1 or TH2) polarity of the immune response. A properly contained (tuberculoid) infection is associated with a TH1 response, while an ineffective immune response, leading to widely disseminated (lepromatous) infection, is associated with a TH2 cytokine profile. The figure shows dot blots in which mRNA samples from the lesions of four patients with the tuberculoid form of leprosy are compared to those of four patients with the lepromatous form, following hybridization with probes specific for the indicated cytokines. Reproduced from P. A. Sieling and R. L. Modlin, *Immunobiology* **191**:378–387, 1994, with permission.

romin antigen skin tests, indicating good specific CMI is present. Their T cells produce IFN-γ and other type 1 cytokines in response to *M. leprae* antigens and thus have activated macrophages capable of killing intracellular leprosy bacilli. The number of *M. leprae* organisms in the lesion is much reduced, and the infection is much more confined than in lepromatous leprosy. The lesions are more organized into granulomas with CD4⁺ TH1, and activated macrophages are present. Although associated with a much more favorable prognosis and much less overall tissue destruction than in lepromatous leprosy, tuberculoid leprosy is still characterized by significant damage to the peripheral sensory nerves. The nerve damage in tuberculoid leprosy is due primarily to the DTH reaction itself, indicative of the balance between protection from more severe infection and harmful effects of immunologically mediated inflammation. Some patients have intermediate disease intensity, with both lepromatous and tuberculoid-type lesions.

The AIDS epidemic has undoubtedly provided the most profound and strongest evidence of the importance of CMI and DTH in human immunity to infection. The characteristic CD4⁺ T-cell destruction in this disease results in the development of opportunistic infections by a broad array of pathogens that are usually controlled by intact DTH responses. In the later stages of AIDS, when CD4⁺ T-cell responses drop below 200 per microliter, a whole host of infectious agents emerge, many of which are not pathogenic in an individual with an intact immune system (Table 16.1). These are referred to as opportunistic infections, reflecting the microbes taking advantage of the decimated immune system, although patients with AIDS also have serious trouble with pathogens that can readily infect healthy people as well. Over three-fourths of patients with AIDS die from an infectious agent other than HIV. What typifies these opportunistic pathogens is the importance of DTH in their control. Not only is the classic DTH-controlled pathogen *M. tuberculosis* seen as a major cause of infection among patients with AIDS, but other related mycobacteria, termed atypical mycobacteria, are also major causes of infection. These soil- and water-borne pathogens are encountered frequently by humans with little consequence when CD4⁺ T cells and DTH are intact due to the ability of resident T cells to activate macrophages to resist infection. Another ubiquitous intracellular organism, *Pneumocystis carinii*, is a common cause of infections in patients with AIDS although fortunately it is relatively well controlled now by excellent diagnosis and treatment. Fungal infections caused by members of the genus *Candida* and *Cryptococcus* can be very devastating in patients with AIDS, as can viral infections caused by herpes viruses like cytomegalovirus and herpes simplex virus. Many of these problematic viral infections in patients with AIDS actually arise from preexisting latent infections often found in many people that in the presence of intact DTH responses are well controlled. Although patients with AIDS are at high risk for infection from a broad range of microbial pathogens, the particularly high susceptibility to pathogens known to be controlled by CD4⁺ T cells and DTH reactions dramatically emphasizes the importance of this immune effector in health and survival.

Nonresolving DTH reactions and granuloma formation

Sometimes activated macrophages and/or CTLs fail to eliminate an invading microbe or even a nonviable foreign antigen that may have been inhaled, ingested, or injected into the skin or other tissue. This can lead to harmful effects from the DTH response, albeit these effects are

Table 16.1 Opportunistic pathogens associated with suppressed immunity

Fungi	Bacteria
Candida albicans	*Mycobacterium* spp.
Cryptococcus neoformans	*Salmonella* spp.
Histoplasma capsulatum	Viruses
Protozoa	Cytomegalovirus
Pneumocystis carinii	Herpes simplex virus
Toxoplasma gondii	

A

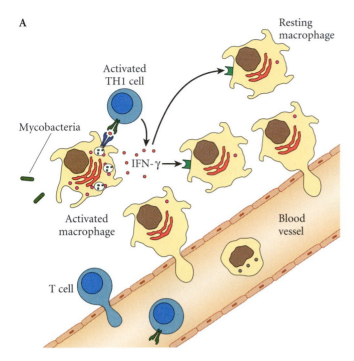

B

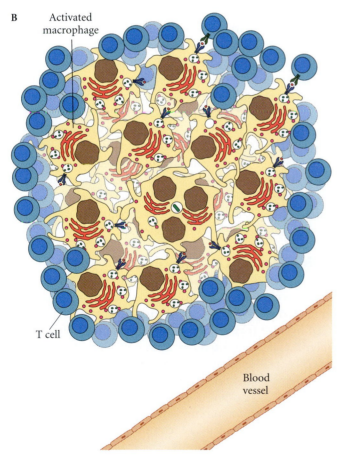

Figure 16.17 The TH1 phenotype correlates with the less severe form of tuberculosis because TH1 cytokines recruit and activate macrophages (**A**), resulting in the formation of a granuloma (**B**) that contains the infection. Specific Th1 T cells are activated by peptide-MHC complexes to secrete cytokines that are chemotactic for cells, including monocytes/macrophages. Other Th1 cytokines, especially IFN-γ, cause the activation of the macrophages in the tissues (**A**). In the chronic form of delayed-type hypersensitivity, an organized arrangement of cells is formed, with the specific T cells on the periphery and activated macrophages in the interior causing tissue damage (**B**). Some macrophages fuse into multinucleated "giant" or "epithelioid" cells.

arguably better than the unchecked progression of infection and disease. In such cases IFN-γ-stimulated expression of additional macrophage products, in conjunction with foreign substances and T-cell signaling via CD40L (CD154) and cytokines, can serve to remodel the local tissue architecture and environment. This is a strategy to wall off and prevent further spread of the antigen, which would be particularly effective against viable microbes. Macrophage-derived TNF-α, IL-1, and chemokines, together with other inflammatory substances, recruit and activate additional neutrophils and monocytes at the infectious site. These cytokines also stimulate fibroblast proliferation (assisted by platelet-derived growth factor) and collagen synthesis (augmented by transforming growth factor β) and deposition. Together with the destruction of normal tissue due to the nonspecific aspects of inflammation and the DTH reaction, especially over a prolonged period, this process results in the remodeling of the original tissue and its replacement with granulomas and/or fibrous tissue.

Granulomas are organized inflammatory tissues characteristic of ongoing DTH reactions that are made in response to chronic infectious or other antigenic stimuli. This obviously occurs because of the failure to completely remove the microbial cells or stimulating antigen. Much of what we know about granulomas has come from the study of *M. tuberculosis* infections. Granuloma formation depends on changes to the activated macrophages as part of chronic stimulation. After their cytoplasmic content increases and granules develop, macrophages undergo further morphologic changes that make them look similar to epithelial cells (Fig. 16.17). These epithelioid macrophages often fuse to form multinucleated syncytia or "giant cells" that surround the source of microbial antigen. T cells are present in a ring around these nodules of epithelioid macrophages/giant cells, and other immune cells may be present, including CD4$^+$ TH2 cells. Whether these classic noninflammatory TH cells limit the extent of tissue damage via their production of type 2 cytokines or actually contribute to the formation and progression of granulomas is a matter of some debate. Clearly, there is a price paid for a chronic DTH reaction that successfully contains a source of antigen that cannot be eradicated: local tissue damage that can range from benign to extensive. An outcome of a nonresolving and extensive chronic DTH reaction is replacement of the normal host tissue with fibrous tissue, leading to scarring and calcification. In tuberculosis, a good deal of the pathology that leads to respiratory problems is due not to the mycobacterial bacilli per se but rather to this chronic form of DTH reaction, with subsequent formation of scar tissue. Other sequelae of the walling off of tuberculosis lesions follow from the physiologic isolation of the center of large granulomas. Probably due both to a diminished blood supply causing a lack of oxygenation and the continuing action of toxic products produced by the activated macrophage/epithelioid-giant cells, the center becomes necrotic and the dead tissue becomes semisolid. This form of the lesion is termed *caseation necrosis* because of the resemblance of the center of the granuloma to cheese. It is in this context of pathology due primarily to CMI, together with chronic DTH reactions to seemingly innocuous antigens (especially experimentally when test antigens are coupled to indigestible latex beads or when complete Freund's adjuvant is employed), that this delayed-type cellular reaction came to be classified as a hypersensitivity.

Cell-Mediated Cytotoxicity

T-cell-mediated cytolysis of target cells, particularly that by MHC class I-restricted CD8$^+$ CTLs, constitutes one of the earliest described and perhaps best mechanistically characterized systems of cytotoxic effector cells. The targets of CTLs, often infected with an intracellular pathogen or transformed into a tumor cell, need to be killed to control the underlying pathologic process. In addition, target cells can be killed by a variety of other effectors, loosely termed K or killer cells. Many of these cells express FcR on their surface so they can become armed with antibody that provides immune-based recognition of foreign antigens. Not all cells expressing FcR are capable of cytotoxic activity. PMNs are highly phagocytic but generally less efficiently cytotoxic. NK cells, discussed extensively in chapter 3, are highly cytotoxic, recognizing aberrant cells either via FcR-bound antibody or by the K-cell receptor system. NK cells are part of a cell type defined by its morphologic properties termed large granular lymphocytes (LGL); typically these cells are about 50% larger than resting lymphocytes and have prominent granules within their cytoplasm. LGL cells are sometimes identified by their function; for example, IL-2-activated LGL cells have been shown to be cytolytic to tumor cells and are designated

lymphokine-activated killer cells. Lymphokine-activated killer cells removed from an individual and expanded in vitro in the presence of IL-2 and then reinfused into cancer patients have shown some promise as an immunotherapy. Along with DTH, immunologically based cytotoxic effector cells form the two mediators of CMI.

CTLs

Biologic Significance

One advantage of a CTL response is the ability to destroy cells infected by viruses or other intracellular parasites and tumor cells when these are present in tissues with many surrounding or nearby normal cells. To limit damage to the surrounding normal tissues, the extensive use of secreted, nonspecific effector molecules is contraindicated as they themselves may be harmful. By focusing the attack on the infected or transformed cell, CTLs with their MHC-restricted TCR recognition structures are well suited to the selective elimination of undesirable cells. As the recognition phase is highly specific due to an extremely diverse TCR repertoire and the lytic reaction is contact dependent and directional, there is little lysis of normal, healthy bystander cells. Protective immunity to many viral infections is thought to require a two-pronged attack: neutralizing antibodies to inhibit the infectivity of cell-free virions and CTLs to destroy the virus-producing cell factories. Some viral infections and tumor cells elicit inflammation and DTH responses involving CD4$^+$ TH1 cells and macrophages, and in some cases the CD4$^+$ cells are cytolytic. Most CD8$^+$ CTLs also produce type 1 cytokines, especially IFN-γ, which not only functions as the key macrophage-activating factor but also can have direct effects on virus-infected and tumor cells. CD4 TH1 cells are also frequently involved in the generation phase of CTL responses.

Induction of CTL Responses

Like all T cells, differentiation to mature CD8$^+$ CTLs initially occurs in the thymus before seeding of the peripheral, secondary lymphoid organs. Although these recent CD8$^+$ T-cell thymic emigrants are not constitutively cytolytic, and hence are more accurately termed precursors of CTLs (pCTLs), they are committed to a lytic functional phenotype characterized by the presence of the CD8 coreceptor. pCTLs do not use a particular subset of variable, differentiation, or joining TCR genes, as the functional TCR repertoires of pCTL cannot generally be distinguished for CD4$^+$ TH cells. The existence of some cytolytic CD4$^+$ cells indicates that expression of CD8 is not absolutely required for development of the lytic effector function of T cells.

Before sensitization, the frequencies of pCTLs specific for a particular antigen are generally quite low, often <1 in 10^5. An exception is the CTL repertoire to an MHC-incompatible antigen, for which the precursor frequency is often a few percent of the $CD8^+$ T cells. To be effective, pCTLs must both expand in number and terminally differentiate into activated effector CTLs. In vivo clonal expansion and differentiation of naive pCTLs can occur as early as 7 to 10 days after the introduction of antigen. Because of the increased starting frequency of pCTLs, allogeneic MHC-specific CTL responses, including transplantation rejection responses, are especially strong. Experimentally, primary antiallogeneic MHC responses can easily be measured by standard, short-term ^{51}Cr-release assays after 4 to 5 days of mixed lymphocyte culture. In contrast, measurement of CTL responses to most microbial antigens requires restimulation with antigen: a secondary or memory in vitro CTL response is typically employed after initial stimulation, or priming, in vivo.

As with activation of all naive T cells, $CD8^+$ pCTLs receive signal 1 through their cell surface TCR molecules following the binding of foreign peptide presented by MHC class I on the surface of the target cell. Most peptides are obtained from newly synthesized protein antigens of viruses, intracellular bacteria or parasites, or tumor cells via proteasome degradation and TAP (transporter associated with antigen presentation) heterodimer transport to the endoplasmic reticulum. Since many infectious viral agents do not readily infect APCs such as macrophages and dendritic cells, receipt of signal 1 only through the TCR and in the absence of costimulation can serve as an anergic instead of inductive signal. Thus, pCTLs need to receive additional costimulatory factors from professional APCs, and also may need help from $CD4^+$ TH cells, to obtain the second set of signals needed for activation and differentiation.

The mechanism of delivery and nature of signal 2 for pCTLs, the types of APCs that can stimulate pCTLs, and the requirement for $CD4^+$ TH cells are not fully resolved. Indeed, it appears that there are multiple mechanisms and pathways that can activate pCTL, some requiring $CD4^+$ cells, some not. Although there appears to be heterogeneity in the requirement for signal 2 among $CD8^+$ CTLs, production of IL-2 (and possibly other cytokines) is critical to drive pCTL expansion. This may come from $CD4^+$ cells or from the CTL itself (Fig. 16.18). Thus, both autocrine and paracrine production of IL-2 can drive the expansion of pCTLs. CTL responses in which the pCTLs are unable to produce enough IL-2 for their own expansion after TCR engagement are more likely to be CD4-dependent responses.

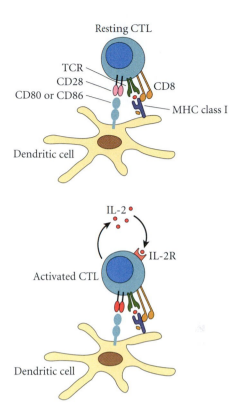

Figure 16.18 Direct activation of a naive $CD8^+$ CTL precursor by a virus-infected DC. (**Top**) The CTL receives signal 1 (TCR-MHC-peptide) and signal 2 (CD28-CD80/86) from the DC. (**Bottom**) This causes the CTL to produce both IL-2 and its receptor (IL-2R), stimulating CTL activation in an autocrine manner.

$CD4^+$ T cells can become involved in pCTL activation by at least two mechanisms. Both involve APCs, principally DCs, with one model proposing that a tricellular, simultaneous interaction of $CD4^+$ TH cells, $CD8^+$ pCTL, and DC is needed and the second proposing that only two cells are needed, $CD4^+$ T cells and DC; this activates the DC and makes it able to provide costimulation to pCTL (Fig. 16.19). But for an MHC class I-restricted response, the DC must present foreign antigen on the class I molecule. One way this could occur is if a microbial agent invaded and grew within the DC, producing antigens for the cytosolic processing pathway involving proteasomes, TAP proteins, and loading of class I molecules. But many viral antigens do not invade and grow in DCs. To present antigens from these pathogens, the DCs must acquire them from their external environment and shunt them to the cytosolic antigen presentation pathway for loading on class I molecules. This can occur in both a TAP-dependent and TAP-independent fashion. Since the DCs can also present these antigens on class II molecules, they have the capacity to stimulate both $CD4^+$ and $CD8^+$ T cells. In some instances, $CD4^+$ TH cells and pCTL interact with the DC

A

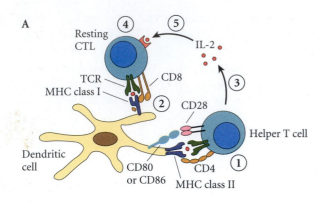

B

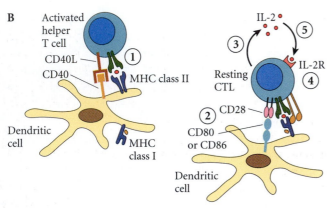

Figure 16.19 TH cells may assist the activation of naive CTLs by two different mechanisms. (**A**) The CTL, TH cell, and DC may form a tripartite complex, in which the DC simultaneously presents antigen to TH cells (1) and CTLs (2). Activation of the helper cell results in production of IL-2 (3), while presentation of antigen to the CTL results in synthesis of the IL-2R (4). Helper cell-produced IL-2 can then bind the CTL IL-2R in a paracrine manner (5), completing activation of the CTL. (**B**) Alternatively, the TH cell may form a bipartite complex with only a DC (1), activating the DC to increase its expression of the CD80 or CD86 costimulatory molecules (2). This activated DC may then be able to stimulate production of both IL-2 (3) and the IL-2R (4) on the CTL, allowing autocrine IL-2 stimulation (5). In either model, but particularly in mechanism B, up-regulated dendritic cell expression of CD80 or CD86 is a key requirement for costimulation via interaction with CD28 on the T cell. An efficient way of up-regulating CD80 or CD86 on dendritic cells is signaling via CD40 after its ligation by CD154 expressed by activated CD4 T helper cells.

at the same time (three-cell model), and in others, they may interact in a sequential fashion (two-cell model). Either way, the pCTL receives IL-2 and other activation factors from both DC and CD4$^+$ T cells to differentiate into effector CTL.

It has also been shown that some CTL responses develop in the absence of CD4$^+$ help. This seems to be dependent on the level of the pCTL. At sufficiently high densities, the pCTL may be interacting with enough DCs in a small microenvironment such that the pCTLs themselves produce enough cytokines for activation to proceed as the level of cytokines exceeds the required threshold. Another possible means for providing signal 2 in the absence of

CD4$^+$ cells may arise when large numbers of CD8$^+$ pCTLs interact with DCs and substitute for CD4$^+$ TH cells, leading to an increase in the level of costimulatory molecules and cytokine production by the DCs themselves. Since experimental data support all of these models for pCTL activation, they likely are all operative, but the specific one utilized in a given situation will depend on individual factors, notably levels of pCTL.

CTL Effector Phase: Lytic Mechanisms

Lysis of target cells by CTLs differs fundamentally from antibody-dependent, complement-mediated lysis, wherein osmotic swelling and subsequent bursting of cells along with physical or chemical injuries lead to cellular *necrosis*. Killing of the target cells by CTLs occurs when the activated CTLs initiate the programmed cell death menu leading to apoptosis. Apoptosis is characterized by cell shrinkage, loss of plasma membrane integrity leading to the appearance of factors normally found only on the cytosolic face of the plasma membrane appearing on the external side of the membrane, and an ordered pattern of fragmentation of nuclear DNA. CTL-mediated cytolysis is best described in the context of a lytic cycle (Fig. 16.20). Five steps in the CTL lytic cycle can be defined:

1. Initial CTL binding to the target cell presenting antigen on MHC class I for CD8$^+$ T-cell lysis or on class II for CD4$^+$ T-cell lysis.
2. Strengthening of the binding of CTL to target via multiple MHC-TCR interactions and CTL activation.
3. CTL introduction of the "lethal hit" via activation of the target cell's program for apoptotic lysis.
4. Recycling of the CTLs to attack additional target cells.
5. Target-cell death once the CTL has detached.

Target-cell binding is probably not initially highly dependent on specific TCR-MHC recognition events. Rather, effector–target-cell conjugate formation relies on a more nonspecific binding mediated by adhesion molecule interactions, especially the β_2-integrin LFA-1 (CD11a/CD18) of the CTL with target cell ICAM-1, -2, and/or -3 ligands. CTL binding to target cells can be readily blocked experimentally by factors that disrupt LFA-1–ICAM-1 interactions, including divalent cation chelating agents such as ethylenediaminetetraacetic acid (EDTA), and by antibodies to LFA-1. Stabilization of conjugate formation is probably necessary because the affinity of the monovalent TCR has typically been estimated to be low. Stabilization of binding also facilitates lysis of target cells bearing only a small number of particular MHC-peptide complexes.

When a sufficient number of specific peptide-MHC complexes have interacted with the CTLs via their TCR,

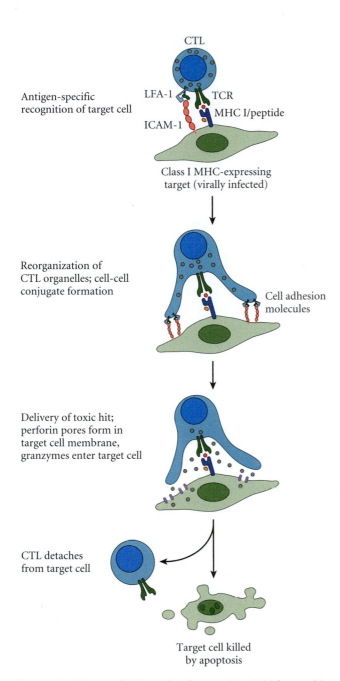

CTL

Antigen-specific
recognition of target cell

LFA-1   TCR

ICAM-1   MHC I/peptide

Class I MHC-expressing
target (virally infected)

Reorganization of
CTL organelles; cell-cell
conjugate formation

Cell adhesion
molecules

Delivery of toxic hit;
perforin pores form in
target cell membrane,
granzymes enter target cell

CTL detaches
from target cell

Target cell killed
by apoptosis

Figure 16.20 Stages of CTL-mediated cytotoxicity. Initial recognition of an infected target cell occurs via the TCR-peptide-MHC class I complex, which induces reorganization of the CTL membranes and organelles toward the area of plasma membrane contact with the target cell. The membrane-bound secretory granules then fuse with the plasma membrane, and perforin, granzymes, and other potentially cytotoxic factors are released directionally toward the target cell. The CTL then detaches, and the target cell is eventually killed by apoptosis. Some CTL factors such as granulysin are also toxic to the microbes infecting the target cell.

CTLs become activated. Signaling proceeds through the TCR-associated CD3 and ζ:ζ homodimers and/or ζ:η heterodimers, along with the participation of CD8 coreceptor-associated signaling. The precise mechanism of CTL activation is not fully defined but is thought to be generally similar to CD4$^+$ T-cell activation. Thus, signal transduction mechanisms leading to gene transcription provide some of the signals needed for the activated CTL to become cytotoxic. In addition, the initial LFA-1 binding further stabilizes and strengthens conjugate formation via enhanced LFA-1 binding, and coupled with the participation of other adhesion molecules such as CD2, CD8, and the TCR, the cytolytic process can proceed.

There are two different primary mechanisms by which CTLs mediate killing of cellular targets, although there is some debate as to the relative utilization of these two pathways. One pathway involves a soluble factor called *perforin* that is released from cytoplasmic granules that first migrate to the cell's plasma membrane and fuse with it to release the perforin. The perforin forms pores in the target cell's membrane, allowing the injection of toxic enzymatic *granzymes* into the target cells. The second pathway is dependent on cell surface interactions between receptor-ligand pairs of the TNF-TNF receptor (TNF-R) families. Expression of the proper receptor on the target cell followed by cellular activation through the death domains associated with the cytoplasmic tails of the TNF-R family members leads to apoptosis. For many CTL activities, the CTL expresses Fas ligand (CD95L) on its surface and the target cell expresses the receptor, Fas (CD95), a member of the TNF-R family, that initiates the apoptotic process.

The perforin-granzyme pathway is the primary mechanism by which CTLs lyse target cells infected with intracellular microbes, including most viruses. These two cytotoxic factors are located in the granules of fully mature CTLs in inactive forms. Upon T-cell activation at the effector phase, the cytoplasmic contents of the CTLs undergo reorganization such that these granules are concentrated near the area of contact of the CTL and target-cell surface membranes where TCR clustering has taken place. Fusion of granule membranes with the CTL plasma membrane results in the localized and directional exocytosis of granule contents to the target cell. Perforin polymerizes in a Ca^{2+}-dependent manner to form channels approximately 16 nanometers in diameter, providing an explanation for the early observation that Ca^{2+} was required for much of the lysis by CTLs to occur. The polymerized perforin channels insert into the plasma membrane of the target cell, but not the effector CTL, to form pores (Fig. 16.21). Perforin has some structural and functional ho-

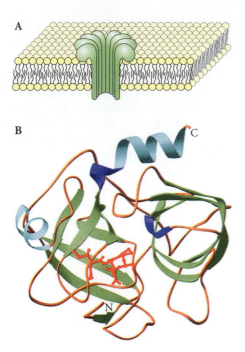

Figure 16.21 Cytotoxicity by CTLs can be caused by the introduction of perforin and granzymes to the target cells. (**A**) One view is that perforin forms stable multimers in the target cell plasma membrane, forming transmembrane pores. Other data suggest that pores are not needed for delivery of mediators of apoptosis and perforin serves merely as a translocator complexed to serglycan, a chondroitan sulfate proteoglycan. Granzyme B enters cells also complexed to serglycan and activates pro-caspase-3, which in turn becomes caspase-3, a key mediator of apoptosis. (**B**) Structure of granzyme B. The three-dimensional structure of human granzyme B compared to caspase-3, key mediators of cell death with cleavage specificity for aspartic acid in P1. From J. Rotonda et al., *Chem. Biol.* **8:**357–368, 2001, with permission.

mology to the terminal components of the membrane attack complex of the complement system, principally C9. Similar to complement-mediated lysis, experimental application of concentrated perforin in the presence of Ca^{2+} to some sensitive target cells in vitro, particularly red blood cells, can cause pore formation sufficient for swelling and osmotic lysis independent of DNA fragmentation. It is thought unlikely, however, that perforin causes lysis by this mechanism in vivo. Rather, a class of three or more serine protease family members, the granzymes, are injected through the perforin channels into the target cell. The granzymes, particularly granzyme B, then activate the programmed cell death pathway, leading to apoptosis of the target cell. Although not all the details of granzyme activation of apoptosis have been defined, a critical event appears to be cleavage of *IL-1 converting enzyme* and other related cysteine proteases (caspases) to induce a cascade of proteases involved in apoptosis. However, other data suggest that perforin may not form membrane pores but rather may promote translocation of granzyme B into the target cell. In CTL

granules, perforin and granzyme B are complexed to serglycan, a chondroitan sulfate proteoglycan, and the perforin-serglycan complex may promote translocation of the granzyme B-serglycan complex into the target cell to activate pro-caspase 3.

The involvement of a CD95-CD95L interaction to initiate the second mechanism of CTL-mediated apoptosis was confirmed in a variety of ways after numerous observations indicated that granule- and Ca^{2+}-independent lysis of target cells could occur. The most compelling evidence was obtained by the use of two mutant mouse strains, *gld* (defective FasL expression) or *lpr* (defective Fas expression), which were spontaneous mutants and not products of transgenic mouse technology. In addition, transgenic perforin-knockout mice provided another experimental system to observe the importance of CD95-CD95L in target-cell lysis in some situations. With these mice it was demonstrated that CTL activity could occur in the absence of intact CD95-CD95L interactions as well as in the absence of perforin production. However, doubly transgenic mice lacking both systems were virtually devoid of CTL activity. CD95L is expressed transiently on activated T killer cells, both $CD8^+$ CTL and those $CD4^+$ TH1 cells that are also cytolytic. Some target cells express Fas, whereas others do not, and the latter can be lysed only by the perforin-granzyme mechanism. A critical event in signaling into the target cell is the FasL-induced trimerization of Fas (Fig. 16.22). Subsequent activation through the death domain of the cytoplasmic tail of Fas sets in motion a series of events, including the protease cascade mentioned above, that culminate in apoptosis of the target cell, including DNA fragmentation. Thus, the two mechanisms of CTL lysis lead to similar ultimate outcomes.

These final steps of apoptotic killing do not require the continued presence of the effector CTL on or near the target cell. This phase may take many minutes to hours for cell lysis to become fully obvious, as compared with the few minutes required for a CTL to bind its target, become fully activated, and deliver the lethal hit. CTLs are not spent or lysed themselves from their encounter with target cells. Rather, CTLs detach from the target cell and can go on to lyse several more targets sequentially via additional rounds of binding and delivery of cytotoxic signals. Although the unidirectionality of the FasL-Fas mechanism is straightforward, the sparing of CTLs engaged in perforin-granule-mediated cytolysis is more problematic, especially considering the highly interdigitating nature of the CTL and target-cell membranes, as observed by electron microscopy. This has led to speculation that CTLs may actively protect themselves from their own killing mechanism. Although some evidence has been provided

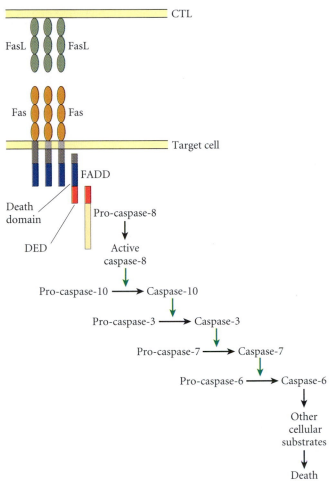

Figure 16.22 Cell signaling pathway following Fas (CD95) ligation. Fas ligation leads to trimerization of Fas, causing recruitment of the adaptor protein FADD (Fas-associated protein with death domain) and pro-caspase-8. FADD and pro-caspase-8 include death effector domains (DED), which are found in proteins with both pro- and anti-apoptotic activity. Pro-caspase-8 is cleaved to its active form (caspase-8), which initiates a cascade of caspase activation events. The terminal caspase (caspase-6) acts on numerous cellular substrates to bring about cell death.

a major homeostatic mechanism contributing to the elimination of most of the clonally expanded, specific effector T cells once they are no longer needed. This phenomenon has been called *activation-induced cell death* and includes both "fratricide," when two activated T cells reciprocally express either Fas or FasL, or "autologous suicide," when a given effector T cell simultaneously expresses both Fas and FasL. Sparing of memory T cells, which presumably do not express Fas, but removal of excess terminally differentiated lymphocytes specific for the inducing foreign antigens allows a return to baseline conditions, normalizes the overall size of the T-lymphocyte pool and lymphoid organs, and thus permits an efficient response to the next set of introduced antigens.

There are other mechanisms of T-cell-mediated cytolysis; however, these cytokine-based mechanisms display neither the high specificity nor the fast kinetics of the perforin-granzyme and FasL-Fas pathways to programmed cell death. Both CD4$^+$ TH1 effector cells and some CD8$^+$ CTLs produce TNF-α and TNF-β/LT that can be cytotoxic to certain cells expressing TNF-R on their plasma membranes. Both soluble and membrane-bound forms of TNF-α and TNF-β contribute to lysis of the target cell by activation of the TNF-R death domains. The high degree of specificity and lack of substantial lysis of innocent bystander cells suggest, however, that soluble TNF-α and TNF-β either play very minor roles or act only locally in CTL-mediated cytolysis. Other properties of TNF can also affect a target cell's viability. Most of the tumor-killing activity of TNF-α is indirect because it induces inflammation and has antiangiogenic effects that prevent the formation of new blood vessels that tumors need to survive. TNF-β binds to the same TNF-R as does TNF-α and thus shares functional activity. In addition to being secreted, TNF-β can associate with an integral membrane protein called LT-β in a heterotrimeric cell surface complex. Secreted homotrimeric TNF-β and the cell surface heterotrimeric form are directly toxic to certain tumor cells by interaction with either the standard TNF-R or a structurally related but different receptor, respectively, and both forms induce a common apoptotic cell death. TNF-α has a lesser ability to cause tumor-cell apoptosis through binding to the standard TNF-R.

A relatively new factor in CTL effector function is a granule molecule referred to as granulysin. This peptide works along with perforin as an antibacterial factor that inserts itself into the outer surface of some bacteria, disrupts the membrane, and kills the target microbe. This is a particularly important finding since before its identification it was unclear how mere lysis of target cells could control an intracellular bacterial infection. Lysis of virally infected cells reduces viral growth and spread, but, if any-

for the existence of such "protectin" molecules, proof of their existence has not been generally accepted. Similarly, a number of studies showed that, whatever the protective mechanism(s), CTLs used as targets in vitro are relatively resistant to killing by other CTLs. This resistance was not absolute, however, and it has also been established that cytolysis of effector CTLs is part of the regulatory mechanisms that decrease for CMI activity following antigen elimination or control.

FasL-Fas interactions among CTLs appear to play an immunoregulatory role to control the overall CTL process. Activated T cells (both CD4$^+$ and CD8$^+$) express Fas and/or FasL during the later stages of an immune response when the source of antigen has diminished. Binding of Fas on these cells and induction of apoptosis may be thing, lysis of a bacterially infected cell would seem to be a good means of spreading the infection as bacteria are not obligate intracellular parasites. Granulysin has also been shown to kill tumor cells, raising the hope that vaccine strategies for tumors could be based, in part, on activating this component of CTL.

ADCC

Heterogeneity of Effector Cells Mediating ADCC

Because ADCC is a broad functional term, it is not surprising that a variety of K cells bearing different FcRs are the effector cells of ADCC. There are FcRs specific for immunoglobulin G (IgG), IgA, and IgE antibodies and their subclasses. NK cells carry out cytolysis of target cells and can have particularly active ADCC capabilities. Their antibody-independent cytotoxic activities are more properly considered components of the innate immune system (see chapter 2). Also, NK cells are of the same lymphoid lineage as CTLs, but NK cells do not use TCR to specifically recognize target cells. Both granulocytes (PMNs and eosinophils) and cells of the monocyte/macrophage lineage are potent mediators of lysis of antibody-coated targets via ADCC. Because PMNs and macrophages are phagocytic and are particularly efficient when the infected cell, tumor cell, or microbe is opsonized by specific antibody, care must be taken to differentiate FcR-mediated enhanced phagocytosis that leads to intracellular digestion

from cellular lysis of antibody-coated targets that does not involve phagocytosis. FcR binding and cross-linking result in signal transduction via the cytoplasmic tails of the transmembrane FcR itself, provoking an entire spectrum of new functions simultaneously in ADCC-effector cells. Many of these functions can lead to the killing of target cells. Regardless of the specific effector cell, class or subclass of antibody, and FcR involved, however, the functions of antibody and FcR in ADCC are clear: bound antibody provides the specificity of the reaction and the corresponding FcR both binds the effector cytotoxic cell to its target and, where applicable, sets in motion an activation cascade that results in delivery of the extracellular lytic machinery of that particular effector cell.

Nature and Specific Roles of Fc Receptors

The low-affinity FcR for IgG, termed the FcγRIIIA receptor (CD16), is expressed by NK cells and by a small subpopulation of monocytes/macrophages (Fig. 16.23). CD16 is anchored to the plasma membrane through transmembrane domains. Surface levels of CD16 can be increased by cytokines, particularly transforming growth factor beta, which can substantially augment the low constitutive expression by monocytes and allow for increased ADCC activity. An isoform of CD16, FcγRIIIB, is found at high density on PMNs and differs from FcγRIIIA in that it is anchored to the PMN surface by a phosphatidylinositol glycan linkage and not transmembrane domains. This lack of transmembrane and cytoplasmic domains makes Fc-

Figure 16.23 A synopsis of several FcRs, which are represented schematically with the CD designations, affinities for antibody, and tissue distributions of the receptors listed underneath.

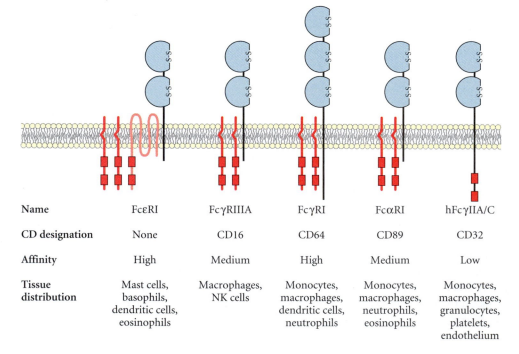

Name	FcεRI	FcγRIIIA	FcγRI	FcαRI	hFcγIIA/C
CD designation	None	CD16	CD64	CD89	CD32
Affinity	High	Medium	High	Medium	Low
Tissue distribution	Mast cells, basophils, dendritic cells, eosinophils	Macrophages, NK cells	Monocytes, macrophages, dendritic cells, neutrophils	Monocytes, macrophages, neutrophils, eosinophils	Monocytes, macrophages, granulocytes, platelets, endothelium

γRIIIB unable to associate with the γ or ζ signaling subunits of transmembrane FcRs. Thus, PMN FcγRIIIB is unable to mediate efficient ADCC, at least of tumor cells. Expression of FcγRIIIB by PMNs can be decreased by shedding or internalization upon PMN activation or by treatment with TNF-α. Because of the moderate affinity of the FcγRIIIA isoform and the low affinity of the FcγRIIIB isoforms for IgG, soluble monomeric IgG is not bound efficiently to cells expressing these FcRs. ADCC is mediated most efficiently when target cells have bound a sufficient density of IgG antibodies or when aggregated IgG is available, so that the avidities of many individual low- or moderate-affinity binding events mediated by FcγRIIIA synergize to provide the needed binding and signaling strength. In addition, low-affinity binding by FcγRIII (and by other low-affinity FcRs, see below) can be augmented when other adhesion molecules expressed by the effector cell (CD2, LFA-1, and CD56) can be used to bind to a target cell.

FcγRII (CD32) consists of a family of receptors that also displays low affinity for IgG antibodies and has several isoforms: types A, B, and C. Monocytes and macrophages can express all three isoforms, whereas PMNs express FcγRIIA and type C. In addition, other cells not capable of ADCC express different types of FcγRII: endothelial cells and platelets express FcγRIIA; B cells express FcγRIIB; and platelets express FcγRIIC. Expression of FcγRIIA on myeloid cells can be augmented by GM-CSF but is inhibited by IL-4 and IL-13. Similar to FcγRIII, the low-affinity nature of the FcγRII isoforms necessitates the binding of only opsonized targets and immune complexes; soluble monomeric IgG molecules are not bound.

FcγRI (CD64) is a high-affinity receptor for monomeric IgG, with an equilibrium dissociation constant (K_d) of 10^{-8} to 10^{-9} M for human IgG1 and IgG3. FcγRI is constitutively expressed by monocytes, macrophages, and DCs, but PMNs also express FcγRI after stimulation with IFN-γ. Exposure to IFN-γ, and to a lesser extent, granulocyte colony-stimulating factor and IL-10, also causes a 5- to 10-fold increase in FcγI cell surface levels on monocytes, macrophages, and DCs. Because of its high affinity for monomeric IgG, FcγRI should be saturated with soluble IgG antibodies in vivo, at least on monocytes in the plasma. This raises questions as to the physiologic role of FcγRI, since in its normal occupied state, binding to opsonized target cells should be inefficient. On the other hand, high-affinity binding of monomeric IgG antibodies by FcγRI allows monocytes/macrophages, unlike ADCC effectors with low-affinity FcγRs, to become "armed" by specific antibody in advance such that a target precoated with antibody is not necessary. Such arming also occurs to a lesser extent with the FcγRIIIA of NK cells.

There are also FcRs for IgA and IgE antibodies. A moderate-affinity FcαR (CD89) is expressed by PMNs, monocytes/macrophages, and eosinophils. Although expressed constitutively, levels of FcαR are substantially increased by exposure to microbial products such as LPS and by cytokines, including IL-1, TNF-α, and GM-CSF. Antibody-coated microbes or infected cells may be either phagocytosed or subjected to ADCC by PMNs and macrophages, and there is evidence for eosinophil-mediated ADCC through FcαR. Although FcαRs can bind to dimeric IgA molecules, receptor cross-linking is required for triggering of these functions, thought to be especially important in warding off infections at mucosal cell surfaces. Two receptors exist for IgE, a high-affinity type I form, which is expressed primarily by mast cells and basophils and at lower levels by eosinophils, certain DCs, and monocytes; and a nonhomologous low-affinity type-II FcεR (CD23) found on B cells, eosinophils, monocytes, macrophages, platelets, Langerhans cells, and possibly T cells. The type 1 FcεR has as its primary function the IgE-mediated release of histamine and other inflammatory mediators of immediate hypersensitivity reactions. FcεRI also may enhance the uptake of IgE-antigen complexes for processing by APCs (DCs) but is not thought to be involved in ADCC. In contrast, in addition to serving as a B-cell differentiation antigen in its FcεRIIA form, FcεRIIB (differing from the A isoform only in its cytoplasmic tail) facilitates ADCC reactions, especially by cytokine-activated eosinophil effectors. Eosinophil-mediated ADCC is particularly effective against helminthic parasites (worms), and immunity or control of worm infections appears to be based on an ADCC-type of killing of these infectious agents. Helminthic parasites often display relative resistance to lysis by PMNs and monocytes/macrophages. The presence of a toxic basic protein specifically in the granules of eosinophils and the induction of IgE antibodies by such parasites are factors that both contribute to this effector function of eosinophils. Specificity is provided by the antibody, toxicity by the granule protein. In addition, expression of FcεRII is increased by IgE and IL-4, which are produced in response to many parasitic infections, and by IFN-γ. Further, IL-5, GM-CSF, and TNF-α activate eosinophils, allowing them to mediate ADCC by both FcεRIIB and FcαR.

Mechanisms of Target Cell Lysis in ADCC

All of the mechanisms found to apply to CTL lysis of targets have been associated with ADCC, but lysis in this context is generally thought to proceed mostly through the perforin-granzyme pathway leading to target-cell apoptosis. Whether cells mediating ADCC also can initiate programmed cell death by a CD95-CD95L interaction is presently unclear. ADCC can lead to phagocytosis instead of a lytic or apoptotic death. Indeed, ADCC can be an effective mediator of immunity to infection due to FcR-mediated opsonophagocytosis of microbial pathogens. Soluble cytotoxic effectors such as TNF may also play a role in ADCC, but this is not supported by convincing data. Eosinophil ADCC of helminthic parasites appears to occur primarily via secretion of the toxic basic granule-derived protein, probably supplemented by production of reactive oxygen and nitrogen intermediates, proteolytic enzymes, and other toxic substances possessed in common with PMNs and monocytes/macrophages. Overall, ADCC mediated by these granulocytic and myeloid effectors may proceed via various combinations of these destructive mediators, resulting in destruction of infected and tumor cells and harmful microbes.

Summary

CMI is a critical component of immune function and is characterized by three specific effector pathways: DTH, mediated primarily by CD4$^+$ T cells; cytolysis, mediated primarily by CD8$^+$ CTL; and ADCC, mediated by a variety of cells possessing various forms of FcR. CMI is primarily important in controlling infections caused by intracellular parasites, which span the spectrum of pathogenic microbes and worms. DTH is activated by immune CD4$^+$ T or NKT cells that specifically recognize either MHC class II-presented peptides or CD1-presented glycolipids, but actual killing of infectious microbes and control of disease are carried out by activated macrophages. The macrophages are activated by cytokines, notably IFN-γ, produced by the CD4$^+$ cells. Failure to clear an infectious stimulus can lead to formation of granulomas that attempt to keep the microbe confined to a single part of a tissue and thus limit its spread. For many viral pathogens, lysis of the cells they infect by CTL, which are generally CD8$^+$ but can on occasion be CD4$^+$, can control viral spread and development of disease. Activation of pCTL can be both dependent and independent of CD4$^+$ T-cell help, but interaction with an activated DC seems to be a requirement for pCTL development into effector CTL. These cells primarily kill targets using perforin and granzymes or by expressing CD95L and binding to CD95, which activates an apoptotic death in the target cell. ADCC is carried out using antibody bound to cell surface FcRs, which are expressed by a broad range of cells, some with ADCC activity and others without this activity. FcRs come in a variety of isoforms and with differing specificities of antibody classes and subclasses, which determine

the specific nature of the ADCC reaction. Cells expressing FcR with low affinity for antibody mediate killing of target cells with high densities of immune complexes, whereas cells with high-affinity FcR can recognize opsonized targets and kill them via cytolysis or phagocytosis. Binding of IgE antibodies to the FcϵRIIB on eosinophils appears to be a critical component of ADCC-induced control of helminthic worm infections. Production of high levels of molecules such as TNF-α and TNF-β can kill target cells expressing TNF-R when secreted by cells that have recognized targets by any of the various mechanisms of CMI. Overall, CMI is a potent and necessary component of immune resistance to a variety of pathogenic microbes, and the loss of CMI function in diseases such as AIDS leads to very high susceptibility to opportunistic infections and their consequences.

Suggested Reading

Barry, M., and R. C. Bleackley. 2002. Cytotoxic T lymphocytes: all roads lead to death. *Nat. Rev. Immunol.* **2**:401–409.

den Haan, J. M., and M. J. Bevan. 2001. Antigen presentation to CD8$^+$ T cells: cross-priming in infectious diseases. *Curr. Opin. Immunol.* **13**:437–441.

Ernst, W. A., S. Thoma-Uszynski, R. Teitelbaum, C. Ko, D. A. Hanson, C. Clayberger, A. M. Krensky, M. Leippe, B. R. Bloom, T. Ganz, and R. L. Modlin. 2000. Granulysin, a T cell product, kills bacteria by altering membrane permeability. *J. Immunol.* **165**:7102–7108.

Harty, J. T., A. R. Tvinnereim, and D. W. White. 2000. CD8$^+$ T cell effector mechanisms in resistance to infection. *Annu. Rev. Immunol.* **18**:275–308.

Ismail, N., J. P. Olano, H. M. Feng, and D. H. Walker. 2002. Current status of immune mechanisms of killing of intracellular microorganisms. *FEMS Microbiol. Lett.* **207**:111–120.

Moody, D. B., and G. S. Besra. 2001. Glycolipid targets of CD1-mediated T-cell responses. *Immunology* **104**:243–251.

Porcelli, S. A., and R. Modlin. 1999. The CD1 system: antigen-presenting molecules for T cell recognition of lipids and glycolipids. *Annu. Rev. Immunol.* **17**:297–329.

Raulet, D. H., R. E. Vance, and C. W. McMahon. 2001. Regulation of the natural killer cell receptor repertoire. *Ann. Rev. Immunol.* **19**:291–330.

Ravetch, J. V., and S. Bolland. 2001. IgG Fc receptors. *Annu. Rev. Immunol.* **19**:275–290.

Rich, R. F., and W. R. Green. 2002. Characterization of the Fas ligand/Fas-dependent apoptosis of antiretroviral, class I MHC tetramer-defined, CD8$^+$ CTL by in vivo retrovirus-infected cells. *J. Immunol.* **168**:2751–2758.

Smyth, M. J., J. M. Kelly, V. R. Sutton, J. E. Davis, K. A. Browne, T. J. Sayers, and J. A. Trapani. 2001. Unlocking the secrets of cytotoxic granule proteins. *J. Leukoc. Biol.* **70**:18–29.

Wang, B., C. C. Norbury, R. Greenwood, J. R. Bennink, J. W. Yewdell, and J. A. Frelinger. 2001. Multiple paths for activation of naive CD8$^+$ T cells: CD4-independent help. *J. Immunol.* **167**:1283–1289.

chapter 17

Mucosal Immunity

Scott Simpson and Lee M. Wetzler

The mucosal surfaces of the body—that is, the surfaces lining the digestive, respiratory, and urogenital systems—have a combined surface area of approximately 300 to 400 square meters (m^2), roughly 200 times larger than the surface area of the skin. Thus, for most pathogens, the mucosal surfaces are the primary site of entry into the host's body. The mucosal immune system consists of both innate defense mechanisms and acquired immunity that protect the mucosa from invading pathogens. As this is the first contact between host and microbe, it is clear that preventing infection at this early stage would be the most propitious means of fighting off disease. Therefore, the mucosal immune response is a key component of the overall system of immunity to infection.

The mucosal immune system consists of an integrated network of anatomic sites, immune effector cells, and tissues, commonly called *mucosa-associated lymphoid tissue* (MALT). This term was derived from observations that mucosal surfaces shared a common lymphoid organization and function. The functions of MALT can be subdivided into three main categories: (i) primary lymphoid development, (ii) induction and amplification of local mucosal immune responses, and (iii) production of the effector mechanisms of local mucosal immunity. The major characteristics of MALT are the predominant production of local immunoglobulin (IgA) and tissue-specific immune-activated mucosal lymphocytes (both T and B cells), which have the ability to enter the circulation but return to the tissue of origin or home to other mucosal tissues. The cellular and architectural makeup of MALT varies among different anatomic sites (Fig. 17.1), and the

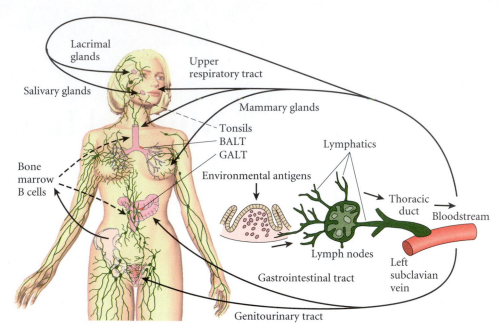

Figure 17.1 Schematic diagram of various MALTs showing the route of entry of ingested antigens and the recirculatory patterns used by some gut leukocytes to populate other MALTs after encounter with antigen.

different types of MALT are sometimes referred to by different names. These include *gut-associated lymphoid tissue* (GALT) of the intestine, *bronchus-associated lymphoid tissue* (BALT) of the lower airways, and *nasopharynx-associated lymphoid tissue* (NALT) of the upper respiratory tract. While most animals have GALT, the presence of BALT and NALT is restricted to some species. For example, most humans do not have BALT of any significance but the NALT is a major component of the mucosal immune system. MALT also exists at anatomic sites such as the mammary, salivary, and lacrimal glands; the genitourinary organs; and the inner ear.

GALT

GALT, the best characterized component of MALT, consists of both highly organized local sites, where lymphocytes collect and are responsible for the inductive phase of the mucosal immune response, and vast diffuse effector sites, where activated cells reside. The inductive sites consist of anatomically discrete single and aggregated lymphoid follicles. Single follicles are present along the entire length of the gastrointestinal (GI) tract (intestine) and are most predominant in the colon and rectum. The aggregated follicles, such as Peyer's patches, are present within the small intestine, appendix, and mesenteric lymph nodes. Dispersed throughout the GALT are many lymphocytes present either as single cells or small collections of multiple lymphocytes. These are referred to as in-

traepithelial lymphocytes (IELs) when they are within the intestinal epithelium itself and lamina propria lymphocytes when they are distributed throughout the lamina propria. The lamina propria is a thin layer of connective tissue that supports the GI epithelium, and together form the mucous membrane. In addition to LP lymphocytes, plasma cells and mast cells are found in the lamina propria.

An additional specialized organ, found at the end of the intestine in chickens, is known as the bursa of Fabricius. This organ is the site of primary B-cell development in birds, a function carried out by the bone marrow in mammals.

Innate Immunity of GALT

Exposure to a pathogen occurs most frequently at the skin or mucosal tissues. For most pathogens, infection (usually associated with frank disease) or colonization (presence of pathogens without signs and symptoms of disease) of a local mucosal site is the first step in infection. MALTs have evolved an elaborate set of protective mechanisms to prevent infection or colonization. These defenses can be categorized as specific and innate. Specific mucosal defense mechanisms consist of both the humoral and cellular immune systems. Innate immunologic mechanisms include physical barriers and factors such as mucus, complement, and destructive enzymes. The nonspecific defense mechanisms of MALT are generally present constitutively and act as a defense against all mucosal pathogens.

Mucosal barrier

Structure and function of the mucosal epithelium

The first line of defense against invading mucosal pathogens is the epithelial surface of the mucosa that demarcates a physical barrier between the body and the external environment. In the GI tract, this physical barrier consists of a single layer of absorptive epithelial cells called enterocytes sealed together by tight junctions that exclude harmful pathogens, peptides, and macromolecules with antigenic potential. The brush border, which dominates the apical membrane of enterocytes, consists of rigid, closely packed microvilli covered with a thick layer of membrane-anchored glycoproteins called the *glycocalyx*. The glycocalyx, which has a negative charge, acts to impede the passage of mucosal pathogens between microvilli and can prevent direct contact with the microvilli. Furthermore, enterocytes can get rid of microorganisms adherent to the microvilli, since portions of microvilli shed continuously from enterocytes as membrane vesicles. Epithelial turnover can also be increased in response to the invasion of harmful mucosal pathogens, thereby shedding any epithelial cells or cells whose apical surface membrane has been colonized.

Tight junctions are a formidable barrier to mucosal pathogens. Under normal conditions the tight junctions are permeable only to water and small ions. However, in response to local events within the epithelium or lumen, the tight junction can open its pore to a radius of 5 nanometers (nm), allowing polypeptides of up to 11 amino acids to pass through. Even when open, the pore size of the tight junctions is still small enough to prevent passage of mucosal pathogens. If the pathogen must invade below the mucosal barrier, it needs a means to traverse the barrier, either by entering cells on the apical side and leaving through the basal or luminal side or by opening up tight junctions to travel between cells.

Antigen uptake and sampling

Pathogens, particulate antigens, or macromolecules are taken up only via a type of highly restricted active vesicular transport across epithelial cells at a site termed the follicle-associated epithelium (FAE) (Fig. 17.2). The FAE is a one-cell-thick layer that forms the interface between the mucosal lymphoid follicle and the lumen of the intestine. The FAE of Peyer's patches is composed primarily of specialized epithelial cells called microfold (M) cells. Antigen uptake via endocytosis can also occur with the intestinal enterocytes. These cells are also capable of constitutive or cytokine-regulated expression of major histocompatibility complex (MHC) class I and/or class II. Enterocytes have been shown to present antigens in vitro; however,

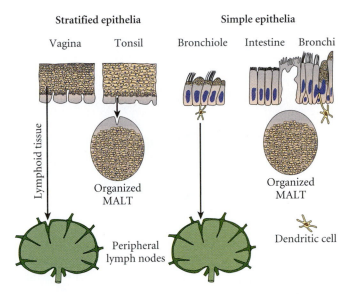

Figure 17.2 Antigens can be sampled at mucosal surfaces and transported to lymphoid tissue by several means. At stratified epithelium, DCs that capture antigen at the mucosal surface can migrate to organized MALT or to peripheral lymph nodes. Such migratory DCs can also sample antigens in the airway epithelia, after which they can migrate to organized MALT or to peripheral lymph nodes. Last, intestine and airways have specialized antigen-sampling cells known as M cells that transport intact antigens across the epithelial layer where the antigens can then encounter the underlying organized MALT. Redrawn from M. R. Neutra et al., *Annu. Rev. Immunol.* **14:**275–300, 1996, with permission.

their role in antigen presentation in vivo has yet to be clearly defined.

M cells, which are specialized for transepithelial transport of antigens across the mucosal barrier, perform an important role in sampling the environment within the GI tract (Fig. 17.3). The basolateral surface of the M cells is deeply invaginated to form a large pocket into which specific subpopulations of lymphocytes migrate. M cells can take up and transport a broad range of sizes and types of luminal antigens and microorganisms, including particles or macromolecules such as native ferritin and toxins; intestinal viruses, including reovirus, poliovirus, and human immunodeficiency virus type 1 (HIV-1); and enteric bacteria, including *Vibrio cholerae* and *Salmonella enterica*. The M cells use multiple mechanisms for the uptake of antigens and microorganisms from the luminal side of the epithelium. Bacteria and large particles are taken up via phagocytosis. Viruses and macromolecules are taken up by absorptive endocytosis through clathrin-coated pits and vesicles. Other types of antigens are taken up through fluid-phase endocytosis. Each of these mechanisms results in the transcytosis of the luminal material to the basal pocket and its subsequent exocytosis. M cells can also take in luminal material via IgA-immune complexes, although M cells lack polymeric immunoglobulin receptors (pIgR).

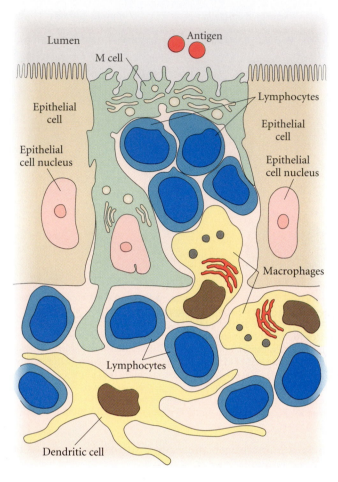

Figure 17.3 M cells are found within the intestinal and airway epithelia and serve the function of transporting antigens (Ag) across the epithelial layer so they can encounter the immune cells of the host. The schematic diagram of an M cell shows the large pocket in its basolateral membrane in which macrophages (Mφ) and lymphocytes (L) reside. DCs are also closely associated with M cells. Antigens in the intestinal lumen contact the apical membrane of the M cell and are transcytosed to its basolateral pocket. Redrawn from M. R. Neutra et al., *Annu. Rev. Immunol.* **14:**275–300, 1996, with permission.

The lysosome content of M cells is also low, allowing them to transport the luminal material to the adjacent lymphocytes without the material undergoing much degradation.

Humoral components of innate immunity in GALT

Mucin
Mucus is a thick viscous layer of glycoproteins that coats the mucosal epithelium, providing an important layer of protection. Mucus consists of a solution of >95% water, ~1% free protein, ~1% dialyzable salts, and ~1% mucin. Mucin molecules of the GI tract are 70 to 80% carbohydrate attached to a protein skeleton varying in size from 1 to several million daltons. Mucin is generated by goblet cells located on the villi and in the crypts of the intestinal surface. Secretion of mucus by goblet cells is stimulated by alterations in the local environment and can occur through either direct or indirect mechanisms. Mucus production can be directly triggered by chemical agents or immune complexes produced during viral, bacterial, or parasitic infections. Alternatively, mucus production can be indirectly triggered by local histamine or cytokine production.

Mucus protects the GI tract in a variety of ways. It acts as a physical barrier, preventing epithelial cells from being damaged by digestive enzymes. It also prevents food and other particulate matter from directly interacting with, and potentially damaging, the mucosal epithelium. Mucus can also trap pathogens and prevent them from reaching the epithelium. This ability is attributed to the similarity of mucin carbohydrate moieties to the glycoproteins and glycolipids present on mucosal epithelial cells themselves. These carbohydrate moieties provide binding sites for pathogens, keeping them trapped within the mucosal layer. Mucin also binds *secretory IgA* (sIgA) via its Fc region, thus trapping pathogens bound to local IgA antibodies. Mucus and associated trapped or bound antigens are eventually expelled from the GI tract by the normal peristaltic movements on intestinal contents. Besides acting as a physical barrier and trap, mucus contains a variety of factors, including lysozyme, peroxidases, and lactoferrin, that are bacteriocidal or can inhibit bacterial growth.

Lysozyme
Human lysozyme is a 14.6-kilodalton (kDa) protein consisting of a single 129-amino-acid chain that is present in milk and other mucosal fluids. The microbial activity of human lysozyme is attributed to its ability to hydrolyze the peptidoglycans of the bacterial cell walls by cleaving the β(1→4) glycosidic bond between *N*-acetylmuramic acid and *N*-acetyl-D-glucosamine (see Fig. 2.3), ultimately resulting in bacteriolysis. Lysozyme also can activate bacterial autolysins and induce bacterial aggregation, thereby resulting in decreased bacterial adherence to mucosal epithelial cells.

Peroxidases
Several forms of human peroxidases are present in mucosal secretions. These enzymes are synthesized in exocrine glands and secreted onto the mucosal surface. Neutrophils and eosinophils also can synthesize these enzymes. Peroxidases protect the mucosal epithelium from pathogens by catalyzing the peroxidation of halides (Cl$^-$, Br$^-$, and I$^-$) and thiocyanate ions (SCN$^-$) to generate reactive products with potent antimicrobial activities that inhibit microbial growth or metabolism. Lacking these ions, the peroxidases can act as catalases to generate

hydrogen peroxide (H_2O_2), which is highly toxic to both the host and mucosal pathogens.

Lactoferrin

Human lactoferrin is an 80-kDa glycoprotein consisting of a single 691-amino-acid chain that binds Fe^{3+} with high affinity (K_a, $\sim 10^{20}$ M). Lactoferrin can be found in exocrine secretions, blood, and leukocytes, and the lactoferrin receptor is expressed on human intestine and brush border membranes. Lactoferrin possesses antimicrobial activity and either can kill most mucosal pathogens or can inhibit their growth by competing with the bacteria for iron. By reducing the level of free iron within the GI tract, lactoferrin deprives the invading bacteria of an essential nutrient. However, some pathogens (e.g., gonococci) take advantage of the presence of lactoferrin and transferrin, expressing specific binding proteins to allow scavenging of iron from these host proteins for utilization by the microbe.

Antimicrobial peptides

Antimicrobial peptides are small proteins (30 to 40 amino acids) that have the ability to kill bacteria, enveloped viruses, and, in some cases, fungi (Fig. 17.4A). The toxic activity of antimicrobial peptides is attributable to their ability to insert into biologic membranes and disrupt their barrier function, leading to the osmotic death of the target microbe (Fig. 17.4B). One class of these molecules is the defensins that exist in a β-pleated-sheet conformation stabilized by three intramolecular disulfide bonds. Defensins are classified as either α-defensins or β-defensins, depending on the arrangement of these disulfide bonds, although a third class of defensins, θ-defensins, has been identified. Although much of the early work on defensins was performed using peptides isolated from neutrophil granules, which produce abundant quantities of defensins, more recent studies have shown that many cell types synthesize these peptides. Several α-defensins are produced by the Paneth cells in the intestinal crypts (located at the bases of the villi), where they may be extremely important in the killing of microorganisms that move into the confined space between villi. Because of their expression in the crypts, α-defensins produced in the intestine frequently are called *cryptdins*. Recent work has led to a greater appreciation of defensins as important components of the innate defense of the gut. Cryptdins are produced in the Paneth cells of the GI tract as a precursor that must be acted on by matrilysin, a matrix metalloproteinase, to produce the mature, active form. In transgenic mice unable to make matrilysin, preparations of peptides from the GI tract had a reduced ability to kill bacterial pathogens. These mice were also more suscepti-

ble to infection by orally administered bacteria. This type of study substantiates the important role of these antibacterial peptides in innate immunity in the GI tract.

Cellular components of innate immunity in GALT

The cellular effectors of innate immunity in GALT are numerous and include virtually all of the myeloid-lineage cell types.

Neutrophils

In virtually all tissues, *polymorphonuclear neutrophils* (PMNs) constitute the first line of defense against bacterial infection. They are highly motile and enter tissues early in the inflammatory response. Neutrophils kill their targets through reactive oxygen species (such as superoxide, peroxide, and hypochlorite), reactive nitrogen species (such as nitric oxide and nitrous acid), lysozyme, lytic enzymes, and defensins and can use these toxic molecules in either phagocytic killing (which occurs within the neutrophil itself following internalization of a microorganism) or through the release of the toxic agents into the extracellular space.

Neutrophils are attracted to sites of infection by formylated peptides produced by bacteria. In the intestine, neutrophils can also be attracted to a site of infection by interleukin-8 (IL-8 or CXCL8) synthesized by the intestinal epithelium in response to infection. Although neutrophils undoubtedly play an important role in host protection in the GALT, the emigration of neutrophils across intestinal epithelium also has been implicated in disruption of the tight junctions of the epithelial barrier, allowing bacterial pathogens access to the submucosal space. Neutrophil accumulation in the intestine constitutes an important protective mechanism, but one consequence of this process may be the ability of a pathogen to take advantage of the disruption of the tight junctions to gain access to the submucosa. Likely at low infectious inocula or microbial levels the PMN response is protective, but if the infectious agent is ingested at a high inoculum or grows to a high level in the GI tract, the PMN response is overwhelmed and the pathogen takes advantage of the disrupted epithelium to move to the submucosal area.

Mast cells

Mast cells (MCs) are best known for their role in the immediate-type hypersensitivity reaction (see chapter 25). However, MCs also are involved in the regulation of many normal physiologic functions. These cells are phenotypically characterized by their granularity and the expression of the high-affinity IgE receptor (FcεRI) and are present

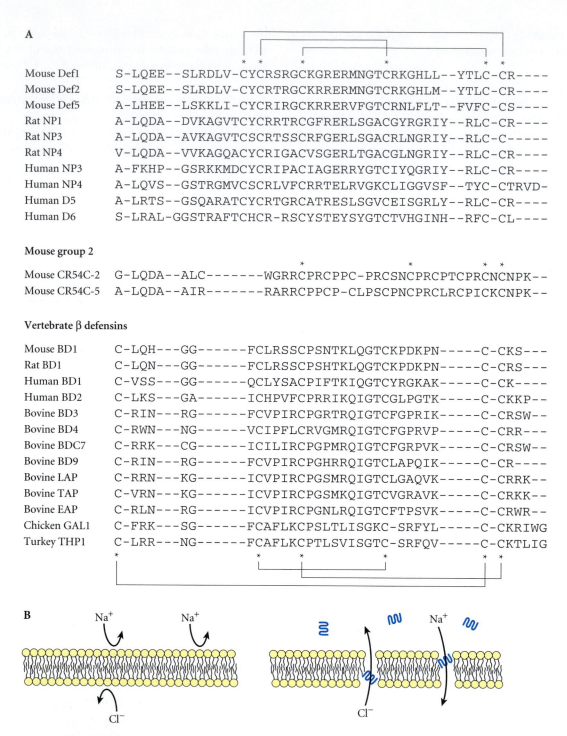

A

Mouse Def1	S-LQEE--SLRDLV-CYCRSRGCKGRERMNGTCRKGHLL--YTLC-CR----
Mouse Def2	S-LQEE--SLRDLV-CYCRTRGCKRRERMNGTCRKGHLM--YTLC-CR----
Mouse Def5	A-LHEE--LSKKLI-CYCRIRGCKRRERVFGTCRNLFLT--FVFC-CS----
Rat NP1	A-LQDA--DVKAGVTCYCRRTRCGFRERLSGACGYRGRIY--RLC-CR----
Rat NP3	A-LQDA--AVKAGVTCSCRTSSCRFGERLSGACRLNGRIY--RLC-C-----
Rat NP4	V-LQDA--VVKAGQACYCRIGACVSGERLTGACGLNGRIY--RLC-CR----
Human NP3	A-FKHP--GSRKKMDCYCRIPACIAGERRYGTCIYQGRIY--RLC-CR----
Human NP4	A-LQVS--GSTRGMVCSCRLVFCRRTELRVGKCLIGGVSF--TYC-CTRVD-
Human D5	A-LRTS--GSQARATCYCRTGRCATRESLSGVCEISGRLY--RLC-CR----
Human D6	S-LRAL-GGSTRAFTCHCR-RSCYSTEYSYGTCTVHGINH--RFC-CL----

Mouse group 2

Mouse CR54C-2	G-LQDA--ALC-------WGRRCPRCPPC-PRCSNCPRCPTCPRCNCNPK--
Mouse CR54C-5	A-LQDA--AIR-------RARRCPPCP-CLPSCPNCPRCLRCPICKCNPK--

Vertebrate β defensins

Mouse BD1	C-LQH---GG------FCLRSSCPSNTKLQGTCKPDKPN-----C-CKS---
Rat BD1	C-LQN---GG------FCLRSSCPSHTKLQGTCKPDKPN-----C-CRS---
Human BD1	C-VSS---GG------QCLYSACPIFTKIQGTCYRGKAK-----C-CK----
Human BD2	C-LKS---GA------ICHPVFCPRRIKQIGTCGLPGTK-----C-CKKP--
Bovine BD3	C-RIN---RG------FCVPIRCPGRTRQIGTCFGPRIK-----C-CRSW--
Bovine BD4	C-RWN---NG------VCIPFLCRVGMRQIGTCFGPRVP-----C-CRR---
Bovine BDC7	C-RRK---CG------ICILIRCPGPMRQIGTCFGRPVK-----C-CRSW--
Bovine BD9	C-RIN---RG------FCVPIRCPGHRRQIGTCLAPQIK-----C-CR----
Bovine LAP	C-RRN---KG------ICVPIRCPGSMRQIGTCLGAQVK-----C-CRRK--
Bovine TAP	C-VRN---KG------ICVPIRCPGSMKQIGTCVGRAVK-----C-CRKK--
Bovine EAP	C-RLN---RG------ICVPIRCPGNLRQIGTCFTPSVK-----C-CRWR--
Chicken GAL1	C-FRK---SG------FCAFLKCPSLTLISGKC-SRFYL-----C-CKRIWG
Turkey THP1	C-LRR---NG------FCAFLKCPTLSVISGTC-SRFQV-----C-CKTLIG

B

Figure 17.4 Antibacterial peptides are proteins of 30 to 40 amino acids that have cytotoxic activity due to their ability to permeabilize membranes. (**A**) Amino acid sequences of antibacterial peptides of several species. See the inside front cover for the amino acid code. Reprinted from A. L. Hughes, *Cell. Mol. Life Sci.* **56:**94–103, 1999, with permission. (**B**) Model for permeabilization of a phospholipid bilayer by antibacterial peptides.

in large numbers in tissues that are constantly exposed to the outside environment, such as the skin and MALT.

MCs mediate a broad range of biologic and immunologic functions, largely as a result of their cellular heterogeneity. In rodents, MCs can be divided into two clearly defined subsets, mucosal (MMC) and connective tissue-type (CMC) MCs, on the basis of the major proteoglycan within their granules. MMCs, which are present within the mucosa of MALT, are characterized by the major granule proteoglycan chondroitin sulfate, whereas CMC granules contain the proteoglycan heparin. Furthermore, MMCs have a very low histamine content, and their development and differentiation are T cell dependent, unlike that of CMCs.

The phenotypic differences between human MC subsets are less defined than those in rodents. Human MCs are derived from CD34$^+$ pluripotent hematopoietic stem cells. However, unlike most hematopoietic cells, MC precursors leave the bone marrow before they are completely mature. The undifferentiated MCs traffic to connective or mucosal tissues as morphologically unidentifiable MC progenitors and complete their differentiation after arriving at the tissue sites. Thus, MC development and heterogeneity are dependent on the anatomic microenvironment where the progenitor MCs undergo final differentiation. Mucosal cells in humans cannot be strictly classified into MMC and CMC. The main criterion for defining human MC subtypes is their neutral protease content and the morphology of their granules. The MC_T subset contains only tryptase, and the MC_{TC} phenotype contains both tryptase and chymase. Moreover, the phenotype of the MC is interchangeable and is influenced by the surrounding microenvironment and local factors. When these human MC subsets were first described, it was suggested that these cells were the equivalents of rodent MMCs and CMCs; however, it has been shown that both subsets (MC_T and MC_{TC}) are present within all tissues. Variable amounts of each subtype are present in each tissue, and the relative number and ratio can vary during disease states. The predominant MCs in the mucosa and submucosa of normal small and large human intestines are the MC_{TC}, while the MC_T are preferentially found in the mucosa in the lung.

Human MCs participate in a broad range of immunologic functions. These cells are involved in the host defense against bacterial and parasitic infections, vascularization, and tissue remodeling. Functionally, the two MC subsets share some activities; however, they also appear to mediate separate immunologic functions. The primary roles of MC_T are host defense and proinflammatory functions. MC_T are found in increased numbers around sites of activated type 2 helper T (TH2) cells. They play a critical role in the clearance of parasites, and their numbers are increased during parasitic infections. The primary role of MC_{TC} is in inflammatory reactions, angiogenesis, and tissue remodeling; they are not involved in immune protection. Their numbers remain unchanged during parasitic infections.

The pleiotropic activity of these cells is attributable to the broad range of immune mediators, both stored (primary mediators) and newly synthesized (secondary mediators), that they can release following cellular activation. The stored mediators include histamine, which stimulates the contraction of intestinal smooth muscle and increases mucus production; heparin, which affects the stability and function of other MC mediators; tryptase, which is mitogenic for fibroblasts and epithelial cells, stimulates the release of IL-8, and increases expression of intercellular adhesion molecule 1 (ICAM-1) on endothelial cells; and chymase, which converts IL-1β to IL-1, proteolytically degrades IL-4, and stimulates secretion from submucosal gland cells. The newly synthesized mediators include the arachidonic acid metabolites prostaglandin D_2, a PMN chemoattractant, and leukotriene C_4, which enhances bronchial mucus production. Following their activation, MCs also generate a plethora of cytokines. The cytokine profile is predominantly TH2-like; however, the activity of the MC cytokines encompasses physiologic, pathologic, and immunologic functions. In vitro, these cells have been shown to generate IL-4, IL-5, IL-6, IL-8, IL-13, granulocyte-macrophage colony-stimulating factor (GM-CSF), tumor necrosis factor alpha (TNF-α), and CCL5 (RANTES, or regulated on activation, normal T cells expressed and secreted), but MC_{TC} do not produce IL-5 and IL-6. These mediators allow MCs to influence other cells within the local environment of the MALT. Moreover, these factors permit two-way communication between MCs and sensory nerves, which allows neuromodulation of both normal gut and lung functions and local immune responses.

Acquired Immunity of GALT

If a mucosal pathogen penetrates the elaborate set of protective defense mechanisms of the mucosal barrier, the mucosal immune system will mount a specific response against the invading pathogen. This response is mediated by the local humoral and cellular immune systems. The fundamental molecular and cellular mechanisms involved in generating a mucosal immune response are similar, if not identical, to the mechanisms required for the generation of a systemic immune response. Thus processing and presentation of antigens to T cells by antigen-presenting cells (APCs), maturation of T cells into effector cells mediating delayed-type hypersensitivity and cytotoxic T lymphocyte (CTL) effectors, and provision of help to B cells to become antibody-secreting plasma cells occur in the GALT in the same way they occur in lymph nodes. However, the mucosal immune system additionally has to produce unique immunologic mechanisms that protect the mucosal tissues without interfering with their essential functions, i.e., respiration or nutrient absorption.

Inductive sites

Acquired immune responses in the GALT are initiated at discrete anatomic locations termed *inductive sites*. Once activated at an inductive site, lymphocytes typically circulate through the body via the blood vessels and then populate various mucosal and nonmucosal tissues. Figure 17.5 lists several important inductive sites, along with the mucosal tissues populated by lymphocytes activated at each inductive site. MALT inductive sites consist of both anatomically discrete single follicles and aggregated lymphoid follicles. Single follicles are present along the entire length of the GI tract and are most predominant in the colon and rectum. Aggregated follicles, such as Peyer's patches, occur within the small intestine, appendix, and mesenteric lymph nodes of the MALT and are also present within the respiratory tract, particularly the NALT.

Peyer's patches

Peyer's patches are scattered throughout the GI tract and are enriched sources of precursors for IgA-producing plasma cells (Fig. 17.6; see Fig. 4.14). Peyer's patches are important in the ingestion of luminal antigens and in the generation of antigen-specific IgA-producing B cells. The greatest number of IgA-positive B cells is found in Peyer's patches.

The Peyer's patch is the classic example illustrating the structure of the FAE. The luminal side of Peyer's patches within the epithelium is demarcated by a large number of M cells that transport antigens in an undegraded form into the submucosa. In the pocket formed on the basal side of the M cell are macrophages and dendritic cells (DCs) that have the potential to process and present the luminal antigens transcytosed by the M cells. However, the primary function of the macrophages is thought to be in the uptake and killing of any incoming mucosal pathogens or ingestion and neutralization of harmful antigens. There also T and B cells residing within the basal fold of the M-cell pocket. Most of the T cells are memory TH cells (CD45RO$^+$ CD4$^+$ TCRα/β$^+$ CD69$^+$), indicating that these cells have been previously activated. It has been suggested that the B cells within the pocket are both memory cells and lymphoblasts undergoing initial activation. Movement of both of these types of B cells into the pocket may allow the initial antigen exposure that activates the lymphoblasts and provides memory B cells with antigen exposure to prolong their production of specific antibody.

The largest component of the Peyer's patch that is located below the M-cell pocket is a follicular area containing mostly B cells surrounded by smaller numbers of T cells concentrated in adjacent sites. B cells within the follicle express naive markers; they are IgM$^+$ and express almost no IgG or IgA. However, as in lymph nodes, antigen-primed B cells along with follicular dendritic cells (FDCs) and T cells organize into a germinal center once activated by antigen. The germinal center is believed to be the site of high-level antibody isotype switching and affinity maturation. The retention and presentation of antigens by the local FDCs are thought to enhance B-cell isotype switching and maturation. Unlike the follicles in systemic lymphoid tissues, Peyer's patch follicles do not generate high levels of antibody-producing cells. IgA-secreting plasma cells are found dispersed throughout the submucosa.

The T-cell zones adjacent to the follicles (parafollicular regions) contain the full complement of T-cell subsets. These regions contain high endothelial venules (HEVs), which permit T cells to circulate through and populate the Peyer's patches. These regions also contain DCs that are essential for antigen-specific activation of the Peyer's patch CD4$^+$ T cells. More than half (~60%) of the T cells present in these zones are CD4$^+$, and their primary role is to selectively enhance IgA class switching and IgA production.

Figure 17.5 Diagram showing the several locations of MALT immune activation (inductive sites) and the spectra of effector sites usually populated by immune cells originally activated at each inductive site.

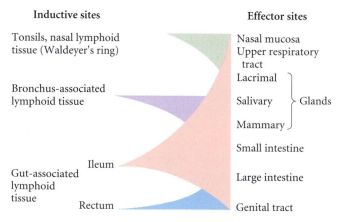

Inductive sites | Effector sites

Tonsils, nasal lymphoid tissue (Waldeyer's ring)

Bronchus-associated lymphoid tissue

Gut-associated lymphoid tissue — Ileum, Rectum

Nasal mucosa
Upper respiratory tract
Lacrimal
Salivary } Glands
Mammary
Small intestine
Large intestine
Genital tract

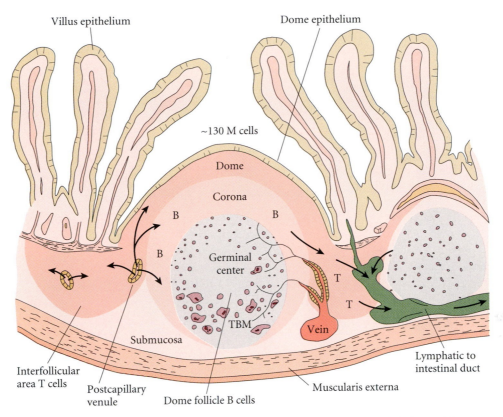

Villus epithelium

Dome epithelium

~130 M cells

Dome

Corona

B   B

B

Germinal
center

T

T

TBM

Vein

Submucosa

Interfollicular
area T cells

Postcapillary
venule

Dome follicle B cells

Muscularis externa

Lymphatic to
intestinal duct

Figure 17.6 Schematic diagram of a Peyer's patch. Each nodule is composed of a follicle (comprising a germinal center, B-cell-rich corona, and T-cell-rich dome), T-cell-rich interfollicular area, and M-cell-containing dome epithelium. The germinal center contains actively dividing lymphocytes and tingible body macrophages (TBM). At the left is a postcapillary venule containing HEV, a site of leukocyte influx. At the right is a lymphatic, a site of leukocyte efflux.

Humoral immunity

B cells

The B cells of the MALT consist of both self-replenishing peritoneal CD5$^+$ B cells (B1 cells) and conventional bone marrow-derived B cells. The Peyer's patches, however, are the major sites of development of IgA$^+$ B cells. Approximately 75 to 80% of the activated B cells within the germinal centers of the Peyer's patch are IgA$^+$, unlike the germinal centers of peripheral lymph nodes, which contain very few IgA$^+$ B cells. Following antigenic stimulation, the B cells undergo cellular differentiation and IgA isotype switching and then must undergo further differentiation to become IgA-secreting plasma cells (Fig. 17.7). The local mucosal T cells provide the B cells with both the costimulatory molecules necessary for cellular activation and proliferation and the cytokines required for cellular differentiation and IgA secretion. The cytokines IL-4, IL-5, IL-6, IL-10, and transforming growth factor beta (TGF-β) generated in the mucosal inductive (Peyer's patches) and effector (lamina propria) sites are biased toward generating a TH2 immune response and play an important role in the differentiation of the IgA-committed B cells into plasma cells. TGF-β promotes immunoglobulin heavy-chain switching to IgA. IL-4 and IL-5 promote both the activation of IgA-committed B cells and the differentiation of IgA$^+$ B cells to plasma cells, and IL-6 promotes high-level secretion of IgA antibody.

The developmental pathways and progenitors of B1 cells are different from those of conventional B cells. B1 cells appear early during ontogeny and arise from progenitor cells in the fetal omentum and liver. Furthermore, these cells are self-replenishing, unlike conventional mucosal IgA plasma B cells, which have a half-life of 5 days. B1 cells comprise about 5% of the peripheral B cells but make up most of the B cells in the peritoneal and pleural cavities. Very few of these cells are present in the peripheral lymph nodes or the Peyer's patches; however, B1 cells can comprise up to 50% of the IgA$^+$ B cells in the lamina propria. The antibody repertoire of the B1 cells is highly restricted. Generally, B1-cell-produced antibodies are

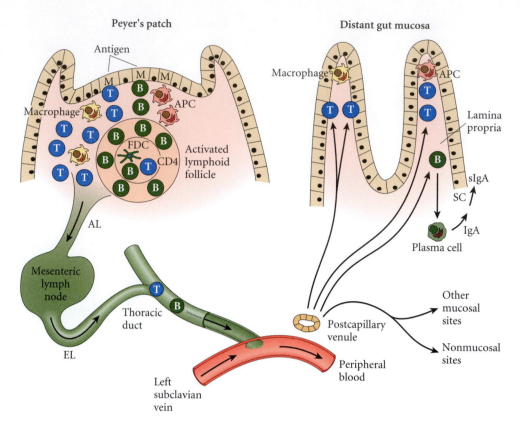

Figure 17.7 Trafficking of B cells and T cells following activation at the Peyer's patch. (**Top left**) Lymphocytes residing at or near an M cell will encounter M-cell-transported antigens and will migrate to a local lymphoid follicle, where activation is facilitated by FDCs. Some lymphocytes activated in this local follicle will enter the lymphatic circulation and are carried via an afferent lymphatic (AL) to a mesenteric lymph node, where further immune activation may occur due to APCs and T cells residing in the lymph node. Activated lymphocytes can then leave the mesenteric node via an efferent lymphatic (EL) and merge with the peripheral blood at the thoracic duct. These peripheral blood lymphocytes can then home to any of a number of mucosal and nonmucosal sites at postcapillary venules. (**Top right**) Lymphocytes activated in the GALT preferentially home back to the intestine, where they reside below the intestinal epithelium and secrete sIgA, which is transcytosed into the intestinal lumen.

low-affinity antibodies encoded by germ line configurations of immunoglobulin genes with broad specificity for common bacterial antigens, such as phosphatidylcholine. The repertoire of B1 cells is established soon after birth. This occurs primarily through positive selection during interaction with common bacterial antigens that are encountered as the GI tract rapidly becomes populated with commensal microorganisms. It is believed that B1 cells provide an essential and early defense against many common mucosal pathogens.

Mucosal immunoglobulins

IgM, IgG, and IgA can be detected in mucosal secretions; however, the most prominent immunoglobulin isotype is IgA. Unlike serum IgA, which is present in monomeric form, the IgA in mucosal secretions (sIgA) exists predominantly as part of a multiprotein complex. sIgA is found in a dimeric form (Fig. 17.8) and in association with two proteins called *J chain* and *secretory component* (SC). Most of the sIgA present in mucosal secretions is derived from local synthesis (i.e., IgA produced at the mucosal site) because of the very high proportion of IgA-producing and IgA-committed B cells in the MALT (Table 17.1).

Structure of IgA and component chains (J chain and SC).

Multiple and single IgA subclasses have been detected in a variety of species. Two IgA subclasses have been described in humans: IgA1 and IgA2. IgA1 comprises 80 to 95% of total serum IgA, and this value is also representative of the proportion of IgA1$^+$ B cells in the bone marrow. The ratio of IgA1 to IgA2 differs within the various mucosal secretions. Since most sIgA is derived from local B-cell synthesis, the ratio of IgA1 to IgA2 reflects the distribution of

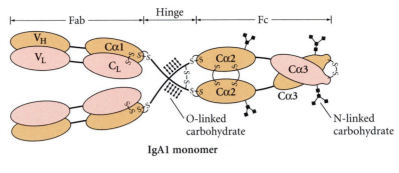

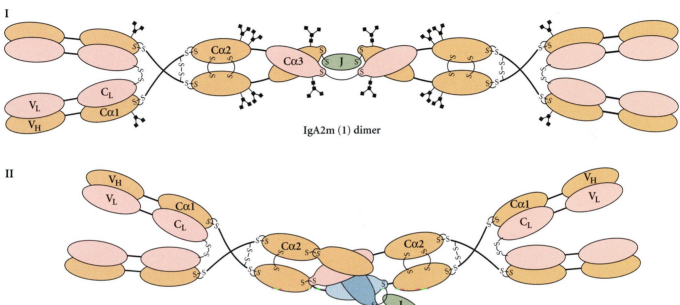

Figure 17.8 Diagram of an IgA1 monomer (**top**) and two different models of the IgA2 dimer (**bottom**). The locations of intermonomer disulfide binds (S-S) and J chain (J) differ between these two models.

the IgA1- and IgA2-producing B cells in the mucosal tissues. IgA1 is the predominant subclass in most mucosal tissues, comprising 30 to 50% of the total immunoglobulin; however, IgA2 is present in equal or greater quantities in the large intestine and female reproductive tract. The local mucosal lymph nodes contain various proportions of IgA1$^+$ and IgA2$^+$ B cells, the ratio being dependent on the precise anatomic location.

Table 17.1 Isotypes and functions of mucosal immunoglobulins

Isotype	Occurrence	Functions
sIgA	Major form of Ig in most secretions of humans and many other mammals	Noninflammatory mucosal protection
sIgM	Second most abundant Ig in most secretions; sIgM compensates for lack of sIgA in IgA deficiency	Probably similar to plasma IgM or sIgA; activates complement
IgG	Normally minor component, but relatively abundant in nasal and respiratory tract secretions; probably transudes from plasma; increased in pathologic, especially inflammatory, conditions	Neutralization; potentially inflammatory; activates complement and phagocytes
IgA (plasma type)	Found in human bile and possibly other secretions; transudes from plasma, or transported by alternative secretion mechanisms	Possibly similar to sIgA, poor complement activation, or inhibitory
IgD	Significant minor component of nasal secretions, milk	Unknown
IgE	Normally insignificant; elevated in atopic allergies and helminthic infections	Adverse hypersensitivity states (atopy); parasite expulsion

One major difference between the two subclasses occurs at the immunoglobulin hinge region. IgA2 lacks a 13-amino-acid segment present in IgA1. This hinge region confers greater flexibility to IgA1 but renders it susceptible to bacteria-derived IgA1-specific proteases. Conversely, the lack of the hinge region in IgA2 confers resistance to these proteases. Both subclasses of IgA in humans are glycosylated. For IgA1, 6 to 7% of the total molecular weight of IgA1 is carbohydrate, and for IgA2, 8 to 10%. The major difference in the glycosylation of the IgA subclasses is the presence of *N*-acetylgalactosamine on IgA1.

Secretory IgA is synthesized in a monomeric form using the same biosynthetic pathways and mechanisms used to produce the other immunoglobulin isotypes. Polymerization of sIgA occurs just before or at the time of cellular secretion, forming dimers, trimers, tetramers, and (rarely) pentamers, in association with the J chain.

The polymeric immunoglobulins, IgA and IgM, are covalently associated with J chain, a 15- to 16-kDa (137 amino acid) glycoprotein. J chain associates with the Fc region of IgM or IgA via disulfide bonding (Fig. 17.8). Expression of the J chain in humans begins at the earliest stages of B-cell differentiation and can be detected in null or pre-B cells. J-chain synthesis is not detected in most of the normal IgA-producing human bone marrow B cells that synthesize monomeric IgA, but high levels of J-chain expression are present in most of the lamina propria IgA-producing B cells that generate polymeric IgA. However, J-chain expression is not restricted to B cells that produce polymeric immunoglobulin. J chains have also been detected in IgG plasma cells isolated from sites of inflammation and in mitogen-stimulated cells. Polymeric immunoglobulin synthesis has been observed in IgM-secreting B cells that have mutated or deleted J-chain genes; however, absence of the J chain seems to skew assembly of the IgM into hexamers. The J chain may not be essential for the initiation of polymerization but may regulate the degree and form of polymerization. The J chain is also essential in the binding of polymeric immunoglobulin to the SC (see below), since IgM polymers that lack J chain fail to bind to this protein efficiently.

As with the J chain, most polymeric immunoglobulin present in mucosal secretions is found in association with the SC protein. SC is an ~80-kDa highly glycosylated protein (22% carbohydrate by mass) that is found either as a free protein or in association with polymeric IgA or IgM in mucosal secretions. SC is a cleaved metabolite of a larger protein receptor (~115 kDa) known as pIgR (Fig. 17.9).

The pIgR is a member of the immunoglobulin superfamily and consists of five extracellular immunoglobulin-like domains, a transmembrane region, and a cytoplasmic

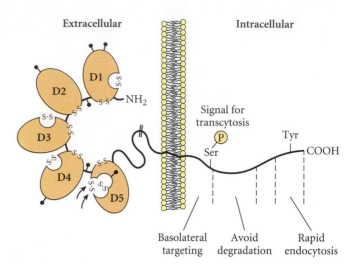

Figure 17.9 Diagram of the pIgR. The extracellular region consists of five immunoglobulin-like domains D1 to D5 and contains the binding site for polymeric immunoglobulin. The intracellular region contains signal sequences for membrane targeting, endocytosis, and transcytosis. The two arrows indicate the binding site for IgA. Ser, serine; Tyr, tyrosine.

tail. Most pIgR expression is restricted to the basolateral surface membrane of epithelial cells. In humans, pIgRs can be detected in all mucosal tissues, with the highest expression on the crypt cells of the large bowel. pIgRs also are present in the gallbladder and portal bile duct of humans; however, in other species pIgRs are expressed on hepatocytes.

The expression of pIgRs is constitutive. However, pIgR expression is increased during mucosal infections. This enhanced expression is believed to be induced by locally generated cytokines. Recombinant interferon-gamma (IFN-γ) causes the accumulation of pIgR mRNA by increasing the transcription as well as the stability of the mRNA. In vitro, TNF-α and IL-4 have also been shown to increase pIgR expression. Together, IFN-γ and TNF-α display an additive effect, whereas IFN-γ and IL-4 exhibit a synergistic effect. IL-4 alone, however, decreases pIgR expression. TGF-β has also been reported to increase pIgR expression in vitro.

Transport of polymeric immunoglobulin. The protection of mucosal surfaces by polymeric immunoglobulin requires that the immunoglobulins be transported from their place of synthesis (usually immediately below the mucosal epithelium) into the mucosal secretions, a process that requires transport of the newly synthesized sIgA across an intact epithelial layer. Such transport is the primary function of the pIgR (Fig. 17.10). The locally synthesized polymeric immunoglobulin binds to the pIgR at the basolateral surface membrane of the epithelial cells. This

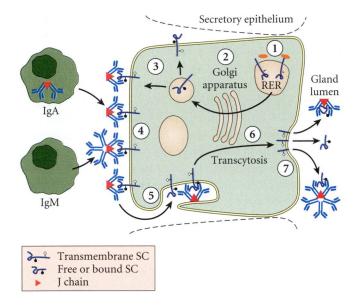

Transmembrane SC
Free or bound SC
J chain

Figure 17.10 Transcytosis of secretory, polymeric immunoglobulin. The pIgR is synthesized in the rough endoplasmic reticulum (RER) (1), glycosylated in the Golgi apparatus (2), and then transported to the basolateral membrane (3). Dimeric IgA or polymeric IgM then binds to the pIgR (4) and is transcytosed from the basolateral membrane of the epithelial cell (5) to the apical membrane (6) and released at the apical membrane (7). During step 6 or 7, the pIgR is cleaved so that the extracellular region of the pIgR (now called SC) remains associated with the immunoglobulin, while the transmembrane and intracellular regions of the pIgR remain on the apical membrane of the epithelial cell.

binding is dependent on the presence of J chain in the immunoglobulin. The K_A of IgM binding to the pIgR is much greater than that for polymeric IgA binding. The initial interaction between polymeric IgA and the pIgR occurs at the first immunoglobulin-like domain of the receptor, resulting in formation of a noncovalent bond. This is followed by a series of subsequent binding interactions that form additional noncovalent bonds. The last binding step is the formation of a covalent disulfide bond between the $C_{\alpha 2}$ region of the IgA and the fifth immunoglobulin-like domain of the pIgR. Upon binding to the pIgR, the IgA is internalized by the epithelial cell via receptor-mediated endocytosis, which occurs through ligand-induced active clustering of the immunoglobulin-pIgR complexes (although unoccupied pIgR can also be endocytosed). Following endocytosis, the pIgR is *transcytosed* to the luminal/apical membrane of the epithelial cell. Sometime during transcytosis, the extracellular domains of the pIgR are proteolytically cleaved from the transmembrane anchor of the pIgR, releasing SC (the name now given to the former extracellular domains of the pIgR) into the local secretions. If the pIgR was bound to polymeric immunoglobulin at the time of transcytosis, the SC remains associated with the immunoglobulin after transcytosis is

complete. After transcytosis of immunoglobulin into the mucosal secretions, SC plays an important role in protecting the immunoglobulin from proteolytic degradation.

Antibody function on mucosal surfaces. Although many immunologists claim that sIgA mediates a broad range of important protective functions (Fig. 17.11), it has been difficult to reconcile these claims with the observation that IgA genetic deficiency is a benign disease in the vast majority of affected individuals. Selective IgA immunodeficiency is the most common type of immunodeficiency in human populations. Certainly a small proportion (10 to 20%) of IgA-deficient individuals have an increased susceptibility to infection and other associated immunologic abnormalities, but the overwhelming majority do not. Those with increased susceptibility to infection likely have other associated immunodeficiencies in addition to IgA deficiency. It has been argued that healthy IgA-deficient individuals compensate for the lack of IgA by increased production of IgM. Although it is true that in IgA deficiency there is more IgM present in mucosal secretions, it is not clear if this immune effector is actually compensating for the missing IgA or is just produced in greater quantity because feedback inhibition mechanisms mediated by IgA antibodies are missing.

In contrast, before modern medical intervention, IgG immunodeficiency was a life-threatening disease that almost always resulted in death due to infection within the

Figure 17.11 IgA can protect mucosal surfaces by three mechanisms. (**A**) Polymeric immunoglobulin can be secreted into a gland lumen to bind luminal antigens. (**B**) During transcytosis, polymeric immunoglobulin can bind and inactivate intracellular viruses. (**C**) Polymeric immunoglobulin that binds to antigen in the submucosal space (to form IgA or IgM ICs) can be transcytosed to the lumen, thus removing the antigen complexed to the immunoglobulin.

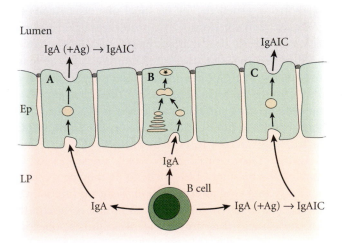

first few years of life, often by pathogens initiating infection at a mucosal surface. Thus, IgG is essential to immunologic resistance to pathogens on mucosal surfaces. Also, IgG is not absent from mucosal surfaces, it is just present proportionately in lower amounts than IgM and IgA. Furthermore, many vaccines that protect against a mucosal pathogen such as influenza and measles virus do so following intramuscular immunization that elicits primarily IgG. IgG-secreting B cells appear to home to mucosal tissues following this vaccination to produce local IgG antibody that mediates protective immunity.

It has also been difficult to reconcile the observation that so much IgA is produced and secreted daily by an individual if it can be dispensed with. While there is no great explanation for why something not essential is produced in such quantities, it must be kept in mind that Darwinian evolutionary forces do not act against neutral phenotypes. Thus, IgA may have been important at some point in evolutionary history, but if its function has been supplanted by other immune mediators such as IgG, the ability to produce IgA may survive even though it does not have an essential function.

Function of sIgA. Even though many individuals live healthy, normal lives without IgA, it is also still possible to use mucosal IgA effectively. Whereas IgM and IgG are essential for mediating local immunity, production of local IgA could also augment resistance to local infection. One function that IgA can mediate is to bind to mucosal pathogens and prevent them from establishing a nidus of infection on a mucosal surface. The SC portion of sIgA is negatively charged. Therefore, sIgA coats the pathogen with an anionic shell that repels it from the negatively charged mucosal membrane. sIgA also can interact with mucin, thereby increasing the likelihood of sIgA-coated pathogens being entrapped within the mucus and ultimately being expelled. The terminal mannose sugars on IgA2 also allow for nonspecific protection against gram-negative bacteria that express mannose-binding lectins and thus become coated with IgA2 antibodies. The mannose sugars on sIgA2 can induce direct agglutination of some enteric bacteria (*Escherichia coli*) that express a mannose-binding surface structure such as a pilus. Thus, there are both antigen-specific and nonspecific molecular mechanisms whereby IgA can be protective.

sIgA can also contribute to virus neutralization by blocking the binding of the virus to its cellular receptor, thus inhibiting viral internalization. If sIgA is internalized into a cell attached to a virus, it can inhibit release of the viral nucleic acid, thus preventing intracellular replication of the virus. IgA-pIgR-containing transcytotic vesicles can intersect and fuse with vesicles in which the viruses are internalized and assembled, inhibiting viral replication and further viral infection. This is one of the few known roles for an antibody working against an intracellular pathogen while it is inside the epithelial cell.

sIgA also has the potential to neutralize pathogen-derived enzymes and toxins. This activity is mediated via blocking of the binding site of the protein to a receptor or by inducing conformational changes in the structure of the protein, rendering it nonfunctional. sIgA can regulate antigen uptake at mucosal sites. It dramatically decreases the uptake of antigenic macromolecules, such as intact luminal food particles in the GI tract. This function is thought to help prevent excessive environmental antigenic challenge and helps reduce the chances of generating an immune or allergy response to ingested food. This idea is supported by the observation that some IgA-deficient individuals have increased uptake of food antigens, circulating food-immunoglobulin complexes, and an increased susceptibility to atopic allergies. sIgA can promote the uptake of antigens into the Peyer's patches via the M cells, which may be important in continued stimulation of local B cells to produce antibody.

sIgA can interact with some nonspecific antibacterial defense mechanisms present in the mucosal secretions. sIgA has been shown to synergistically help the antibacterial activity of lactoferrin, possibly by blocking alternative iron-uptake channels on bacteria that are necessary for microbial growth. It has also been suggested that sIgA and lactoferrin can form complexes. Lactoperoxidase has been shown to bind to sIgA, presumably at its Fc region. This interaction helps stabilize lactoperoxidase and enhance its enzymatic activity.

For many years there was some debate as to whether IgA can activate complement; it now appears that when this activity is detected, it is mostly an artifact. IgA lacks the C1Q-binding motif present on IgG required for activating the classical complement pathway. Reports that IgA can activate complement through the alternative complement pathway (ACP) abounded for a while but were ultimately shown to be due to artificial cross-linking of denatured human serum or colostral IgA that can activate the ACP. Native monomeric or polymeric IgA-antigen complexes fail to activate the ACP. The inability to activate complement may be an extremely important feature of sIgA. It allows inhibition of microbial or food-antigen interaction with the fragile mucosal tissues without inducing inflammation, thus preventing any damage to the mucosal surface.

Metabolism of IgA. The predominant mechanism for the clearance of IgA-containing immune complexes from the circulation is hepatocyte endocytosis. In most species this occurs primarily via receptor-mediated endocytosis utilizing the pIgR. However, human hepatocytes lack the pIgR and therefore must use alternative receptors for IgA uptake and clearance. One of these receptors is the asialoglycoprotein receptor (ASGP-R), which binds both monomeric and polymeric IgA1 at the O-linked oligosaccharide of the IgA1 hinge region. Uptake of IgA1 by hepatocyte ASGP-R usually results in the delivery of IgA1 to degradative lysosomes; however, some endocytosed IgA can be transcytosed into the bile. In humans, endocytosis by ASGP-R represents the major mechanism for clearance of serum IgA1 by the liver.

The mucosal epithelium also participates in the clearance of IgA-containing immune complexes (IgA-ICs) that form within the lamina propria. This might occur when a mucosal antigen or pathogen traverses the epithelial barrier, which can occur readily during infection. The pIgR transports IgA-ICs that reach the basolateral side of the epithelium to the apical side, where the IgA-IC is secreted into the lumen (Fig. 17.11). During transcytosis, the IgA remains complexed to the antigen and the immune complexes are not proteolytically degraded. Moreover, monomeric IgA or IgG associated with the IgA-ICs are also transcytosed along with the complex. This mechanism provides an anti-inflammatory process for the removal of locally formed immune complexes. Last, Kupffer cells (liver macrophages) also contribute to the clearance of immune complexes via FcR-mediated phagocytosis.

Microbial evasion of sIgA. As the immune system has evolved its defense mechanisms in response to the constant barrage of mucosal pathogens that the host continuously encounters, these pathogens have often evolved a variety of means of evading the host's defensive mechanisms, particularly sIgA. Proteases that cleave IgA1, termed IgA proteases, are produced by a limited group of bacteria that can successfully colonize or invade the human mucosa. This group includes the three major causes of bacterial meningitis and some respiratory tract, ear, and urogenital pathogens such as *Neisseria gonorrhoeae*. The IgA1 proteases cleave at the hinge region of IgA1, resulting in the generation of monomeric Fab fragments and Fc or Fc_2-SC fragments. However, the importance of these proteases in microbial virulence has not been established. Workers studying clients of a sexually transmitted disease clinic in the southern United States failed to detect IgA protease in infected secretions of individuals with gonorrhea. More convincingly, human volunteers experimentally given a strain of *N. gonorrhoeae* unable to make the IgA protease nonetheless were susceptible to infection. Thus it may be that the production of an IgA protease by these mucosal pathogens is merely coincidental. Alternately, degradation of IgA1 may be insufficient to provide much of an advantage for a mucosal pathogen. Mucosal tissues often contain a large proportion of the immunoglobulin subclass IgA2, which lacks the extended hinge region of IgA1 and is thus resistant to IgA proteases. In addition, SC confers protease resistance to sIgA from both host and bacterial enzymes present in mucosal secretions such that microbial proteases may have only limited activity on mucosal IgA.

Cellular immunity

APCs

Several types of APCs are present within the MALT and play a critical role in inducing and regulating local mucosal immune responses. These cells include macrophages, DCs, and B cells, which can take up antigens from the local environment, process them through an endosomal (exogenous) pathway, and present the processed peptides complexed with MHC class II. The professional APCs are present throughout MALT and reside largely in the Peyer's patches, lamina propria, and the local draining lymph nodes in the GI tract. Some intestinal epithelial cells (IEC) express MHC class II and can activate MHC-restricted T cells.

Many macrophages are found concentrated in a thick band in the region immediately beneath the luminal epithelium. These cells are also usually present in the villus core and the subepithelial space in the crypt of the small bowel. Some are also found under the dome of Peyer's patches as well as within them. The intestinal macrophages express high levels of HLA-DR, CD11b, CD11c, and CD68, indicating that they are activated. Unlike many other monocytes and macrophages, these cells are largely CD14⁻. Functionally, most of the intestinal macrophages phagocytose and degrade antigens; however, they are weak or inactive accessory cells. Since most of these are found outside of the inductive sites, such as Peyer's patches, they likely do not need to have accessory cell function. Human intestinal macrophages cannot stimulate a primary T-cell response, a function of local DCs. In some species intestinal macrophages regulate primary responses by inhibiting the effects of the local DCs. In the lung, human alveolar macrophages are also suppressive and can inhibit local DC function. However, the human intestinal macrophages can stimulate secondary T-cell responses. It has been suggested, on the basis of their distribution and function, that mucosal macrophages primarily act as a first line of defense by nonspecifically degrading any invading luminal antigens.

Dendritic cells reside largely in the interstitium of the mucosal surface. Two subsets of DCs have been characterized in the GI tract. The first group includes the classical DCs that are esterase-negative, acid phosphatase–negative, FcR-negative, and fibronectin-nonadherent. These DCs express high levels of HLA-DR and have dendritic extensions engaged in T-cell interactions. The second subset of DCs are located in the Peyer's patches and are interdigitating cells also known as *veiled cells*. Phenotypically, DCs express high levels of HLA-DR and very low levels of CD68 and are $CD14^-$. The distribution of DCs in the GI mucosa is similar to that of Langerhan's cells in the skin and forms a reticular network throughout the lamina propria and beneath the basement membrane of the colonic crypts. Functionally, intestinal DCs are potent stimulators of primary T-cell responses. Intestinal DCs can take up and present luminal antigens to naive cells and are potent immunostimulators of primary T-cell responses. In mice, DCs have been shown to regulate TH1 and TH2 cytokine profiles by a mechanism that is dependent on the tissue of origin of the DC. Peyer's patch DCs stimulate an antigen-specific TH2 response, and splenic DCs induce an antigen-specific TH1 response. On the basis of the function and distribution of the intestinal DCs, it has been suggested that the primary role of these cells is to act as cellular immune adjuvants by stimulating local mucosal T-cell responses against any invading luminal antigens.

B cells are abundant throughout the GI tract and the MALT and the antigen-presenting properties of these cells have been well characterized; however, their role as mucosal APCs has not been evaluated.

The predominant nonprofessional APCs in the MALT are the IECs. In addition to their role in fluid, electrolyte, and nutrient absorption and in sIgA-based transport, IECs are important in regulating cellular immune responses. Intestinal epithelial cells constitutively express MHC class II on both their basolateral and apical surfaces. Most class II expression is localized to IECs in the small bowel; however, some colonic IECs also express class II molecules. Intestinal epithelial cells express both HLA-DR and HLR-DP, although HLA-DR is expressed at higher levels. Expression of HLA-DQ has not been detected on IECs.

In vitro, IECs have been shown to present both typical protein antigens and bacterial superantigens to T cells.

IECs from normal noninflamed intestine preferentially stimulate $CD8^+$ T cells, which are present in high numbers and have unique phenotypic characteristics within the GI tract. Furthermore, IECs from inflamed intestine can effectively stimulate $CD4^+$ T cells due to expression of higher levels of MHC class II molecules. It has been suggested that nonclassical restriction elements (CD1/class 1B) are involved in $CD8^+$ intestinal T-cell–IEC interactions. This proposal is based on the observations that monoclonal antibody to MHC class I or class II failed to block stimulation of T cells by IECs; however, monoclonal antibody to CD1d blocked IEC allostimulation of T cells. There are five members of the CD1 family in humans, CD1a through CD1e. CD1d is expressed predominantly on IECs. This restricted expression of CD1d by IECs suggests a role for CD1d as the restriction element for resident $CD8^+$ IELs. Neither the expression of B7 nor that of ICAM-1 costimulatory molecules has been detected on IECs derived from either normal or inflamed intestine. However, IECs can activate T cells, indicating that an alternative costimulation mechanism may be involved in the activation of resident $CD8^+$ intestinal T cells and IELs. The costimulatory molecule CD58 (LFA-3) is expressed on IEC, and blocking antibodies to CD58 (but not to B7) have been reported to inhibit activation of $CD4^+$ T cells in the intestine.

An additional property shared by IECs and professional APCs is the ability to generate a variety of cytokines that regulate a broad range of immunologic activities. In vitro, IECs have been shown to generate the cytokines IL-6, IL-10, and TGF-β, which can modulate T-cell function and generate IL-8 in response to bacterial invasion. IECs have also been documented to produce GM-CSF, which enhances macrophage antigen presentation by stimulating phagocytosis and enhancing expression of MHC class II.

LP T cells

Intestinal T cells are found as both IELs and LP T cells present, respectively, within the epithelial layer or lamina propria. LP T cells are distributed diffusely throughout this tissue in the GI tract. The highest density of LP T cells is at the interface with the intestinal epithelium and in close proximity to the crypts. Most LP T cells are thymus derived. After leaving the thymus, naive T cells enter the mucosal follicles, such as the Peyer's patches, where they encounter antigen. Following antigen stimulation, the LP T cells leave the mucosal follicles, reenter the circulation, and subsequently home to the lamina propria or other mucosal tissues (Fig. 17.1). About 70% of LP T cells express VLAα$_4$β$_7$, which allows them to migrate or home to mucosal tissues. Some LP T cells also express VLA$\alpha_E\beta_7$; however, this homing receptor is preferentially expressed by CD8$^+$ LP T cells (88% of CD8$^+$ LP T cells versus 36% of CD4$^+$ LP T cells).

T cells comprise anywhere from 40 to 90% of the lymphocytes in the human lamina propria. Of the LP T cells, 65 to 85% are CD4$^+$. These cells are predominantly $\alpha\beta$ T-cell receptor (TCR) positive ($\geq$95%), whereas only ~3% of the LP T cells use the $\gamma\delta$ TCR. LP T cells are primarily memory cells. Approximately 50% of the CD8$^+$ LP T cells express the costimulatory ligand CD28, which is associated with cytolytic function. The LP T cells also express low levels of CD29 and CD11a/CD18 and slightly elevated levels of CD2.

The phenotype and functional characteristics of freshly isolated LP T cells also suggest that these cells are activated. Elevated numbers of CD69$^+$, MHC class II$^+$, CD71$^+$, and CD25$^+$ LP T cells are present in the lamina propria. In the peripheral blood, ~3% of the T cells are CD25$^+$; however, 6 to 29% of the T cells in the lamina propria express CD25. The increased expression of CD25 also correlates with enhanced responsiveness to stimulation with low doses of IL-2 and the generation of elevated levels of IL-2.

It is thought that the main functional role of CD4$^+$ LP T cells in humans is to provide help to the local mucosal B cells for immunoglobulin synthesis. This supposition is based on the observation that LP T cells from nonhuman primates fail to proliferate when antigenically stimulated but participate in the generation of an antigen-specific B-cell response. LP T cells provide B-cell help through the generation of a variety of cytokines. The cytokine profile of the LP T cells is predominantly TH2-like. However, LP T cells also can generate TH1 cytokines. Human LP T cells have been shown to generate high levels of IL-4, IL-5, IL-2, and IFN-γ following activation, with a ratio of IL-5- to IFN-γ-generating LP T-cells of 3:1. Perforin- and granzyme-positive CTLs have been identified in normal, noninflamed human small intestine and colon, and LP T-cell cytotoxic activity has been observed experimentally. Recently, the LP T cell has become an intense focus of investigation for its potential role in the etiology of inflammatory bowel disease.

Receptor signaling in LP T cells appears to differ from that in peripheral blood T cells, prompting the suggestion that LP T cells may represent a subset of memory cells that have either altered surface receptors or postreceptor signaling mechanisms that allow them to be stimulated via different activation signals. This premise is based on the observation that LP T cells, unlike peripheral blood CD45RO$^+$ T cells, exhibit diminished proliferative re-

sponses following antigen stimulation. However, proliferative responses and cytokine production following crosslinking of CD2 and CD28 are either unaffected or enhanced. Furthermore, CD3 stimulation of LP T cells results in cessation of calcium flux and low inositol-1,4,5-trisphosphate production as compared with that in CD3-stimulated peripheral blood T cells. The altered responses of LP T cells have been attributed to soluble factors, such as TGF-α or IL-7, generated in the intestinal mucosa. The hyporesponsiveness of LP T cells to antigen-specific stimulation in the GI tract would prevent the clonal expansion of T cells specific for harmless dietary or endogenous bacterial antigens, thus preventing any pathologic inflammation of the intestine.

IELs

IELs constitute a large pool of T cells within the GI tract, averaging 1 IEL for every 10 IECs. In the human small bowel, there is 1 IEL for every 5 IECs, and this ratio falls to 1:20 in the colon. Unlike LP T cells, most IELs do not recirculate, and they can be found on the basement membrane between IECs. Virtually all IELs express the integrin VLA$\alpha_E\beta_7$. The ligand for this addressin is E-cadherin, which is expressed on IECs and allows the IELs to migrate into the intestinal epithelial layer and probably also accounts for the retention of these cells at this tissue site. The highest density of IELs is in the vicinity of mature IECs at the mid-villus region. IELs located within the epithelial layer are predominantly (80 to 90%) cytotoxic T cells expressing a memory phenotype, CD3$^+$ CD8$^+$ CD45RO$^+$. The CD4$^+$ IEL subset is located predominantly in the lamina propria.

Most IELs in humans express the $\alpha\beta$ TCR, while 5 to 15% express the $\gamma\delta$ TCR. $\gamma\delta$ TCR$^+$ IELs, like $\alpha\beta$ TCR$^+$ IELs, express CTL markers or morphology; 30 to 50% of $\gamma\delta$ TCR$^+$ IELs are CD8$^+$, although most $\gamma\delta$ TCR$^+$ IELs are CD4$^-$ CD8$^-$ (double-negative) CTLs. A significant percentage (40%) of the $\gamma\delta$ TCR$^+$ IELs also express the natural killer (NK) cell markers CD16 and CD56. IELs have a granular morphology, and the intracytoplasmic granules contain acid phosphatase, β-glucuronidase, α-naphthyl, acetate esterase, perforin, and granzyme. The IEL lysosomes also contain the CTL/NK-cell-restricted protein TIA-1. TIA-1 is an RNA-binding protein that can enter permeabilized cells and cleave DNA. Because of this activity, TIA-1 is thought to participate in the induction of apoptosis of target cells. In vitro, IELs have been demonstrated to exhibit CTL activity. However, the function of CD8$^+$ $\alpha\beta$ TCR$^+$ or $\gamma\delta$ TCR$^+$ IELs in mucosal immunity remains largely unresolved. It has been proposed that the $\gamma\delta$ TCR$^+$ IEL may have a role in the immunologic surveillance of mucosal surfaces by eliminating infected or damaged IECs via interactions with heat shock proteins. One mechanism by which this may be accomplished is by the nonclassical MHC-like proteins MICA and MICB. MICA and MICB are nonpolymorphic MHC proteins that are recognized by the γδ TCR, leading to killing of the MICA- or MICB-expressing target cell. Given that expression of MICA and MICB on target cells is greatly increased during and after physiologic stress, this mechanism of target-cell recognition may represent a general response aimed at killing target cells likely to be infected with virus or to be precancerous.

In situ, few IELs synthesize DNA and very few have high mitotic activity, indicating that these cells do not replenish themselves within the intestinal epithelial layer. That IELs have low-level proliferation in vivo is supported by the observations that freshly isolated IELs from normal uninflamed intestine do not express the activation markers CD25 (IL-2R) or CD71 (transferrin receptor). Furthermore, IELs demonstrate only weak proliferation following either mitogenic or antigenic stimulation, even in the presence of IL-2 or IL-4. IELs, however, can be stimulated to proliferate and produce IL-2 via activation through CD2. On the basis of these observations, it has been suggested that the cellular activation pathways that IELs use may differ from those used by peripheral blood T cells.

Human αβ TCR$^+$ IELs have an extremely limited TCR repertoire, stemming from extremely limited V_α and V_β gene-segment usage. A similar phenomenon seems to occur with γδ TCR$^+$ IELs; 60 to 70% of freshly isolated human γδ TCR$^+$ IELs were found to utilize the $V_\delta 1$ and $J_\delta 1$ gene segments and to express the corresponding receptor. Evidence also indicates that γδ TCR$^+$ IELs throughout the human GI tract are oligoclonally derived (derived from the expansion of a relatively small population of T cells). It has been hypothesized that the restricted TCR repertoire of the IELs indicates that these mucosal cells recognize a very limited number of antigens.

In mice, CD8$^+$ αβ TCR$^+$ IELs are MHC class I restricted, a fact supported by the observation that this IEL population is absent in β$_2$-microglobulin-knockout mice. However, CD8$^+$ γδ TCR$^+$ IELs are still present in these mice, suggesting that restriction elements other than MHC class I may be involved in the differentiation and development of this population of cells. One alternative restriction element for γδ TCR$^+$ IELs is CD1d, an MHC class Ib molecule expressed on IECs. CD1d has been demonstrated in vitro to be sufficient to allostimulate CD8$^+$ T-cell proliferation.

It has been suggested that the GI tract functions as a primary lymphoid organ, supporting the development and maturation of lymphoid cells. This hypothesis is based primarily on data from studies in mice demonstrating that IELs can develop via an extrathymic pathway. A series of elaborate experiments using transgenic and knockout mice showed that there are two distinct populations of CD8$^+$ IELs: (i) a thymus-dependent population that expresses the CD8αβ heterodimer and has a broad αβ TCR repertoire and (ii) a population that expresses the CD8αα homodimer and develops within the GI tract independent of the thymus. Expression of the RAG gene, an indicator of T-cell development in the thymus, has been detected within the human intestinal epithelium. Furthermore, some evidence demonstrates that the GI tract can positively and negatively select developing T cells, suggesting that the GI tract could functionally substitute for the thymus.

Mucosal lymphocyte homing

Following antigen stimulation, some of the Peyer's patch B cells and T cells enter the efferent lymphatics where they travel to the thoracic duct and then enter the systemic circulation. From the circulation they can populate distant MALT effector sites, such as the lamina propria, glandular tissue, and the respiratory and reproductive tracts (Fig. 17.7). It has been estimated that in rats and mice approximately 10^8 to 10^9 lymphocytes are exchanged between blood and the intestinal lymph each day. A critical component of lymphocyte homing to the MALT, in both humans and other species, is the receptor-ligand-specific interaction between homing receptors on circulating mucosal lymphocytes and the vascular addressins on endothelial cells that permit migration of the lymphocytes into a tissue. These receptor-ligand interactions provide the specificity for organ-specific homing patterns. The lymphocyte-endothelial cell interactions involve multiple receptors that participate in a complex series of receptor-ligand binding events (see Fig. 4.4 to 4.6). The pattern of expression of homing receptors is regulated on both the lymphocyte and tissue endothelial cell by factors such as cellular activation, cytokine secretion, cell type, and state of the cellular maturation and differentiation. Moreover, these homing receptors can bind multiple, different ligands providing the specificity of the homing response by the coordinated use of several ligand-receptor pairs. Lymphocytes that were initially activated at a given mucosal site exhibit preferential homing back to the mucosal site of origin; however, these cells can also home to other mucosal sites.

One critically important homing receptor is CD62L (L-selectin), which is expressed on naive B and T

(CD45RA$^+$) cells. CD62L allows naive cells to enter into the various lymphoid tissues such as the Peyer's patches via the HEV. The endothelial ligands for CD62L are the addressin glycosylation-dependent cell adhesion molecule 1, a sulfated proteoglycan composed of a complex sialylated carbohydrate linked to a protein backbone and CD34. CD62L expression is decreased following antigenic stimulation and is expressed at very low levels on activated CD45RO$^+$ T cells. Once activated, the lymphocytes leave the lymph node, enter the thoracic duct, and then enter the bloodstream. Memory and effector lymphocytes fail to efficiently reenter the lymph nodes and Peyer's patches because they express very low levels of CD62L. These cells, however, express high levels of leukocyte function-associated antigen 1 (LFA-1), CD44, and very late antigen 4 (VLA-4). The ligands for these homing receptors are present on the endothelium in peripheral tissues. Some endothelial cells constitutively express the appropriate receptor whereas others do so after exposure to proinflammatory cytokines.

A particular combination of ligands and receptors determines the homing pattern of a lymphocyte to a mucosal or peripheral tissue. The interaction of LFA-1, also known as CD11a/CD18, with ICAM-1 illustrates this point. LFA-1–ICAM-1 interactions not only increase the strength of the binding of activated lymphocyte to the endothelial cell to potentiate homing to peripheral and mucosal tissues but also serve as an accessory molecule in the lymphocyte-HEV binding leading to entry of naive cells into lymph nodes. Other examples of receptor-ligand interactions mediating different patterns of lymphocyte migration are also known. Expression of CD44 and VLA-4 is increased on memory B cells and T cells and is thought to play a role in mucosal homing. CD44, a polymorphic single-chain proteoglycan that binds to hyaluronate, also serves as an accessory molecule for HEV binding. Besides mucosal homing, CD44 is involved in leukocyte adherence and T-cell activation. VLA-4, a member of the integrin family, is a heterodimeric protein consisting of an α and a β chain. One member of the VLA-4 family, VLA α_4/β_7, plays a critical role in mucosal lymphocyte homing. The ligand for VLA α_4/β_7 is the mucosal addressin cell adhesion molecule 1 (MAdCAM-1), which is expressed on the endothelium of HEV of Peyer's patches, mesentery lymph nodes, and the flat-walled venules of the mucosal lamina propria. MAdCAM-1 is a member of the immunoglobulin superfamily and consists of three immunoglobulin-like domains. MAdCAM-1 can be modified by the attachment of glycosaminoglycans, which may enable it to interact with CD44. VLA α_4/β_7 can also bind to the extracellular matrix protein fibronectin. VLA

α_E/β_7, another member of the VLA-4 integrin family, is found expressed on IELs and allows these cells to migrate deep into the mucosal epithelium. The ligand for VLA α_E/β_7 is the addressin E-cadherin expressed on the local mucosal epithelial cells.

Not all of the activated mucosal lymphocytes leave the MALT to home to other tissues. Some are retained at the mucosal site of activation. Retention within the local mucosal tissues is due to the expression of several surface molecules that can bind the cells to extracellular matrix proteins present in the MALT. The adhesiveness of several integrins, such as LFA-1 and VLA-4, is enhanced following antigen recognition and other stimuli such as cytokines, which can increase the adherence of the mucosal lymphocytes to the extracellular matrix and other cells within the activation site. Overall, the activated lymphoid cells within an induction site are a combination of cells that migrate into the site from other inductive sites as well as cells activated at that local site.

Factors Regulating the Mucosal Immune Response: Oral Tolerance

Oral tolerance, first described in 1911, refers to the development of a state of systemic immunologic hyporesponsiveness or nonresponsiveness to an antigen that is administered orally. Such tolerance is a crucial component of the normal immune response following mucosal exposure to antigen. The GI tract is continually exposed to an enormous load of luminal antigens, dietary and bacterial. Oral tolerance allows for decreased systemic immune responses to a variety of harmless luminal antigens that could overwhelm the mucosal and systemic immune system or divert them away from their primary role of generating protective immune responses to invading pathogenic microbes.

Oral tolerance is an antigen-specific immune regulatory mechanism, and its induction is dependent on several factors. These factors include the dose of the administered antigen, the type of immune response being assayed, the duration of the challenge, the time after administration of the fed antigen that the immune response is evaluated, the history of previous exposure to the antigen either mucosally or systemically, the age of the subject, and the microflora within the GI tract. Oral tolerance is not mediated by a single immunologic mechanism; the primary mechanisms are active suppression, clonal anergy, and clonal deletion. The major factor determining the mechanism induced is the dose of the orally fed antigen. Low doses of fed antigen induce suppression; higher doses induce clonal anergy and/or deletion (Fig. 17.12). However, oral routes of immunization are also known:

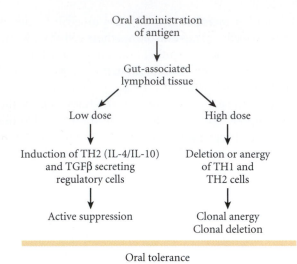

Figure 17.12 Mechanisms of oral tolerance induction.

oral vaccines for polio and typhoid fever are highly effective. What determines whether an orally administered antigen will be immunogenic or suppressive is not fully understood.

Airway Immunity: BALT

Many immunologic publications refer to the BALT consisting of lymphoid aggregates distributed throughout the larger passageways of the respiratory tract, with additional lymphocytes distributed within the subepithelial spaces. However, classic BALT has only been demonstrated in rats and rabbits. In humans, these organized lymphoid structures are rarely found in the lung but are commonly found in the upper respiratory tract and consist of the tonsils and adenoids. They are referred to as NALT. In some pathologic conditions in humans a BALT-like structure can develop around the air passages in the lung. The NALT and GALT lymphoid follicles have a common structural organization, and both tissues are characterized by specialized antigen-sampling structures, suggesting a functional role for NALT similar to that of GALT. This local mucosal immune system in the upper respiratory tract (the tissues above the tracheal opening) allows for production of specific immune effectors that promote the removal or elimination of any viral or bacterial pathogens that challenge the respiratory mucosa without damaging the mucosal surface or impairing the gas exchange in the lung. In addition, the lower respiratory tract (the lungs and other tissues below the tracheal opening) has additional innate immune mechanisms that contribute to maintenance of sterility within the lung.

Innate Immunity in the Respiratory Tract: the Alveolar Epithelium

The respiratory system has evolved a sophisticated first line of defense designed to decrease the inhalation of particulates, including bacteria and viruses, or to eliminate them if they enter the lung. Most ambient macroscopic particles are filtered out of the inhaled air by the mouth and nose; however, small particles (<2 to 3 micrometers [μm] in diameter) can travel to the lower respiratory tract. The large bronchi, which are the first structures derived from bifurcations of the trachea, are designed to drive or force any inhaled particulates into the mucus-covered walls of the airway, where the particles can subsequently be removed. Mechanical barriers and reflex mechanisms, including coughing and sneezing, operate in the respiratory tract to remove any inhaled pathogens.

The alveolar epithelial layer performs a variety of functions in the lung, including secretion of antimicrobial factors, ciliary clearance of mucus, and generation of inflammatory chemokines and cytokines that attract inflammatory and phagocytic cells into the lung. The epithelium is composed of three cell types: type I and type II alveolar epithelial cells and Clara cells. Type I alveolar epithelial cells are responsible for gas exchange, and type II cells and Clara cells generate the lung secretions. Lung secretions consist of a complex mixture of constituents that play critical roles in protecting the lung epithelium and clearing inhaled particulates. Pulmonary secretions consist of an underlying sol phase and an upper gel phase. The sol phase, which is in direct contact with the epithelial cells, is well hydrated to provide a low resistance that allows unimpeded movement of cilia. The upper gel phase contains mucin and other complex glycoproteins that make the secretions sticky, allowing them to trap macroparticles. Particles forced against the airway wall become trapped in the mucus, which is then transported by coughing or by movement of cilia on airway epithelial cells to the mouth, where it is swallowed or expectorated. Several factors that prevent bacterial adherence or growth also are present in the lung secretions. sIgA transcytosed by the alveolar cells and local IgG prevents invading pathogens from adhering to the lung's epithelium. In addition, local antibodies can block viral replication intracellularly (Fig. 17.11). The airway secretions also contain the iron-scavenging proteins transferrin and ferritin, which are derived from serum, and lactoferrin, which is generated by the alveolar epithelial cells. The alveolar epithelial cells also secrete lysozyme and some complement components that are bacteriocidal.

The epithelial barrier also plays a vital role in the inflammatory processes in the lung. Alveolar epithelial cells generate a variety of chemokines that mediate a broad range of chemotactic and immunologic activities. Cytokine production can be stimulated directly from epithelial cells when they interact with particulates or pathogens or indirectly via cytokines derived from particulate-stimulated alveolar macrophages. Upon stimulation, the alveolar epithelial cells express a variety of integrins, including ICAM-1, that allow the infiltration or retention of lymphocytes, leukocytes, and monocytes. Similar to what is observed in GALT, large numbers of neutrophils are found in the airway during acute or chronic infection. Stimulated epithelial cells also can promote the survival of the local inflammatory cells via the generation of cytokines and other factors.

Acquired Immunity in the Respiratory Tract: Inductive Sites

In species like rats and rabbits that produce an actual BALT, particles present in the airstream are forced against the airway wall due to the diversion of the airflow at the dichotomous branching points of the large bronchi. Cells of the BALT take up the luminal particles present at these impact sites and around the bifurcations preceding the major bronchial divisions (Fig.17.13). The overlying epithelium of the BALT contains M cells that are phenotypically and functionally similar to Peyer's patch M cells; however, the layer is less specialized and is heavily infiltrated with lymphocytes. Structurally, the BALT is comparable to Peyer's patches, but the structural and functional divisions of the BALT lymphoid follicles are less discrete than those of Peyer's patches. The BALT is found associated with efferent lymphatic vessels and normally consists of one follicle. Germinal centers are normally seen in the BALT only after antigenic stimulation. The parafollicular regions of the BALT contain primarily T cells, whereas plasma cells are found around the periphery. APCs in the BALT are predominantly alveolar macrophages and DCs and are distributed throughout the BALT. Like Peyer's patch APCs, the APCs of BALT can take up and process the luminal antigens and can then either initiate local immune responses or traffic to the local draining lymph nodes. Less organized lymphocyte aggregates are also present within the airway.

Less is known about the inductive sites in the NALT, which is the primary inductive site for human respiratory immune responses. The tonsils and adenoids seem to be organized into follicles with T-cell zones, B-cell zones, and the potential to form germinal centers. Dendritic-like cells are involved in antigen presentation. In addition to the tonsils and adenoids, other structures within the upper respiratory tract can collect lymphocytes and allow orga-

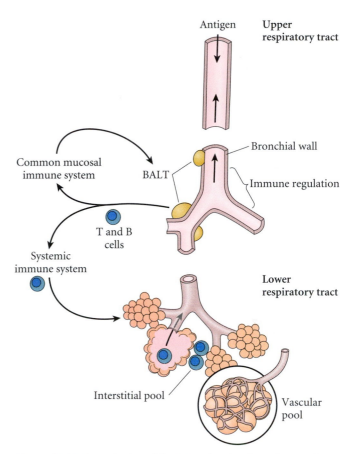

Figure 17.13 Organization of the BALT showing the pathways of lymphocyte recirculation and points of exchange between the mucosal and systemic immune systems.

nized immune-response follicles to form. Thus, tonsillectomy and adenoidectomy can be carried out when indicated without major compromise to the immune system.

Humoral Immunity: B Cells and Immunoglobulin

IgA is the predominant isotype of antibody in the upper respiratory tract, trachea, and major bronchi. IgA constitutes 10% of the total proteins in upper respiratory secretions, and ~67% of the sIgA is the IgA1 subclass. IgG comprises only ~1% of the antibody in bronchial secretions, and IgE is present only in trace amounts. In the smaller bronchi and the alveoli, however, IgG is the predominant antibody isotype. IgG antibodies play an important role in lung defense, since deficiencies in either IgG2 or IgG4 are associated with bronchiectasis, a progressive dilation of the bronchi or bronchioles as a consequence of inflammation. IgG1 and IgG2 comprise 65 and 28%, respectively, of the IgG present in the alveolar lavage fluid, while IgG3 and IgG4 comprise ~2 and ~6%, respectively.

In the lung, T cells outnumber B cells by at least 10:1, and in the alveoli, B cells are only 5% of the total lymphocytes. Aggregates of B cells in association with T cells can be found located adjacent to visceral pleura and sometimes near blood vessels. B cells and plasma cells are also found in the submucosa of the respiratory tract and in the alveoli and interstitium. However, it appears these cells arise in lymphoid tissues outside the lung. This view is supported by the observation that the appearance of antigen-specific B cells following intratracheal immunization is preceded by the appearance of these cells in regional lymph nodes, spleen, and blood. Memory B cells are retained at the sites of previous immune responses within the lung and can be activated locally with antigenic stimulation.

Cellular Immunity

Antigen presentation

Pulmonary macrophages are found within various sites in the lungs (alveoli, the interstitium, and the pleural cavity) and, within each site, are heterogeneous with respect to size, differentiation or maturity, and surface phenotype. Alveolar macrophages are the most abundant non-parenchymal cells in the lung, numbering 15 billion to 30 billion cells (there are ~5 to 10 times more macrophages than lymphocytes in the lung). Alveolar macrophages are drawn into the lung via the local production of CC chemokines, such as macrophage inflammatory protein 1 (MIP-1), MIP-2, and macrophage chemoattractant protein 1 (MCP-1), which are generated by type II alveolar epithelial cells and resident macrophages. A primary role of alveolar macrophages is removal of any small particles, normally ≤ 3 μm in diameter, that reach the alveolar spaces. In addition to ingesting and destroying particles and pathogens, these cells play other vital roles in lung defense, including antigen presentation and accessory cell function and maintenance of lung homeostasis.

Alveolar macrophages are not effective APCs and can induce only weak antigen-specific T-cell proliferation. Evidence indicates that this activity is mediated through both cellular contact and soluble factors. Activated alveolar macrophages generate a variety of factors that can inhibit lymphocyte proliferation, including superoxide anions (O_2^{-}), leukotrienes, prostaglandins, vitamin D metabolites, nitric oxide, TGF-β, and IL-Rα. The inability to induce T-cell proliferation may also be attributed to the lack of expression of CD80 and CD86 by alveolar macrophages. These cells also express lower levels of LFA-3 and generate lower levels of IL-1 compared with other macrophages. Reports also have indicated that alveolar macrophages have decreased antigen uptake and processing ability. Several studies also have shown that alveolar macrophages can strongly inhibit the APC function of pulmonary DCs and that this effect can be lessened by pretreatment of the DCs with GM-CSF.

Although alveolar macrophages can dampen antigen-specific T-cell proliferation, these cells do not inhibit T-cell activation and antimicrobial functions, indicating a role during the effector phase of the local immune response. Alveolar macrophages can stimulate calcium mobilization by T cells, expression of CD25 (IL-2R), and production of IL-2. Furthermore, alveolar macrophages can participate in the generation of T-cell-dependent, antigen-specific antibody responses, an activity related to the ability of alveolar macrophages to induce the production of cytokines by T cells. These observations indicate that alveolar macrophages can stimulate T-cell effector functions while simultaneously inhibiting T-cell proliferation and expansion.

Alveolar macrophages play a vital role in the recruitment and activation of other immune cells to the lung. Through the production of a plethora of chemoattractants, including LTB-4, IL-8, MCPs, and MIPs, alveolar macrophages can recruit PMNs, eosinophils, monocytes, and lymphocytes into the lung. The alveolar macrophages generate a variety of proinflammatory cytokines (e.g., IL-1, IL-8, and TNF-α) that can activate most local immune cells and the alveolar epithelial cells. These observations indicate that the role of alveolar macrophages is to remove any potential antigenic stimuli from the lung and to prevent the generation of any unnecessary immune responses that could damage the lung or prevent it from working properly.

As in the GALT, DCs have an important role in regulating and inducing local mucosal immune responses in the lung. Networks of DCs are interlaced throughout the alveolar epithelium, interstitium, septa, and BALT or NALT. The interdigitating processes of these cells reach almost to the bronchial lumen, perhaps enabling them to sample antigens directly. These cells are extremely mobile and, after antigenic stimulation, can migrate to local lymph nodes or central lymphoid organs. DCs constitutively express high levels of MHC class I and class II and express all the costimulator molecules (CD80, CD86, ICAM-1, LFA-1 [CD11a], LFA-3 [CD59], CD11c, CD18, and CD29) necessary for T-cell activation and proliferation and also express CD1. In humans, some populations of DCs express CD1c and under some conditions express CD1b, whereas other subpopulations express primarily CD1a. Unstimulated alveolar DCs are weak T-cell stimulators; however, once activated, these cells are the most potent APCs in the lung. Activated DCs also generate several cytokines, including IL-1, IL-6, IL-8, IL-12, TNF-α, and MIP-1, which can modulate the function of local inflammatory cells and the immune response. It has been suggested, based on the observations that lung DCs are ideally situated in the lung to sample antigens that penetrate alveolar epithelium and are potent T-cell stimulators, that these cells play a vital role in initiating local immune responses against any invading pathogens.

The alveolar epithelium is largely impermeable to antigens; however, some evidence indicates that both type I and type II alveolar epithelial cells can endocytose and/or phagocytose particles present in the airway. In vivo, alveolar epithelial cells express relatively low levels of MHC class II; however, expression is increased following cellular stimulation (i.e., cytokines, IFN-γ). In inflammatory lung diseases, such as asthma or chronic bronchitis, elevated expression of MHC class II on alveolar epithelial cells is observed regularly. In vitro, these epithelial cells can stimulate allogeneic T-cell proliferation, although it is not known whether they can participate in self-MHC-restricted stimulation of pulmonary T cells in vivo.

Although B cells are generally classified as professional APCs and are distributed throughout the lung, their role as APCs in the lung remains incompletely understood.

T cells

An estimated 4×10^8 lymphocytes are found on the epithelial surface of the human lung, and >95% are T cells. CD4$^+$ and CD8$^+$ T cells are present in the lung at a ratio of ~2:1, which is comparable to that in peripheral blood. T cells are also the predominant lymphocytes (70 to 95% of the lymphocytes) in the interstitium and alveoli. Lung T cells are 95% $\alpha\beta$ TCR$^+$, with the remaining T cells $\gamma\delta$ TCR$^+$. There may be preferential expression of certain TCRs on lung T cells. For example, there is evidence that lung T cells preferentially express the *TRAV12-1* gene in patients with sarcoidosis, a granulomatous disease with major manifestations of activated cellular immune responses in the lung.

Unlike in the GALT, the initial steps for generating a primary immune response in the lung occur outside the lung. Alveolar macrophages and DCs take up and transport antigens that enter the lung to regional and central lymph nodes. Naive T cells at these sites are activated and subsequently circulate to the lung, where they are retained. At least two integrins, VLA-4 and LFA-1, have been implicated in the homing of T cells to inflammatory sites in the lung. Lung T cells express lower levels of VLA α_4/β_7 than do peripheral blood T cells and higher levels of VLA α_E/β_7 than peripheral blood T cells. Accordingly, VLA α_4/β_7 antibodies can block T-cell homing to the GI tract but fail to block T-cell homing to the lungs.

Lung T cells are primarily memory cells, with 70 to 99% of T cells present on the epithelium and in the pleural fluid being CD45RO$^+$. Bronchoalveolar lavage T cells obtained from healthy lungs display normal antigen-specific proliferative responses to a broad range of pulmonary- (e.g., mycobacteria) and nonpulmonary (e.g., tetanus toxoid)-derived antigens, indicating that circulating peripheral T cells also can migrate to, or circulate through, the lung. A significant number of pulmonary T cells have an activated phenotype; ~7% are HLA-DR$^+$ and ~20% are CD25$^+$ (1 to 10% positive for α chain and 5 to 20% positive for β chain). These cells produce higher levels of IL-2 following TCR activation and respond more rapidly and have greater proliferative responses following antigenic stimulation. In studies that examined cytokine production of lung T-cell clones, the cytokine patterns were similar among the various clones; however, unlike T-cell clones generated from peripheral blood, most lung T-cell clones generated both IFN-γ and IL-4. These results indicate that most T cells within the lung are TH0 memory lymphocytes (committed to neither the TH1 nor the TH2 phenotype) that can generate a variety of cytokines with a broad range of immunologic functions.

Despite the predominantly TH0 phenotype of lung CD4$^+$ T cells, their primary role is to help B cells. Experimental evidence indicates that these cells are involved in generating local antibody responses that can be detected in the lung following local immunization with T-cell-dependent antigens. CTL activity mediated by local CD8$^+$ T cells and NK cells can also be detected in the lung. Recent evidence indicates that lung CD8$^+$ T cells may play an important role in protection against mucosal viral pathogens such as HIV or adenoviruses.

Urogenital Tract Immunity

The immune system of the urogenital tract (UGT) shares several fundamental characteristics with the GALT, although there are key differences, i.e., the UGT does not contain any organized lymphoid tissues, M cells, or goblet cells. However, the UGT immune system forms an effective barrier against invading pathogens. Moreover, in females, sex hormones, such as estradiol and progesterone, appear to influence the mucosal immune response in the UGT, which consists of both innate and acquired defense mechanisms.

Innate Immunity of the UGT

A prominent innate feature of the UGT is the effective barrier the epithelium forms to protect against the invasion of mucosal pathogens. The UGT epithelium consists of two cell types, squamous and transitional epithelial cells, and its structure permits large volume changes and the ability to withstand the pH and osmolality of urine without altering the barrier function. Additional innate factors include mechanical, bacteriocidal, and anti-adhesive defense. Urine flow provides effective bacterial clearance of the UGT, and urine is also bacteriocidal for some mucosal pathogens. This bacteriocidal activity is governed by several factors, including concentration of urea and ammonia, pH, and osmolality. The epithelial cells of the urinary tract and bladder have also been known to produce defensins, which also are generated in other mucosal sites. The role of defensins in the immune protection of the UGT, however, is not understood. UGT epithelial cells also generate a variety of proinflammatory cytokines, including IL-1 (α and β), IL-6, and IL-8, following bacterial stimulation.

Like the GALT, the mucosal secretions in the UGT contain a variety of factors that block bacterial adherence to tissue. One component of the UGT secretions is the Tamm-Horsfall glycoprotein (uromodulin) that is generated by luminal cells in the nephron and is found at the epithelial surface as high-molecular-weight aggregates. Tamm-Horsfall glycoprotein is believed to substitute for the mucins generated by the goblet cells in other MALT sites. Tamm-Horsfall glycoprotein has specific sugar residues that inhibit the binding of certain types of bacteria by providing a binding site for the bacterial surface proteins. This can competitively block bacterial adherence to UGT epithelial cells. Tamm-Horsfall glycoprotein also may play a role on PMN-bacterial interactions within the UGT, since it can bind to these cells and stimulate enhanced phagocytic activity.

Acquired Immunity of the UGT

Specialized antigen-transporting epithelial cells have not been observed in the uterus or any other part of the UGT. Uterine epithelial cells can endocytose antigen; however, the antigen is trafficked to lysosomes where it is ultimately degraded and not presented on MHC proteins. Vaginal and cervical epithelia are permeable to antigens, allowing them to enter the submucosa for uptake by the local APCs. Lymph nodules have been noted in the endometrium; however, they are rare. These nodules are largely T-cell aggregates, although in some aggregates, B cells are present within formed germinal centers and a surrounding mantle zone. A few nodules have also been identified in the oviduct and the cervix, but none have been observed in the vagina. It is thought that these nodules may be induced during infection; however, their role in the local mucosal immune response remains unresolved. Lymphatic vessels are also present within the en-

dometrium and the myometrium that allow trafficking of antigen-stimulated APCs to the local genital lymph nodes.

The UGT possesses a normal population of APCs. DCs are present in the stratified epithelium of the vagina and cervix. These DCs extend into the lumen, allowing the cells to sample the luminal antigens. Once these cells capture antigen, they can traffic to the local draining lymph nodes where they can activate T cells. Macrophages also are present in the UGT and are the most prominent APCs in the penile urethra. Moreover, uterine and vaginal endothelial and stromal cells have been shown to stimulate T cells via MHC class II-restricted antigen presentation and ICAM-1 and LFA expression.

The primary components of the humoral immune system in the UGT are the pIgR-expressing epithelial cells and the local antibody-producing cells (plasma cells). Plasma cells are distributed throughout the UGT. B cells are common in the oviduct, and IgG$^+$ and IgA$^+$ B cells are present in the fallopian tubes. Significant numbers of IgM$^+$, IgG$^+$, and IgA$^+$ B cells are also present in the cervix. It is interesting that IgA$^+$ plasma cells are rare or absent in the uterus. Secretory and monomeric IgA is present in UGT secretions; however, unlike other MALT sites, IgG is the predominant isotype in the mucosal secretions, with a ratio of IgG to IgA ranging from 2:1 to 10:1. Although plasma cells are broadly distributed throughout the UGT, some secreted IgG and IgA are serum-derived. The sIgA is transported into the lumen of the UGT via pIgRs, which are widely expressed on UGT epithelial cells. The IgG passes directly across the UGT epithelium, although it is not clear how it crosses the epithelial layer. It has been suggested that it may be accomplished by slow leakage through the epithelial layer or by intracellular transport. CD4$^+$ and CD8$^+$ T cells are present throughout the UGT; however, unlike peripheral blood T cells, CD8$^+$ T cells outnumber CD4$^+$ T cells in the UGT. There are numerous T cells in the stroma of the cervix. In the urinary tract, CD8$^+$ T cells are distributed within the epithelial layer and CD4$^+$ T cells are located in the urethral lamina propria. CD8$^+$ T cells are the primary T cells in the endometrium and are scattered through the stroma or in aggregates. These cells are also present within the vaginal epithelium. IELs have been observed in the vagina, cervix, uterus, and oviduct.

Little is known about the role of UGT CD4$^+$ T cells. Experimental data indicate that these cells are involved in generating local antibody responses, since antigen-specific antibodies can be detected in UGT secretions following vaginal or uterine immunization with T-cell-dependent antigens. CTL activity can be detected throughout the UGT and is mediated by both the local CD8$^+$ T cells and the IELs. Recent evidence indicates that the UGT CD8$^+$ T cells may play an important role in providing immune protection against mucosal viral pathogens such as herpes simplex virus or HIV.

Damage to Mucosal Sites by the Immune Response

The protective mechanisms that defend mucosal sites from colonization or invasion by microorganisms are essential for health and survival since this is the route of entry of inhaled, ingested, or sexually encountered pathogens. Infection of these tissues results in pathology that can be immediately life-threatening: pneumonia in the lung, vomiting and diarrhea in the GI tract, an inability to expel urine in the UGT. But the inflammatory responses that result from immune attack on pathogens can also injure these mucosal tissues, compromising their basic function. To prevent extensive damage, the tissues of the MALT engage in responses such as having IELs provide help to B cells while undergoing minimal cellular activation themselves, and IgA antibodies that retain the ability to bind foreign agents but lack the ability to activate the complement cascade. Nonetheless, prolonged inflammation in these mucosal tissues often occurs, giving rise to many chronic human diseases such as Crohn's disease in the GI tract, sarcoidosis in the lung, and pelvic inflammatory disease in the UGT. Thus, in spite of the fact that many of the immune responses that occur in the MALT are specialized to provide protection to the host while simultaneously minimizing potentially damaging inflammatory events, the inability to resolve an infectious or pathologic process leading to inflammation can often cause extensive tissue damage. Balancing the ability to destroy or remove the constant barrage of foreign antigens that assault our mucosal tissues continuously without causing undue and injurious inflammation is a major task of mucosal immunity.

Summary

The surface area of the mucosa in a human adult is approximately 300 to 400 m^2, roughly 200 times greater than the surface area of the skin, and is the primary site of invasion for most pathogens. The mucosal immune system, which consists of both innate defense mechanisms and acquired immunity, protects the mucosa from invading pathogens. The mucosal immune system consists of an integrated network of tissues, inductive sites, and effector cells and molecules, commonly termed the MALT. The MALT consists of a variety of tissues, including the intestine, bronchial tree, nasopharyngeal area, mammary gland, salivary and lacrimal glands, genitourinary organs, and the inner ear. The MALT has three main roles: (i) primary lymphoid development; (ii) induction and amplification of local mucosal immune responses, which occur within highly organized local inductive sites such as the Peyer's patches; and (iii) effector mechanisms of local mucosal immunity mediated within vast diffuse effector sites such as the lamina propria. The MALT is characterized by the selective production of local IgA, which is attributed primarily to the generation of IL-4, IL-5, IL-6, IL-10, and TGF-β by the local TH2 cells within the mucosal inductive and effector sites. It is also characterized by the ability of the mucosal lymphocytes to preferentially home to mucosal tissues. Mucosal homing is mediated via the mucosal homing receptor VLAα$_4$/β$_7$, an integrin that is expressed on mucosal lymphocytes. The ligand for VLAα$_4$/β$_7$ is the vascular addressin MAdCAM-1, which is expressed on the endothelium of HEVs of Peyer's patches, mesentery lymph nodes, and the flat-walled venules of mucosal lamina propria. Together, these homing receptors help regulate the mucosal immune effectors and integrate them with the components of other tissues of the host.

Suggested Reading

Boyton, R. J., and P. J. Openshaw. 2002. Pulmonary defences to acute respiratory infection. *Br. Med. Bull.* **61**:1–12.

Brandtzaeg, P. 2001. Nature and function of gastrointestinal antigen-presenting cells. *Allergy* **56**:16–20.

Freihorst, J., and P. L. Ogra. 2001. Mucosal immunity and viral infections. *Ann. Med.* **33**:172–177.

Guy-Grand, D., and P. Vassalli. 2002. Gut intraepithelial lymphocyte development. *Curr. Opin. Immunol.* **14**:255–259.

Kraehenbuhl, J. P., and M. R. Neutra. 2000. Epithelial M cells: differentiation and function. *Annu. Rev. Cell Dev. Biol.* **16**:301–332.

Nagler-Anderson, C. 2001. Man the barrier! Strategic defences in the intestinal mucosa. *Nat. Rev. Immunol.* **1**:59–67.

Nagler-Anderson, C., and H. N. Shi. 2001. Peripheral nonresponsiveness to orally administered soluble protein antigens. *Crit. Rev. Immunol.* **21**:121–131.

Neurath, M. F., S. Finotto, and L. H. Glimcher. 2002. The role of Th1/Th2 polarization in mucosal immunity. *Nat. Med.* **8**:567–573.

Neutra, M. R., N. J. Mantis, and J. P. Kraehenbuhl. 2001. Collaboration of epithelial cells with organized mucosal lymphoid tissues. *Nat. Immunol.* **2**:1004–1009.

Russell, M. W., and J. Mestecky. 2002. Humoral immune responses to microbial infections in the genital tract. *Microbes Infect.* **4**:667–677.

chapter 18

Immunity to Bacterial Infections

Gerald B. Pier

Bacteria and Disease

Many diseases reported from the earliest recorded history of humanity are now known to have been due to bacterial infections. Since the promulgation of the germ theory of disease by Louis Pasteur, Robert Koch, and other famous bacteriologists of the 19th century, tremendous progress has been made in understanding what types of bacteria cause diseases and how to identify and classify them. Christian Gram in 1884 developed the Gram stain to generally classify bacteria as either gram positive or gram negative, reflecting different properties of their cell surfaces that determined the bacterial cells' ability to retain or lose a dye complex made of crystal violet and iodine (Fig. 18.1). Gram-positive bacteria retain the dye and their outer surface is a rigid cell wall; gram-negative bacteria do not retain the dye and their outer surface is actually a protein-, lipid-, and polysaccharide-studded phospholipid membrane termed the outer membrane. In the first half of the 20th century, hospital wards were filled with people sick with pneumonia, meningitis, diarrhea, and other bacterial diseases. The discoveries of Alexander Fleming, Howard Florey, and Ernst Chain about the antibacterial effect of penicillin led to the Nobel Prize for the three of them in 1945, and the discovery by Selman Waksman of streptomycin, the first antibiotic effective against tuberculosis, similarly led to a Nobel Prize for him in 1952. The introduction of these effective antibacterial agents advanced the practice of medicine dramatically. Although these drugs and other antibiotics markedly changed the reasons for hospital admissions after World War II, they hardly eliminated bacterial pathogens as serious threats to life and limb.

The molecular biology revolution of the last half of the 20th century led to major advances in our understanding of the molecular and cellular bases for the

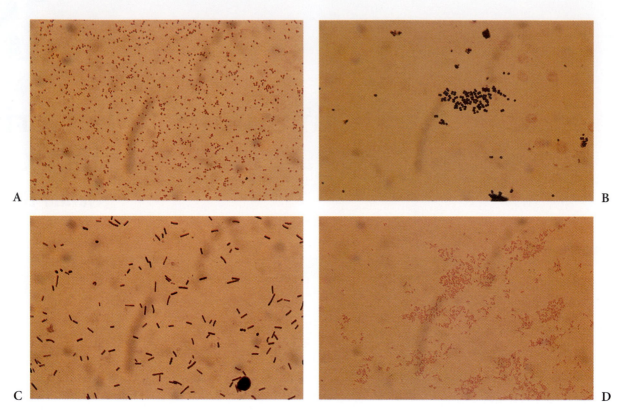

Figure 18.1 Gram stains showing gram-positive (**B and C**) and gram-negative (**A and D**) bacteria. (**A**) A *Moraxella* sp.; (**B**) *Staphylococcus aureus*; (**C**) a *Clostridium* sp.; (**D**) *E. coli*.

ways in which bacteria cause diseases, and this century similarly saw the development of numerous important vaccines to prevent serious bacterial infections. Overall, immense progress has been made in preventing and treating bacterial infections, yet some of the most daunting challenges in the practice of medicine are still related to the problems presented by bacterial infections. Indeed, in the less-developed countries, bacterial diarrhea remains one of the major causes of death during the first year of life, and in developed countries, serious bacterial infections remain a principal cause of extended hospital stays and death. In addition, there is the continuing problem of new infections, such as Legionnaires' disease, caused by newly discovered bacterial pathogens, or established pathogens producing new types of infections such as menstrual toxic shock syndrome, which emerged with the development of certain types of high-absorbency tampons in the early 1980s. Furthermore, previously recognized diseases not initially thought to be due to an infectious agent are, in fact, now being found to be due to infectious agents, i.e., gastric ulcers and *Helicobacter pylori*. A particularly frightening recent development has been the emergence of bacterial pathogens that are resistant to almost all useful antibiotics. A new generation of

vaccines and immunotherapies may be needed to control bacterial infections. Critical to the development of these therapies is an understanding of how bacterial infections occur and how the immune system handles these invaders.

Bacterial Diseases: Many Infectious Agents and Many Diseases

Bacteria can infect virtually any part of the body and cause disease due to the growth of the microbe in a tissue, elaboration of bacterial factors that are harmful to the host, and elicitation of an inflammatory response that is part of both the pathologic disease process and the recovery process leading to development of acquired immunity (Fig. 18.2). In reality, the different species of bacteria that commonly cause disease in animals and humans often have strong preferences for infecting specific body sites. It is thus helpful to classify bacterial diseases on the basis of tissue site of infection, e.g., skin, respiratory, gastrointestinal, central nervous system, or genitourinary. Numerous different types of bacteria can cause lung infections leading to pneumonia; similarly, gastrointestinal bacterial infections leading to stomach distress, vomiting, diarrhea, etc., are also caused by a number of different pathogens.

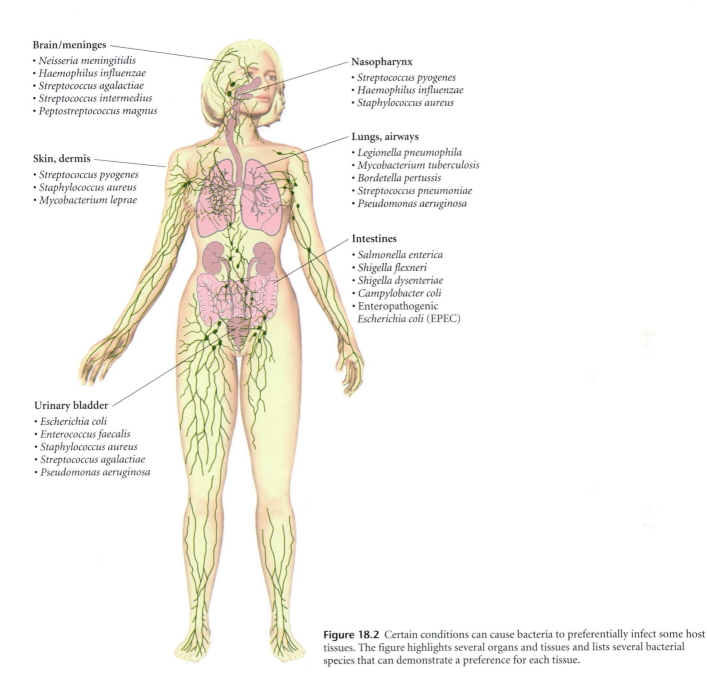

Brain/meninges

- *Neisseria meningitidis*
- *Haemophilus influenzae*
- *Streptococcus agalactiae*
- *Streptococcus intermedius*
- *Peptostreptococcus magnus*

Skin, dermis

- *Streptococcus pyogenes*
- *Staphylococcus aureus*
- *Mycobacterium leprae*

Urinary bladder

- *Escherichia coli*
- *Enterococcus faecalis*
- *Staphylococcus aureus*
- *Streptococcus agalactiae*
- *Pseudomonas aeruginosa*

Nasopharynx

- *Streptococcus pyogenes*
- *Haemophilus influenzae*
- *Staphylococcus aureus*

Lungs, airways

- *Legionella pneumophila*
- *Mycobacterium tuberculosis*
- *Bordetella pertussis*
- *Streptococcus pneumoniae*
- *Pseudomonas aeruginosa*

Intestines

- *Salmonella enterica*
- *Shigella flexneri*
- *Shigella dysenteriae*
- *Campylobacter coli*
- Enteropathogenic *Escherichia coli* (EPEC)

Figure 18.2 Certain conditions can cause bacteria to preferentially infect some host tissues. The figure highlights several organs and tissues and lists several bacterial species that can demonstrate a preference for each tissue.

Sexually transmitted bacterial diseases disrupt the normal function of the genitourinary tract. Meningitis, an inflammation of the meninges covering the brain and spinal cord, can also be caused by an array of bacterial pathogens.

It is also well established that some infectious bacteria are more promiscuous in regard to their ability to infect many different tissues. *Staphylococcus aureus*, the common cause of "staph" infections, can initiate disease in almost any body tissue. *Streptococcus pyogenes*, the cause of "strep throat," can also infect the skin, and some very potent strains of this bacterium can give rise to necrotizing fasciitis, the so-called "flesh-eating" disease. However, this organism does not cause gastrointestinal disease nor is it considered to be capable of typical sexual transmission. These examples are in contrast to some bacterial infectious agents highly restricted to infecting very specific tissues: *Vibrio cholerae*, the cause of cholera, infects only the human gastrointestinal tract and is essentially never seen to cause infections elsewhere under natural conditions.

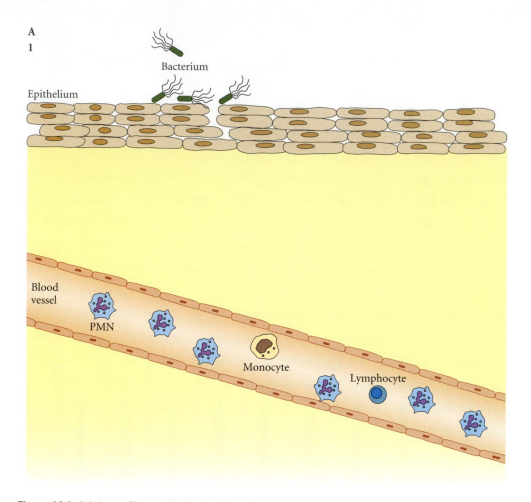

Figure 18.3 (A) Steps of bacterial infection. (**1**) Infection begins with attachment of the bacterium to a host tissue. Persistence and growth of the bacterium at this site are termed *colonization*. (**2**) Invasion of the bacterium into deeper host tissues, together with the elaboration of toxic substances by the bacterium, can result in injury to host cells and tissues (p. 429). (**3**) Inflammation at the site of invasion can be initiated by antibody binding to bacteria, by complement activation on the bacterial surface, or by wound healing mechanisms such as the plasmin system or the kinin system (p. 430). In all of these cases, components C3 to C5 of the complement system can be activated to generate soluble split products called *anaphylatoxins* (fragments C3a, C4a, and C5a) that alter vascular permeability and activate local macrophages and neutrophils. (**B**) A picture of a "hypothetical" bacterium showing different factors that promote colonization, entry, and then progression to disease (p. 430). Alginate can promote colonization by adhering to host tissues. LPS and the pilus promote persistence of the bacterium by creating resistance to complement and phagocytosis, respectively. The type III secretion system is used by the bacterium to deliver bacterial enzymes and toxins into host cells. Many bacteria secrete toxins that can injure host tissues or diminish host immune responses. Such toxins may include signaling proteins, proteases, and superantigens.

An understanding of the biologic basis for how bacteria cause disease and the immunologic basis of resistance to bacterial pathogens requires insight into several basic factors that together direct the initiation and outcome of bacterial infections. The interaction of bacteria with the host is frequently thought to consist of three stages: bacterial entry and colonization of host tissues, bacterial invasion and growth in host tissues along with the elaboration of toxic substances, and the inflammatory response of the host (Fig. 18.3A). These stages reflect the more traditional concepts of *infection* (presence of bacteria in a host) and *disease* (reaction to the infection). Even though these terms are often used interchangeably, when signs and symptoms of disease are present, the term disease and not infection should be used. Signs refer to responses measurable in both animals and humans, such as temperature increases, whereas symptoms indicate being able to report how one feels during an illness and are thus limited to humans beyond infancy (perhaps excepting crying and other nonverbal indications infants have of indicating distress).

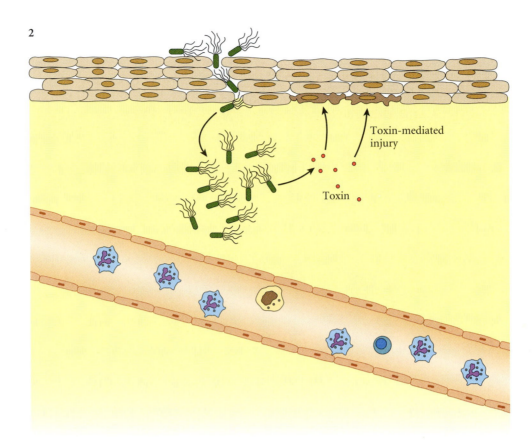

2

Toxin-mediated injury

Toxin

Figure 18.3 *(continued)*

Many organisms may infect an individual without causing significant disease, hence the need for distinguishing between infection and disease.

Pathogenicity is the term used to indicate the potential ability of a microbial pathogen to cause disease or elicit significant inflammation consistent with disease; an organism might have a high or low pathogenic potential. The pathogenic potential of a given organism is dependent on the quantitative and qualitative production of myriad factors by the bacterium and referred to as *virulence factors*. These virulence factors may be classified as those that promote bacterial colonization and infection, usually molecules on the bacterial surface (Fig. 18.3B), and those that cause progression of the infection to an actual state of disease. Virulence factors can disrupt host cellular function due to secreted toxins or toxic bacterial metabolites. In addition, the host's inflammatory response to infection can contribute greatly to the observed disease and its attendant signs and symptoms. A successful immune response by the host at any of these stages of infection has the potential to abort or attenuate the resultant disease, whereas an inappropriate or ineffective immune response resulting in prolonged inflammation and tissue damage can be part of the ongoing disease process.

Innate Immunity and Bacterial Infection

Innate immune effectors (see Fig. 2.1) clearly function as major mediators of resistance to bacterial infection (Table 18.1). In fact, the vast majority of bacteria encountered by a mammalian organism are readily dealt with by the innate immune system. High numbers of bacteria are found on human skin and in the upper respiratory tract, the gastrointestinal tract, and the female genital tract, yet most the time these *commensal organisms*, essentially the normal or usual strains of bacteria residing in or on a host, are without pathologic effects—they do not cause disease. The physical and physiologic barriers that prevent bacterial entry or destroy them quickly after infection due to the enzymatic and protein effectors of the innate immune system represent a major first line of defense against any bacterial organism. Prominent players in this regard are lysozyme, proteases, antimicrobial peptides, and iron-sequestering proteins. Breaching this defense, such as occurs with skin wounds, greatly increases susceptibility

3

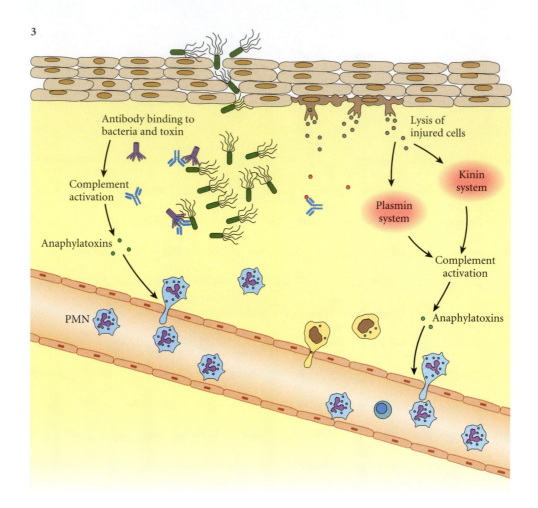

Antibody binding to
bacteria and toxin

Complement
activation

Anaphylatoxins

PMN

Lysis of
injured cells

Kinin
system

Plasmin
system

Complement
activation

Anaphylatoxins

B

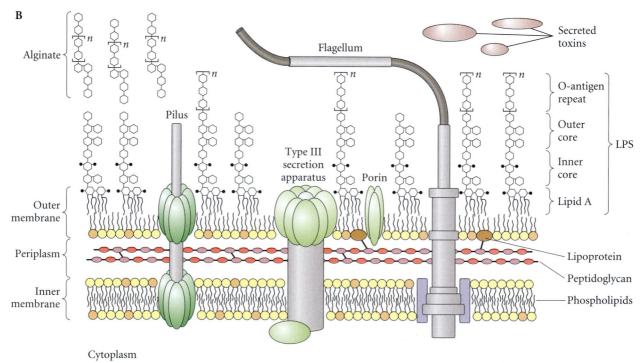

Alginate

Pilus

Flagellum

Secreted
toxins

Type III
secretion
apparatus

Porin

O-antigen
repeat

Outer
core

LPS

Inner
core

Lipid A

Outer
membrane

Periplasm

Inner
membrane

Cytoplasm

Lipoprotein

Peptidoglycan

Phospholipids

Figure 18.3 *(continued)*

Table 18.1 Innate immune effectors mediating resistance to bacterial infection

Type of mechanism and examples
Physical and physiologic barriers
Skin, sebum, mucosal epithelial cells, mucus, and mucous flow
Enzymatic and protein effectors
Lysozyme, proteases, antimicrobial peptides, iron-sequestering proteins, complement
Recognition of PAMP
TLRs
TLR2 and peptidoglycan and glycopeptides
TLR4 and LPS
TLR5 and bacterial flagella
TLR9 and CpG DNA
Endocytic pattern recognition molecules
Mannose receptor/scavenger protein
CR3
Soluble collectins
Conglutinin
Mannose-binding lectin
Surfactant proteins A and D

to infection. Complement is also very important in innate immune resistance to infection (see chapter 5), both on mucosal surfaces and in the blood. Individuals with deficiencies in the early components of complement, particularly C3, are more susceptible to bacterial infection. Phagocytes are critical to resistance to bacterial infections, and in situations where there is diminished phagocytic activity or diminished ability to kill ingested bacteria, there is enhanced occurrence of bacterial infection.

The Toll-like receptors (TLRs) along with endocytic and soluble pattern-recognition molecules that bind to conserved bacterial structures such as lipopolysaccharide, peptidoglycan, flagella, components with mannose, and other similar bacterial products activate inflammation and promote opsonization, clearly important in early responses to bacterial pathogens (see chapter 2). Recognition of these common components made by multiple different bacterial pathogens by the host's TLRs induces cellular changes of immune cells, including monocytes, macrophages, epithelial and endothelial cells, and especially dendritic cells. TLR signaling in dendritic cells induces maturation and release of cytokines, including interleukin-12 (IL-12) and tumor necrosis factor alpha (TNF-α), that enhance the innate immune function of macrophages and also form a link with the acquired immune response by aiding in the activation of T cells by the dendritic cells that have thus been matured. Immature dendritic cells are able to take up and process antigen whereas mature dendritic cells have increased expression of peptide-loaded major histocompatibility complex (MHC) on their surface along with increased levels of the costimulatory molecules CD80 and CD86 (B7-1 and B7-

2). This enhances the ability of these matured dendritic cells to present antigen to T cells and induce their activation. Other than initiating innate immune response to pathogen-associated molecular patterns (PAMP), recognition of PAMP by TLRs allows an improved acquired immune response to these pathogens.

Much of what we know about molecular mechanisms of innate immunity comes from studies of human disease and animal models where increased susceptibility to bacterial infection occurs. Humans with congenital deficiencies in CD18, which is the β_2 chain of the heteromeric molecules that combine with CD11 to form integrins, are more susceptible to bacterial infection because of lack of leukocyte function-associated molecule 1 (CD11a/CD18) and complement receptors (CD11b/CD18 and CD11c/CD18). They have a disease termed leukocyte-adhesion deficiency. Chronic granulomatous disease is due to an inability of phagocytes to produce a proper oxidative burst to kill ingested bacteria, resulting in enhanced bacterial infections. Humans with deficiencies in mannose-binding protein, which promotes innate opsonization of numerous bacterial organisms, have greater occurrences of bacterial infections. Mice lacking TLR4 have enhanced resistance to lipopolysaccharide (LPS)-mediated endotoxic shock but greater susceptibility to oral infection due to *Salmonella* bacteria. Clearly, the signaling from the bacterial LPS via TLR4 is important in initiating an early, innate immune response to the infectious pathogen. These few examples illustrate the critical role of innate immune effectors in resistance to bacterial infection since loss of function of these innate immune effectors greatly increases the risk from bacterial infection.

Many important pathogenic bacteria such as *Mycobacterium tuberculosis* grow inside host cells, principally tissue-associated macrophages, and are referred to as intracellular pathogens (Table 18.2). At the innate level, natural killer (NK) cells are primary mediators of resistance to these infections. NK cells are important for recognizing infected cells and eliminating them along with their load of pathogenic bacteria. Recent studies have implicated specific NK-cell receptors (see chapter 3) in recognition, lysis, and killing of *M. tuberculosis* that had been inside infected monocytes. Hundreds of millions of

Table 18.2 Bacterial pathogens that can escape humoral immune mechanisms, survive intracellularly, and require activated phagocytes or CTLs for successful elimination

Listeria monocytogenes	*Brucella* species
Nocardia asteroides	*Chlamydia* species
Mycobacterium tuberculosis	*Mycoplasma* species
Mycobacterium leprae	

individuals in the world have active tuberculosis, and many more are exposed to the microbe, but usually only about 10% of exposed individuals go on to develop disease. One component that might account for the determination of susceptibility or resistance to infection has been the ability of NK cells to destroy infected alveolar macrophages early in the course of infection.

Immune System Function and Resistance to Bacterial Infections

The major function of the immune system is to attenuate the ability of microbial pathogens to cause disease and eventually eliminate pathogenic foreign substances, microbes, and their associated toxins from host tissues. A number of mechanisms intrinsic to innate, antibody-mediated, and cell-mediated immune effectors are used in eliminating pathogenic bacteria. As is well known, the first critical function of the immune system is to recognize a parasite as foreign. But even this simple, obvious step can be difficult in regard to some bacterial infections, as a subset of bacteria have surface determinants that are similar to those found on mammalian cell membranes, causing the organism to appear as a self antigen to the immune system of an infected individual. These bacterial surface structures are often the critical ones against which an immune response must be made for acquired immunity to control the bacterial pathogen effectively. On the other hand, all bacterial surfaces contain at least some proteins and polysaccharide determinants that are immunogenic and often, but not always, these antigens can be targets of protective immune effectors.

Immunity to bacterial pathogens that cause damage principally by infecting and growing in body fluids and tissues but not inside cells, the extracellular pathogens, is primarily dependent on the presence of antibodies (Fig. 18.4). These antibodies provide protective immunity by mediating the killing of live organisms, through opsonophagocytosis or the promotion of complement-mediated bacteriocidal activity or by neutralizing the activity of various bacterial toxins. Antibacterial antibodies may potentially prevent adhesion of bacteria to host tissues, but this effect is not well demonstrated as being operative in human infection. For those bacteria such as *M. tuberculosis* that reside inside cells, cell-mediated immunity plays a critical role in the host's resistance to infection (Fig. 18.5).

The situation with regard to immunologic protection against bacterial pathogens has grown more complex as our understanding of how these microbes survive within an infected host grows. It is now being appreciated that many traditional "extracellular" bacterial pathogens actu-

ally are capable of invading host cells and residing in intracellular compartments, raising the possibility that cell-mediated immune effectors contribute, in part, to immunity to infection against these pathogens. In addition, intracellular pathogens may be released from cells they have previously invaded, giving them an extracellular stage and making them potentially susceptible to antibody-mediated immune effectors. In responding to a bacterial infection, both cell-mediated immune effectors and antibodies are made to many pathogens because of the involvement of CD4$^+$ T cells in coordinating both the antibody response and the production of delayed-type hypersensitivity and cytotoxic T-lymphocyte cellular effectors. Although immunity to a specific pathogen has often been

Figure 18.4 Mechanisms of immunity to extracellular bacteria mediated by antibodies. (A) For gram-negative bacteria, binding of antibodies and complement can result in opsonization via Fc receptors or CR expressed by macrophages or neutrophils (1). Antibody binding can also activate complement via the classical pathway, resulting in membrane attack complex (MAC) formation (2) and opsonization via complement receptors. Antibodies bound to the bacterium can also trigger antibody-dependent cell-mediated cytotoxicity (ADCC) as neutrophils bearing Fc receptors and CR release proteases, nucleases, lipases, and reactive oxygen intermediates (ROIs) (3). (B) For gram-positive bacteria, MAC formation is ineffective in killing bacteria due to the presence of the thick bacterial cell wall; however, opsonization (1) and ADCC (2) are still effective.

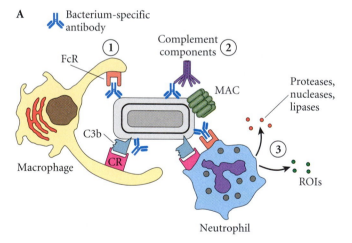

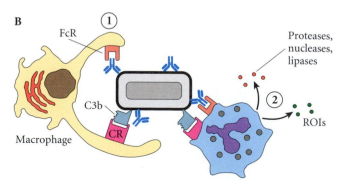

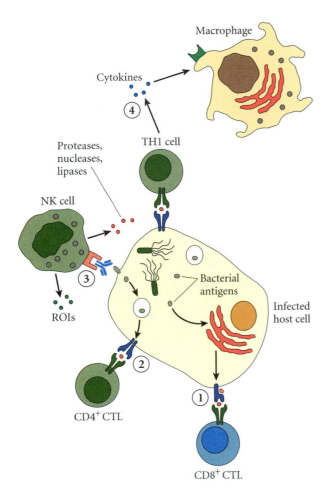

Figure 18.5 Mechanisms of immunity to intracellular bacteria mediated by cell-mediated immunity. (1) Bacterial antigens present in the cytoplasm of an infected host cell can be processed via the endogenous presentation pathway and presented to CD8+ CTLs on MHC class I. (2) Bacterial antigens present in endosomes of an infected host cell can be processed via the exogenous presentation pathway and presented to CD4+ CTLs on MHC class II. (3) Bacterial antigens present on the surface of an infected cell can be bound by antibodies and targeted for killing by NK cells using ADCC. (4) Some CD4+ T cells that recognize bacterial antigens complexed with MHC class II may be TH1 cells, which may be capable of initiating a DTH reaction resulting in the activation of macrophages, which may kill bacteria and infected host cells via proteases and reactive oxygen intermediates (ROIs).

associated with a specific type of immune effector—T-helper type 2 (TH2)-dependent antibody responses to prevent pneumonia caused by *Streptococcus pneumoniae* and TH1-dependent CD4+ T-cell-mediated DTH to prevent tuberculosis due to *M. tuberculosis*—recent results suggest that for some pathogens a mixed TH1 and TH2 response may be needed for optimal immunity. For example, *H. pylori*, which causes stomach ulcers, infects about one-half of the world's population and resides in the stomach principally within the mucus lining the stomach wall. But 20% or so of the organisms are also found within the gastric epithelial cells of the stomach. Ongoing

attempts at developing vaccines to prevent *H. pylori* infection indicate a mixed TH1 and TH2 response may be optimal for full immunity, perhaps needed to deal with both the intracellular and extracellular organisms found in the infected area of the stomach.

Role of Complement and Antibody

Studies of the effect of antibody and complement in the serum have told us the most about protective immunity against extracellular bacterial pathogens (Table 18.3). Complement and antibodies mediate their antibacterial effect by two major mechanisms: opsonophagocytosis and direct bacterial lysis (Fig. 18.4). Opsonophagocytosis is key to immunity to gram-positive bacteria and gram-negative organisms that cannot be killed by the lytic pathway of complement. Critical to opsonic killing is the coating of bacteria with both antibody and complement opsonins that can also bind to Fc receptors and complement receptors (CR) on phagocytic cells. Antibody classes differ in their ability to bind to Fc receptors so the immunoglobulin isotype can be a factor in the efficiency of opsonophagocytosis. Specific complement protein fragments, notably C3b and C3bi (a subfragment of C3b), bind avidly to CR1 and CR3 present on many phagocytic cells. One aspect of immunity to bacterial infection is the need for these opsonins to be available to the Fc and CR on phagocytes. Many bacterial pathogens avoid opsonophagocytosis by coating themselves with an outer capsule that interferes with the ability of antibody and complement opsonins bound to the microbial surface below the capsule to interact with receptors on phagocyte membranes. Initial attraction of phagocytic cells to areas of infection is mediated by chemotactic proteins such as the complement split products C3a and C5a, as well as cytokines such as IL-8. As long as the phagocytic cell can access the specific opsonins on the bacterial surface, it can ingest and destroy the microorganisms by using intracellular antibacterial enzyme systems.

Complement-mediated bacteriolysis is the operative form of immunity to some gram-negative bacteria. Susceptibility to classic bacterial spinal meningitis (meningococcal infection) is related to an inability of the host's serum to mediate killing of the infecting strain. Individuals with mutations in genes encoding the terminal components of complement are incapable of forming membrane attack complexes, and even when they develop specific antibody to the meningococcal bacterial cell, they are still at risk for developing meningitis because of the abnormal functionality of their complement system.

Because of its polymeric structure, immunoglobulin M (IgM) is capable of initiating complement activation even

Table 18.3 Common extracellular bacterial pathogens that are cleared by humoral immune effectors and examples of their common disease manifestations

Gram-positive bacteria	Gram-negative bacteria
Streptococci	*Neisseria meningitidis*
Strep throat, scarlet fever, skin and soft tissue infections	Spinal meningitis
Pneumococci (*Streptococcus pneumoniae*)	*Haemophilus influenzae*
Pneumonia, meningitis, bacteremia	Pneumonia, bacteremia, meningitis
Staphylococci	*Legionella pneumoniae*[a]
Toxic shock syndrome, skin and soft tissue infections, food poisoning, pneumonia, abscesses, endocarditis	Legionnaires' disease
Corynebacterium diphtheria	*Bordetella pertussis*
Diphtheria	Whooping cough
Bacillus anthracis	Gram-negative enteric bacteria, including *Escherichia coli, Klebsiella pneumoniae, Enterobacter,* and *Serratia* spp.
Anthrax	Local tissue infection, bacteremia, urinary tract infection
Clostridium tetani and *Clostridium botulinum*	*Pseudomonas aeruginosa*
Tetanus and botulism	Local tissue infection, particularly in the lung, bacteremia, urinary tract infection
	Salmonella enterica serovar Typhi[a]
	Typhoid fever
	Shigella dysenteriae, S. flexneri, S. boydii, S. sonnei
	Shigellosis, sometimes bacillary dysentery
	Vibrio cholerae
	Cholera
	Yersinia pestis[a]
	Plague
	Bacteroides fragilis
	Intraabdominal infection

[a]These organisms also have an intracellular component to their infection and may also require cell-mediated immunity as an adjunct to full immunity.

if only a single IgM molecule is bound to a bacterial surface antigen. In contrast, IgG is monomeric and therefore can activate complement only when the surface density of the IgG binding to antigen is high enough to allow one C1q component to simultaneously bind two neighboring IgG molecules on the bacterial surface (see Fig. 5.6). IgM is the most efficient isotype for complement-mediated killing of bacteria, activating lytic or phagocytic mechanisms. IgG antibodies arise somewhat later during the immune response, and although IgG is less efficient than IgM at mediating complement activation, IgG antibodies usually have a higher affinity for the bacterial antigens, which is another correlate of effective immunity. It has become increasingly clear over the past few years that high-affinity antibodies most effectively mediate protection from bacterial infections. Indeed, it appears that many humans have naturally occurring antibodies to many bacterial antigens, but these are usually of a low affinity and hence the antibodies are not very effective during serious infection.

In some circumstances, antibodies alone can mediate phagocytosis and have shown to be mediators of immunity by their ability to protect complement-deficient mice from experimental infection. In these cases, Fc receptors on phagocytic cells that bind to the Fc portion of IgG and IgA allow for complement-independent opsonization of the infecting microbe, leading to effective phagocytosis and killing. The opsonic capacity of an antibody molecule

depends on its isotype as the various classes (and subclasses) of immunoglobulin differ in their ability to be bound by Fc receptors. In humans, the subclasses IgG1 and IgG3 are usually the most efficient opsonizing antibodies. In contrast, Fc receptors for IgM are not present on most phagocytic cells; thus IgM-mediated phagocytosis and protection are usually completely dependent on the presence of complement. An Fc receptor for IgA (CD89) can promote phagocytosis of organisms opsonized by antibody of this isotype, but IgA is not thought to activate complement in most in vivo settings.

Cell-Mediated Immunity and Bacterial Infection

Acquired immunity to intracellular bacteria may involve both CD4$^+$ T cells carrying out DTH reactions (T$_{DTH}$ cells) or CD8$^+$ T-cell-directed cytotoxicity. In both of these cases bacterial pathogens are killed either within the infected cells or following release from the infected cell after it has been lysed. Although antibodies are not generally thought to be primary mediators of immunity to intracellular bacterial pathogens, antibodies theoretically may attach to the surface of an intracellular pathogen and prevent intracellular invasion or antibody may neutralize the effect of toxins that are secreted outside infected cells. One example of antibody-mediated immunity to an intracellular bacterial pathogen is the ability of antibody to the *Listeria monocytogenes*-secreted toxin known as listeriolysin to neutralize bacterial growth inside infected macrophages. T$_{DTH}$ cells are usually CD4$^+$ and work by secreting cytokines that activate MHC class II-positive macrophages and similar cells to the point where the infected cell can kill pathogens residing within them. CD8$^+$ T-cell cytolysis may be most important for killing nonmacrophage cells that bacterial pathogens have invaded, although they also can be cytolytic for MHC class II-positive cells because these cells also express MHC class I. The importance of T lymphocytes in the control of intracellular bacterial pathogens has been pointedly shown by the high level of disease due to these pathogens that occurs in patients with AIDS with reduced CD4$^+$ T-cell activity, which also affects development of functional CD8$^+$ cytotoxic T cells.

Cytokines and Chemokines in Cell-Mediated Immunity to Bacteria

At the molecular level, cytokines and chemokines are critical factors in cell-mediated immunity to intracellular bacterial pathogens. Cytokines function both to attract phagocytic cells to the site of infection and to activate them. Usually this is due to secreted bacterial products. Bacterial pathogens that can escape antibody-mediated immune effector mechanisms, survive intracellularly, and require activated phagocytes for successful elimination include those causing tuberculosis, leprosy, brucellosis, and listeriosis.

The most critical cytokine mediating intracellular killing of many pathogenic microbes is interferon-gamma (IFN-γ), which engenders enhanced bacteriocidal activity of infected phagocytic and nonphagocytic cells. Studies of mice deficient in production of IFN-γ or its receptor show this cytokine is critical for mediating immunity to intracellular bacterial pathogens such as mycobacteria, salmonellae, listeriae, and rickettsiae. Mice unable to make IFN-γ or its receptor or have their IFN-γ neutralized by antibody are much more susceptible to infection with these pathogens. IFN-γ can be produced by many different cells of the immune system: T cells, NK cells, and macrophages.

Another important cytokine in cell-mediated immunity is TNF-α. This cytokine can work in concert with IFN-γ to activate cells to enhance their ability to kill infecting pathogens. TNF-α also promotes migration of phagocytic cells into the circulation from the bone marrow. Other cytokines found to play important roles in killing of intracellular bacteria are IL-1, IL-6, IL-8, IL-12, and IL-18. IL-12 and IL-18 are well known to promote IFN-γ production along with TNF-α secretion and phagocyte production of nitric oxide (NO), which directly mediates bacterial killing.

Chemokines also play a role in activating killing mechanisms in infected cells, often by inducing production of NO. Chemokines CCL3 (MIP-1α), CCL4 (MIP-1β), and CCL5 (RANTES) can increase killing of organisms inside cells by promoting generation of NO. The chemokines CXCL9, CXCL10, and CXCL11, which all bind to chemokine receptor CXCR3, may have an antimicrobial activity that directly kills intracellular bacterial pathogens. Chemokine production can be enhanced by cytokines such as IFN-γ and TNF-α.

Host Response to Bacterial Infection

The inflammatory response of the host is critical to the interruption and resolution of the infectious process but is often responsible for the signs and symptoms of disease. Bacterial infection promotes a complex series of host responses involving the complement, kinin, and coagulation pathways as well as activation of the acquired immune responses, notably antibody and T cells activated in response to intracellular bacteria. Most likely the initial recognition of a foreign pathogen involves activation of complement, and the generation of molecules such as C3a and C5a initiates inflammation. This response leads to changes in endothelial membranes whereby receptors for inflammatory cells are produced on the luminal side of the blood vessel, causing these cells to adhere to the endothelium and to migrate through them to the site of infection (see Fig. 5.11). Factors such as IL-1, IL-6, and TNF-α are then produced, leading to fever, muscle proteolysis, and other effects that comprise the quantitatively measurable signs and subjectively reported symptoms of disease.

Immunity at Mucosal Surfaces

Since the initial site of entry and attachment of bacteria is usually a mucosal surface, a great deal of emphasis has been placed on the mucosal immune system as an important mediator of resistance to infection. Local antibodies are usually the major determinants of successful resistance to infection at the mucosal surface. IgA is found in the highest concentrations in mucosal secretions and is thought to function in immunity by binding to bacterial surface antigens and preventing the cells from attaching to their targets on epithelial cells. However, although this idea is widely touted, it has not been possible to definitively show that this mechanism of protective immunity is operative on the mucosal surface of a living animal. The molecular mechanism whereby IgA prevents bacterial attachment to host receptors is inferred only from in vitro studies. IgA cannot activate complement, and while the CD89 IgA Fc receptor is expressed on phagocytes residing on mucosal surfaces, the contribution of this pathway to mucosal immunity is not well documented by rigorous experiments. IgG and IgM are also present on mucosal surfaces, and these two can have effects not only in blocking adherence of microbes to host tissues but in activating complement and mediating bacteriocidal and opsonic killing. Convincing data demonstrating that IgA has a major role in resistance to infection in vivo are limited. This somewhat heretical statement is supported by the observation that congenital IgA deficiency is common, and many of these individuals do not show any signs of enhanced susceptibility to bacterial infection. However, it is obvious that preventing bacterial entry and attachment would be the most effective mechanism of immunity, attacking the infectious inocula early on and limiting the development of disease. Therefore, finding ways to generate effective immunity on a mucosal surface, regardless of the antibody class mediating immunity, is of obvious importance. One means to engender such immunity is to vaccinate with immunogens applied to a mucosal surface. Oral vaccines for enteric infections and antigens either inhaled or delivered as nose drops for respiratory infections may be superior to injected vaccines.

Immunity at mucosal surfaces is difficult to study because of the need for invasive means to obtain samples from the respiratory, gastrointestinal, and genitourinary tracts for evaluations. Furthermore, while excellent molecular and cellular tools exist to document the importance of complement activation and opsonophagocytosis in immunity to infection, similar tools do not exist for documenting how antibodies such as IgA might function. Whether opsonic killing by IgG and IgM along with complement occurs routinely at a mucosal surface is unclear as it is not certain if there is a sufficient level of these effectors present at the beginning of an infection. However, both phagocytes and complement can be quickly mobilized from the blood and possibly the local tissues to deal with pathogens on mucosal surfaces that have overcome innate immune defenses. Data supporting a role for opsonic IgG in resistance to mucosal colonization have recently been obtained following the introduction of a conjugate vaccine for *Haemophilus influenzae* type b. Systemic immunization with the conjugate vaccine was effective in reducing colonization of the oropharyngeal mucosal surfaces, indicating that the immune effectors generated by the vaccine were present in the oropharynx at a sufficient level to promote bacterial killing.

The Study of How Bacteria Cause Disease: Bacterial Pathogenesis

Critical to an understanding of how the immune system recognizes, responds to, and eliminates pathogenic bacteria is insight into the basic process of infection and disease. This involves deriving knowledge of the molecular architecture of the bacterial surface, its interaction with the host, and the host immune response. Virtually all of the advances made in comprehending bacterial diseases and designing effective antimicrobial and vaccine-based strategies to treat or control these infections have come from examining the structures of bacterial cells, particularly their outer cell walls and membranes, the toxins and metabolites they secrete, and the protein, lipoprotein, glycolipid, and polysaccharide structures they make to promote colonization and disease and help the microorganism avoid host defenses. Thus, delving into this area, known as the study of bacterial pathogenesis or bacterial virulence, provides the underpinning needed to understand mechanisms of immunity operative against bacterial infections.

Cell Wall Structure of Gram-Positive and Gram-Negative Bacteria

Gram-positive bacteria

Gram-positive organisms are defined as those bacteria that have a typical lipid bilayer cytoplasmic membrane surrounded by a rigid cell wall that provides the bacteria with their characteristic shape, differentiates them from eukaryotic cells, and allows them to survive in osmotically unfavorable environments (Fig. 18.6). The cell wall is composed primarily of peptidoglycan (Fig. 18.7), which is a polymer of *N*-acetylglucosamine and its lactyl ether, *N*-acetylmuramic acid, with peptide side chains covalently bound to the lactyl group. The peptide chains consist of alternating D- and L-amino acids and usually are linked to each other by a pentaglycine bridge that binds a terminal D-alanine on one peptide substituent to the penultimate L-lysine on a neighboring peptide. Variations in this basic structure have been described for a number of bacterial genera.

Teichoic and lipoteichoic acids

In addition, the cell walls of gram-positive bacteria contain teichoic acids, which are phosphate-linked polymers of sugar alcohols such as ribitol or glycerol and can be further substituted by different components (Fig. 18.8). Lipid tails can anchor some of these to the cytoplasmic membrane, giving rise to lipoteichoic acids. Some organisms have teichoic acids in which the glycerol or ribitol phosphate polymer is linked directly to *N*-acetylmuramic acid in the peptidoglycan. The various substituents on teichoic acids often are responsible for the biologic and immunologic properties associated with disease caused by pathogenic gram-positive bacteria.

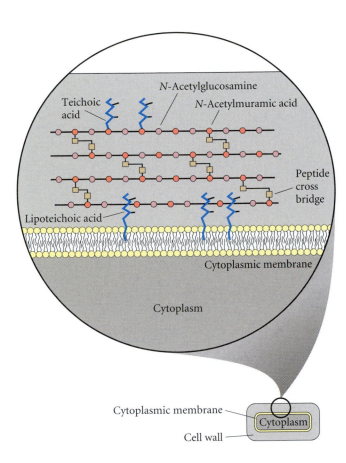

Figure 18.6 Schematic structure of the gram-positive bacterial cell wall. The wall consists of a peptidoglycan layer composed of liner copolymers of N-acetylglucosamine and N-acetylmuramic acid, cross-linked to each other by oligopeptide cross bridges. Teichoic acids and lipoteichoic acids (anchored at N-acetylmuramic acid and in the plasma membrane, respectively) are thought to play a role in regulating the breakdown of the cell wall that occurs during cell division.

Surface polysaccharides and capsules

Most pathogenic gram-positive bacteria that can invade host tissues, such as the blood, have additional extracellular structures, often composed of polysaccharide, that either are part of the cell wall or represent an extracellular substance surrounding the cell, known as a capsule (Fig. 18.9). Streptococci can be differentiated into over 20 serogroups on the basis of polysaccharides that make up part of the cell wall. Many of these serologic differences also correspond to different streptococcal species. The major species of streptococcus that infect humans, the group A streptococci, which cause local infections such as pharyngitis (strep throat) or can spread throughout the host to cause a systemic or disseminated infection, are

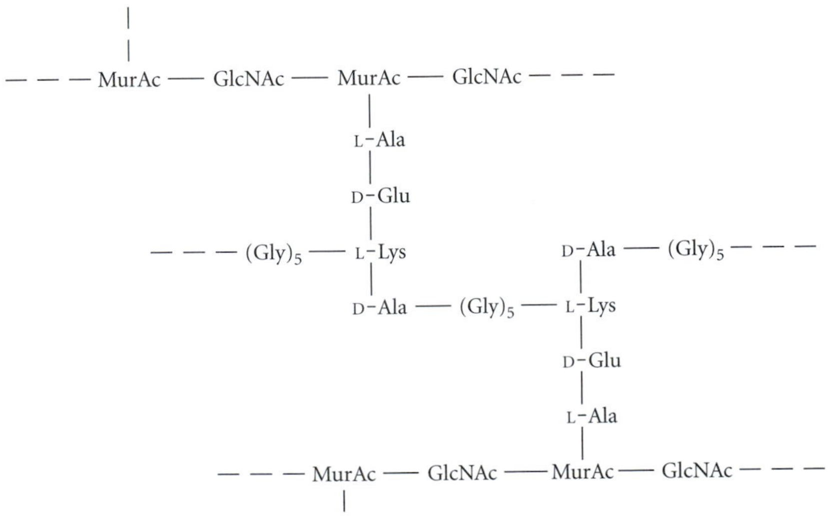

Figure 18.7 Peptidoglycan. The schematic structure of the peptidoglycan layer of the cell wall of *S. aureus* shows the polysaccharide backbone composed of alternating N-acetylmuramic acid (MurAc) and N-acetylglucosamine (GlcNAc) residues linked β-1,4 with a tetrapeptide bridge emanating from the MurAc residue and composed of L-alanine (L-Ala), D-glutamate (D-Glu), L-lysine (L-Lys), and D-alanine (D-Ala). The tetrapeptide bridges are then cross-linked with a pentaglycine peptide [(Gly)5]. Variations in peptidoglycan structure are common among gram-positive bacteria.

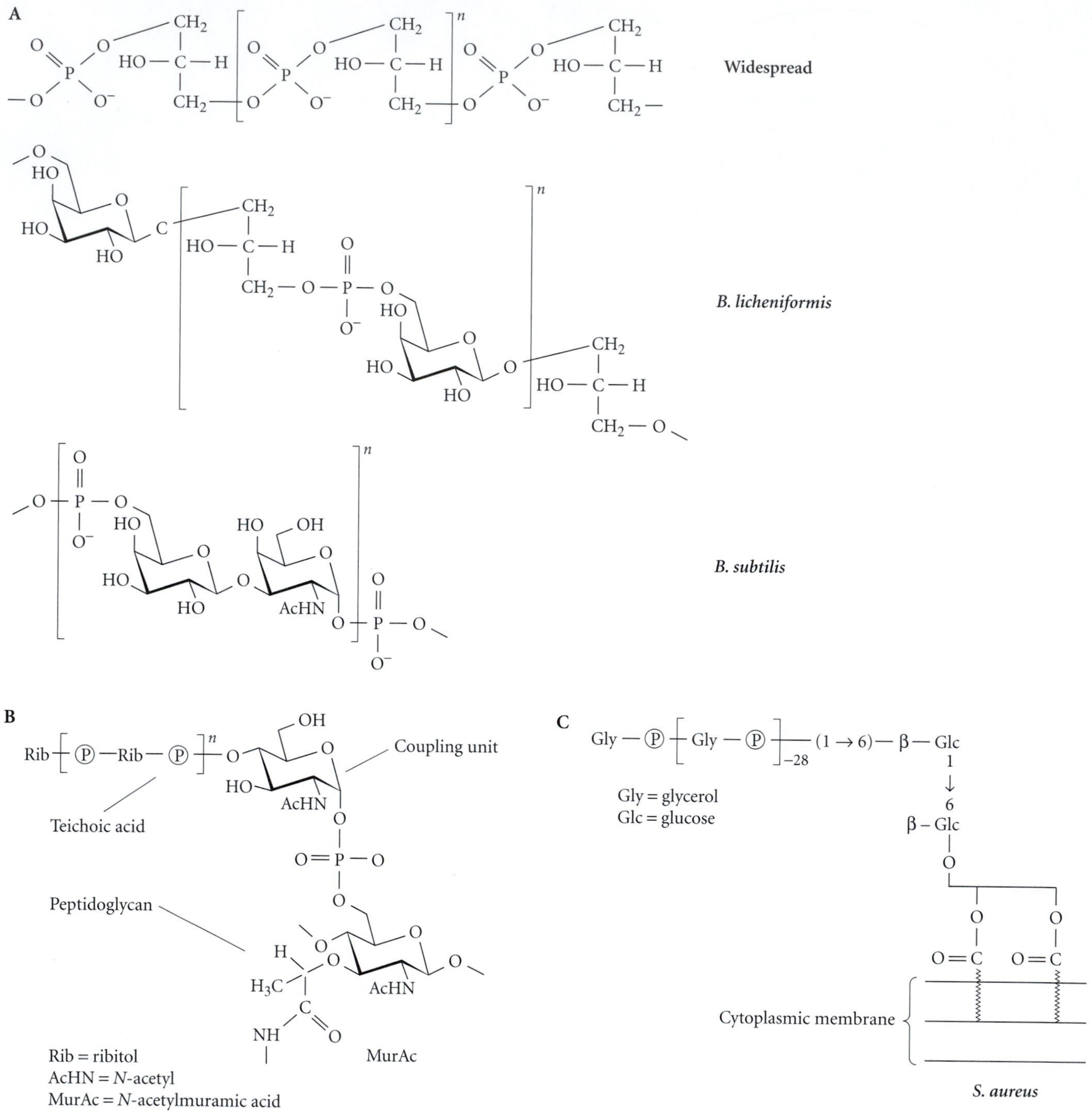

A

Widespread

B. licheniformis

B. subtilis

B

Rib—(P)—Rib—(P)ₙ

Teichoic acid

Peptidoglycan

Coupling unit

Rib = ribitol
AcHN = N-acetyl
MurAc = N-acetylmuramic acid

C

Gly—(P)—Gly—(P)₋₂₈—(1 → 6)— β— Glc

Gly = glycerol
Glc = glucose

β – Glc

Cytoplasmic membrane

S. aureus

Figure 18.8 Teichoic acids. Representation of the structures of teichoic acids found in the cell walls of gram-positive bacteria. (**A**) A generic structure for teichoic acids (**top**). This is a repeat unit of the three-carbon sugar glycerol linked to each other by phosphate groups and is referred to as a glycerol teichoic acid. Variations in this basic structure are frequently found, such as the use of ribitol, a five-carbon sugar alcohol, in place of glycerol. The teichoic acid of *Bacillus licheniformis* (**middle**) contains a glucose-glycerol disaccharide linked via phosphate groups whereas the teichoic acid of *Bacillus subtilis* (**bottom**) is a glucose-*N*-acetylglucosamine disaccharide linked by phosphate groups. (**B**) Teichoic acids are linked directly to *N*-acetylmuramic acid in the peptidoglycan. This type of teichoic acid uses ribitol (Rib) instead of glycerol and is coupled via an amino sugar and phosphate groups (coupling unit) to *N*-acetylmuramic acid in the peptidoglycan. (**C**) The structure of lipoteichoic acid from *S. aureus*, showing the linkage of a typical glycerol-teichoic acid to a glycolipid through a glucose disaccharide. The lipid is then anchored in the bacterial cytoplasmic membrane.

A

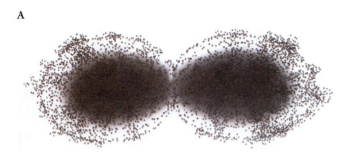

B

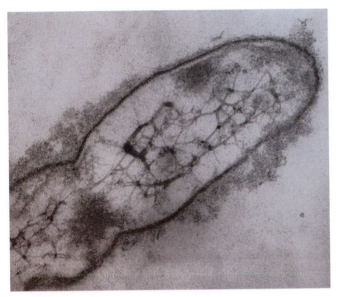

Figure 18.9 Bacterial capsules. Electron micrographs of the capsule surrounding the outer cell wall layer of a gram-positive *(Staphylococcus epidermidis)* (**A**) and a gram-negative *(P. aeruginosa)* (**B**) bacterium are shown. The outer capsule layer is visualized with specific antibodies raised to the purified antigen. (**A**) The antibody binding to the capsule has been detected with a secondary IgG conjugated to ferritin, producing an electron-dense black dot where the secondary antibody binds to the primary antibody bound to the capsule. (**B**) The capsule was made sufficiently electron dense with antibody to the capsule alone to see the fuzzy outer layer of variable thickness.

surrounded by an extracellular coat of a hyaluronic acid polysaccharide. Since hyaluronic acid is a normal constituent of mammalian tissues, this antigen is not immunogenic and is not the target of protective immunity against group A streptococci. However, the streptococcus that causes classic bacterial pneumonia, often referred to as the pneumococcus, is surrounded by an extracellular polysaccharide capsule that is the key antigenic target for protective antibodies. The presence or absence of the pneumococcal capsule was the critical factor associated with one of the most important discoveries in all of biology: that of M. S. Avery, C. M. MacLeod, and M. McCarty in 1944, who showed that DNA was the cellular constituent that carried genetic information. They used pneumococci lacking a capsule in their studies and showed they could transfer the genetic information for making a capsule with DNA but not with other cellular components. Capsular polysaccharides also are found among staphylococci.

Gram-negative bacteria

Outer components of the gram-negative bacterial cell

Gram-negative bacteria possess a cytoplasmic membrane and a peptidoglycan cell wall similar to that of gram-positive bacteria, although the cell wall of gram negative bacteria is thinner than that of gram-positive bacteria. In addition to these structures, gram-negative bacteria are characterized by the presence of an outer membrane that surrounds the cell wall and is covalently linked to it. This linkage occurs between the tetrapeptides of the peptidoglycan layer and a lipoprotein that is embedded in the outer membrane (Fig. 18.10). Also embedded in the outer membrane are proteins (called outer membrane proteins) that function to maintain the integrity of the outer membrane, regulate the diffusion of molecules into the cell, and act as receptors for proteins such as siderophores that scavenge iron and possibly other molecules critical for bacterial growth. Embedded within the outer membrane is the LPS, which is a major component of virulence and a major target for humoral immunity during bacterial infection. For many pathogenic gram-negative bacteria, there is also an extracellular polysaccharide capsule layer that is a target for humoral immunity and the antigen used in several successful vaccines.

LPS

As its name implies, LPS is composed of a glycolipid covalently linked to a carbohydrate structure (Fig. 18.11). LPS is embedded in the outer membrane, via the glycolipid backbone, known as lipid A, with the polysaccharide portion protruding from the cell surface. Lipid A is the biologically active component of LPS, inducing many host inflammatory effectors such as TNF-α and IL-1, leading to production of acute-phase proteins, fever, hypotension, etc. Lipid A contains both sugars and lipids, and the nature and arrangement of the lipids determine the ability of the molecule to provoke inflammatory responses. For example, lipid A from some gram-negative bacteria such as *Escherichia coli* is toxic whereas the lipid A from *Bacteroides fragilis*, a component of the normal gut microbiota, is biologically inactive. The lipid As from these two microbes have different fatty acid components. Attached to the lipid A is a short oligosaccharide known as the *inner core*. In many important bacterial pathogens, the inner

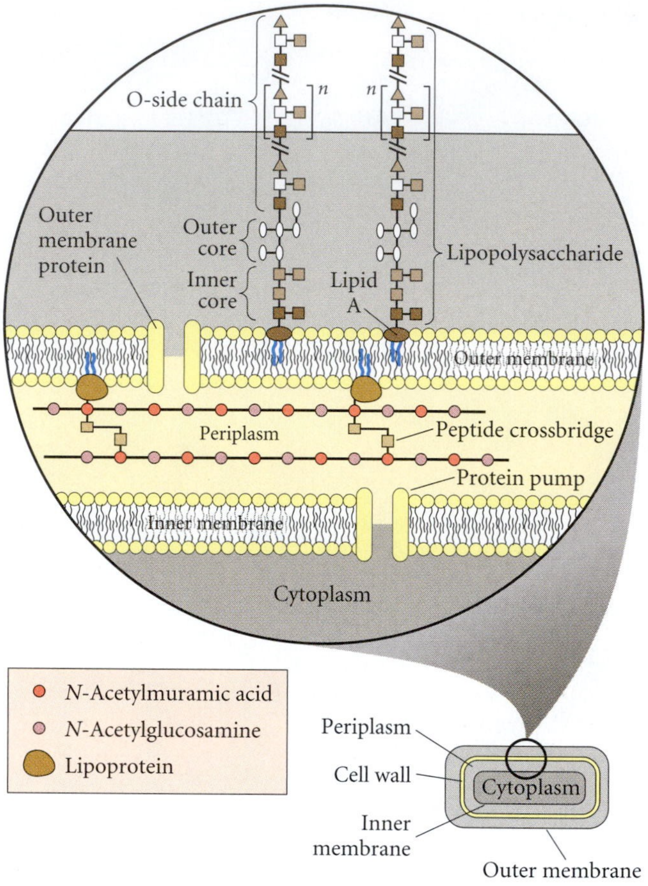

Figure 18.10 Schematic representation of the outer surface structure of a gram-negative bacterium. The characteristic structure of the gram-negative bacterial surface is a double membrane with the space between the membranes, called the periplasm, containing a thin cell wall composed of peptidoglycan. Both membranes contain numerous integral and peripheral proteins that carry out numerous functions, including transport of molecules across the membranes. The outer membrane is anchored to the cell wall by lipoproteins that are embedded in the outer membrane and are covalently coupled to the cell wall. The outer leaflet consists entirely of LPS rather than phospholipid (for clarity, the diagram shows only two LPS molecules). The LPS composition of the outer membrane renders the bacterial surface resistant to phospholipases. The hydrophobic anchor of LPS is a unique molecule called lipid A.

core is composed of a disaccharide or trisaccharide of an unusual sugar called 2-keto-3-deoxyoctonate. Additional sugar substituents are linked to the inner core, forming a *complete core* that is somewhat conserved among related gram-negative pathogens. Attached to the core are the O

polysaccharide side chains, which, when present, confer serologic variability to different strains within a species and protect the cell from host proteins such as lytic complement components. O polysaccharides can be composed of a variety of monosaccharides, ranging from the

Figure 18.11 Schematic representation of the LPS found in the outer membrane of gram-negative bacteria. Man, mannose; Rha, rhamnose; Gal, galactose; GlcNAc, N-acetylglucosamine; Glc, glucose; Hep, L-glycero-D-mannoheptose; KDO, 2-keto-3 deoxyoctonate; GlcN, glucosamine. The precise monosaccharide composition of the LPS core and O side chain varies among bacterial species and serovars.

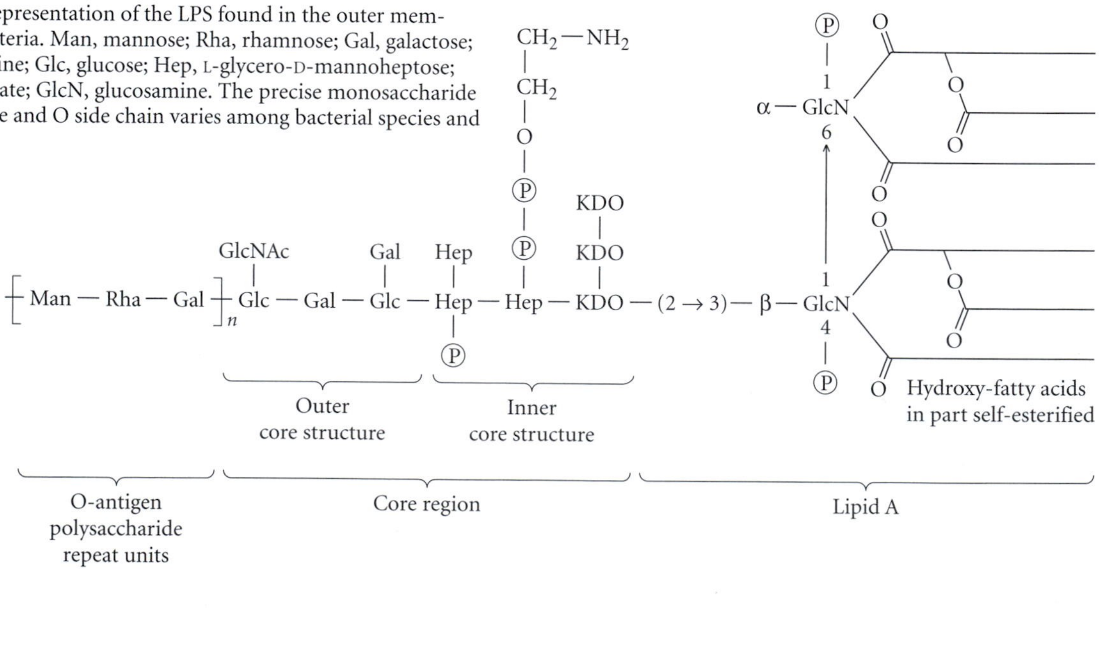

common pentoses and hexoses to more complex and un-usual structures such as pseudaminic acid (5,7-diamino-3,5,7,9-tetradeoxynonulosonic acid) found in some strains of *P. aeruginosa* and in *Shigella* type 7 LPS. These sugars can be substituted by a variety of groups, such as formyl, acetyl, and hydroxy-butyryl side chains; amino acids or peptides; or phosphate groups. This high level of chemical variability is thought to be key to bacterial pathogenesis, because each variation in a basic structure is potentially capable of altering the ability of an antibody to bind to the bacteria to promote its killing. For example, one reason that a person might get food poisoning due to salmonellae more than once during his or her lifetime is that these bacteria can produce hundreds of different O polysaccharides. An infection caused by one strain will elicit the production of antibody to a specific O polysac-charide, but these antibodies will not prevent infection by a strain with a chemically, and hence immunologically, distinct O polysaccharide.

Pili

Pili or fimbriae extend through the outer membrane into the external environment, appearing in electron micro-graphs as hair-like projections that may be confined to one end of the organism (polar pili) or be distributed more evenly over the surface, with up to several hundred per cell (Fig. 18.12). These structures are potential targets for an immune response, so knowledge of their structure and function is an important component for understand-ing immunity to bacterial infections. An individual cell may make multiple pili with different functions. Most pili are composed of a major pilin protein subunit with a molecular weight of 17,000 to 30,000 that polymerizes to form the pilus. Some pili, such as the galactose disaccha-ride (gal-gal)-binding pili of *E. coli*, have additional pro-teins critical for pilus function located at the pilus tips. To date, the major function attributed to pili is that of medi-ating binding of bacteria to host tissues. For *Neisseria gon-orrhoeae*, the cause of gonorrhea, to infect a human host, it must use its pili to attach to epithelial cells that line the urethra. It has been shown that only *N. gonorrhoeae* that expresses pili causes disease in humans.

Flagella

Flagella are long appendages that are attached to either one or both ends of the bacterial cell (polar flagella) or are distributed over the entire cell surface (peritrichous flag-ella) (Fig. 18.12). Flagella enable a cell to swim about and are composed of a polymerized or aggregated basic pro-tein, in this case called flagellin. Flagellin polymerizes in a tight helical structure, thus forming the main flagellar structure, and is serologically variable among different bacterial species. Bacteria known as spirochetes, which cause diseases such as syphilis and Lyme disease, have fil-aments similar to flagella that run along the long axis of the center of the cell. These organisms swim by rotating around this filament. Other species of bacteria are able to glide over a surface in the absence of obvious motility structures such as flagella.

Initial Stage of Bacterial Infection: Colonization of Host Surfaces

Bacterial pathogens usually enter our bodies through the mucosal and skin surfaces, including the respiratory, ocu-lar, gastrointestinal, and genitourinary tracts. Skin can be an important site of bacterial colonization, particularly for staphylococci, and direct inoculation of pathogens into the host via or through the skin is always a risk factor for subsequent disease. Occasional diseases, such as swim-mer's ear, which usually is caused by *P. aeruginosa*, can oc-cur via colonization of the auditory canal. Successful col-onization usually requires bacterial adherence to the mucosal surface. In this regard, infection and coloniza-tion can be used interchangeably; however, infection usu-ally is reserved for pathogenic organisms, whereas colo-nization is used for organisms that do not necessarily cause disease but can in certain circumstances (i.e., breaches of innate immune systems due to skin break-down, other immune deficiencies, etc.). Adherence is

Figure 18.12 Transmission electron micrograph of a piliated strain of *P. aeruginosa*. Each cell possesses hundreds of pili (small arrows), which promote aggregation of the bacteria. Also visible is a flagellum (large, open arrows) that is folded under the cell. Flagella are longer and have a larger diameter than pili. In this example, there is only one flagellum, known as a polar flagellum, as it emerges from the cell at one end, or pole.

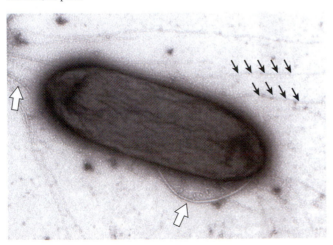

most often attributed to the pili, surface polysaccharides, lipoteichoic acids, and protein adhesins exposed on the cell surface, although any microbial surface structure has the potential to mediate adherence to host tissues. Host targets for bacterial adherence are either the epithelial cells that line mucosal tracts or the mucous layer itself. In the latter case, the bacteria must circumvent the host's normal ability to clear the mucus-coated bacterial cells. Such circumvention is thought to occur in states such as ciliary dyskinesis in the respiratory tract (in which the epithelial cilia, which normally propel mucus up and out of the airway, either cease beating or beat in an unsynchronized fashion) or chronic *P. aeruginosa* colonization of the respiratory tract in individuals with cystic fibrosis.

It now appears that an individual bacterial cell expresses multiple, often serologically variable, adhesins and uses these during the various stages of colonization. For example, most strains of *E. coli* express type 1 pili, whose binding to host tissues is inhibited by D-mannose (suggesting that the pili function by binding to mannose carbohydrates on host tissues). These pili appear to help the organisms bind to mucus. Strains of *E. coli* causing kidney infections (pyelonephritis) express a different adhesin, the Pap or P pilus, which mediates binding to digalactose residues on globosides of the human P blood groups. Adherence here is due to minor components of the pilus proteins found only on the tip of the pilus structure. *E. coli* that causes diarrheal disease expresses receptors for enterocytes on the small bowel, along with other receptors termed *colonization factors*.

Other bacterial structures involved in adherence to host tissues are found among organisms such as staphylococci and include proteins that bind host structures such as fibrin, fibronectin, laminin, and collagen. These likely promote the normal colonization of the nares and skin by these bacteria. Fibronectin appears to be a commonly used receptor for various pathogens, with a particular sequence in fibronectin, Arg-Gly-Asp (RGD), being critical to binding. Surface lipoteichoic acids promote adherence of streptococci to mucosal surfaces. The mucoid exopolysaccharide or alginate capsule of *P. aeruginosa* promotes binding of mucoid strains to respiratory mucins. Both coagulase-negative and coagulase-positive staphylococci have emerged as important pathogens, owing to their ability to colonize prosthetic devices and catheters commonly used in medical care. The surface capsular polysaccharide of these organisms promotes binding to the prosthetic material and renders the bacteria resistant to many antibiotics and immune effector mechanisms of the host.

Although it appears that interruption of the colonizing ability of a bacterial pathogen by production of antibody specific to the microbial adhesins is a potential strategy for immunologic intervention, there is little evidence that this mechanism of immunity is operative or contributes to high-level host resistance to infection. Part of the problem is that there are multiple adhesins on a given bacterial cell, so a number of different antibodies would need to be present to achieve good inhibition of colonization. The antigenic variability of bacterial adhesins is another factor that hinders the effectiveness of the host's immune response. Organisms can evade the protective immune response to surface antigens by varying the amino acid sequence of the pertinent epitopes and essentially "evade" the response by no longer expressing the specific epitopes the immune response (be it antibody mediated or cell mediated) recognizes. Bacteria have set up elaborate systems for antigenic variation of surface structures like pili or other adhesins for this very purpose. Although antibodies can be produced with a high affinity for an antigen, if the antibody to a microbial adhesin is of a lower affinity than is the ligand for the adhesin, it could be difficult for the antibody to interrupt colonization. Finally, surface adhesins can be targets for opsonophagocytic antibody, and differentiating whether a particular antibody works in an in vivo setting by inhibiting adherence or mediating opsonic killing is difficult. Although much research is being directed toward identifying bacterial adhesins needed for colonization and using them as potential vaccines, there are no existing vaccines for human diseases based on interrupting a bacterial adhesin-host ligand interaction.

Tissue Invasion and Disease

Invasion of bacteria into deeper mucosal tissue layers may occur via intracellular uptake by epithelial cells or by a paracellular route, whereby bacteria traverse between epithelial cells by interrupting junctions between adjacent cells. Among virulent strains of *Shigella* that can cause a severe form of diarrhea known as dysentery, outer membrane proteins and LPS are critical for bacterial invasion of epithelial cells and multiplication. Bacteria that cause gonorrhea and meningitis penetrate by poorly understood mechanisms into mucosal cells before disseminating into the blood. Staphylococci and streptococci elaborate a variety of extracellular enzymes such as hyaluronidase, lipases, nucleases, and hemolysins that are probably important in breaking down cellular and matrix structures and giving the bacteria access to deeper tissues and blood. Organisms that colonize the gastrointestinal tract frequently can translocate through the mucosa into the blood and, in situations of inadequate host defenses, cause bacteremia. *Yersinia enterocolitica* causes some forms of diarrhea and is capable of invading the mucosal epithelium because of the activity of the invasin protein. Invasin tightly binds β1-integrin proteins on epithelial cell membranes and in doing so causes the epithelial cell membrane to wrap around the bacterial cell (thus causing internalization of the bacteria by the epithelial cell). Some bacteria such as *Brucella* (the cause of brucellosis) and *Salmonella* (the cause of enteric fever) can be carried from a mucosal site to a distant site by phagocytic cells such as polymorphonuclear leukocytes or macrophages that ingest, but fail to kill, the bacteria. Failure of these phagocytes to kill the ingested bacteria is due to a variety of bacterial defense mechanisms that interfere with phagolysosome function. Obviously, bacteria have evolved many different ways of getting into a host, remaining there, and then spreading to other parts of the body to cause disease.

A number of important pathogens cause disease without further invading host tissues. One of these pathogens of recent note is enteropathogenic *E. coli* (EPEC). EPEC adheres tightly to the apical plasma membrane of its host's intestinal epithelium by inducing the formation of "pedestals" (also called "attaching and effacing lesions") on the epithelial cell surface. Pedestals are elevated regions of plasma membrane that contact the EPEC cell and result in a strong interaction between the membrane and the bacterium. EPEC triggers pedestal formation in its host's epithelium by delivering a signaling molecule from the bacterial cell directly into the host cell via a specialized bacterial secretion system termed the type III secretion system. Injection of bacterial proteins and toxins into the host cell causes the cytoskeleton of the cell to reorganize and form pedestals. Other examples of pathogens that cause disease through local tissue infection are *Bordetella pertussis* (whooping cough), *V. cholerae* (cholera), *Clostridium tetani* (tetanus), *Clostridium botulinum* (botulism), *Corynebacterium diphtheriae* (diphtheria), *M. tuberculosis* (tuberculosis), and *Mycobacterium leprae* (leprosy).

Some pathogens can cause both local disease, such as pharyngitis and epiglottitis, skin ulcerations, and diarrhea, and disease due to tissue invasion. Progression of some bacterial diseases from local commensal colonization to disseminated infection sometimes requires a breach in host tissues to cause deeper infections, such as peritonitis due to *Bacteroides fragilis* or other intestinal organisms. These microbes are normally part of the commensal microflora of the gastrointestinal tract, but when this tissue is ruptured by something like a burst appendix or intestinal trauma, they can enter the peritoneum and cause severe disease. In this case, bacterial factors are not critical for invasion, but tissue injury is. Commensal mi-

croflora can also cause disease when the makeup of this "normal" flora is altered due to antibiotic therapy, for example. Then normally non-disease-causing organisms can overgrow and cause disease. Examples include *Clostridium difficile* antibiotic-associated infectious colitis and yeast vaginitis.

As for the colonization factors, immunologic effectors that interrupt or neutralize invasion factors have not been generally found to promote high-level resistance to spread of organisms and subsequent pathology. Again, this is likely due in part to the multitude of factors that many pathogenic bacteria can use to invade tissues. Some animal studies have suggested that neutralization of the type III secretion mechanism has potential to protect against infection, but these studies are in an early stage. However, there is no extant vaccine used in humans predicated on neutralization of an invasive activity of a bacterial pathogen.

Disease

Disease is a complex phenomenon resulting from the colonization, invasion, and toxin elaboration by bacteria and the subsequent immune response of the host. It is interesting that many bacterial factors that cause diseases in mammals also cause disease in plants, worms, fungi, and fruit flies. Toxin elaboration is one of the best-characterized molecular mechanisms of bacterial pathogenesis, while host factors such as IL-1 and IL-6, TNF-α, kinins, inflammatory proteins, products of complement activation, and mediators derived from arachidonic acid metabolites (leukotrienes) and cellular degranulation (histamine) readily contribute to the severity of disease. The interplay of these factors will dictate the severity of the disease, which may range from mild to severe even among individuals infected with the same microorganism. One of the major factors that attenuate the course of disease is host immune responses, which often account for the discrepancy in disease severity among different individuals.

Toxins

Some of the first bacterial diseases to be understood were those due to toxin-elaborating organisms. Diphtheria, botulinum, and tetanus toxins are responsible for the disease associated with local *C. diphtheriae*, *C. botulinum*, and *C. tetani* infections, respectively. Enterotoxins produced by *E. coli*, *Salmonella*, *Shigella*, and *V. cholerae* contribute to diarrheal disease caused by these organisms. Staphylococci, streptococci, *P. aeruginosa*, and *Bordetella* species elaborate a variety of toxins that cause or contribute to disease in the host; these toxins include toxic shock syndrome toxin (TSST; cause of toxic shock syndrome), en-

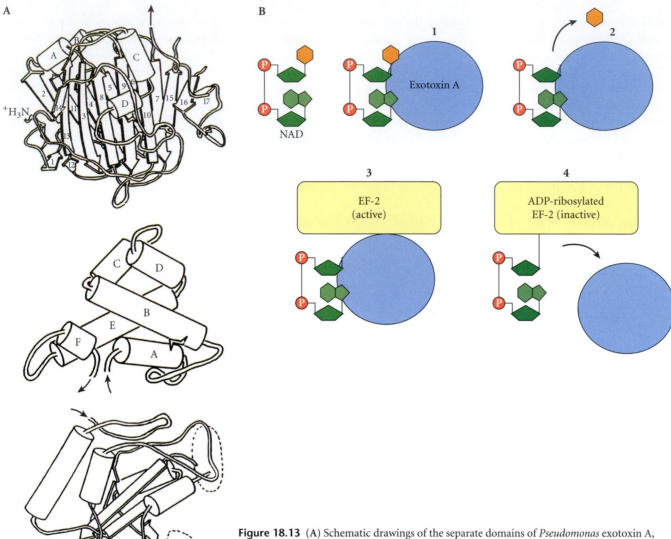

Figure 18.13 (A) Schematic drawings of the separate domains of *Pseudomonas* exotoxin A, separately oriented to give illustrative views: domain I (**top**), including residues 1 to 252 and 365 to 404; domain II (**middle**), including residues 253 to 364; and domain III (**bottom**), beginning at residue 405. The dotted lines in domain III indicate regions where electron density is difficult to trace. Reprinted from V. S. Allured et al., *Proc. Natl. Acad. Sci. USA* **83**:1320–1324, 1986. (**B**) The mechanism of action of exotoxin A. The toxin binds to nicotinamide adenine dinucleotide (NAD) (**1**) and releases the nicotinamide moiety to leave ADP-ribose on the toxin (**2**). The toxin then approaches active elongation factor 2 (EF-2) (**3**) and catalyzes the transfer of the ADP-ribose to EF-2, resulting in a cessation of protein synthesis in the eukaryotic cell (**4**).

terotoxins (diarrheal diseases), erythrogenic toxin (streptococcal infections), scarlatinal toxin (scarlet fever), exotoxins A, S, T, and U (associated with pseudomonal infections), and pertussis toxin (whooping cough). A number of these, such as cholera, diphtheria, and pertussis toxins; *E. coli* heat-labile toxin; and *P. aeruginosa* exotoxins A, S and T, have adenosine diphosphate (ADP)-ribosyltransferase activity whereby the toxins enzymatically catalyze the transfer of the ADP-ribosyl portion of nicotinamide

adenine diphosphate (NAD) to target proteins and inactivate them (Fig. 18.13).

The staphylococcal enterotoxins, TSST-1, and streptococcal pyogenic exotoxins are classic superantigens that stimulate a large proportion of their host's T lymphocytes in a relatively nonspecific manner (see Fig. 8.14). This stimulation can occur without processing of the protein toxin by antigen-presenting cells (APCs). Part of this process involves stimulation of the APCs to produce IL-1 and

TNF-α, which have been implicated as the cause of many of the clinical features of diseases such as toxic shock syndrome and scarlet fever.

Neutralization of some of these bacterial toxins is highly effective in preventing disease, but usually only when the toxin is the major or sole cause of the pathology. Thus, neutralizing antibody to diphtheria, tetanus, and botulinum toxins is highly protective, and the diphtheria and tetanus vaccines routinely administered to humans work by provoking the production of neutralizing antibodies. In the case of enterotoxins, neutralization of the toxin usually reduces the severity of the pathologic changes associated with disease but does not always completely prevent it. For example, neutralization of the enterotoxin produced by *V. cholerae*, termed cholera toxin, reduces the volume of diarrhea fluid made during infection but does not completely prevent diarrheal disease. Although some of the ADP-ribosylating toxins, such as *P. aeruginosa* exotoxin A, are toxic when administered in purified form, antibody to these toxins seems to play only a minor role in resistance to infection and disease. Toxins that are injected directly into a mammalian cell via the type III secretion system are not available to antibodies for neutralization.

Endotoxin

The lipid A portion of gram-negative LPS has potent biologic activities that cause many of the clinical features of gram-negative bacterial sepsis. These include fever, muscle proteolysis, uncontrolled intravascular coagulation, and shock. This effect appears to be mediated by production of IL-1, TNF-α, and perhaps IL-6 by mononuclear cells. These molecules have potent hyperthermic activity, which is exerted via their effects in the hypothalamus; increase vascular permeability; alter endothelial cell activity; and induce these cells to procoagulant activity. Numerous therapeutic strategies aimed at neutralizing the effects of endotoxin are under study, but the difficulty of this strategy in achieving success is underscored by recent therapeutic failures. These strategies include antibodies to lipid A, soluble receptors to TNF, and administration of the IL-1 receptor antagonist that blocks the binding of IL-1 to its cellular receptor.

A new appreciation for endotoxin and for its role in the host immune response has recently been kindled by the elucidation of a signaling cascade that allows the host's immune cells to utilize bacterial LPS as a potent costimulatory signal for initiation of an immune response. This process involves the coordinated action of several host proteins. Endotoxin (or LPS), which may be present on a bacterial surface or may be released from bacteria, is bound by a host serum protein called LPS-binding protein (LBP). This complex of LPS and LBP is a functional ligand for the host membrane proteins CD14 and TLR4 in association with MD2. TLR4 is a transmembrane protein that initiates a signaling cascade in the host's immune cells (see Fig. 2.7). This has many consequences: one is reduction of the activation threshold for immune cells for stimulation by other conventional antigens and another is generation of a potent cascade of cytokines that are needed to resist infection but if overproduced lead to severe pathology and sometimes death.

Bacterial Invasion

Some diseases are most likely caused by the presence of bacteria in tissue sites where they do not belong. Invasion of the blood by gram-negative rods gives rise to sepsis and bacteremia without obvious involvement of secreted exotoxins, although endotoxin is very important. Pneumococcal pneumonia is attributed primarily to the growth of the organism in the lung and to the attendant inflammatory response of the host, with little evidence for an important role for bacterial toxins in this disease. Bacteremia and invasion of the meninges by meningitis-producing organisms such as *N. meningitidis*, *H. influenzae*, *E. coli* K1, and group B streptococci appear to be due to the ability of these organisms to get into these tissues and multiply. Most of the tissue destruction here is the result of bacterial growth and host inflammation.

Bacterial Virulence Factors: How They Thwart Host Immunity

Virulence factors are the panoply of proteins, glycolipids, carbohydrates, teichoic acids, peptidoglycan, metabolites, enzymes, and toxins that bacteria use to cause disease. Many of these work by thwarting host defenses. Proteins, enzymes, and toxins can destroy or impede the function of lymphocytes and granulocytes. Glycolipids like LPS and cell wall structures such as teichoic acids and peptidoglycan can overstimulate inflammation, making normal defenses ineffective. Carbohydrates, particularly the long O side chains on LPS and capsular polysaccharides, prevent phagocytosis. Many of these can cause activation of the complement system, depleting the host of this critical immune effector. Enterotoxins and other bacterial superantigens easily disrupt the normal immune response, overactivating inflammation and host responses, which leads directly to disease and pathology. Counteracting these factors, usually with antibody, allows the host to modulate their effect and promote effective immunity. It has been appreciated since the beginning of the age wherein microbes were shown to be responsible for infections, starting in the 1870s, that proteins and toxins were major factors causing disease. More recent work has focused on several important virulence factors whose mode of action is being defined at the molecular and cellular level, which is starting to lead to new vaccines and immunotherapies.

Surface Polysaccharides and Proteins and Bacterial Survival

For organisms to invade host tissues effectively, particularly the blood, they must avoid the major host defenses of complement and phagocytic cells (Fig. 18.14). This is achieved most frequently through the presence of cell surface polysaccharides, either as capsular polysaccharides or as long O polysaccharide antigens characteristic of the smooth LPS of invasive gram-negative bacteria. These molecules appear to prevent the activation and/or deposition of complement opsonins or to limit access to these molecules of phagocytic cells that have receptors for complement op-

Figure 18.14 Bacteria evade complement-mediated killing by a number of mechanisms. (**A**) The presence of capsule or calyx outside the bacterial cell can prevent activated complement components (such as C3b) from attaching to the bacterial cell wall or outer membrane. (**B**) The presence of long or bulky surface components (green) on the surface of the bacterium can prevent complement receptors on phagocytes from binding activated complement components (such as C3b) that are attached to the bacterial surface. (**C**) Expression of certain surface proteins (for example, a CD59-related protein produced by *Borrelia burgdorferi*) diverts the activation of the MAC away from the bacterial membrane. (**D**) Bacteria express some enzymes (such as elastase) that can cleave, inactivate, or cause the disassembling of the activated complement components. (**E**) The outer membrane may be resistant to insertion of the C5b67 complex. (**F**) Secreted inhibitors of complement (SIC) bind to complement complexes C5b67 and C5b678, preventing membrane insertion.

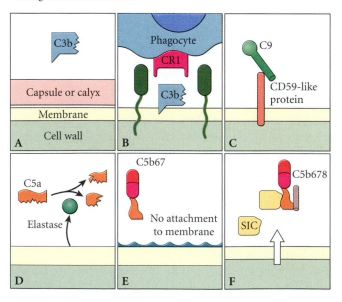

sonins. M proteins of group A streptococci convey resistance to phagocytic activity in blood, likely by binding the complement regulatory protein, factor H, which downregulates complement deposition on the organism. Some bacteria such as *Brucella, Yersinia, Listeria, Francisella,* and *Mycobacterium* spp. resist destruction inside phagocytic cells. Even in the absence of an obvious bacteremic phase, such as in shigellosis, the production of a smooth LPS is critical for bacterial pathogenesis and disease.

Biofilms, Quorum Sensing, and Bacterial Pathogenesis

A mechanism of bacterial pathogenesis that has recently received a great deal of attention is the ability of populations of bacteria to establish a cell-to-cell communication network using soluble factors. The network often results in a bacterial *biofilm,* an organized growth of many microbial cells in a microcolony. Communication among the cells occurs by *quorum sensing,* indicative of a time when an infectious bacterial inoculum has reached a critical mass, or quorum, and the cells within the biofilm can detect and respond to each other. This type of communication is used by many species of bacteria for maintaining organized growth in the environment and is also crucial for survival of some pathogenic bacteria in and on hosts. Formation of a community of microbes or biofilm is part of many infectious disease processes, including the formation of dental plaque and its attendant pathology of cavities. When populations of bacteria reach a certain size, the concentration of small-molecular-weight signaling molecules, often in the form of peptides or acyl-homoserine lactones (homoserine amino acid molecules substituted with fatty acids of different lengths), increases to the point such that bacterial receptors bind these signaling molecules. This results in gene transcription from the bacterial chromosome and the production of virulence factors.

A well-studied quorum-sensing system is used by *P. aeruginosa,* an important pathogen of immunocompromised hosts and patients with cystic fibrosis. After initial attachment of *P. aeruginosa* to a surface, the organisms spread on the surface, a process that requires pili, then grow into a small microcolony, followed by accumulation of homoserine lactones to levels sufficient to activate gene transcription leading to formation of a biofilm (Fig. 18.15). In patients with cystic fibrosis, there is a large buildup of *P. aeruginosa* cells into microcolonies, and the homoserine lactone molecules are readily detectable in lung fluid obtained from infected patients. However, another critical component of *P. aeruginosa* infection in patients with cystic fibrosis is the elaboration of a viscous polysaccharide capsule which is similar in structure to al-

A

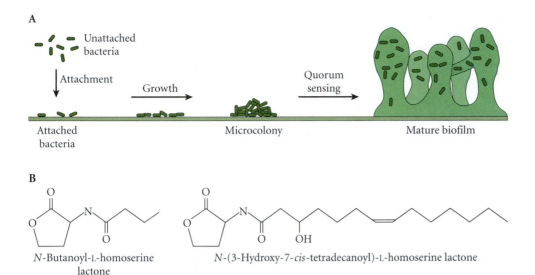

B

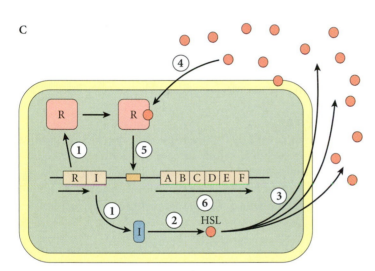

Figure 18.15 (A) Diagram of the biofilm-maturation pathway of *P. aeruginosa*. Unattached cells that approach a surface may attach. Attached cells will proliferate on a surface and use specific functions to actively grow into microcolonies. The high-density microcolonies differentiate into mature biofilms using an intercellular communication mechanism called quorum sensing. (B) Quorum sensing is mediated by small soluble molecules called *autoinducers*. Most autoinducers are homoserine lactones such as *N*-butanoyl-L-homoserine lactone and *N*-(3-hydroxy-7-*cis*-tetradecanoyl)-L-homoserine lactone. (C) Mechanism of quorum sensing. As bacteria grow, they simultaneously produce (1) a transcriptional regulator (R) and a biosynthetic enzyme (I) that synthesizes (2) the homoserine lactone (HSL). The HSL diffuses out of the bacterial cell (3). As the bacterial cell density increases to a critical point, the concentration of extracellular HSL will exceed that of the intracellular HSL, and the HSL will begin to accumulate in the bacterial cells (4) and bind to R. The HSL-R complex can bind to a genetic response element (5), thus activating transcription of critical bacterial genes (6). Panel A is reprinted with permission from M. R. Parsek and E. P. Greenberg, *Proc. Natl. Acad. Sci. USA* **97**:8789–8793, 2000.

ginate made by seaweed. Production of this alginate is not dependent on the quorum-sensing system, but it is likely that the two factors together are needed for establishing and maintaining lung infection in patients with cystic fibrosis, a process that can last for 20 to 30 years in some patients before their lungs are totally destroyed and they succumb to the infection. While it is possible that the small-molecular-weight quorum-sensing molecules may be targets for neutralization by the immune system, a more likely scenario for therapy involves the identification of drugs that inactivate these critical signaling systems.

Mechanisms of Secretion of Microbial Virulence Factors

For many pathogenic bacteria to infect a host effectively, they must neutralize the immune response, both innate and adaptive, long enough for infection to be established. One prominent mechanism for accomplishing this neutralization is the secretion of factors that render host cells incapable of initiating effective immune responses. A number of important gram-negative pathogens use a specific mechanism, referred to as type III secretion, to deliver proteins into host cells. The mechanism of type III secretion is conserved among organisms, but the various molecules they deliver can be quite different. One of the best-studied type III secretion systems is used by *Yersinia pestis*, the causative agent of bubonic plague, or Black Death. In the 13th and 14th centuries, this disease devastated European populations, with estimates as high as 33% of the population dying of this disease. The proteins for the *Y. pestis* type III secretion system are contained on a 70-kilobase (kb) bacterial plasmid, a self-replicating genetic element inside the bacterial cell that is independent of the chromosome. To prevent disease from *Y. pestis*, the host must make substantial amounts of IFN-γ and TNF-α. These are produced, in part, by the interaction of the bacterial LPS with the host's LPS-binding protein, CD14, and TLR4 (Fig. 18.16). To cause disease, *Y. pestis* must prevent the host from initiating this signaling pathway. Secretion of effector proteins to prevent the host from eliminating *Y. pestis* organisms is carried out by 29 proteins that form the Ysc channel, which allows bacterial factors to be secreted out of the bacterium. The bacterial effector proteins, referred to as Yops, and their secretion from the bacterial to the host cell cytosol is assisted by chaperones known as the Ysc proteins. The Ysc channel allows three additional bacterial proteins that form the translocator complex to produce a pore in the host cell's plasma membrane to deliver the Yop effectors. These effectors have a variety of activities, including phosphotyrosine phosphatase, inactivation of molecules that control the host cell's ability to move and properly adhere to other cells at the site of infection, and prevention of translocation of the transcription factor nuclear factor κB (NF-κB) to the nucleus. This latter event is needed for optimal secretion of IFN-γ and TNF-α. Some of the molecular factors involved in the pathogenesis of *Y. pestis* infection are shown in Fig. 18.17. A promising vaccine candidate for controlling plague includes the LcrV component of the translocators, which, as a purified protein vaccine, has protected mice against infection. An analogous approach for preventing infections due to *P. aeruginosa* has used this organism's homolog of LcrV, termed PcrV, as a successful vaccine in animal experiments.

Bioterrorism and Bacterial Pathogens

The anthrax outbreak that occurred in the United States in the fall of 2001 generated a strong interest in further understanding how the bacterial agents of bioterrorism cause disease and how the public can be protected. The U.S. Centers for Disease Control and Prevention (CDC) has categorized numerous bacterial pathogens into classes indicative of their potential threat (Table 18.4). As with all other diseases, understanding the virulence factors elaborated by these organisms and how they can be counteracted by the immune system will form the central core of the types of vaccines and immunotherapies that will be developed to lessen the threat of bioterrorism and biowarfare.

Four bacterial pathogens are listed as category A agents, along with smallpox and viral causes of hemorrhagic fevers. These four pathogens provide a nice overview of the immunologic effectors that mediate many of the molecular mechanisms of resistance to infection.

Anthrax

Anthrax, caused by the gram-positive sporulating bacillus *Bacillus anthracis*, causes disease by producing three major virulence factors: edema toxin, lethal toxin, and a capsular polysaccharide. Anthrax can be acquired or spread through the skin (cutaneous anthrax), the respiratory

Figure 18.16 Effects of *Yersinia* Yops proteins on inhibition of the inflammatory response needed to resist infection. Normally, proinflammatory factors such as bacterial LPS, bound to the LBP, interact with receptor CD14 and coreceptor from the Toll-like family. This leads to phosphorylation cascades (tyrosine kinases and mitogen-activated protein kinase kinase [MAPKK]), resulting in the activation of mitogen-activated protein kinases (MAPKs) and of the IκB kinase (IKK) kinase, which acts on the inhibitor of NF-κB (IκB). Phosphorylation of (IκB) is followed by its degradation, and NF-κB migrates to the nucleus and activates transcription of proinflammatory cytokines, including TNF-α. Two of the translocated Yop proteins, termed YopP (in *Y. enterocolitica*) or YopJ (in *Y. pestis*), prevent the activation of the two phosphorylation cascades and thus block the release of TNF-α. This Yop protein also induces macrophage apoptosis through the activities of the caspase (Casp) proteins. Reprinted with permission from G. R. Cornelis, *Proc. Natl. Acad. Sci. USA* **97:**8778–8783, 2000.

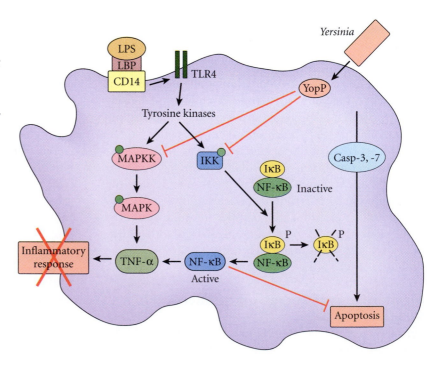

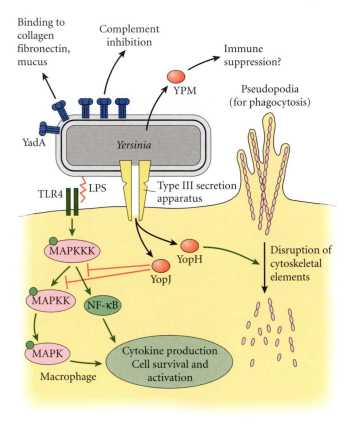

Figure 18.17 Some of the molecular factors involved in the pathogenesis of *Y. pestis* infection. The YadA homotrimeric protein anchored to the outer membrane of the bacterium serves as an adhesin, allowing the bacterium to bind to host molecules such as collagen, fibronectin, and mucus. YadA also inhibits complement activation by the classical pathway. *Yersinia* species secretes a superantigen called YPM (*Yersinia pseudotuberculosis*-derived mitogen) that may promote bacterial survival in the host by impairing immune function. The interaction of host macrophages with gram-negative bacteria usually results in activation of the macrophage when TLR4 on the macrophage surface binds bacterial LPS. TLR4 signaling proceeds via the MAPK pathway. *Yersinia* prevents macrophage activation through the YopJ protein, which is delivered into the macrophage cytoplasm by the bacterial type III secretion apparatus, and inhibits the MAPK pathway. The type III secretion apparatus is composed of Ysc and translocator proteins. YopH is another protein that is delivered into the macrophage cytoplasm by the type III secretion apparatus. YopH inhibits phagocytosis by disrupting cytoskeletal elements.

tract (inhalation anthrax), and the gastrointestinal tract (gastrointestinal anthrax). If untreated, all three forms are potentially fatal. Immunity to anthrax can be engendered by vaccination against a component common to both the edema and lethal toxins called *protective antigen*. Current injectable anthrax vaccines work primarily be eliciting antibody to protective antigen. The capsule is made up of poly-D-glutamic acid; as such, the D-glutamic acid polymer is not terribly immunogenic due to the inability of APCs to degrade the D form of the amino acid polymer chain.

Plague

The causative agent of plague, *Y. pestis*, causes three forms of disease in humans: bubonic plague, pneumonic plague, and septicemic plague. Bubonic plague is acquired from the bites of fleas that have fed on infected rats and is not spread from person to person. Septicemic plague occurs when the organism enters the blood, but this too is not transmissible. Pneumonic plague, however, occurs with lung infection and is a highly transmissible infection. Plague, as noted above, causes disease by a large number of mechanisms, with toxins secreted by the type III secretion system playing a prominent role. *Y. pestis* also produces a protein capsule. A plague vaccine consisting of inactivated bacteria was licensed in the United States in 1911, but its efficacy is uncertain. The protein capsule has been shown to be a highly efficacious vaccine in animals and likely will be developed as one component of a comprehensive

Table 18.4 Microorganisms classified according to their potential threat of bioterrorism and biowarfare[a]

Biological diseases and agents
Category A[b]
Anthrax (*Bacillus anthracis*)
Botulism (*Clostridium botulinum* toxin)
Plague (*Yersinia pestis*)
Smallpox (variola virus)
Tularemia (*Francisella tularensis*)
Viral hemorrhagic fevers (Ebola, Marburg, Lassa, and Crimean-Congo hemorrhagic fever viruses)
Category B[c]
Brucellosis (*Brucella* species)
Epsilon toxin of *Clostridium perfringens*
Glanders (*Burkholderia mallei*)
Q fever (*Coxiella burnetii*)
Ricin toxin from *Ricinus communis* (castor beans)
Staphylococcus enterotoxin B
Category C[d]
Hantaviruses
Multidrug-resistant tuberculosis
Nipah virus
Tick-borne encephalitis viruses
Tick-borne hemorrhagic fever viruses
Yellow fever

[a]Full information: http://www.bt.cdc.gov/Agent/Agentlist.asp.

[b]Category A diseases and agents are pathogens that are rarely seen in the United States and the economically developed countries. They pose a risk to national security, can be easily disseminated or transmitted from person to person, cause high mortality, have the potential for major public health impact, might cause public panic and social disruption, and require special action for public health preparedness.

[c]Category B diseases and agents are agents that are moderately easy to disseminate, cause moderate morbidity and low mortality, and require specific enhancements of diagnostic capacity and enhanced disease surveillance.

[d]Category C diseases and agents are agents include emerging pathogens that could be engineered for mass dissemination in the future because of availability, ease of production and dissemination, and potential for high morbidity and mortality and major health impact.

plague vaccine. LPS antigens are also candidates for inclusion in a plague vaccine. Antibodies to these antigens likely will promote opsonic killing of the bacteria.

Tularemia

Tularemia is another serious bacterial infection with bioterroist potential caused by an organism named *Francisella tularensis*. It is usually transmitted to people from infected animal carcasses or insect bites but can be spread in contaminated water or food or via inhalation from the air. Person-to-person transmission of *F. tularensis* does not appear to occur. Fortunately, this organism rarely makes its way into human populations, but its ability to survive under harsh conditions in the environment makes it a potential threat. It is difficult to get tularemia from ingestion, but inoculation into the skin or aerosol inhalation can readily cause infection in most humans with low doses of the microbe. Little research has been done on this organism to understand mechanisms of immunity to its virulence factors. It is a facultative intracellular pathogen, and cell-mediated immunity likely plays a critical role in immune resistance. Immunity depends on production of TNF-α and IFN-γ by either $CD4^+$ or $CD8^+$ cells. An experimental intradermal vaccine of live, attenuated organisms is available but not licensed, and its efficacy is not known.

Botulism

Botulism is caused by a very potent toxin secreted by the spore-forming, gram-positive, anaerobic bacterium called *C. botulinum* that is commonly found in soil. Botulinum toxin is one of the most potent toxins known. The most common cause of botulism is from contaminated food, where spores of this organism germinate in sealed food containers under anaerobic conditions and elaborate the toxin. Food-borne botulism is very serious, not only for the rapidity with which the toxin works and its potential to paralyze muscles needed for breathing, but also because additional cases can occur from individuals who eat similarly contaminated food. Infants are susceptible to botulism when spores from contaminated food, such as honey, germinate in their gastrointestinal tract. Wounds can also be infected by *C. botulinum* whose spores germinate in the wounded tissue and produce toxin. Immunity to botulism is clearly mediated by toxin-neutralizing antibodies, a supply of which is kept by the CDC for use with small numbers of cases. With proper supportive care, such as mechanical ventilation, people can recover from botulism, but this takes a long time and is expensive. Curiously, widespread use of a vaccine for botulism may meet resistance as minute

doses of the toxin, known as Botox, are being used as a treatment for cosmetic disorders. A vaccine could render this therapy ineffective.

Antigenic Targets Involved in Protective Immunity

Antigenic Targets of Immunity for Extracellular Pathogens

The most effective antigens for obtaining protective immunity due to antibody and complement activation are bacterial surface structures. Antibody and complement opsonins buried below the surface are generally not accessible to Fc and complement receptors on the surface of phagocytes and function poorly, if at all, in opsonization and protection. Thus, most humans have antibodies in their serum that react with common bacterial antigens such as peptidoglycan, teichoic acid, and conserved portions of LPS. Although these antibodies may play an important role in protecting otherwise healthy individuals from the occasional organism that gains access to their blood, they do not seem to offer adequate protection under circumstances where a more serious threat of infection exists. In these instances, antibodies to cell surface structures, particularly capsules and LPS O side chains, offer the best level of protective immunity.

Polysaccharide antigens make up the majority of bacterial capsules that are targets for protective immunity. For many years it was thought that binding of these oligosaccharide epitopes to antibody involved four to seven sugar moieties. Recently, it has become clear that conformational epitopes are produced by polysaccharides and these are recognized by protective antibodies. Since the repeating-unit oligosaccharide structure of some bacterial capsular polysaccharides mimics the oligosaccharide moieties of mammalian tissues, the ability of host antibodies to bond to a conformational epitope expressed only by polymeric forms of the polysaccharide may provide a mechanism by which the immune system recognizes a bacterial capsule as foreign. Many bacterial polysaccharides are immunogenic in animals and human subjects and are effective as vaccines or as components of vaccines. However, polysaccharide-protein conjugate vaccines have generally superior immunogenicity. The presence of conformational epitopes may provide an explanation for how a polysaccharide can be effective as a vaccine but not produce antibodies cross-reacting with host tissues.

To appreciate the importance of bacterial capsules and surface antigens in protective immunity, one needs only to look at the antibacterial vaccines that have been developed or are being developed. Successful capsular polysaccharide and polysaccharide-protein conjugate vaccines against pneumococcal pneumonia, spinal meningitis due to *N. meningitidis*, typhoid fever due to *Salmonella enterica* serovar Typhi, and invasive infection caused by *H. influenzae* are available. Other capsular polysaccharide vaccines under development include those to prevent infection of newborns with group B streptococci, infection with *P. aeruginosa* in patients with cystic fibrosis, peritonitis due to *Bacteroides fragilis* infection, and sepsis due to *E. coli* and *Klebsiella* species. The O polysaccharides of LPS are targets for protective immunity in infection due to enteric pathogens such as *E. coli* and *Shigella* species and against *Klebsiella* species and *P. aeruginosa* and may be important components of vaccines against *V. cholerae*, *B. pertussis*, and other gram-negative pathogens.

Antigenic Targets for Intracellular Bacterial Pathogens

What has been elusive in the field of cell-mediated immunity to intracellular bacterial pathogens has been finding specific antigenic targets that induce protective immunity. This may not be so critical for an intracellular pathogen. Any antigen, whether on the bacterial surface or within the bacterial cell, that initiates T-cell immunity can cause secretion of cytokines and activation of phagocytic cells. Also, cytotoxic T lymphocytes (CTLs) can destroy infected target cells. The CTLs appear to have antimicrobial factors, such as granulysin, that can directly kill bacteria. Other mechanisms of bacteriocidal action include generation of oxygen radicals and other toxic substances within activated macrophages and release of defensins and similar antibacterial polypeptide factors from granules. While activated phagocytes, particularly macrophages, are clearly better equipped to eliminate intracellular bacteria, we are just beginning to understand the genetic, molecular, and cellular factors that interact to provide protective immunity in this setting.

Protection against Bacterial Exotoxins

Toxic substances elaborated by bacteria are frequently a major cause of disease and are targets for humoral immunity when the bacterial cell itself does not need to be killed. In most of these situations, immunity is effected by the presence of neutralizing antibodies. These usually function by binding directly to the toxin and preventing it from attaching to its cellular receptor or inactivating the toxin's enzymatic activity. Among the first successful active and passive immunotherapies against bacterial disease was the successful treatment of diphtheria in the 1890s. This early work paved the way to the development of a wide variety of vaccines that neutralize bacterial toxins responsible for disease. Active immunization with toxoids of diphtheria and tetanus has markedly decreased the incidence of these diseases, particularly in the developed countries. Passive immunotherapy with specific antibodies to toxins responsible for toxin-based bacterial diseases has been successful in treating anthrax, diphtheria, tetanus, and botulism. Vaccines against organisms whose virulence is mediated only partially by toxin have not been completely effective, even when antibodies to toxins are present, because of the presence of additional bacterial factors that contribute to the disease process. Therefore, vaccines with only partial efficacy include those against *V. cholerae* and *E. coli* enterotoxins, *P. aeruginosa* exotoxin A, and *B. pertussis* toxin, although fairly good success with a vaccine composed of a toxoid of the latter preparation has been reported in some countries.

Summary

There are many molecular mechanisms whereby bacterial pathogens cause disease in humans and other animals. Some bacteria, such as *C. diphtheriae*, secrete a toxic protein that poisons mammalian cells. Other bacteria, such as *N. meningitidis* and *H. influenzae*, cause disease simply because they are able to access and grow in a certain tissue of their host where toxic and other destructive effects from bacterial metabolism damage tissues and organs. Last, in some of the latter cases, it is not the growth of the microorganism per se that causes disease, but the activation of the host's own immune effector mechanisms that damages innocent bystander host tissues.

The molecular mechanisms employed by bacterial pathogens to colonize, invade, infect, and disrupt the host are both numerous and diverse. Each phase of the infectious process involves the interaction of a variety of bacterial and host factors in a manner that can lead either to resolution or to disease. Recent recognition of the coordinate genetic regulation of the elaboration of bacterial virulence factors when organisms go from the environment to the mammalian host emphasizes the complex nature of the host-parasite interaction. Fortunately, many diverse factors must come into play to allow the pathogen to succeed in causing disease, and thus a large number of potential therapeutic approaches for interrupting this process can be investigated and developed to provide effective strategies for preventing and treating bacterial infections.

The immune effector mechanisms that are needed to combat bacterial infection successfully vary, depending on the location of the bacterium within the host, the structural properties of the bacterial cell, and the mechanisms by which the bacterium causes disease. Extracellular bacteria can usually be killed solely by the action of antibodies and complement proteins, while these same immune effectors are ineffective against bacteria that reside within cells of the host. Many gram-negative bacteria can be directly lysed by the action of complement proteins, while the outer, thick cell wall of gram-positive organisms protects them from the lytic action of complement; gram-positive bacteria must therefore be killed by opsonophagocytic mechanisms. Bacteria that cause disease by proliferating in the tissues of their host must be killed to prevent or reverse disease. In contrast, disease caused by toxin-producing bacteria can sometimes be prevented simply by antibody-mediated neutralization of the toxin. All of these are important considerations that affect the ongoing development of antibacterial treatments and vaccines.

Suggested Reading

Bassler, B. L. 2002. Small talk. Cell-to-cell communication in bacteria. *Cell* 109:421–424.

Beeching N. J., D. A. Dance, A. R. Miller, and R. C. Spencer. 2002. Biological warfare and bioterrorism. *Br. Med. J.* 324: 336–339.

Beutler, B. 2002. Toll-like receptors: how they work and what they do. *Curr. Opin. Hematol.* 9:2–10.

Bhatnagar, R., and S. Batra. 2001. Anthrax toxin. *Crit. Rev. Microbiol.* 27:167–200.

Casadevall, A. 2002. Passive antibody administration (immediate immunity) as a specific defense against biological weapons. *Emerg. Infect. Dis.* 8:833–841.

Cornelis, G. R. 2000. Molecular and cell biology aspects of plague. *Proc. Natl. Acad. Sci. USA* 97:8778–8783.

Dehio, C., S. D. Gray-Owen, and T. F. Meyer. 2000. Host cell invasion by pathogenic Neisseriae. *Subcell. Biochem.* 33:61–96.

Galan, J. E. 2001. Salmonella interactions with host cells: type III secretion at work. *Annu. Rev. Cell Dev. Biol.* 17:53–86.

Green, D. W. 2002. The bacterial cell wall as a source of antibacterial targets. *Expert Opin. Ther. Targets* 6:1–19.

Hunter, C. A., and S. L. Reiner. 2000. Cytokines and T cells in host defense. *Curr. Opin. Immunol.* 12:413–418.

Lyczak, J. B., C. L. Cannon, and G. B. Pier. 2002. Lung infections associated with cystic fibrosis. *Clin. Microbiol. Rev.* 15:194–222.

Wilson J. W., M. J. Schurr, C. L. LeBlanc, R. Ramamurthy, K. L. Buchanan, and C. A. Nickerson. 2002. Mechanisms of bacterial pathogenicity. *Postgrad. Med. J.* 78:216–224.

Immunity to Viruses

Edward Barker

Viruses and Disease

Viruses are noncellular, submicroscopic entities whose genomes consist of one of two types of nucleic acids (RNA or DNA) and that replicate inside living cells. Using the synthetic machinery of the host cell, viruses create specialized elements called *capsids* that allow their genome to be transferred to other cells efficiently. Unlike other intracellular organisms, viruses are completely dependent on the cellular metabolism of the host for reproduction, since they are not metabolically self-sufficient. Therefore, they are classified as *obligate intracellular parasites*. This obliges the virus to utilize the host cell efficiently and to possess replicative mechanisms that result in viral survival and propagation. Some viruses survive and propagate for months to years mainly within an individual host whereas others have short survival times in an individual and propagate by moving rapidly from an infected to a naive or nonimmune host. Animal and human hosts must be able to scrutinize their tissues closely for viral infections and be able to respond rapidly using both innate and acquired immune systems. Otherwise, they are at risk for virus-induced cellular and tissue destruction, loss of normal tissue function, and development of disease due to the viral infection. Numerous viral diseases of humans are known; Table 19.1 lists a few viral infections associated with human disease.

Many of the signs (measurable responses such as temperature) and symptoms (being able to report how one feels during an illness and thus limited to humans beyond infancy) of viral infections are well known due to the ubiquity of viruses in our environment and the common occurrence of viral infections throughout life. Viral infections of the respiratory tract account for almost one-half of all acute illnesses. Children have more than six of these infections in their first year of life on average, whereas adults usually have three to four per year. Acute viral respiratory infections produce signs such as fever (actually unusual during the common

453

Table 19.1 Some common diseases caused by viruses in humans

Virus family	Virus	Diseases
Herpesviridae	Herpes simplex virus type 1	Cold sores
	Epstein-Barr virus	Infectious mononucleosis, Burkitt's lymphoma
	Varicella-zoster virus	Chicken pox, shingles
Poxviridae	Variola virus	Smallpox
Hepadnaviridae	Hepatitis B virus	Hepatitis
Papovaviridae	Papillomavirus	Warts
Orthomyxoviridae	Influenza virus	Respiratory diseases
Togaviridae	Rubivirus	Rubella
Paramyxoviridae	Mumps virus	Mumps
	Morbillivirus	Measles
	Respiratory syncytial virus	Respiratory diseases
Rhabdoviridae	Lyssavirus	Rabies
Retroviridae	HIV	AIDS
Coronaviridae	SARS virus	SARS

cold but more common with other viral respiratory infections such as influenza), increased secretion of fluids (rhinorrhea), sneezing, and coughing. Symptoms include sore throats, often the first thing noticed as a cold develops, malaise, and headache. Viruses are also common causes of gastrointestinal illness, and in less developed countries, this type of infection is a significant cause of mortality in infants and young children. In infants, the major cause of viral gastroenteritis is rotavirus infections, which manifest from mild diarrhea in most cases to severe dehydration, which can be fatal. In adults, most of the viral gastroenteritis is due to Norwalk and related viruses, and is usually characterized by the abrupt onset of nausea, cramps, vomiting, and diarrhea. This usually resolves in 24 to 48 hours.

Tissue Tropism and Viral Infections

Most of us have firsthand experience with viral infections and know that many of these infections lead to diseases in specific organs and tissues. We expect the cold and flu viruses to cause signs and symptoms of disease in the respiratory tract; the pox viruses to cause lesions on the skin; the herpesviruses to cause lesions on oral and genital mucosal tissues; and the rabies virus to replicate within and disrupt the normal function of the central nervous system. Viruses that principally affect specific tissues have a propensity or tropism to grow in cells that are primarily found in their target tissues. This property not only accounts for the close association of disease manifestations with site of viral replication but also for the highly restricted species specificity that many viruses have. Measles and smallpox viruses only infect humans, poliovirus

higher primates. But influenza virus can infect a broad range of mammalian and avian species. Immune effectors that prevent or resolve viral infections must interfere with the virus's getting to its target tissues to replicate or must eventually stop it from growing in the target tissue in order to recover from the infection.

Some viruses move from their site of entry in the body where they may undergo limited replication to the target tissue by migrating via the blood, lymphatics, or even inside phagocytic cells. Measles virus initially replicates in the epithelial cells of the respiratory tract, then spreads through the blood to the cells of the reticuloendothelial system where the leukocytes can become infected. Multiple body systems, including the skin and respiratory tract, become sites of viral growth and tissue damage. Immune reactions to the virus growing in the endothelial cells lining the blood vessels in the skin produce the rash characteristic of measles, whereas virus growing in the respiratory tract produces cough and coryza (inflammation of the nose and throat). In a scenario such as this there are multiple means for the immune system to prevent measles infection: inhibition of the initial growth in the respiratory tract, inhibition of viral spread through the blood, and inhibition of viral growth at systemic sites.

No simple means exists for classifying viruses according to the human diseases they produce, since several different virus types can cause the same clinical disease. For example, hepatitis can be caused by infection of liver cells by the yellow fever virus, which uses RNA to encode its genetic information, or by hepatitis B virus, which uses DNA to encode its genetic information. A variety of viruses cause infections of the central nervous system leading to paralysis or death in humans, such as encephalitis viruses, poliovirus, and rabies virus.

The Course of Viral Infections and Development of Disease

The use of the diagnostic methods to determine the presence of a specific virus in a diseased animal or human and the monitoring of clinical signs and symptoms that occur during the infection have made it possible to describe the course of many virally caused diseases. Generally, three approaches are taken to diagnose viral infections: (i) isolation of virus in culture from specimens obtained from the infected host, followed by laboratory identification of the virus; (ii) direct identification of viral components from cells of the infected tissues or fluid specimens of the host, usually by detection of viral antigens; and (iii) demonstration in the infected host of a significant increase in serum antibodies to a virus or its components during the course of illness. Polymerase chain reaction methods using virus-specific primer sequences have recently been used to directly detect viruses in clinical specimens. This has been useful for delineating the level of human immunodeficiency virus (HIV) infection in patients with acquired immunodeficiency syndrome (AIDS).

Most viral infections are acute in nature, in that they cause a sudden onset of signs and symptoms of short duration (less than 1 month). However, a few viruses are able to cause a latent infection where the virus genetic information remains inside a host cell's nucleus and only produces symptoms long after the initial infection has cleared. For example, chicken pox is caused by varicella-zoster virus, which can be recovered many years later from "shingles" lesions; this is possible because the varicella-zoster virus remains dormant in the ganglia of some individuals who have recovered from chicken pox. The virus is thought to be held in check by the immune system of its host during this latency period but begins to replicate when the host is later exposed to a variety of physical or pharmacologic insults that cause immunosuppression.

Humans have been also been found to harbor viruses without developing signs, symptoms, or disease. Epstein-Barr virus, the causative agent of infectious mononucleosis (acute infection) and Burkitt's lymphoma (a type of B-cell cancer), is often carried asymptomatically. In such cases, antibodies to Epstein-Barr virus can be found in the sera of infected individuals despite their lack of symptoms. In other examples, the infected host can transmit the virus to uninfected individuals, even in the absence of virus-like illness or symptoms. An example of this is seen in individuals with asymptomatic chronic hepatitis B or HIV infections.

Slow viruses are another type of virus that can lead to illness only several years after the initial infection. Many neurologic diseases are a consequence of slow-virus infections. The pathogenesis of the infection follows the integration of the DNA of the slow virus into the host cells and the production of virus surface antigens. Immunologic responses to these antigens then cause destruction of the tissue, leading to disease symptoms; note that, in this case, the host's immune response to the viral infection, not the infection per se, is the cause of disease. Thus, for viral diseases it is critical to appreciate when the immune response of the host is important for the resolution of infection or the exacerbation of infection.

Emergence of New Viral Diseases

Over the past few decades it has become abundantly clear that the high and rapid replication rate of viruses frequently leads to new viral strains with high virulence for humans and animals of economic importance. The most obvious example is HIV, which probably first infected humans in the 1950s but emerged in the 1980s to become a major pathogen. By the early 21st century HIV infection and AIDS became one of the most common causes of death due to an infectious agent. The influenza pandemic in 1918 and 1919 killed tens of millions of people, including many young adults, yet we still do not understand why this variant of the influenza virus was so virulent. Uncommon viruses such as Ebola virus can emerge as serious human pathogens when there is increased contact between humans and animal reservoirs, with subsequent spread to other humans. Modern transportation facilitates viral spread into new places as exemplified by the emergence of infection with West Nile virus in the United States, which probably entered the country in infected mosquitoes carried on an airline flight from the Middle East where the virus was endemic. Within only 3 to 4 years, this virus spread from its initial focus in the northeastern United States to the entire country. In the spring of 2003 a new form of a coronavirus, previously mostly known as a cause of the common cold in humans, but more severe infections in animals, emerged in the eastern People's Republic of China, causing severe acute respiratory syndrome (SARS). The virus likely infected humans from a reservoir in wild animals such as palm civets that are eaten as a delicacy in some parts of China. Airline travel allowed this infection to spread to other cities, notably Toronto, Canada. Although initial responses to identify and control the disease in its earliest phases were slow, a subsequent rapid worldwide response contained the disease within a few months. However, the possibility of reemergence in the future, particularly in winter, when coronavirus infections are more common, remains a major threat. Overall, the ability of viruses to infect virtually any type of cell, from bacterial to human, their rapid generation times, large number of particles produced, and often high mutation rates make them the preeminent pathogen able to generate new variants, and thus new infectious diseases, in very short periods.

Innate Immunity and Viral Infections

Mechanistically the innate immune system plays a key role in resistance to viral infections. Many people feel a "cold coming on" but then do not get much more symptomatic. This likely reflects, in part, the activation of innate immune effectors, although antibody could also contribute to this state. Viral replication rapidly stimulates innate immunity (see chapter 2). *Interferons* were discovered as antiviral factors, and when type I interferons bind to receptors on cells they initiate a cascade of events that makes the cell stop synthesizing proteins, thus preventing further production of viral proteins (see Fig. 2.10). Interferons also stimulate production of Toll-like receptor 3, which then responds to double-stranded RNA, the genetic material of many important pathogenic viruses, allowing infected cells to produce inflammatory signals that initiate host immunity. Natural killer (NK) cells can recognize virally infected cells and kill them via cytotoxicity, interrupting production of new viruses. Complement proteins can disrupt the membranes of some viruses that exit from the cells they infect by "budding" from the host cell membrane, thereby coating themselves with a piece of the membrane. Such enveloped viruses can be lysed by the membrane attack complex of the complement system (see Fig. 5.4). Some viruses can be coated by complement opsonins for destruction by phagocytes. Obviously, many components of the innate immune system are essential for protecting animals and humans from viral pathogens.

Interferon

Interferons exist in two forms (type I and type II), which are unrelated biochemically and use different receptors, although they both have antiviral effects (Fig. 19.1). The

Figure 19.1 Interferon can control viral infections by binding to receptors on cells infected with the virus or on neighboring uninfected cells and prevent further spread of the virus. The binding of interferon to its receptor inhibits synthesis of viral protein by induction of DAI (double-stranded RNA-activated inhibitor of translation; also called RNA-dependent protein kinase, or PKR). Upon interaction with its receptors, interferon can increase the expression of MHC class I molecules, which enhances the destruction of infected cells by CTLs and prevents uninfected cells from being killed by NK cells. Upon interaction with specific receptors on NK cells, interferon can increase their capacity to kill virus-infected cells that have decreased MHC class I molecules on their surface and/or are coated with antiviral antibodies.

type I interferons (IFN) exist as three classes, α, β, and κ. IFN-α consists of 15 subtypes, with an 85% homology in the genes for the different subtypes. IFN-β is a product of a single gene expressed in many cell types after viral infection. IFN-κ is expressed only by keratinocytes. The type II interferon, IFN-γ, is produced only by activated lymphocytes during immune responses.

IFN-γ binds to specific receptors on cells and activates a *Janus family* of tyrosine kinases, which in turn can phosphorylate signaling proteins known as the *signal transducers and activators of transcription* (STAT). The binding of phosphorylated STAT, in addition to other transcription factors, to the promoter of several genes induces the synthesis of antiviral proteins such as 2′,5′-adenylate synthetase, which can be activated by double-stranded RNA, present during some viral infections. In addition, ribonucleases that cleave RNA and decrease synthesis of viral protein are activated. Binding of interferon to its receptor on uninfected cells can induce a small family of the host cell's guanosine triphosphatases (GTPases) called Mx; these GTPases have potent antiviral activity. The introduction of genes encoding for Mx proteins into cells normally susceptible to a virus can make them resistant to infection. Mx proteins inhibit viral replication by two mechanisms. First, cytoplasmic Mx protein can prevent the transport of viral ribonucleoproteins into the nucleus of the host cell, preventing assembly of the nucleocapsid. Second, nuclear Mx protein directly inhibits viral polymerase activity.

A somewhat different approach to inhibiting viral replication is taken by type I interferons, which induce production by host cells of a protein called DAI (double-stranded RNA-activated inhibitor of translation; also called RNA-dependent protein kinase). DAI is a kinase that, when activated by binding to double-stranded RNA, phosphorylates eIF-2, locking it in an inactive state (see Fig. 2.6). Thus, interferon prevents the synthesis of new viruses by inhibiting *all* protein synthesis in the host cell.

Interferons also can act against viruses by increasing the expression of major histocompatibility complex (MHC) class I molecules on the cell surface. This increases the likelihood of an infected cell being recognized and killed by cytotoxic T lymphocytes (CTLs). In addition, interferon increases the expression of TAP transporter proteins and the LMP-2 and LMP-7 components of proteasomes. Both are involved in processing antigen for MHC class I presentation to CD8[+] T cells. In an indirect way, interferon may also increase killing of virus-infected cells by NK cells, since NK cells are nonspecifically activated following exposure to interferons.

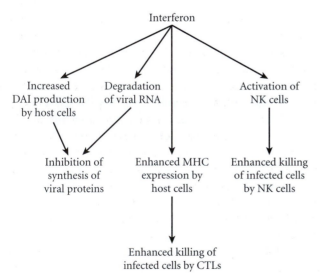

NK cells

The control of virus early in infection is dependent on NK cells, since this cell population is present before conventional, primary T-cell responses develop (primary acquired responses by B cells and T cells usually require about 2 weeks to begin). A clear example of the role of NK cells in controlling viral infection is during herpesvirus infections. Removal of NK cells in animals infected with this virus has been shown to result in an increase in replication of the virus. The NK cells mediate control of viruses in two ways: (i) by inducing apoptosis of the infected cells following the release by NK cells of cytoplasmic granules containing perforin and granzymes or through increased expression of FasL, which triggers Fas on the infected cells; and (ii) by producing and releasing interferons (Fig. 19.2). It is notable that the first of these two mechanisms is virtually identical to the killing mechanisms of CTLs. However, unlike CTLs, NK cells do not recognize specific viral antigens. Rather, NK cells recognize their targets by the *two-receptor model*. The two-receptor model states that NK cells initially recognize their target cells by binding ubiquitous carbohydrates on the target cell surface but are prevented from killing healthy, uninfected cells because of the ability of the NK cell's *killer inhibitory receptors* to recognize the MHC class I molecules on the target cell surface and to trigger a negative signal (see Fig. 16.6). This process is an effective means of controlling viral infection because some viruses decrease the expression of MHC class I

Figure 19.2 NK cells can control viral infections in several ways. (i) MHC class I molecules on the surface of the infected cells are downmodulated by the virus to evade killing by CTLs. This reduction in the expression of MHC class I triggers the NK cells to kill the infected cells though their ability to induce apoptosis. (ii) NK cells, through their Fc receptors, recognize the infected cells coated with antiviral antibodies and destroy them via perforin/granzymes or Fas-Fas-L interactions through the mechanism of ADCC. (iii) NK cells produce increased amounts of IFN-γ following exposure to IL-12 (produced by antigen-presenting cells during antiviral immune responses). IFN-γ can then bind to receptors and control or prevent the production of virus.

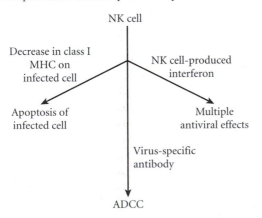

molecules in order to evade CTL responses. In doing so, however, the virus-infected cell becomes a viable target for NK-cell killing. Infected cells bound by antiviral antibodies can be killed by NK cells by another mechanism known as *antibody-dependent cell-mediated cytotoxicity* (ADCC) (see Fig. 16.2). NK cells destroy virus-infected cells coated with antiviral antibodies when the antibody bound to the cell surface of the infected cell interacts with Fc receptors on the NK cells. NK cells expressing the Fc receptor Fc-γRIII (CD16) recognize the immunoglobulin G1 (IgG1) and IgG3 subclasses of antiviral antibodies in humans. The interaction of antibody with the Fc receptor triggers the NK cells to become cytotoxic.

Viruses and Acquired Immunity

Because viruses are fairly simple biologic entities, possessing both small size and small genomes, their capacity to cause infection and disease is more limited than that of biologically more complex pathogens such as bacteria and protozoan parasites. In many cases, host resistance to viral infection is fairly well understood, and our comprehension of these immune mechanisms has been exploited to produce a number of successful vaccines. Antibody to antigens on the viral surface is sufficient to prevent infection by viruses that cause smallpox, polio, measles, mumps, rubella, chicken pox, hepatitis A and B, and influenza, to name some for which successful vaccines have been made. These viruses are highly infectious, meaning they can propagate rapidly by spreading to nonimmune hosts. However, the simple genetic composition of a virus can also permit changes in surface antigens and avoidance of host antibody responses due to rapid changes in the viral genome. HIV is now the preeminent example of this type of virus. Although biologically and genetically simple by comparison to other organisms, viruses nonetheless have potent means to evade the immune response, indicating that their genetic constitution is sufficient for them to be adept at confounding and frustrating both innate and acquired immunity.

Cell-mediated immunity also can be a critical component of immunity to viral infections, but this effector arm appears to be more important for resolution of viral infections. Thus, in an infected individual development of CTLs recognizing viral peptides on MHC class I of infected cells augments the inhibition of viral growth and spread, thus limiting further infection and halting disease progression. Delayed-type hypersensitivity reactions appear important for immunity to herpes simplex virus, poxviruses, and possibly HIV. As in many settings both cell-mediated immunity and antibody work together to prevent and resolve viral infections, a process likely highly beneficial to a mammalian host as it provides multiple means to combat viral infections.

Antibody-Mediated Antiviral Responses

The biologic function of antibodies directed to viral antigens is to bind to the viral particles and their products to facilitate their removal from the body. Moreover, cells that are infected by the virus can be destroyed by antibodies either through the use of complement or by the induction of ADCC (Fig. 19.3). The antiviral antibodies directed to antigens on the viral surface, referred to as envelope or capsid antigens, are the most effective in controlling and clearing viral infections, although antibodies to other viral components, such as enzymes involved in replication or proteins found in the core of the virus particle, also are present in the host and may be beneficial. The viral antigens that elicit antibody responses are usually proteins; however, occasionally antibodies are produced to carbohydrates that are attached to viral glycoproteins. The fact that most epitopes on viral antigens are found on proteins means that a virus

can escape binding by antibody present in an infected host through mutation of the viral gene that encodes the antigen. The most dramatic illustration of this tactic is provided by the influenza virus, which is capable of repeatedly infecting the same host in spite of vigorous immune responses to the virus. Such repeated infection can take place because the two most immunodominant antigens of the virus, hemagglutinin (HA) and neuraminidase (NA), are highly variable due to the high mutation rate of the genes that encode them. Similarly, HIV is able to evade its host's antibody responses by rapid changes to the gene that encodes the gp160 protein, which is made up of two components, the gp41 membrane protein and the immunodominant gp120 surface glycoprotein.

Protection of the host from systemic viral infection usually involves antiviral antibodies of the IgG and IgM classes. Since IgM is the first isotype of antibody made in response to an antigen, the appearance of IgM antiviral antibodies is generally indicative of a new or recent viral infection. IgA antibodies also may play a role in antiviral immunity, since they are typically found in secretions of

Figure 19.3 Antibody-dependent control of viruses. Antibodies directed to viral epitopes can control HIV infection in several ways. (**A**) The antibodies (blue) can prevent a viral ligand (green) from binding to the host-cell receptor (red) and entering the host cell. (**B**) If a virus succeeds in infecting a cell, the antibody (blue) can recognize viral antigens (green) on the membrane of the infected cell. This can lead to lysis of the infected cell through the activation of complement (red) (**1**) or by ADCC (**2**) by activating NK cells expressing Fc receptors (purple), which in turn can induce the infected cell to undergo programmed cell death (apoptosis).

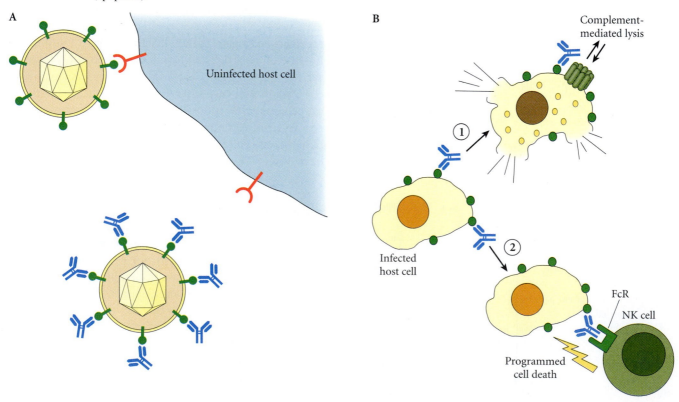

the mucosal surfaces, which represent a common point of entry into the host of many viral pathogens. Although it is possible to protect a mucosal surface from viral infection by having local IgA present, antibodies of the IgG and IgM isotypes are also detected in fluids lining the epithelial surfaces and doubtless play a role in the protection of these sites. Indeed, correlates of protection against infections of mucosal and epithelial surfaces such as those caused by influenza virus and poliovirus are with levels of serum IgG and not local IgA. These findings suggest that although IgG is present at quantitatively lower amounts in mucosal fluids when compared with IgA, the IgG may be the more important effector of immunity.

The entry of viruses into host cells is initiated by binding of protein *ligands* on the virus to *receptors* on the surface of the host cell. Binding of antibody to viral ligands can prevent this crucial molecular interaction from occurring and prevent the virus from entering the host cell. This ability of antibodies is known as *neutralization* (Fig. 19.3). Another mechanism of neutralization is interference with the fusion of the viral outer envelope with the cell membrane of the host, an event that has to occur for the virus to enter the cell. Neutralization of virus particles following extracellular binding of antibody may not occur until the viral-antibody complex is inside the host cell. Here the antibody prevents the release of the viral nucleic acid without which the virus cannot replicate.

Complement can assist antibodies in neutralizing virus by coating them, thus magnifying the neutralizing effect of antibodies. Complement also can lyse enveloped viruses or virus-infected cells that express viral antigens (Fig. 19.3). The former may be of special importance, in that enveloped virions are unable to fix the damage to their membrane because they lack the necessary repair machinery. Complement on a viral surface can be activated through either the classical pathway or the alternative pathway.

In some instances, antiviral antibodies may not be beneficial to the host. For example, antibodies can strip viral antigens from the surface of the infected cell, making the cell invisible to the cellular immune responses. Antibodies may block the interaction of CTLs with the antigen or increase the rate of infection of cells expressing antibody (Fc) or complement receptors. Moreover, antibody may help transfer virus from cells bearing Fc or complement receptors to permissive cells interacting with them.

Cellular Antiviral Immune Responses

Antiviral cellular immune responses are required to inhibit the further spread of virus in the infected cells and are essential for clearing the host of virus once infection has been established.

CTLs

The first clear evidence that T cells can recognize viruses came in 1974, when it was found that CTLs from a virus-infected animal could kill cultured cells infected with the same virus but not cultured cells infected with an unrelated virus. Once a CTL has recognized a viral peptide bound to an MHC molecule on the surface of the target cell, its function is the destruction of that infected cell before the latter releases new virus particles. This response must be precise enough to spare uninfected cells adjacent to the infected cells, thus inflicting minimal tissue damage while eradicating the infected cells. Both $CD8^+$ and $CD4^+$ CTLs can kill infected cells that express viral antigens in the context of MHC class I and class II molecules, respectively.

CTLs kill their target cells by one of two pathways. One mechanism is the release by the CTL of pore-forming proteins at the site of the CTL–target-cell interface. The pore-forming peptides, when aggregated, form a transmembrane channel on the surface of the infected cell, allowing CTL proteases called *granzymes* to enter the infected cell. These granzymes cleave proteins in the infected cells, thus inducing the cells to undergo apoptosis (see Fig. 16.21). Another mechanism by which CTLs induce cell death is through the interaction of membrane-bound Fas ligand (FasL) to its receptor, Fas, that is located on the surface of the target cell (see Fig. 16.22). Expression of FasL on CTLs is enhanced following activation and upon degranulation. This interaction of FasL on CTLs with the Fas receptor leads to apoptosis of the infected cell.

Antiviral CTL responses generally occur in four phases (Fig. 19.4): an induction phase, an activation-induced cell-death phase, a silencing phase, and a memory phase. During the induction phase, $CD8^+$ precursor CTLs proliferate and differentiate, with a substantial increase in the number of $CD8^+$ cells, usually leading to an inversion of the CD4 to CD8 ratio from 2:1 to 1:2. This increase in $CD8^+$ cells occurs soon after infection because viruses replicate in cells and present viral antigens through MHC class I molecules, thereby stimulating a strong antiviral immune response. The differentiated CTLs are then able to carry out cytotoxic activity against targets cells. Although the response is virus specific, T cells with a low affinity for viral antigen and for cross-reactive antigens also are induced during this induction phase.

The next phase in CTL response during viral infection is activation-induced cell death (AICD). During this phase, CTLs that have been activated by viral antigens are induced to undergo apoptosis. The mechanism underlying this pathway may involve Fas-FasL interaction on the CTL surface. The silencing phase in the CTL response involves a loss of AICD but the continuation of apoptosis in

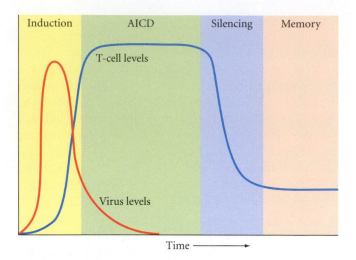

Figure 19.4 Stages of the response of CTLs to viruses. During an acute viral infection, the antiviral CTL response generally occurs in four phases: an induction phase, an AICD phase, a silencing phase, and a memory phase. During the induction phase, CTL precursors that can recognize specific antigens expressed by the virus develop into effector cells that replicate and are capable of responding to infected cells expressing the viral antigens and of destroying them. This leads to a decline in virus levels in the host. This stage is followed by the AICD stage, in which the CTL responding to another encounter with the viral antigen is programmed to die. This stage is marked by a plateau in the number of CTLs. The silencing phase is marked by a decrease in the number of CTLs. Despite this loss of a large number of virus-specific CTLs, some of these cells not only remain viable but also continue to be stable in the final phase of CTL responses, the memory phase. These memory cells are in a resting state but still have the ability to recognize specific viral antigens and to become reactivated when the host encounters the virus again.

virus-specific CTLs. The purpose of the AICD and silencing phases is to bring an end to the immune response once the antigen has been cleared and to return the host's immune system to its normal state. Despite this loss of a large number of virus-specific CTLs, some of these cells remain not only viable but also stable in the final phase of CTL responses, the memory phase. These memory cells, although mostly dormant, still have the ability to recognize specific viral antigens, proliferate, and lyse infected cells upon reencounter with the same viral antigen.

Antiviral cytokines produced by CD8+ cells

CD8+ cells also may eliminate infected cells through an increase in the production of cytokines, such as tumor necrosis factor beta (TNF-β), which can bind to receptors on the infected target cells and eliminate the virus by inducing programmed cell death of the infected cell. The mechanism by which programmed cell death is initiated by the TNF receptor is similar to that initiated by the Fas protein upon its binding to Fas-L. In addition, production of IFN-γ is enhanced after triggering the T-cell receptor

(TCR)-CD3 complex and can directly inhibit virus replication, increase MHC expression on the target cell surface, and activate other antiviral effector cells (see below).

CD8+ cells from individuals infected with HIV can control the replication of the virus in infected cells by a noncytotoxic mechanism that is independent of any known cytokine and may involve an uncharacterized factor known as the CD8+ cell antiviral factor. Unlike the anti-HIV CTL responses, this CD8+ cell anti-HIV function is not restricted by MHC molecules expressed on the infected cells. The cell antiviral factor is able to control HIV replication by terminating transcription of viral RNA. Loss of this antiviral activity in the CD8+ cells of HIV-infected individuals correlates with a change from an asymptomatic state to the development of AIDS.

Structural Properties of the Virus

The Capsid

The structural organization of the virus includes a capsid that encloses the genetic material. The genetic material and the capsid together are known as the *nucleocapsid* (Fig. 19.5). The role of the capsid is to protect the genetic material of the virus from host-derived nucleases. Capsids are made up of protein subunits assembled into simple geometric shapes and are typically helical, isometric, or cone shaped, with the exception of the capsid of poxviruses, which has a more complex structure (Fig. 19.6). Under the electron microscope, the helical capsid structure appears as a rod that has a hexagonal or rounded contour and contains a central channel. The proteins of the helical capsid assemble in a repeating manner, producing a helix in which the nucleic acid is coiled. The isometric capsid structure appears to be a regular icosahedron (i.e., a 20-sided polyhedron) surrounding the viral nucleic acid.

The Envelope

In some viruses, the capsid may be surrounded by a phospholipid bilayer acquired from the host cell as the virus buds from the cell (Fig. 19.5 and 19.6). The acquisition of an envelope provides protection against proteases and allows the virus to leave the host cell without damaging the cell. The virus envelope can be derived from either the cytoplasmic or nuclear membrane of the host cell. For example, herpesviruses replicate in the nucleus, where the viral nucleocapsid is made and assembled. When this virus buds from the cell, it acquires its envelope from the nuclear membrane. In some instances, host-cell proteins are present on the surface of the viral envelope. These host proteins can make the virus "appear" to be self in origin and

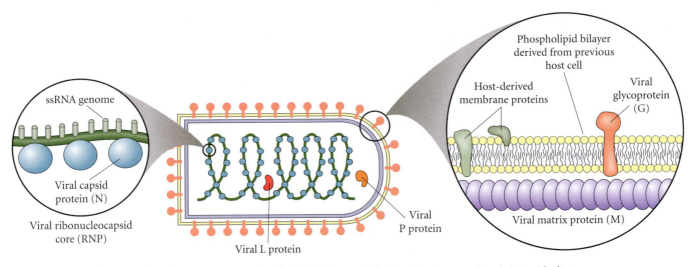

Figure 19.5 Schematic cross-section of a rhabdovirus particle. The virus is an enveloped virus with glyco-proteins and matrix proteins embedded in the lipid bilayer. The viral capsid protein, together with the nega-tive-sense single-stranded (ss) RNA, makes up the ribonucleocapsid core, which forms a helix structure. L and P are viral proteins that, when complexed together, form functional enzymes necessary for viral replication.

can therefore be very important for viral evasion of its host's immune response. During assembly of the virus, the capsid proteins interact with the cell membrane of the host through the use of viral matrix proteins embedded in the membrane. Other viral proteins embedded in the viral envelope can act as ligands for receptors on the surface of the host cell and can later mediate infection of new host cells.

Viral Nucleic Acid

The genetic information of a virus comes in a variety of forms of either RNA or DNA (Fig. 19.7). These forms include single-stranded or double-stranded RNA chains. The single-stranded RNA either can encode protein (*positive* or *sense* strand) or not (*negative* or *antisense* strand). If the viral genome is antisense, a complementary (sense) strand must be made before viral proteins can be synthesized. RNA can exist in the virus as monocistronic segments or polycistronic strands. For RNA viruses to replicate, they must carry a gene encoding an RNA-dependent RNA polymerase, since mammalian cells do not produce an enzyme with this activity. Negative-stranded RNA virions must carry the RNA polymerase into the cell so that they can begin to propagate upon entry into the cell.

Although chromosomal DNA is double stranded in almost all living organisms, DNA from some viruses is single stranded, existing in either a linear or circular form (Fig. 19.7). In viruses with double-stranded DNA, the DNA can take the form of a circular molecule, a linear complex, or a linear complex with the ends covalently linked or can consist of a linear DNA strand containing proteins bound to the free ends of the viral DNA (Fig. 19.7).

Viral DNA synthesis begins at the *origin of replication* on the viral template, where special initiator proteins must bind and attract the DNA replication enzymes of the host cell. Since DNA-dependent DNA polymerase requires a primer, replication of linear forms of viral DNA is difficult. Some viruses have adapted by circularizing their DNA or by having covalently linked ends, terminal repeats, or specialized proteins that serve to prime DNA polymerase directly.

Some RNA viruses encode an RNA-dependent DNA polymerase, or reverse transcriptase (RT), which uses the viral RNA as a template to make a complementary DNA strand. These are referred to as retroviruses, of which HIV is the best-known member. RT protein is commonly synthesized before assembly of a new virion, and the RT packaged into the viral capsid along with the viral RNA genome. When the single-stranded RNA of the retrovirus enters a cell, the RT protein that is brought into the host cell with the virus begins to make a copy of the viral RNA strand into a DNA strand to form a DNA-RNA hybrid. The same enzyme, recognizing this DNA-RNA complex, begins to degrade the RNA strand, making the DNA strand available for the synthesis of a second DNA strand. Together with a viral protein that promotes integration of this newly formed double-stranded DNA, known as an integrase, the two ends of the new DNA are inserted into virtually any site of the host cell's chromosome. The next step of the infectious process involves the production of a large number of viral RNA molecules after transcription of the integrated viral DNA by the host cell's DNA-dependent RNA polymerase.

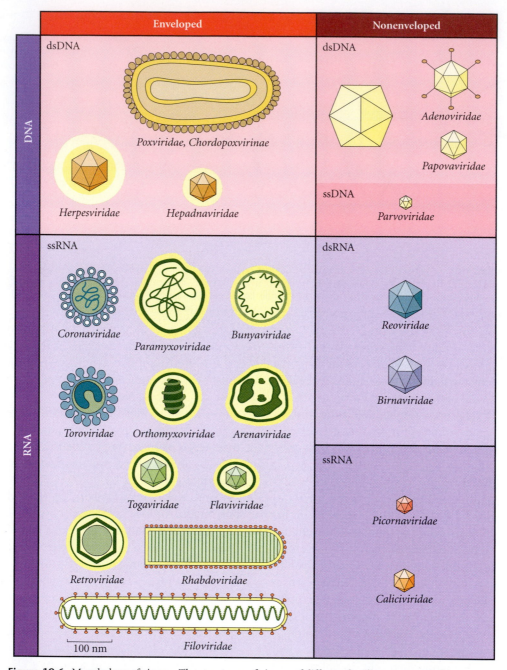

Figure 19.6 Morphology of viruses. The structures of viruses of different families are separated into groups on the basis of whether they are enveloped or nonenveloped and whether their genome is RNA or DNA. ds, double-stranded; ss, single-stranded. Redrawn from J. A. Levy et al., *Virology,* 3rd ed. (Prentice Hall, Englewood Cliffs, N.J., 1994), with permission.

Replication of the Virus

In general, the replication cycle of a virus involves the following steps: adsorption, entry, exposure of the viral genome to the host cell's metabolic machinery, production of viral proteins and genome, assembly of the virus components, and exit from the host cell (Fig. 19.8). Although the events that occur during virus replication are unique to the type of virus and host cell, all the steps described above must take place for viruses to propagate. Viral infection leads to rapid cell death (cytocidal or acute infection), long-term production of virus (chronic infection), or dormancy (latent infection).

The entry of a virus into the host cell requires its interaction with molecules on the cell surface termed *receptors*. Under normal circumstances, these receptors trigger

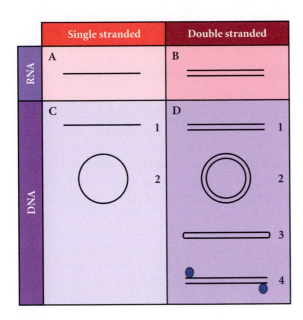

	Single stranded	Double stranded
RNA	**A**	**B**
DNA	**C** 1 2	**D** 1 2 3 4

Figure 19.7 Different forms of viral DNA and RNA. Viral RNA can exist in either a linear single-stranded (**A**) or double-stranded (**B**) form. Viral DNA can exist as a single-stranded (**C**) or double-stranded (**D**) form in either a linear (**1**) or circular form (**2**). Double-stranded DNA may also exist in a linear form with covalently linked ends (**3**) or have covalently linked terminal proteins (**4**).

Figure 19.8 Steps in infection of a cell by rhabdovirus. (1) Virus attaches to its receptor on the host cell. (2) Virus enters the cell by endocytosis of the cytoplasmic membrane. (3) The viral envelope fuses with the endosome membrane, and the nucleocapsid enters the cytoplasm. (4) Uncoating of the nucleocapsid occurs. (5) The negative-sense viral RNA is transcribed into a positive-sense viral RNA. N, NS, M, G, and L are mRNAs encoding various viral protein components (see Fig. 19.5 for precise definitions). (6) The positive-sense RNA serves as a template for the viral genome. (7) The negative-sense RNA becomes incorporated into a new nucleocapsid. (8) The nucleocapsid joins with the matrix protein at the host cell membrane. (9) The virus buds from the cell.

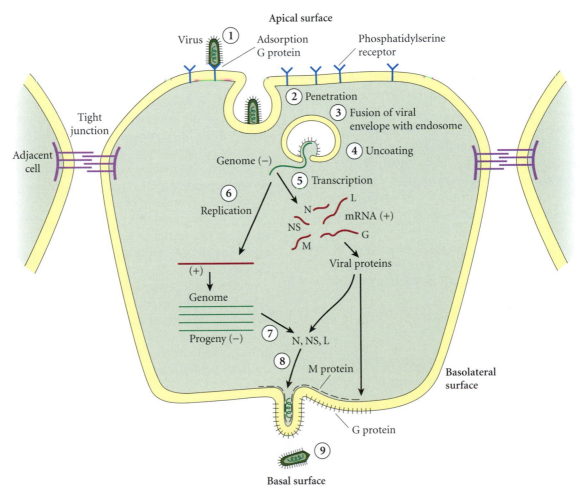

physiological functions upon binding to their cognate ligands. Such functions can include cell adhesion, regulation of cytoskeletal architecture, nutrient acquisition, or cell activation. An immunologically relevant example of such an interaction is the binding of the secreted cytokine interleukin-2 (IL-2) to its cellular receptor (the IL-2 receptor), leading to the immunologically important result of T-cell activation. However, viruses can mimic certain ligands and thereby bind to receptors on their host's cells, an ability accounting for the specificity of most viruses for certain cell types of their host. Several of these are listed in Table 19.2.

Upon interaction with the receptor, a virus can enter the cytoplasm of the host cell by the process of endocytosis. With nonenveloped viruses, the capsid is digested on the cell surface by proteolytic enzymes, and the viral genome is then transported into the cell. With enveloped viruses, the membrane of the virus fuses with the host-cell membrane and the viral capsid enters the cell, where it is degraded by intracellular proteolytic enzymes, releasing the viral genome into the host-cell cytoplasm.

The entry of the viral genome into the host cell usually results in replication of virus (although replication may not occur until after a long latency period). The genome of many viruses, primarily negative-strand RNA and some DNA viruses, can replicate only by using their own replication enzymes (brought into the cell or synthesized in the host cell). In other cases, viruses use the host cell's replication enzymes. Viral mRNA is made next and is then translated to produce viral proteins. Viruses at this stage are wholly dependent on the host cell (e.g., ribosomes, transfer RNA, and amino acid pools). The virus is then assembled, after which the virus particle is released from the cell, either through the process of budding (where the virus particle can acquire its envelope) or lysis of the host cell, allowing release of nonenveloped viruses. Whether the host cell is lysed following virus replication also may depend on events in the host cell during virus production. For example, cells in early mitosis that are infected with polioviruses are not lysed; however, if these

same host cells are infected when they are not dividing, they will be destroyed following the production of virions.

Host-Cell Response to Viral Infections

Cytopathic effect

The most easily recognizable pathologic effect of viral infection is the destructive or cytocidal effect characterized by extensive damage to many host-cell organelles. Other cytopathic effects include an imbalance of ions across the host cell's plasma membrane, causing an influx of water and a ballooning of the membrane. The cytopathic effects observed during viral infections usually occur late in the replication stage of the virus. Cells infected with poliovirus have been shown to release lysosomal phospholipases into the cytoplasm, leading to the disruption of the plasma membranes and eventually to death of the cell.

Virus-infected cells can also be induced to die by apoptosis. Although cytotoxic lymphocytes and the removal of host-cell growth factors can induce apoptosis in these infected cells, programmed cell death can occur after infection even in the absence of cytotoxic cells and in the presence of abundant amounts of growth factors. Therefore, apoptosis is thought in some cases to be a direct response of the host cell to viral infection. This event may be aimed at initiating an acquired immune response to the virus.

Intracellular inclusions

Another feature of viral infections is the formation of massive *inclusion bodies* in either the nucleus or cytoplasm of the infected cell. Inclusion bodies are discrete foci of viral activity made up of viral particles clustered together or aggregations of cellular products that form as a result of virus production. The staining pattern and location of these bodies vary depending on the type of virus infecting the cell. For example, the cytoplasm of poxvirus-infected cells contains basophilic inclusions that represent clusters of many virus particles. The nuclei of virally infected cells can contain crystalline arrays of virions. Disruption of the mitotic spindle apparatus in cells infected with some types of viruses produces crescent-shaped bodies in their cytoplasm. Another feature of infected cells can be the formation of extra and irrelevant cellular membranes. Therefore, numerous types of changes can occur throughout a cell during viral growth, and these changes are often directly related to disruption of cell function and development of disease.

Cell fusion

Some viral infections result in the formation of giant host cells containing several nuclei that all share a common cytoplasm. The multinucleated giant cell is generally referred to as a *syncytium*. Some viruses produce a fusion

Table 19.2 Host-cell receptors for some human-pathogenic viruses

Virus	Receptor
Lyssavirus	Acetylcholine receptor
HIV	CD4, CCR, CXCR chemokine receptors
Variola virus	Epidermal growth factor receptor
Epstein-Barr virus	CD21
Rhinovirus	CD54
Influenza virus	Glycophorin A receptor

Table 19.3 Defense mechanisms used by viruses against immune responses

Antivirus mechanism	Defense strategy of virus	Virus	Effector molecule
Apoptosis	Homolog of *bcl-2* gene product	Epstein-Barr virus	BHRF1
Interferon	Interfere with interferon	Poxvirus/E3L	
	Shut off viral protein production		
	Shut off IFN-γ production	Epstein-Barr virus	BCRF1
Antibody	Reassortment of viral genes	Influenza virus	
Antigen presentation	TAP inhibition	Herpes simplex virus	ICP47
	MHC class I suppression	CMV	US11
Oxidative stress response	Antioxidant	Molluscum contagiosum virus	MCO66L

factor, which is one of the proteins found in the outer portion of the virus, that can lead to the formation of a syncytium. This fusion factor interacts with glycoproteins or glycolipids on a neighboring host cell and causes the cells to fuse. This process may be a way for viruses to spread directly from one host cell to another without the need for an extracellular viral intermediate. Syncytium formation may also be the result of inappropriate activity of viral envelope proteins that are intended to mediate infection of new host cells following budding of new virions from the current host cell.

Effect on host-cell metabolism

Inhibition of the host's protein synthesis would be an obvious cause of cellular damage, but the way in which this is carried out varies among viruses. A number of viruses cause a rapid and complete cessation of the production of host proteins; others gradually inhibit the host's cellular protein synthesis. The latter inhibition is usually the result of competition between viral mRNA and host mRNA for the limited supply of host ribosomes. Some viruses can prevent further synthesis of host protein by disrupting host mRNA synthesis whereas others may interrupt protein synthesis by disrupting ribosomal RNA synthesis. A slow decrease in host-cell DNA synthesis can occur in many viral infections as an indirect effect of cessation of RNA and protein synthesis throughout the infected cell. Replicating viral particles need to commandeer the host cell transcription and translation machinery in order to produce progeny virions, so changes in host-cell protein synthesis are often seen as a consequence of viral infection.

Evasion of Host Antiviral Immune Defenses

For viruses to propagate efficiently within their host cells they must do so before their reproduction is halted by the immune response. Many viruses have developed mechanisms to modulate the host's defense system. These evasion mechanisms include assumption of a state of dormancy or latency, the regulation of molecules involved in apoptosis and antigen presentation, or disruption in the production of antiviral cytokines (Table 19.3). Moreover, mutations in viral antigens can prevent the virus from being recognized by the TCR or immunoglobulin and prevent destruction of the infected cell.

Dormancy and the Proviral State

The viral particle or virion exists outside the host cell and is the end product of a process within the cell that involves the replication and expression of the viral genome, synthesis of viral proteins, and assembly of these viral proteins and genetic material into complete virus particles. Some viruses can avoid clearance by the immune system by inserting their genomes into the host chromosome and remaining dormant. In these cases, the dormant viral genome is referred to as a *provirus*. Proviruses can exist for extended periods, sometimes causing no observable signs of disease at all and other times resulting in pathologic effects such as immunosuppression and production of tumors. Human papillomavirus often causes benign warts in different parts of the body, but it can also become dormant in the female genital epithelium and eventually produce dysplasias (disrupted tissue appearance) and even cervical cancer. It is the purpose of the Papanicolaou (Pap) test to detect these changes so early medical intervention can be used to treat this situation.

Many viruses can assume the dormant or latent state even in the presence of a host immune response. For example, most individuals make good immune responses to herpes simplex virus, but it can remain latent in neuronal cells where only a limited number of viral genes are transcribed and translated. But in the face of poorly defined stimuli the virus can be reactivated, leading to lesions on the lips, mouth and face (cold sores), or genitalia (genital herpes) most commonly, but potentially anywhere in the body along a mucosal or visceral surface. In all of these respects, both the virus and host are faced with a difficult balancing act. The virus must avoid being detected and destroyed by its host's immune effectors until it has carried out its prime function of replicating to produce progeny virions that can infect new host cells or new hosts. The host must utilize both innate and acquired immune mechanisms to limit viral entry into cells where they can replicate, limit viral spread from infected to uninfected cells, limit tissue destruction and resultant pathology that produces the signs and symptoms of disease, and try to either completely eliminate the virus or confine it to a tissue where only occasional reactivation can occur.

Inhibition of Antiviral Humoral Immunity

Viruses have adapted to be capable of escaping antibody- or complement-mediated destruction. For example, human cytomegalovirus (CMV) encodes a unique Fc receptor. Since a single antibody cannot simultaneously bind the CMV Fc receptor and CD16 on the surface of NK cells, the CMV Fc receptor can competitively inhibit ADCC of NK cells. A herpes simplex virus gene can encode for soluble complement receptors capable of binding to complement components and inactivating them before the complement proteins can bind to the virus. Poxviruses also can evade destruction by complement through the production of viral proteins that inhibit the complement activation cascade.

One other mechanism that allows viruses to escape antiviral antibodies is the alteration of viral antigens. This alteration occurs not only in antigens recognized by antibodies but also in those recognized by TCRs on CTLs. Neutralizing antibodies to the major surface proteins on the influenza virus envelope, HA and neuraminidase NA, enable the host to prevent infection or to decrease further spread. To avoid these antibodies, the influenza virus has developed two ways of changing its surface antigens (see Fig. 21.3 and 21.12). The first, known as *antigenic drift*, is caused by point mutations in the genes encoding HA and NA. Usually, every 2 to 3 years, variants in influenza virus develop point mutations in genes that enable them to avoid neutralization by antibodies present in the general population. Thus, individuals who are resistant to an old variant of the influenza virus are susceptible to the new variant. However, this mutation tends to result in only mild disease and dissemination since antibodies can still recognize HA and NA epitopes that have not been altered. The second mechanism, known as *antigenic shift*, occurs when the segmented RNAs encoding HA and NA are reassorted between different viral strains infecting the same cells (this is possible because the genome of influenza virus actually consists of eight separate pieces of RNA). The change leads to the inability of the existing anti-influenza antibody of the host to recognize the new surface antigens. In these instances, severe disease results since preexisting immunity of the host is rendered essentially useless.

Evasion of Cellular Antiviral Immune Responses

Interference with presentation of viral antigen on the MHC molecule

Since CTLs can prevent virus production by eliminating infected host cells before progeny are produced (and thereby interrupt the spread of virus to other cells), viruses have adapted means of decreasing the presentation of their own antigens by the host's MHC class I and class II molecules. For example, the cytosolic protein ICP47 (infected cell polypeptide 47) from herpes simplex virus can bind to TAPl/TAP2 complexes and prevent the transport and association of peptide antigens with an MHC class I molecule. US11, a gene product of human CMV, can dislocate newly synthesized MHC class I molecules from the endoplasmic reticulum to the cytosol of the infected cells, where they are acted on by *N*-glycanases and proteasomes (see Fig. 12.5). The *BZLF2* (*Bam*HI <u>Z</u>-region <u>l</u>eftward-oriented open reading <u>f</u>rame <u>2</u>) gene of Epstein-Barr virus encodes a type II membrane glycoprotein expressed late in infection. This protein binds to MHC class II molecules and interferes with binding of viral peptide antigen to the MHC. Viruses can also modulate MHC expression by decreasing host protein synthesis. The ability of viruses to inhibit cytokine production also may affect MHC expression indirectly, since cytokines such as TNF-α and IFN-γ can increase expression of MHC class I and class II.

Cytokines and soluble cytokine receptors encoded by viruses

Although cytokines are soluble mediators produced during immune activation in the host, viruses possess genes encoding cytokines that can decrease immune responses. For example, the *BCRF1* (<u>Bam</u>HI <u>C</u>-region <u>r</u>ightward-oriented open reading <u>f</u>rame <u>1</u>) gene of the Epstein-Barr virus encodes a 17-kilodalton (kDa) protein that binds to the IL-10 receptor and carries out functions similar to those of IL-10. This has been shown to decrease the production of IFN-γ and thus decrease the antiviral effects of this cytokine. Poxviruses also encode soluble receptors for IFN-γ, TNF-α and -β, and IL-10, enabling them to prevent these cytokines from binding to their receptors on NK cells and CTLs involved in controlling the virus.

Not only do cytokines made by viruses decrease cellular immune responses, they also can enhance infection. For example, variola virus encodes an 18-kDa protein growth factor that binds to the epidermal growth factor receptor and mediates mitogenesis. This enables the virus to induce hyperplasia at the infection site and facilitate its own spread.

Several viruses have acquired the ability to prevent the interferon-induced shutdown of protein translation. Poxviruses, for example, produce the E3L protein, which binds to double-stranded RNA and competes with the double-stranded RNA-dependent kinase DAI. Since DAI kinase cannot bind to double-stranded RNA, it is unable to phosphorylate and inactivate eIF-2. Another method by which poxviruses subvert interferon activity is by encoding the protein K3L, which acts as a competitive substrate for DAI kinase because of its significant amino acid homology to eIF-2.

Regulation of apoptosis

Apoptosis can occur in virus-infected cells following infection and is a major mechanism by which CTLs kill virus-infected target cells. Viruses have adapted ways of preventing apoptosis. For example, the *E1B/19K* gene product of adenovirus, which is expressed relatively early in infection, can prevent apoptosis induced by TNF or Fas. The *E1B/19K* gene product is a homolog of the *bcl-2* gene product and functions to protect cells from a variety of apoptosis-inducing factors. A similar virus-encoded gene product, BHRF1, has been found in Epstein-Barr virus. These same viral products that protect the virus against CTL-mediated destruction also may lead to the immortalization of some virus-infected cells, a pivotal step toward virus-induced tumorigenesis.

Regulation of oxidative stress

Viruses have the ability to avoid damage by peroxides or oxygen metabolites (oxidative stress elements) produced by phagocytic cells at sites of inflammation. For example, molluscum contagium virus, a poxvirus that leads to benign tumor-like skin lesions in individuals with AIDS or other immunodeficiencies, produces a protein (MC066L) that is 74% homologous with human glutathione peroxidase. This selanoprotein (so named because it requires selenium as a cofactor) can protect infected cells from death induced by hydrogen peroxide, and in doing so, protect the virus, which the host cells harbor.

Summary

Viruses are intracellular pathogens with genomes consisting of RNA or DNA enclosed within a protein capsid that is, in some cases, surrounded by a lipid membrane. The sole purpose of the virion is to propagate itself by using the host cell's machinery to replicate and express the viral genome, synthesize viral proteins, and assemble these viral proteins and genetic material into complete, new virus particles. The end result of this replication process usually leads to death of the host cell, to tissue damage, and eventually to disease. Although viruses are generally cytopathic, some viral infections lead to chronic production of virus, dormancy, or in some cases, oncogenesis. To bring about control of the viral infection, the host invokes the production of interferon, which can abrogate virus production or assist in the immune response to the virus. These immune responses consist of neutralizing antibodies, which not only prevent viruses from entering the host cells but also destroy infected cells by complement and ADCC. NK cells and CTLs also are involved in controlling viruses through their ability to induce the death of the infected cells or through the production of interferon. Viruses, however, are able to escape these immune responses by expressing products that inhibit the function of these immune effectors.

Suggested Reading

Grandvaux, N., B. R. tenOever, M. J. Servant, and J. Hiscott. 2002. The interferon antiviral response: from viral invasion to evasion. *Curr. Opin. Infect. Dis.* **15**:259–267.

Greber, U. F. 2002. Signalling in viral entry. *Cell. Mol. Life Sci.* **59**:608–626.

Jung, M. C., and G. R. Pape. 2002. Immunology of hepatitis B infection. *Lancet Infect. Dis.* **2**:43–50.

Klasse, P. J., and Q. J. Sattentau. 2002. Occupancy and mechanism in antibody-mediated neutralization of animal viruses. *J. Gen. Virol.* **83**:2091–2108.

Klenerman, P., M. Lucas, E. Barnes, and G. Harcourt. 2002. Immunity to hepatitis C virus: stunned but not defeated. *Microbes Infect.* **4**:57–65.

Russell, J. H., and T. J. Ley. 2002. Lymphocyte-mediated cytotoxicity. *Annu. Rev. Immunol.* **20**:323–370.

Sieczkarski, S. B., and G. R. Whittaker. 2002. Dissecting virus entry via endocytosis. *J. Gen. Virol.* **83**:1535–1545.

Taniguchi, T., and A. Takaoka. 2002. The interferon-alpha/beta system in antiviral responses: a multimodal machinery of gene regulation by the IRF family of transcription factors. *Curr. Opin. Immunol.* **14**:111–116.

Weiss, R. A. 2002. Virulence and pathogenesis. *Trends Microbiol.* **10**:314–317.

Zinkernagel, R. M. 2002. Anti-infection immunity and autoimmunity. *Ann. N. Y. Acad. Sci.* **958**:3–6.

chapter 20

Immunity to Parasitic and Fungal Infections

Judith E. Allen and Leo X. Liu

All infectious microorganisms are parasites in the broadest sense because they depend on the host animal for essential nutrients and impart some degree of harm to that host. By convention, however, parasitic infections refer to those caused by protozoa and helminths. Protozoan and helminthic parasites pose a tremendous threat to animal and human health, particularly in the developing world (Table 20.1). Every year several hundred million people contract malaria, the most serious human protozoan disease, and close to 1 million children die of *Plasmodium falciparum* malaria in Africa. More than 1 billion people harbor intestinal nematode parasites, and some 200 million people worldwide are affected by schistosomiasis, a fluke disease transmitted by snails. In economically advanced countries such as the United States, protozoan parasites such as *Toxoplasma gondii* and *Cryptosporidium parvum* have emerged as important opportunistic pathogens in patients with acquired immunodeficiency syndrome (AIDS).

Eukaryotic parasites are distinguished from most bacterial and viral pathogens by their complex genomes and life cycles and the long duration of chronic infections in the host. Every parasite has a complex life cycle, undergoing sequential stages that may develop in soil or water, arthropod vectors, and one or more mammalian hosts. The parasite typically undergoes radical morphologic and biochemical changes as it develops from one stage to the next. Each developmental stage expresses unique molecules, and this antigenic complexity has direct implications for the nature of immune responses in parasitic infections. Host specificity is another striking characteristic of parasites: in most cases, a given protozoan or helminthic parasite can develop fully in only one or

Table 20.1 Major parasitic infections of humans

Disease	Major species	Areas of endemicity	Infections (millions)	Mode of transmission	Site of parasitism	Duration of infection (yr)	Immunopathology
Protozoa							
Malaria	*Plasmodium falciparum, P. vivax, P. ovale, P. malariae*	Worldwide in tropics and subtropics	300	*Anopheles* mosquito bite	Erythrocytes	1–2	+
Leishmaniasis, visceral	*Leishmania donovani*	India, China, Africa	<1	Sand fly bite	Macrophages	Lifelong	+
Leishmaniasis, cutaneous	*Leishmania major*, others	Worldwide in tropics and subtropics	12	Sand fly bite	Macrophages	Lifelong	−/+
Trypanosomiasis, African (sleeping sickness)	*Trypanosoma brucei*	Sub-Saharan Africa	<1	Tsetse fly bite	Bloodstream	Months	−
Trypanosomiasis, South American (Chagas' disease)	*Trypanosoma cruzi*	Latin America	20	Reduviid bug bite	Blood, muscle	Lifelong	++
Toxoplasmosis	*Toxoplasma gondii*	Worldwide	>100	Infective stages in cat feces, undercooked meat	Many cell types	Lifelong	−
Helminths							
Intestinal nematodes							
Ascariasis (roundworms)	*Ascaris lumbricoides*	Worldwide in tropics and subtropics	1,000	Infective eggs in fecally contaminated soil	Small intestine	1–2	−/+
Hookworm	*Ancylostoma duodenale, Necator americanum*	Worldwide in tropics and subtropics	900	Infective larvae in fecally contaminated soil	Small intestine	2–3	−/+
Trichuriasis (whipworm)	*Trichuris trichiura*	Worldwide in tropics and subtropics	500	Infective eggs in fecally contaminated soil	Colon and cecum	5	+
Tissue nematodes							
Lymphatic filariasis	*Wuchereria bancrofti*	Worldwide in tropics and subtropics	>100	Mosquito bite	Lymphatics	>10	++
Onchocerciasis (river blindness)	*Onchocerca volvulus*	Sub-Saharan Africa, Central and South America	20	Blackfly bite	Subcutaneous	>10	++
Trematodes							
Schistosomiasis	*Schistosoma mansoni*	Africa, Arabia, South America, East and Southeast Asia	>200	Infective cercariae from freshwater snails	Mesenteric veins	>10	++
	S. japonicum	East Asia			Mesenteric veins		
	S. haematobium	Africa, Middle East			Vesical plexus veins		
Cestodes							
Cysticercosis (tissue)	*Taenia solium* (pig tapeworm)	Worldwide	>10	Infected pork	Subcutaneous tissues, brain	Lifelong	+

a few mammalian host species. Finally, many parasites undergo both intracellular and extracellular replicative stages, placing additional demands on host immune resistance to infection.

Protozoan parasites are unicellular, and their small size permits them to be either intracellular or extracellular parasites. Protozoa reproduce asexually by binary fission. Protozoan parasites, like bacterial pathogens, replicate either outside of or directly within the host. Thus, even a single bite from a malarious mosquito, for example, can ultimately result in severe sickness or death from malaria. Helminthic parasites, on the other hand, are large multicellular worms that are almost exclusively extracellular parasites of the blood, tissues, or intestinal tract. Helminths reproduce sexually; thus, a single infectious helminth egg or larva develops into only a single adult worm. For a large "worm burden" to develop in the body of the host, repeated exposure to infectious larvae or eggs is required. Thus, people heavily infected with helminthic parasites have usually lived for a long time in the area of ongoing transmission.

Infections with protozoa and helminths are typically chronic (often lasting for the remainder of the lifetime of the host), with the onset of disease symptoms in many instances developing years after the initial infection. The remarkable longevity of many parasites is due to the diverse mechanisms they have evolved to counteract or evade host immune responses. What we understand about human immune responses to parasites is derived largely from animal models and in vitro systems. Although the immunology of parasitic infections is not completely understood, it is clear that host immune responses to parasitic infections are very different from those to conventional microbial pathogens. In many cases, long-term immunity to viral and bacterial pathogens can be achieved after only a single exposure. No such sterilizing immunity exists to protozoan and helminthic parasites, against which immunologic protection is rarely (if ever) complete. Furthermore, inappropriate immune responses observed in some individual host animals can lead to immunopathologic tissue damage that typifies some parasitic diseases, such as schistosomiasis and lymphatic filariasis. For parasitic infections, in particular, an important distinction between *infection* and *disease* must be kept in mind: infection occurs each time the host is exposed to the infective stage of the parasite, but clinical disease occurs only in individuals in whom deleterious numbers of parasites or ineffective (or inappropriate) immune responses develop. In an area of high endemicity, virtually everyone may be infected with malaria or intestinal helminths, but only a minority of

the population at any given time suffers clinical symptoms. Thus, a long-lasting infection, accompanied by some degree of immunopathology, characterizes most parasitic infections. These features clearly pose a formidable challenge for the development of vaccines against parasites, and indeed, no vaccine has yet been fully developed against any human parasitic infection.

Protozoal Infections

The most serious and intensively studied protozoal infections include malaria, leishmaniasis, trypanosomiasis, and toxoplasmosis (Table 20.1).

Malaria: a Serious Blood-Borne Protozoal Infection

Malaria is a leading cause of death worldwide, especially among young children in tropical and subtropical countries. Of the *Plasmodium* species that cause disease in humans, *P. falciparum* can be rapidly fatal if untreated, whereas the other species cause an acute febrile illness that is only rarely life-threatening. Malarial sporozoites, after they are inoculated by an infective anopheline mosquito bite, invade and replicate in the liver, emerging as merozoites that establish an infectious cycle within red blood cells (Fig. 20.1). Disease symptoms in malaria are due to the intra-erythrocytic cycles of infection that result in high fevers, anemia, and cerebral disease. Cerebral malaria, an acute infection in the central nervous system, leads to disorientation, delirium, and coma and is the most common cause of death in falciparum malaria.

The complex life cycle of the malarial parasite (Fig. 20.1) provides many opportunities for the immune system to respond to and control this infection. However, protective immunity does not develop after a single episode of infection. Only after many years of repeated exposure to infectious mosquito bites does an individual apparently become more resistant or "immune" to reinfection, as manifested by the presence of fewer parasites in the bloodstream and fewer episodes of fever and other signs of clinical disease. Children living in areas where the parasite is highly endemic are infected at a very young age and do not develop a protective immune response despite repeated exposure to malarious mosquito bites. As these children get older they still become infected, but the number of clinical episodes declines. Only in adulthood, after years of exposure, is there a substantial reduction in the number of parasites in the blood. Less exposure to infective mosquitoes cannot explain the lower number of infections in adults; thus, it is presumed that older individuals have some acquired immunity. In areas where

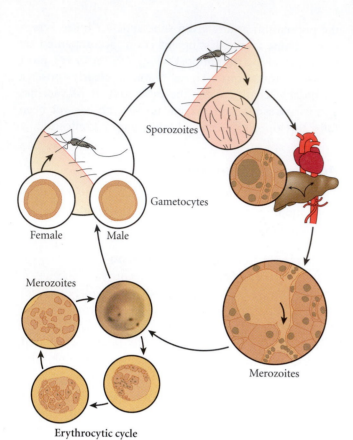

Erythrocytic cycle

Figure 20.1 Life cycle of malaria parasites. Malaria is transmitted by the bite of the female anopheline mosquito, which injects the sporozoite stage of *Plasmodium* species into the bloodstream. Sporozoites invade the liver, where they divide extensively without inducing a host inflammatory response. Eventually the infected liver cell ruptures, releasing merozoites into the bloodstream, where they invade erythrocytes and continue asexual division within the erythrocyte. Infected erythrocytes then lyse, releasing more merozoites to continue ongoing erythrocytic cycles of infection. Some of the merozoites develop into sexual stages (gametocytes) that are ingested by the mosquito, in which sexual development of the parasite proceeds, giving rise to infective sporozoites that are transmitted to the next host when the infected mosquito takes a second blood meal. Extensive hemolysis leads to severe anemia and splenomegaly. *P. falciparum* is particularly virulent because it can infect a high proportion of erythrocytes and cause cerebral disease due to microvascular occlusion. An antigenically variant family of *P. falciparum* proteins expressed on the erythrocyte cell surface mediate adherence of infected erythrocytes to postcapillary venule endothelium (see section on immune evasion by parasites, antigenic variation), which causes cerebral malaria. The circle containing a photo shows a photomicrograph of a *P. falciparum* trophozoite.

transmission of malaria is low, no significant immunity develops in any age group. The difficulty in developing strong immunity to malaria is due in large part to the tremendous strain diversity of the malaria parasite and the remarkable level of antigenic variation by individual parasite proteins.

Leishmaniasis: a Cutaneous and Visceral Intracellular Protozoal Infection

Protozoa of the genus *Leishmania* parasitize macrophages in the skin and visceral organs. In the Old World *Leishmania major* and in the Western Hemisphere *Leishmania mexicana* and other species cause cutaneous skin ulcers, which can result in unsightly permanent scars when the subcutaneous tissue also is involved. Visceral leishmaniasis (also called kala-azar) is a debilitating and progressive infiltrative infection with *Leishmania donovani* of the liver, spleen, and bone marrow. Leishmaniasis is transmitted by the bite of a sandfly (Fig. 20.2). The infective

Figure 20.2 Life cycle of *Leishmania species*. Leishmaniasis is an infection of rodents, canines, and other mammals, including humans. *Leishmania* species are transmitted by the bite of an infected female sand fly. The infective-stage promastigotes enter the bite wound, activate complement, and are rapidly taken up by local macrophages. Within the phagolysosome of the macrophage, the promastigotes transform into amastigotes that replicate by binary fission within the cell, eventually filling the cytoplasm. Upon rupture of the infected macrophage, the released amastigotes are taken up by new macrophages. Amastigotes are engulfed from the infected mammal by the bite of another sand fly, develop into promastigotes within the insect's gut, migrate to the insect salivary glands, and are deposited on the skin of another host when the sand fly takes its next blood meal. The photograph shows a cutaneous ulcer due to *L. major*.

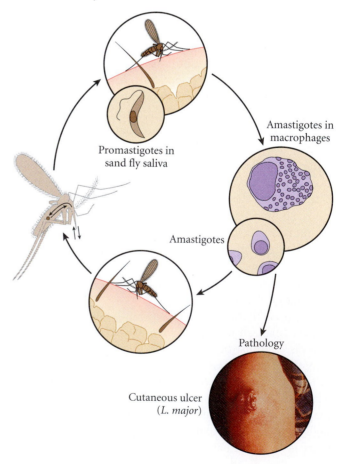

Promastigotes in sand fly saliva

Amastigotes in macrophages

Amastigotes

Pathology

Cutaneous ulcer
(*L. major*)

promastigotes are incorporated into macrophages, where they transform into amastigotes that live and multiply within endolysosomal vacuoles.

Cutaneous leishmaniasis (also called Oriental sore) is probably the only major human parasitic infection for which there appears to be immunity to reinfection. Individuals whose initial lesions have healed are permanently protected from developing new ulcers in the future despite ongoing exposure to biting sand flies. This phenomenon has been appreciated since ancient times by villagers in areas of high endemicity in the Middle East, who practice the custom of deliberately inoculating an inconspicuous body area (such as the underarms) with infective material to prevent future facial disfigurement by the natural infection. As with many other intracellular infections, cell-mediated immunity seems to be the most important mechanism of resolving the infection, with little if any role for antibodies. *Leishmania* antigens are presented to the host's T cells on major histocompatibility complex (MHC) class II proteins, a feature thought to be due to the unique endosomal location of the intracellular parasite. Leishmaniasis has been intensively studied in murine models, which have demonstrated that CD4$^+$ T helper type 1 (TH1) effector lymphocytes are the most critical components of acquired, protective cell-mediated immunity. These T cells produce cytokines that are necessary for the activation of macrophages, which in turn destroy intracellular parasites by producing nitric oxide and reactive oxygen intermediates.

Trypanosomes: Tissue and Blood Protozoan Parasites

Another intracellular protozoan, *Trypanosoma cruzi*, causes Chagas' disease, a very serious problem in South and Central America. *T. cruzi* is transmitted to humans by reduviid bugs when *T. cruzi* trypomastigotes present in the insect's feces enter the human host through breaks in the skin (the insect bite) or mucous membranes and subsequently infect macrophages and other human cells (Fig. 20.3). Intracellular multiplication proceeds until the host cells rupture, releasing additional parasites (amastigotes) that spread to other cells or through the bloodstream (as trypomastigote forms). The parasite infects a wide variety of cells, including muscle and nerve cells as well as macrophages. As with leishmaniasis, activation of macrophages and generation of nitric oxide are critical for parasite killing. Cytotoxic T cells, specific antibody, and complement also help to control *T. cruzi* infection by destroying infected host cells or directly killing the parasite. Unfortunately, antigens of *T. cruzi* cross-react with human cardiac muscle and mesenteric nerve

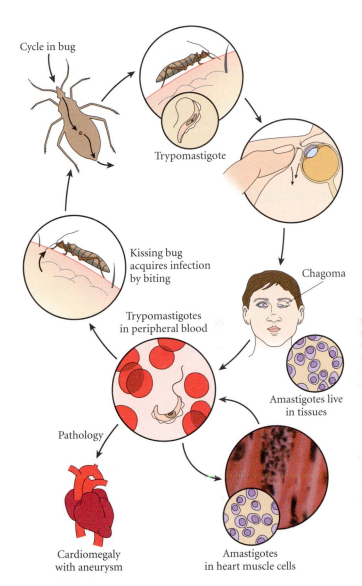

Figure 20.3 Life cycle of *T. cruzi*. *T. cruzi* is transmitted among various mammalian hosts by hematophagous reduviid bugs native to parts of Central and South America. An infected bug defecates while feeding, discharging infective trypomastigotes in the feces. The trypomastigotes enter the bite wound, mucous membranes, or conjunctivae and infect a wide variety of cells. An indurated inflammatory lesion (chagoma) often appears at the site of the bite and parasite entry. Within host cells the trypomastigotes transform into amastigotes, replicating until the host cells rupture to release additional parasites. Trypomastigotes in the circulation can be ingested by reduviid bugs during a blood meal, thereby continuing the parasite life cycle. Chagas' disease can also be transmitted by blood transfusion because of the stages in the bloodstream. Early in the disease, heavy infection of the cardiac muscle occasionally causes acute heart failure and sudden cardiac death. The pathogenesis of chronic Chagas' disease is not well understood, but myocardial inflammation, fibrosis, and atrophy can develop with few or no detectable parasites. In some patients, focal inflammation and destruction of the myenteric nerve plexus of the gut result in loss of peristalsis and enormous dilatation of the esophagus or colon. The photomicrograph shows amastigotes.

antigens. Therefore, immune reactions directed to parasite antigens eventually result in severe damage to the host tissues. Although the acute phase of Chagas' disease is often asymptomatic, chronic infection can lead to serious and fatal cardiac arrhythmias, cardiomyopathy, or megacolon.

African trypanosomiasis, also known as sleeping sickness, is an important disease throughout equatorial Africa. Unlike the intracellular protozoan parasites mentioned thus far, *Trypanosoma brucei* has a strictly extracellular existence. These hemoflagellates are transmitted by the bite of the tsetse fly and also are found in wild animals, particularly antelope, which can serve as reservoirs for the transmission of trypanosomiasis to humans and domestic cattle. The disease is characterized by intermittent fevers associated with the emergence of new antigenic forms of the parasite in the bloodstream. Although the surface glycoproteins of the trypanosome are very immunogenic, an elegant mechanism of antigenic variation allows the trypanosome to survive in the host. Invasion of the central nervous system leads to coma and a universally fatal outcome if untreated.

Toxoplasmosis: an Important Zoonosis

The intracellular pathogen *Toxoplasma gondii* has a very broad host specificity, such that this parasite can infect and become encysted in the tissues of virtually any warm-blooded animal. The definitive host is the cat (both domestic and wild) where parasite sexual development occurs in the small intestine (Fig. 20.4). Other mammals, including humans, can become infected when they eat the eggs deposited in cat feces or eat undercooked meat from an infected animal. The parasite has a tropism for neural tissue and normally remains encysted in the central nervous system. Infection is very common, and it is estimated that over a third of the world's population has been exposed. Although the infection is generally asymptomatic, there are two groups of people who are at significant risk for disease: immune-compromised individuals and pregnant women. Toxoplasmosis in immune-compromised individuals became a significant problem at the advent of the AIDS epidemic in the 1980s, and toxoplasmic encephalitis remains a leading cause of death among individuals infected with human immunodeficiency virus (HIV). Infection of pregnant women is an important public health issue, as a primary infection during pregnancy can lead to infection of the fetus, causing abortion or congenital disease, including mental retardation and blindness.

Helminthic Infections

Parasitic helminths are taxonomically divided into nematodes (roundworms), trematodes (flukes), and cestodes (tapeworms). Depending on the species, infective stages of these multicellular worms may be either invasive larvae or ingested eggs that soon hatch to release larvae. The adult worms typically live for many years in specific host anatomic niches, such as the bloodstream or gut, producing eggs or larvae as "evacuation" stages that exit the body for subsequent transmission to other hosts. All of these stages have the potential to stimulate limiting or deleterious host immune responses. The most serious helminthic parasites from a global human health perspective are schistosomes, filarial nematodes, and intestinal nematodes (Table 20.1).

Schistosomiasis: a Blood Fluke Infection Transmitted by Freshwater Snails

Schistosomiasis in humans is caused by several *Schistosoma* species, whose highly immunogenic eggs, when deposited in local tissues, trigger chronic inflammation and subsequent immunopathologic reactions that are largely responsible for the clinical disease. Humans become infected when cercariae from infested snails penetrate the skin (Fig. 20.5). The adult worm pairs live for a decade or more in abdominal veins or blood vessels of the bladder, producing eggs that, when not expelled, lodge in the bowel wall (*Schistosoma mansoni* and *Schistosoma japonicum*), bladder wall (*Schistosoma haematobium*), or liver (all three species). Over the long and fecund lifetime of the adult worms, a very large number of eggs become lodged in these tissues. The T-cell-mediated host reaction to these eggs results in the formation of granulomas, which in turn produce the pathologic consequences of hepatic fibrosis (liver scarring) and portal hypertension (high blood pressure in the liver vein) or bladder and urinary tract fibrosis.

As with many parasites, there is little evidence for protective immunity to schistosomes. Most infected people, when treated with drugs that eradicate existing parasites, are still susceptible to reinfection with cercariae. However, epidemiologic studies indicate that in areas where schistosomes are endemic, adults are less likely than children to become reinfected, not because of reduced exposure but because of lowered susceptibility to infection. This decreased susceptibility in adults may be due to a selective immunity to the waterborne infective larvae that does not eliminate the adult worms already in the body. This concept of "concomitant immunity" hypothesizes that the adult worms induce immune responses that are protective against the infective larvae but not against the

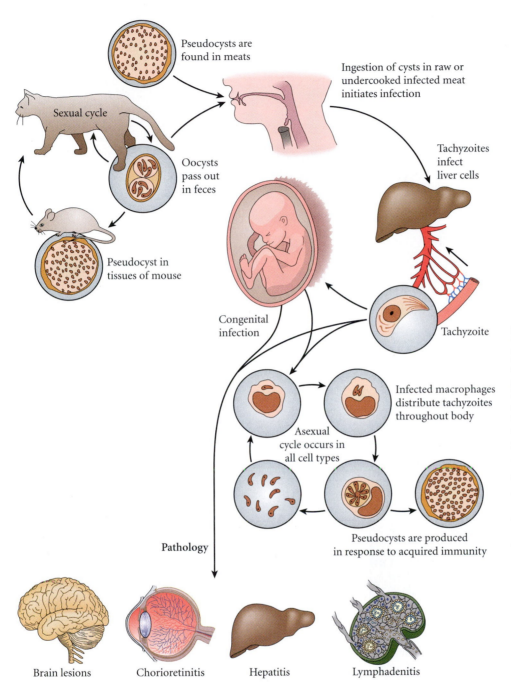

Figure 20.4 Life cycle of *T. gondii*. The family *Felidae* is the definitive host, and sexual stages of the parasite are found in the epithelial cells of the gut, and oocysts are shed in the feces. In the intermediate host (any mammal or bird), the parasite undergoes asexual division in one of two stages. The tachyzoite is rapidly dividing and can infect any nucleated cell. In the absence of a T-cell response, unrestricted growth of tachyzoites will kill the host. Normally, in the presence of a competent immune system, the tachyzoite stage is cleared from the tissues while the more slowly dividing form of the parasite, the bradyzoite, persists within pseudocysts. An active T-cell response to the parasite is required to prevent reemergence of the virulent tachyzoites from pseudocysts. There are three routes of transmission: (i) horizontal transmission via oocysts (i.e., cat to rodent), (ii) horizontal transmission via tissue cysts (i.e., rodent to cat or pig to human), and (iii) vertical transmission (congenital infection) via tachyzoites.

adult schistosomes. The adult schistosome therefore survives its host's immune response by diverting that response toward a different life stage of the schistosome.

Filariasis and Onchocerciasis: Intravascular and Tissue Nematode Infections

Filarial nematodes cause two serious immunopathologic diseases in humans, lymphatic filariasis and onchocerciasis. Lymphatic filariasis is a mosquito-transmitted infec-

tion caused by *Wuchereria bancrofti* and *Brugia* species (Fig. 20.6). The infective larvae develop into thread-like adult worms that reside in the lymphatic vessels. Adult female filarial worms produce microfilariae that circulate in the bloodstream and are ingested by a mosquito vector to continue the parasite's life cycle. Lymphatic filariasis is characterized by damage to the lymphatic vessels, with episodic lymphatic inflammation, pain, and fever. The presence of adult worms in the lymphatic vessels can lead

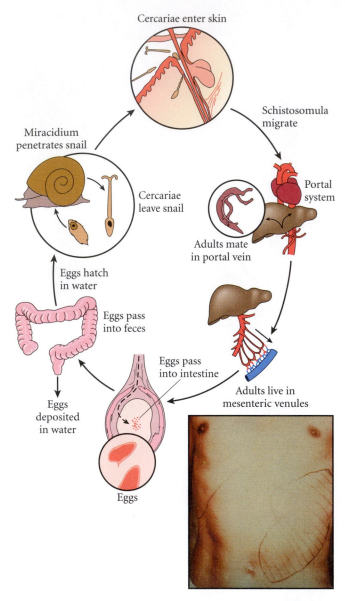

Figure 20.5 Life cycle of *S. mansoni*. Humans become infected with schistosome parasites by standing or swimming in fresh water infested with schistosome-infected snails. Infective schistosome larvae called cercariae emerge from infected snails and actively penetrate human skin. In the skin, the larvae of *S. mansoni* and *S. japonicum* transform into schistosomules, which migrate to the lungs and the portal vein, where the developing male and female schistosomes pair, settle in the mesenteric veins, and mature into adult worms. In these blood vessels, the female adult worm lives tightly ensconced within a longitudinal canal of the male worm and continuously produces eggs. Although most *S. mansoni* and *S. japonicum* eggs are passed out in the feces, others are carried retrograde by the portal venous system to the liver, where they become trapped in the portal triad. The life cycle of *S. haematobium* differs in that the adult worms of this species live in the bladder veins, and eggs of *S. haematobium* are expelled primarily in the urine, but some lodge in the bladder wall. Schistosome eggs passed in the feces or urine hatch in fresh water to release miracidia that infect snails and develop into infective larvae. The photo shows a patient with an enlarged spleen and liver due to *S. mansoni* infection.

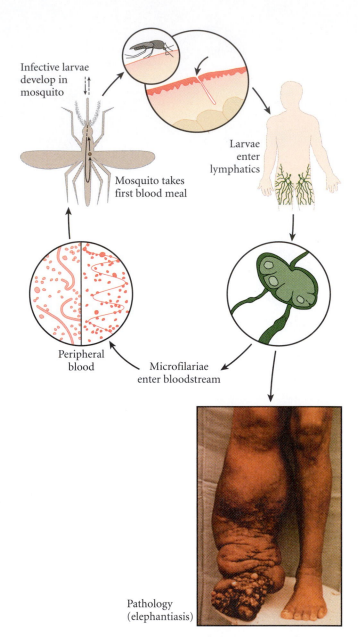

Figure 20.6 Life cycle of *W. bancrofti*. Lymphatic filariasis is caused primarily by *W. bancrofti* and to a lesser extent by *Brugia malayi*. The infection is transmitted by *Culex*, *Anopheles*, and *Aedes* species of mosquitos, which deposit infective larvae in the bite wound. The infective larvae migrate to the lymphatic vessels and lymph nodes, where they mature into adult worms. The offspring of adult worms are microfilariae, which enter the bloodstream. To complete the life cycle, microfilariae are ingested by another mosquito vector, in which they develop into new infective larvae. Chronic inflammation and lymphatic vessel damage can cause the gross lymphedema and skin changes of elephantiasis.

to lymph stasis and eventually to elephantiasis, with gross enlargement of the limbs, scrotum, or breast. The precise cause of lymphatic lesions is unknown but is likely due to the combined effects of mechanical damage and immune-mediated inflammatory responses. Onchocerciasis is an important cause of severe eye disease and dermatitis in areas of endemicity in Africa and Central America. *Onchocerca volvulus* is transmitted by black flies that breed in fast-flowing waters; thus, "river blindness" is the popular name for the disease. Adult *O. volvulus* worms reside in subcutaneous nodules, and the microfilariae migrate in the subcutaneous and ocular tissues. Unlike lymphatic filariasis, in which lymphatic damage is due primarily to the adult parasites, onchocercal disease is caused by immune responses to the circulating microfilariae.

As with schistosomiasis, it has been difficult to establish the existence of protective immunity to filarial parasites, and an individual human host can be infected countless times. However, the intensity of infection (i.e., the total number of worms harbored in the body) does decline with age in both lymphatic filariasis and onchocerciasis. This age-dependent reduction in worm burden suggests that partial protection may be acquired over time. Specific T-cell responses to the adult worms are actively suppressed during infection in individuals with circulating microfilariae. This parasite antigen-specific immunosuppression, while allowing the parasites to survive, also slows the development of immune-mediated tissue damage. In some individuals, this parasite-specific immunosuppression is lost, T-cell responses to worm antigens become vigorous, and tissue damage and loss of function develop. Furthermore, microfilariae are generally no longer detectable. These observations strongly suggest that immune-mediated responses are a primary cause of the pathology associated with filariasis.

Intestinal Nematodes Infect One-Fourth of the World's People

Intestinal nematodes have an enormous public health impact in developing countries, in part because of the vast number of people—more than 1 billion—infected with *Ascaris lumbricoides*, hookworm, or *Trichuris trichiura* (Table 20.1). Although these infections do not cause overt clinical problems in the majority of cases, disease can arise from massive infections or an inappropriate immune response. These gut parasites have relatively simple life cycles, with no intermediate host or vector, and are transmitted via infective eggs in contaminated food and water or by penetration of the skin by larvae found in feces-contaminated soil. Some of these species (such as *Trichuris*) develop entirely within the gut (Fig. 20.7),

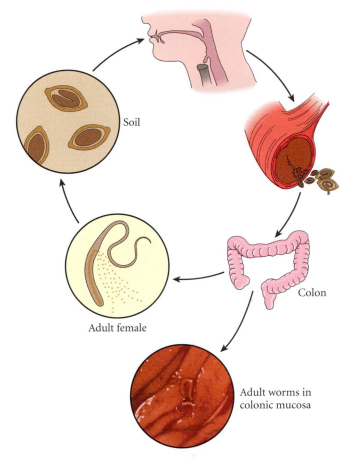

Figure 20.7 Life cycle of *T. trichiura*. Trichuriasis is transmitted directly by a human fecal-oral route with no intermediate vector. Adult whipworms (so called because of their broad posterior section and thin tapering anterior section) live in the colon and cecum. Adult female worms release thousands of unembryonated eggs daily, which pass via the feces and embryonate in the soil. Infection is acquired when infective eggs from the soil are accidentally transported to the mouth via unclean hands or contaminated food or water and are swallowed. After ingestion, the embryonated eggs hatch in the small bowel, releasing larvae that mature and then migrate to the large bowel.

whereas others (*Ascaris* and hookworms) migrate as larvae through the lungs and other tissues. *Trichinella spiralis*, a tissue nematode, is transmitted when a carnivorous mammalian host consumes larvae encysted in infected meat. *Trichinella* larvae mature to adult worms in the gut, and newborn larvae migrate via the bloodstream, where they penetrate and become encysted in striated (skeletal) muscle cells. All of these helminthic parasites provoke a polarized immune response, with dramatic expansion of the CD4$^+$ TH2 lymphocyte subpopulation. The TH2 cytokines, interleukin-4 (IL-4), IL-9, and IL-13, are important for expelling nematodes from the gut. However, the relative importance of these cytokines and the effector mechanisms they mediate vary considerably between nematode species.

Immune Responses in Parasitic Infections

T Cells and Cytokines Regulate Immune Responses in Parasitic Infections

T cells are critical in the control of all parasitic infections. Despite an apparent absence of protective immunity that protects against reinfection, the cell-mediated arm of the immune system is required to control parasitic infections. In particular, CD8$^+$ T cells and macrophages activated by CD4$^+$ cells can be effective in mediating control of protozoan parasites. T cells also are required for the production of high-affinity, parasite-specific antibodies involved in complement activation and antibody-dependent cellular cytotoxicity (ADCC). Genetically deficient mice that lack both B and T cells or athymic mice that have few T cells are unable to control infections and develop overwhelming parasite burdens that can be fatal. T-cell-mediated immunity is important not only in controlling natural infection but also in determining the host range of a pathogen. For example, mice are normally resistant to infection with human filarial parasites and destroy the incoming larvae. However, human filarial parasites can fully develop into adult worms in athymic mice that lack T cells.

For many parasitic diseases, the development of tissue injury, and hence clinical symptoms, often is due to inappropriate, rather than insufficient, immune responses to the parasite. Although CD8$^+$ and CD4$^+$ T cells and the cytokines that they produce are necessary for the control of parasitic infection, T cells are also frequently the most important factor in disease progression and immune-mediated injury (Table 20.2). The experimental dissection of immune responses resulting in disease resolution versus disease progression in parasitic infections led to the important discovery that the immune system can generate polarized and cross-regulating subsets of TH cells.

TH-cell subsets and their cytokines regulate immune responses to parasites

The expansion of TH1 or TH2 cells in response to infection is dependent on both the nature of the invading organism and the genetics of the host. The importance of host genetics is most dramatically demonstrated in studies of inbred mouse strains in which differences in genetic background can determine whether an infection is harmless or lethal. The functional importance of these TH-cell subsets was first demonstrated in a mouse model of infec-

Table 20.2 The potential role of T-cell subsets in parasitic diseases

Parasite	T-cell subset(s)	Potential function in disease[a]
Protozoa		
Leishmania major (murine)	TH1	Protection
	TH2	Exacerbation
Trypanosoma cruzi	CD8$^+$	Protection
Plasmodium		
Liver stage	CD8$^+$	Protection
Cerebral	TH1	Immunopathology
Toxoplasma gondii	CD8$^+$, TH1	Protection
Helminths		
Schistosoma mansoni (murine)	TH1	Protection
	TH2	Immunopathology
Trichuris muris	TH2	Protection
	TH1	Exacerbation

[a]The association of specific T-cell subsets with disease outcome derives from animal models and is not always mutually exclusive and generally is not as clear-cut in human infections.

tion with *Leishmania* where induction of the TH1 subset leads to disease resolution, whereas induction of the TH2 subset leads to disease progression. As more infectious diseases have been studied and their protective immune responses characterized, it has become apparent that activation of TH1 lymphocytes is usually necessary for destruction of protozoa.

In striking contrast to unicellular infections, infection with multicellular helminths results in an induction of the TH2 lymphocyte subset. This is characterized by an increase in the numbers of eosinophils and mast cells and heightened immunoglobulin E (IgE) levels in individuals who are infected with parasitic worms. This TH2 bias has been most thoroughly studied in murine models of infection but is also seen in humans infected with schistosomes or filarial nematodes, in whom there is an expansion of TH2 cytokine-producing cells. For helminths that reside in the tissues, it is not yet evident whether this induction of a TH2 response most benefits the host or the parasite. The situation with gut nematodes is more clear-cut where numerous experimental models have demonstrated that TH2 cytokines are necessary for clearance of the parasites from the gastrointestinal tract.

IL-12: a cytokine that initiates the TH1-dependent cell-mediated immune response

IL-12 is produced by phagocytic cells and B cells in response to infection with protozoan parasites and is the critical component in the early response to infection that drives TH1 cell expansion and production of interferon-gamma (IFN-γ) (Fig. 20.8). IL-12 directly stimulates the production of IFN-γ by T cells and natural killer (NK)

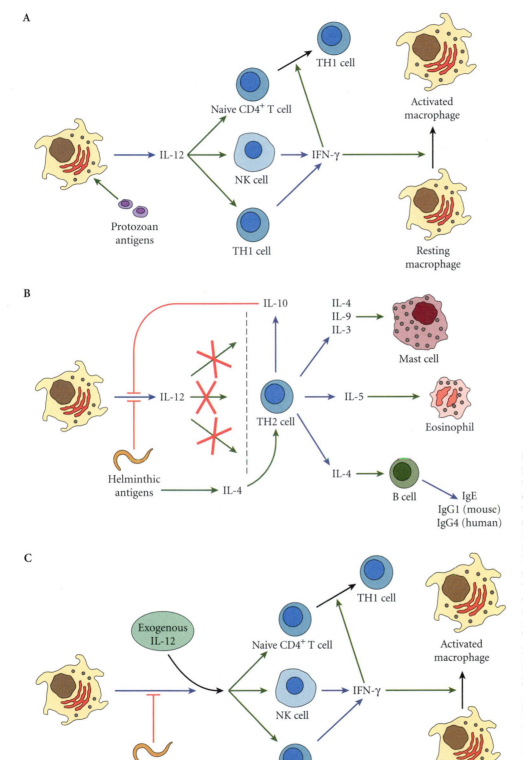

Figure 20.8 IL-12 and parasite infection. (**A**) Early in infection with intracellular parasites, IL-12 is produced by phagocytic cells and induces the production of IFN-γ by NK cells and T cells. This early production of IFN-γ may help control infection by immediately activating macrophages. In addition, IL-12 and the IL-12-driven cytokine IFN-γ favor the development of parasite-specific TH1 cells, in addition to inducing the production of high levels of IFN-γ by already differentiated TH1 cells. (**B**) This early production of IL-12 is functionally analogous to the early induction of IL-4 synthesis by helminthic parasites, which drives TH2 development. That helminthic parasites do not induce production of IL-12 may contribute to the development of TH2 as a default pathway. (**C**) If IL-12 is added early during helminthic infection, the normal induction of TH2 cells is prevented, and responses such as IgE synthesis and eosinophil production are significantly reduced.

cells. For intracellular protozoan parasites, IFN-γ is the major cytokine responsible for disease resolution because of its capacity to activate macrophages. For example, mice that are treated with antibodies that block IL-12 die during the acute phase of infection with *T. gondii*. Antibodies that block IFN-γ also increase susceptibility to disease. Similarly, some strains of mice are genetically susceptible to disseminated *L. major* infection because of their propensity to mount a TH2-type response (which is nonprotective) to infection. However, if these mice are treated with recombinant IL-12 during the early stages of *L. major* infection, they not only are cured of the infection but also remain resistant to reinfection (Fig. 20.9). Under these conditions, cotreatment with blocking antibodies to IFN-γ abrogates the protective effects of IL-12. Cell-mediated immune resistance to intracellular parasites is likely predicated on production of IL-12, which then induces the production of IFN-γ and activation of macrophages, responses that ultimately result in control and elimination of the parasites. Generally, however, helminthic infections do not induce the production of IL-12, perhaps because of the extracellular location of parasitic worms. The absence of IL-12 may favor the polarization of the immune response toward the TH2 cell subset in helminthic infections.

IL-4 initiates the TH2 response to helminthic infections

Elevated levels of IgE and eosinophils in blood and tissues, as well as mast-cell hyperplasia, are the hallmarks of helminthic infection and are induced by cytokines of the TH2 subset. The critical factor responsible for inducing the TH2 subset is the cytokine IL-4. To differentiate into TH2 cells, naive T cells must encounter IL-4 in the microenvironment where antigen is first recognized. Although this finding provided a clue as to what molecular signal determines when a TH2 response will occur, it also posed a more perplexing question: where does the initial dose of IL-4 come from at the beginning of the primary immune response? A distinct population of T cells designated as NK1.1$^+$ T cells has been identified as a likely source of early IL-4 production. NK1.1$^+$ cells have a limited T-cell receptor repertoire and may recognize nonpeptide antigens common to many helminth species. However, numerous other cell types, including γδ T cells, mast cells, basophils, and eosinophils, can produce IL-4

Figure 20.9 Murine leishmaniasis model. Experimental models of *Leishmania* infection have provided the most dramatic illustrations of the impact of TH-cell subsets on disease outcome. Susceptible BALB/c or resistant C57BL/6 mice when inoculated in the footpad with *L. major* develop a local swelling at the site of infection. In BALB/c mice, the *Leishmania* parasites disseminate throughout the body and the mice die by 8 weeks postinfection. However, in C57BL/6 mice, infection remains localized and the footpad swelling heals. These mice are resistant to reinfection. Susceptible BALB/c mice produce high levels of IL-4 and little IFN-γ in response to parasite antigen, while the reverse pattern is seen with the resistant C57BL/6 mice. Susceptible mice can be made resistant by the addition of antibody to IL-4 within the first few days of infection. In addition, normally resistant mice develop disseminated disease if given antibody to IFN-γ. Antibody to IL-4 blocks the induction of TH2 cells that downregulate protective TH1 responses, while antibody to IFN-γ blocks the ability of TH1 cells to activate macrophages.

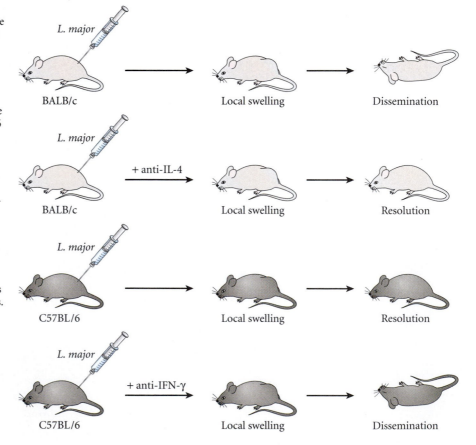

and may also be important sources of early IL-4. Once fully differentiated, TH2 cells take over as the sources of IL-4, IL-5, IL-6, IL-9, and IL-13. These cytokines stimulate the production of mast cells, eosinophils, and IgE and are therefore responsible for the immunologic manifestations of helminthic infection. It is not yet known exactly what helminth-derived signals or antigens trigger the initial IL-4 response necessary for induction of TH2 cells.

Although IL-4 is undoubtedly the critical initiator of TH2 responses, infection of IL-4-deficient mice with the rodent gastrointestinal nematode *Nippostrongylus brasiliensis* has demonstrated the existence of an IL-4-independent pathway of TH2 development. In the absence of IL-4 it is likely that IL-13 can initiate TH2 responses. IL-13 has numerous overlapping functions with IL-4 because they can both utilize the same receptor, and both cytokines activate the transcription molecule STAT6, which is essential for their function.

Cross-regulation of TH-cell subsets

It has long been observed that immune responses to infections such as leprosy and leishmaniasis can fall into two distinct patterns corresponding to TH1 or TH2 responses. In cases of infection with intracellular parasites, these two response patterns correlate with good and poor prognosis, respectively. TH1- and TH2-type immune responses demonstrate tight cross-regulation, such that the initiation of one type of response inhibits the initiation of the other. This cross-regulation has provided the explanation for the mutually exclusive nature of immune responses to leprosy and leishmaniasis.

IL-10 and TGF-β decrease both TH1- and TH2-type responses during parasite infection

IL-10 is often considered a TH2 cytokine because it can be produced by TH2 cells and inhibits TH1 responses. In addition, the production of IL-10 early in an immune response will promote the development of TH2 responses by suppressing the TH1 response. However, it is becoming increasingly apparent that IL-10 can be produced by a large variety of cells, including the regulatory subpopulation of TH cells, and is a potent negative regulator of both TH1 and TH2 responses. This regulatory activity may be partly due to its ability to inhibit antigen-presenting cell function. This may be particularly important in the context of parasitic diseases where suppression of inflammatory responses is essential to prevent the damage associated with chronic infection.

The production of IL-10 has been observed during many parasitic infections and can play a critical role in disease outcome. Macrophages activated during infection with a protozoan parasite have the capacity to kill the parasite, but those same macrophages can trigger a potent inflammatory response that is damaging to the surrounding host tissue. The role that IL-10 plays in maintaining this critical balance between disease and protection is illustrated in mouse models of *T. gondii* infection. The production of IL-10 early in infection diminishes the effectiveness of IFN-γ-mediated macrophage activation and allows the parasite to survive and establish a chronic infection. However, IL-10-deficient mice, although effectively able to kill the parasite, die from an overwhelming inflammatory response to infection. Thus, the outcome of a parasitic infection might be governed not only by whether a certain cytokine is produced, but perhaps also by the timing of the cytokine's expression.

Both human and murine studies of helminth infection strongly suggest that IL-10 is important to prevent tissue damage associated with the chronic nature of these infections. In individuals infected with the filarial parasites that cause elephantiasis and river blindness, the production of IL-10 is correlated both with higher infection levels and reduced disease manifestations. In schistosomiasis, chronic disease is associated with granulomas that form around the parasite eggs. These granulomas contain large numbers of macrophages and eosinophils and though largely mediated by TH2 cells, TH1-type responses can contribute to the tissue destruction. Murine models have demonstrated that IL-10 downregulates both IL-5 and IFN-γ, significantly reducing liver damage associated with the granuloma.

Transforming growth factor β (TGF-β), a cytokine produced by activated monocytes, regulatory T cells, and other inflammatory cells, also has the capacity to reduce certain TH1 responses and can act synergistically with IL-10 to inhibit macrophage effector functions. In malaria infection, tissue damage and disease are associated with the overproduction of proinflammatory cytokines such as tumor necrosis factor alpha (TNF-α). In contrast, severity of disease is inversely correlated with TGF-β, and this cytokine appears to be essential to prevent severe immunopathology. As with IL-10, TGF-β helps maintain the balance between protection and disease. There is also evidence that parasites induce the production of TGF-β to promote their own survival.

Both IL-10 and TGF-β can be produced by antigen-specific T cells that do not produce TH1 or TH2 cytokines. These cells, termed regulatory T cells or sometimes TH3 cells, are likely to be critical components in the controlled suppression of immune responses during chronic infection with both intracellular and extracellular parasites.

TH-Cell Subsets Control Disease Outcome in Leishmaniasis

Cytokine profile analysis has demonstrated that the poor cell-mediated response and high levels of antibody frequently observed during *Leishmania* infection result from activation of the TH2 subset. In contrast, a high degree of cell-mediated immunity, associated with very strong delayed-type hypersensitivity reactions (see Fig. 16.9) and parasite clearance, is due to TH1-derived cytokines.

The direct roles of IFN-γ and IL-4 in disease resolution and progression, respectively, have been demonstrated by experiments in which animals were treated with blocking antibodies directed to these cytokines. BALB/c mice are highly susceptible to *Leishmania* infection because of their propensity to mount a nonprotective TH2 response to this pathogen. BALB/c mice, however, can resolve *Leishmania* infection if they are treated with antibodies to IL-4 at the time of infection. C57BL/6 mice naturally mount a protective TH1 response to *Leishmania*, and the protective response of these mice can be ablated by the administration of blocking antibody to IFN-γ within the first 10 days of infection (Fig. 20.9). Protection also is conferred by the adoptive transfer of *Leishmania*-specific TH1 cells, whereas transfer of TH2 cells exacerbates disease. IL-4 mediates disease progression by directly inhibiting the activation of macrophages by IFN-γ and by directing the differentiation of *Leishmania*-specific T cells into the TH2 phenotype. These TH2 cells produce IL-10, which acts synergistically with IL-4 in blocking IFN-γ production by TH1 cells. The murine *Leishmania* model provides the most vivid illustration of the cross-regulatory properties of TH-cell subsets and continues to provide an ideal model to investigate the factors that regulate TH1 and TH2 cell differentiation in vivo.

It is important to note that although the murine model of leishmaniasis presents a clear-cut case for the beneficial effects of TH1 cytokines, excessive TH1 responses (or TH2 responses) can be problematic for the infected individual, as is apparent in human cases of leishmaniasis—individuals who generate strong antiparasitic cell-mediated responses can develop disfiguring lesions at the site of infection. Thus, the delicate balance between protection and disease is repeatedly illustrated in the study of parasitic infection.

TH2 Responses Control Infection with Intestinal Nematodes

The dramatic induction of TH2-derived responses during helminthic infection is likely to represent a mechanism that has evolved to control infection with multicellular parasites. In the case of intestinal nematode infections, it

is evident that TH2-derived responses are critical for elimination of worms from the gut. This was first demonstrated with *Trichuris muris*, a cecal parasite of the mouse that serves as a model for human infection with the whipworm *Trichuris trichiura*. *Trichuris* develops entirely within the gut without a tissue-migrating phase or intermediate host (Fig. 20.6). Most inbred strains of mice infected with *Trichuris* are resistant to infection and expel the parasite before adult worms become established in the intestine. Some strains, however, are not capable of expelling the parasite and harbor long-term chronic infections. In vitro cytokine analyses of the lymph nodes draining the gut demonstrate a direct correlation between the expansion of TH2 cells and the elimination of the parasite. In vivo, mice that are normally susceptible to infection become resistant if they are depleted of IFN-γ. In addition, mice that are normally resistant to infection become susceptible if they are given antibodies that block IL-4 function (Fig. 20.10). Thus, in contrast to leishmaniasis, TH2 responses in trichuriasis are associated with parasite

Figure 20.10 Murine *Trichuris* model. Experimental infection with the intestinal helminth *T. muris* provides a clear example of the ability of TH2 cells to mediate disease resolution. By 20 days postinfection, resistant BALB.K mice have expelled all the worms from the gut (**top right**). In contrast, the susceptible B10.BR mice establish a chronic infection and are incapable of expelling worms at any time point (**top left**). A strikingly different pattern of cytokine secretion is seen in these two strains. The resistant mice produce high levels of TH2 cytokines, which are detectable when parasites are cleared from the intestine. The susceptible mice produce low levels of TH2 cytokines but high levels of the TH1 cytokine IFN-γ soon after infection. Antibodies that block IL-4 cause BALB.K mice to establish chronic worm infection (**bottom right**), while antibodies that block IFN-γ help B10.BR mice to expel the worms (**bottom left**).

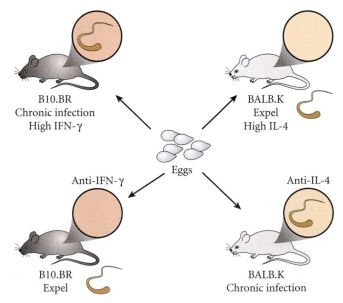

B10.BR
Chronic infection
High IFN-γ

BALB.K
Expel
High IL-4

Anti-IFN-γ

Eggs

Anti-IL-4

B10.BR
Expel

BALB.K
Chronic infection

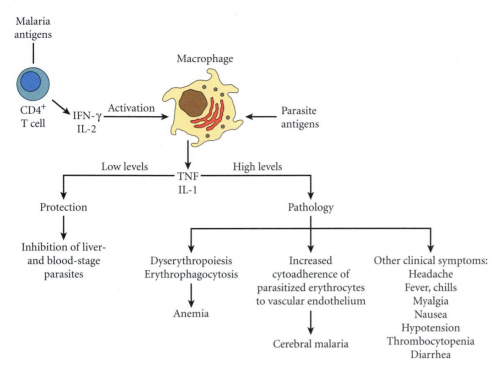

Figure 20.11 TNF and severe malaria. Large quantities of IL-1 and TNF believed to be important in pathogenesis are produced in people infected with *P. falciparum*. These cytokines, when administered exogenously, can reproduce the fever and nonspecific symptoms of malaria in humans. Overproduction of TNF is thought to be responsible for many of the life-threatening and severe pathologies associated with complicated malaria, including high fevers, hypoglycemia, and cerebral malaria. RBCs parasitized by *P. falciparum* adhere to small venule endothelial cells, causing microvascular occlusion. Parasites sequestered in brain vessels may stimulate local production of high levels of IL-1 and TNF. NO produced by cerebral endothelium in response to high levels of IL-1 and/or TNF may be directly responsible for neurologic symptoms of malaria by interfering with neurotransmission. Adapted from Fig. 14.3 (p. 317) of K. S. Warren (ed.), *Immunology and Molecular Biology of Parasitic Infection* (Blackwell Science, Boston, Mass., 1993).

elimination, whereas TH1 responses are associated with disease exacerbation. *T. muris* provided the first clear-cut example of the requirement for TH2-type responses in mediating protection. These studies have been extended to several other intestinal nematodes, and the requirement for TH2-type responses in worm expulsion is a universal feature of nematode species that inhabit the gut. However, the specific TH2 cytokines that are needed (i.e., IL-4, IL-5, IL-9, or IL-13) differ significantly and reflect the distinct effector mechanisms that mediate expulsion of different parasite species. This emphasizes that different types of immune response (TH1 or TH2) are better suited to combating different infectious agents.

The Interplay between TH1 and TH2 Responses during Parasitic Infection

Although murine models of leishmaniasis and the intestinal nematode infections provide striking examples of the importance of polarized TH-cell responses in disease outcome, the functional roles of TH1 and TH2 in many parasitic infections are considerably more complex.

Malaria

Immunity to falciparum malaria is very slow to develop; however, it appears that immunity to disease can develop more rapidly than immunity to infection. Studies with mice and humans suggest that responses mediated by both TH1 and TH2 cells play different but equally critical roles in controlling infection and disease. Immunity to the sporozoites that are injected by the mosquito is mediated by antibody that prevents infection of the hepatocytes, while CD8[+] cells can destroy the parasite once they have entered the liver cells. Production of IFN-γ by the CD8 cells, rather than direct lytic activity, is responsible for controlling parasite replication. It is also likely that IFN-γ-producing CD4[+] TH1 cells are important in controlling the liver stage of infection. However, the erythrocytic cycle of the malaria parasites commands the most attention. At this stage, exponential growth of the parasite takes place and the symptoms of disease accompanying infection occur. At this stage of infection, TH1 cells produce proinflammatory cytokines that promote macrophage activation and the destruction of infected red blood cells (RBCs). In addition, as the infection progresses, TH2 cells drive the production of specific antibody, which blocks reinvasion of more RBCs, mediates destruction of infected RBCs through complement activation, and enhances uptake by macrophages through Fc receptors.

In *P. falciparum* infection, the overproduction of TH1-type cytokines, although important in parasite control, is associated with the life-threatening complications of cerebral malaria (Fig. 20.11). Cerebral malaria was originally thought to occur because parasitized RBCs adhere to the vasculature of the brain and cause physical blockages that limit oxygen supply. Although parasite adherence is certainly an important factor in generating tissue damage, it is now believed that parasite sequestration in the brain leads to the production and release of proinflammatory cytokines. TNF-α appears to be the critical cytokine in mediating development of brain lesions and, not surprisingly, IL-10 is essential for preventing more severe damage to the brain tissue.

Schistosomiasis

Although high levels of IgE and eosinophils are key features of schistosomiasis in both humans and animals, their role in acquired immunity is not clear, and it has been difficult to demonstrate that these responses provide a benefit to the host. Studies of human populations and some in vitro experiments suggest that IgE and eosinophils are important for killing the parasites and protecting the host from disease. In contrast, studies of mice suggest that these responses are not relevant to parasite clearance and that TH1-derived cytokines are more important in the establishment of protective immunity. This highlights the complexity of the host-parasite interaction and demonstrates the difficulties in interpreting observations made in animal studies as they apply to human disease.

IgE and eosinophils may be protective in human infection

In vitro, schistosome-specific IgE, when combined with eosinophils, can kill larval schistosomes via ADCC, but whether this is also true in vivo is not known. Population-based epidemiologic studies, conducted in Africa, of reinfection with *S. haematobium* have shown a strong association between high levels of parasite-specific IgE and resistance to reinfection. Levels of IgE specific for adult worm antigens were low in children, who were readily reinfected, but high in adults, who remained uninfected. These studies controlled for differences in exposure to water, where exposure to the infective cercariae occurs. The TH2 cytokine IL-4 increases the synthesis of IgE, whereas the TH1 cytokine IFN-γ decreases its production. People who are exposed to *S. haematobium* but remain uninfected produce more IL-4, while infected individuals produce more IFN-γ in response to parasite antigen. In addition, IL-5, which is critical for the generation of eosinophilia, is produced in larger quantities by individuals who are resistant to reinfection.

TH1 responses to schistosome larvae are protective in mice

Studies of mice infected with *S. mansoni* have demonstrated that there is an initial TH1 or TH0 cytokine response early in infection, followed much later by a TH2-type response that occurs only after the worms have reached sexual maturity. When naive mice are given a single immunization with irradiated schistosome larvae, they develop a high level of resistance to a subsequent challenge infection. The attenuated larvae migrate to local lymph nodes, some getting as far as the lung, but do not progress to adulthood and egg production. The cytokine response elicited by the irradiated larvae is predominantly TH1-like. When these immunized mice are challenged with a natural infection, the incoming parasites are rapidly killed in the lung. In vivo studies with neutralizing antibody have shown that the protective immune response is dependent on IFN-γ. If mice infected with *S. mansoni* are treated with neutralizing antibodies to IL-4 and IL-5, their previously high blood levels of IgE and eosinophils drop to background levels, but the mice are still resistant to reinfection. Therefore, in direct contrast to epidemiologic studies of humans, it appears that in the mouse model TH1 responses are critical for control of infection, whereas the development of TH2 responses is ineffective in or irrelevant to such protection. It is important to recognize that mice do not express the high-affinity Fc receptor for IgE on eosinophils and thus the data from mice may not be directly relevant to the situation in humans. However, it illustrates that the induction of TH1-type responses can confer protection to incoming schistosome larvae. Because TH2 responses induce the lesions associated with infection, vaccination strategies that target a protective TH1 response may be worth consideration.

Disease in schistosomiasis is due to a TH2-directed granulomatous response to worm egg antigens

Disease following schistosome infection results from the host inflammatory response to the parasite eggs and consists of a TH-cell-dependent granuloma surrounding the egg. The granuloma consists of T cells, B cells, macrophages, fibroblasts, and a large number of eosinophils. In experimental mouse models, the intensity of the granulomatous inflammation peaks at 7 to 8 weeks and then subsides, with shrinkage of egg granulomas. Early responses to the egg antigens are of both the TH1 type and TH2 type (Fig. 20.12A), with a subsequent shift to a long-lasting TH2 response (Fig. 20.12B). The importance of the TH2-type responses in causing egg-associated tissue damage is demonstrated in studies in which treatment of mice with the TH1-driving cytokine IL-12 diminishes severity of the disease. Paradoxically, other evidence suggests that IL-10 produced by TH2 cells, B cells, and macrophages during granuloma formation is the major factor in the reduction of the granuloma size and associated pathology. IL-10

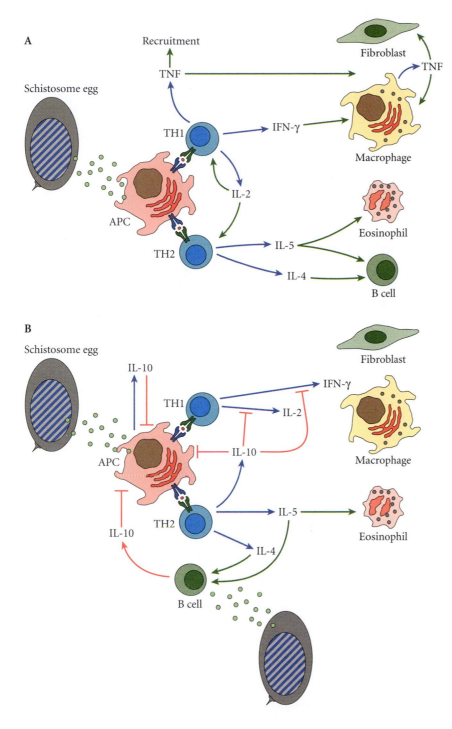

Figure 20.12 TH1/TH2-cell differentiation induced by *S. mansoni* eggs. The protective TH2 pattern of cytokine secretion in schistosomiasis begins only when the adult worms start to deposit eggs. However, the immune response that generates the egg granuloma is highly complex and involves a dynamic interplay between TH-cell subsets and a variety of inflammatory cells, including both activated macrophages and eosinophils. (**A**) The T-cell-dependent inflammatory response to the eggs is initially a mixed TH1 and TH2 response. TNF-α produced by both egg-specific T cells and macrophages recruited into the site is a key cytokine in the full development of the egg granuloma. (**B**) With time the overall inflammatory response subsides and the granuloma becomes fully TH2 mediated. Slow release of soluble egg antigens may be responsible for the shift to TH2 responses. Among these antigens are the Lewis^x trisaccharide, which stimulates (red arrow) a specific subset of B cells to proliferate and produce large quantities of IL-10. IL-10 can downregulate the expression of costimulatory molecules on antigen-presenting cells (APCs) and is the cytokine most responsible for the downmodulation of granuloma size that occurs over time.

reduces the expression of the costimulatory molecules CD80 and CD86 on the local macrophages. Presentation of egg antigens in the absence of these CD28 costimulatory molecules leads to T-cell anergy, thus reducing the intensity of the inflammatory response generated against egg antigens.

It is now known that schistosome eggs can drive the immune response dramatically toward the production of TH2 cytokines. The potency of this TH2 stimulus is demonstrated by the *bystander effect* of immunization with schistosome eggs. An antigen that normally elicits TH1 cytokines following immunization will instead elicit TH2 responses, such as specific IgE, if coinjected with schistosome eggs. Schistosome eggs can also decrease existing TH1 responses. Glycoproteins present on the schistosome egg surface are the most immunoreactive components of the schistosome egg surface. Oligosaccharides derived from these egg glycoproteins contain the Lewis^x trisaccharide, which stimulates large quantities of host IL-10. The Lewis^x trisaccharide and related structures are expressed by other pathogens as well as by certain metastatic tumors that are known to elicit high levels of IL-10.

Immune Effectors in Parasitic Infections

Macrophages and Nitric Oxide Are Critical for Parasite Killing

The macrophage is the most important cytokine-activated cell in the control and elimination of parasites. Nitric oxide (NO) appears to be the main mechanism by which macrophages kill parasites. NO-related products produced by activated macrophages (see Table 2.1) are cytotoxic or cytostatic for malaria parasites, *Leishmania*, *T. cruzi*, *Toxoplasma*, schistosomes, and the pathogenic fungus *Cryptococcus neoformans*. IFN-γ is an important cytokine in this respect because it can activate the respiratory burst (see Fig. 3.5) that generates NO. Other cytokines, particularly TNF-α, can act synergistically with IFN-γ to enhance NO production by increasing the levels of the enzyme-inducible nitric oxide synthase (iNOS). The cytokines TGF-β and IL-10 inhibit NO production by macrophages.

The murine leishmaniasis model most clearly illustrates the importance of NO production in the control of parasite infection. Mice with targeted disruptions of the gene for IFN-γ or its receptor cannot control replication of *Leishmania* and succumb to a fatal infection (Fig. 20.9). Macrophages from these knockout mice are unable to produce NO. Similarly, mice with a targeted disruption of the iNOS gene still develop a strong TH1 response to *L. major*, with high levels of IFN-γ and low levels of IL-4, but are highly susceptible to infection compared with highly resistant wild-type control animals. Finally, in normally resistant wild-type mice, the administration of drugs that block the NO production also permits unrestricted parasite growth. Collectively, these experiments demonstrate that IFN-γ is required to control *Leishmania* infection because of its ability to induce NO production by macrophages.

The NO pathway is also important in the killing of extracellular helminths. Larval stages of most helminth parasites can be killed in vitro by IFN-γ-activated macrophages. Many parasites including filarial nematodes have evolved numerous strategies to counter oxidative attack, suggesting this is an important means of immune attack

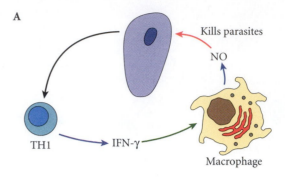

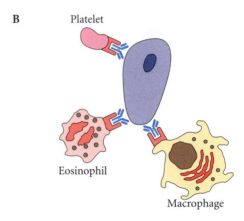

Figure 20.13 Immune effector mechanisms involved in killing of schistosome larvae. (**A**) Direct killing by cytokine-activated macrophages. In the mouse model, infective schistosome larvae (schistosomulae) induce an initial TH1 response with secretion of IFN-γ, which activates macrophages to produce NO, which in turn kills the parasites. (**B**) In ADCC, a foreign organism is coated by specific antibody, which then binds effector cells that kill the pathogen. In vitro, schistosomulae of *S. mansoni* can be killed by a combination of eosinophils and antibodies from infected patients. IgE antibodies promote this reaction by binding to specific Fc receptors on the eosinophil surface. Eosinophils adhering to the antibody-coated schistosomulum degranulate and release reactive oxygen intermediates and other toxins that kill the organism over about 24 hours. Platelets and macrophages possess similar cytotoxic properties in vitro. Whether ADCC plays a major role in actual clinical immunity is unknown, however, and a protective role for eosinophils or IgE in human helminthic infections in vivo is supported only by circumstantial evidence and epidemiologic studies.

in vivo. More direct evidence exists for schistosome larvae that elicit predominantly TH1 responses: macrophages activated by the TH1 cytokine environment are able to kill the larvae in an antibody-independent manner. Reactive nitrogen oxides produced by IFN-γ-activated macrophages have been implicated as the primary mechanism by which TH1 cytokines mediate this larval killing (Fig. 20.13). In mice vaccinated with irradiated larvae, a large proportion of incoming schistosome larvae are killed at the lung stage of development. The lung may be a major site of schistosome killing because TH1 cytokines induce NO production by vascular endothelial cells in this tissue.

Cytotoxic CD8⁺ T Cells Help Control Intracytoplasmic Protozoan Parasites

Cytotoxic CD8$^+$ T cells have long been recognized as the most important effector cells in the control of viral infection. As with viruses, the antigens of many intracellular protozoans (e.g., *T. cruzi*) can be processed via the endogenous antigen-presentation pathway and are therefore also potential targets for CD8$^+$ T cells. The importance of CD8$^+$ cells in *T. cruzi* infection has been demonstrated in mice that lack MHC class I molecules. These mice cannot control the growth of *T. cruzi* and, unlike normal mice, die during the acute phase of infection. Similarly, CD8$^+$ cells play a decisive role in resistance to both primary and secondary infection with *T. gondii*. In contrast, *Leishmania* parasites reside in a late endolysosomal compartment not accessible to MHC class I presentation; thus, CD8$^+$ cells are not major players in immunity to leishmaniasis.

In the case of malaria, the sporozoite enters the liver and invades hepatocytes within minutes after inoculation by the mosquito bite. Mice can be immunized against challenge with *P. falciparum* by live sporozoites that have been irradiated and hence cannot replicate. This immunity is directed at the liver stage of the malarial parasite and requires both CD8$^+$ cells and IFN-γ (Fig. 20.14). Production of NO by hepatocytes is believed to play an important role in this immunity to the liver stage of infection; indeed, it is thought that CD8$^+$ cells and IFN-γ protect the host by inducing the enzyme iNOS in the liver. Although all stages of the malaria parasite are susceptible to killing by NO, NO-mediated cytotoxicity at the liver stage is the critical mechanism of protection in mice vaccinated with irradiated sporozoites. A protective role for CD8$^+$ cells against malaria in humans has been more difficult to ascertain. However, epidemiologic evidence collected among West African children suggests that there is a correlation between the MHC class I allele HLA-B53 and protection against both cerebral malaria and severe

Figure 20.14 Immunity to the liver stages of malaria parasites. Vaccination of laboratory animals with irradiated sporozoites can provide protection against reinfection in experimental models. This immunity is T cell dependent and is due to the development of antibodies to the invading sporozoite and to cell-mediated immunity to the pre-erythrocytic liver stages (merozoites). The latter involves cytotoxic T cells that lyse the infected hepatocytes and the generation of cytokines that mediate resistance. In addition to killing directly, T cells produce IFN-γ, which inhibits growth of the parasite within the liver cells. Other lymphokines, such as IL-6, TNF, and IL-1, also inhibit intracellular development of the parasite. IL-6 can be produced directly by liver cells in response to IFN-γ, TNF, and IL-1. IL-6 and IFN-γ exert their effect on parasite development by inducing the production of NO by infected hepatocytes and by Kupffer cells (liver macrophages). These cytokines can also induce the expression of MHC class II molecules on hepatocytes, thereby allowing lysis by CD4$^+$ cells and by CD8$^+$ MHC class I-restricted cells. IL-6 along with IL-1 and TNF induces hepatocytes to release C-reactive protein (CRP), which can bind to the sporozoite and inhibit the early stages of development.

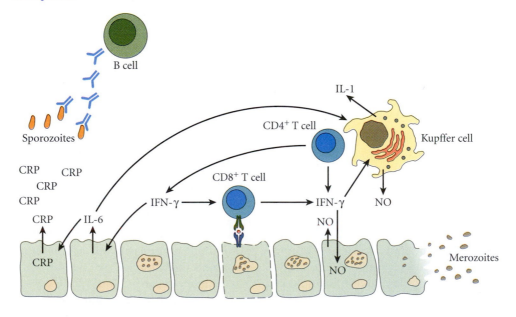

anemia. The B53 allele may exert a protective effect by presenting liver-stage parasite antigens to cytotoxic CD8$^+$ T cells.

Antibodies and Immunoglobulin Isotypes in Parasitic Infections

Neutralizing antibodies in combination with antibody-mediated activation of complement are important effectors of host defenses against bacteria and some viruses. Host antibodies to specific parasite antigens are easily detectable in most protozoan and helminthic infections. However, parasites have evolved several mechanisms to subvert antibody action and complement activation. Cell-mediated immunity, not antibody, is the dominant mode of protection against protozoan parasites, especially intracellular parasites. But antibodies are the most important mechanism of killing African trypanosomes, which are purely extracellular parasites. Antibody also can contribute to the control of infection with intracellular parasites by acting on extracellular stages. For example, antibody may limit invasion of liver cells by malarial parasites as well as control the erythrocytic stage of infection (Fig. 20.14). Larval schistosomes can be coated in vitro with specific IgE antibodies. Effector macrophages, eosinophils, and even platelets can then bind to the parasites through the IgE Fc receptor to facilitate cellular degranulation and killing of the worm (Fig. 20.13). This ADCC mechanism has been repeatedly demonstrated in vitro as a potential mechanism for helminth killing but has yet to be proven operative in vivo.

The roles of the individual isotypes of antibody in helminthic infections are not fully understood. IgE is the prime mediator of immediate-type hypersensitivity (allergic) reactions through its binding to the high-affinity IgE receptor on the membrane of basophils and mast cells. Highly elevated serum concentrations of IgE are characteristic of helminthic infections, yet infected individuals only rarely exhibit allergic symptoms. This may be due to the concomitant high levels of IgG4. IgG4 can form small immune complexes with parasite antigens, thus decreasing the amount of soluble parasite allergen available to the IgE-coated mast cells. These two immunoglobulin subclasses are both synthesized in response to production of IL-4 and IL-13 but are independently regulated by factors that have not yet been defined. IL-10 may play a role here as it has been shown to preferentially induce IgG4 production. IL-10 production is a common feature of chronic helminth infection, and this cytokine probably has multiple roles in preventing allergic inflammation in addition to its influence on IgG subclass.

In schistosomiasis, low worm burdens of *S. mansoni* and *S. haematobium* have been epidemiologically linked to high IgE levels, while susceptibility to high burdens is correlated with increased levels of antibody of other isotypes, particularly IgG4. IgG4 may function as a type of "blocking" antibody to compete with IgE binding to worm antigens and thus minimize damage due to IgE-mediated immunopathology. Relative susceptibility or resistance to infection may thus depend on a balance between protective IgE responses and IgG4-blocking antibodies. In the case of lymphatic filariasis, many infected individuals have no apparent symptoms but have high levels of circulating microfilariae, while others have cleared microfilariae from the bloodstream but have developed signs of chronic lymphatic disease. It is interesting that individual hosts with circulating microfilariae but few symptoms have extremely high levels of IgG4 and low levels of IgE. In contrast, this ratio of antibody isotypes is reversed in elephantiasis, a major clinical manifestation of lymphatic filariasis. The fact that individuals who develop elephantiasis have a low burden of microfilariae suggests that the IgE response, not the parasitic organism, is playing a causal role in the lymphatic immunopathology which is characteristic of this chronic infection (Fig. 20.15).

Mast Cells and Goblet Cells in Intestinal Nematode Infection

Although it has been established that TH2 cytokines are required for the expulsion of nematodes from the gut, it has been more difficult to define the effector cells on which these cytokines act. It is now apparent that multiple TH2-cell-driven effector pathways exist in the intestine and that parasites vary in their susceptibility to particular host defense mechanisms. Our knowledge of TH2 cytokines suggested that the key effectors would be antibody, eosinophils, and mast cells. Surprisingly, in experimental model systems, neither eosinophils nor antibodies have proven necessary. However, in some infections, (e.g., *Trichinella spiralis*) antibody is required for the more rapid expulsion of parasites sometimes observed upon secondary infection.

The mucosal mast cell is critical for the expulsion of some (e.g., *Strongyloides* spp. and *Trichinella*) but not other (e.g., *Trichuris* and *Nippostrongylus*) intestinal nematodes. Mast cells bind IgE to their surfaces via the high-affinity FcεR, and the dramatic increase in IgE levels following infection with gut nematodes may be an important part of parasite-directed mast-cell degranulation and mediator release. Besides the usual toxic effect that these mediators would have on any pathogenic organism, they also trigger gut motility and the production

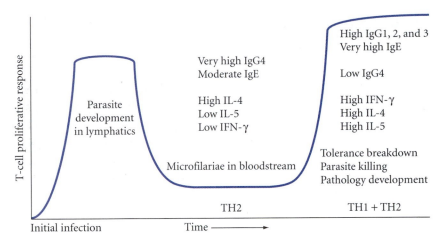

Figure 20.15 Cytokine and antibody profiles during lymphatic filariasis. Lymphatic filariasis presents as a wide spectrum of clinical situations in different patients, ranging from individuals with a high number of parasites but few clinical symptoms to those with chronic disease but few detectable parasites. The nature of the immune response in these individuals is equally diverse. Following infection with filarial nematodes, early immune responses are consistent with a TH1 profile. However, with the appearance of parasite microfilariae in the bloodstream, TH2 cytokines become dominant, with a rapid disappearance of T-cell proliferative responses and a striking increase in synthesis of parasite-specific IgG4. The induction of T-cell tolerance to the parasite is most apparent in the TH1 subset. In individuals with developed disease, this tolerance is broken, and responses of both the TH1 and TH2 types increase dramatically. Thus, both increased cell-mediated responses and extremely high levels of serum IgE have been implicated in pathogenesis. However, it should also be noted that both TH1 and TH2 responses to filarial antigens are present in individuals who are immune to reinfection; therefore, both types of TH response may be important in host protection as well as pathogenesis. Redrawn from Maizels and Lawrence, *Parasitol. Today* 7:271–275, 1992, with permission.

of mucin glycoprotein by intestinal goblet cells. Hypersecretion of mucus may block mucosal contact and nutrient uptake by the parasite. This increase in fluid secretion in combination with increased peristalsis may be sufficient to flush out the worm.

In the absence of mast cells, similar effects on gut physiology can occur. Interestingly, expulsion of another gut nematode, *N. brasiliensis*, does not require mast cells and is more dependent on IL-13 production than IL-4 levels. This is apparently due to the fact that IL-13 is a potent inducer of goblet cell hyperplasia and suggests that mucin secretion is a key component in expelling *N. brasiliensis*. Importantly, IL-4, when injected directly into mice, is able to induce gut motility and fluid secretion. These apparently direct effects of TH2 cytokines on gut physiology may explain why some parasites can be expelled in the absence of mast cells.

Eosinophils

Eosinophilia is a universal feature of infection with helminths, and it has long been assumed that these potent cytotoxic cells are important in mediating destruction of large multicellular pathogens. Surprisingly, however, there is little evidence to support a role for eosinophils in mediating expulsion of gut parasites. There is considerably greater evidence to suggest that

eosinophils can fulfill their cytolytic function on larval stages of parasites that migrate through the tissues. This has been most evident in vaccination studies, in which eosinophils, probably by binding specific antibody through their Fc receptors, seem to be capable of destroying the incoming larvae of a challenge infection. Eosinophils may also be a critical part of the aggressive innate response directed against parasitic larvae that are entering a host for which they are not adapted. Parasites that have coevolved with a particular mammalian host will have developed mechanisms to avoid or circumvent this response to establish infection.

Immune Evasion by Parasites

Parasites have evolved a variety of sophisticated mechanisms to evade effective host immune responses (Table 20.3). Seclusion within a host cell can render intracellular pathogens inaccessible to immune surveillance. Many parasites produce molecules that inhibit nonspecific host effector mechanisms such as complement. Parasites also may shield themselves with host-derived molecules or display an ever-changing repertoire of surface antigens to elude antibody-mediated destruction. Perhaps most importantly, parasites can induce host cells to take on an immunosuppressive role.

Table 20.3 Some mechanisms of parasite immune evasion

Mechanism	Parasite example(s)
Antigenic variation	*Trypanosoma brucei* *Plasmodium* merozoites
Evasion from macrophages	
Prevention of lysosome- phagosome action	*Toxoplasma gondii*
Prevention of lysosomal toxic action	*Leishmania* amastigotes
Escape into cytoplasm	*Trypanosoma cruzi*
Resistance to complement lysis	*Leishmania, T. brucei,* *T. cruzi, Taenia solium*
Immune suppression	Filariae
Surface and secreted antioxidant enzymes	Parasitic nematodes, schistosomes

Intracellular Parasitism: Seclusion from the Immune System

Infection of and replication within host cells allow intracellular protozoan parasites to avoid many of the immune defense mechanisms of the host, particularly the combined effects of antibody and complement. Paradoxically, many of these parasites reside in macrophages, the professional phagocyte specialized to kill foreign organisms. Different protozoans have evolved independent strategies to avoid destruction within the cell.

Leishmania promastigotes (inoculated into the mammalian host following an infective sand fly bite) activate serum complement and become opsonized with C3b. This coating of C3b triggers the uptake of the promastigotes into the macrophage without triggering the cell's respiratory burst. The phagosome containing the parasite fuses with the lysosome to form a late endolysosomal compartment. To survive within this hostile environment, the parasite produces antioxidant enzymes and inhibitors of lysosomal enzymes.

T. gondii infects not only macrophages but also many other cell types in an uptake process actively controlled by this protozoan. Unlike *Leishmania*, *Toxoplasma* parasites avoid destruction by preventing fusion of the phagosome with the lysosome and live permanently in a unique parasitophorous vacuole, a specialized structure within the cytoplasm that is entirely segregated from the endocytic system of the host cell. The parasite thereby avoids exposure to lysosomal enzymes and an acidic environment.

T. cruzi, the causative agent of Chagas' disease, can invade a variety of cell types at the site of the bite of the reduviid triatomid bug. Unlike most intracellular bacteria or protozoa that enter the host cell by classical phagocytosis, the infective trypomastigote of *T. cruzi* enters by a distinct mechanism. The trypomastigote attaches to the surface of the host cell, then triggers a calcium-dependent clustering of lysosomes at that site of attachment, after which it rapidly fuses with the lysosome and enters the cell. Within hours the vacuole around the parasite is lysed and *T. cruzi* escapes into the cytoplasm, thereby avoiding destruction by lysosomes. Inside the cytoplasm the amastigote stage replicates before transformation into trypomastigotes, which are released by the cell into the bloodstream to infect more cells.

All helminthic parasites of humans live in extracellular spaces, with one notable exception: *T. spiralis*. Larvae migrate from the gut, through the bloodstream to the periphery, where they penetrate striated (skeletal) muscle cells. The *Trichinella* larva radically transforms the muscle cell into a specialized nurse cell that protects and provides nutrients for the parasite. Larvae survive in the nurse cells for the lifetime of the host, awaiting transmission to the next carnivorous host.

Parasites Produce Antioxidant Enzymes

Oxygen radicals exist as natural by-products of aerobic existence, and mammalian tissues contain oxygen-scavenging enzymes for protection against the damaging effects of these molecules. Activated leukocytes, including eosinophils, neutrophils, macrophages, and platelets, produce hydrogen peroxide, superoxide ions, and hydroxyl radicals that are toxic to pathogens. Parasites, in turn, use their own oxygen-scavenging enzymes to protect themselves from host attack and generally contain far higher concentrations of these enzymes than does the surrounding host tissue. The major antioxidant enzymes are superoxide dismutase, catalase, and glutathione peroxidase. Superoxide dismutase is the most widely studied and is produced in extraordinarily large amounts by some parasites. All protozoan and helminth parasites examined so far contain at least one of these antioxidant enzymes.

Parasites Survive by Interfering with the Complement Cascade

Leishmania promastigotes are completely covered by a carbohydrate-rich surface known as a glycocalyx that is largely composed of lipophosphoglycan (LPG) containing repeating disaccharide units that increase in number during the development of the parasite in the insect. This elongated LPG binds complement, thereby assisting in the directed entry of the parasite into macrophages via complement receptors expressed on the macrophage plasma membrane. At the same time, the parasite avoids complement-mediated cell damage by virtue of the extreme length of the LPG polymer: the lytic C5b-9 complex forms too far away from the parasite membranes to cause significant damage.

Stages of *T. cruzi* parasites that live within the mammalian host are resistant to complement-mediated lysis. Amastigotes are protected from the lytic C5b-9 complex by virtue of their intracellular location, whereas the bloodstream trypomastigotes prevent assembly of the complement cascade-amplifying enzyme C3 convertase by expressing a molecule analogous to mammalian decay-accelerating factor (DAF), which blocks assembly and accelerates the decay of C3 convertase (see Fig. 5.15). Schistosome larvae accomplish the same ends by acquiring DAF directly from human erythrocytes. Schistosomes insert the host DAF into their surfaces by adsorbing the lipid anchor of DAF into their own outer lipid bilayer in quantities sufficient to inhibit complement-dependent damage.

Infestation of the central nervous system with the tissue cyst of *Taenia solium*, the pig tapeworm, can cause seizures and other serious neurologic symptoms. This helminth produces factors that inhibit complement pathways, as well as sulfated carbohydrates that activate complement at a great distance from the parasite. Paramyosin, produced by *T. solium,* prevents initiation of the classical complement pathway by inhibiting complement component C1. Paramyosin has been isolated from numerous helminthic parasites and has potential as a vaccine candidate.

Antigenic Variation

There are many examples of antigenic variation by a pathogen as a mechanism for avoiding an effective host immune response. However, none is as dramatic as that of *T. brucei*, the protozoan agent that causes African sleeping sickness. The entire surface of this hemoflagellate parasite is covered with a dense protein coat that consists of a single antigen known as the variant surface glycoprotein (VSG). In 1910, R. Ross and D. Thomson noted that there were regular fluctuations in the number of bloodstream parasites, corresponding to febrile episodes in patients suffering from sleeping sickness (Fig. 20.16). It is now known that each wave of parasitemia comprises primarily a clonal population of parasites expressing a single VSG. The parasitemia declines when the host immune response (in the form of antibodies to the current VSG) destroys this group of parasites. However, a parasite with a new VSG on its surface, which is not susceptible to antibody clearance, replaces the previous population of parasites. Each parasite contains nearly 1,000 genes encoding different variants of VSG and through an elaborate mechanism of regulation and translocation, these genes are activated one at a time to effect antigenic variation. Gene switching occurs at low spontaneous rate, and thus at any one time point there will be a parasite that can escape (at least temporarily) recognition by the immune system.

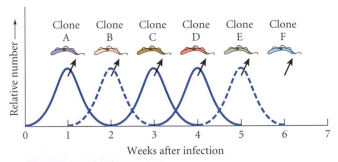

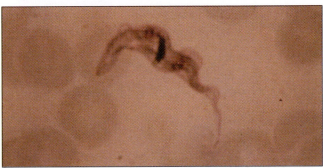

Figure 20.16 Antigenic variation in African trypanosomes. African trypanosomiasis (sleeping sickness) is characterized by successive waves of parasite proliferation in the bloodstream, the result of antigenic variation in the parasite population. The peaks of parasitemia are observed in mice infected experimentally with a single clone of *T. brucei* as well as in natural infections in humans. Each wave is due to a new antigenic variant of the parasite (e.g., clone A, B, or C) that expresses a new VSG. Each decline is a result of a specific antibody response to that VSG. A few individual trypanosomes survive by expressing a different VSG, thus giving rise to a new wave of clonal parasites. The photo is of a blood smear showing a trypanosome.

Of the four species of *Plasmodium* that cause human disease, *P. falciparum* is responsible for nearly all of the mortality attributable to malaria. Erythrocytes infected with maturing *P. falciparum* trophozoites adhere to microvascular endothelial cells and disappear from the peripheral circulation. Such retention in vascular beds allows the parasite, safely sequestered within the RBC, to escape destruction by the spleen, which usually removes abnormal erythrocytes from the circulation. Furthermore, cytoadherence of parasitized erythrocytes to cerebral blood vessels contributes to the life-threatening complication of cerebral malaria. It is now known that *P. falciparum* secretes a large protein, known as PfEMP1 (*P. falciparum* erythrocyte membrane protein 1), that forms knob-like structures on the surface of the erythrocyte membrane and mediates the binding of the infected RBC to a variety of endothelial surface receptors (Fig. 20.17). Infected individuals respond to a given malarial infection by producing isolate-specific antibodies to the parasite-derived proteins on the surface of the erythrocyte. However, like the trypanosome VSG family, the PfEMP1

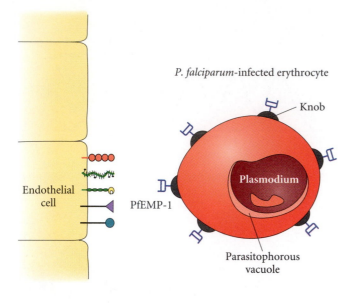

P. falciparum-infected erythrocyte

Knob

Plasmodium

PfEMP-1

Endothelial cell

Parasitophorous vacuole

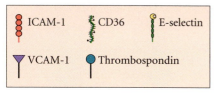

ICAM-1   CD36   E-selectin

VCAM-1   Thrombospondin

Figure 20.17 *P. falciparum* erythrocyte membrane proteins (PfEMP1) mediate both antigenic variation and cytoadherence in *P. falciparum* malaria. Erythrocytes parasitized by *P. falciparum* express a variant antigen from the PfEMP1 family, which is concentrated on surface knobs and mediates attachment of the infected erythrocyte to the vascular endothelium. Different PfEMP1 proteins likely mediate binding to different endothelial cell surface receptors, including intercellular adhesion molecule 1 (ICAM-1), vascular cell adhesion molecule 1 (VCAM-1), E-selectin, CD36, and the matrix protein thrombospondin. The high frequency with which antigenic variants of PfEMP1 arise in the parasite population allow new antigenically variant malarial parasites to escape antibody-mediated immune destruction.

group of proteins display a striking degree of antigenic variation. The genes that encode these proteins (*var* genes) make up 2 to 6% of the parasite genome and switching between variants occurs at a very high rate. Emergence of new antigenic variants in the parasite population allows the infection to become chronic and explains why blood infection can be established even in previously infected individuals.

Parasites Can Exploit Host Cytokines

The most extreme means by which parasites subvert the immune system is by taking advantage of their host's cytokine regulatory network. In the case of *S. mansoni*, eggs trapped in host tissues are enveloped in a granuloma whose formation is dependent on the inflammatory cytokine TNF-α. Amazingly, adult schistosomes respond to TNF-α by dramatically increasing their egg output. The

schistosome parasite thus exploits a host immunoregulatory molecule, produced in response to infection, to enhance its own life cycle.

T. cruzi, an obligate intracellular parasite, infects most cell types by adhering to specific receptors on the membrane of host cells. However, the parasite also requires activation of the TGF-β signaling pathway before it can invade the cytoplasm of host cells. Infection with *T. cruzi* induces the expression of TGF-β by host cells. Since TGF-β typically functions as a regulatory cytokine (decreasing both TH1 and TH2 cells), this induction of TGF-β has a dual benefit for the parasite of inhibiting immune effector mechanisms and promoting the parasite's entry into the host cell. Other successful parasites can regulate the immune responses of their host by either preventing the induction of the appropriate proinflammatory cytokines or by inducing the production of immunosuppressive cytokines. Examples of this abound in the literature and include the ability of both *Leishmania* and *T. gondii* parasites to enter host macrophages without inducing IL-12, the capacity of schistosome egg carbohydrates to induce IL-10, and the induction of TGF-β by *Leishmania*, *T. gondii*, and *T. cruzi*.

Immunology of Fungal Infections

General Features of Fungal Infections

Fungi are eukaryotic organisms normally found in nature as free-living species that live on dead organic material. Whereas the vast majority of fungi are harmless, a small number of fungal species can cause human diseases, called mycoses, which range from relatively common superficial infections to rare but life-threatening systemic diseases, particularly in immunocompromised hosts. Although serious fungal infections are rarer than bacterial, viral, or parasitic infections, they are often very difficult to treat because of the lack of highly effective, safe antifungal drugs. One effective agent, amphotericin B, exists for the treatment of the systemic mycoses but frequently has serious adverse effects.

Fungal pathogens, although eukaryotic, differ dramatically from classical parasites. Most significantly, with the exception of some dermatophytes (fungi that cause infection of the skin), fungi are not dependent on interaction with the mammalian host for survival. Fungi are ubiquitous in nature, growing in the soil, on vegetation, and in bodies of water, and only cause disease by accidentally infecting humans. Fungi occur in two forms: as unicellular yeasts and as molds that grow in branching chains called *hyphae*. The most pathogenic fungi include molds of the genus *Aspergillus* and the dimorphic genera *Cryptococcus*

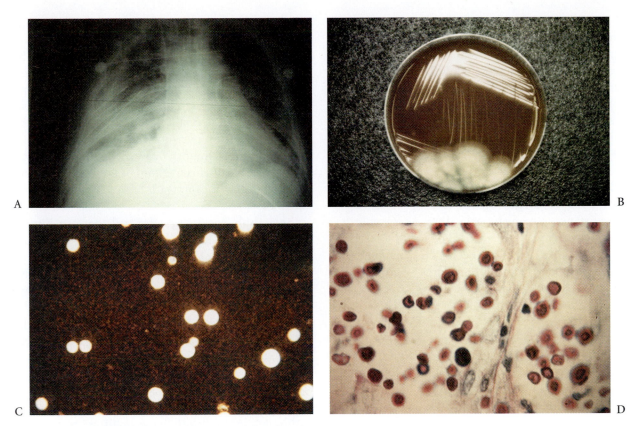

Figure 20.18 Systemic mycoses. Some fungal species grow only as molds; others grow only as yeast forms. Species that can grow in either form are known as dimorphic fungi and include many of the clinically important opportunistic fungal pathogens. Generally, these species grow in mycelial forms or as mold at room temperature but as yeast in the human body. (**A**) Invasive pulmonary aspergillosis in a patient with leukemia. (**B**) Growth of an *Aspergillus* sp. on an agar culture plate. (**C**) *C. neoformans* yeast cells in the spinal fluid of a patient with AIDS with cryptococcal meningitis. Slide is stained with India ink to highlight the yeast capsule. (**D**) Yeast cells of *C. neoformans*, stained with periodic acid-Schiff stain, in the liver of a patient with disseminated cryptococcosis. Some of the yeast cells have characteristic narrow-based buds.

and *Histoplasma*, which grow as molds in nature or on cell culture plates but are yeast-like budding cells in infected human tissue (Fig. 20.18).

Diseases caused by fungi can be classified into three clinical groups: superficial, subcutaneous, and systemic mycoses. The superficial mycoses are the most common and include infections of the skin, hair, and nails such as athlete's foot and ringworm. These dermatophyte infections are chronic, with a relatively mild localized inflammatory response. Also included in this group are infections of the mucosal surfaces with *Candida albicans*. Although *C. albicans* is normally present in the mouth, vagina, and intestinal tract, its overgrowth can occur in individuals who are immunosuppressed or undergoing antibiotic therapy. Subcutaneous mycoses are generally caused by puncture wounds and are characterized by localized abscesses. The most serious fungal infections are the systemic mycoses, including histoplasmosis,

cryptococcosis, and coccidioidomycosis, which usually begin as lung infections and are acquired by inhaling the spores of free-living fungi. Most infections are asymptomatic or cause a mild influenza-like illness but occasionally disseminate to other tissues and are invariably fatal without treatment. The systemic mycoses are far more likely to cause disseminated disease in individuals with impaired immune systems, including patients undergoing high-dose corticosteroid therapy or cancer chemotherapy and patients with AIDS. *C. albicans* also can disseminate in individuals who are iatrogenically immunosuppressed, particularly if they have chronic foreign bodies such as intravenous and indwelling catheters.

Immunity to Fungal Infections
Natural resistance to fungi
Natural or innate resistance mechanisms that do not require induction of a specific immune response are a

critical component in preventing the establishment and development of most fungal infections. These innate mechanisms, which include the physical barriers of the skin and mucous membranes, chemical factors in serum and skin secretions, and both phagocytic and nonphagocytic cells, are extremely effective in humans and are one of the reasons most fungal infections are mild or self-limiting. However, when these mechanisms prove insufficient, T-cell-mediated immune response is required for effective control.

Effector cells in fungal infections

Natural resistance to many fungal pathogens is highly dependent on the action of professional phagocytic cells. Although intracellular killing can occur, most fungi are attacked extracellularly because their large size precludes uptake by these cells. Of the phagocytic cells, neutrophils are the most effective killers of fungal organisms. They are particularly important in the control of infection with the opportunistic pathogens *Candida* and *Aspergillus*, as evidenced by the development of overwhelming infection with these pathogens in individuals who have acquired or hereditary neutrophil defects. Neutrophils are not normally present in high numbers in the tissues but are drawn to the site of infection by chemotactic factors produced directly by the fungus or by activation of complement via the alternative pathway. Fungi also can stimulate the production of cytokines such as IL-1 and TNF-α that increase the expression of adhesion molecules on the local endothelium, thereby enhancing infiltration of neutrophils to the site of infection.

Neutrophils kill fungal pathogens using both oxygen-dependent and oxygen-independent toxic mechanisms. The oxygen-dependent mechanisms involve the generation of toxic components via the oxidative burst or the release of granules containing myeloperoxidase, an enzyme involved in generating hypochlorous acid. The oxygen-independent mechanisms include serine proteases and defensins (antimicrobial peptides). Although highly effective in the destruction of most fungal pathogens, neutrophils are ineffective against some species, perhaps because of factors that are produced by yeasts that inhibit neutrophil function or, as in the case of *C. neoformans*, because the capsule surrounding the microorganism prevents binding to neutrophil receptors.

Alveolar macrophages are the first line of cellular defense against infection with inhaled spores of fungi that can cause respiratory disease. Purely opportunistic fungi such as *Aspergillus* spp. are readily destroyed by alveolar macrophages. However, *Coccidioides immitis* and *Histoplasma capsulatum*, both of which can become established in normal healthy individuals, are resistant to killing by macrophages. In the case of *C. immitis*, the infective particle is taken up by the phagocyte but is not killed because the phagosome does not fuse with the lysosome. *H. capsulatum* is a facultative intracellular fungus that can grow within the macrophage. If macrophages are not activated, they are less potent at killing fungi than are neutrophils. Thus, the role of macrophages in resistance to fungal infection is more important in acquired immunity, where they become an effective tool of the specific immune response following activation by TH1-cell-derived cytokines.

A nonphagocytic effector cell that can limit fungal growth is the NK cell. Although usually associated with the destruction of tumor cells, NK cells can act against fungi in two different ways. NK cells can kill directly by releasing cytolysin-containing granules in the vicinity of the cryptococcal cell wall, as has been shown with *C. neoformans*. They also can kill indirectly if they are stimulated by mycotic (fungus-derived) agents to produce cytokines such as TNF and IFN-γ, which activate local macrophages to kill the organism.

Acquired immunity to fungal infections

Although innate immune mechanisms are critical for the control of fungal infections, they are at times insufficient to limit the growth of fungal pathogens. In these cases, the specific arm of the immune system is required to prevent full-blown infection and life-threatening disease, as demonstrated by the increased susceptibility to fungal infection of individuals undergoing immunosuppressive therapy or individuals with AIDS. In addition, murine models of immunodeficiency have shown the importance of an intact immune system in preventing fatal disease.

Protective immunity to pathogenic fungi that can cause systemic disease is critically dependent on the interaction between pathogen-specific CD4$^+$ T cells and macrophages. There is little evidence that antibodies are a critical factor in the resolution or control of these infections. For example, during infection with *C. immitis*, the spectrum of disease states ranges from benign self-limited infection to a disseminated fulminant infection. The former is associated with strong T-cell reactivity and low levels of antibody, whereas progressive coccidioidomycosis is characterized by depressed T-cell proliferative responses and strong B-cell responses. The importance of T cells and the limited value of humoral responses have also been observed in protective immune responses elicited to other pulmonary fungal pathogens, such as *H. capsulatum*. This dichotomy is directly analogous to that of the protozoan parasite *Leishmania*, where the induction of

TH1 responses is critical for disease resolution, while TH2 responses lead to exacerbation of disease.

The role of TH1 and TH2 cytokines in disease resolution has been evaluated in murine models of candidiasis, coccidioidomycosis, and histoplasmosis. Treatment of mice with blocking antibody against IFN-γ leads to progressive infection with *C. albicans* in mice that were previously immune. In addition, mice treated with antibody to IL-4 recover from an otherwise lethal inoculum of *C. albicans*. In studies of coccidioidomycosis, mice resistant to disease produce higher levels of IFN-γ than do susceptible mice when challenged with *C. immitis*. In contrast, susceptible mice manifest predominantly an IL-4 response to infection. The protective role of IL-12 has been illustrated in murine studies with *H. capsulatum*. Naive mice require IL-12 to generate an effective immune response to *H. capsulatum* and die if given neutralizing antibody to IL-12 at the time of infection. Consistent with studies on protozoal infection, if neutralizing antibody is given later in infection, it has no effect on survival. Further, if mice are given IL-12 (or neutralizing antibody to IL-4) at the time of infection, protection is enhanced. The effects of IL-12 are directly related to its ability to induce IFN-γ as the protective effects are abrogated when mice are treated with anti-IFN-γ. These studies demonstrate the importance of TH1 activation and IFN-γ production in protective immunity and further demonstrate that the TH2 cytokine IL-4 is detrimental to the host during the course of infection.

The importance of neutrophils in antifungal immunity may go beyond their direct cytotoxic activities and may be related to their capacity to produce IL-12. Production of IL-12 by neutrophils on exposure to fungal pathogens may be a key factor in influencing the development of TH1 cells. The importance of TH1 lymphocytes lies in their ability to activate macrophages, since the latter have a poor ability to destroy yeast unless specifically activated. TH2 responses and IL-4 permit disease to progress by dampening TH1 cells and by directly preventing the activation of macrophages. Studies with *C. neoformans* have demonstrated that, as with protozoan parasites, the induction of NO is the primary killing mechanism of activated macrophages. In the case of *H. capsulatum*, the NO chelates iron, depriving the fungal pathogen of an essential nutrient.

Immunity to dermatophytes

Immunity to dermatophyte infections differs from immunity to systemic mycoses because dermatophytes are not opportunists but organisms adapted to colonization of human skin, nails, and hair and are incapable of invading living tissue. However, the specific immune response is still important in disease control, as persons with immunologic defects are the most likely to develop chronic infection. Furthermore, there is an inverse correlation between the severity of the inflammatory response to infection and the chronicity of infection. Thus, infections that result in highly inflammatory lesions are almost always self-limiting, whereas infections with little inflammation can persist for long periods. The induction of TH1 versus TH2 responses may determine the outcome of these infections as well. Individuals who generate immediate-type hypersensitivity (i.e., TH2-dependent) responses to dermatophyte antigens appear to develop chronic disease and are unable to elicit the delayed-type hypersensitivity (TH1-dependent) response seen in individuals who clear the infection.

The association of chronic dermatophytoses with atopy has led to the suggestion that dermatophyte antigens are important allergens. However, the role of fungal antigens in asthma and other serious allergic conditions remains to be clearly proven. A more clear-cut role for fungal organisms in allergic disease is illustrated by allergic bronchopulmonary aspergillosis. This disease occurs in individuals who are hypersensitive to *Aspergillus fumigatus* and have activated TH2 cells and asthma-like symptoms. Allergic bronchopulmonary aspergillosis provides another striking example of the importance of regulatory cytokines in all forms of disease whether TH1 or TH2 mediated. On exposure to *A. fumigatus*, IL-10 is responsible for reducing lung inflammation and airway hyperresponsiveness by limiting the extent of both TH1 and TH2 cell activation.

Summary

Eukaryotic parasites, including protozoa and multicellular helminthic worms, have life cycles that require residence within a host organism or organisms. Some of these parasites are intracellular, residing within host cells such as macrophages, while others are extracellular and reside in various tissues of their host such as the gut. From the standpoint of the parasite, the goal of infection is to simply survive for a period of time sufficient to allow propagation of the parasite and its transmission to additional host animals. To accomplish this goal parasites have evolved numerous elaborate strategies to circumvent or forestall their host's innate and acquired immune responses. These strategies include deliberate seclusion within the cells of their host, inactivation of immune effector molecules, and dysregulation of the host's cytokine network. Because of these numerous evasion tactics, immune responses against these parasites are seldom effective. In some cases, protective immunity can be achieved after a very long period of exposure to the parasite. In other cases, the protective immune response is nullified by antigenic variation by the parasite. These strategies employed by the parasite provide clues for what will be required of future attempts at the creation of successful vaccines.

While not strictly dependent on their human host for sustenance, fungal organisms can also parasitize human hosts and other mammals. Ubiquitous in nature, funguses are usually effectively dealt with by the host's innate and acquired immune responses and therefore present serious threats only in cases of immune compromise. Some fungal infections, however, are extremely superficial, and because of this, are frequently able to establish chronic infection because they do not elicit a potent immune response.

Suggested Reading

Beeson, J. G., and G. V. Brown. 2002. Pathogenesis of *Plasmodium falciparum* malaria: the roles of parasite adhesion and antigenic variation. *Cell. Mol. Life Sci.* **59:**258–271.

Behm, C. A., and K. S. Ovington. 2000. The role of eosinophils in parasitic helminth infections. *Parasitol. Today* **16:**202– 209.

Carruthers, V. B. 2002. Host cell invasion by the opportunistic pathogen *Toxoplasma gondii. Acta Trop.* **81:**111–122.

Claudia, M., A. Bacci, B. Silvia, R. Gaziano, A. Spreca, and L. Romani. 2002. The interaction of fungi with dendritic cells: implications for T$_H$ immunity and vaccination. *Curr. Mol. Med.* **2:**507–524.

Crameri, R., and K. Blaser. 2002. Allergy and immunity to fungal infections and colonization. *Eur. Respir. J.* **19:**151–157.

Denkers, E., and R. T. Gazzinelli. 1998. Regulation and function of T-cell-mediated immunity during *Toxoplasma gondii* infection. *Clin. Microbiol. Rev.* **11:**569–588.

Engman, D. M., and J. S. Leon. 2002. Pathogenesis of Chagas heart disease: role of autoimmunity. *Acta Trop.* **81:**123–132.

Kennedy, M. W., and W. Harnett. (ed.). 2001. *Parasitic Nematodes: Molecular Biology, Biochemistry and Immunology.* CABI Publishing, Wallingford, Oxon, United Kingdom.

Lawrence, C. E. 2003. Is there a common mechanism of gastrointestinal nematode expulsion? *Parasite Immunol.* **25:** 271–281.

Lilic, D. 2002. New perspectives on the immunology of chronic mucocutaneous candidiasis. *Curr. Opin. Infect. Dis.* **15:**143–147.

Maizels, R. M., and M. Yazdanbakhsh. 2003. Immune regulation by helminth parasites: cellular and molecular mechanisms. *Nat. Rev. Immunol.* **3:**733–744.

Malaguarnera, L., and S. Musumeci. 2002. The immune response to Plasmodium falciparum malaria. *Lancet Infect. Dis.* **2:**472–478.

Markell, E., W. A. Krotoski, and D. T. John. 1998. *Markell and Voge's Medical Parasitology,* 8th ed. W. B. Saunders and Co., Philadelphia, Pa.

Pearce, E. J., and A. S. MacDonald. 2002. The immunobiology of schistosomiasis. *Nat. Rev. Immunol.* **2:**499–511.

Rogers, K. A., G. K. DeKrey, M. L. Mbow, R. D. Gillespie, C. I. Brodskyn, and R. G. Titus. 2002. Type 1 and type 2 responses to *Leishmania major. FEMS Microbiol. Lett.* **209:**1–7.

Sacks, D., and A. Sher. 2002. Evasion of innate immunity by parasitic protozoa. *Nat. Immunol.* **3:**1041–1047.

Zambrano-Villa, S., D. Rosales-Borjas, J. C. Carrero, and L. Ortiz-Ortiz. 2002. How protozoan parasites evade the immune response. *Trends Parasitol.* **18:**272–278.

Vaccines and Vaccination

Gerald B. Pier

At the end of the 20th century, the U.S. Centers for Disease Control and Prevention cited vaccination as the number one public health achievement of that century. This surpassed reductions in motor vehicle accidents, control of infectious diseases, and the decline in deaths from cardiovascular disease, including stroke, as a public health achievement. The impact of vaccination on disease can be readily appreciated from the reductions in the occurrences of many illnesses that were rampant in the early part of the 20th century (Table 21.1). The elimination in 1977 of smallpox as a human disease must rank as one of the major achievements of modern medicine. The impending elimination of paralytic polio further emphasizes how effective vaccines can be in preventing infectious diseases. Vaccine development and production encompass many medically related activities, ranging from basic research in microbiology and immunology to pharmaceutical development to the economics of vaccine production and effectiveness. Obviously, understanding the essential role of the immune system in vaccine development dictates that immunology form a solid foundation for the advances made in vaccinology. Indeed, the success of vaccines in infectious diseases has prompted interest in this method of disease control for many diverse areas that involve immunology, including allergy, autoimmune diseases, and cancer, along with interest in using vaccines as a method of contraception or even potentially to prevent diseases such as Alzheimer's disease.

Table 21.1 Decrease in cases of vaccine-preventable diseases in the United States through 1998 as reported by the U.S. Centers for Disease Control and Prevention[a]

Disease	No. of cases		
	Baseline[b]	1998	Reduction (%)
Smallpox	48,164	0	100
Diphtheria	175,885	0	100
Pertussis	147,271	7,405	95
Tetanus	1,314	41	97.9
Paralytic polio	16,316	0	100
Measles	503,282	100	100
Mumps	152,209	666	99.6
Rubella	47,745	364	99.3
H. influenzae type b	20,000	63	99.7

[a]Reported in *Morb. Mortal. Wkly. Rep.* **48**:243–248, 1999.
[b]Baseline = 20th-century annual prevaccine infection rate.

Early and Defining Issues in Vaccine Development

The basic immunologic principle of *memory* and its role in protection against infection has been known for centuries, although the molecular and cellular factors for immunologic memory have only recently been defined. Nonetheless, writings of individuals such as Hippocrates indicated knowledge of resistance to multiple infections of the same sort. During the outbreak of pneumonic plague or "Black Death" in 14th century Europe that reportedly killed up to 33% of the population, one job that befell the survivors of plague was to retrieve and bury the bodies of individuals who had died from the disease because it was known that the survivors would not become ill again. Smallpox represented a particularly devastating human disease, and a practice now known as *variolation* was undertaken first in Asia, then later in Europe to deliberately give individuals smallpox in the hope of reducing the lethality of the disease. In this procedure, which originated in China and was used more commonly around 1700 in Europe, cotton swabs containing dried matter from smallpox lesions were placed into the nostrils as a means of preventing smallpox. Also, as smallpox lesions can be quite disfiguring, such inoculations could prevent facial disfigurement. This may have been another consideration for undertaking this somewhat dangerous practice.

One of the most famous milestones in medicine and vaccine development came in 1796, when Edward Jenner, a London physician, reported that he had inoculated an 8-year-old boy with material derived from the pus of milkmaids who had cowpox, a usually benign disease. The inoculated boy was then later challenged with material taken from an active smallpox lesion. The boy did not become ill with smallpox. Interestingly, although Jenner is given the credit for this discovery, this practice was not uncommon in the English farmlands of the 18th century. A farmer named Benjamin Jesty noticed around 1774 that smallpox did not "take" in farm workers who had cowpox, and he therefore inoculated his wife and daughters with lesions containing cowpox (although no deliberate challenge was used here). This observation motivated Jenner to carry out his experiment. Jenner did communicate his finding to the physicians of his day, prompting the adoption of cowpox inoculation as a means of preventing smallpox, although at the time, the concept of a virus, antibody, or other immunologic effector had not yet been developed. Jesty was eventually recognized by the British government, but well after Jenner had described his experiment and gained considerable fame from it.

While vaccination against smallpox grew in the 19th century, with some cities, such as New York, developing the beginnings of a public health infrastructure with requirements for vaccination, true advances did not come until the last quarter of the 19th century with the discovery of microbial causes of infectious diseases and the fundamental molecules of the immune system. Louis Pasteur in Paris found that he could use weakened strains of microorganisms to prevent diseases, demonstrating this principle for anthrax in cattle and rabies in humans. Emil Adolf von Behring and Shibasaburo Kitasato were able to use new information about microbiology and immunology to develop serum therapy for diphtheria. In the early part of the 20th century, vaccines for tetanus and diphtheria were developed, as were serotherapies for many other infectious diseases. One of the pioneering advances was the production of specific antisera against the agent of pneumococcal pneumonia (*Streptococcus pneumoniae*), which allowed Maxwell Finland, generally regarded as the father of modern infectious disease practice, to treat patients at Boston City Hospital in the pre-antibiotic era. Interestingly, the development of antibiotics and their widespread use after World War II resulted in a downturn of interest in vaccines, as antibiotics were viewed as the basis for the end of infectious diseases. This prediction, of course, was never realized, and the increasing problems of antibiotic resistance have prompted, to some degree, a resurgence in vaccine research and development.

Basic Concepts of Vaccination
Types of Protection
An individual can become immune to a microbial pathogen by one of two pathways: by developing an immune response following infection or immunization, a

process called *active immunization*, or by being given antibodies induced in other humans or animals or derived in the laboratory, a process called *passive immunization* (Table 21.2). Active immunization offers the benefit that it can induce cell-mediated immune responses in addition to antibody-mediated immunity. Histocompatibility barriers and the problem of graft-versus-host diseases presently preclude transferring T cells from an immune to a nonimmune individual. Therefore, passive immunization cannot be used to transfer cell-mediated immunity (CMI). However, this is done frequently in laboratory experiments with inbred strains of animals, where no histocompatibility barriers prevent the adoptive transfer of T cells among different individual animals within the inbred strain.

Serotherapy with horse antiserum (passive immunization) was the basis for von Behring's and Kitasato's work, but this type of therapy often was confounded by the development of *serum sickness* a few weeks after treatment. Serum sickness is due to the recipient's immune response to foreign proteins in the horse serum. However, at the time, with no alternative therapy, this was better than dying of the infectious disease. Today, horse antiserum is only used in dire need (postexposure, when active disease is already present or imminent) and when no other alternative exists. Worldwide, horse antiserum is currently used to treat only botulism, diphtheria, tetanus, and rabies. Use of serum from humans immunized against an infectious agent circumvented some of the problems of using animal sera for serotherapy, but serum had to be given in large amounts, generally precluding it as a practical form of therapy. In the 1970s a method was developed to purify and concentrate serum immunoglobulin G (IgG) and inject it intravenously. The possibility of contamination with serious blood-borne pathogens such as hepatitis and human immunodeficiency virus (HIV) diminished the enthusiasm for this approach, although intravenous IgG was never found to be a vector for viral diseases. Human immune serum has recently become

available for tetanus and rabies but is not yet available everywhere. These two human antisera have supplanted horse antiserum in situations where passive immunotherapy is indicated. Recently, the technology to produce human monoclonal antibodies in the laboratory has developed to the point where these reagents are being tested, and some even marketed, for treatment of disease.

Active immunization with a suitable vaccine is the preferred means of inducing immunity to a microbial pathogen, as this route produces not only protective immunity but also immunologic memory in the recipient. However, inducing the proper type of immunity via active vaccination can be challenging. Vaccines consisting of killed bacterial or fungal cells usually do not make for a good vaccine, and only in some instances, such as with the inactivated polio vaccine, do killed viral particles make a good vaccine. There are several important requirements for a vaccine that underlie all aspects of development, testing, and production of a vaccine.

Defining Antigenic Targets of Immunity

Most microbes present a variety of antigenic targets to the immune system, but usually only a small minority of these are targets for protective immune responses (Table 21.3). One classic way of defining protective antigens has been to compare responses in infected individuals during infection, using serum or cells obtained in the acute phase of the infection, and again weeks to months later as the patient is convalescing from the infection. Oftentimes the levels of antibodies or cellular responses to protective epitopes will rise in this circumstance. However, antibodies to many other antigens could increase as well, so there is little to distinguish protective antigens useful in vaccine design from nonprotective antigens.

Certain classes of antigens are, however, often associated with protective immune responses. When a toxin is the predominant factor causing diseases, as in tetanus and diphtheria, antibodies to the toxic entity mediate immune protection. For antibody-mediated responses to whole

Table 21.2 Comparative mechanisms for inducing active or passive immunity

Type of immunity	Method of delivery	Therapeutic targets
Passive immunity	IV-IgG	Kawasaki syndrome, immune thrombocytopenia purpura
	Human immune globulin	Postexposure prophylaxis in nonimmune individuals: measles, rabies, tetanus
	Monoclonal antibodies	Cancer cells, immune cells involved in graft rejection
	Animal antitoxins	Animal and insect bites
	Transplacental IgG	Agents against which mother is immune
Active immunity	Natural infection	Individual infecting pathogen
	Vaccination	Variety of pathogenic microbes: measles virus, mumps virus, rubella virus, hepatitis viruses, polio virus, *Clostridium tetani* (tetanus agent), *Corynebacterium diphtheriae* (diphtheria agent), influenza virus, *H. influenzae* type b, pneumococcus, varicella-zoster virus (chicken pox agent), smallpox virus, rabies virus

Table 21.3 Microbial antigens that can be targeted for vaccine development

Type of organisms	Antigenic target	Mechanisms of immunity	Example
Bacteria	Toxins	Neutralization of toxin	Tetanus
			Diphtheria
	Capsular polysaccharides	Opsonophagocytic killing	Pneumococcal pneumonia
		Bacteriocidal killing	Meningococcal infections
	Surface proteins	Opsonophagocytic killing	Streptococcal infections
		Transmission blocking	Lyme disease
Viruses	Capsid coat protein	Neutralization of infectivity	Measles, mumps, rubella
	Internal core antigens	CMI	HIV gp24
			Influenza virus nucleoprotein
Fungi	Capsular polysaccharide	Opsonophagocytic killing	*Cryptococcus* infections
	Surface proteins	Unknown	*Candida* infections
Protozoan parasites	Surface proteins	Antibody-mediated neutralization	Malaria
		CMI	Malaria

microbial cells, surface antigens are usually protective. Prominent proteins on the surface of a virus often induce protective immunity: the hemagglutinin of influenza, measles, and mumps viruses; the surface capsid proteins of poliovirus; and the hepatitis B surface antigen. For bacterial and some fungal infections, surface capsular polysaccharides are obvious targets of protective antibody. Successful vaccines for *Haemophilus influenzae* type b infections, meningococcal meningitis (caused by *Neisseria meningitidis*), and pneumococcal infection (caused by *S. pneumoniae*) are all predicated on incorporation of purified capsular polysaccharide antigens into the vaccine. For CMI, protective antigens are often much more difficult to determine, as they could be present anywhere in the microbial cell (not just on the microbial surface) and are effective only if they can be processed and presented by antigen-presenting cells (APCs) to appropriate T cells.

Requirements for a Safe Vaccine

The basic requirements for an effective vaccine are listed in Table 21.4. The vaccine must be safe, immunogenic, induce the proper type of immunity in the recipient, have a practical duration, avoid induction of significant immunosuppression, and have an acceptable cost-benefit ratio. *Cost* includes as its components both the monetary resources required to produce and deliver the vaccine and any health risk that is associated with its use. *Benefit* clearly refers to the protection afforded to the recipient by the vaccine but can also include benefits provided on a

Table 21.4 Properties of an effective vaccine

Safe	Effective duration
Immunogenic	Nonimmunosuppressive
Host responds with proper type of immunity	Cost vs benefits
	Relative risks of vaccine vs infection

population scale, such as reduced medical costs associated with no longer needing to cure individuals of the disease that the vaccine prevented. For example, vaccines consisting of killed microbial cells or viral particles are inexpensive to produce, so the cost is low, but so are the benefits: they are frequently undesirable because they cause serious side effects in recipients (i.e., are not very safe), are often poorly immunogenic, fail to elicit the proper type of immune effector in the recipient, and provide only a short period of immunity. In contrast, the measles-mumps-rubella (MMR) vaccine is somewhat expensive, but when used in a large number of children in a given country, is highly effective in preventing these three diseases.

Safety is a prime factor in vaccine development. Some effective viral vaccines are composed of inactivated particles, including polio, influenza, hepatitis A, and rabies virus vaccines. Live, attenuated microbes are often safe and immunogenic but have the potential to revert to full virulence or cause diseases in immunocompromised individuals. Purified components such as cloned viral antigens (e.g., those of hepatitis B virus) or isolated bacterial capsular polysaccharides (e.g., those of *S. pneumoniae* and *H. influenzae*) often make for excellent and safe vaccines but can be expensive to produce and have other problems important for consideration as a vaccine product. Although killed bacterial vaccines for diseases such as cholera (caused by *Vibrio cholerae*), plague (caused by *Yersinia pestis*), whooping cough or pertussis (caused by *Bordetella pertussis*), and typhoid fever (caused by *Salmonella enterica* serovar Typhi) have been around for a while, these vaccines tend to be associated with quite a bit of toxicity and can be limited further by their poor efficacy in preventing diseases over the long term. Immunization of infants against whooping cough with a killed vaccine was highly effective in preventing disease, but the toxicity of the killed whole-cell vaccine interfered with ready acceptance of this vaccine by parents. This problem led to the development and use of an acellular pertussis vaccine composed of purified bacterial components and inactivated toxins that is much less toxic. Live, attenuated viral vaccines (e.g., oral polio vaccine, measles, mumps, rubella, and chicken pox) offer potent immunity, but the fact that these are live pathogens means that some individuals, usually those with underlying immunocompromise, become ill in response to the vaccine strain of the virus. This type of problem with the oral, live polio vaccine led to the recommendation that the inactivated polio vaccine be used for immunizing babies. Chemically treated *toxoids* of proteins such as diphtheria and tetanus toxin, which retain their immunologic properties but lose their toxic properties, are highly successful vaccines, but not all toxins are easily inactivated and not all toxins retain their immunogenicity when inactivated. More recently, genetically modified toxins lacking critical residues for toxicity but otherwise retaining immunogenicity have been developed and tested with encouraging results.

Immunogenicity is another prime consideration for a vaccine, requiring that the host respond with the proper type of immunity. Use of purified components requires that they retain the desired properties during purification and that the host can mount an immune response to them. Some vaccine materials, such as bacterial capsular polysaccharides, must be of a large molecular size (e.g., >100,000 daltons) to be immunogenic (Fig. 21.1), and many of these are not immunogenic in children under the age of 2 years, the individuals most in need of vaccines. Recent advances in conjugation of polysaccharides to protein carriers have led to the development of a highly successful vaccine for *H. influenzae* type b, which has virtually eliminated this common cause of infection and meningitis in children younger than 2 years of age. As is typical for hapten-carrier immunogens, the protein carrier is be-

Table 21.5 Types of effector mechanisms known to be involved in immunity to microbial pathogens that would need to be elicited by a vaccine

Effector mechanisms	Type of pathogen targeted	Mediators of immunity
Opsonophagocytic killing	Bacteria Fungi Some viruses	IgG and IgM antibody Complement Phagocytes
Microbicidal killing	Bacteria Viruses?	IgM and IgG antibody Complement
Mucosal immunity	Bacteria	IgA, IgG, and IgM antibody
	Viruses	Complement for IgG and IgM
	Fungi Protozoan parasites Helminthic parasites	Mucosal phagocytes IgE antibody Eosinophils
DTH	Bacteria Fungi Some viruses Protozoan parasites Helminthic parasites	CD4$^+$ T cells Activated macrophages Cytokines
Cytotoxic cells	Some bacteria Viruses Fungi Protozoan parasites Helminthic parasites	CD8$^+$ T cells NK cells Eosinophils Cytokines Antibody for antibody-dependent cell-mediated cytotoxicity

lieved to convey a T-cell-dependent signal to the B cell responding to the polysaccharide, enhancing differentiation and proliferation of B cells into plasma cells. Although inactivated polio, influenza, hepatitis, and rabies vaccines represent successful killed viral vaccines, killed particles make for poor vaccines for many viral pathogens. Hence, live, attenuated strains must be developed, rigorously tested for safety, and analyzed to ensure the development of the proper type of immunity.

Thus, it is important to know which type of immune effector needs to be provoked by a vaccine for induction of *protective immunity*. Unfortunately, this knowledge is rarely available before vaccine development. Multiple factors may be involved in protective immunity (Table 21.5). Immune effectors must often have specific biologic properties; if complement fixation is key to immunity, a vaccine must elicit antibodies of the proper isotype (IgM, IgG1, and IgG3). The anatomic site of infection also plays a role; vaccines against pathogens that enter and replicate primarily on mucosal surfaces need to induce local immunity, whereas vaccines to prevent blood-borne or lymphatic spread of a pathogen need to elicit systemic immunity. While IgA antibodies induced by local immunization are often thought to be key components of immunity on a mucosal surface, vaccines such as inactivated

Figure 21.1 Correlation of the immunogenicity of a bacterial polysaccharide antigen with its molecular size. Pools made of the largest polymers, which averaged ~450 kDa in size, were able to induce an IgG immune response, whereas pools made of polymers with an average size of ~100 kDa or ~10 kDa did not.

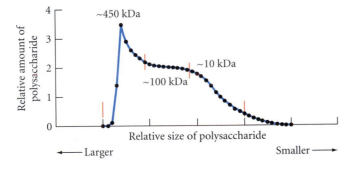

polio and influenza viruses that are injected into the muscle or skin are highly effective in preventing gastrointestinal or lung infections. The basis for this immunity appears to be local production of IgG and other antibodies at a mucosal site, which can be effectively stimulated by systemic immunization.

Other considerations relevant to vaccine development reflect compromises between the need for vaccine-induced immunity and the limitations of the vaccine itself. For example, some poorly immunogenic vaccines might require an adjuvant for maximal immunogenicity, but only one adjuvant is currently approved for human use: precipitated aluminum salts (alum). While newer, nontoxic adjuvants for human use are under development, one can envision a situation whereby a fair amount of toxicity from an adjuvant would be acceptable if that were the only means of preventing the spread of a serious disease. The duration of the immunity is also important but relative; the ideal vaccine should provide lifelong immunity comparable to that provided by the natural infection. However, there are exceptions to this. Travelers going to an area where cholera or plague is endemic might be willing to use a vaccine with a short duration that protected them during their period of travel. However, such a vaccine would be of little use to individuals residing in areas where infection is endemic. Problems with immunosuppressive properties of vaccines, notably measles vaccine, have been observed at times, and it is of course critical that a vaccine not render an individual more susceptible to other diseases. One possibility for a mechanism of measles virus-induced immunosuppression is the observation that two viral proteins, the nucleoprotein and surface hemagglutinin, bind to receptors on cells important in immune responses: Fcγ receptors and CD46. These interactions have been reported to reduce the activation of dendritic cells (DCs), decrease the production of interleukin-12 (IL-12), and promote loss of antigen-specific T-cell proliferation.

Immune Recognition of Pathogens

Basic Considerations

As with all immunologic phenomena, certain basic properties of vaccine antigens that are targets for protective antibodies need to be met. First, the target antigen must be seen by the host's immune system as foreign. Since many pathogenic organisms mimic host antigens to avoid immune recognition, this condition might not always be met. For example, group B *N. meningitidis*, a major cause of bacterial meningitis, coats itself with a capsular polysaccharide that is identical to an oligosaccharide found on the host's own neural tissue. In this case the capsule of this organism, normally a prime target for protective antibody, is not immunogenic. Similarly, group A *Streptococcus* coats itself in hyaluronic acid, a major tissue component of mammalian organs, preventing induction of immune responses. In other cases, the immune response must often be directed at specific epitopes on an antigen. For some pathogens the immunodominant epitopes do not elicit protective immunity, notably problematic with viruses such as HIV and other organisms that cause chronic infections. One proposed mechanism for persistence of chronic infection in an immunocompetent host involves the chronic lung infection with *Pseudomonas aeruginosa* in individuals with cystic fibrosis (CF) (Fig. 21.2). When the chronic infectious state emerges, the organism produces massive amounts of a capsular polysaccharide chemically related to seaweed alginate. However, the bacterial polysaccharide is acetylated and presents at least two different epitopes to the immune system. One epitope involves portions of the molecule containing acetylated hydroxyl groups of the sugar components and the other involves portions with nonacetylated sugars. The former epitopes are specific to the pathogen, whereas the latter epitopes are shared with seaweed alginate. Possibly because seaweed alginate is commonly added to food, most humans, including patients with CF before infection, have antibody to the epitopes shared between the bacterial polysaccharide and seaweed alginate. However, these antibodies do not protect against chronic *P. aeruginosa* infection and, in fact, appear to prevent the production of antibodies to the acetylated epitopes in most individuals when they are vaccinated with the acetylated bacterial polysaccharide. Thus, patients with CF are unable to produce a protective antibody response against *P. aeruginosa* infection because of the failure of their immune system to mount an antibody response to a particular epitope on a bacterial surface polysaccharide antigen.

The variety of potential immune effectors that can be elicited by an infectious agent does not mean that all of them are effective in providing protection. As noted above, a vaccine antigen must provoke the proper type of immune response. Although we generally consider antibody to be the predominant effector of immunity to extracellular pathogens and cell-mediated effectors to be operative against intracellular pathogens, many organisms have both extra- and intracellular phases. Knowing the proper type of effector mechanism of immunity greatly facilitates vaccine development. Alas, this is rarely the case, as effective vaccines for most pathogens have been developed principally by empiric methods, with an understanding of

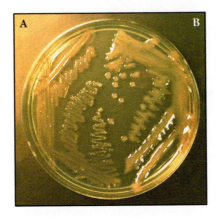

Figure 21.2 Demonstration of the specificity of protective antibodies to different antigenic epitopes. Patients with cystic fibrosis initially become infected with environmental strains of *P. aeruginosa* (**A**). Within a year or so the organisms undergo a phenotypic change to become mucoid (**B**). This change is due to the overproduction of an extracellular polysaccharide chemically related to seaweed alginate, a polymer of randomly linked mannuronic (or M residues) and guluronic (or G residues) acids (**C**). *P. aeruginosa* alginate differs from seaweed alginate due to the addition of acetate groups to the mannuronic acid residues by the bacterium. Antibodies that have been found to be protective against infection recognize epitopes with acetate on them, whereas most chronically infected patients produce only antibodies to epitopes lacking acetate and are thus unable to control the infection.

the type of effective immunity being subsequent to vaccine development. Viruses are classic intracellular pathogens, and $CD8^+$ cytotoxic T lymphocytes (CTLs) appear to be major mediators of immunity in this situation. However, most of the effective viral vaccines in use appear to work by eliciting antibody responses that prevent the initial infection of a cell by a virus. This may reflect a primary role for antibody neutralization in prevention of viral diseases and an important role for $CD8^+$ T cells in resolution of disease. The causative agent of typhoid fever, *S. enterica* serovar Typhi, lives within host macrophages. One might expect that immune resistance to this infection would be based on $CD4^+$ T-cell-mediated immunity acting via the delayed-type hypersensitivity (DTH) pathway. However, a highly effective vaccine for this infection consists of the capsular polysaccharide of the organism that elicits opsonizing antibody and prevents the blood-borne dissemination of the organism. Developing a vaccine for HIV infection or even just the progression of the infection to clinical acquired immunodeficiency syndrome (AIDS) is of paramount importance in the field, but understanding of the immunologic basis for immunity to HIV infection and progression to AIDS is still incomplete. Of equal importance is a vaccine for malaria, but since the organism that causes the disease, *Plasmodium falciparum*, has both an extracellular and

an intracellular phase to its life cycle, there is evidence for the efficacy of both antibody and CMI against these infections. One approach is to engender both types of immune effectors, but the question still remains as to which epitopes are the best vaccine candidates. While the immune effectors likely to be protective against many organisms can be inferred from the types of infections they cause, the many exceptions and poorly understood mechanisms by which immune responses limit the disease caused by pathogenic microbes leave vaccine development still more an empiric, than rational, science.

Genetic, physiologic, and immunologic variability among mammalian hosts is increasingly being recognized as a potential influence on whether a proper immune response will be made to a vaccine by most individuals in a population. At a very basic level, the vaccinee must be physiologically healthy enough to respond to the vaccine. One consequence of malnutrition is an immunodeficient state, leading to problems with vaccine efficacy in parts of the world with poor nutrition. An individual who does not have a major histocompatibility complex (MHC) protein that can present a protective peptide epitope to a T cell, or who lacks clones of T cells that can respond to the peptide-MHC combination, may not mount an effective immune response to a vaccine.

For many animals, particularly humans, immune systems are not fully formed at birth. Maturation of the immune response is often necessary before a vaccine will be immunogenic in infants.

An important consideration for resistance to an infectious agent is the level of immunity manifest by most members of the community, so-called *herd immunity*. For a pathogen that is transmitted from human to human, the chain of infection cannot be sustained if enough individuals are immune to the pathogen. Individuals lacking their own immunity will nonetheless be at a low risk for infection because most of the individuals in the community are immune. The percentage of individuals in a population who need to be immune to provide herd immunity is not clearly known for most pathogens but is generally estimated to be around 75%. The good news about herd immunity is that not every individual in a community has to be vaccinated in order to prevent a disease. However, this can lead some individuals to avoid vaccinating themselves or their children, relying on herd immunity for protection and leaving it to others to as-

sume the risks of vaccination, which fortunately are very low. But if too many people take this stance, herd immunity could decline to nonprotective levels.

Parasite Evasion or Neutralization of Host Immune Effectors

Even in the presence of host immunity, some microbes are able to employ sophisticated mechanisms to avoid natural or vaccine-induced immunity. This capability provides a great challenge to vaccine development. Perhaps the most common microbial mechanism for evading host defenses is antigenic variation, wherein a given microbe may produce up to hundreds, or even thousands, of distinct surface antigens and effective immunity is needed against many, if not all, of these antigens. This is one major barrier to vaccines against agents such as rhinoviruses, which cause the common cold, or against HIV. Influenza virus undergoes antigenic shifts and drifts from year to year, necessitating a new vaccine for each set of yearly variants (Fig. 21.3). Fortunately, only a few variants predominate each winter during flu season, but predicting the variants that will pre-

Figure 21.3 (A) Antigenic drift occurs when small changes in protective epitopes render antibody produced from a prior vaccine (antibody 2 [green]) ineffective against new epitopes (dark red), while some preexisting antibodies (antibody 1 [blue]) remain but are not fully effective against the new virus. (B) Antigenic shift occurs when influenza viruses from two different species infect a cell of an animal and exchange genetic information. Again new epitopes (blue) that avoid binding to any of the preexisting antibody induced by a prior vaccine can be produced.

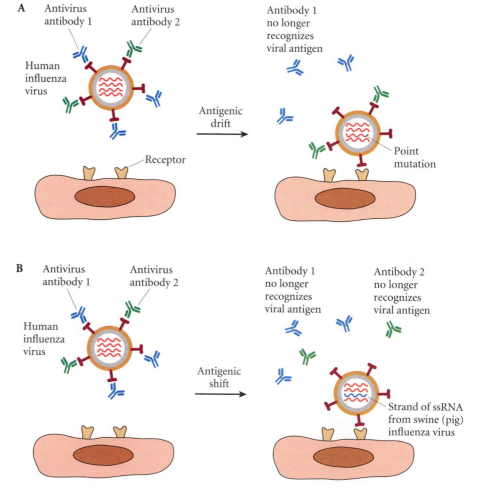

dominate needs to be done at least a year in advance in order to manufacture enough flu vaccine to meet demands. *S. pneumoniae*, which causes pneumococcal pneumonia, is able to make over 100 different surface capsular polysaccharides, the major targets of protective antibody. Developing a vaccine containing this number of components would not be feasible; however, 23 of these variants cause over 90% of the disease, so a vaccine with this limited number of individual polysaccharides has been manufactured.

Many microbes try to avoid host immune effectors by a variety of mechanisms. Secretion of possible decoy antigens to intercept host effectors and prevent them from getting to the microbe has been proposed as a potential avoidance mechanism. Some microbes make proteases that destroy host immune effectors, such as an IgA protease made by many bacteria that cause infections on mucosal surfaces. However, no definitive role for this protease in avoidance of host immune effectors has been shown. Many microbes are able to live both intracellularly and extracellularly in a host. It has been proposed that an organism might avoid protective antibody by hiding inside host cells. Such a situation would require an effective vaccine to elicit both antibody and CMI.

Vaccine Components and Vaccination Strategies

Antigenic Targets and Delivery Vehicles

In addition to the very important decision of what antigen(s) to use for a vaccine, choosing the form in which the antigen will be delivered is also critical. The successful human vaccines developed to date include purified and protein-conjugated capsular polysaccharides of bacteria, inactivated toxins (toxoids), recombinant protein antigens (hepatitis B), killed and attenuated bacterial cells and viral particles, and immune serum for passive protection, such as rabies immune globulin for postexposure prophylaxis (i.e., passive immunization). Experimental vaccines (i.e., those tried only in animals or that are in early studies in humans) include anti-idiotype vaccines, peptide-based vaccines, DNA-based vaccines, antigen presentation from infected or transfected APCs, and immunization with live, recombinant, attenuated viruses and recombinant bacterial cells expressing vaccine antigens for other organisms. Also, inclusion of adjuvants (see chapter 8 and Table 8.1) and purified cytokines or cytokine genes is central to some vaccine development efforts.

Anti-Idiotype Vaccines

Although interest in this approach has waned somewhat from earlier enthusiasm, there are nonetheless excellent examples of the potential utility of this strategy. According to the *idiotypic network theory*, the variable region of an antibody molecule represents a completely novel molecular epitope, which a host animal cannot have encountered previously and to which it therefore cannot be tolerant. This antibody will therefore elicit an *anti-idiotype* antibody specific for the first antibody's antigen-binding site. Since this anti-idiotype antibody is complementary to the first antibody's antigen-binding site, it should mimic the three-dimensional shape of the original antigen (which was also complementary to the first antibody's antigen-binding site) (Fig. 21.4A). The initial antibody to the vaccine target is referred to as antibody 1, and the anti-idiotype antibody as antibody 2. Since the idiotope determinants on antibody 2 are mimics of epitopes on the initial antigen, antibody 2 could be used in place of antigen as a vaccine. This strategy would be particularly useful for immunizing against toxic antigens that could not be safely detoxified, antigens that are more difficult and expensive to purify than the anti-idiotype antibody, and antigens that are poorly immunogenic, such as purified polysaccharides, which would be replaced by more immunogenic protein epitopes. This could be accomplished by one or several anti-idiotype antibodies making up the vaccine. Limitations on this strategy are the suboptimal immunogenicity of the idiotope determinants; the concern about using mouse monoclonal antibodies in these situations, which would induce anti-mouse antibodies in the recipients; and the concern about using human monoclonal antibodies for fear of inducing an autoimmune response to conserved epitopes on antibody molecules.

Peptide-Based Vaccines

Synthetic or recombinant peptides mimicking known protective B- or T-cell epitopes on pathogens could be delivered safely. Peptide vaccines suffer from the poor immunogenicity of purified peptides in the absence of strong adjuvants, but this problem can be overcome by coupling the peptides to a solid matrix support or formulating immunostimulating complexes (ISCOMs) (Fig. 21.4B). One critical prerequisite for peptide vaccines is the need to identify protective T- and B-cell epitopes that are immunogenic in most humans. The T-cell epitopes would be expected to vary considerably, depending on an individual's HLA type, so the vaccine would need to contain peptides universally immunogenic when presented by the highly polymorphic MHC proteins found in human populations. Another consideration would be to ensure that a peptide vaccine does not contain epitopes that would make an individual's T cells anergic to activation. Studies

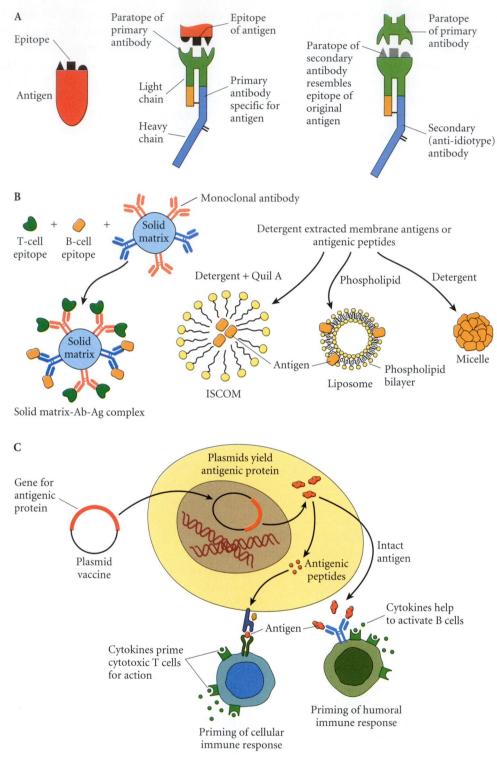

Figure 21.4 Principles of some of the newer vaccination strategies being evaluated for vaccinating against disease. (**A**) The use of anti-idiotype antibodies as surrogate antigens. (**B**) Multivalent vaccines that can combine multiple vaccine epitopes in one vaccine. Such vaccines also can incorporate vaccine antigens in a liposomal or micellar structure that can fuse with membranes to deliver antigens to within the cells. (**C**) DNA vaccines allow activation of both helper and cytotoxic T cells and B cells.

with peptide agonists and antagonists clearly indicate that closely related peptides have very different abilities to effect T-cell responses (see Fig. 14.10). Peptides usually require strong adjuvants to be immunogenic, and even when antibody that is specific to the pathogen develops, it is often of low affinity or of the wrong isotype. In addition, it is thought that peptides do not generally mimic conformational B-cell epitopes and that few protective antibodies are directed at linear B-cell epitopes. Nonetheless, some conserved, linear peptide determinants of important pathogens have been identified and could form the basis for an effective peptide vaccine. Conjugation of the peptide to a carrier protein is another strategy that could enhance the immunogenicity of peptide epitopes.

DNA Vaccines

One of the more promising strategies that have been developed recently is that of DNA vaccines, which are based on the finding that injecting a mammal with DNA that encodes a microbial protein can elicit both T-cell responses and antibody responses to the foreign protein (Fig. 21.4C). The DNA is usually a recombinant bacterial plasmid into which the gene for the microbial antigen has been inserted and placed under the control of a strong promoter that transcribes genes in mammalian cells. Injected DNA is taken up by host cells, the recombinant protein is produced and recognized as foreign by the immune system, and T- and B-cell responses are generated. How the injected DNA makes its way to the nucleus of the host cell for transcription into mRNA has not been determined. Also, as most DNA vaccines are injected into muscle, it is not clear if the muscle cells produce the protein and process and present it on MHC class I molecules or if the DCs in the tissues are the initiators of immunity.

DNA vaccines can potentially be produced inexpensively and offer many conveniences relative to protein-based or whole-organism vaccines. For example, DNA vaccines can be distributed widely without the need for equipment such as refrigerators, since DNA plasmids are stable at ambient temperatures. Second, multivalent vaccines can easily be produced by incorporating multiple genes (encoding multiple bacterial proteins) into one plasmid. Third, DNA vaccines can be delivered through the skin via a "gene gun," obviating the need for needles and syringes. Drawbacks include the limitation that DNA vaccines are useful only when the protective antigen or antigens are protein in nature. In addition, the need to use strong mammalian promoters to drive gene expression raises the potential that these promoters might recombine with the host's DNA and activate undesirable genes such

as oncogenes. Last, if the DNA itself is immunogenic, there is the potential for the development of a lupus-like autoimmune condition.

Despite these drawbacks, there is great enthusiasm for this approach, as DNA vaccines have the ability to induce production of a natural protein without modification or denaturation and to sustain an immune response because of long-lived antigen production. Provoking both cell-mediated and humoral immunity is another advantage of DNA vaccines. Numerous animal studies have documented the potential efficacy of DNA vaccines, and human trials have already started. Specific infectious agents targeted include HIV, hepatitis B virus, influenza virus, and human papillomavirus (associated with cervical cancer), and a variety of other pathogens. In addition, DNA vaccines are being considered for use as cancer vaccines, as vaccines to prevent autoimmune diseases, and as antifertility agents.

Adjuvants

Adjuvants are substances that, when cointroduced along with an antigen, enhance the immunogenicity of that antigen (see chapter 8 and Table 8.1). Although adjuvants have long been known to potentiate immune responses, only one adjuvant, aluminum salts or alum, has been approved for use in human vaccines. Despite its safety, alum is not an ideal vaccine adjuvant. Immune responses stimulated by alum tend to be strongly polarized to a TH2 cytokine profile, favoring production of antibodies, particularly of the IgA and IgE isotypes, at the expense of CMI. The modes of action of some adjuvants are noted in Table 8.1. However, the molecular and cellular mechanisms that initiate the actions are not precisely defined and are probably variable among different types of adjuvants (Table 21.6). Most adjuvants provoke inflammatory responses due to cytokine and chemokine release (Fig. 21.5). Other factors induced by adjuvants, such as heat shock proteins, may also play a role by recruiting inflammatory cells to the site of antigen/adjuvant injection or by activating T cells, as has been shown for the stress-induced, nonclassical MHC proteins MICA and MICB. Enclosing antigens in lipid vesicles such as liposomes or in ISCOMs composed of adjuvant compounds has worked effectively in animal systems to enhance immunogenicity of vaccine antigens. These lipid-enclosed antigens may also be delivered intracellularly by fusion of the lipid shell of the vaccine and the plasma membrane of the host cell, entering the endogenous antigen-processing pathway and potentiating CD8$^+$ cytotoxic T-cell responses.

One factor recently appreciated to be common to many adjuvants is their ability to activate DCs through a variety of

Table 21.6 Mechanisms of action of some adjuvants[a]

Concept of action	Examples of adjuvants	Key event(s)
Facilitation of antigen uptake, transport, and presentation by APCs	ISCOMs, Quil A, Al(OH)$_3$, liposomes, cochleates, poly(lactic/glycolic acid)	Antigen localization in the lymph node
Depot effect	Oil emulsions, Al(OH)$_3$, gels, polymer microspheres, nonionic block copolymers	Prolonged antigen presentation
Alert/activate initial responding cells	Complement, CpG-rich motifs, LPS (monophosphoryl lipid A), mycobacteria (muramyl dipeptide), yeast extracts, cholera toxin, ISCOMs?	Signaling of PRRs on innate immune cells[b]
Danger signal	Oil-emulsion surface-active agents, Al(OH)$_3$, IFNs, heat shock proteins, hypoxia, etc.	Tissue destruction/stress
Recombinant signal 2	Cytokines, costimulatory molecules	APC polarization, T- and B-cell help

[a]Modified from V. E. Schijns, *Curr. Opin. Immunol.* **12:**456–463, 2000, with permission.
[b]PRR, pattern-recognition receptors; HSPs, heat shock proteins.

means, particularly the Toll-like receptors (TLRs) (see Table 2.2 and Fig. 2.7). Microbial components such as lipoarabinomannan, peptidoglycan, lipopolysaccharide (LPS), and zymosan (yeast cells) have long been known to be potent adjuvants. The recent appreciation that these molecules signal through TLRs has advanced our understanding of how some adjuvants work (Fig. 21.6). TLRs are expressed promi-nently on DCs and likely work by potentiating their responses to antigens, allowing lower doses of antigen to be effective immunogens. One adjuvant that has shown great promise is oligonucleotide DNA with a sequence motif common in bacteria but rare in mammals. This motif, known as the CpG motif, is recognized by TLR9 and causes cellular activation and cytokine/chemokine production, as

Figure 21.5 Visualization of the essential steps of different concepts of adjuvanticity. (**1**) Facilitation of antigen transport, uptake, and presentation by antigen-capturing and -processing cells in the lymph node draining the vaccine injection site. (**2**) Repeated or prolonged release of antigen to lymphoid tissues (depot effect). (**3**) Signaling via pattern-recognition receptors (PRRs) activates innate immune cells to release cytokines necessary for upregulation of costimulatory molecules. (**4**) Danger signals from stressed or damaged tissues alert the APCs to upregulate costimulatory molecules. (**5**) Note that signaling by recombinant cytokines or costimulatory molecules mimics classical adjuvant activity. Steps 3, 4, and 5 allow signal 2 as well as signal 1 from APCs. Reprinted from V. E. Schijns, *Curr. Opin. Immunol.* **12:**456–463, 2000, with permission.

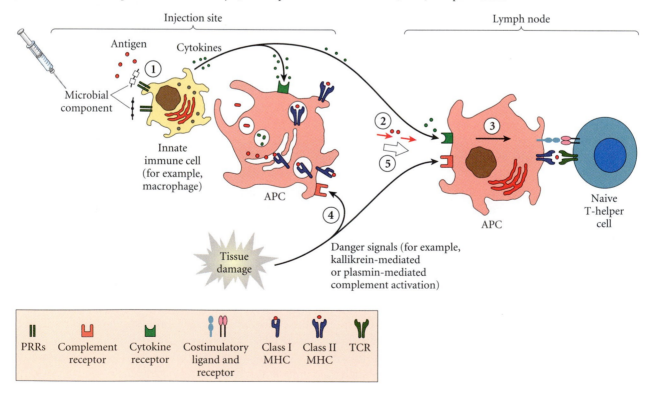

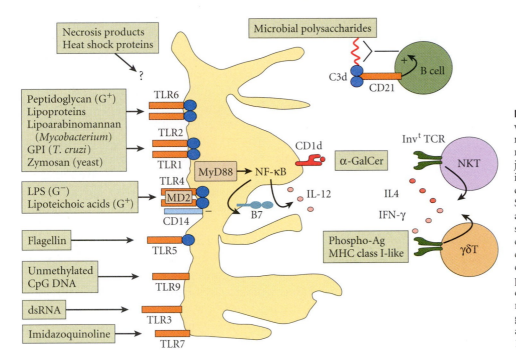

Figure 21.6 Pathways whereby adjuvants activate cells. TLRs transduce signals following recognition of specific microbial structures known to have adjuvant activity. Immune response modifier drugs such as imidazoquinoline can also activate DCs through TLR7. Soluble complement factors can tag antigens with C3d and improve the response of B cells to the antigen. NK T cells that express an invariant T-cell receptor (Inv⁺ TCR) and respond to glycolipid antigens, such as α-Gal-Cer, presented by CD1 MHC-like molecules can secrete cytokines that augment immune cell responses to coexisting antigens. Reproduced from A. Bendelac and R. Medzhitov, *J. Exp. Med.* **195**:F19–F23, 2002, with permission.

do the other TLR molecules responding to bacterial and viral factors. This CpG motif can be incorporated into recombinant DNA vaccines to enhance immunogenicity, or oligonucleotides that contain this motif can be mixed with vaccine components to enhance immunogenicity.

In addition to the TLRs, other pathways of adjuvant activity have been described. Some adjuvants activate complement, leading to the deposition of complement breakdown products onto the antigen. This occurs commonly with carbohydrate antigens. The covalently linked complement fragments, such as C3d, promote binding of the antigen to CD21 on B cells, lowering the threshold for cellular responses to the antigen. It has recently been noted that some antiviral compounds such as imidazoquinoline have adjuvant properties and activate cells via TLR7. A recently described adjuvant activity involves presentation of a glycolipid antigen, α-galactosylceramide, to natural killer (NK) T cells (see chapter 3). These cells respond to glycolipid antigens presented by CD1 MHC-like molecules and express an invariant T-cell receptor molecule that mediates this response. When presented with very low amounts of α-galactosylceramide, NK T cells respond by secreting high levels of cytokines that can influence and activate neighboring DCs. One adjuvant property of α-galactosylceramide is its ability to stimulate CD8⁺ CTL responses to non-living antigens. CD8⁺ T-cell responses are usually made to antigens such as viral proteins that are synthesized by a cell and presented on MHC class I via the endogenous or cytosolic presentation pathway.

Cytokines known to activate immune responses are another new class of potential adjuvants. In particular, inclusion of either IL-12 protein or the gene for IL-12 in DNA vaccines can drive an immune response toward a type 1 helper T-cell (TH1) response if this is desired. Similar skewing of the response toward a TH2 bias can occur with IL-4. Interferon-gamma (IFN-γ), granulocyte-macrophage colony-stimulating factor, and IL-2 have all been evaluated as cytokine adjuvants. It is likely that combinations of cytokines will be found to be optimal for enhancing immune responses to vaccine agents.

Several microbial products have also been used extensively as adjuvants. Two prominent ones are active or detoxified fragments of cholera toxin and heat-labile toxin, closely related molecules involved in the production of diarrhea. These molecules bind to GM1-ganglioside, a glycosphingolipid found ubiquitously on the cell surface of mammalian cells, and to other gangliosides. These toxins are composed of a toxic A subunit and nontoxic B subunit, the latter of which contains most of the adjuvant activity. Interestingly, the B subunit of the heat-labile toxin seems to be a better adjuvant than the related B subunit of cholera toxin. These toxins and toxoids have been used extensively in animal research involving the development of vaccines delivered onto a mucosal surface, the gastrointestinal and respiratory tracts most notably. However, their mechanism of action is not well understood. The B subunits increase expression of cell surface activation markers on APCs, notably the level of

MHC class II and the costimulatory CD80 and CD86 molecules. DCs can mature from precursors in the presence of these toxins and subsequently stimulate naive T cells to become activated. Since the crystal structures of both cholera and heat-labile toxins have been determined, it is expected that nontoxic recombinant proteins will be made that retain strong adjuvant properties and minimal toxicity.

Antigen Production in Infected or Transfected Mammalian Cells

Expression of a protective antigen in mammalian APCs, particularly DCs, represents a vaccine strategy of high potential. Since DCs are the key intermediaries between antigens and lymphocytes, concentrating antigen in these cells could help focus the immune response toward the production of the desired protective effector cells and molecules. Animal and human cells can be transfected in vitro with DNA to express a vaccine antigen and then reintroduced into the original donor to stimulate immune responses. In addition, inclusion of other adjuvant compo-

nents, such as CpG DNA motifs, in the DNA vaccine vector increases immunogenicity. These strategies are being pursued with DCs and macrophages as APCs (Fig. 21.7). One promising strategy is to transfect DNA encoding the production of CD40L into cells, which enhances their ability to stimulate immune cell responses. Alternately, DCs can be exposed to microbial antigens; allowed to ingest, process, and present the antigen on MHC molecules; and then be introduced into a recipient to induce immunity. This process avoids exposure of the whole, live subject to the immunizing material and yet delivers the vaccine directly to the most potent APCs known to induce immune responses. In addition, if autologous cells are used, then HLA type would not be a concern. Numerous animal studies have indicated that transfected or infected DCs can elicit protective immune responses. However, some additional aspects of this vaccine strategy need to be better understood, particularly how to optimize maturation of DCs once they have ingested antigen. Immature DCs ingest antigen most efficiently, but lymphocyte activation requires DC maturation that results in presentation of T-cell epitopes on MHC class I and class II molecules and production of costimulatory molecules such as CD86. In addition to being studied for immunization against microbial pathogens, DCs are being studied intensively for delivery of antigens protective against tumor cells.

Live, Recombinant Vector Vaccines

The powerful understanding that we now have in the area of microbial pathogenesis has permitted the deliberate creation of attenuated strains of viruses and bacteria that can be used to deliver antigens whose expression comes from recombinant DNA placed into the organism's genome or carried on a plasmid. Typically, viral or bacterial strains used for such purposes are genetically modified such that genes essential for eliciting disease are removed while genes necessary for the ability of the microbe to grow and replicate are left intact. The oral polio vaccine and the MMR vaccines are naturally attenuated strains that have almost all of the desired properties of a vaccine. Using molecular genetic techniques to create safe, attenuated microbial vectors for delivery of vaccine antigens builds upon this well-established principle. In particular, organisms such as *Salmonella* spp. and poxviruses into which large amounts of foreign DNA can be inserted are undergoing intense investigation for their vaccine capabilities (Fig. 21.8). However, live vaccines always have the potential for causing disease in a small number of recipients, mostly those with dysfunctional immune systems, and there is a possibility that the vaccine strain could reacquire virulence traits and become pathogenic.

Figure 21.7 Transfection of macrophages with costimulatory molecules and microbial antigen can elicit protective immunity. Mice were vaccinated with cells expressing CD40L and the gp63 antigen from *Leishmania* (L-gp63). Mice were injected with irradiated cells expressing both CD40L and gp63 (open squares) or with cells expressing gp63 alone (solid circles). Vaccinated mice were challenged with 5×10^5 *Leishmania amazonensis* promastigotes in the footpad 1 week after the final booster injection. Immunization with L cells expressing CD40L and microbial antigen resulted in reduced immunopathology, as determined by a footpad swelling response. In addition, the mice immunized with cells expressing CD40L and gp63 had lower levels of parasites in the infected tissues (**inset**). Reprinted from G. Chen et al., *Infect. Immun.* **69:**3255–3263, 2001, with permission.

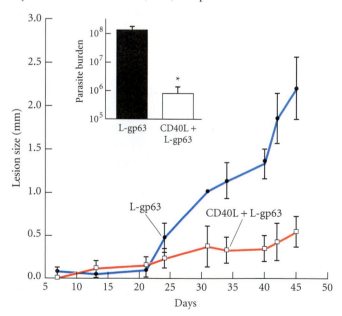

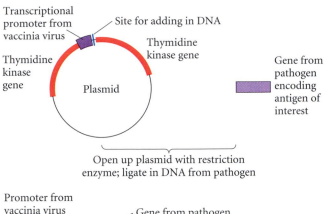

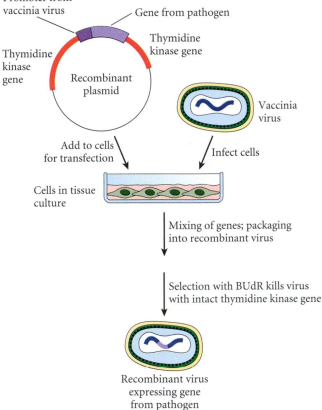

Figure 21.8 Construction of a viral vector vaccine containing DNA encoding a protective antigen from another organism. A DNA plasmid from a poxvirus engineered to contain a viral promoter in the middle of the nonessential thymidine kinase gene is used as a recipient for pathogen DNA. This DNA is inserted into the plasmid under the control of a viral promoter. When the recombinant plasmid is mixed with live virus in cell culture, some of the viral particles will recombine with the plasmid DNA and incorporate the pathogen DNA and the interrupted thymidine enzyme. Exposing cell cultures to bromodeoxyuridine (BUdR) kills the virus particles with intact thymidine kinase genes and selects for the particles with the pathogen antigen DNA interrupting the viral thymidine kinase gene.

Reverse Vaccinology

The information gained from the sequencing of the genomes of many microbes has made it possible to predict the types of antigens that might be present on the surface of the organism and to then prepare recombinant proteins for evaluation for immunization. Whereas traditional approaches to vaccine development relied on established biochemical, serologic, and microbiologic methods, reverse vaccinology takes an entirely new approach (Fig. 21.9). Using the genome sequence of an organism, computers can be used to predict which genes encode proteins that have motifs likely to be exposed on the organism's surface. Through polymerase chain reaction technology, a large number of recombinant proteins can be made quickly and expressed and evaluated as vaccine candidates by using in vitro serology or convalescent sera from patients. Usually a range of 10 to 30 proteins will be viable candidates after about 18 months of evaluation, which is a much larger number of vaccine candidates than could be found in a similar time frame by conventional methods.

Route of Vaccination

A successful vaccine invokes an immune response by interacting with various cells of the immune system and triggering those cells to become activated and generate effector and memory cells specific for the vaccine antigens. For this outcome to occur, it is desirable that the vaccine antigens be introduced into an anatomic site where they are very likely to encounter immune cells and tissues that will maximize the efficiency of the immune response (for example, lymph nodes). Therefore, the anatomic route by which a vaccine is introduced is a critical factor determining the outcome of vaccination.

Most current vaccines are introduced by intramuscular injection. This route of introduction offers several benefits over other routes (for example, intravenous) of administration. Antigens that are deposited in muscle tissue can form persistent precipitates that are dissolved and reabsorbed relatively slowly, effectively increasing the length of time during which the recipient's immune system encounters the vaccine antigens. In contrast, intravenously introduced antigens are frequently cleared rapidly (usually over a period of days or even hours) and therefore cannot stimulate the immune system for very long.

Muscle tissue, like many other solid tissues, is filled with DCs, which are efficient APCs. These DCs routinely survey solid tissues for antigens and transport those they encounter to regional lymph nodes, where they can display the antigen to T lymphocytes. Therefore, vaccine

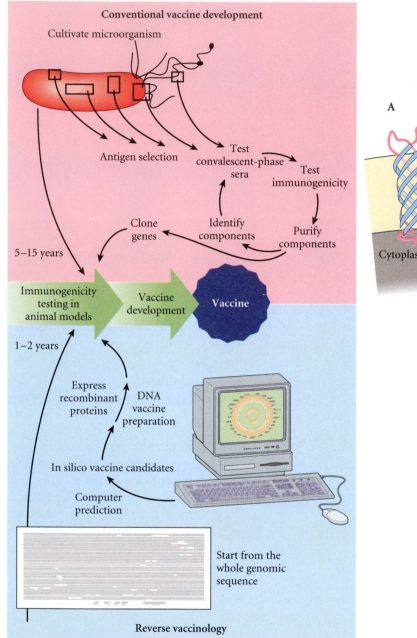

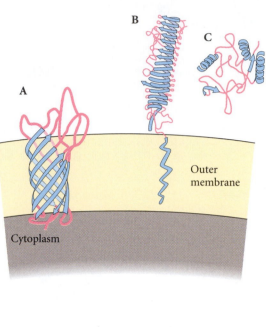

Figure 21.9 Comparison of traditional methods used to develop vaccines and reverse vaccinology technology. This new technique relies on computer predictions of surface antigens based on structural characteristics, which can quickly lead to the preparation of a recombinant protein or DNA vaccine for evaluation. Application of this strategy for development of vaccines against group B *N. meningitidis* identified, within an 18-month period, 25 surface-exposed proteins that have vaccine potential. Many of these proteins were different from the conventional outer membrane proteins embedded in the organism's outer layer or secreted, which usually were too variable to be good vaccine candidates. Instead, the newly identified proteins were membrane-anchored lipoproteins (**A and B**) or secreted proteins (**C**). Reprinted from R. Rappuoli, *Vaccine* **19**:2688–2691, 2001, with permission.

antigens deposited in muscle are likely to be efficiently processed and presented to the immune system. In contrast, antigens introduced intravenously are most likely to be processed and presented by circulating resting B cells. Although B cells can be efficient APCs after they are activated, resting B cells are ineffective as APCs since they do not express the B7 costimulatory protein. In fact, resting B cells that present antigen are more likely to anergize T lymphocytes than activate them, causing the recipient's immune system to tolerate the vaccine antigens instead of responding to them.

Last, muscle tissue is an attractive route for vaccine introduction because it is readily accessible. Injecting antigens into a large muscle such as the deltoid is a quick, easy, and reproducible way to introduce antigens into vaccinees.

Bacterial Vaccines

Modern vaccine research is rooted in our current, detailed understanding of immune mechanisms and proceeds by a rational application of these principles to achieve the desired state of immune protection. Progress in bacterial vaccine development comes from understanding the importance of different antigenic epitopes on the microbial surface and the ability of these epitopes to elicit an effective immune response in vaccinated individuals. The effectiveness of the elicited response depends not only on the magnitude of the response but also on the range of immune mechanisms that are activated during the response.

For many bacterial pathogens, opsonophagocytic killing mediated by antibodies, complement, and phagocytes is the major means of eliminating a microorganism and controlling infection. The outer capsular polysaccharide or protein coats that protect many bacterial pathogens from phagocytosis in the absence of specific antibodies are ideal vaccine candidates as they elicit protective, opsonic antibodies (Fig. 21.10). Lysis of gram-negative bacteria by antibody and complement alone is effective in vitro in killing some bacterial strains, but this mechanism of immunity has been firmly established only for resistance to neisserial infections, i.e., meningococcal (bacterial meningitis) and gonococcal (gonorrhea) infections. This was discovered through observations that individuals with genetic deficiencies of the terminal components of the complement membrane attack system are subject to recurrent neisserial infections. Oftentimes lytic antibodies also promote opsonic killing, making it difficult to determine which immune mechanism is more important in host protection. Gram-positive bacteria such as *Staphylococcus aureus* and *Streptococcus pyogenes* cannot

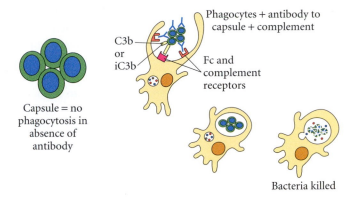

Figure 21.10 Major immunologic mechanism mediating protective immunity to bacterial pathogens is antibody to the cell surface capsule. Capsules protect bacterial pathogens from host defenses; to overcome the resistance of the bacteria to phagocytosis, antibodies to the capsule need to be elicited.

be lysed by complement because of the lack of an outer membrane as found in gram-negative bacteria. Here, opsonophagocytosis is the predominant mechanism of effective immunity.

When the major cause of disease is a toxin, neutralizing antibody directed against the toxin provides protection. Many bacterial toxins work by having two domains, one involved in binding the toxin to a cellular target and the other having the cytotoxic activity that is manifested after the toxin is internalized by a host cell. Here, effective vaccines usually work by preventing the toxin from binding to the cell so that the toxic portion is unable to do its destructive work inside the cell.

For bacteria that cause infections and disease primarily due to intracellular residence, CMI is the major mediator of protection. Many studies have suggested that CD4$^+$ T$_{DTH}$ cells are major effectors of immunity to intracellular pathogens, working by activating macrophages through cytokines that then allow the activated macrophage to kill either resident or newly internalized microbial cells. However, CD8$^+$ CTLs probably contribute to this process as well. One mechanism whereby CD8$^+$ cells might function has been suggested by studies showing that the granules of these cells contain antimicrobial factors, such as granulysin, that can actually kill bacteria on their own.

Finally, the immune effector, be it antibody or T cell, must be delivered to the anatomic site of infection to engender phagocytic activity, toxin neutralization, or killing of intracellular microbes. Since many bacterial pathogens cause infections at or on mucosal surfaces, it is often thought that IgA antibody is important in local immunity. However, IgA immunodeficiency is the most common type of immunodeficiency and the vast majority of these individuals do not suffer from recurrent infections. Recent evidence suggests that IgG antibodies, although present in lesser amounts than IgA on mucosal surfaces, may nonetheless be the major class of antibody involved in protection. While IgA immunodeficiency is mostly a benign condition, IgG immunodeficiency, prior to modern medical interventions to alleviate this condition, was always a fatal genetic disease, with death due to recurrent and uncontrollable infections, many initiated from mucosal sites. Many intracellular pathogens, such as salmonellae, listeriae, and *Mycobacterium tuberculosis*, enter macrophages in gastrointestinal or lung tissues, and effective immunity to these pathogens requires the accumulation of T cells at the site of infection. This appears to be a property of antigen-activated immune T cells that migrate to the site of infection, as opposed to naive T cells that do not remain in specific tissues but migrate through the body via the lymphatic and blood circulations.

Types of Bacterial Vaccines

Toxoids

Among the earliest successful vaccines for diseases caused by bacteria were those that targeted the toxins causing tetanus and diphtheria. These vaccines were made by treating bacterial culture supernatants with detoxifying agents, such as formaldehyde, to inactivate the toxin while retaining its antigenic and immunogenic properties. Recently, molecular genetic techniques have been used to accomplish this goal. This approach was applied to a component of the acellular pertussis vaccine, consisting of pertussis toxin. Other toxins, such as those involved in diarrheal diseases, may be amenable to a recombinant DNA approach for detoxification with retention of immunogenicity. Some diseases, such as menstrual toxic shock syndrome, are caused by a toxic factor produced by a bacterium, e.g., *S. aureus*, but because of the rarity of the disease, there is no obvious need for a vaccine for this disease.

Diphtheria and tetanus toxoids are now given routinely to children in many parts of the world and have resulted in a dramatic reduction in the incidence of disease (Table 21.1). Tetanus toxoid boosters also are given to older children and adults following trauma or injury, as levels of antibody to the toxin decline over time. Booster doses for diphtheria prevention are recommended once every 10 years for adults for comparable reasons. The importance of maintaining an effective vaccine program for these diseases was highlighted by the outbreak of diphtheria experienced after the breakup of the Soviet Union in the newly independent states that had been part of that country. Before the breakup, efficient public health measures kept immunity to diphtheria high; afterward, the breakdown in the public health infrastructure allowed many newborns to go unvaccinated. In 1990, there were 1,436 reported cases of diphtheria in the newly independent states; in 1995, there were more than 50,000 cases. Initiation of a vigorous vaccination program brought the number of cases down to 2,720 by 1998. Thus, loss of vaccination coverage allowed for a large increase in disease, and reinstitution of vaccination brought the disease back under control.

Capsular polysaccharides

Most major human bacterial pathogens coat themselves with an extracellular layer of polysaccharide that serves to prevent the organism from being eliminated by opsonophagocytic or lytic killing (Fig. 21.10). Overcoming this bacterial mechanism of resistance to immunity requires the generation of antibodies to the polysaccharide. These antibodies work by coating the bacterial surface with opsonic antibodies and opsonic complement fragments. When these opsonins are on the bacterial outer surface, Fc receptors and complement receptors on the surface of phagocytes can ingest and kill the pathogenic microbe. However, many, but not all, purified polysaccharide antigens tend to be poorly immunogenic in children under the age of 2 years, the major population at risk for bacterial infections. As noted above, conjugation of these polysaccharides to protein carriers has proved tremendously successful in making these vaccines immunogenic and effective in protecting young children against infection.

A major problem with capsular polysaccharide vaccines is the tremendous structural, and hence serologic, variability in the antigens along with the poor immunogenicity of some of them. *S. pneumoniae* makes over 100 different capsular types. Since ≥90% of the infections are caused by about 23 different types, a 23-valent vaccine is feasible and has been produced and used. *N. meningitidis* makes a more limited number of capsule types, but since the serotype B antigen is not immunogenic, this organism remains a serious cause of meningococcal meningitis even where vaccines for other serotypes are used. One of the reasons for the serologic variability in capsular polysaccharides is the great number of ways that monosaccharides can link to each other to form an epitope, as compared with the number of ways amino acids can link together to form peptide epitopes. For example, three identical hexose monosaccharides have the potential to link together to form up to 384 different trisaccharide repeat units; three identical amino acids can form only one epitope. Another concern about capsular polysaccharide-based vaccines is the potential to select strains making capsules not included in a particular vaccine. Studies with the recently developed seven-valent conjugate vaccine for pneumococcal infection in young children have shown the potential for emergence in vaccinated individuals of strains that do not express one of the vaccine antigens.

Surface proteins

There are many examples of bacterial surface proteins that provide protection in animal studies, but so far few of these have been made into effective human vaccines. One notable example is the recently developed but then discontinued vaccine for Lyme disease, which consists of a lipoprotein designated *outer surface protein A* (OspA). Interestingly, OspA is not expressed by the Lyme disease spirochete (*Borrelia burgdorferi*) during human infection but rather in the *Ixodes* tick vectors that deliver the organism to humans when ticks feed on them. Antibodies in the blood of vaccinated individuals bind to the Lyme disease organism during tick feeding and inactivate the spirochete before it can be transmitted to human hosts. However, in 2001 the vaccine was removed from the market because of unacceptable toxicity and side effects.

Pili, prominent appendages of bacteria that stick out from the surface and are involved in twitching motility and interactions with host tissues, often have been successful in preventing infections in animals challenged with human pathogens. There is a successful pilus-based vaccine used in farm animals to prevent neonatal diarrhea, but there appears to be a great deal of variability in the serologic properties of pili of human pathogens. Flagella are used by gram-negative bacteria for motility and have also been successful in animal studies of potential human vaccines. Several trials of flagellar vaccines are currently under way in humans, but no definitive results are yet available. The organism that causes streptococcal pharyngitis, i.e., "strep throat," and other serious diseases such as rheumatic fever, is coated with a highly serologically variable protein called M protein. This antigen is a target for protective immunity, but it has been difficult to make a vaccine out of this material because of its serologic variability and potential to provoke toxic autoantibodies. Almost all bacteria express numerous surface proteins that are being evaluated as vaccines. These include outer membrane proteins of gram-negative bacteria and surface proteins of gram-positive bacteria that bind to host factors such as collagen, fibrinogen, and other tissue components.

We lack adequate insight into the mechanisms by which antibodies to these surface proteins provide protective immunity. Such insight is critical for vaccine development, as one needs to know early on that a vaccine candidate is capable of eliciting the proper type of immunity in a recipient. For factors involved in bacterial adherence to host tissues or cells, such as pili and surface appendages of gram-positive bacteria that bind to host factors, it has been proposed that antibodies prevent the bacteria from binding to the host, which is viewed as a necessary early step in the infection process. While in vitro studies readily affirm this principle, there is little evidence that such a mechanism is operative in vivo. Neutralization of bacterial motility by antibodies to flagella may underlie protective immunity induced by this antigen, but again, in vivo studies confirming this mechanism of action have not been readily produced. A problem in understanding the mechanism of action of antibodies to all of these entities is that they all may depend on opsonophagocytic antibodies in addition to antibodies that have other properties, making it difficult to know if one property, or a combination of properties, underlies protective immunity.

Killed whole bacterial cells

Killed whole bacterial cells were among the earliest vaccines developed, and killed cells for prevention of cholera, typhoid fever, whooping cough, anthrax, and plague have existed for some time. These vaccines all are associated with high toxicity and limited duration of immunity. The vaccine for whooping cough, consisting of killed, whole cells of the causative agent, *B. pertussis*, was used for decades. Although it was clearly successful at preventing disease, the real and imagined toxicity of this vaccine limited its acceptance in the United Kingdom in the 1970s, and there was a marked increase in the disease since the vaccine was not used extensively. The killed whole-cell pertussis vaccine was given to children at 2, 4, and 6 months of age and, particularly after the first dose, appeared to make the infants restless and slightly feverish for 24 to 48 hours. Fortunately, a newer type of vaccine with much less toxicity, the acellular pertussis vaccine, has now supplanted the older, killed whole-cell vaccine. Similarly, the killed whole-cell vaccine for typhoid fever, often given to health care workers and soldiers, has been supplanted recently by two better vaccines: an attenuated strain taken orally and either a purified capsular polysaccharide or a conjugate of this antigen linked to a protein carrier. Various cholera vaccines delivered orally have recently been produced or are under evaluation. The plague vaccine is used mostly by individuals potentially in contact with diseased animals, such as veterinarians, and soldiers who might be in areas where plague is endemic or at risk for exposure from biologic weapons. Newer vaccines for this organism consisting of purified outer coat antigens are under development. Overall, killed whole bacterial cell vaccines have had only limited success in preventing infection and disease.

Live, attenuated bacterial vaccines

As success with live, attenuated viral vaccines grew, so did interest in a similar strategy for producing bacterial vaccines. The most widely used vaccine in the world is, in fact, a live, attenuated strain of *Mycobacterium bovis*, termed BCG for bacillus Calmette-Guérin, that is used for prevention of human tuberculosis caused by *M. tuberculosis*. BCG vaccine has been given to more than 1 billion people in the world and is also used as an immunotherapeutic agent in cancers, such as bladder cancer, where its stimulatory properties appear to augment host immunity to the cancer. An enormous amount of controversy surrounds the use of this vaccine. One problem is the tremendous genetic plasticity of the BCG vaccine organism, and various strains have undergone major genetic changes over the years, meaning that different BCG vaccine strains are used in the world, and some may be more effective than others. As a corollary of this, BCG vaccine appears to be more effective in some parts of the world than in others and may be more effective against tuberculosis in young children than in adults. BCG vaccine may be better at offering protection against dissemination of the bacterium from the lung to other tissues (referred to as miliary tuberculosis) than at providing protection against lung infection. Another problem is that the vaccine, because it is live, can cause serious infections in immunocompromised individuals. The reason for the widespread use of this vaccine is that, in nonimmunocompromised hosts, the vaccine is safe to give at birth. In many parts of the world this may be the only time a child comes in contact with health care workers, making it opportune to use BCG vaccine at this stage. Also, because of the tremendous worldwide impact of tuberculosis, there is a major need for strategies to limit the consequences of this widespread infection.

Salmonella species have been another major focus of research in the field of live, attenuated vaccines. *Salmonella* possesses several attributes that make this genus attractive as vaccine candidates. First, salmonellae are normally enteric pathogens, initiating infection by invading the epithelial layer of the small intestine. Because of this route of infection, salmonellae are natural candidates for the development of vaccines intended to generate mucosal immunity. Thus, immunity that is generated in response to an engineered, attenuated *Salmonella* vaccine could be useful for protecting against any of a large number of diseases whose causative agents invade the body by an oral route. Another feature of salmonellae that makes them excellent

candidates for live, attenuated vaccine vehicles is their natural ability to infect immune cells such as macrophages in the intestine. While normal pathogenic salmonellae use this ability to infect and disable their host's macrophages, an engineered vaccine strain of *Salmonella* might be useful for delivering vaccine antigens to these APCs with high efficiency. Attenuated *Salmonella* vaccine strains have been developed by introducing mutations into the bacterium that diminish its overall growth. Several strains have been attenuated through the introduction of auxotrophic (nutritional) defects, which slow the growth of the bacterium by preventing it from synthesizing needed biomolecules such as amino acids. More recently, M. J. Mahan and coworkers created an attenuated strain by mutating the DNA adenine methyltransferase (Dam) gene, which is essential for DNA repair. One problem common to all attenuated vaccine strains is the possibility of reversion to a virulent phenotype. For this reason, most attenuated vaccine strains are introduced through deletion of the essential gene, rather than through point mutation, as the latter can revert to the normal sequence through a secondary mutation.

One of the hopes for safe, live, attenuated vaccines is that they not only may be inexpensive and easy to deliver to large populations but also may be genetically engineered to express protective antigens from other organisms. The development of a live, attenuated oral vaccine for typhoid has spurred investigations into how bacteria can be rendered harmless by genetic manipulation but still maintain sufficient properties to provoke an immune response. This is not that easy: the more attenuated the strains, the less immunogenic they seem to become; however, if properties are retained to provide efficient immunity, the organism often contains residual and unacceptable toxicity. Also, a high level of assurance that the organism will not revert to an infectious and toxic phenotype must be provided. It is hoped that, with the advent of the modern genomics era and with the DNA sequences of many bacterial pathogens now known, genes will be found that can be inactivated to render the organism harmless but immunogenic.

Successful Bacterial Vaccines

Although we need vaccines for many important bacterial pathogens, the growing list of successful vaccines is highly encouraging and provides a road map for future vaccine development (Table 21.7). The most successful vaccines are toxoids for preventing diphtheria and tetanus, along with vaccines containing purified capsular polysaccharides, usually conjugated to a carrier protein. In the 1980s, the most common cause of meningitis in children was infection with *H. influenzae* type b. The development by the

Table 21.7 Bacterial vaccines developed to date

Disease	Causative organism	Vaccine constituents	Efficacy
Diphtheria	*Corynebacterium diphtheriae*	Inactivated exotoxin	>95%
Tetanus	*Clostridium tetani*	Inactivated toxin	>95%
Meningitis and sepsis	*Haemophilus influenzae* type b	Polysaccharide-protein conjugate	>90%
	Neisseria meningitidis	Purified polysaccharide	90% for 2- to 3-yr-olds
		Polysaccharide-protein conjugate	In development
Pneumonia and sepsis	*Streptococcus pneumoniae*	Purified polysaccharide	60% for >2-yr-olds
		Polysaccharide-protein conjugate	>95% for sepsis
Whooping cough	*Bordetella pertussis*	Acellular components including inactivated toxin and adherence factors	80–90%
Typhoid fever	*Salmonella enterica* serovar Typhi	Inactivated whole cells	50–70% (short-lived)
		Live, attenuated strain	50–70%
		Purified polysaccharide	>70%
		Polysaccharide-protein conjugate	>75%
Plague	*Yersinia pestis*	Inactivated bacteria	Uncertain
Anthrax	*Bacillus anthracis*	Inactivated avirulent bacteria	Uncertain
Tuberculosis	*M. tuberculosis*	Live, attenuated BCG	Controversial; best protection against disseminated disease
Cholera	*Vibrio cholerae*	Inactivated bacteria	50% (short-lived)

early 1990s of a capsular polysaccharide-conjugate vaccine that could be given to infants has resulted in the virtual elimination of this disease in areas where this vaccination is widespread. One of the commercially available conjugate vaccines for *H. influenzae* incorporates a protein isolated from the outer membrane of the bacterium that causes one form of spinal meningitis, designated *N. meningitidis,* as a carrier. This particular conjugate vaccine is more immunogenic than similar vaccines using a different carrier protein. The protein used to produce this more immunogenic conjugate vaccine had been shown not only to enhance T-cell help for B cells making antibody to the capsular polysaccharide but also has adjuvant activity. The adjuvant activity may be different from that of others in that it appears to work by preventing apoptosis of immune cells responding to the capsular polysaccharide and thus prolonging their ability to secrete antibody. More recently, a similar type of conjugate vaccine for preventing pneumococcal pneumonia has been developed and licensed for use in infants, as has a polysaccharide-protein conjugate vaccine for prevention of typhoid fever. Because of the success of these vaccines, a conjugate vaccine containing capsular polysaccharides of various strains of *N. meningitidis* that cause meningococcal meningitis may soon be available.

Difficulties with Bacterial Vaccines

Efforts to develop antibacterial vaccines have in many cases encountered practical obstacles. These obstacles can generally be categorized into one or two groups: lack of immunogenicity of bacterial antigens and lack of protective efficacy of the resulting immune response. Lack of immunogenicity is frequently attributable to the fact that many bacteria enshroud themselves in a thick carbohydrate layer called a *capsule*. The thickness of the capsule shields the underlying bacterial antigens from the antigen receptors of the host, and the capsule is itself poorly immunogenic. Most capsules are poorly immunogenic because they are composed of carbohydrate and therefore cannot be recognized by most T lymphocytes. Without T-cell help, B cells that are activated do not undergo affinity maturation or isotype switching and do not form any memory cells upon activation. To address this issue, many bacterial vaccine laboratories have turned to the use of *conjugate vaccine* strategies, in which a carbohydrate antigen of interest is chemically conjugated to an immunogenic protein antigen that is capable of activating T cells. Some bacterial capsules go one step further to avoid provoking an immune response in their host, by structurally resembling their host's endogenous carbohydrates. For example, group A *Streptococcus* produces a capsule that consists of hyaluronic acid, a carbohydrate commonly found in the connective tissues of humans. This capsule has been shown to have antiphagocytic properties and will seldom invoke an immune response because of its chemical similarity to the host's hyaluronic acid.

Another factor that inhibits the effectiveness of antibacterial vaccines is the ability of many bacterial species to vary the antigens they express. This can occur by the activation and inactivation of certain bacterial genes (quantitative changes in expression) or by alteration of the nucleotide sequences of expressed genes (qualitative changes in genes). Quantitative changes in gene expression levels occur under many circumstances during bacterial growth. *Bacillus* species generate reproductive spores that express different antigens than the actively growing form of the bacterium. Bacteria that are actively growing continuously regulate their gene expression in response to availability of nutrients and their growth phase. In addition, bacteria that infect humans express a different pattern of genes after they establish infection than they did before they infect their host (the genes that are switched on are called *in vivo expressed genes*). For all of these reasons, the bacteria that invade and grow in a host's tissues may express different antigens than the bacteria that originally entered the host. An immune response generated to one set of bacterial antigens may not be effective against a bacterium expressing a different set of antigens.

Viral Vaccines

Similar to the early stages of antibacterial vaccine development, several early vaccines against viral pathogens were successful despite a lack of detailed knowledge of immune function. The classic example of this was the development of the smallpox vaccine at the end of the 18th century, which has essentially eradicated the disease in the present day. Today, antiviral vaccine development is driven by our understanding of viral replication and antiviral immune mechanisms. The replicative cycle of viruses dictates that viral structural proteins be synthesized inside infected host cells, where they are subject to degradation via the cytosolic antigen processing pathway and presentation on MHC class I proteins. The protective potential of antiviral CTLs is therefore obvious. Interestingly, however, the major correlate of immunity with almost all extant vaccines is neutralizing antibody,

not antiviral CTLs. Neutralizing antibodies can function by numerous mechanisms, including masking critical docking proteins to prevent virus–host-cell interactions, and initiation of the classical complement cascade. Thus, one major property of a successful viral vaccine is that it induces the development of antibodies that prevent the virus from getting into a host cell or replicating within that cell. To date, successful vaccines have been targeted at viruses with relatively limited antigenic and serologic diversity, or at least a variability that changes slowly over time (Table 21.8). A vaccine for the common cold would be desirable, but with hundreds of different serologic types of rhinoviruses in circulation, developing a vaccine against all of these types would be daunting. A vaccine for HIV infection is undoubtedly a top priority, but the tremendous antigenic variation this organism undergoes during infection presents a formidable challenge to vaccine development. Some recent studies suggest that HIV infection may be more amenable to immunologic control via cytotoxic CTLs, but targeting this immune effector mechanism for vaccine development remains controversial.

Viral antigens that are targets of neutralizing immune effectors are usually large glycoproteins encoded by the viral genome (protective antigens are usually not host proteins whose expression is induced due to infection). Essentially all viral antigens require T cells for immunogenicity, potentially accounting for the hypersusceptibility of T-cell-deficient individuals to viral infections. Antibody, CTLs, and antibody-dependent cell-mediated cytotoxicity have all been implicated as mechanisms of immunologic resistance to viral infection (Fig. 21.11). While antibody seems to play the predominant role in vaccine-induced immunity, other immune effectors may be augmentative or needed when antibody immunity wanes.

Table 21.8 Viral vaccines developed to date

Disease	Type of virus	Vaccine constituents	Efficacy (%)
Smallpox	Variola virus	Vaccinia virus	100
Polio	Picornavirus	Oral: live, attenuated virus	>95
		Inactivated virus particles	>95
Hepatitis A	Picornavirus	Killed virus	>90
Hepatitis B	Hepadnavirus	Recombinant antigen	>80
Influenza	Orthomyxovirus	Inactivated virus	~50–70
Measles (rubeola)	Paramyxovirus	Live, attenuated virus	>95
Mumps	Paramyxovirus	Live, attenuated virus	>90
Rubella (German measles)	Togavirus	Live, attenuated virus	>95
Chicken pox (varicella)	Varicella-zoster virus	Live, attenuated virus	>80
Rabies	Lyssavirus	Inactivated virus	100
Yellow fever	Flavivirus	Live, attenuated virus	>90
Japanese encephalitis	Flavivirus	Inactivated virus	>90

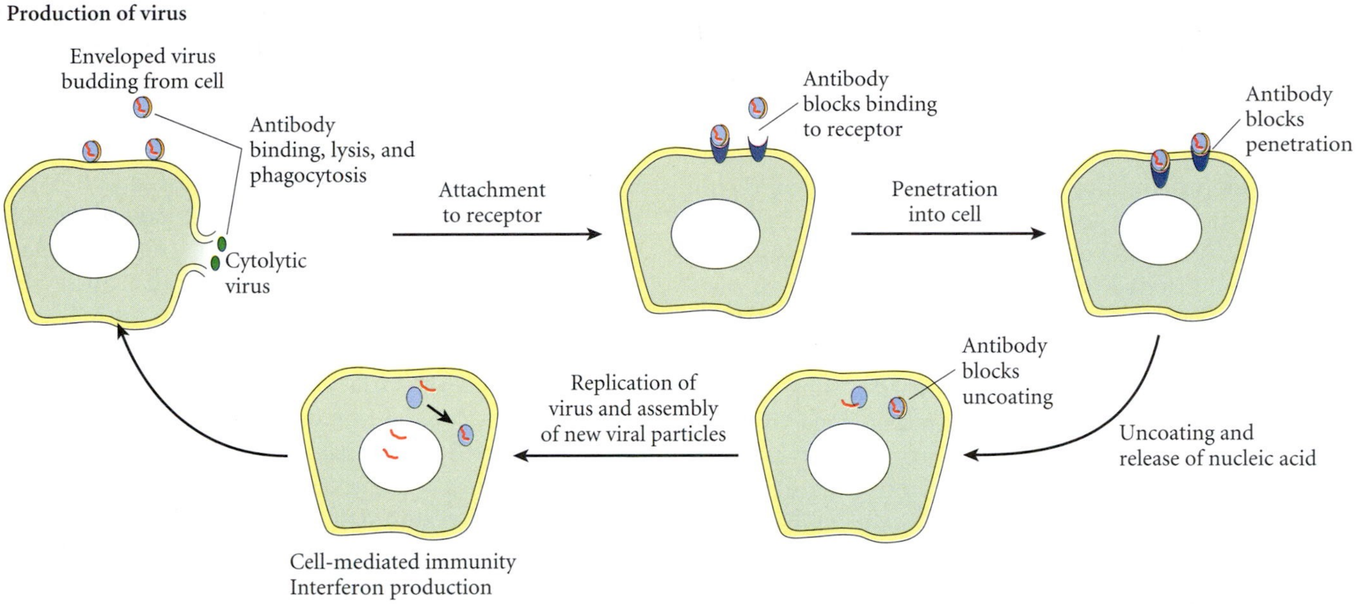

Production of virus

Figure 21.11 Replicative cycle of a virus and potential points of possible function of immune effectors. Viruses leaving a cell as either an enveloped particle, via budding, or a nonenveloped particle, via cytolysis, could be neutralized by antibody binding and complement activation or phagocytosis. Antibodies also can block viral receptors from binding to targets, prevent penetration, or prevent uncoating. Once viral replication is initiated in another cell, cell-mediated processes such as cytolytic T cells, antibody-dependent cellular cytotoxicity, and interferons could participate in preventing further production of virus.

Antibodies can disrupt many stages of the viral life cycle, including viral adsorption to a target cell, fusion of the viral surface with the cellular surface, release of viral nucleic acid into the host cell cytoplasm, and replication of the viral genome. Some antigens elicit protective immunity via one of these mechanisms, but full immunity may be due to the provocation of a combination of different neutralization mechanisms by the vaccine. Specific epitopes on viral surface molecules are often major targets for protective antibody, while antibodies specific to internal epitopes are not capable of inducing antibody production since they are "hidden" in the interior of the virion. Complement may assist in immunity to a virus, since enveloped viruses that bud from host cells enclosed in a host membrane may be lysed by complement. Both enveloped and nonenveloped viruses are subject to phagocytosis following opsonization by antibody or complement split products.

The role of CD8$^+$ CTLs in immunity to viral infection is predicated on the ability of these cells to recognize and lyse infected cells. Recent studies suggest that granules in cytotoxic cells contain antiviral peptides and proteins that directly kill the virus. However, the role of CTLs in primary immunity to virus infection is not as well established as some think. It has been proposed that CTLs may be needed for resolution of a primary infection while anti-

body is important for preventing the initiation of a subsequent infection. Even if this is the case, one could still argue that antibodies are not the only immune effectors that a successful vaccine needs to generate. Understanding immune effectors to HIV has been a goal for over 20 years in attempts to develop a vaccine. Studies in some individuals infected with HIV who do not go on to develop AIDS (so-called long-term nonprogressors) suggest that CTLs may play a key role in limiting viral replication. CTLs may also be critical during the infectious but asymptomatic part of HIV infection, where rapid viral replication is balanced by effective host immunity.

NK cells have been shown to contribute to immunity in several animal models of antiviral vaccination. As described in chapter 3, NK cells are lymphocytes that do not rearrange their genes for T- and B-cell antigen receptors. NK cells can eliminate pathogens by a variety of mechanisms. One may be to bind antibody to surface Fc receptors that target the cytotoxic NK cells to infected cells, inducing apoptosis in the infected cells. Another key component is induction of IFN-γ, which elicits an antiviral state in cells exposed to the IFN. Unlike CTLs and memory B cells, NK cells do not have a memory phenotype, meaning that any vaccine-induced effector mechanism that involves these cells must include an entity such as antibody molecules, which can be produced in an antigen-specific fashion and can benefit from the process of immunologic memory.

Types of Viral Vaccines

Viral surface proteins

Both enveloped and nonenveloped viruses have on their surface proteins that are used for binding to the cells of their host. In the case of enveloped viruses, such surface proteins are inserted into the plasma membrane of the virus's host cell during synthesis of new viral particles. Budding of new virions from the infected host cell gives each new virion a membrane envelope containing the viral surface antigen. In the case of nonenveloped viruses, the surface antigens are part of the virus's protein capsid. Because host cell attachment is a crucial step of infection, these viral surface proteins are attractive candidates for vaccine antigens. Purified surface antigen of hepatitis B virus (HBsAg) is currently used as a vaccine. Protective levels of anti-HBsAg antibodies are usually attained after three intramuscular injections of the vaccine.

Antibodies specific for viral surface proteins can confer protection by various mechanisms. The mere binding of the antibody to the viral surface protein can prevent the virus from binding to its host-cell receptor. Depending on the isotype of anti-surface protein antibody, the antibody may be able to opsonize the virus for phagocytosis or activate the classical complement cascade. Activated complement proteins can further opsonize the virus, can disrupt the envelope of some viruses, or can enshroud the virus in a thick complement protein coat that prevents the virus from binding to its host cell. Also, some viral surface proteins undergo conformational shifts upon binding to the host cell. The conformational shifts are sometimes essential for the fusion of the viral envelope with the host cell plasma membrane. Binding of antibody to surface proteins can inhibit these conformational shifts, thus preventing virus entry into the host cell.

The surface protein complex of HIV consists of two proteins called gp41 and gp120. gp41 is a transmembrane protein found in the envelope of HIV, and gp120 is a soluble protein found on the outside of the virus attached to gp41. gp120 binds to the two host cell receptors for HIV: CD4 and a chemokine receptor. Upon binding of gp120 to these receptors, gp41 undergoes a conformational shift that exposes a critical *fusigenic* domain of the protein, which causes the viral envelope to fuse with the host cell membrane. The gp41-gp120 complex has been the focus of intense study as a potential vaccine antigen. So far, the results of these studies have been disappointing. HIV has a very high mutation rate that results in frequent changes in the structure of gp120. Antibodies produced in response to vaccination with one form of gp120 protein are frequently not protective after the virus undergoes mutation.

Killed or inactivated viral vaccines

Some viral vaccines, notably the inactivated poliovirus vaccine developed by Jonas Salk in the 1950s, work well when killed virus is inoculated into a human vaccinee. Hepatitis A and rabies can be prevented with a killed viral vaccine as well. The vaccine against infection with hepatitis B virus is based on a recombinant protein antigen expressed on the viral surface. However, most other successful viral vaccines are predicated on the development of live, attenuated strains that undergo some limited replication in the host without causing disease. This is likely due to the need to stimulate host responses that occur in association with viral replication and suggests some contribution of CTLs to the efficacy of viral vaccines, since only live, replicating virus would likely stimulate CD8$^+$ cells due to presentation of endogenous viral antigens via MHC class I molecules. Since neutralizing epitopes on viral proteins may be induced during maturation in a specific host, production of viral vaccines in cells of a nonhuman host may not produce a vaccine strain with the proper neutralizing epitopes.

Live, attenuated viral vaccines

The Sabin oral poliovirus vaccine was an early example of a live, attenuated vaccine (after use of live vaccinia virus to prevent smallpox), and because the orally ingested vaccine strains were subsequently excreted into the environment, this vaccine had a side benefit of spreading vaccine strains into the community with the potential for naturally vaccinating many individuals. A consequence of this approach has recently emerged, where the elimination of polio from many parts of the world has left the vaccine strains as the predominant ones in some communities, and rare cases of polio in compromised hosts due to vaccine strains have been reported. Recent recommendations for polio vaccination have reverted to endorsing the use of the inactivated vaccine as the initial immunogen in infants to prevent polio due to a vaccine strain. Many other viral vaccines used routinely today are live, attenuated strains, including vaccines to prevent measles, mumps, rubella, and varicella (chicken pox) infections. Although these vaccines are usually not given until a child is 1 year of age, potentially minimizing the threat of infection in immunocompromised hosts who may not have been diagnosed prior to this age, there are still cases of disseminated infection due to the vaccine reported in young children.

Recombinant vector vaccines

Attenuated viruses can be used as vehicles for the delivery of recombinant vaccine antigens, much in the same way that attenuated bacteria can be used for such purposes. Vaccinia virus, used as a vaccine to prevent smallpox, can also be used as a vector for delivering recombinant vaccine antigens. Vaccinia has several advantages for this type of application. The genome of the virus is sufficiently large (approximately 200,000 base pairs) that it can tolerate the insertion of large pieces of genetic material without impairing viral replication or assembly. Also, the virus is easy to deliver to a vaccinee. Introduction of the virus into a small cut or abrasion on the skin is usually sufficient.

Successful Viral Vaccines

Some of the most spectacular advances in public health due to the use of vaccines have been the result of successful viral vaccines (Table 21.1). Smallpox was eliminated from the human population by the end of the 1970s through vigorous vaccination plans. While this was no mean feat, it was possible because smallpox is exclusively a human pathogen with no animal or environmental reservoir. Mass campaigns for polio vaccination have succeeded in eliminating this disease from many parts of the world, and it is expected that it too will be eliminated by 2010. In countries where MMR vaccine has been used, the incidence of these diseases has declined by more than 99%. Elimination of measles is the next goal for worldwide public health vaccination programs. However, this process is hampered by the need for the current vaccine to be kept refrigerated, which is not possible in many parts of the world lacking an electrical supply. Indeed, the development of solar-powered refrigerators may be as consequential for elimination of measles virus as was development of the vaccine.

Difficulties with Viral Vaccines

There are major immunologic and virologic hurdles to developing viral vaccines. Antigenic variability among viruses is often high, meaning that a successful vaccine frequently requires many components to ensure that the virus does not escape its host's immune response through mutation. Moreover, it is often difficult to isolate sufficiently attenuated, replicative forms of a virus. For many viral vaccines, we have a poor understanding of what constitutes protective immunity to the virus. For example, it was once thought that neutralizing antibodies to HIV proteins would be present in the genital tract of professional sex workers who are repeatedly exposed to HIV. However, neither mucosal IgA nor IgG has been detected in many of these individuals. Illnesses produced by viral infections are highly variable and encompass acute, chronic, latent/dormant, and recurrent but subclinical disease. These different disease states likely rely on different immunologic mechanisms for their manifestation. It is thought that most individuals harbor Epstein-Barr virus for most of their life but that it is effectively controlled by immunity to this virus. Thus, effective immunity is not based on elimination of this virus but on controlling its ability to replicate and produce disease.

Antigenic variation in influenza virus

While many viruses produce a tremendous amount of serologic variability at all times, influenza viruses tend to circulate throughout the world with a limited number of serologic variants. These variants are produced by two mechanisms: antigenic drift and antigenic shift (Fig. 21.3). *Antigenic drift* is the more common but more subtle mechanism for generating variation. From year to year, point mutations accumulate in the genes encoding the viral surface hemagglutinin and neuraminidase antigens, potentially producing epitopes not recognized by preexisting antibodies (Fig. 21.12). Thus, antigenic drift underlies the need for yearly influenza vaccination. To produce a new supply of influenza vaccines each year, manufacturers need to identify at least a year in advance (to account for the long time required to produce such a large quantity of vaccine) which type of drift is likely to emerge in the following fall/winter flu season. *Antigenic shift* occurs

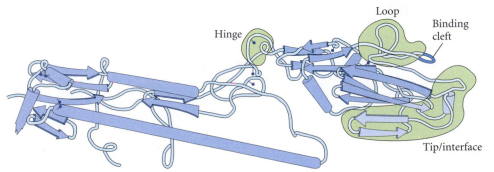

Loop

Hinge

Binding cleft

Tip/interface

Figure 21.12 Structure of the hemagglutinin of influenza virus. The binding cleft anchors the virus to sialic acid residues on host cells. In the areas designated as the tip, the loop, and the hinge, amino acid changes accumulate to produce antigenic drift. Within these regions are amino acids that change with the highest frequency. The crystal structure is from I. Wilson et al., *Nature* **289**:366–373, 1981, with permission.

when influenza viruses from different host species, such as swine and humans, both infect another species such as migratory waterfowl. When two disparate viruses infect the same cell, the viral nucleic acids, which consist of eight single-stranded RNAs, can undergo a reassortment to produce a hybrid virus with major antigenic changes. This type of antigenic change occurs more rarely and in the past has been associated with cycles that correlate with the presence of a large number of nonimmune individuals younger than 17 to 20 years old. These individuals have not been previously exposed to the new variant of influenza and thus are susceptible to infection to these new virus variants. Attempts to control emergence of antigenically unique strains of influenza virus have focused on surveillance of farm animals such as chickens, which are often the first to get infected with new strains. In 1997, a new variant of influenza virus caused severe infection in chickens in Hong Kong that was transmitted to humans, prompting the elimination of all chickens in Hong Kong to control the emergence of this new strain. In January 2004, the same variant caused human influenza in Vietnam and Thailand.

Safety of Viral Vaccines

As many of the currently licensed or available vaccines for viral infections use live, attenuated virus particles, safety is of paramount importance in the development of viral vaccines. As noted earlier, while attenuated strains are safe for immunocompetent individuals, immunocompromised hosts are frequently vulnerable to infection by attenuated viruses. Even when an attenuated vaccine performs well in preclinical and clinical trials and appears to be safe during these trials, rare events can occur that are not detected until after the vaccine passes the trial period. A vaccine to prevent one form of infantile diarrhea caused by rotavirus was withdrawn within 2 years of its licensing date because of the development of intussusception, an intestinal obstruction whereby a segment of the bowel inserts itself into a more distal part of the bowel. It was esti-

mated that to detect this rare complication, more than 100,000 infants would have had to be studied during prelicensing testing, an obviously unfeasible clinical trial.

Vaccines for Fungal Infections

Fungal pathogens have become major causes of infectious diseases during the past few decades, along with the significant increase in the proportion of individuals with underlying immunodeficiencies (such as AIDS) among hospitalized patients (see chapter 20). These findings have indicated that CMI is critical for immunity to fungal infections (although some fungi, such as cryptococci and *Candida albicans*, show a susceptibility to antibody-mediated immunity). In parts of the world some fungal infections can cause serious diseases in otherwise healthy people. As complex organisms, existing as both haploid and diploid cells and growing in mycelial or yeast forms, fungi present a plethora of antigens to the immune system that are potential targets for vaccine development. Often fungi are found in one form in the environment from which they are acquired and in another form in the infected mammalian host. This means that the antigenic epitope that stimulates an immune response during the initial infection may no longer be expressed after the fungal infection has become established. As fungal pathogenesis is not that clearly defined in many instances, it is difficult to know which form of the organism to target with a vaccine. In addition, vaccines for these infections are presently being evaluated primarily experimentally in laboratory settings, although some immunotherapeutic reagents for cryptococcosis are in early clinical trials (Table 21.9).

Fungal Diseases Targeted by Current Vaccine Research

Histoplasmosis

Histoplasma capsulatum causes histoplasmosis, which is manifested primarily as a lung disease in those parts of the world where this fungus is endemic. Laboratory vac-

Table 21.9 Fungal vaccines under development

Disease	Etiologic agent	Immune effectors	Vaccines in development
Histoplasmosis	*Histoplasma capsulatum*	Cell mediated	H glycoprotein (β-glucosidase), HIS-62 (heat shock protein), cell wall and cell membranes
Coccidioidomycosis	*Coccidioides immitis*	Cell mediated	Enzyme, spherule outer wall extract, alkali-soluble antigen, water-soluble antigen, urease
Blastomycosis	*Blastomyces dermatitidis*	Cell mediated	WI-1 surface adhesin
Cryptococcosis	*Cryptococcus neoformans*	Humoral	Capsular polysaccharide, melanin
Candidiasis	*Candida albicans*	Humoral Cell mediated	Mannan, mannoprotein Enolase
PCP	*Pneumocystis carinii*	Humoral Cell mediated	Major surface glycoproteins

cines for this pathogen have focused on surface glycoproteins termed H and M proteins, cell wall proteins, and heat shock proteins. Immunity appears to be primarily through a TH1 cell-mediated immune pathway. The particular efficacy of a given vaccine candidate in animals may depend on the route of infection. For example, the H glycoprotein does not protect against systemic *H. capsulatum* infection but does protect against pulmonary infection. As it is likely that complex organisms such as fungi express different antigens in different tissues they infect, an effective vaccine may need to contain a variety of different antigens for these different disease manifestations.

Coccidioidomycosis

Coccidioidomycosis is caused by *Coccidioides immitis*, which lives in the soil, particularly in arid regions of North, Central, and South America, and causes infections in about 40% of the people who inhale wind-borne arthrospores. In host tissues these grow as spherules containing endospores. Coccidioidomycosis is primarily a lung infection, which tends to be self-limiting. A serious but rare manifestation is dissemination outside the thoracic cavity. Individuals who recover from coccidioidomycosis appear to have life-long immunity to reinfection, indicative of a protective response that appears mostly to be a CD4$^+$ DTH (T$_{DTH}$) response. Thus, vaccine development is feasible and has focused on protection against lung infection. A vaccine based on formaldehyde-killed spherules was tested in the 1970s, but doses were limited due to toxicity. At tolerable doses the spherule vaccine was not protective. More recent laboratory work has focused on the potential vaccine efficacy of outer wall proteins and soluble extracts from the spherules, a recombinant 48-kilodalton (kDa) T-cell-reactive protein, a urease, and a heat shock protein.

Blastomycosis

Blastomycosis is due to the dimorphic fungus *Blastomyces dermatitidis*. Infection occurs by inhalation and results in a pneumonia that is self-limiting in some patients. Most individuals have a chronic infection. Again, a T$_{DTH}$ response seems to be protective. Laboratory studies point to a cell surface adhesin termed WI-1 as an antigen that can elicit protective immunity in mice. Also, strains of *B. dermatitidis* lacking the WI-1 antigen are nonpathogenic for mice and could potentially be used as a live, attenuated vaccine effective in protecting the animals against lethal pulmonary infection by provoking immune response to antigens other than WI-1.

Cryptococcosis

Cryptococcosis has been studied extensively because its causative agent, *Cryptococcus neoformans*, expresses capsular polysaccharides like many bacterial pathogens. Four serotypes, designated A, B, C, and D, are known, with types A and D being responsible for most human disease. Several monoclonal antibodies and conjugate vaccines consisting of the capsular polysaccharide complexed to tetanus toxoid have been investigated in early human trials. Many cases of cryptococcosis occur in immunocompromised patients, especially patients with AIDS, suggesting an important contribution of CD4$^+$ cells to immunity. However, cryptococcosis also occurs in pigeon handlers because of the long-term survival of the fungus in pigeon droppings to which the handlers are constantly exposed. The capsule is composed of a backbone of mannose substituted with xylose and glucuronic acid, referred to as glucuronoxylomannan. Serologic differences are due to the number of xylose side chains and degree of O acetylation. Inducing protective immunity by either the purified glucuronoxylomannan or a conjugate vaccine has been problematical due to the complexity of the serologic structure of the glucuronoxylomannan and immunologic responses to it (Fig. 21.13). Certain antibodies to glucuronoxylomannan are protective in animal models while others are not. Variability in both the epitopes on the target antigen and by the usage of variable-region genes of different antibodies contributes to this complicated situation. As few as two changes in amino acids in the antibody V$_H$ region may account for the difference between a protective and nonprotective antibody to the capsular polysaccharide. In animals, some antibodies are protective when given passively at certain doses but actually enhance infection when given at higher doses. Such a problem will complicate development of vaccines using glucuronoxylomannan, as a given individual may have a predilection to respond to a nonprotective epitope and produce nonprotective antibody. Another potential antigen is a melanin-like substance, and antibodies to this material have shown partial protective efficacy in animals (Fig. 21.13). One possible solution is the use of peptide antigens as molecular mimics of protective epitopes, perhaps as part of a conjugate vaccine using melanin as a carrier, so that only antibodies of the desired specificity and idiotype are produced. Passive therapy with antibodies directed at multiple antigens may also enhance protective efficacy.

Candidiasis

Candidiasis is caused by members of the genus *Candida*, with *C. albicans* the most common species causing human disease. Candidiasis can be a local infection on the skin or

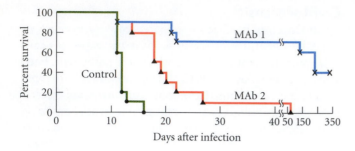

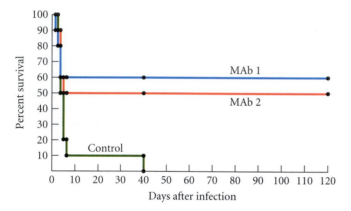

Figure 21.13 Survival curves of mice treated with monoclonal antibodies (MAbs) to different cryptococcal antigens. (**Top**) Two different monoclonal antibodies reactive to the capsular polysaccharide prolonged survival, with one antibody clearly better than the other in providing survival from infection. (**Bottom**) Two different monoclonal antibodies to the melanin antigen also resulted in prolonged survival following infection. Reprinted from J. Mukherjee et al., *Infect. Immun.* **60:**4534–4541, 1992 (top), and A. L. Rosas et al., *Infect. Immun.* **69:**3410–3412, 2001 (bottom), with permission.

mucous membranes, and breaks in the skin and mucous membranes can lead to infections of deeper tissues. Because this fungus is normally found in the human gastrointestinal tract, it commonly colonizes implanted medical devices, where it can cause bloodstream infections. A prophylactic or therapeutic vaccine for this increasingly common infection would be highly desirable, but only laboratory studies have been conducted. Several candidate vaccines, including members of the aspartyl proteinase (Sap2) family, the 65-kDa mannoprotein (MP65) antigen, and heat-killed cells delivered intranasally along with an adjuvant, have shown some efficacy in animal studies. Interestingly, infections with *Candida* species are common in patients with AIDS who have low CD4$^+$ cell counts, suggesting that these cells play a critical role in immunity and that provoking a T$_{DTH}$ response would be a goal of vaccine development. The results with some experimental vaccines tested in animals support this view, while other experimental results in animals indicate that antibodies to the mannoprotein can reduce colonization levels in infected tissues.

Pneumocystis carinii infection

Infection with *P. carinii* emerged in the early part of the AIDS epidemic as a prominent cause of pneumonia, designated PCP for *P. carinii* pneumonia. Although *P. carinii* was initially considered to be a parasite, it is now recognized as a fungus. The frequent occurrence of PCP in patients with AIDS implicates CMI as a major immune effector. An antigenic group of proteins termed the major surface glycoprotein, consisting of a family of proteins with molecular weights between 90 and 140 kDa, is immunogenic and elicits both humoral and cellular immunity in animal studies. These proteins also serve an adhesin function, although it is not known if antibodies can inhibit adherence of *P. carinii* to lung tissues.

General Strategies for Future Development of Vaccines for Fungal Infections

Since no human vaccine for a fungal infection is currently available, there are no paradigms to define a general strategy for development of this field. Fungal infections are common in immunodeficient patients, particularly those with T-cell immunodeficiencies, yet numerous animal studies suggest that antibodies to fungal antigens are protective. Fungal antigens are quite diverse, with no obvious type of antigen known to represent a class of protective antigens such as bacterial capsular antigens or viral outer surface antigens. Progress in vaccine development for these important pathogens will likely be slow for the foreseeable future until better correlates of immunity are established and protective antigens are identified.

Vaccines for Parasitic Diseases

Parasitic diseases are among the most common causes of severe infections, with a high degree of associated mortality (see chapter 20). The two major classes of parasites that infect humans and animals are protozoan parasites and helminth worms. Protozoa are single-cell organisms and often grow both inside and outside cells of infected humans. The major protozoan parasites of humans include *Plasmodium* species that cause malaria, *Trypanosoma* species that cause sleeping sickness, *Leishmania* species that have a variety of disease manifestations, and *Toxoplasma gondii* that causes toxoplasmosis. In addition, many protozoan parasites cause less severe infections, including amebiasis due to *Entamoeba histolytica*; babesiosis, which is transmitted to humans by tick bites; and intestinal infections such as giardiasis, cryptosporidiosis, and trichinosis. Helminth worms are large, multicellular organisms that obviously are extracellular and present a large mass of foreign tissue for the immune system to react to. Over 1 billion people are infected by tissue nematodes such as *Trichinella spiralis*, which causes trichinosis, and by intestinal nematodes, including roundworms, hookworms, pinworms, and whipworms. Filarial worms that infect the skin and lymphatic tissues are also major causes of disease, infecting 100 million to 200 million individuals. Two of these, *Onchocerca volvulus* and *Loa loa*, can cause severe eye infections. Trematodes, or flukes, are another class of helminthic worms that includes the agents of schistosomiasis, which is thought to infect over 200 million people worldwide. Although schistosomal infections do not provoke significant clinical disease in many cases, its common occurrence makes vaccine development a high priority.

Protozoan Diseases Targeted by Current Vaccine Research

Malaria

A malaria vaccine would represent a major milestone in vaccine development and public health, and a concerted effort is being directed toward this goal. Malaria infects 100 million to 300 million people, causes 1 million to 3 million deaths each year, and is endemic in over 100 countries, with a total population of 2.5 billion people. However, as for all protozoan parasites, significant barriers hinder the development of malaria vaccines. These barriers, including the complex life cycle of the plasmodia and their high level of antigenic variation, have made it difficult to determine the contribution of humoral immunity and CMI to the control of this pathogen. Such information is vital for vaccine design and testing. Also, many individuals have a partial immunity, being susceptible to infection and carrying parasites in their blood but having reduced disease symptoms. Nonetheless, even a partially effective vaccine could result in a large decrease in the suffering exacted by malaria.

Understanding protective immunologic mechanisms is a key part of vaccine development; thus, the major challenge in developing a malaria vaccine is to gain insight into these factors. Malaria sporozoites are initially extracellular organisms as they are injected from mosquito saliva into the host's blood. Within a short time, they enter the liver and take up an intracellular residence in hepatocytes (see Fig. 20.1). Thus both antibody and cellular immunity are likely important in these different stages. Merozoites are released from the liver and enter erythrocytes, causing the host to become parasitemic and symptomatic. Because erythrocytes lack MHC antigens, non-MHC-restricted immune resistance would have potential relevance here. Release of merozoites from infected erythrocytes continues the cycle, and some of these merozoites differentiate into gametocytes. Ingestion of gametocytes during another mosquito bite passes the infection on to subsequent individuals when they are bitten by the infected mosquito.

Some success in producing immunity to malaria has been attained. Allowing mosquitoes containing irradiated, killed sporozoites to repeatedly feed on volunteers resulted in protection of six of nine volunteers subsequently exposed to mosquitoes that contained live sporozoites. Although the study demonstrated an important principle, there is no practical way to use this strategy for billions of people. A major protein on the surface of the sporozoite, the circumsporozoite protein, contains a repetitive B-cell epitope that has shown some success in eliciting protective immunity, but only when very high antibody titers are achieved. A vaccine containing this antigen in a strong adjuvant gave short-term protection, waning by 6 months, in African volunteers. There are protein antigens on the surface of merozoites and on infected erythrocytes that are also targets of protective immunity. A major drawback to these vaccines is the antigenic variability of the proteins. Interestingly, antibody to this variant antigen is thought to provide partial immunity once an individual responds to a large number of the variant epitopes. Finding a conserved, protective epitope on the variant antigens is a potential strategy, but this approach is in the early stages.

Merozoite surface protein 1 (MSP-1) has shown promise for 2 decades, and an antigenic cocktail in an experimental vaccine called Spf66 showed some early efficacy, which, unfortunately, was not replicated in later field trials. MSP-1, along with other proteins, is a likely component of some of the next generation of malaria vaccines to be tested. Induction of antibody and T-cell responses to malaria antigens expressed on the surface of infected erythrocytes and hepatocytes is likely going to be based on the use of DNA vaccine delivery systems. Many different vaccine components are being pursued for use against malaria (Table 21.10). As the genome sequence of the malaria parasite was completed at the end of 2002, it is now hoped that new targets for vaccine development will be identified.

Trypanosomiasis

One form of trypanosomiasis is caused by *Trypanosoma cruzi* infection, leading to Chagas' disease. Usually Chagas' disease is self-limiting, leaving patients in a state of chronic infection but without symptoms. Some individuals develop life-threatening systemic infections. The parasite is transmitted in the feces of the reduviid bug, and in-

Table 21.10 A selection of *P. falciparum* antigens as targets for parasite-neutralizing immune response[a]

Antigen	Mol wt (10³)	Antigenic diversity	Potential targets for[b]	Location[b]
PfEMP1	250–300	Extensive	Cytoadherence Ab	RBC surface
Pf332	280	No	ADCI, inhibitory Ab	RBC surface
RIFINS	27–45	Yes	NK cell	RBC surface
MSP-1	230	Extensive	Inhibitory Ab	MS
MSP-2	45–55	Extensive	Inhibitory Ab	MS
MSP-3	50	Yes	ADCI	PV, MS-associated
GLURP	220	No	ADCI	PV, MS-associated
Pf155/RESA	155	No	Inhibitory Ab	Dense granules
AMA-1	80	Yes	Inhibitory Ab	Rhoptries
EBA-175	175	Yes	Inhibitory Ab	Microneme

[a]Reprinted from A. Bolad and K. Berzins, *Scand. J. Immunol.* **52:**223–239, 2000, with permission.

[b]Ab, antibody; ADCI, antibody-dependent immunity; RBC, red blood cell; MS, merozoite surface; PV, parasitophorous vacuole.

fection results when the parasite enters the host through breaks in the skin, mucosa, or conjunctiva (see Fig. 20.3). Another form is due to *Trypanosoma brucei*, and infection with this organism causes sleeping sickness, or African trypanosomiasis. The parasites are transmitted by the bite of the tsetse fly. All vaccine development work for these parasites is experimental. A crude, soluble extract of *T. cruzi* protects mice against infection, and IFN-γ has been shown to be a critical mediator of immunity. Several recombinant and purified proteins, along with DNA vaccines encoding these proteins, have also shown efficacy against infection in animals. A singularly large challenge to vaccine development arising from chronic trypanosomiasis is the antigenic shift of the variant surface glycoprotein (VSG) (see Fig. 20.16). VSG covers most of the organism's surface during bloodstream infection. Thus, antigenic shifts in VSG allow waves of parasitemia to occur, because an effective antibody response to one variant, although promoting clearance of that variant, also selects for another variant. One parasite may have more than 1,000 antigenically distinct VSG genes. The antibodies to the VSG antigens render the trypomastigote form of the organism sensitive to lysis by complement; in the absence of such antibody, the trypomastigotes are resistant to complement-mediated lysis. As with many other pathogens, exact correlates of protective immunity that can be used to guide vaccine development are not fully defined for the trypanosomes.

Leishmaniasis

Leishmaniasis is caused by a number of species of protozoan parasite of the genus *Leishmania*. The sandfly is the vector that transmits the promastigote form to a new host (see Fig. 20.2). The disease can range from a local skin infection that usually resolves (cutaneous leishmaniasis), to a mucocutaneous spread of infection, to a systemic infec-

tion involving parasites inside macrophages throughout the body (visceral leishmaniasis). Strong data support the role of TH1-directed immune response in resolution of infections with *Leishmania*. Vaccine candidates include killed protozoal cells, usually mixed with an adjuvant; genetically modified, live, attenuated cells; DNA vaccines encoding recombinant proteins such as cysteine proteinases; and purified proteins. One interesting approach tested in mice used a cell line transfected with the leishmaniolysin, or gp63 protease antigen, along with the CD40 ligand (CD40L) (Fig. 21.7). CD40L induces IL-12 production by APCs, a key step in eliciting immunity to *Leishmania*. Other approaches, such as the use of cytokine adjuvants to enhance TH1 responses, are also under development. At present the development of an effective vaccine is limited by incomplete knowledge about which antigens are protective and the long-term safety of the various vaccine candidates under consideration and uncertainty about whether the use of drugs may be more feasible than vaccination for disease control.

Toxoplasmosis

The obligate intracellular parasite *T. gondii* can produce acute or chronic infection. These usually do not provoke symptoms in immunocompetent hosts. Transmission is through contact with cat feces or ingestion of undercooked meat. Infection via the gastrointestinal route elicits IgA responses that can be diagnostic of infection. Both humoral and cellular responses are part of the normal reaction to infection, but protective immunity is best correlated with CMI. Lytic CD8[+] T cells are likely important effectors of immunity, and cytokines produced by T cells, such as IFN-γ and tumor necrosis factor alpha, appear critical for mediating immunity.

As with most vaccines for parasites, vaccines for toxoplasmosis are all experimental. Purified and recombinant proteins, such as surface antigen 1 (SAG1), granule antigen 1 (GRA1), GRA7, and rhoptry protein 2 (ROP2; rhoptries are apical organelles that release their contents during the invasion process), elicit partial or full protection in animals. DNA vaccines directed against these antigens have also shown efficacy in animal studies. Further advances in vaccine development should come from a greater understanding of the biochemistry of infection and genetics of *T. gondii*.

Vaccines for Other Parasites

Many other important parasitic protozoa and helminths would be on a list of vaccines needed to promote public health. All of these represent complex organisms with multiple phenotypes, with complicated genomes, and for which we have an incomplete understanding of the underlying immunity that an effective vaccine would need to elicit. For example, the helminthic parasites of the *Schistosoma* genus elicit a high level of IgE antibody during human infection, but experimental evidence suggests a need for a CD4$^+$ T-cell-based protection following immunization with experimental antigens. Usually antigens on the surface of the parasitizing form of the worm represent potential vaccine targets, and recombinant and DNA-vaccine forms of these antigens are all under study. The multiple challenges for vaccine development could not be better exemplified than in the attempts to develop vaccines for parasitic infections. The key will be to identify correlates of immunity and antigens that elicit protective immunity but do not exacerbate disease.

Passive Immunization

The strategy of passive immunization encompasses the use of exogenously made human or animal antibodies, either polyclonal or monoclonal, to protect against infection and disease. The first Nobel Prize in medicine was awarded to Emil von Behring in 1901 for his work on serum therapy, particularly for treating diphtheria. Thus passive immunization was one of the earliest benefits to emerge from the study of immunology. Many advances were made during the 20th century, most notably the development of a process to purify and safely administer via the intravenous route large quantities of the IgG fraction of antibody, means to produce safe vaccines to give to individuals whose serum can be used for passive therapy, and the development of monoclonal antibodies that can potentially be produced in large quantities for use in passive therapy. Even nonimmune intravenous IgG preparations (IVIgG) have found uses in treating immunodeficiency diseases and diseases such as immune thrombocytopenia purpura

and Kawasaki syndrome, a systemic condition of unknown etiology seen mostly in children. The mechanism of protection in these situations is not understood. Immune globulin derived from large pools of human plasma and fractionated by cold-ethanol precipitation, or hyperimmune IVIgG prepared from plasma of volunteers immunized with certain vaccines, has demonstrated efficacy in numerous situations but usually is reserved for administration to individuals shortly after their likely exposure to an infectious agent, so-called postexposure immunization (Table 21.11). An individual bitten by a potentially rabid animal will be given antirabies immune globulin along with rabies vaccine as part of the postexposure treatment. Passive therapy reagents are available for postexposure immunization against measles; hepatitis A and B and non-A, non-B hepatitis; botulism; tetanus; diphtheria; cytomegalovirus infection; and varicella. These important reagents are all based on the same strategy described by von Behring in his Nobel Prize presentation speech (http://www.nobel.se/medicine/laureates/1901/behring-lecture.html). Passive immunization is also effective for treating bites from venomous spiders and insects and is given within 72 hours of birth to prevent sensitization of mothers whose erythrocytes lack the Rh antigen (Rh-negative) to the Rh antigen on erythrocytes of their fetuses when paternal genes encode for production of the Rh antigen.

Passive therapy does have some drawbacks. One major concern is the potential for transmitting blood-borne infectious agents, particularly since the passive reagents

Table 21.11 Passive immunotherapeutic reagents available for postexposure prophylaxis

Disease(s)	Reagent
Botulism	Equine botulism antitoxin
Measles	Standard human immune globulin (high titers of antibody in most individuals)
Rubella	Standard human immune globulin (high titers of antibody in most individuals) but only for pregnant women in first trimester of pregnancy; efficacy unreliable
Tetanus	Human tetanus immune globulin
Rabies	Human rabies immune globulin
Hepatitis A; non-A, non-B hepatitis	Normal human immune globulin
Hepatitis B	Human hepatitis B immune globulin, usually for neonates born to infected mothers to prevent neonatal transmission
Spider toxins	Horse antivenin
Snake toxins	Antivenins developed to be specific to the particular snake toxin

often are made from the blood of many individuals. Fortunately, current practices for purifying and treating immune globulins and IVIgG have been highly successful in preventing transmission of infectious agents. Some sera contain IgG isohemagglutinins, antibodies directed at red cell antigens. These could cause an anemic reaction in a recipient. Another concern is an allergic or even anaphylactic reaction to the components of the passive reagent. This is of concern particularly in individuals with natural IgA immunodeficiency. Trace amounts of IgA in IVIgG preparations have been known to provoke antibodies to IgA in deficient individuals, and these antibodies can cause severe reactions with subsequent administration of immune globulins. Other allergic reactions can develop because of the complex nature of the passive reagents. The passive reagent itself might have harmful antibodies, such as those to the cells of the recipient. Serum sickness is another complication of passive therapy. This occurs about 2 weeks posttreatment, when the recipient responds with antibody to foreign antigens in the passive reagent. The formation of immune complexes between the passively administered antibodies and the recipient's newly synthesized antibodies is thought to be a component of the serum sickness reaction. These immune complexes can become deposited in highly vascularized tissues such as the intestine or kidneys and initiate destructive inflammatory reactions through the local activation of complement.

Summary

The development of vaccines has been, and continues to be, one of the greatest accomplishments in modern medicine. Many basic principles and immunologic concepts have been elucidated to facilitate vaccine development. Still, the diversity of microbial pathogens, the antigens they produce, and the types of immune responses that need to be elicited by a vaccine present formidable challenges. A large number of strategies for producing vaccines have emerged from biomedical research, including toxoids; purified antigens; killed microbial particles; live, attenuated organisms; anti-idiotype antibodies; and peptide and DNA vaccines. Vaccine development can be augmented by the use of adjuvants, including nonspecific and specific stimulators of immune activity. More sophis-

ticated adjuvants such as recombinant cytokines or DNA vaccines that encode both protective antigens and cytokine adjuvants are on the horizon. Use of DCs to deliver antigens holds promise for a safe and effective means of eliciting immunity to almost any pathogen. Vaccine development is often limited by the great serologic diversity of protective epitopes expressed within a species of pathogenic microbe, as well as by our incomplete understanding of immune correlates of protection. Passive therapy also has shown efficacy in prevention and even treatment of some infectious diseases, and newer technologies involved in production of human monoclonal antibodies likely will increase the range of diseases that are amenable to therapy by passive reagents. Continued research into the immunologic basis for protective immunity to infection will be a key component of future vaccine development, as will continued research into the molecular basis for microbial pathogenesis.

Suggested Reading

Bendelac, A., and R. Medzhitov. 2002. Adjuvants of immunity: harnessing innate immunity to promote adaptive immunity. *J. Exp. Med.* **195:**F19–F23.

Coombes, B. K., and J. B. Mahon. 2001. Dendritic cell discoveries provide new insight into the cellular immunobiology of DNA vaccines. *Immunol. Lett.* **78:**103–111.

Gregersen, J. P. 2001. DNA vaccines. *Naturwissenschaften* **88:**504–513.

Handman, E. 2001. Leishmaniasis: current status of vaccine development. *Clin. Microbiol. Rev.* **14:**229–243.

Hull, H. F. 2001. The future of polio eradication. *Lancet Infect. Dis.* **1:**299–303.

Nalin, D. R. 2002. Evidence based vaccinology. *Vaccine* **20:**1624–1630.

Obaro, S., and R. Adegbola. 2002. The pneumococcus: carriage, disease and conjugate vaccines. *J. Med. Microbiol.* **51:**98–104.

Ogra, P.L., H. Fade, and R. C. Welliver. 2001. Vaccination strategies for mucosal immune responses. *Clin. Microbiol. Rev.* **14:**430–445.

Orme, I. M. 2001. The search for new vaccines against tuberculosis. *J. Leukoc. Biol.* **70:**1–10.

Pappagianis, D. 2001. Seeking a vaccine against *Coccidioides immitis* and serologic studies: expectations and realities. *Fungal Genet Biol.* **32:**1–9.

Rappuoli, R. 2001. Conjugates and reverse vaccinology to eliminate bacterial meningitis. *Vaccine* **19:**2319–2322.

Richie, T. L., and A. Saul. 2002. Progress and challenges for malaria vaccines. *Nature* **415:**694–701.

IMMUNE SYSTEM DYSFUNCTION: DEFICIENCIES

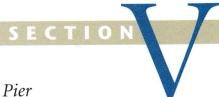

SECTION V

chapter 22

Immunology and AIDS

Saskia Boisot and Gerald B. Pier

Etiology and Epidemiology of AIDS

Although discovered relatively recently, human immunodeficiency virus type 1 (HIV-1) has had a tremendous impact on many dimensions of science and society. Since the identification of HIV as the cause of the acquired immunodeficiency syndrome (AIDS) in the early 1980s, tens of millions of persons have been infected. HIV-1 is particularly prevalent in sub-Saharan Africa, where the virus probably originated in humans after crossing the species barrier from chimpanzees, and its expansion throughout the world has been explosive. Three major groups of HIV-1, designated M (main), O (outlier), and N (non-M, non-O), appear to have arisen from three independent crossings of HIV-like viruses from chimpanzees into human populations, notably from chimpanzees in western equatorial Africa where it is believed the various HIV groups originated. The group M viruses are divided into subtypes, designated A to D, F1, F2, G to J, and K. All of these subtypes originated from a common group M ancestor, which is believed to have existed before 1940 and forms a branching point on a phylogenetic tree. Organisms that are derived from a common ancestor and share common features form a *clade*. The related virus HIV-2 causes a similar, but less virulent, syndrome of immunodeficiency. HIV-2 is most closely related to a type of simian immunodeficiency virus that occurs in sooty mangabeys, a primate species found in western Africa, where the highest prevalence of HIV-2 occurs. Although HIV-2 can cause a disease similar to that of HIV-1, the generally milder course of HIV-2 infection and limited spread of this isolate have resulted in much less study than has occurred with HIV-1.

After initial infection with HIV-1, there is usually an acute flu-like illness that develops within several weeks, but after this most individuals are clinically asymptomatic for years. An average of 10 years passes before an untreated individual develops AIDS, although this can be as short as 2 years and as long as 20 years. AIDS is a syndrome of immunodeficiency that is marked by declining levels of $CD4^+$ lymphocytes and the development of various opportunistic infections and malignancies. To eventually combat this scourge, the immunologic processes underlying infection by the virus, the immune damage caused by infection, and the host's immune responses to infection will need to be understood in fine molecular details.

Understanding the ways in which HIV infection is transmitted among humans has been a major component of disease prevention, as this understanding underlies many preventive strategies ranging from education to vaccination. Transmission of HIV-1 generally occurs via three major routes: sexual contact, exposure to blood or blood products, and perinatal infection. Particular types of sexual exposures carry a relatively high risk (1 per 100 exposures) compared with other types of sexual contact. The risk of transmission by female-to-male heterosexual contact is substantially lower (1 per 1,500). Direct infusion of infected blood or blood products carries a particularly high risk of infection. Since the introduction of screening procedures, transmission of HIV-1 via transfusion has become very rare in countries that screen the blood supply (transfusion-associated risk is estimated at about 1 per 450,000 transfusions in the United States). Transmission via illicit intravenous drug use, however, remains a common mode of infection. Perinatal infection (vertical transmission from mother to fetus or neonate) carries a risk of about 1 in 3 without intervention. In areas that can afford diagnosis and antiretroviral therapy, perinatal infections have been reduced dramatically. Vertical transmission, however, remains a large problem in many parts of the world where such therapies are unavailable.

Diagnosis of HIV-1 infection usually is determined by demonstrating the presence of virus-specific antibodies, although recent molecular technologies permit the identification of virus-specific RNA in plasma. For antibody diagnosis, an enzyme-linked immunosorbent assay followed by a confirmatory immunoblot is used to establish the diagnosis and has a high degree of sensitivity and specificity for chronically infected individuals. During acute infection, however, a false-negative result may be obtained before an antibody response develops (typically less than 3 months after initial exposure). In this case, direct measurement of viral p24 antigen or viral nucleic acid sequences in plasma can confirm infection.

HIV
Virus structure

HIV-1 belongs to the viral genus *Lentivirus* of the family *Retroviridae*. The structure of this virus (Fig. 22.1) is similar to that of other lentiviruses. It is spherical and consists of a capsid surrounded by an envelope of host cell-derived membrane and membrane components. The bullet-shaped capsid is composed of the $p24^{gag}$ protein (Gag), the most plentiful protein in the virion, and contains two duplicate strands of RNA that are the viral genome. In close association with the RNA are the nucleocapsid proteins p7 and p9 and the enzymes reverse transcriptase, RNase H, integrase, and protease. This core is coated by a host cell-derived lipid membrane, which is acquired by the nascent virion as it buds from an infected cell. Lining the inside of this membrane is the matrix for the viral structure, which is composed of the p17 outer core, or Gag, protein.

The outer surface of the membrane is studded with envelope glycoproteins, each of which consists of two components, gp41 and gp120. The gp41 component is a transmembrane protein that binds to the external gp120 protein noncovalently through hydrophobic interactions. The gp41-gp120 unit exists on the viral surface in trimers and is responsible for the binding and fusion of virions to target cells for infection. The average virion surface contains about 72 of these structures. These proteins of the viral envelope are heavily glycosylated through the addition of complex-carbohydrate side chains by cellular enzymes during passage through the endoplasmic reticulum (ER) and the Golgi apparatus. The purpose of these carbohydrate side chains may be evasion of antibody responses in the host.

Life cycle of HIV

The life cycle of HIV-1 (Fig. 22.2A and 22.3) is typical of that of other retroviruses in general details. Free virions bind to host target cells via specific interactions of the viral envelope with receptors on the target cells, allowing membrane fusion and entry of the viral capsid. Inside the host cell, the viral RNA genome is reverse transcribed to DNA and integrated into the host-cell genome. Cellular factors of the host are then used to produce viral RNAs and proteins. Viral proteins and RNA genomes are packaged and assembled to produce progeny virions that bud off the host cell, completing the replicative cycle.

Viral binding and entry

Entry of HIV-1 into $CD4^+$ cells is a complex process that involves the interaction of several proteins. The virus requires at least two receptors on its target cell: the CD4 molecule and a *coreceptor*. Chemokine receptors (G-

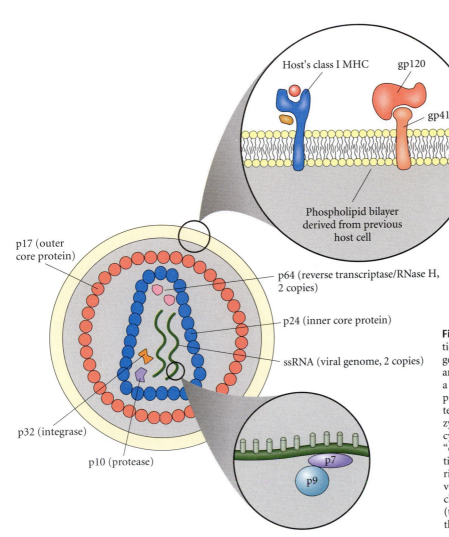

p17 (outer core protein)

Host's class I MHC

gp120

gp41

Phospholipid bilayer derived from previous host cell

p64 (reverse transcriptase/RNase H, 2 copies)

p24 (inner core protein)

ssRNA (viral genome, 2 copies)

p32 (integrase)

p10 (protease)

p7

p9

Figure 22.1 Structure of the HIV virion. The infectious particle contains duplicate strands of viral RNA genome in tight association with the viral proteins p7 and p9 (**bottom**). This RNA complex is packaged into a bullet-shaped capsid (composed of the viral protein p24) along with viral enzymes integrase (p32), protease (p10), and two copies of RT (p64). These enzymes play important roles in the viral infectious cycle. The viral capsid is further enclosed within an "outer core" composed of viral p17 protein. This entire particle is enclosed in a membrane envelope derived from the virus's most recent host cell. This envelope contains many host proteins (e.g., host's MHC class I) as well as the viral proteins gp41 and gp120 (**top**), which are important for docking and entry of the virion with its host cell.

protein-associated transmembrane receptors whose usual role is to signal for chemotaxis and cellular activation) serve as the coreceptor in concert with CD4. Various strains of HIV-1 utilize different chemokine receptors, possibly determining which cells can be infected. When the virus infects a cell, the viral envelope glycoprotein gp120 first binds CD4 on the target cell. This binding induces a conformational change in gp120, exposing a binding site for the chemokine receptor. Then gp120 binds the chemokine receptor, further changing its conformation to expose the associated gp41. By a poorly understood process, gp41 then mediates fusion of HIV-1 with the target-cell membrane, whereupon the viral core is released into the cytoplasm.

Integration

Once the virus has entered the target cell, the viral RNA is reverse transcribed to DNA. The viral RNA-dependent DNA polymerase (reverse transcriptase [RT]) first synthe-sizes a single strand of DNA complementary to the viral RNA. RNase H degrades the remaining viral RNA, allowing synthesis of the second strand of DNA and yielding double-stranded viral DNA. This viral DNA then migrates to the nucleus and undergoes noncovalent circularization by association of the long terminal repeat sequences (LTRs). Viral integrase mediates random integration into the host's chromosomal DNA, yielding the provirus.

Expression

The viral LTR serves as the promoter for viral gene expression. A number of factors influence expression of viral genes and proteins acting as regulators and enhancers of viral gene expression. One HIV gene, *tat*, is known to be an important positive regulator of transcription of all other HIV genes through its interaction with the LTR. Transcription further relies on host-cell transcription factors; numerous factors have been shown to act upon the LTR, increasing HIV gene transcription. The most clearly

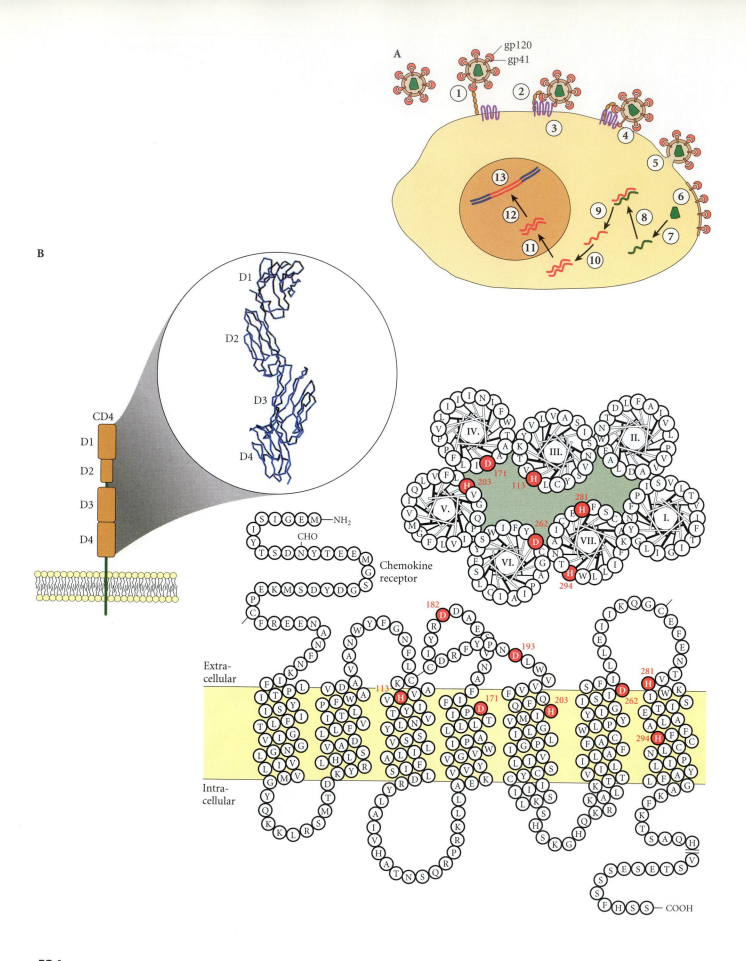

described of these are NF-κB and nuclear factor of activated T cells (NF-AT). Both of these transcription factors attach to binding sites in the LTR. Expression of HIV-1 in infected CD4+ lymphocytes is thus dependent on cellular activation that leads to nuclear translocation of these required transcription factors. The NF-κB protein is an inducible transcription factor expressed in T cells and macrophages. NF-κB is abundantly present in the cytoplasm of resting T cells, where it is bound to its cytoplasmic inhibitor (inhibitor of κB [IκB]). Upon cellular activation, IκB is degraded and the active NF-κB is translocated to the nucleus. By comparison, NF-AT is synthesized de novo following T-cell activation. In addition, cytokines may affect cellular activation, probably by influencing the activity of factors such as NF-κB, and therefore affect the amount of viral expression in infected cells.

Infected cells that are not activated, such as resting memory T lymphocytes, may contain proviral DNA that is not expressed because of a lack of cellular transcription factors necessary for viral expression. Thus, HIV-1 may be carried by a long-lived cell type in a quiescent state (a *latent reservoir*). Once such T cells encounter their target antigen, however, cellular activation would occur and lead to viral expression and replication.

Processing, assembly, and release

The component proteins of HIV-1 are expressed from different mRNA species derived from the proviral DNA. A 55-kilodalton precursor protein that will be cleaved to yield all of the viral core proteins is synthesized from an mRNA transcript that encodes the entire precursor protein. This precursor is myristylated at the N terminus and is cleaved by the viral protease into the final Gag protein subunits p17, p24, p7, and p9. The p17 protein retains the myristylated N terminus and binds to the inner glycoprotein envelope, giving it an important role in guiding viral

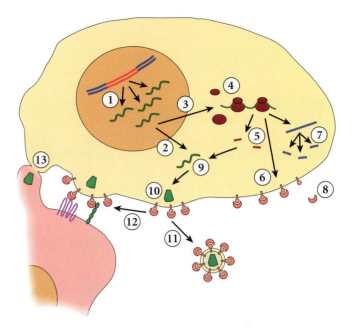

Figure 22.3 HIV activation and replication. Integrated prophage is transcribed by host RNAP II (**1**) from promoters located in the virus's LTRs (Fig. 22.4). These viral transcripts either are exported from the nucleus to be assembled into new phage particles (**2**) or are translated into viral proteins in the cytoplasm (**3 and 4**). Some viral proteins are synthesized as mature proteins that will be assembled into nascent viral capsids (**5**), others such as the gp41-gp120 complex are transported to the host cell membrane (**6**), and still others are translated as precursor proteins that require proteolytic cleavage to be converted to their mature form (**7**). On the host cell surface, some gp120 protein can spontaneously dissociate from gp41 (**8**); this soluble gp120 protein has been implicated in some aspects of HIV pathogenesis. Assembly of new viral particles proceeds as single-stranded viral RNA is complexed with viral p7 and p9 proteins (**9**) and is then packaged into a capsid composed of viral p24 and p17 proteins (**10**). Nascent viruses either can bud from the host cell membrane to produce new, infectious virions (**11**) or, alternatively, can bind directly to CD4 receptors of neighboring host cells before budding occurs (**12**). In the latter case, virus can be spread from one infected host cell directly to another host cell without generating a virion intermediate (**13**). In the diagram, the second host cell is depicted in pink (rather than yellow) for clarity, although the two host cells may, in fact, be the same type of cell.

Figure 22.2 (**A**) Infection of a host CD4+ cell by HIV (see Fig. 22.1 for identification of structures). The initial interaction of the virion with its host cell is the binding of viral gp120 with host cell CD4 protein (**1**). This induces a conformational shift in gp120 that exposes the chemokine-binding site (**2**), which subsequently interacts (**3**) with the host cell's chemokine receptor CXCR4 (on CD4+ T cells) or CCR5 (on monocytes). This second interaction triggers conformational shifts in gp41 that expose the fusigenic domain of gp41 (**4**), initiating virion-host-cell fusion (**5**) and introducing the viral capsid into the host cell (**6**). The viral capsid is dissembled, freeing the viral genome (**7**). Viral RT then synthesizes a complementary DNA strand using the single-stranded viral genome RNA as a template (**8**), and then degrades the original RNA strand, leaving a single-stranded DNA copy of the viral genome (**9**). Host-cell enzymes then synthesize a complementary DNA strand, making the viral genome into double-stranded DNA (**10**), which enters the nucleus with the help of the viral Vpr protein and inserts into the host cell's DNA via the action of viral integrase enzyme (**11**). (**B**) Diagrams of the HIV receptor, CD4 (**top**), and coreceptors, the chemokine receptors CCR5 and CXCR4 (**bottom**) on T lymphocytes. (**Top**) Diagram of the CD4 glycoprotein. HIV binds to the D1 and D2 domains, which form a rigid unit. The crystal structure of the D1 and D2 chemokine receptor family is at the right. (**Bottom**) Diagram of the chemokine receptor family of receptors, showing bound ligand (red). The cylinders represent transmembrane-spanning regions, of which there are seven. Reprinted from J. H. Wang, *Proc. Natl. Acad. Sci. USA* **98**:10799–10804, 2001 (**A**), and L. O. Gerlach et al., *J. Biol. Chem.* **276**:14153–14160, 2001 (**B**), with permission.

cores to budding sites in the infected cell. The p24 protein is the major structural protein comprising the viral capsid. An intermediate p15 protein is cleaved from the C terminus of the precursor. This intermediate is further cleaved into the final p7 and p9 proteins, which associate with the viral RNA in the mature virion.

The Pol protein that is a full-length precursor to the RT, RNase H, protease, and integrase proteins is translated from a transcript that contains most of the coding sequence for Gag in addition to the sequence for Pol. This transcript is produced at a frequency about 5% that of the full-length Gag transcript and is translated in a different reading frame. The Pol protein is also processed by the viral protease to form the mature final proteins. These proteins are packaged into the core of new virions.

The gp160 Env precursor protein is translated from a single viral RNA transcript. It is cleaved by cellular enzymes within the Golgi apparatus into the mature gp120 and gp41 subunits. The gp120 protein comes from the N terminus of the precursor and is posttranslationally modified by glycosylation at approximately 24 sites.

The complete virion is then assembled at the cytoplasmic side of the host-cell plasma membrane. The newly assembled viral cores bud through the surface of the plasma membrane of the infected cell, carrying an envelope composed of both host-cell membrane components spiked with viral envelope proteins.

Viral Tropism

Individual strains of HIV-1 prefer to infect specific cell types, notably CD4$^+$ T cells or monocytes, a phenomenon that was an unexplained observation until 1996. Although HIV-1 was known to require the presence of the human CD4 molecule on the surface of the target cell (Fig. 22.2B, top), CD4 alone was not sufficient for viral entry; it was therefore postulated that coreceptors were needed on the cell surface. This was further supported by the observation that certain cell types such as laboratory immortalized CD4$^+$ T-cell lines and monocytes could be infected by some strains of HIV-1 but not others, suggesting they bore different coreceptors for HIV-1. In general, viral isolates were categorized into two phenotypes: "M-tropic" isolates, which were able to replicate in primary monocytes but not in immortalized T-cell lines, and "T-tropic" isolates, which were able to replicate in immortalized T-cell lines but not in monocytes.

The discovery of chemokine receptors as coreceptors for HIV-1 led to an explanation for these observations on cellular tropism. These are transmembrane receptors that contain an N terminus extracellular domain, seven membrane-spanning regions, and a C terminus intracellular

signaling domain that interacts with G-proteins (Fig. 22.2B, bottom). The usual role of these receptors is to interact with chemokines. For the vast majority of HIV-1 isolates, the chemokine receptors CCR5 and/or CXCR4 serve as coreceptors. Strains of virus may therefore be functionally classified as CCR5-tropic, CXCR4-tropic, or dual-tropic. These classifications have been found to correlate with the phenotypic categories of M-tropic (CCR5) and T-tropic (CXCR4), as monocytes bear CCR5 and immortalized T-cell lines bear CXCR4. Chemokine receptors in addition to CCR5 and CXCR4 have been found to be capable of facilitating viral entry, and the list is growing. Generally, these other receptors are used in addition to CCR5 and/or CXCR4.

The significance of the use of viral coreceptors is unclear. Receptor use determines which cells are susceptible to infection by a particular virus, which may determine which cells are targeted in vivo. Early in infection, HIV strains that use the CCR5 chemokine receptor predominate, and this is associated with the asymptomatic phase of infection. Later, viral isolates emerge that use the CXCR4 or both receptors, and this is associated with development of clinical AIDS. Activated CD4$^+$ lymphocytes, which are thought to be the key cells targeted by HIV-1, bear both CCR5 and CXCR4. The strains of HIV-1 isolated from the brains of individuals late in infection, for example, often use CCR3.

The most striking finding regarding the use of chemokine receptors by HIV-1 is the high degree of resistance of some CCR5-deficient individuals to infection despite repeated exposures to the virus from high-risk behaviors. These persons are homozygous for a 32-base-pair (bp) deletion in the CCR5 gene that truncates CCR5 and renders them functionally CCR5-deficient. This mutation has an allelic frequency of about 10% in the white population (and therefore a frequency for homozygotes of about 1%) and is not found in persons of Asian or African descent. This mutation in the CCR5 gene appears to have arisen in Europe about 700 years ago, but why it is found at such a high frequency in carriers is unclear. One intriguing, but highly speculative, thought is that this deletion conferred resistance to some other infectious disease, such as plague, and coincidentally provided resistance to infection when HIV emerged as a pathogen. Homozygotes with the 32-bp deletion in CCR5 appear immunologically normal yet relatively resistant to HIV infection. The fact that their CD4$^+$ lymphocytes are resistant to M-tropic virus yet fully susceptible to T-tropic virus in vitro is evidence for the central role of M-tropic virus in the establishment of infection in vivo. There is also some evidence that heterozygotes for this mutation, although susceptible to infection, may progress to AIDS more slowly. Unlike CCR5, homozygous deletion of CXCR4 is lethal in utero, at least in transgenic mice.

Animal Models of HIV Infection

A major impediment to the study of HIV infection is that this virus exclusively infects and causes AIDS in humans. HIV can cause infection in chimpanzees, but they do not go on to develop AIDS-like illnesses. Along with the high cost and endangered-species status of the chimp, it is not a very good model for HIV infection. Instead, what has been extensively used is infection of rhesus monkeys with simian immunodeficiency virus (SIV), a cousin of HIV. SIV is naturally found in certain species of monkeys in the wild, but it generally is not harmful to its natural host. Rhesus monkeys are not natural hosts of SIV but are highly susceptible to infection and develop an AIDS-like illness with a pathogenesis similar to HIV. Some hybrid strains of SIV and HIV, called SHIVs, have been developed in the lab that contain genes from HIV spliced into the SIV background. The SHIVs also cause infection and AIDS-like illness in rhesus monkeys. This model has become the laboratory standard for investigating the pathogenesis of HIV and AIDS and the development of new drugs and vaccines, and it is considered to share enough similarity with human AIDS to be highly useful for the types of studies needed to develop better treatments and potential cures for HIV infection. However, it must be kept in mind that this model, like all animal models, is not a perfect mimic of human disease and findings in the SIV model have to be carefully corroborated with human studies. Other models under development include production of transgenic mice expressing human receptors for HIV and studies in some other systems of related im-

munodeficiencies, such as the feline immunodeficiency virus infection in cats, which can provide important insights into human HIV infection.

The Viral Genome

The genome of HIV-1 is approximately 9.8 kilobases long and consists of genes for several structural proteins and genes for regulatory factors (Fig. 22.4). The structural genes encode the Gag, Pol, and Env proteins, which are typical components of all retroviruses and play well-defined roles in determining the structure and life cycle of the virus. The genome also contains several regulatory genes that are unique to lentiviruses and in some cases found only in HIV-1. The purposes of these regulatory elements are numerous, ranging from transcriptional regulation to immune evasion; many of their functions remain to be elucidated.

Viral Structural Genes

HIV-1 contains the three major genes for structural proteins typical of retroviruses: *gag*, polymerase (*pol*), and envelope (*env*). These code for the proteins that form the virus structure and perform the replicative functions described above. In general, these genes are translated into precursor proteins that then undergo cleavage and processing to form the mature subunit proteins used for virus assembly.

LTRs

As with other retroviruses, the HIV-1 genome is flanked by two LTRs, each consisting of unique 3′ (U3), repeat (R), and unique 5′ (U5) regions. The 5′ LTR is present at the 5′ end of all viral mRNAs and contains nucleotide se-

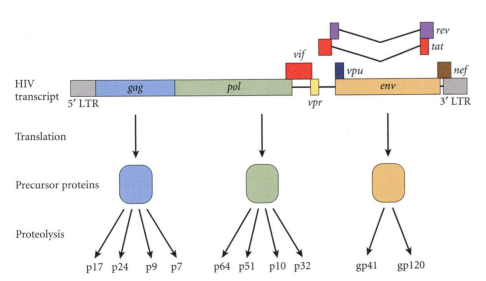

Figure 22.4 Organization of HIV genetic coding regions. The HIV genome is approximately 10 kilobases long and contains genes for nine primary translation products. The coding regions of *vif*, *vpu*, *nef*, *rev*, and *tat* overlap reading frames of other HIV genes. The *rev* and *tat* genes have two exons that must be joined by splicing before translation. The primary translation products for the *gag*, *pol*, and *env* genes are precursors that must be proteolytically processed to generate mature viral proteins.

quences that provide the signals required for transcription. These sequences include a binding region for host cellular RNA polymerase II (RNAP II) holoenzyme complex and the coding region for an RNA structure that binds to the *trans*-activator (Tat) protein and is called the *trans*-activating responsive sequence (TAR). These control viral transcription. The 3′ LTR contains signals for posttranscriptional polyadenylation of the initial mRNA transcript, allowing the mRNA to be transported to the cytoplasm for translation.

Tat

Tat is a protein of approximately 86 amino acids that contains two functional domains. The N-terminal region is a cofactor-binding domain required for the recruitment of cyclin T (CycT). The C-terminal region is an arginine-rich RNA-binding motif that is responsible for the interaction of Tat with its responsive element in the 5′ LTR. This region also acts as a localization signal to target Tat to the nucleus, thus forming a nuclear localization sequence (NLS).

Tat is essential for efficient transcription of all viral genes through a novel mechanism (Fig. 22.5). Independently of Tat, the host cellular RNA-P II complex can bind the proviral DNA sequences at the 5′ LTR promoter and initiate transcription, but transcription elongation is inefficient after production of a short stretch of RNA. The initially transcribed 5′ RNA sequence includes a 59-nucleotide hairpin-loop structure critical for Tat function known as TAR. TAR in turn, contains a "bulge" responsible for binding Tat and a "loop" that can bind CycT. Tat binds the bulge structure on TAR and serves to recruit CycT, which binds to both Tat and the loop. In turn, CycT can then direct cyclin-dependent kinase 9 (CDK-9) to phosphorylate the C-terminal domain of RNAP II, and this provides the crucial signal that then permits processive elongation of the nascent RNA molecule.

The reason for the Tat requirement as a mechanism for transcription of viral genes is unclear. Most other retroviruses undergo efficient RNA elongation without any such viral cofactor. Speculation exists about whether this mechanism improves efficiency of viral transcription in activated T cells or is a control mechanism to allow viral latency (lack of expression) in infected cells for the purpose of immune evasion.

Regulator of virion protein expression (Rev)

Rev is a protein of approximately 116 amino acids that is required for export of HIV-1 RNA transcripts from the nucleus to the cytoplasm. Rev has two functional domains, which mediate its initial import to the nucleus af-

ter translation, RNA binding, and export of the RNA transcripts to the cytoplasm after RNA binding. The N-terminal region of Rev contains an arginine-rich sequence believed to serve both as an NLS for unbound Rev and as a motif for RNA binding. The C-terminal region contains a leucine-rich sequence that is a nuclear export signal for Rev bound to viral RNA transcripts. Thus, Rev acts as a shuttle for carrying HIV-1 RNA from the nucleus to the cytoplasm.

This shuttle function is important for the expression of HIV-1, allowing the relatively small genome of the virus to have multiple overlapping reading frames. Under normal circumstances, cells export only fully spliced cellular mRNAs. This normal regulation of export of RNA transcripts is accomplished by a poorly understood mechanism whereby the presence of an intact splice site in mRNA inhibits the export of the transcript. This is advantageous

Figure 22.5 Regulation of transcription of HIV mRNA. (**A**) Transcription proceeds normally until RNA polymerase (Pol) II crosses the region of HIV containing the TAR sequence. (**B**) TAR RNA forms a large hairpin-loop secondary structure that stalls further transcription. (**C**) Binding of the Tat and CycT proteins to the TAR loop structure helps recruit CDK-9, which phosphorylates the RNA polymerase. (**D**) This phosphorylation event relieves transcription repression, allowing transcription to proceed.

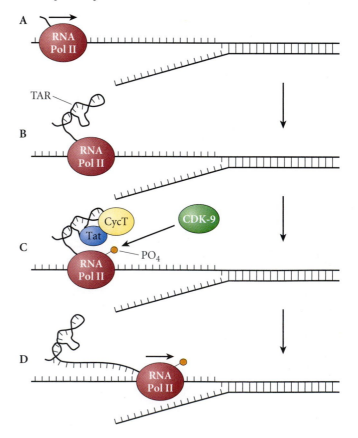

to the cell because it allows only fully spliced mRNAs to enter the cytoplasm for translation; therefore, immature transcripts containing undesirable introns are not exported. Unlike host cellular transcripts, the HIV-1 genome uses alternative splicing to allow the formation of several different gene products from the initial RNA transcript. As such, most HIV mRNAs (with the exception of *tat*, *rev*, and *nef*) contain sites that have not been spliced. Because HIV-1 uses the same cellular enzymes for RNA processing and thus the same splice-site sequences as the host cell, most HIV-1 transcripts are inhibited from nuclear export by normal cellular pathways. The Rev protein allows for specific export of the unspliced viral RNAs, which would otherwise be retained and degraded in the nucleus.

Rev in the cytoplasm binds to a nuclear import protein (importin β) that carries it into the nucleus. There, Rev encounters viral transcripts containing the Rev-responsive element, which is a 243-nucleotide RNA stem-loop structure that binds Rev. Additional Rev molecules are then recruited to form a multimer structure, which then recruits cellular exportin 1 and Ran-guanosine triphosphate (GTP) to target the entire complex for export to the cytoplasm. There, Ran guanosine triphosphate-activating protein causes GTP hydrolysis, leading to the dissociation of exportin 1 and Ran-guanosine diphosphate from Rev and the release of the RNA. The free Rev is then available for shuttling back to the nucleus.

Nef

Nef is an approximately 206-amino-acid protein that has been found to have numerous effects on infected cells. Its presence is not required for viral replication in vitro, and early studies suggested it might be a negative regulator of viral transcription, hence its misnomer as a "negative factor." Nef is now known to have several potentially important roles in the pathogenesis of HIV-1 infection.

Decreased amounts of the CD4 molecule on the surface of infected cells are a clearly defined effect of Nef. As a receptor for HIV-1 gp120, cell surface CD4 would be expected to form complexes with newly synthesized gp120 and thus potentially interfere with the release of virions. As such, reduction of cell surface CD4 appears to be an important function mediated by HIV-1 involving at least three mechanisms: intracellular binding of CD4 by newly synthesized envelope; degradation of intracellular CD4 mediated by another viral protein, Vpu; and active endocytosis of cell surface CD4 mediated by Nef. Nef appears to act as a connector between CD4 and the endocytic machinery of the cell, probably through direct binding to a dileucine motif within the cytoplasmic tail of CD4. Nef then appears to interact with the cellular adapter protein

2 complex to target CD4 to clathrin-coated pits for endocytosis and degradation in lysosomes.

Nef also appears to enhance virion infectivity through a mechanism independent of decreasing cell surface CD4. The mechanism for this effect is as yet unknown. Virions formed in the presence of Nef are more efficient at completing proviral DNA synthesis and are thus more infectious than are virions formed in its absence. This enhancement is conferred in the process of virion assembly; Nef has been shown to be packaged into virions at low efficiency, although the significance of this observation is unclear. Independent expression of Nef in target cells infected with HIV mutants lacking the *nef* gene does not reconstitute the lost infectivity of virions produced in the absence of viral Nef.

Decreased expression of cell surface major histocompatibility complex (MHC) class I is a function of Nef that is presumed to play a role in the escape of infected cells from immune recognition. The mechanism for this process is poorly understood. Loss of cell surface MHC class I is not as efficient as that of CD4. Specific sequences in the tail of MHC class I appear to be required for removal of MHC class I from the cell surface, although the mechanism is distinct from that of binding to the dileucine motif of CD4. As with CD4, MHC class I appears to be endocytosed and transported to lysosomes for degradation.

Cellular signal transduction and activation appear to be affected by Nef, although there is controversy about the precise effects and mechanisms. In various experimental systems, Nef has been reported either to enhance or to inhibit cellular signaling. It has been suggested that Nef binds a cellular protein involved in activation and thus may serve to modulate cellular activation, although this is highly speculative.

Virion protein R (Vpr)

Vpr is a 96-amino-acid protein that is packaged into HIV-1 in a molar amount similar to that of Gag. Specific sequences at the center of Vpr allow it to interact with the C-terminal region of Gag for packaging into virions. At least two functions have been identified for Vpr: nuclear import of the viral preintegration complex and induction of cell cycle arrest.

Many viruses are limited to infecting dividing cells because of a dependence on the normal breakdown of the nuclear membrane during mitosis to access the chromosomes of the host cell. By contrast, HIV-1 and other lentiviruses can infect nondividing cells, an ability that is dependent on access to the nuclear import pathway. Although this process is poorly understood, HIV-1 appears to be capable of accessing the nucleus by at least two processes. The first involves the viral matrix protein, which contains an NLS that is rich in basic amino acids and dependent on importin. The second involves Vpr, which does not have a typical NLS motif and works through an importin-independent pathway that is not yet clearly defined. Vpr-mediated transport may be related to direct interaction of Vpr with nucleoporins and requires the first 70-amino-acid sequence of the Vpr N terminus.

Vpr has also been found to induce an arrest in the G2 phase in HIV-1-infected cells. The precise mechanism of this effect is not known. The progression of cells from phase G2 to mitosis is dependent on the mitotic (CDK) complex, which includes the catalytic subunit p34^{cdc2}. The activity of p34^{cdc2} requires association with cyclin B and its phosphorylation by a cyclin-activating kinase. This process is further regulated by phosphorylation at specific sites on p34^{cdc2} by the protein kinase Wee1, which prevents premature activation, and by dephosphorylation of the same sites by the protein phosphatase CDC25C, which permits subsequent progression to mitosis. Cells expressing Vpr have markedly reduced CDK activity, but this does not seem to be mediated by direct interaction of Vpr with CDK. Vpr may act along an unknown regulatory cascade that controls the phosphorylation states of Wee1 (active hypophosphorylated state) and CDC25C (inactive hypophosphorylated state), which in turn affect CDK. The purpose of cell cycle arrest is not known; it would seem disadvantageous to preclude the survival of chronically infected cells in vivo. Experimental evidence indicates that LTR-driven viral transcription may be enhanced during phase G$_2$, however, and that this may result in a net gain in viral production, considering the likely rapid immune clearance of infected cells in vivo.

Viral protein U (Vpu)

Vpu is an integral membrane protein with N-terminal transmembrane and C-terminal cytoplasmic domains. This protein associates with internal cellular membranes in oligomeric form. It has at least two proposed functions: induction of degradation of CD4 and enhancement of virion release.

Like Nef, Vpu plays a role in decreasing expression of CD4, which is important to the efficient production of HIV-1 envelope proteins on the surface of infected cells. The mechanism is distinct from that of Nef, however. In the ER, the cytoplasmic tail of Vpu binds to a specific sequence in the cytoplasmic tail of CD4 distinct from that recognized by Nef and targets the bound CD4 to an ER-associated protein-degradation pathway. After binding to CD4, Vpu recruits the cellular factor h-βTrCP to the ER membrane. The h-βTrCP protein in turn serves to recruit Skp1, which

targets CD4 for ubiquitin-mediated proteolysis, probably in the proteosome. Vpu then appears to be recycled.

Vpu also facilitates the release of virions from infected cells, independently of its effects on CD4 expression. This function appears to depend on sequences in the N terminus of the protein, as opposed to the interaction with CD4. Mutation of Vpu results in decreased release of virus and increased release of intracellular viral particles, suggesting that Vpu somehow promotes budding and release of virions. How this occurs is unknown.

Virion infectivity factor (Vif)

Vif is a protein found in most lentiviruses that promotes virion infectivity, although the mechanisms are poorly understood. The expression of Vif appears to be highly conserved in vivo and to be necessary for pathogenic infections of macaques with SIV, suggesting an important role for viral replication in vivo. In vitro, Vif is required for virions to be infectious in primary CD4$^+$ T cells and in some immortalized CD4$^+$ cell lines, although Vif-deficient viruses can replicate in other immortalized cell lines. This seems to be related to effects on viral assembly and maturation. Vif is incorporated into the viral core, and Vif-deficient virions appear to have an abnormal core structure.

Pathogenesis

The study of the pathogenesis of HIV-1 infection has been aided greatly in recent years by improved methods of viral detection and a clearer understanding of the dynamics of the interactions between virus and host. Whereas infection was once thought to be marked by a long period of viral latency followed by reappearance of active replication at the onset of clinical deterioration, it has now become clear that the entire course of infection is characterized by the interplay of continuous dynamic viral replication and host responses. The typical course of infection (Fig. 22.6) may be considered in several stages on the basis of the evolution of virologic and host parameters, including the concentration of virus in the blood, CD4$^+$ lymphocyte counts, and antiviral immune responses.

Acute Infection

Infection of a host begins with exposure to HIV-1. In the case of mucosal exposure to the virus, it is thought that the professional antigen-presenting tissue dendritic cells (DCs) are the first cells to be infected. DCs and Langerhans cells are CD4$^+$ and can be infected with HIV-1 in vitro. Recently it has been shown that the C-type lectins expressed by these cells (see Fig. 2.9) are used to internalize HIV and transport the virus to the lymph nodes. The

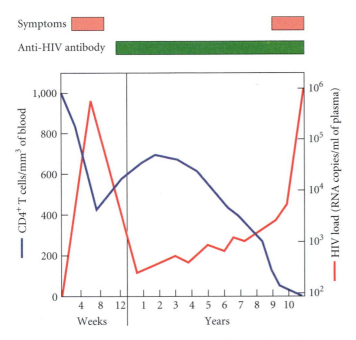

Figure 22.6 Immunopathogenesis of HIV infection. The pathogenesis of HIV has two stages. The early stage of infection takes place within the first several weeks of infection and presents as a flu-like syndrome (which is usually not recognized as HIV infection). This is a viremic state marked by a temporary decrease in the number of circulating CD4$^+$ T cells. After several weeks, the viral load is controlled by the host's immune response, and the number of CD4$^+$ T cells slowly recovers to almost normal levels. This marks the beginning of an asymptomatic latent period, which usually lasts up to about 10 years. Later in this asymptomatic period, the number of CD4$^+$ T cells begins to decline gradually. Eventually, the CD4$^+$ cell count becomes low enough to compromise host immunity. The viral load rapidly escalates at this time, and the host also may begin to experience opportunistic infection by other bacterial, viral, and fungal pathogens.

uptake of HIV by the DCs via C-type lectins and CD4 does not result in infection of the DCs as defined by viral replication; the DCs are said to promote a "transinfection" since they serve as conduits to transport HIV to T cells. Lymphocytes clustered with DCs become highly activated, which drives vigorous replication of HIV-1 at these sites. Infection then spreads systemically.

During this acute phase of infection, there is a rapid spike in viral replication that usually occurs 3 to 6 weeks after initial exposure. The level of plasma viremia can reach tens of millions of virions per milliliter of blood. Concurrent with this viral spike is an acute nadir in the number of circulating CD4$^+$ lymphocytes. This explosive rate of infection is most likely due to a lack of protective immune responses during this initial period, with unopposed viral replication and destruction of lymphocytes. During this period, no antiviral immune responses are detectable. Clinically, approximately 60% of individuals develop a nonspecific mononucleosis-like illness. Common

symptoms are fever, pharyngitis, lymphadenopathy, headache, rash, nausea, and diarrhea. Antibody testing for HIV-1 is negative because humoral immune responses have not yet developed, although infection may be detected by blood tests for p24 antigen or viral RNA/DNA. This illness is self-limited and often goes undiagnosed.

Within weeks, plasma viremia drops, CD4$^+$ T cells reach near normal concentrations, and a quasisteady state is reached. The mechanism for the resolution of the acute phase of infection is not clear, although it is believed that the development of HIV-1-specific cellular immunity plays an important role. The decline in the level of viremia coincides temporally with the development of these responses, although antibody responses do not develop until later, suggesting that cellular immunity partially contains viral replication.

Chronic Asymptomatic Infection

The quasisteady state reached after acute infection is marked by relatively stable levels of viremia and near-normal CD4$^+$ T-cell counts. The number of CD4$^+$ T cells decreases very gradually during this time, and the infected individual is relatively asymptomatic. This period was once thought to be one of quiescence, but it has become clear in recent years that the observed stable viral and cellular parameters of this phase are actually the result of a dynamic equilibrium. For many individuals, the older methods of detection of HIV infection, such as p24 enzyme-linked immunosorbent assay and quantitative cultures, were not sensitive enough to detect virus in their blood during chronic infection, leading to the mistaken conclusion that virus was not replicating. More sensitive polymerase chain reaction-based methods of detection, however, have shown that the majority of individuals have stable viremia during this chronic phase. Researchers have determined that the measured amount of circulating virus, although fairly constant, is actually the result of vigorous ongoing production and destruction of virus. Similarly, CD4$^+$ T cells are produced and cleared in large numbers.

The rates at which virus and cells are produced and destroyed have been calculated for individuals treated with drugs, which can at least temporarily stop viral replication in infected individuals. If it is assumed that the drugs stop viral production without affecting viral clearance, clearance can be measured directly by observing the decline in viremia after initiation of therapy. Because production and clearance should be equal in a steady state, the rate of viral production is assumed to be equal to the measured rate of clearance. Similarly, it is assumed that the drugs stop destruction of CD4$^+$ T cells, and the rate of cellular loss is approximated by measuring the increase in concentration of these cells after the initiation of drug therapy. Such studies have shown that viral replication is quite vigorous: approximately 10^{10} viral particles are produced and cleared daily. Further calculations based on these data indicate that the life cycle of virus is approximately 1.2 days and that free virions have a half-life of approximately 0.3 days. $CD4^+$ T cells also turn over rapidly, with approximately 10^{10} produced and cleared daily and with a half-life of infected cells of approximately 2.2 days.

This chronic phase of infection typically lasts years, with progression to AIDS occurring, on average, approximately 10 years after infection in untreated persons. During this time, there is a very gradual decrease in the number of $CD4^+$ T cells and an increase in the level of viremia. For poorly understood reasons, an "inflection point" is reached and the decline in $CD4^+$ T cells and increase in viremia are accelerated. There is a tight inverse correlation between the set point of viremia established after acute infection and the duration of the asymptomatic phase; this may indicate that better immune control of viral replication leads to more durable immune responses. The level of viremia is thus an important prognostic indicator of risk for progression.

Late Infection

After the chronic asymptomatic phase of infection, there is a rapid and progressive decline in the number of $CD4^+$ T cells and an increase in viral load. This accelerated phase usually begins after the $CD4^+$ T-cell count has dropped to approximately 500 cells per cubic millimeter (mm^3). With this decline, clinical symptoms such as fevers, sweats, lymphadenopathy, and weight loss often develop. Furthermore, the risk of various opportunistic infections rises, especially as the $CD4^+$ T-cell count drops below 200 cells/mm^3, with the eventual development of AIDS, leading to death, without treatment. The cause for this progressive failure of the immune system is unclear. Loss of immune containment of HIV-1 infection itself is thought to play an important role in the accelerated depletion of $CD4^+$ cells. One interesting observation is that the phenotype of the circulating virus often changes (in about 50% of infected individuals) from M-tropic (which is the predominant phenotype in almost all individuals beginning in primary infection) to T-tropic. Whether this "switch" is the cause or an effect of immunocompromise is not known. The phenotype of the circulating lymphocytes also changes in late disease, with the strong T helper type 1 (TH1) bias of early infection changing to the TH2 phenotype; again, the cause of this phenomenon is not known. This change may reflect a failure and loss of virus-specific cellular immunity, which is TH1 specific.

Immune Defects Due to HIV-1 Infection

With progression to AIDS after infection, global failure of the immune system ensues. Numerous defects of immunity have been identified in infected individuals, but the precise mechanisms of immune damage remain unclear. Given the central role of $CD4^+$ T lymphocytes in coordination of the acquired immune system, the loss of these cells is probably the chief factor leading to the immunosuppression associated with AIDS.

Functionally, almost all aspects of immunity are affected as the disease progresses. There is a conspicuous loss of cellular immunity and an increased susceptibility to intracellular pathogens such as mycobacteria and viruses. Humoral immunity is dysregulated, with loss of specific antibody responses. The components of the innate immune system are also affected. In particular, monocytes/macrophages can be directly infected by HIV-1, and polymorphonuclear leukocytes are probably secondarily affected by loss of other cell types. On the gross level, damage to the lymphoreticular system is visible on pathologic examination. In later disease, the structure of lymph nodes is perturbed, with eventual complete loss of architecture. Nodes in the latest stages of disease are fibrotic and lack lymphoid and antigen-presenting cells.

$CD4^+$ T Lymphocytes

The most clearly defined immune deficit is loss of $CD4^+$ T lymphocytes. Both naive (CD45 RA^+) and memory (CD45 RO^+) phenotypes are depleted. Several mechanisms have been proposed to explain the occurrence of $CD4^+$ lymphopenia in HIV-1 infection (Table 22.1), but the basic question of how the virus effects the depletion of $CD4^+$ T cells in infected individuals remains without a definitive answer.

Loss of $CD4^+$ T lymphocytes occurs as a direct consequence of infection. Necrotic death of cells due to viral infection may provide an explanation for some of the cell loss. Apoptosis of infected cells is another proposed mechanism to explain $CD4^+$ T-cell loss; programmed cell death has been noted in infected cells in vitro, although its cause is not understood. Aberrant signaling caused by binding of gp120 to CD4 or an intracellular viral protein may induce apoptosis. Tat and Vpr have been reported to induce apoptosis. Finally, clearance of infected cells by the immune system (cytotoxic T lymphocytes [CTLs] or antibody-dependent cytolysis) may be another reason for depletion of $CD4^+$ T cells.

Several bystander mechanisms may contribute to cell loss. Infected cells can form syncytia with other $CD4^+$ T cells; the gp120 expressed on the infected cell surface can bind to neighboring uninfected cells and result in cell-cell

Table 22.1 Mechanisms of leukopenia caused by chronic HIV-1 infection

Type of infection	Cellular effect	Molecular bases
Direct infection	Necrosis	
	Apoptosis	Aberrant signaling by gp120
		Viral protein (Tat, Vpr?)
	Immune clearance	Cytotoxic T cells
		Antibody-mediated
Bystander cell loss	Syncytium formation	
	Free gp120 binding	Aberrant signaling
		Immune clearance (antibody)
	Superantigen	
Decreased production	Stem cell infection	
	Thymocyte gp120 binding	
	Loss of antigen-presenting cells	

fusion. Multinucleated giant syncytia are observed in vitro, but not in vivo, raising questions about the physiologic relevance of this observation. Free gp120 released from virions or infected cells is another potential cause of bystander cell death. Suggested mechanisms involved in the killing of CD4$^+$ T cells by gp120 include apoptosis due to aberrant signaling after CD4 binding, mediation of the binding of anti-gp120 antibody to cells and thus their sensitization to antibody-dependent cellular cytotoxicity or antibody-dependent complement-mediated cytotoxicity, and interference with T-cell receptor (TCR) binding to the MHC class II-antigen complex. Finally, the selective loss of CD4$^+$ T lymphocytes with certain TCR β chains has been interpreted as suggesting a possible mediation of cell loss by a viral superantigen.

Mechanisms of decreased cell production also have been proposed. Thymocytes or pluripotent stem cells may be susceptible to infection, leading to decreased production of CD4$^+$ lymphocytes and other cells. Binding of free gp120 to thymocytes may interfere with the selection of CD4$^+$ lymphocytes during thymic ontogeny. Dysfunction and/or loss of antigen-presenting cells could lead to decreased generation or proliferation of CD4$^+$ effector cells.

Antigen-Presenting Cells
Defects in antigen presentation may play an important role in immunosuppression due to infection. Professional antigen-presenting cells (monocytes/macrophages and myeloid DCs) are directly susceptible to infection, and their numbers decrease in vivo with the progression of clinical disease. In vitro, perturbations of monocyte/macrophage antigen-presenting functions (phagocytosis, chemotaxis, cytokine production) are observed. Although productively infected immature DCs appear to be capable of normal maturation and stimulation of T cells, the progressive loss of DCs probably contributes to an inability to generate and maintain cellular immune responses.

B Lymphocytes
B-cell function is also markedly altered, even during the asymptomatic phase of infection. B-cell hyperreactivity is a hallmark of HIV-1 infection; most infected individuals demonstrate a polyclonal hypergammaglobulinemia. Terminal differentiation of B cells to antibody-secreting plasma cells appears to occur in the absence of the usually required signals, leading to nonspecific polyclonal activation. The mechanisms causing this dysfunction are unknown. The potential consequences of this nonspecific activation include autoimmunity (due to unregulated production of autoantibodies), impaired antibody-isotype switching (from primary IgM to secondary IgG), inability to respond to specific antigens, and a high incidence of B-cell lymphomas due to chronic activation.

CD8$^+$ T Lymphocytes
Cellular immune responses are markedly impaired in late disease; probably multiple factors are involved. Induction and maintenance of CD8$^+$ cell responses are highly dependent on the helper function of CD4$^+$ T cells and therefore responses wane with loss of CD4$^+$ T cells. The loss of DCs, which play a key role in generating and coordinating both CD8$^+$ and CD4$^+$ lymphocyte responses, is likely to be a significant contributing factor as well. Some studies have suggested that activated CD8$^+$ cells transiently express CD4 and can therefore be infected by HIV-1; whether this possible infectibility plays a role in CD8$^+$ cell dysfunction or depletion in vivo is not known.

Other Cell Types
Pluripotent stem cells can be infected in vitro with HIV-1. What role this plays in vivo is unclear; however, loss of stem cells due to infection could certainly contribute to depletion of all of the above-mentioned cell types. Natural killer cells appear to have decreased cytolytic function with disease progression, although their numbers are not

markedly diminished. Neutrophils can exhibit defective phagocytic function and impaired chemotaxis.

Immune Responses to HIV-1 Infection

Immune responses to HIV-1 infection have been an area of intense interest and study. The observation that most infected individuals maintain a healthy, asymptomatic state for many years after infection suggests that there may be immune responses that contain the infection but that eventually fail. Understanding the mechanisms of such protective immunity might allow the design of therapies that augment or prolong antiviral immunity in infected persons or a preventive vaccine. Candidates have emerged in the search for protective antiviral immune responses: virus-specific cytolytic T-cell responses, $CD8^+$ lymphocyte-derived cytokines, and virus-specific antibodies.

Role of $CD4^+$ T Cells

Destruction of $CD4^+$ T cells is the hallmark of HIV infection and AIDS, but the role these cells play in immune resistance to progression of infection is just beginning to be investigated. Individuals who do well in spite of being HIV infected possess both $CD4^+$ and $CD8^+$ T cells that respond to HIV antigens. Indeed, since loss of $CD4^+$ T-cell function precedes the widespread destruction of these cells by HIV, it may be that $CD4^+$ cells are critical for maintaining effective immunity carried out by $CD8^+$ CTL. Studies of long-term nonprogressors who remain healthy in spite of being HIV infected show that many of these individuals have HIV-specific $CD4^+$ immune T cells that respond to antigens such as the p24 viral glycoprotein. Other studies have indicated that patients who make an effective response to drug therapy also produce $CD4^+$ T-cell responses to HIV antigens that contribute to control of viral load. Increasingly it is being accepted that an effective immune response to HIV includes viral-specific $CD4^+$ T cells, likely functioning as helper cells to initiate and maintain CD8 CTLs.

HIV-1-Specific CTLs

$CD8^+$ MHC class I-restricted CTLs have emerged as an important component of the immune response to HIV-1 infection. These killer cells have TCRs that bind to a specific HIV peptide of about nine amino acids (epitope). The epitope is generated in the infected cell from a translated protein that has been processed by the proteasome in the infected cell, transported by the transporter associated with processing complex, and presented with a specific MHC class I molecule on the cell surface (Fig. 22.6; also see Fig. 12.1). After this specific binding, the CTL ly-

ses the target cell through the release of various enzymes (lytic pathway) and the triggering of programmed cell death (apoptotic pathway). Virus-specific CTLs have been shown to play important roles in controlling and resolving viral infections such as influenza and cytomegalovirus and thus are a natural candidate for immunity in HIV-1 infection.

Several clinical correlations suggest that HIV-1-specific CTL activity has a protective role. Many infected individuals have vigorous virus-specific CTL responses, which are unprecedented for other chronic viral infections. These responses can be of remarkable breadth; up to 14 different recognized viral epitopes have been observed to elicit immune responses in a single infected individual. The onset of this activity is temporally correlated to the decrease in viremia during primary infection, before the development of neutralizing antibodies, suggesting that CTLs contribute to the control of viral replication in vivo. Some studies have found that a waning of CTL responses correlates with disease progression, although these results are controversial. Recent data have shown that antiviral CTL activity is inversely correlated with the viral load in plasma, supporting the hypothesis that these cells suppress viral replication in vivo. Finally, some studies have suggested that some multiply exposed but uninfected individuals (needle stick-exposed health-care workers, sexual partners of infected persons, and prostitutes in epidemic areas) have detectable CTL responses in the absence of antibody responses, suggesting that infection may have been aborted by cellular immunity.

In vitro studies have added further evidence that CTLs are protective. HIV-1-specific CTLs have been shown to lyse acutely infected cells with high efficiency and early in the viral life cycle, potentially before the production of progeny virions. In coculture experiments, CTLs are potent inhibitors of HIV-1 replication, and under some conditions are capable of sterilizing viral cultures. These activities are dependent on recognition of the infected cells by TCRs and are therefore antigen specific and MHC class I restricted. Studies of viral inhibition by CTLs in vitro have demonstrated that at least two potential pathways account for this effect. As would be expected, direct cytolysis of infected cells has an important role in suppressing viral replication. This appears to be the dominant, more potent mechanism. A second mechanism involves the release of cytokines. When activated by TCR recognition of a target cell (or nonspecifically by lectins or CD3 binding in vitro), CTLs release numerous cytokines. Some of these are suppressive for HIV-1 replication in vitro, including the chemokines RANTES, MIP-1α, and MIP-1β, which are ligands of CCR5 and therefore inhibit the entry of M-tropic strains of virus that bind CCR5. Other non-CCR5-binding cytokines that suppress viral replication have been observed and additional factors likely remain to be identified.

Antiviral Cytokines

In vitro studies of the cytokines released by $CD8^+$ lymphocytes have generally revealed that several substances may have activity against HIV-1 (Table 22.2). In addition to release of chemokines that bind CCR5 and block entry of certain strains of HIV-1, another cytokine, termed CD8 cell-derived antiviral factor (CAF), has been found that acts after viral entry at the level of inhibition of LTR-mediated transcription. The exact identity of CAF remains unknown. Controversy has surrounded the identity of the $CD8^+$ cells that produce CAF; some investigators have stated that these cells are separate "noncytolytic" lymphocytes and not CTLs. Recent evidence suggests, however, that CTLs may produce such antiviral soluble factors, including the nonchemokine substance(s). It is probable that production of these antiviral factors is not limited to a particular subset of noncytolytic $CD8^+$ cells. The role of such factors in vivo remains to be determined.

The identification of RANTES, MIP-1α, and MIP-1β as blockers of HIV-1 binding to CCR5 has led to an intensive search for other such chemokine factors that act on CCR5 and CXCR4. MCP-2 is another ligand for CCR5 that can block HIV-1 cellular entry in vitro. This chemokine does not appear to be produced by $CD8^+$ lymphocytes. The search for ligands of CXCR4 has revealed two factors, termed SDF-1α and SDF-1β, that can bind CXCR4 and block cellular entry of T-tropic strains of HIV-1 in vitro. These are also not produced by $CD8^+$ cells. A new $CD8^+$ cell-derived chemokine, macrophage-derived chemokine, has been proposed to block both M-tropic and T-tropic strains of HIV-1; however, this chemokine does not appear to bind either CCR5 or CXCR4, and the demonstration that macrophage-derived chemokine has antiviral effects is highly controversial.

In addition to using CCR5 or CXCR4 for cell entry, different strains of HIV-1 have been found to be capable of utilizing a growing list of other chemokine receptors for entry. In general, ligands for these receptors are able to block viral entry through these receptors. Because it is presumed that the virus usually uses CCR5 or CXCR4 to enter cells in vivo, the significance of these other receptors and chemokines is unclear.

Antiviral Antibodies

Antibodies that recognize a variety of HIV-1 proteins are produced in response to infection. Those that have activity against viral replication in vitro (neutralizing antibodies) usually appear after viremia has already decreased during primary infection, suggesting that they are not responsible for the reduction in viremia. Most neutralizing antibodies are specific for gp120 and presumably act by interfering with the binding of gp120 to target cells. Neutralizing antibodies specific for gp41 have also been described.

Some studies have suggested that the antiviral humoral response may be more pronounced in individuals with long-term, nonprogressing infection, but again these conclusions are controversial. Experimental evidence demonstrates that the therapeutic benefit conferred by the transfer of pooled immunoglobulin from seropositive donors to other infected individuals is variable. Most studies have shown that neutralizing antibodies tend to be much more effective against laboratory strains of HIV-1 than against primary isolates from patients. Overall, the degree to which neutralizing antibodies contribute to immune protection against HIV-1 infection in vivo is unknown.

Evasion of Immune Responses by HIV-1

Despite the generation of potent immune responses to HIV-1, the virus persists and ultimately overwhelms the immune system in most, if not all, infected individuals. The immune response during the asymptomatic stage may be viewed as one of effective containment of the virus. Indeed, it is now fairly certain that loss of effective containment is the event that leads to progression to symptomatic AIDS. As there is no defining factor, occurrence, or other event that is known to trigger loss of effective immune containment, it has been difficult to know the molecular and cellular basis for progression to AIDS. Several mechanisms whereby HIV-1 may evade host immunity are likely to contribute to the persistence of and eventual failure to contain virus.

Escape from Antiviral Cytokines

Whether HIV-1 is suppressed by cytokines in vivo and responds to this pressure is not known. It has been suggested that the switch of viral phenotype from M-tropic

Table 22.2 Secreted factors that inhibit HIV-1 infection

Factor	Example	Mechanism
Chemokines	RANTES, MIP-1α, MIP-1β, MCP-2	Competition with virus for binding to CCR5 viral coreceptor
	SDF-1α, SDF-1β	Competition with virus for binding to CXCR4 viral coreceptor
Other secreted factors	CAF	Inhibition of LTR-mediated viral transcription

(CCR5-using) to T-tropic (CXCR4-using) during late disease may indicate escape from the inhibitory effects of CCR5-binding chemokines RANTES, MIP-1α, and MIP-1β. However, the early predominance of M-tropic virus even in individuals exposed to T-tropic strains argues against this point. It is also not clear if competitive binding of chemokines and HIV to receptors plays any role in viral inhibition in vivo. Thus, while observed experimentally in cell culture, chemokine inhibition of viral entry, replication, and infection is not known to be a major mechanism of resistance to HIV infection.

Escape from Neutralizing Antibodies

The development of effective neutralizing antibodies to HIV-1 is hindered by at least two mechanisms. It is believed that the functionally important sites for viral neutralization on gp120 are conformationally protected from binding to antibodies. This may explain why a CD4-induced conformational change in gp120 is required for exposure of the chemokine-receptor binding site. In the native state the CD4-binding epitope is not available for antibody binding. Another means whereby gp120 evades binding to antibodies is glycosylation; gp120 is heavily glycosylated, reducing its immunogenicity. Experimental evidence in the SIV model indicates that alteration of the envelope to prevent glycosylation in vivo results in a much more efficient generation of neutralizing antibodies. Furthermore, there is a high rate of reversion in vivo to favor glycosylation of the envelope of the mutant SIV, suggesting a selective advantage for the glycosylated phenotype.

Free virus may be protected from the effects of neutralizing antibodies or antibody-mediated clearance in general by becoming trapped in the extracellular matrix of follicular DCs (FDCs) in lymph nodes. Virions held by FDCs are thought to remain viable for years and are inaccessible to antibodies, making FDCs a potential reservoir for latent virus.

Escape from CTLs

HIV-1 may utilize any of many potential mechanisms to evade recognition by CTLs (Table 22.3). Any perturbation of the sequence of events leading to binding of a virus-specific CTL with the appropriate epitope-MHC complex on the target cell may contribute to viral escape. Thus, any interference in the processes of generating the correct epitope, presenting the epitope, targeting of the infected cell by the CTL, and maintaining the CTL response may play an important role in the failure of immunity.

The sequence of the epitope is crucial for recognition by CTLs, and sequence variation is thought to be an important means of viral escape from extant host immunity. Mutations in either of the two anchor residues can prevent binding of the epitope to the MHC class I molecule, resulting in lack of presentation at the cell surface. Similarly, single amino acid changes within the epitope can inhibit binding of the TCR to the peptide-MHC complex. The mutation rate of HIV-1 is high because its RT lacks a proofreading domain, allowing for a great deal of sequence variation to be generated in viral nucleic acids. Mutations in recognized epitopes have been documented in primary and chronic infection, although it is more difficult to document such mutations in chronic infection. It is unclear why such escape mutations are not observed more commonly in chronic infection, although one possible explanation is that epitopes that can be changed at low cost to viral fitness are altered early, leaving only recognized epitopes that are conserved.

Other epitope mutations may affect recognition by CTLs indirectly. Mutation of an epitope can lead not only to loss of recognition but also to antagonism of recognition of the original epitope, presumably by competing for TCR binding but failing to activate the CTL to kill the infected target. Such mutations have been reported in clinical isolates of HIV-1. Another theoretical means of escape is a mutation in the epitope or its flanking sequences that interferes with processing in the proteosome or transport by the transporter associated with processing complex. Such mutations have not been observed in clinical isolates of HIV-1 to date.

Direct viral effects on infected cells are another means of escaping detection by CTLs. MHC class I expression is decreased on infected cells, an effect mediated at least in part by Nef. In vitro, cells infected with Nef-competent strains of HIV-1 appear to be less susceptible to lysis by CTLs than are those lacking Nef, suggesting that Nef functionally impairs the ability of CTLs to recognize infected cells. Evidence supporting the role of Nef in vivo includes the finding that disease progression tends to be much slower in individuals infected with *nef*-deleted HIV-1. Also, macaques experimentally infected with *nef*-deleted SIV usually have an asymptomatic infection and more pronounced CTL responses, but eventually go on to develop illness.

Table 22.3 Mechanisms by which HIV-1 evades host immunity

Mechanism	Arm of immunity affected
Prevention of T-cell help	CTLs and B cells
Antigenic drift	CTLs and B cells
Reduction of MHC class I expression	CTLs
Latent reservoir	All
Infection of immune-privileged sites	All

An important mechanism of HIV-1 persistence is the "latent reservoir," which is composed of resting memory $CD4^+$ T cells that contain integrated provirus that is not expressed as infectious virions. Although most activated infected cells die, a small percentage may survive and revert to a resting memory phenotype. Lacking cellular activation factors, the provirus is not expressed and the infected cell does not present viral antigens for recognition by CTLs. Upon reactivation of the memory cell, however, the virus can then be expressed and complete the replicative cycle. It has been shown that this reservoir is probably seeded during primary infection and has a half-life of at least several years.

Infection of cells in immune-privileged sites is another potential mechanism underlying HIV evasion of host immunity. Several anatomic sites are relatively protected from inflammation: for example, the central nervous system. These are areas where CTLs might have poor penetration and thus a reduced ability to clear infected cells, such as microglia in the brain. It is not clear to what extent such reservoirs play a role in vivo in the progression to AIDS.

Loss of virus-specific CTLs may provide an explanation for the late failure of immunity. In the face of ongoing viral replication, terminally differentiated CTLs must be constantly generated from a dividing pool of memory cells. Limited regenerative capacity could lead to "clonal exhaustion" of these cells over years of infection. This has been shown to occur in murine models of chronic viral infection. Measurement of the length of $CD8^+$ telomeres, however, suggests that these cells undergo massive turnover in HIV-1-infected persons. Telomere length, which decreases progressively with cellular division, is markedly reduced in the $CD8^+$ cells of these persons.

Perhaps the most striking deficit involving cellular immunity to HIV-1 is in the area of virus-specific $CD4^+$ lymphocytes. This is believed to be a key defect that may explain the inability of CTLs to contain infection. The generation and maintenance of CTL responses require "help" from $CD4^+$ lymphocytes, as do many other immune responses. Almost all individuals with chronic HIV-1 infection have a notable lack of virus-specific $CD4^+$ T cells. A very small subset of patients with slow or nonprogressing infection, however, have virus-specific helper $CD4^+$ T cells. The presence of these cells may explain the superior long-term ability of these patients to contain viral replication. Recent studies have suggested that HIV-1-specific help is lost in almost all individuals during acute infection, most likely because the virus targets activated $CD4^+$ T cells. In response to the new antigens of HIV-1 during primary infection, virus-specific $CD4^+$ T cells are probably highly activated and deleted by infection, leading to loss of help for CTLs. Thus, the virus may ensure its persistence by damaging the helper responses needed by virus-specific CTLs.

Pharmacologic Therapy for HIV-1 Infection

Therapeutic advances made since recognition of AIDS in the early 1980s have had a substantial impact on the morbidity and mortality associated with HIV-1 infection. The earliest successes were improvements in the diagnosis, treatment, and prophylaxis of otherwise unusual infections commonly associated with the immunodeficiency, such as *Pneumocystis carinii* pneumonia. In time, drugs that targeted HIV-1 itself were developed, the first being zidovudine (ZDV [AZT]). All the early agents were nucleoside analog inhibitors of viral reverse transcriptase. Although these drugs seemed extremely potent in vitro, initial results in vivo were very disappointing. Clinical benefits such as an increase in $CD4^+$ T-cell counts were transient, and patient survival was minimally affected. In retrospect, these early efforts of testing drugs individually were doomed to failure because of the rapid development of drug resistance. The high mutation rate and vigorous viral replication readily selected drug-resistant mutants.

In the mid-1990s, new classes of drugs were developed and combination drug therapy (to minimize drug resistance) became the standard strategy. This led to potent and prolonged control of viral replication in some patients. Despite these successes, it has become clear that a cure is not likely to be achieved with drug therapy alone; the drugs are not able to affect virus in compartments such as the memory T-cell latent reservoir. Furthermore, multidrug resistance has become increasingly common.

Nucleoside RT Inhibitors

Nucleoside RT inhibitors were the first class of drugs to be developed for treatment of AIDS. These compounds are analogs of nucleosides and are phosphorylated within the cell to their active form. In the process of reverse transcription by viral RT, chain formation is terminated when the drug is incorporated instead of the normal nucleotide, preventing the production of viral DNA. Hydroxyurea, a chemotherapeutic agent, has been used as an adjunctive therapy to deplete the intracellular nucleotide pool and therefore encourage phosphorylation of the antiviral nucleoside inhibitors.

When these drugs are used individually, resistance develops rapidly through mutations in RT that reduce the binding of the drug. Nucleoside inhibitors are a fairly diverse class of drugs, and cross-resistance is limited. Nucleoside RT inhibitors are a mainstay of combination antiretroviral therapy; many standard regimens use a purine and a pyrimidine analog together with a third agent such as a protease inhibitor or non-nucleoside RT inhibitor.

Nonnucleoside RT Inhibitors

Nonnucleoside RT inhibitors also interfere with the function of RT but are not nucleoside analogs. They bind a site distinct from the nucleotide-binding site of the enzyme, interfering with its function. As with nucleoside RT inhibitors, nonnucleoside RT inhibitors act early in the viral life cycle, preventing the production of proviral DNA just after infection of the target cell. Again, resistance develops rapidly when these drugs are used alone. Unlike the nucleoside RT inhibitors, the nonnucleoside RT inhibitors are a closely related group of drugs and the degree of cross-resistance is high.

Protease Inhibitors

As a class, the protease inhibitors target the viral protease, which is required for processing the viral precursor proteins into their mature forms. Virions formed in the absence of viral protease activity are nonviable. Protease inhibitors interfere with protease function, thereby acting later in the viral life cycle than RT inhibitors. The protease inhibitors are a closely related group of drugs, and there is a moderate degree of cross-resistance.

Future Antiviral Drugs

Other stages of the viral life cycle are potential targets for intervention. For example, the specific interactions required for viral entry may be vulnerable to inhibitors. Modified chemokines or small-molecule blockers of chemokine receptors targeted at CCR5 and/or CXCR4 are being investigated as agents to prevent binding of virus to chemokine receptors. Another area of interest is viral fusion via gp41, which can be suppressed by agents in vitro. A recently approved fusion inhibitor drug for HIV, enfuvirtide, is a peptide that blocks viral entry into cells.

Viral Fitness, Viral Resistance, and Viral Evolution

The ability of a successful pathogen like HIV-1 to replicate within a given environment is measured as *viral fitness,* which is influenced by both microbial and host factors. For the virus, fitness is determined by multiple factors, including its ability to replicate within a host, the ability to find the appropriate host cells to divide in (viral tropism for host cells), and having a mutation rate that allows it to avoid host immune responses and drug treatments. Since the infected individual is mounting an immune response to the virus, host factors also affect viral fitness. In addition to immunologic responses, the availability of target cells for viral replication and other host genetic factors will also determine the viral fitness in an individual host. In the presence of antiviral drugs, host immune effectors, and similar antiviral host factors, the virus is pressured into finding ways to continue to infect and replicate within the host. *Viral resistance* represents the microbe's ability to change in response to exogenous pressures, and in general, the more resistant viruses have a higher degree of fitness. However, this is a complex situation; for example, in the presence of antiviral drugs a variant may arise that is resistant to the drug but has decreased replicative capacity when compared to the nonresistant parental strain. This change is often seen among the earliest drug-resistant HIV-1 variants that arise during antiretroviral therapy. So often there is a trade-off between acquiring a needed genetic capacity for survival under a given environmental pressure such as antiviral drugs and reductions in other properties that contribute to higher viral fitness.

The natural host responses to HIV and the use of pharmacologic therapies to treat infection affect the *evolution* of the virus within an infected person. Following the emergence of drug-resistant strains with reduced replicative capacity, other mutations will arise that compensate for the reduced viral replicative capacity. Selection pressures will favor mutations leading to greater replicative capacity, and if drug therapy continues, then the virus must also continue to be drug resistant. For example, during treatment with protease inhibitors, resistant HIV mutants will emerge that produce a protease with amino acid changes close to the substrate-inhibitor binding site, thus preventing inhibitor binding. But these strains have reduced replicative capacity. To compensate, additional mutations can accumulate in the protease gene that increase the enzymatic activity of the protease, which in turn enhances the ability of the virus to replicate. How natural immunity and pharmacologic therapy affect viral evolution will have a major impact on the design and use of future anti-HIV drugs and vaccines.

Potential Vaccines and Immunotherapies for HIV-1 Infection

Manipulation of the immune system offers several lines of potential future strategies for prevention of or therapy for HIV-1 infection. Effective immunoprophylaxis that prevents infection with a vaccine leading to sterile immunity offers the best hope for curbing the virus on a global level; antiretroviral drugs are prohibitively expensive for many parts of the world and are not curative. Vaccines that prime the immune system to better resist HIV infection and progression are another major strategy being pursued. Because damage to the immune system is a key to both the pathogenicity and persistence of HIV-1 infection, immunotherapy focused on reconstituting or enhancing immune responses following infection is another logical goal. Most of the attempts at human HIV vaccines have been based on empirical approaches without the intent of generating a specific type of immune effector. This is because effectors mediating solid protection against HIV infection are not known. But there has been progress, and in 2002 several HIV vaccine trials were under way.

Vaccination

Although there is no compelling evidence to show that immune responses can prevent initial infection, which would be key to generating solid immunity to HIV, some studies in animal models have suggested that full-fledged infection resistance may be possible. Formalin-inactivated SIV vaccination has protected monkeys from challenge with infectious SIV. Chimpanzees have been protected from HIV-1 challenge in different studies by vaccination with recombinant gp120, passive infusion of a gp120 V3 loop-specific monoclonal antibody, and vaccination with combinations of whole inactivated virus, recombinant proteins, and peptides. DNA vaccines have also been protective in both the SIV-macaque and HIV-1–chimpanzee models. However, the field is filled with cautionary tales about the long-term utility of vaccine candidates relying on a live vector. One of the most suggestive demonstrations of a potential HIV vaccine occurred in rhesus monkeys immunized with attenuated SIV (*nef*-deleted, alone or in combination with deletions of other accessory genes). However, it was later found that *nef*-deleted SIV caused infection in neonatal monkeys. More importantly, it is not known if these animal models are relevant for predicting efficacy in humans and what types of immunity are required to prevent infection.

Approaches to vaccination that are under consideration include the use of passive immunization with antiserum (presumably lacking infectious virus), whole inactivated virus, recombinant proteins, peptides, DNA vaccines, recombinant viruses or bacteria expressing HIV antigens, and live, attenuated virus. Passive immunization obviously provides only antibodies. Some approaches induce primarily antibody and CD4$^+$ lymphocyte helper responses (whole inactivated virus, recombinant proteins) since they supply exogenous proteins that are processed for presentation to B cells and CD4$^+$ cells. Peptides, which are designed to represent commonly recognized MHC class I-restricted epitopes, induce primarily CTL re-

sponses. Approaches that induce cellular expression of HIV-1 proteins (DNA vaccines, recombinant viruses, and live, attenuated virus) produce proteins that are processed for both MHC class I and class II presentation and are therefore capable of generating virus-specific antibody, helper, and CTL responses.

Human trials of recombinant gp160 vaccines have been disappointing but are nonetheless the focus of some of the more advanced clinical trials. High concentrations of neutralizing antibody responses have been generated, but the antibodies tend to be effective only against laboratory strains of HIV-1, showing a narrow spectrum of activity. Vaccine failures have been reported, with infection occurring despite vaccination. Recombinant poxvirus vaccines have been shown to generate both cellular and humoral immune responses, although these are weak compared with those in naturally infected individuals. Trials of DNA vaccines are also under way and have shown promising results in rhesus monkey trials. Although a live, attenuated vaccine would be most likely to generate strong responses, there are obvious safety concerns.

Immune Reconstitution and Immunotherapies

A wide variety of approaches, ranging from therapeutic vaccinations to gene therapy, have been proposed to bolster immunity in infected individuals. The major goal is repair of the immune damage associated with HIV-1 infection. Strategies include augmentation of antiviral immune responses, generation of virus-resistant cells, and replacement of cells lost in HIV-1 infection.

Recent advances in antiretroviral therapy have made it possible to suppress viral replication to concentrations undetectable in many individuals. The capability for self-renewal of the immune system after prolonged suppression of infection is not well understood and is an area of active study. Evidence suggests that at least some degree of reconstitution occurs; clinically, immunity against various opportunistic infections has been noted to return in patients previously heavily immunosuppressed. Observation of the CD4$^+$ lymphocyte pool after treatment has revealed a fairly rapid increase in memory T cells and a more gradual increase in naive T cells that continue over many months or years, indicating the possibility that the immune system may recover the ability to make new responses to antigens. In general, however, chronically infected individuals who are treated do not generate CD4$^+$ helper T-cell responses specific for HIV-1, which are likely to be a critical component of antiviral immunity. Some data suggest that loss of these helper responses may be prevented by treatment during acute infection, before seroconversion, but the clinical significance of these findings remains to be determined.

Vaccination of infected individuals may be a way of improving antiviral immunity. Passive immunization, recombinant gp160 vaccination, and peptide vaccination are among approaches that have been considered to either reinforce or broaden immune responses. A key barrier may be the consumption of activated CD4$^+$ T cells that respond to vaccines, such as virus-specific helper cells generated in response to recombinant viral proteins. Adjuvant use of combination antiretroviral therapy to suppress viral replication or other therapies to prevent cellular infection may play important roles.

Ex vivo expansion and subsequent reinfusion of autologous cells are another strategy that has been considered. Reinfusion of expanded autologous virus-specific CD8$^+$ CTLs has been attempted to improve antiviral immunity, with no apparent benefit, probably suggesting the need for other supporting elements, such as CD4$^+$ T-cell help. Reinfusion of expanded CD4$^+$ T cells has also been proposed to repair the deficits caused by infection. Whether expanded CD4$^+$ T cells from an infected individual would contribute a functionally useful repertoire is an important consideration for such an approach.

The use of cytokines to augment immunity is a concept that has reached the point of clinical trials. Interleukin-2 (IL-2) therapy has been tried in patients, with the goal of providing missing "help" and improving cellular immune responses. Increases in CD4$^+$ T-cell counts have been noted after treatment of infected individuals with IL-2. IL-2 has also been considered for use with combination antiretroviral therapy as a means of activating the latent reservoir.

Gene therapy is another tactic that may have applications in HIV-1 infection. Redirection of T cells with recombinant HIV-1-specific TCRs has been considered as a means of producing immunity to the virus. Another idea has been to transduce cells, particularly stem cells, with antiviral genetic constructs, in hopes of allowing immune reconstitution with cells resistant to infection. Genetic constructs that have been tested in vitro include antisense inhibitors, decoys for *tat* binding, intracellular antiviral antibodies, and ribozymes to cleave viral RNA. A common barrier to institution of all these approaches is the transduction of stem cells; most available vectors are inefficient at transducing slowly dividing cells such as stem cells.

Summary

HIV-1 is a retrovirus that chronically infects CD4$^+$ cells, including helper T cells and cells of the monocyte/macrophage lineage. Infection proceeds through several stages: an acute initial phase characterized by rampant, unopposed viral proliferation (which may or may not exhibit a flu-like constellation of symptoms); a chronic, asymptomatic phase characterized by a dynamic equilibrium between viral proliferation and immune system-mediated viral destruction; and a progressive, symptomatic late phase characterized by degradation of the host's immune responses, expansion of viral load, and the onset of immune suppression and opportunistic infections. As an RNA retrovirus, HIV-1 has a replicative cycle that includes reverse transcription of its RNA genome to DNA, followed by integration of this DNA intermediate into the chromosomes of its host cell. This integrated provirus can then either be transcribed to produce new viral RNA genomes or remain dormant for an undetermined length of time likely to extend to a scope of years. The HIV genome encodes many regulatory proteins that modulate the virus's replication. This aspect of the virus's replication is still incompletely understood.

Since its appearance in the early 1980s, HIV-1 has been the focus of intense study aimed at interfering with viral infection or replication or at the generation of protective immunity to the virus. Whereas the former strategy has yielded promising results in the form of combination drug therapy, the latter strategy has thus far been unsuccessful. Both of these therapeutic strategies need to overcome the tremendous capacity of HIV-1 for hypermutation, which results from its lack of proofreading activity during reverse transcription. This hypermutation allows the virus to randomly generate variants of itself that can evade the action of potential therapies: drugs that inhibit the RT enzyme can become ineffective if the RT mutates so as to no longer bind the drugs, and antibodies that recognize the virus's surface glycoprotein become inactive if the epitopes recognized by the antibodies are mutated. Combination multidrug therapy has temporarily provided a solution to this problem, since the application of several antiviral drugs requires that a viral variant become simultaneously resistant to all of the component drugs. Still, multidrug resistance is beginning to emerge among clinical isolates of this virus, and so new therapies, perhaps based on the generation or the maintenance of immunity, will likely be needed in the future.

Suggested Reading

Blankson, J. N., J. E. Gallant, and R. F. Siliciano. 2001. Proliferative responses to human immunodeficiency virus type 1 (HIV-1) antigens in HIV-1-infected patients with immune reconstitution. *J. Infect. Dis.* **183**:657–661.

Center, D. M., H. Kornfeld, T. C. Ryan, and W. W. Cruikshank. 2000. Interleukin 16: implications for CD4 functions and HIV progression. *Immunol. Today* **21**:273–280.

Chinen, J., and W.T. Shearer. 2002. Molecular virology and immunology of HIV infection. *J. Allergy Clin. Immunol.* **110:**189–198.

Garnett, G. P., L. Bartley, N. C. Grassly, and R. M. Anderson. 2002. Antiretroviral therapy to treat and prevent HIV/AIDS in resource-poor settings. *Nat. Med.* **8:**651–654.

Greene, W. C., and B. M. Peterlin. 2002. Charting HIV's remarkable voyage through the cell: basic science as a passport to future therapy. *Nat. Med.* **8:**673–680.

Ho, D. D., and Y. Huang. 2002. The HIV-1 vaccine race. *Cell* **110:**135–138.

Mascola, J. R., and G. J. Nabel. 2001. Vaccines for the prevention of HIV-1 disease. *Curr. Opin. Immunol.* **13:**489–495.

Moylett, E. H., and W. T. Shearer. 2002. HIV: clinical manifestations. *J. Allergy Clin. Immunol.* **110:**3–16.

Piguet, V., and D. Trono. 2001. Living in oblivion: HIV immune evasion. *Semin. Immunol.* **13:**51–57.

Turville, S. G., P. U. Cameron, A. Handley, G. Lin, S. Pohlmann, R. W. Doms, and A. L. Cunningham. 2002. Diversity of receptors binding HIV on dendritic cell subsets. *Nat. Immunol.* **3:**975–983.

Yoshizawa, I., Y. Soda, T. Mizuochi, S. Yasuda, T. A. Rizvi, T. Takemori, and Y. Tsunetsugu-Yokota. 2001. Enhancement of mucosal immune response against HIV-1 Gag by DNA immunization. *Vaccine* **19:**2995–3003.

chapter 23

Clinical and Genetic Perspectives in Primary Immunodeficiency Disorders

Jeff M. Milunsky and Stephen I. Pelton

The hallmark of immunodeficiency syndromes is the enhanced susceptibility to infection, as manifested by more frequent illness, disease due to uncommon pathogens or even to commensal organisms that rarely cause infections, or clinical disease that is less responsive to standard antimicrobial therapy. Affected individuals are also at greater risk for malignancies. The great majority of immunodeficiencies, both in children and adults, are *secondary*, meaning that they are the consequences of impairment of the immune system caused by malnutrition, malignancy, cytotoxic drugs, or chronic disease. *Primary immunodeficiencies*, in contrast, are associated with inherited defects. The clinical manifestations of primary and secondary immunodeficiencies are similar, reflecting the nature of the immune defect rather than its cause. During the past two decades, the identification and detailed investigation of the acquired immunodeficiency syndrome (AIDS) have not only heightened our awareness of immunodeficiency, but have expanded our understanding of the relationship between specific immune defects, opportunistic pathogens, and clinical syndromes.

For many years the discussion of immunodeficiency diseases was primarily limited to clinical descriptions of disease courses. The explosive development of molecular techniques during the past two decades has enabled identification of specific functional defects that underlie immunodeficiency (Table 23.1). The discovery and cloning of the genes responsible for these defects have enhanced our understanding of disease pathogenesis. In the past 5 years, almost 25 newly recognized host-defense genes have been identified and cloned. Prenatal diagnosis, early intervention such as bone marrow transplantation, and new advances in therapeutic agents such as cytokines (e.g., granulocyte colony-stimulating factor)

553

Table 23.1 Molecular defects associated with immunodeficiency

Defective protein	Name of deficiency	Phenotype
Growth factors and receptors		
IL-2	SCID	T-cell activation not possible
IL-7, IL-7R[a]	SCID	No T-cell maturation
γc	SCID	No T-cell or B-cell maturation
Regulatory/activational receptors		
CD40, CD40L	Hyper-IgM syndrome	No T-cell-dependent humoral responses, no class switching
Cellular metabolism		
PNP, ADA	SCID	No T-cell or B-cell maturation
phox, MPO	CGD	Inefficient phagocytic killing
Cell adhesion molecules		
CD18 (β2 integrin)	LAD	Leukocytes cannot extravasate
Antigen presentation machinery		
TAP-1/2	Bare lymphocyte syndrome	Low expression of MHC class I
Transcription factors		
CIITA, RFX	Bare lymphocyte syndrome	No expression of MHC class II
DNA recombination and repair		
RAG-1/2, DNA-PK, XRCC4, ligase-IV	SCID	No V(D)J recombination
Complement proteins		
C3		Susceptibility to infection by all bacteria
C4, C2		Immune complex disorders owing to poor clearance of complexes
C5, C6, C7, C8, C9		Susceptibility to infection by gram-negative bacteria

[a]IL-R, interleukin receptor; γc, common gamma subunit of IL-2 cytokine receptor subfamily; phox, phagocyte oxidase; MPO, myeloperoxidase; DNA-PK, DNA-dependent protein kinase.

offer great promise for treating and even curing these diseases. Future possibilities include gene-transfer therapies that would target the specific genetic defect in an infant's hematopoietic stem cell, allowing the engineered stem cell to reconstitute the patient's white blood cells with functionally normal cells. Indeed, in April 2002, a report of genetic correction of X-linked severe combined immunodeficiency in four of five male infants by retroviral gene transfer was published.

Immunodeficiency disorders may manifest solely as recurrent infection of a given tissue or anatomic site or may be encountered as part of a syndrome with many other features. Autosomal dominant, autosomal recessive, and X-linked recessive modes of inheritance have all been described. However, the identification and characterization of the genetic basis for a disorder may be hindered by any of several factors. For example, identification of an immunodeficiency as X-linked may not be obvious if the number of cases due to de novo mutations in the X chromosome is significant, since the frequent occurrence of affected males in the absence of any history of affected male relatives would obscure the X-linked basis of the disorder. Autosomal recessive immunodeficiency conditions are rare except when consanguinity is involved or descendants from a limited ancestry have children (known as a "founder effect" in the field of population genetics). Last, for the majority of the recognized host-defense genes, all occurrences of disease are not caused by a single common mutation but rather by any of a great variety of mutations, making genetic screening difficult. Advances in the technology of gene-mutation detection will facilitate these analyses in the future.

Basic Defects Leading to Immune Dysfunction

There are several ways to look at the molecular and cellular basis for immunodeficiency. One is to examine the basis for a specific defect in development or function, whether it is phagocytic, humoral, cellular, combined, or associated with immunologically important proteins such as complement. A large number of such defects are known (Table 23.1 and Fig. 23.1). Another is to take a more clinical focus in order to provide greater insight into the clinical manifestations of defects in host immune function and the overlapping clinical manifestations resulting from specific defects. We will first describe some basic defects leading to a range of immunodeficiency diseases, then look at different clinical manifestations of a variety of these and other immunodeficiency diseases. A key feature of understanding immunodeficiency, as well as normal immune system function, is to identify the molecular and cellular defects giving rise to an immunodeficient state. These basic defects are the targets for clinical intervention.

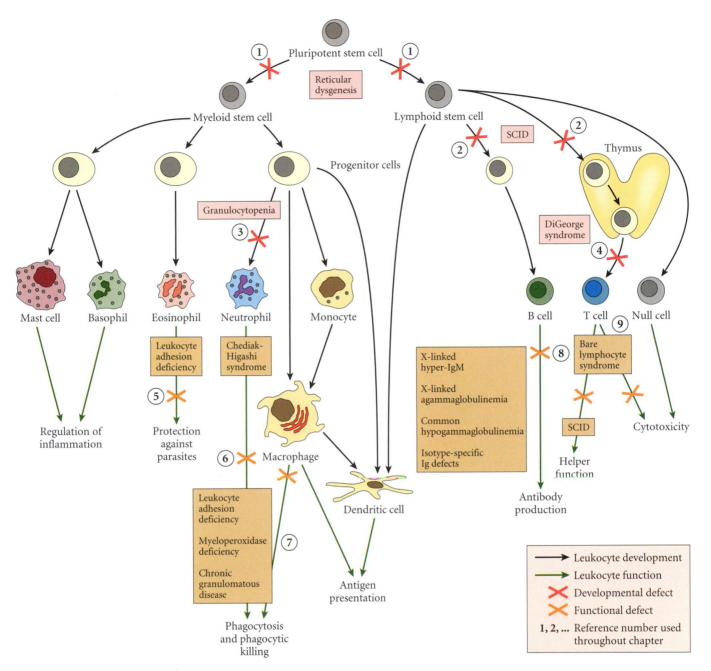

Figure 23.1 Diagram of leukopoiesis, indicating the locations of developmental or functional defects associated with immunodeficiency. The names of some immunodeficiency syndromes are given in pink boxes (for developmental defects) or orange boxes (for functional defects). Note that some defects (for example, LAD) affect the function of more than one cell lineage. Also note that some classes of immunodeficiency (for example, SCID) can result from either developmental defects or functional defects.

Defects in Lymphocyte Development and Function

The development of lymphoid stem cells into mature T and B cells involves many steps, and if the development is halted at any of these steps, the resulting immunodeficiency can be based on nonfunctional T cells, B cells, or both. Such conditions usually lead to *severe combined im-*

munodeficiency (SCID). A number of genetic defects give rise to SCID (Fig. 23.2 and label 2 in Fig. 23.1). Defects that affect lymphoid stem cell development can be based on deficiencies in production of key factors needed for development or defects in metabolism resulting in accumulation of toxic metabolites in the developing cells. If the lymphoid stem cell cannot generate rearranged T-cell re-

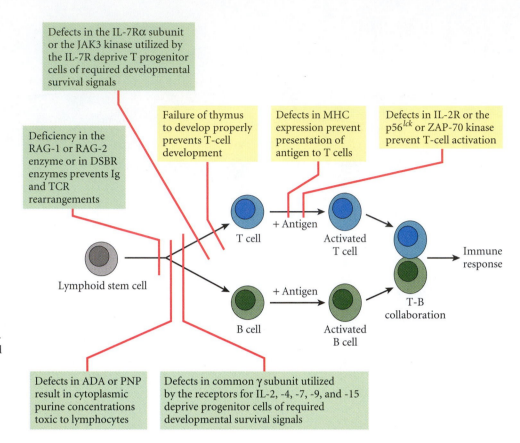

Defects in the IL-7Rα subunit or the JAK3 kinase utilized by the IL-7R deprive T progenitor cells of required developmental survival signals

Deficiency in the RAG-1 or RAG-2 enzyme or in DSBR enzymes prevents Ig and TCR rearrangements

Failure of thymus to develop properly prevents T-cell development

Defects in MHC expression prevent presentation of antigen to T cells

Defects in IL-2R or the p56*lck* or ZAP-70 kinase prevent T-cell activation

Lymphoid stem cell

T cell

+ Antigen

Activated T cell

Immune response

B cell

+ Antigen

Activated B cell

T-B collaboration

Defects in ADA or PNP result in cytoplasmic purine concentrations toxic to lymphocytes

Defects in common γ subunit utilized by the receptors for IL-2, -4, -7, -9, and -15 deprive progenitor cells of required developmental survival signals

Figure 23.2 Flow chart of lymphocyte development and function, indicating the locations of developmental or functional defects that result in SCID. Some of the defects that are shown (yellow boxes) only affect T cells directly, but result in a SCID phenotype due to an inability of helper T cells to help B cells.

ceptor (TCR) and immunoglobulin gene rearrangements due to defects in the recombination-activation (*RAG*) genes or the double-stranded break repair (*DSBR*) genes, then mature T and B cells cannot be produced. Some individuals with SCID due to mutations in either *RAG-1* or *RAG-2* make a small amount of functional protein and thus have some V(D)J recombination in their lymphocytes. This gives rise to a set of improperly regulated, oligoclonal T cells that reach the periphery and give rise to symptoms similar to graft-versus-host disease. The disease is called Omenn syndrome and is fatal unless treated early. Most of the patients become severely ill in the first few weeks of life. Interestingly, individuals with the same genetic defect in the *RAG* genes associated with classic SCID where no T cells develop, as well as Omenn syndrome, where some T cells develop, have been identified. This indicates that genetic factors other than defects in the *RAG* genes may be critical for the different clinical manifestations of *RAG* gene defects.

Since DNA rearrangements are critical for proper B- and T-cell development, other cases of SCID are due to defects in DNA repair and metabolism. *Ataxia telangiectasia* (AT) is a multisystem disorder affecting the brain, skin, and immune system. It is an autosomal recessive disorder with varying degrees of severity, owing to the degree

to which T-cell function is compromised. The disease is due to a defective protein called ATM, which is involved in fixing damaged DNA. These patients also have other diseases due to their inability to repair injured DNA, including cancers, endocrine abnormalities, liver problems, and retarded growth.

Toxic metabolites from improper nucleotide synthesis can build up in early lymphoid progenitors in patients lacking the enzyme *adenosine deaminase* (ADA) or *purine nucleoside phosphorylase* (PNP). These toxic metabolites prevent maturation of lymphoid stem cells, particularly T cells. ADA deficiency was the first genetic disease for which gene therapy was tried, using both delivery of genes to the patients and extracting their stem cells and correcting them by retroviral transfer of the *ADA* gene. Another therapy for these deficiencies is to provide the enzyme encased in polyethylene glycol, which is taken up by the lymphoid cells and used to correct the buildup of toxic metabolites.

Cytokine binding and signaling are key to emergence of T and B cells. One major form of X-linked SCID is due to defects in production of the common gamma cytokine receptor subunit utilized by receptors for interleukin-2 (IL-2), -4, -7, -9, and -15. This is the genetic defect that the "boy in the bubble" had. The γ chain interacts with the

JAK3 kinase for signal transduction, and patients with a defective JAK3 kinase have a form of SCID similar to X-linked SCID. In X-linked SCID B cells are normal in number but defective in antibody production. To distinguish between the need for the common γ chain in B-cell development or B-cell response to antigen, investigators have looked at healthy female carriers of this defect to determine if their B cells have inactivated the X chromosome with the wild-type or mutant copy of the gene. In females, only one of the two X chromosomes in a cell is active. Naive B cells had mostly, but not totally, inactivated the defective chromosome, indicating a need for the cytokine receptors using the γ chain in the proper development of most B cells. However, when antigen-activated, isotype-switched memory B cells were looked at, they all had inactivated the defective chromosome, indicating an absolute need for the γ chain in B-cell responses. Since the γ chain is part of the IL-4 receptor needed for B-cell activation, it seems likely that this aspect of B-cell responses is critical for antibody production.

Defects more specifically localized to IL-7 production, receptor binding, and signaling inhibit T-cell development by failing to provide survival signals. If the thymus fails to develop as an organ, then T cells also cannot develop. This occurs in DiGeorge syndrome, or congenital thymic dysplasia (label 4 in Fig. 23.1). As T-cell maturation requires interaction with major histocompatibility complex (MHC) proteins presenting self peptides, defects in MHC protein production will inhibit T-cell development. Also, anything that prevents proper IL-2-mediated activation of T cells will lead to a T-cell immunodeficiency.

ZAP-70 is a protein tyrosine kinase expressed exclusively in T cells and the related natural killer cells. A deficiency in ZAP-70 kinase results in low numbers of T cells because of the blockage of their maturation in the thymus and defects in TCR signaling.

Bare Lymphocyte Syndrome

Bare lymphocyte syndrome is an immune deficiency resulting from failure to produce MHC class I or class II molecules (Fig. 23.3 and label 9 in Fig. 23.1). Bare lymphocyte syndrome, another recessive form of SCID, accounts for approximately 5% of patients with SCID. The defect is expressed not only on lymphocytes or cells of lymphoid origin but on all affected cells and results in an inability to mount a full immune response. Most of the genes involved are inherited in an autosomal recessive fashion. The most common type of bare lymphocyte syndrome is due to a failure to synthesize MHC class II molecules, which would compromise antigen presenta-

tion (Fig. 23.3B). The result is an inability to positively select CD4$^+$ cells in the thymus and therefore few functional CD4$^+$ cells are present. This results in a SCID phenotype. The genes for the MHC class II molecules are generally intact, and the disease is due to defects in transcriptional components of the MHC class II gene complex. To produce class II molecules, several transcriptional activators are needed. One of these is a transcription factor called class II transactivator (CIITA). Individuals with the most common type of bare lymphocyte syndrome, referred to as complementation group A, do not make this transcription factor, which thus limits the production of class II molecules. A rarer form of MHC class II deficiency occurs in individuals unable to produce regulatory factor X (RFX), a transcription factor that normally binds to a portion of the promoter involved in transcription of class II genes. RFX is composed of three polypeptides named RFXANK (also referred to as RFX-B), RFX5, and RFXAP. Individuals with homozygous deficiencies in the genes for these polypeptides fall into bare lymphocyte syndrome complementation groups B, C, and D, respectively. Often they have reduced levels of MHC class I proteins as well, as RFX plays a role in transcription of the class I genes. This disorder is most frequent among individuals of Mediterranean ancestry and has been treated successfully by bone marrow transplantation.

Other forms of bare lymphocyte syndrome are due to failure to produce adequate amounts of MHC class I but adequate amounts of MHC class II (Fig. 23.3C). This is usually due to defects in the genes encoding the transporter associated with antigen processing (*TAP1* or *TAP2*) and not to effects in genes for MHC class I. Affected individuals have few CD8$^+$ αβ T cells due to lack of sufficient expression of MHC class I to promote CD8$^+$ T-cell selection. They do, however, have normal numbers of CD8$^+$ γδ T cells. Lack of MHC class I does not result in as severe an immunodeficiency as one might expect. For example, viral infections are not a major problem with these patients even though CD8$^+$ T cells play a role in controlling viral growth. This may be due to the important role of antibody in control of viral infections. Another possibility is that there may be TAP-independent means to load MHC class I proteins with peptides, allowing for a reduced but sufficient response to viral infection.

Defects in Phagocytic Killing

Phagocytosis of foreign microbes is a key component of immune resistance to infection, and defects in this element of the immune response can have devastating consequences. Ingestion of a foreign microbe into a phagosome is followed by fusion with a lysosome containing

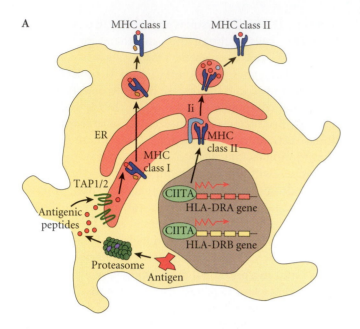

A

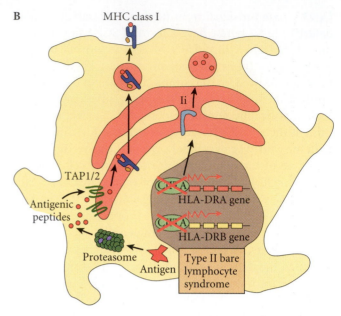

B

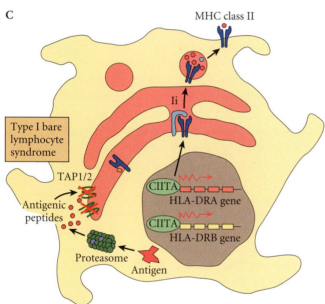

C

Figure 23.3 Bare lymphocyte syndrome (BLS). (**A**) Diagram of trafficking and peptide loading by MHC class I (MHC I) and class II (MHC II) in a normal antigen-presenting cell. (**B**) The more common type of BLS, BLS (MHC II), usually results from a failure to synthesize MHC class II due to a defect in the transcription factor CIITA. MHC class I is still produced and loaded with peptide normally. (**C**) A less common form of BLS, BLS (MHC I), is characterized by normal synthesis of MHC class I but greatly reduced membrane expression of MHC class I due to a defect in TAP. TAP deficiency results in an inability to load antigenic peptides onto MHC class I, causing the class I proteins to be retained in the endoplasmic reticulum (ER). Ii, invariant chain.

hydrolytic enzymes and other factors that damage or kill the microbe (Fig. 23.4). Accompanying this process is the production of toxic metabolites of oxygen (the oxidative burst) needed to kill microorganisms. A family of reduced nicotinamide adenine dinucleotide phosphate (NADPH) oxidase enzymes known as p22, p67, and p91, along with the myeloperoxidase enzyme, are needed in these reactions to produce the oxidative burst, and defects in their production or function prevent an adequate microbicidal response in the phagocyte. Common manifestations of these defects are chronic granulomatous diseases and myeloperoxidase deficiency (label 7 in Fig. 23.1). Under-

lying the phagocytic process is the proper movement of the phagosomes and lysosomes through the cell to meet up and fuse. In Chediak-Higashi syndrome (label 6 in Fig. 23.1) the lysosomes fail to fuse properly with the phagosomes but rather fuse with each other, producing a large number of vacuoles in the cytoplasm of the phagocyte.

Leukocyte Adhesion Deficiency

Another critical component of immune function is the proper movement of leukocytes around the body to orchestrate immune reactions. Defects in the ability of leukocytes to get to where they are needed to interact with

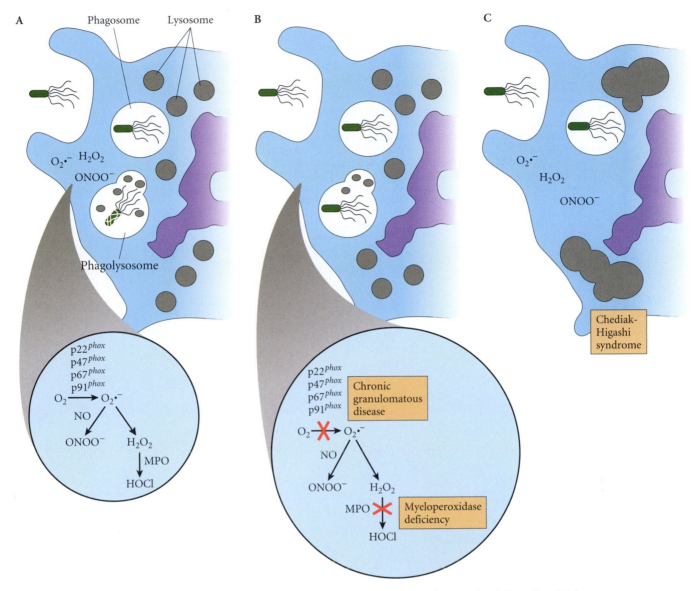

Figure 23.4 Defects in phagocytic killing. (A) In a normal phagocyte, phagocytosis of a bacterium is followed by a fusion of the phagosome with a lysosome (large black circles) to form a phagolysosome. In the phagolysosome, hydrolytic enzymes (small black circles) damage ingested bacteria. Simultaneously, a family of NADPH oxidases (p22, p67, and p91) and myeloperoxidase (MPO) enzymes become activated to produce the oxidative burst, resulting in the production of toxic oxygen intermediates such as superoxide ($O_2^{\bullet-}$), peroxynitrite ($ONOO^-$), hydrogen peroxide (H_2O_2), and hypochlorous acid (HOCl), which also participate in microbial killing. (B) Some phagocytic defects, such as CGD and myeloperoxidase deficiency, result from defects in the enzymes needed for the oxidative burst. Without the oxidative burst, hydrolytic enzymes in the phagolysosome are insufficient for microbial killing. (C) Chediak-Higashi syndrome results from a defect in the regulation of lysosome trafficking and fusion. As a result, most lysosomes in a Chediak-Higashi syndrome phagocyte prematurely fuse with each other, resulting in giant, nonfunctional lysosomes. In these phagocytes, the oxidative burst occurs normally, though it alone is insufficient for microbial killing in the absence of phagosome-lysosome fusion.

other cells can result in ineffective responses. One well-known immunodeficiency in this regard is leukocyte adhesion deficiency (LAD) (Fig. 23.5 and label 7 in Fig. 23.1). Normal movement of leukocytes through the blood and into inflamed tissues requires a number of important factors. One of these factors is the production of integrin proteins of the CD11/CD18 groups that mediate high-affinity binding of white blood cells to the vascular endothelium, which occurs before the diapedesis of the cell into the tissue. The LAD syndrome is caused by deficiency

Figure 23.5 LAD. (A) In a normal individual, leukocytes are able to leave the circulation and enter solid tissues by a multistep process of extravasation. This involves the following steps: (1) low-affinity rolling adhesion mediates by mucin-selectin interactions; (2) signaling via chemokines such as IL-8; (3) conversion of leukocyte integrin proteins to their high-affinity form via a G protein-dependent signal upon binding to IL-8; (4) high-affinity binding of leukocyte to vascular endothelium, leading to leukocyte arrest; and (5) diapedesis. (B) In an individual with LAD, rolling (I) and signaling via IL-8 (II) still occur normally, but a defect in leukocyte integrin proteins (III) prevents high-affinity leukocyte-endothelium interactions. Therefore, leukocytes never arrest on the endothelium and detach from the latter (IV).

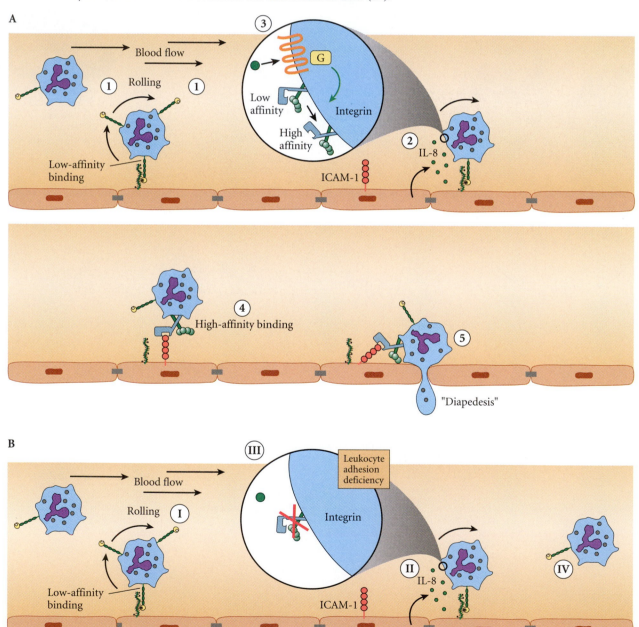

of the integrin common β_2 subunit (CD18) caused by mutations in the gene on chromosome 21q22.3. Individuals lacking high-affinity integrins fail to produce a functional immune response. Problems in LAD include altered chemotaxis of cells, a defect in their spreading, and random migration. T cells in patients with LAD do not become properly activated due to inefficient interactions with antigen-presenting cells. Other aspects of LAD include failure to produce complement receptors. This leaves the patient unable to properly opsonize and kill bacterial pathogens such as staphylococci. Most individuals with this autosomal recessive disease fail to produce the three α and four β chains of the integrin proteins and are severely affected. Some produce reduced amounts and are somewhat healthier clinically.

Reticular Dysgenesis

The most severe form of SCID, reticular dysgenesis, is due to an uncommon defect in bone marrow stem cells of unknown etiology and autosomal recessive inheritance (label 1 in Fig. 23.1). Since the defect lies in the hematopoietic stem cell, reticular dysgenesis results in deficiency of all lineages of red and white blood cells and thus causes severe immunodeficiency with early presentation and poor prognosis unless bone marrow transplantation can be performed. Thus far, no specific genetic defect has been identified.

Clinical Manifestations of Immunodeficiency

Manifestations of immune dysfunction frequently target the respiratory tract, skin, and gastrointestinal tract or are associated with invasive (systemic) infectious disease (Table 23.2). Many defects may present as major manifestations in one anatomic area and minor manifestations in other organ systems. Each section will discuss clinical presentation, functional deficits, genetic implications, diagnostic testing, and potential therapeutic interventions. AIDS will be discussed as appropriate; however, the focus will be on primary immunodeficiencies since human immunodeficiency virus (HIV) and AIDS are covered in detail in chapter 22.

Clinical Aspects of SCID Syndrome

SCID syndrome (SCIDS) can be defined as any immunodeficiency that affects more than one lineage of leukocyte; however, in most cases, the principal lineages affected are the lymphoid B and T cells (Fig. 23.2 and label 2 in Fig. 23.1). Patients with SCIDS demonstrate marked lymphopenia and anergy (nonresponsiveness) of their

Table 23.2 Common clinical manifestations of primary immune deficiency

Bacterial infections
Invasive bacterial disease
Recurrent or prolonged respiratory tract illness including recurrent otitis and/or sinusitis
Bronchiectasis
Lung, hepatic, or splenic abscess
Gingivitis
Recurrent cutaneous abscesses
Viral infections
Disseminated varicella
Recurrent herpes zoster
Paralytic polio due to vaccine strain (oral polio vaccine)
Chronic enteroviral meningoencephalitis
Giant cell pneumonia secondary to measles or measles vaccine virus
Severe Epstein-Barr virus disease
Fungal infections
Mucocutaneous candidiasis
PCP

lymphocytes to antigens. Levels of immunoglobulins, response to immunizations, and proliferative responses to mitogens in vitro are minimal. Lymph nodes are usually hypoplastic (underdeveloped), and dysplasia (malformation) of the thymus is nearly universal.

The T-cell abnormalities in cell-mediated deficiencies are profound, and infection with opportunistic pathogens is therefore the hallmark of these diseases. In addition, the children may present with failure to thrive, recurrent bacterial infections similar to those seen in X-linked agammaglobulinemia (XLA), or chronic diarrhea and malabsorption. Chronic cutaneous candidiasis, as well as chronic hepatitis due to cytomegalovirus or disseminated herpesvirus infections, may also occur.

A clinical presentation of SCIDS can result from any of numerous genetic defects that negatively affect the maturation or survival of B and T lymphocytes. Since B-cell activation is usually dependent on T-cell help, defects affecting T cells can give a SCIDS-like phenotype even if the maturation and survival of B cells are unaffected. In addition to defects in the *RAG* and *DSBR* genes leading to SCIDS, a defect in the gene encoding CD44, a cell-adhesion receptor important for the interaction of developing lymphocytes with stromal cells in primary lymphoid organs, results in deficient lymphocyte maturation and thymic hypoplasia (Nezelof syndrome).

ADA deficiency

ADA deficiency was the first genetic defect associated with SCIDS and accounts for approximately 30% of cases. Patients with the autosomal recessive disorder have characteristic skeletal abnormalities of the ribs and hips, with prominence of the costochondral junctions of the rib cage and a dysplastic pelvis. More than 30 mutations of the ADA gene have been catalogued, allowing correlations between genotype and phenotype. Prenatal diagnosis by DNA and enzyme analysis is available.

The mainstay of treatment of ADA deficiency has been transplantation with HLA-matched bone marrow; however, success has been achieved with haploidentical, T-cell-depleted transplants. Also, prenatal diagnosis is available, and two in utero transplants have been successful to date, with postnatal evidence of functional engrafted T cells. Therapy has also been attempted via enzyme replacement and gene replacement. The attempts at enzyme replacement have coupled ADA enzyme to polyethylene glycol to increase membrane permeability to the enzyme. One of the first gene-therapy protocols involved two ADA-deficient children. The low efficiency of gene transfer into hematopoietic stem cells remains the most severe limitation of retroviral gene therapy for this disorder. Improving retroviral vectors has been suggested as a possible means of overcoming this hurdle.

PNP deficiency

PNP deficiency accounts for approximately 4% of patients with SCIDS. Apart from recurrent infections beginning in the first year of life, about one-fourth of patients present with neurologic problems ranging from spasticity to mental retardation. Curiously, although PNP deficiency results in generalized immune suppression, about one-third of patients with PNP-SCIDS have autoimmune manifestations, ranging from hemolytic anemia (complement-mediated lysis of red blood cells due to the production of autoantibodies that recognize surface antigens on the red cells) to systemic lupus erythematosus (complement-mediated destruction of host tissues following deposition of complexes of DNA- and DNA-specific autoantibodies). The reason for increased risk of autoimmunity is not entirely understood. It may be related to the known (i) greater resistance of memory B cells than naive B cells to suppression and (ii) preferential use by the memory subpopulation of B cells of certain immunoglobulin V_H gene families, which may predispose toward autoreactivity.

Bare lymphocyte syndrome

Bare lymphocyte syndrome accounts for approximately 5% of patients with SCIDS. Affected individuals suffer from a variety of bacterial, viral, and opportunistic infections, primarily of the respiratory and gastrointestinal tracts, and they may have protracted bouts of diarrhea associated with infection with *Candida albicans* or *Cryptosporidium parvum*. Similar to PNP-SCIDS, bare lym-

phocyte syndrome is associated with an autoimmune condition, primary sclerosing cholangitis, which is an obstruction of the common bile duct secondary to inflammation and fibrosis of the liver.

HIV infection

HIV specifically infects CD4 lymphocytes, adversely affecting both their number and function. Over time, T-cell deficiency predominates in the clinical picture, and persistent thrush, chronic diarrhea, and susceptibility to opportunistic pathogens such as *Pneumocystis carinii*, cytomegalovirus, and *Cryptosporidium* become manifestations of severe immune depletion. Clinically, these patients resemble those with SCIDS.

DiGeorge syndrome

DiGeorge syndrome (label 4 in Fig. 23.1) is a developmental fetal defect involving the third and fourth fetal pharyngeal arches. The syndrome is characterized by thymic aplasia or hypoplasia, hypoparathyroidism, and cardiac malformations (Fig. 23.6). Variable degrees of immunodeficiency involving both T- and B-cell defects may be as severe as those in SCIDS. The majority of patients with DiGeorge syndrome have a microdeletion of chromosome 22q11.2, detectable by fluorescent in situ hybridization. Microdeletions of 22q11.2 have also been seen in patients with velocardiofacial syndrome (a genetic defect similar to DiGeorge syndrome that features cleft palate, heart defects, and facial abnormalities) and isolated conotruncal (pertaining to division of the heart chambers during embryogenesis) cardiac defect. There is genetic heterogeneity for DiGeorge syndrome, with a minority of patients having a microdeletion of chromosome 10p13-p14.

Figure 23.6 DiGeorge syndrome. A thymic shadow is absent in the anterior-posterior chest radiograph.

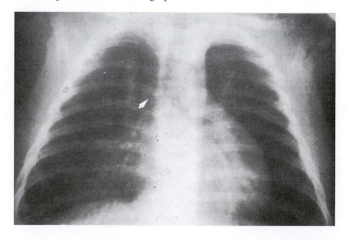

Wiskott-Aldrich syndrome

Wiskott-Aldrich syndrome is a rare X-linked recessive disorder characterized by recurrent pyogenic infection, thrombocytopenia, and eczema. Serum immunoglobulin M (IgM) concentrations are low, but IgA and IgE concentrations are higher than normal and the total IgG concentration is usually within the normal range. Individuals affected with this syndrome do not make antibodies to polysaccharide antigens and have poor immune responses to protein antigens. The number of T cells progressively decreases over time, and in vitro assays measuring lymphocyte proliferative responses demonstrate weak responses, especially to CD3-specific antibodies. This phenotype is explained by the role of the Wiskott-Aldrich syndrome protein (WASP) as an adapter protein for signaling mediated by the TCR. Thus, in affected individuals, the size of the initial T-cell pool is normal because T-cell maturation is unaffected. However, the T-cell pool steadily decreases because of the inability of the patient's T cells to become activated, expand, and form memory populations. Thrombocytopenia is prominent during infancy, with the onset of eczema in the first 1 to 2 years. As a child, the patient may experience increased susceptibility to sepsis pneumonia, chronic viral infections, autoimmune disease, and opportunistic pathogens. Those surviving are at an increased risk for lymphoreticular malignancies, especially non-Hodgkin's lymphoma. More than 110 different mutations in the WASP gene have been found. Prenatal diagnosis is available for families with a known mutation or by linkage analysis. The treatment of choice is HLA-matched bone marrow transplantation.

Invasive Bacterial Disease: Bacteremia and Sepsis

Early-onset invasive bacterial disease

Invasive bacterial disease is common among children because of their frequent environmental exposure to respiratory pathogens, as in day care facilities; their naive immune systems, which lack immunologic memory; and the diminished barrier protection afforded by their skin (especially in premature infants). Although episodes of neonatal invasive disease are frequent, the enhanced susceptibility of neonates is primarily physiologic, for the three reasons given above. However, congenital granulocytopenia (a reduction in the number of granulocytes, usually referring to neutrophils) may manifest during early infancy as omphalitis (inflammation of the navel), invasive bacterial disease, and/or perianal abscess (Table 23.3). Congenital granulocytopenias are due to a defect in growth and/or differentiation of granulocytes that results in their decreased production by the bone marrow re-

Table 23.3 Clinical manifestation of granulocyte defects

Defect	Clinical symptoms
Granulocytopenia	Omphalitis
	Perianal abscess
	Hepatic abscess
	Invasive bacterial disease
Granulocyte killing defect	Lung, splenic, or hepatic abscess
	Suppurative lymphadenitis
	Fungal or commensal pathogens (usually lung)
	Recurrent cutaneous abscesses
	Gingivitis

flected systemically in granulocyte concentrations of <1,500 cells per cubic millimeter (mm^3).

Congenital granulocytopenias either arise sporadically or are inherited as autosomal dominant or recessive traits (label 3 in Fig. 23.1). Several rare autosomal disorders include congenital granulocytopenia as a characteristic feature. Kostmann syndrome is a congenital agranulocytosis condition that stems from maturational arrest of myeloid cells at the promyelocyte stage and is associated with susceptibility to bacterial infections and some cancers. Schwachman-Diamond syndrome, a congenital disorder with autosomal recessive inheritance, includes granulocytopenia, failure to thrive, and pancreatic insufficiency. Reticular dysgenesis (label 1 in Fig. 23.1) is a very severe immunodeficiency caused by a defect in bone marrow stem cells that results in pancytopenia (a reduction in the number of all types of hematopoietic cells). Cyclic granulocytopenia, an autosomal dominant disorder caused by a defect in the gene encoding the neutrophil elastase enzyme (which is hypothesized to perturb hematopoiesis), typically manifests as alternating cycles of normal granulocyte counts that last about 3 weeks, followed by granulocytopenia that lasts approximately 1 week that is caused by a failure of granulocyte maturation. Isoimmune granulocytopenia (granulocytopenia due to the killing of the fetus's granulocytes by maternal antibodies to fetal granulocyte antigens) has been described in the setting of maternal deficiency of CD16 expression. Since the mother's cells do not express CD16, her immune system sees any CD16 present on the surface of fetal granulocytes as nonself, resulting in maternal production of isoimmune antibody to CD16-bearing fetal granulocytes.

Therapeutic approaches to preventing infection are often specific for the identified genetic defect, although broad-based therapies are sometimes used (e.g., transfusions of irradiated leukocytes are thought to be essential in children with overwhelming infection). Growth factors such as granulocyte colony-stimulating factor and granulocyte-macrophage colony-stimulating factor may be beneficial for the prevention of chronic and recurrent infection in patients surviving early infancy and are usually successful at interrupting the cyclical nature of the neutropenia. Bone marrow transplantation has been attempted in patients who do not respond to this type of therapy. For isoimmune disease, intravenous immune globulin (IVIG) decreases the destruction of granulocytes.

Invasive bacterial disease in infants and children

Sepsis due to the common pediatric respiratory pathogens *Streptococcus pneumoniae* and *Haemophilus influenzae* type b is often the presenting manifestation in children with critically low levels of IgG (<200 milligrams per deciliter [mg/dl]) (Table 23.4). Most often these infants are well for their first 3 to 6 months of life, until the decay of transplacentally acquired maternal IgG. The first identified immunodeficiency disease of this type was Bruton's XLA, a blockage of B-cell differentiation caused by a defect of B-cell-specific Bruton tyrosine kinase (BTK) (label 8 in Fig. 23.1). The BTK protein couples the pre-B-cell receptor present on developing B cells to nuclear events needed for B-cell growth and differentiation (see Fig. 7.24A). These patients are susceptible to invasive bacterial infection and chronic enteroviral meningoencephalitis (inflammation in the meninges of the brain) and are at risk for paralytic polio if immunized with live oral polio vaccine (because of the inability of their immune system to kill the attenuated poliovirus). One reason for a recent decision in the United States to use inactivated polio vaccine in infants for their primary series of polio immunizations instead of the oral vaccine is to prevent accidental infection with the vaccine strain in immunodeficient babies.

The gene encoding BTK has been localized to chromosome Xq22 and was cloned in 1993. Since then, several hundred different mutations in BTK have been catalogued. The majority of these mutations result in premature termination codons and/or translational reading frame shifts. About one-third are de novo mutations. Analysis of these mutations has been greatly facilitated by the establishment of a BTK mutation database. Databases of this sort make it possible to correlate genotype and phenotype, identifying mutations that are associated with a mild versus a severe clinical course. Prenatal diagnosis and carrier detection are possible via genetic linkage analysis but are best completed by assaying for specific known mutations in the BTK gene. In the absence of data on the specific mutation possessed by an affected family, female carriers can be identified as having nonrandom inactivation of the X chromosome.

Diagnosis of XLA is made by identifying extremely low levels of IgG (<100 mg/dl) and the absence of IgM and IgA. Low numbers of circulating mature B cells are found by flow cytometry. Treatment is immunoglobulin replacement with pooled IVIG. Doses between 350 and 600 milligrams per kilogram (mg/kg) are required every 2 to 4 weeks. Even with replacement IVIG, patients may still experience complications such as chronic lung disease, including bronchiectasis, which is the persistent dilation of bronchi as a result of chronic infection or inflammation (Fig. 23.7), and chronic and recurrent arthritis possibly due to *Ureaplasma urealyticum*.

The mode of inheritance of the hyper-IgM syndrome (label 8 in Fig. 23.1), which is characterized by increased serum levels of IgM and the absence or critically low levels of serum IgG, IgA, and IgE, may be X-linked, dominant, or autosomal recessive, depending on which gene is defective in an affected individual. The primary clinical manifestations resemble those of XLA. In addition, *P. carinii* pneumonia (PCP) (Fig. 23.8), autoimmune cytopenias, and an enhanced risk for gastrointestinal cancers and uncontrollable plasma cell infiltration of abdominal organs have been observed in patients with the hyper-IgM syndrome. This syndrome is differentiated from XLA by the presence of normal numbers of B cells on flow cytometry and increased serum IgM. The X-linked form of the disease is the most common form and results from a mutation in the gene encoding CD154 (the CD40 ligand [CD40L], also called gp39). This ligand is expressed on T cells and triggers B-cell isotype switching of antibody production upon interaction of CD154 with the B-cell protein CD40. Thus, although these patients' B cells can be activated, no isotype switching can occur, explaining the overrepresentation of IgM in these patients' serum. Prenatal diagnosis and carrier detection are accomplished primarily by linkage analysis. A rapid whole-blood flow-cytometry procedure for the diagnosis of X-linked hyper-IgM syndrome and identification of the carriers is now available. Successful cures by bone marrow transplantation have been achieved.

Table 23.4 Clinical manifestations of B-cell defects

Immune defect	Clinical manifestations
Reduced IgG (<200 mg/dl)	Invasive bacterial disease
	Recurrent respiratory tract disease (upper and lower)
	Paralytic polio secondary to vaccine strain (oral poliovirus vaccine)
	Chronic enteroviral meningoencephalitis
	Autoimmune disease
Diminished IgA and/or IgG subclass concentrations	Recurrent otitis and/or sinusitis
	Bronchiectasis

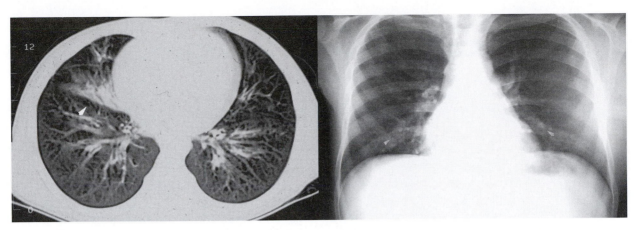

Figure 23.7 Bronchiectasis. (**Left**) A computed tomographic scan confirms chronic pneumonia/bronchiectasis in the right lower lobe. (**Right**) A chest radiograph of 12-year-old boy showing chronic right lower lobe infiltrate (arrowheads) consistent with bronchiectasis.

Hyper-IgM syndrome can also be inherited in dominant and autosomal recessive forms. Even though the causative genetic lesion is distinct for each form of the disease, the clinical syndrome arises from the same cellular defect (lack of isotype switching by B cells). Autosomal recessive hyper-IgM syndrome is caused by a mutation in the gene encoding CD40. A dominant mutant allele for CD154 containing an RNA splicing defect recently was described. The aberrantly spliced form of the CD154 protein forms multimers in the cytoplasm with CD154 encoded by the wild-type allele and prevents the wild-type CD154 from being properly placed in the plasma membrane. Thus, even though this form of hyper-IgM syndrome is X-linked, the phenotype is expressed in a dominant fashion, since even a heterozygous female (possessing one normal copy of the CD154 gene) fails to express cell surface CD154.

Although HIV specifically infects CD4 lymphocytes and adversely affects both their number and function, B-cell dysfunction occurs early and widely in HIV infection, probably because of a deficit of T-cell cytokines. These patients are deficient in IgG and have an increased incidence of bacteremia, especially due to encapsulated organisms.

Increased Susceptibility to Invasive and Recurring Neisserial Disease

Complement proteins are critical for bacterial lysis, recruitment of phagocytic cells, and amplification of the inflammatory process. Since the terminal components (C5, C6, C7, and C8) produce membrane attack complexes that lyse gram-negative bacteria (such as *Neisseria* and *Haemophilus* species) (see chapter 5), patients with defects in these proteins experience an increased rate of relapse and recurrence of meningococcemia, meningococcal meningitis, and disseminated gonococcal infection. Deficiencies in terminal complement proteins have an autosomal recessive pattern of inheritance.

Complement proteins C3, C3b, and iC3b are important opsonins for recognition of bacterial pathogens by phagocytes that express complement receptors 1 and 3. C3 deficiency increases susceptibility to meningitis, bacteremia, pneumonia, and peritonitis, especially with gram-positive pathogens such as *Staphylococcus aureus* and *S. pneumoniae* (Table 23.5). Since the opsonic forms of component C3 are actually the proteolytic split products C3b and iC3b, a similar, hypersusceptible phenotype is observed in individuals with deficiencies in the protein factor I, which cleaves C3b to iC3b.

Figure 23.8 PCP. Diffuse interstitial disease with nodularity suggests PCP.

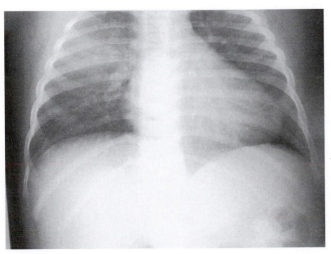

Table 23.5 Clinical illness in association with complement deficiency

Immune defect	Clinical syndrome
C5, C6, C7, or C8 deficiency	Meningococcal sepsis or meningitis
	Disseminated gonococcal syndromes
C3 deficiency	Invasive bacterial disease due to encapsulated pathogens

Table 23.6 Clinical manifestations of T-cell deficiency or dysfunction

Defect	Clinical manifestation
Decrease in T-cell number or function	PCP
	Mucocutaneous candidiasis
	Disseminated varicella
	Recurrent herpes zoster
	Measles pneumonia
	Disseminated BCG infection
	Disseminated *Mycobacterium avium-M. intracellulare* infection

Assays for total hemolytic complement are widely available and are used for initial diagnosis of suspected complement deficiencies. The presence of each of the nine complement components at >50% of normal concentrations is necessary for normal results in the total hemolytic complement assay. If screening for total hemolytic complement identifies an abnormality, the individual complement proteins should be measured. The rapid turnover of complement proteins impedes the usefulness of replacement therapy. Therefore, antimicrobial prophylaxis and immunization with *Haemophilus*, pneumococcal, and meningococcal vaccines are indicated as preventive strategies.

Respiratory Tract Infection

The respiratory tract is a common portal of entry for bacterial and viral pathogens. Host defense mechanisms, including local and serum antibody, cellular immunity, complement, and phagocytic cells, help limit invasiveness and bring about eventual recovery. It is not surprising that respiratory illnesses that are rare among normal individuals are more common in individuals with defects in one or more components of the immune system.

Respiratory Infection with Opportunistic Pathogens

Infection with the opportunistic pathogen *P. carinii* is clear evidence of a deficit in host defenses. Before the HIV epidemic, this organism (classified somewhat controversially as a fungus that cannot grow outside human bodies) had only caused a handful of recorded infections. However, during the HIV epidemic this pathogen became a major cause of PCP. Experience with HIV infection has permitted definition of the CD4 level in adult blood at which risk for PCP increases dramatically (<200 CD4 cells/mm^3). The establishment of such a threshold for infants has been more difficult, and clinical evidence from infants with primary immunodeficiency syndromes such as hyper-IgM syndrome (label 8 in Fig. 23.1) suggests that both deficits in T-cell function and deficits in T-cell number contribute to susceptibility to PCP. SCIDS is the prototype immunodeficiency syndrome (label 2 in Fig. 23.1)

associated with the occurrence of PCP (Table 23.6 and Fig. 23.8). In 1981 it was reported that 31 (27%) of 115 patients with SCIDS had at least one episode of PCP.

Recurrent or Prolonged Respiratory Tract Infection

IgA deficiency

Isolated IgA deficiency (label 8 in Fig. 23.1) is the most commonly observed immunodeficiency, with a prevalence between 1 in 400 and 1 in 1,000 individuals. Although the majority of patients are asymptomatic, about 10 to 20% of IgA-deficient individuals have increased susceptibility to sinopulmonary and gastrointestinal infections (Table 23.4). The genetics of IgA deficiency is complex. Autosomal dominant and recessive inheritance has been described in some families. Between one-third and one-half of individuals with chromosome 18 deletion also have IgA deficiency. However, there is a discordance of IgA deficiency in identical twins. Therefore, there is a strong environmental component for the determination of serum IgA level. A failure to switch to IgA-producing B lymphocytes or impaired survival of such cells may be an important molecular mechanism for IgA deficiency.

IgG-subclass deficiency

IgG-subclass deficiency (label 8 in Fig. 23.1) has been associated with a spectrum of recurrent respiratory infections (Table 23.4). The manifestation usually is frequent infections. IgG1 and IgG3 reach adult levels by the end of the first year of life, but IgG2 and IgG4 do not achieve adult levels until late in the first decade. Studies of children with deficiencies in IgG subclasses revealed that all had recurrent otitis and sinusitis (ear and sinus infections, respectively), most had at least one episode of pneumonia, and 50% had recurrent asthma. In another study, almost 25% of nonallergic children with chronic wheezing and cough had an IgG-subclass deficiency. Diagnosis of IgG-subclass deficiency requires measurement of specific subclasses, since the total IgG concentration is frequently normal because deficiencies in IgG2, IgG3, or IgG4 are reflected only as a small portion of the total IgG. Establishing the diagnosis is difficult, since concentrations of IgG2 and IgG4 are related maturationally, and low levels in the first several years of life therefore may normalize during the second decade.

Transient hypogammaglobulinemia of infancy

Transient hypogammaglobulinemia of infancy (THI) is an extreme exaggeration of the normally observed decline in IgG after birth. In THI, IgM and IgA levels are normal but the IgG level is depressed. IgG levels usually are between 200 and 400 mg/dl and increase slowly to within the normal range after the first 2 years of life. It is hypothesized that a delay in B-cell maturation is responsible for the failure to achieve normal IgG concentrations early in life. Clinically, children with THI usually suffer from mild, but more frequent, respiratory infections and rarely require specific therapy. On occasion, prophylactic antibiotics may be appropriate to prevent recurrent disease.

Common variable immunodeficiency

Common variable immunodeficiency (CVID) includes a group of late-onset variable defects in B- and T-cell function and regulation. Although families with autosomal recessive inheritance of CVID have been described, in the majority of families, the role of heredity remains undefined. The presence of a susceptibility locus within the HLA gene cluster on chromosome 6 has been suggested. In addition to experiencing recurrent sinopulmonary infections, patients with CVID have recurrent herpes simplex and herpes zoster infections and increased susceptibility to enteroviral infection and to *Giardia lamblia* infestation. They also have a high incidence of lymphoreticular malignancies and gastric carcinoma. Patients frequently have diffuse lymphadenopathy (enlarged lymph nodes) and splenomegaly (enlarged spleen). Diagnosis is based on decreased IgG and often decreased IgA and IgM concentrations. No intrinsic B-cell defect has been identified, and currently the leading hypothesis is that CVID is due to inadequate B-cell stimulation rather than to intrinsic B-cell failures.

AT

Between 1 in 100,000 and 1 in 40,000 individuals develop AT. At least 70% develop immunodeficiency, with 50% experiencing recurrent sinopulmonary infection, often leading to the development of bronchiectasis and chronic lung disease. Variable immunologic abnormalities are observed, including IgA deficiency, low IgG2 levels, and T-cell defects. Abnormal T-cell function usually is seen as absent or delayed hypersensitivity and as a reduced response to mitogens in vitro. Patients typically have persistent production of alpha-fetoprotein. The AT gene is located on chromosome 11q22-q23, and mutation leads to defects in DNA repair. These patients have a significantly increased risk of malignancy, especially breast cancer and lymphoma. Clinically, the cerebellar degeneration that results in progressive ataxia (loss of muscular coordination) and development of oculocutaneous telangiectasias (dilation of blood vessels of the eyes) usually precedes the onset of immunodeficiency. There is presently no effective therapy for this disorder.

Complicated Pneumonia: Lung Abscess and Empyema

A lung abscess is an area of necrotic material distinguished from pneumonia by the destruction of parenchymal tissue and the presence of cavitation, as well as by a large burden of bacterial pathogens (Fig. 23.9). The pathogenesis of lung abscesses represents either aspiration of bacteria from the nasopharynx or hematogenous (i.e., via the blood) dissemination of bacteria to lung parenchyma. Today, lung abscesses are uncommon and are found primarily in adults secondary to aspiration or in children with underlying deficits in immune function. Empyema (the accumulation of pus in a body cavity) represents a complication of pneumonia with the presence of purulent pleural effusion and chemical or microbial evidence of severe inflammation. Both these complications of respiratory tract infection occur more frequently in patients with neutrophil dysfunction. Inability of neutrophils to actively phagocytose and kill bacterial pathogens may result in recurrent lung abscess and/or empyema (Table 23.3).

Figure 23.9 Lung abscess. A chest radiograph shows early abscess cavities (arrowheads).

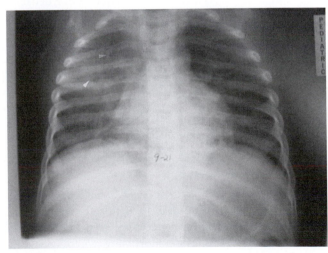

Chronic granulomatous disease

Chronic granulomatous disease (CGD) (Fig. 23.4 and label 7 in Fig. 23.1) is now recognized as the most frequent host defect associated with recurrent or multiple lung abscesses in children. This is a spectrum of disorders characterized by defective oxidative metabolism and intercellular killing. Ninety percent of children manifest symptoms by age 2 years. Clinically recurrent or multiple hepatic or splenic abscesses and suppurative lymphadenopathy may occur in addition to the respiratory tract complications. *S. aureus* is the single most common bacterial pathogen, although fungal infections with *Candida* and *Aspergillus* species are also frequent. Pulmonary infection with *Aspergillus*, *Nocardia* species, *Burkholderia cepacia*, or *Serratia marcescens* should alert the clinician to the potential of a phagocytic killing defect.

CGD can be inherited either as an X-linked or autosomal recessive disorder. The impairment of phagocytic killing of ingested microorganisms is due to defects in any of four genes encoding enzymes of the cytochrome oxidase system necessary for the production of superoxide anions. The more severe and more common cases of X-linked recessive CGD (two-thirds of cases) result from defects in the *CYBB* gene (encoding the heavy chain of cytochrome *b*) located on chromosome Xp21.1. Individuals with less severe symptoms may have the autosomal recessive CGD caused by a defect in one of three oxidase genes located on chromosomes 1, 7, and 16, respectively. Prenatal diagnosis of this disorder is available. The failure of phagocytes to demonstrate intracellular staining in the nitroblue tetrazolium assay is diagnostic. The mainstay of treatment has been antibiotic prophylaxis (trimethoprim-sulfamethoxazole) and bone marrow transplantation.

Glucose-6-phosphate dehydrogenase deficiency

Individuals whose erythrocytes are deficient in glucose-6-phosphate dehydrogenase (G6PD) typically have episodes of hemolytic anemia as a result of exposure to certain drugs and foods. This X-linked trait also leads to a profound deficiency of G6PD in leukocytes that is associated with a phagocytic bacteriocidal defect resulting from subnormal respiratory bursts. The clinical presentation can be similar to that of CGD. However, individuals whose G6PD activity is 25% of normal have not shown an unusual susceptibility to infection.

Myeloperoxidase deficiency

Myeloperoxidase deficiency (Fig. 23.4 and label 7 in Fig. 23.1) can either be acquired or inherited as an autosomal recessive disorder. Its prevalence is between 1 in 2,000 and 1 in 4,000 individuals. The majority are generally healthy but have delayed granulocyte killing activity and may suffer recurrent candidal infections. Several mutations have been identified in the myeloperoxidase gene on chromosome 17q22-23.

Job's syndrome

Job's syndrome (hyper-IgE syndrome) can be identified in patients with at least two of the following three characteristics: recurrent staphylococcal subcutaneous abscesses, staphylococcal pneumonia with cyst formation, and increased levels of IgE (>2,000 international units per milliliter [IU/ml]). It has been suggested that a defect of immune regulation may be the basis for this syndrome. Autosomal dominant inheritance is likely. Patients often have hyperextensible joints, scoliosis (abnormal curvature of the spine), and multiple fractures, and almost all have delayed loss of their primary dentition. Relative macrocephaly (disproportionately large head), a prominent forehead with deep set eyes, a broad nasal bridge, a long philtrum (area between the nose and the upper lip), and prominent jaw characterize their facies. Clinically, the IgE levels may decline over time and even be normal in some patients.

Skin Manifestations of Immune Deficiency

Recurrent cutaneous abscesses (pyoderma) alone or in combination with gingivitis, candidal diaper or mucocutaneous disease, or perianal abscess may suggest impaired leukocyte function (Table 23.2). In addition, chronic otitis media (middle ear infections) and recurrent respiratory tract infections may be part of the clinical syndrome. Serious defects in phagocytic function are reported in 2 of 100,000 individuals and represent about 20% of patients with congenital immunodeficiency syndromes. Secondary phagocytic deficits due to diabetes mellitus or to alcohol or drug use are seen more commonly but primarily in adult patients.

LAD

LAD (Fig. 23.5 and label 5 in Fig. 23.1) is a rare autosomal recessive disorder in which leukocytes fail to mobilize or migrate to sites of tissue injury. Adjunctive clinical features include delayed separation of the umbilical cord and perirectal abscesses, as well as recurrent staphylococcal and gram-negative bacterial infections. Diagnosis is made by the demonstration by flow cytometry of a deficiency in CD18 on phagocytes and of reduced adhesion to activated endothelial cells. In the severe form (type 1) of LAD, the CD18 molecule is completely absent. Without a bone marrow transplant, most of those affected will die during infancy or early childhood. Those patients with a partial absence (type 2 LAD) of the CD18 molecule have a better prognosis, usually surviving into adulthood. Replacement of the defective β-subunit (CD18) in the patient's myeloid precursor cells by gene therapy may be possible in the future.

Chediak-Higashi Syndrome

Chediak-Higashi syndrome (Fig. 23.4C and label 6 in Fig. 23.1) is characterized by partial oculocutaneous albinism, recurrent pyrogenic infections, increased bleeding tendency, and progressive neurologic deterioration. A defect in the *LYST* gene on chromosome 1, causing faulty lysosomal assembly, results in a defect in degranulation and in giant cytoplasmic granules. An accelerated lymphomatous phase occurs in approximately 85% of patients. During this accelerated stage, 90% of patients are granulocytopenic and anemic. Frequently, the function of their natural killer cells is profoundly decreased. Chediak-Higashi syndrome is suspected in the presence of partial albinism and neurologic impairment. Review of white blood cell morphology demonstrates giant granules within leukocytes.

Other Disorders of Leukocyte Mobility

Several other disorders of leukocyte mobility, including type 1B glycogen storage disease and mannosidosis, are known. Neutropenia, impaired neutrophil migration, and recurrent infection, especially with *S. aureus*, are prominent features of type 1B glycogen storage disease. Other features include hepatomegaly (enlarged liver), fasting hypoglycemia, lactic acidosis, short stature, hyperlipidemia, and hepatomas. Mannosidosis is an autosomal recessive lysosomal storage disease caused by a deficiency of acidic α-mannosidase enzyme. Typical features include coarse facies, psychomotor retardation, hepatosplenomegaly (enlargement of the liver and spleen), hearing loss, dysostosis multiplex (bone malformation), and recurrent soft tissue infections. A defect in chemotaxis and phagocytosis in neutrophils has been described. The gene for α-mannosidosis (lysosomal α-mannosidase) has been cloned, and many mutations have been identified, with clinical manifestations ranging in severity from a milder form displaying a constellation of the above-mentioned symptoms to a severe, early-onset form resulting in death during infancy. Successful bone marrow transplantation has been reported, with improvement in the bony manifestations, nonprogression of the cognitive dysfunction, and complete resolution of recurrent sinopulmonary disease and organomegaly.

Diagnostic evaluation of phagocyte function includes the use of an in vitro Boyden chamber (a closed chamber containing a filter with micron-sized pores through which leukocytes can migrate) to assess chemotaxis. Flow cy-

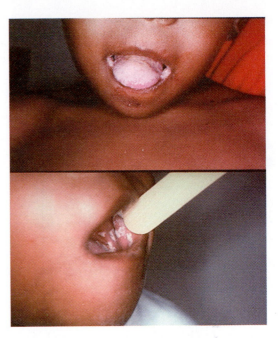

Figure 23.10 Mucocutaneous candidiasis. Fungal plaques are seen on the inner lining of the cheek and coating the tongue.

tometry is used to identify deficiencies in cell surface receptors. Opsonophagocytic activity (the ability of the leukocytes to phagocytose and kill microorganisms) also is measured directly.

Mucocutaneous Candidiasis

Mucocutaneous candidiasis is a spectrum of diseases involving persistent or recurrent candidal infections of mucous membranes, skin, and/or nails (Fig. 23.10 and Table 23.2). A common feature of the diseases that are due to an identified immune defect is an alteration in T-cell number or function (e.g., cytokine production). Persistent oral candidiasis is also an especially prominent feature of progressive HIV infection. Mucocutaneous candidiasis is often a prominent feature of SCIDS, DiGeorge syndrome, and immunodeficiencies specific to candidal antigens. In the latter, patients lack cellular immunity to *Candida* species that manifests as decreased production of the cytokine migration inhibitory factor by T cells following in vitro stimulation.

Oral Manifestations of Immune Deficiency

Periodontitis and gingivitis are common in individuals with genetic, developmental, or acquired disorders involving either phagocyte deficiencies or functional abnormalities of neutrophils (Table 23.3). Defective neutrophil chemotaxis is thought to represent a major pathologic mechanism in individuals with periodontitis syndromes. The molecular pathogenesis of juvenile periodontitis syndrome remains unclear. Severe gingivitis also is seen in patients infected with HIV and patients with severe malnutrition, viral illnesses, or unusually severe complications of vaccination with live virus vaccines.

Viral Illnesses or Vaccine Complications of Unusual Severity

Viral illnesses that are relatively common among normal individuals may be more severe, disseminated, prolonged, or recurrent in individuals with certain immunodeficiency syndromes. X-linked lymphoproliferative disease is an X-linked recessive disorder characterized by severe or fatal mononucleosis, acquired hypogammaglobulinemia, or malignant lymphoma in affected males exposed to infections with Epstein-Barr virus. Fatal infectious mononucleosis occurs in 67% of patients. The responsible *SH2D1A* gene has been cloned, and prenatal diagnosis is available by direct mutation analysis. Bone marrow transplantation and infusion of cord blood stem cells have been used in affected males.

Infection with measles virus or immunization with live measles vaccine has resulted in giant cell pneumonia in patients with SCID and comparable T-cell deficiencies (Table 23.6). Varicella-zoster virus, which causes the mild disease chicken pox in healthy individuals, can cause disseminated infections with pulmonary and hepatic complications in individuals with T-cell deficiency or HIV infection. Herpes zoster (a disorder that occurs upon reactivation of a latent varicella-zoster virus infection; also called *shingles*) also appears more frequently in children with this class of immunodeficiency.

Chronic enteroviral meningoencephalitis and paralytic polio following immunization with oral polio vaccine have been observed in patients with severe IgG deficiencies such as XLA and CVID. Progressive and disseminated bacillus Calmette-Guérin (BCG) infection following immunization with BCG vaccine (live bacterial vaccine for prevention of tuberculosis) has also been reported to occur in children with SCID.

Summary

Defects in innate and acquired immunity are characterized by increased susceptibility to infections by pathogens, both common and uncommon and those that never cause disease in the normal host. The majority of these immunodeficiencies are secondary, due to an impairment of the immune system through malnutrition, drugs, infections, etc. However, many important immunodeficiency diseases mainly affect children and are due to genetic defects and disease manifestation at an early age. Defects in innate immunity include poor production or lack of production of neutrophils or phagocytes, defects in phagocyte activity due to defects in the production of antimicrobial substances like oxygen radicals (CGD and myeloperoxidase deficiency), defects in cell adhesion and chemotaxis (LAD), and so forth. The major defects in acquired immune function include total lack of production of B and/or T cells (SCID and RAG defects), B-cell dysfunction resulting in a decrease in or a lack of production of antibodies that aid in protection from infections (common hypogammaglobulinemia, hyper-IgM syndrome, etc.), defects in antigen presentation and recognition of foreign antigens (bare lymphocyte syndrome), and so forth. Defects in metabolism can also result in faulty B- and T-cell production from lymphoid stem cells (ADA deficiency, PNP deficiency, etc.).

Clinical manifestations of immunodeficiency are most often seen as increased susceptibility to infection. Mucosal, skin, and oral surfaces are the most affected due to their intimate contact with the environment where they serve as a source of entry for pathogens. Many immunodeficiencies also involve other systems, including the neurologic and endocrine systems. Clinical presentations are the result of effects of infection and organ dysgenesis and can encompass failure to thrive, developmental abnormalities, and symptoms severe enough to lead to death. A number of therapeutic approaches have been successfully developed to treat immunodeficiency, including replacement of missing factors (ADA or IVIG), gene therapy, bone marrow transplantation, and supportive care treating the symptoms of the disease. Science and medicine have come a long way from having to keep babies born with SCIDS in a sterile environment, and continued improvements in modern medical therapies will have a major impact in reducing the consequences of immunodeficiency.

Suggested Reading

Buckley, R. H. 2001. The hyper-IgE syndrome. *Clin. Rev. Allergy Immunol.* **20:**139–154.

Buckley, R. H. 2002. Primary cellular immunodeficiencies. *J. Allergy Clin. Immunol.* **109:**747–757.

Bunting, M., E. S. Harris, T. M. McIntyre, S. M. Prescott, and G. A. Zimmerman. 2002. Leukocyte adhesion deficiency syndromes: adhesion and tethering defects involving beta 2 integrins and selectin ligands. *Curr. Opin. Hematol.* **9:**30–35.

Cunningham-Rundles, C. 2001. Physiology of IgA and IgA deficiency. *J. Clin. Immunol.* **21:**303–309.

Etzioni, A. 2002. Novel aspects of hypogammaglobulinemic states. *Isr. Med. Assoc. J.* **4:**294–297.

Fischer, A. 2002. Primary immunodeficiency diseases: natural mutant models for the study of the immune system. *Scand. J. Immunol.* **55:**238–241.

Khan, W. N. 2001. Regulation of B lymphocyte development and activation by Bruton's tyrosine kinase. *Immunol. Res.* 23:147–156.

Kirkpatrick, C. H. 2001. Chronic mucocutaneous candidiasis. *Pediatr. Infect. Dis. J.* 20:197–206.

Kokron, C. M., F. A. Bonilla, H. C. Oettgen, N. Ramesh, R. S. Geha, and F. Pandolfi. 1997. Searching for genes involved in the pathogenesis of primary immunodeficiency syndromes: lessons from mouse knockouts. *J. Clin. Immunol.* 17:109–126.

Lekstrom-Himes, J. A., and J. I. Gallin. 2000. Immunodeficiency disease caused by defects in phagocytes. *N. Engl. J. Med.* 343:1703–1714.

Leonard, W. J. 2001. Cytokines and immunodeficiency diseases. *Nat. Rev. Immunol.* 1:200–208.

Puck, J. M. 1999. Prenatal diagnosis of primary immunodeficiency diseases, p. 563–580. *In* A. Milunsky (ed.), *Genetic Disorders and the Fetus,* 4th ed. Johns Hopkins University Press, Baltimore, Md.

Reith, W., and B. Mach. 2001. The bare lymphocyte syndrome and the regulation of MHC expression. *Annu. Rev. Immunol.* 19:331–373.

Yang, K. D., and H. Hill. 2001. Granulocyte function disorders: aspects of development, genetics and management. *Pediatr. Infect. Dis. J.* 20:889–900.

chapter 24

Cancer and the Immune System

Lisa H. Butterfield, Stephen P. Schoenberger, and Jeffrey B. Lyczak

Cancer can be considered as a disease resulting from the progressive cellular expansion of a single cell whose progeny have escaped from normal regulatory mechanisms controlling cell division and homeostasis. At first glance, cancer appears to be a vast and bewildering array of diseases, with as many different types of cancer as there are types of cells in the body (Table 24.1). There are, in fact, over 100 different types of cancer known, and subtypes of these disease states can be found within specific organs. As methods for the treatment and prevention of infectious and cardiovascular diseases improve, cancer is emerging as the leading cause of death in industrialized countries (Fig. 24.1). Although conventional cancer treatments such as surgery, chemotherapy, and radiation have greatly enhanced patient survival, manipulation of the immune response to cancer cells to promote their destruction remains an important and increasingly realistic goal for physicians. Immunological control of cancers could conceivably play a role in the eradication of primary tumors and disseminated metastases as well as the residual cancer cells that remain after conventional treatment regimens. The ideal result of immunotherapy would be the specific eradication of cancer cells with minimal damage to normal host cells. However, almost by definition a tumor cell has escaped immunologic recognition and progressed to cancer because the affected patient's immune system did not control tumor growth. Attainment of the goal of effective immunotherapy for tumors requires an understanding of how the immune system both fails to respond to cancer cells and has the potential to respond and the ways in which this response can be strategically manipulated.

Table 24.1 Nomenclature of several types of cancer

Normal tissue	Benign tumor[a]	Malignant tumor[b]
Blood vessels	Angioma	Angiosarcoma
Bone	Osteoma	Osteosarcoma
Cartilage	Chondroma	Chondrosarcoma
Epithelium	Papilloma	Carcinoma
Glandular epithelium	Adenoma	Adenocarcinoma
Liver hepatocytes	Hepatoma	Hepatocarcinoma
Skeletal muscle	Rhabdomyoma	Rhabdomyosarcoma
Smooth muscle	Leiomyoma	Leiomyosarcoma

[a]Benign tumors are anatomically restricted to their original tissue site.
[b]Malignant tumors are capable of spreading (metastasis) to distant sites.

Figure 24.1 Cancer deaths in the United States, comparing the period from 1950 to 1969 with the period from 1970 to 1994. Data are for white males of all ages, are grouped according to county, and are expressed as the number of cancer-related deaths per 100,000 person-years. The vertical black bar in the center of each graph shows the nationwide average of cancer-related deaths. Data are from the National Cancer Institute's Atlas of Cancer Mortality, which can be viewed at http://www3.cancer.gov/atlasplus/.

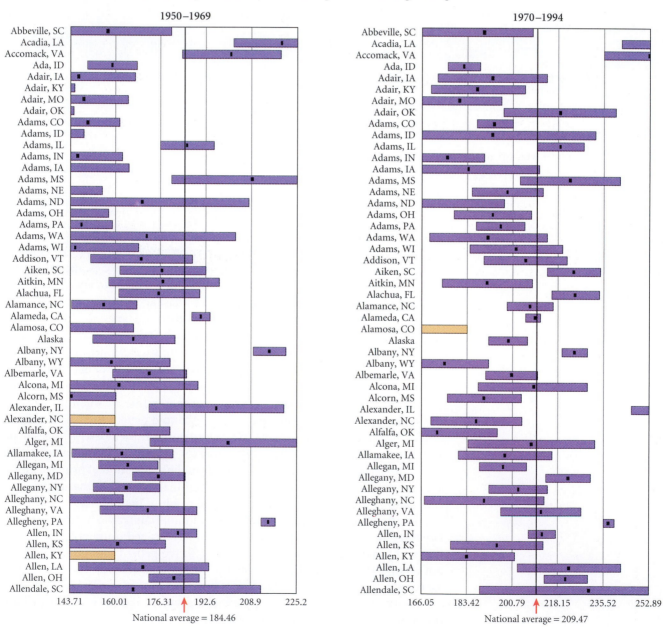

Cancer Is a Disease of Genes

Through intensive research efforts over the past 25 years, cancer is now understood as a series of defects in the molecular machinery that governs proliferation and homeostasis in nearly all cell types. Normal cellular growth within an organism is kept in balance by various regulatory circuits that govern the rate at which cells divide, differentiate, and die. Some of these regulatory circuits are intrinsic to the cell whereas others are coupled to the signals that cells receive from their surrounding microenvironment (Fig. 24.2). Cancer arises through a process termed *neoplastic transformation* that occurs when a

Figure 24.2 Schematic diagram of a typical eukaryotic cell showing the factors or conditions that regulate its growth. Exogenous factors, stimuli, or cues are shown in black type. Growth inhibitory factors and events are shown with red arrows. Growth stimulatory factors and events are shown with green arrows. TNF-R, tumor necrosis factor receptor; CAM, cell adhesion molecule; FAK, focal adhesion kinase; RB, retinoblastoma tumor suppressor protein; TF, transcription factor.

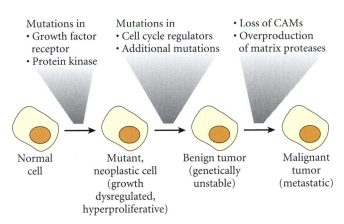

Figure 24.3 The multistep process of tumorigenesis. The cell, which is originally normal (at the left), undergoes several genetic changes in a stepwise fashion. Each genetic change results in a phenotypic alteration that favors unregulated growth, exemption from apoptotic signals, genetic instability, and metastasis (ability to spread from its original tissue site to other remote tissues of the host).

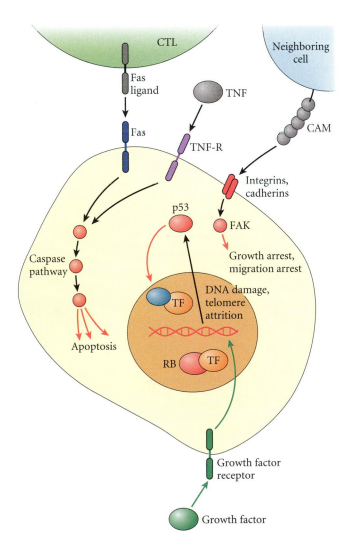

cell undergoes a series of genetic alterations and acquires the capability to escape these regulatory mechanisms. This process is thought to occur in a discrete stepwise process involving the age-related incidence of four to seven stochastic events that drive the transformation of a normal cell into highly malignant clonal derivatives (Fig. 24.3). This process is similar to a Darwinian model of evolution, in that each genetic change confers a growth advantage that leads to overrepresentation of the altered cell. The successive and heritable nature of cellular transformation events is supported by histological analyses of precancerous lesions revealing cells that appear to represent intermediate steps in the pathway between normal and transformed cells.

Another known situation that establishes a genetic basis for cancer comes from studies that have identified certain mutant forms of normal genes that predispose individuals to be at a greater risk for a given type of cancer. For example, women have a 10% lifetime risk for developing breast cancer, but among these patients are a small percentage with mutations in one of two genes, *BRCA1* and *BRCA2*, that greatly increase the risk of developing breast cancer. However, even carrying a high-risk mutation in the *BRCA* genes does not inevitably lead to breast cancer as 20 to 30% of women with mutant genes never develop this disease. Thus there are clearly modifier genes that can counteract the negative effects of the mutant genes. Other genetic predispositions to cancer include colon cancer associated with the adenomatous polyposis coli gene on chromosome 5; hereditary nonpolyposis colon cancer associated with DNA mismatch repair genes on chromosomes 2, 3, and 7; melanoma associated with the

CDNK2A gene on chromosome 9; testicular cancer associated with the *TCG1* gene on the X chromosome; and the Li-Fraumeni multiple cancer syndrome arising from mutations in the *TP53* gene on chromosome 17.

Genetic Changes in Transformed Cells

Modern molecular biology has allowed the vast catalog of different cancers described over the past century to be represented by an equally broad spectrum of cancer genotypes. Although the genetic defects permitting such autonomous growth are numerous, certain molecular themes have become apparent, allowing these defects to be organized into classes, according to what growth-regulatory mechanism is affected (Table 24.2). Any defective gene whose altered function promotes the conversion of a normal cell to a tumor cell is termed an *oncogene*. The normal version of the same gene is termed a *proto-oncogene* to denote that the gene is capable (through mutation) of giving rise to a cancer-causing oncogene. Figure 24.4 depicts several ways that a proto-oncogene can be converted to an oncogene. Conversion can occur by either point mutation, frameshift mutation, or chromosomal translocation. The consequences of these genetic events can either be loss of the gene's original function, enhancement of its original function, or a change in the gene's rate of transcription. In some cases, the proto-oncogene is a growth-promoting gene, and through either increased transcription or increased activity of its protein product, the oncogene causes unregulated cell division. An example of this is the Src protein tyrosine kinase shown in Fig. 24.4A. In other cases, the proto-oncogene normally serves a role in preventing or delaying cell division, and a loss-of-function mutation in the oncogene removes this regulatory mechanism, resulting in inappropriate cell division. Proto-oncogenes that fall into this category are sometimes referred to as *tumor-suppressor genes* or *anti-oncogenes*. An example of a tumor suppressor gene is the p53 protein, which normally functions to arrest the cell division cycle while DNA repair is proceeding, ensuring that existing mutations will be corrected and chromosomal integrity restored before DNA synthesis proceeds.

Another way that tumor cells attain the ability to proliferate in an uncontrolled fashion is by becoming independent of the growth signals on which normal cells are dependent. Many of the oncogenes associated with cancer act by mimicking normal growth signals in various ways (Table 24.3). This can occur by increased expression of soluble growth factors or growth factor receptors that can lead to autocrine stimulation of cell division. Cancer cells often have alterations in the downstream cytoplasmic signaling components of growth factor receptors, leading to the constitutive transmission of growth signals, even in the absence of the actual growth factor. Examples of this type of change are the numerous point mutations found in *ras* oncogenes that lead to their constitutive activation and the genetic translocations that lead to chronic myelogenous leukemia (CML). CML is due to a chromosome translocation known as t(9;22), which results from movement of the breakpoint cluster region (*bcr*) on chromosome 22 to the c-*abl* gene on chromosome 9. This translocation gives rise to what is known as the Philadelphia chromosome. The protein product of this fusion, the Abl tyrosine kinase, appears to be necessary for oncogenic transformation of CML cells. The wild-type c-Abl tyrosine kinase does not transform cells. A major advance in cancer chemotherapy has recently occurred with the licensing of Gleevec (also referred to as STI571 or imatinib mesylate), which is a small molecule that specifically inhibits the tyrosine kinase activity of the Bcr-Abl fusion protein.

The ability of a cancer cell's growth program to be freed from its dependence on environmental signals does not in itself guarantee expansive growth. Work by Leonard Hayflick and colleagues in the 1960s revealed that cells in culture have a finite replicative potential and enter a nonproliferative "senescent" state after having achieved a certain number of doublings (referred to in some older literature as the "Hayflick number"). Cellular senescence can

Table 24.2 Biochemical basis for stimulation of cell growth by oncogenes

Oncogene	Proto-oncogene product	Normal function of proto-oncogene	Alteration in oncogene
v-*src*[a]	c-Src[a]	Protein tyrosine kinase	Constitutively active
v-*erb*B	EGF-R	Growth factor receptor with intrinsic kinase activity	Does not contain growth factor binding domain; kinase domain is constitutively active
v-*sis*	PDGF	Growth factor	Overexpression
Ha-*ras*	Ras	Signaling molecule	Constitutively active
v-*abl*	Abl	DNA-binding kinase; inhibitor of transcription	Loss of inhibitory activity
myc	Myc	Transcription factor	Overexpression

[a]"v-" indicates a viral analog of the gene; "c-" indicates a normal cellular version of the gene.

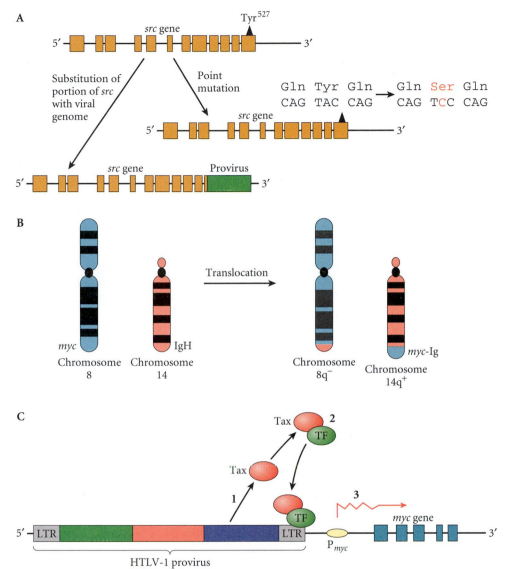

Figure 24.4 Conversion of a normal proto-oncogene to a cancer-promoting oncogene can result from changes in expression of the proto-oncogene or from alterations in the activity of the protein encoded by the proto-oncogene. **(A)** The *src* proto-oncogene encodes a protein tyrosine kinase. Point mutation at the 3′ end of the gene results in loss of the tyrosine at position 527 (Tyr^{527}) that is crucial for negative regulation of the kinase's enzymatic activity. The regulatory tyrosine also can be lost by insertion of viral DNA that interrupts the *src* gene coding sequence prior to Tyr^{527}. In either case, the mutant form of the kinase is constitutively active. **(B)** The *myc* proto-oncogene encodes a transcription factor that helps regulate cell division and cell death. Chromosomal translocation between the q arm of chromosome 8 and the q arm of chromosome 14 places the *myc* gene in the middle of the Ig heavy chain locus, enhancing transcription of the *myc* gene in B cells. This results in dysregulated cell division and the formation of B lymphomas. **(C)** Insertion of the human T-lymphotropic virus type 1 (HTLV-1) provirus near the *myc* proto-oncogene causes overexpression of *myc*, driven by strong enhancer elements in the viral long terminal repeats (LTRs). The virus encodes a protein called Tax (1) that activates (2) several host cell transcription factors (TF). The activated TFs then enhance transcription (3) from the nearby *myc* promoter (P$_{myc}$ [yellow oval]) by binding to the proviral LTR.

be overcome by disabling anti-oncogenes such as p53 and pRB, thus allowing the cells to proceed through additional rounds of division. Because this dysregulation uncouples cell division from the normal mechanisms of DNA repair, the progeny of these cells accumulate chromosomal abnormalities. These cells can reach a state called "crisis," which is characterized by the large-scale cell death and the rare emergence of an *immortalized* variant that acquires

Table 24.3 Characteristics acquired during emergence of a tumor cell

Characteristics	Mechanism	Genetic example(s) of mutations and effects of cell growth
Growth signal independence	Mimic normal signals via altered signaling components	Src, Ras: constitutive signaling; Her-2/Neu: initiates signal without ligand p53; RB: cell cycle proceeds despite DNA damage
Release from antiproliferative signals	Loss of function of regulatory proteins	Fas: cell does not respond to pro-apoptotic signals
Acquire blood supply	Activate local angiogenesis	Vascular endothelial growth factor Angiomodulin
Spread to other anatomic sites (metastasis)	Degrade extracellular matrix Downregulate cell adhesion molecules Modification of cell adhesion apparatus	Plasminogen activator, matrix metalloproteinase Integrins CD44, focal adhesion kinase

the capacity for limitless replicative potential. The molecular basis for cellular immortalization in cancer cells is thought to be their ability to maintain the length of the structures called *telomeres* that are found at the ends of chromosomes. Telomeres consist of several thousand repeats of a short 6-base-pair (bp) sequence that are progressively shortened by 50 to 100 bp with each successive cell division. Once telomeres are reduced in length to below a crucial threshold length, they can no longer protect the chromosomes from end-to-end fusions with other chromosomes, and this may underlie the many karyotypic aberrations associated with crisis. Telomeres are normally maintained by an enzyme called *telomerase*, which catalyzes the addition of hexanucleotide repeats to the ends of telomeric DNA. Telomerase is not expressed in senescent normal cells, but numerous tumor samples have been found to express this enzyme at high levels, suggesting that cancer cells exploit this enzyme for their own benefit.

Liberated from cellular senescence and capable of autonomous proliferation, the growing tumor mass requires a supply of oxygen and nutrients to sustain its growth, a need which becomes progressively more urgent as the mass of the tumor increases. The process of *angiogenesis* leads to the formation of blood vessels and capillaries within a tissue and is carefully regulated by counterbalancing negative and positive signals. Some of these signals are mediated by soluble factors interacting with their receptors that are able to either promote or inhibit blood vessel growth. Others involve the interaction of cellular proteases with integrin

molecules as well as elements of the extracellular matrix and can mediate the mobility of vascular endothelial cells. The ability of solid tumors to induce angiogenesis seems to stem from several factors (Fig. 24.5). First, the physical expansion of the tumor per se can activate the thrombin cascade by causing local tissue injury. This enzymatic cascade increases vascular permeability, activates matrix metalloproteases, and triggers production of vascular endothelial growth factor (VEGF). Second, some tumors can themselves produce VEGF, enhancing the angiogenic process. The ability of an incipient cancer to activate the "angiogenic switch" from vascular quiescence to sustained angiogenesis appears to represent an important step in the tumorigenic process. The work of Judah Folkman and colleagues has demonstrated that a tumor's dependence on angiogenesis can be exploited for therapeutic purposes, a finding that has led to the development of novel drugs that control the bioavailability of pro- and antiangiogenic factors and thereby inhibit tumor growth.

For cancer cells to thrive and expand, the increased growth rate must be matched by a decrease in the rate at which they die. The removal of cells in vivo normally occurs through programmed cell death or apoptosis, which acts the same in nonhematopoietic cells as it does in hematopoietic cells such as lymphocytes. Apoptotic cells and their remains are ultimately engulfed by phagocytes. Escape from apoptosis is emerging as a key feature of cancer, with mounting evidence coming from both animal studies and clinical human tumor biopsies. Studies with

Figure 24.5 Solid tumors induce angiogenesis and direct new blood vessels to grow into the tumor, providing the tumor with nutrients and waste removal. Growing tumor masses stimulate angiogenesis by causing local tissue injury (1), thus activating the thrombin cascade (2). Thrombin activates endothelial cells and platelets (3) to produce matrix metalloproteases (MMPs), VEGF, and tissue factor (TF). VEGF directs growth and elongation of vascular endothelium (4). MMPs dissolve extracellular matrix (ECM) components to allow growth of new vascular endothelium (5). TF stimulates further production of thrombin, setting up a positive feedback loop (6). Some tumors secrete VEGF to enhance this process (7). Reprinted from D. E. Richard et al., *Oncogene* 20:1556–1562, 2001, with permission.

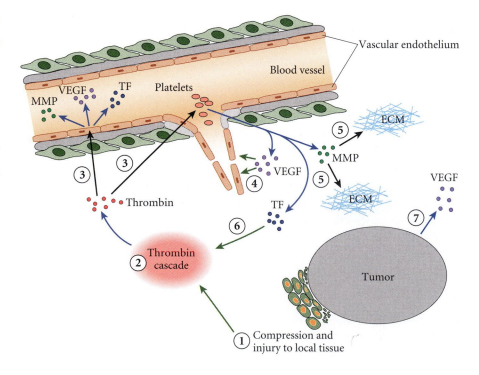

mice have revealed that apoptosis pathways can be interrupted in tumor cells at several levels. In some cases, the tumor cells lose expression of a surface receptor protein that normally receives signals initiating apoptosis. Tumor cells that have lost expression of the CD95 (Fas) are not capable of responding to the protein CD95L (Fas ligand [FasL]), which cytotoxic T lymphocytes (CTLs) use to induce apoptosis of their targets. In other cases, the biochemical signaling pathway that mediates apoptosis is either disabled or dysregulated to favor survival of the tumor cell. In Burkitt's lymphoma, a tumor derived from lymphocytes, the transformed cells overexpress the antiapoptotic protein Bcl-2. These cells are highly resistant to several cytotoxic mechanisms.

Most tumors arise by the neoplastic transformation of a cell in a solid tissue and are therefore initially confined to a discrete anatomical location. In many cases, however, cells from the tumor acquire the ability to detach from the tumor mass and invade adjacent tissues and distant sites in a process called *metastasis*. These distant colonies are called *metastases* or *secondary tumors* and account for over 90% of human cancer deaths. Metastasis allows tumor cells to expand to new areas where nutrients and space are not limiting and frequently results in the growth of tumor masses in other tissues or organs whose normal function is disrupted as a result of tumor growth. The metastatic spread of cancer is a complex, incompletely understood process involving changes in the expression of genes that tether a cell to its surroundings, such as integrins, tissue homing molecules, and extracellular proteases. Sometimes the newly formed metastases can conscript normal host tissue into the metastatic process by utilizing factors they produce such as matrix-degrading proteases or growth factors to promote tumor growth.

The Immune Response to Cancer

It has been more than 100 years since Paul Ehrlich first suggested that tumors could be destroyed by immune mechanisms. On the basis of this proposition, scientists began studying the interaction between immune cells and tumors in hopes of amplifying antitumor immunity as a means of treating cancer. Early experimental studies of the immune response to tumors focused on the outgrowth versus rejection of tumor fragments transplanted between outbred mice. Tumor rejection in these cases was thought to reveal the existence of tumor-specific antigens and suggested that the immune system could be used to control cancer. However, in the 1930s Peter Gorer showed that the rejection observed in these experiments was actually directed against the dissimilar major histocompatibil-

ity complex (MHC) antigens on the graft and could not be distinguished from tissue rejection in general. It was only when inbred strains of mice became available that critical investigation into the immunogenicity of tumors could be undertaken. Tumors from one mouse would usually grow in a second mouse if the two mice were of the same strain and hence shared MHC antigens, since the tumor would be seen as "self tissue" by the genetically identical recipient mouse (Fig. 24.6A). However, if the recipient mouse was of a different strain and MHC type than the donor mouse, the tumor would be rejected by the recipient mouse. In the 1940s and 1950s, chemical carcinogens were used to induce tumors that could be excised (i.e., surgically removed), inactivated for growth, and then used as vaccines to immunize other mice of the same strain type. These studies demonstrated that sometimes such tumors expressed antigens (called *tumor-specific antigens* [TSAs]) that could invoke protective immunity and prevent vaccinated mice from acquiring the same type of tumor at a later time (Fig. 24.6B). It was later shown that this protective immunity could be induced within an individual animal and, importantly, could be transferred from a vaccinated mouse to a naive (unvaccinated) mouse by lymphocytes obtained from the immunized donor. The TSAs expressed by mutagen-induced cancers appeared to be unique to each tumor in that immunization with a given tumor able to confer protection from challenge with the identical tumor could not protect animals from challenge with morphologically similar tumors derived from a separate site even when the second tumor was induced by the same chemical agent. Subsequent studies in the 1960s showed that some virally induced tumors express TSAs that are identical to those expressed by other tumors induced by the same virus but are distinct from the TSAs expressed by tumors induced by other viruses. We now know that such virus-specific TSAs are actually products of the viral genome that are expressed in every cell infected by a given virus. Target antigens have been identified at the molecular level for a variety of tumors. The existence of tumor-specific antigens and their immunogenicity are key factors determining the usefulness of immunotherapy against any given tumor.

Mechanisms of Antitumor Immunity
Classes of Tumor Antigens

The molecular identification of tumor antigens has provided important insights into the immune response to cancer and remains a key factor in the development of antitumor immunotherapies. Antigens that are unique to a tumor represent a molecular target that the immune system

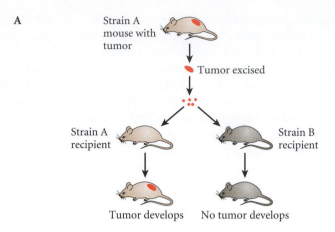

Figure 24.6 Use of inbred mouse strains to demonstrate antigen-specific immune protection against transplanted tumors. (**A**) A tumor transplanted from one mouse to another will usually grow in the recipient mouse if the donor and recipient mice are of the same strain, since the tumor will appear as self tissue to the immune system of the recipient. However, the transplanted tumor will always be rejected by the immune system of the recipient mouse if the donor and recipient are of different strains. (**B**) Chemically induced tumors sometimes express antigens that are the result of mutagenesis and are unique to each tumor (TSAs). Killing tumor X from mouse 1 allows it to be used as a vaccine. If tumor X expresses a TSA, then a mouse vaccinated against tumor X will subsequently be protected against challenge with live cells from tumor X. This protection is antigen specific, since the vaccinated mouse is not protected from challenge with live cells from tumor Y.

can use to recognize and specifically destroy a tumor. These antigens are classified according to their pattern of expression on tumor cells and on normal, nontransformed cells.

TSAs

TSAs are the ideal antigenic targets for an immune-based cancer therapy. An immune response against such an antigen holds the promise of attacking the tumor while sparing normal, healthy cells. TSAs are formed anytime a protein produced by the tumor cells is qualitatively altered so that the protein has a sequence unique to the tumor. One example of this would be a tumor cell protein produced from a gene harboring one or more point mutations. Another example would be viral proteins in a virally induced tumor. Since cancer is characterized by genomic instability, it is not unlikely that a tumor cell will eventually begin to produce a gene product that is unlike any expressed by

normal host cells. From the standpoint of antitumor immunotherapy, TSAs are attractive because of their uniqueness. Even other cells that bear mutations in the same protein as the tumor are extremely unlikely to bear the *exact same* mutations. This benefit, however, is also a liability. Since TSAs are unique to each newly arising tumor, it cannot be assumed that any one tumor expresses a therapeutically useful TSA, and so the presence of TSAs must be determined on a case-by-case basis.

An interesting type of TSA expressed by T-cell and B-cell cancers is represented by the idiotype antigenic determinants on the T-cell receptor or the membrane immunoglobulin expressed by the tumor cells. Leukemias and lymphomas are typical manifestations of lymphoid cell cancers. It has been possible to remove the tumor cells and make anti-idiotypic antibodies and CTLs against tumor-specific idiotopes and use these to treat the cancer.

However, as there are no other known cell types that produce any type of surface epitope analogous to idiotopes, it is likely that targeting of these types of TSAs will be limited to lymphoid cancers.

TAAs

In many cases, a tumor will possess no unique antigens that the host's lymphocytes can recognize or will possess such antigens but fail to express them at a high enough level for antigen-specific recognition to occur. In such cases, tumors may be recognized by the immune system on the basis of quantitative changes in their protein expression profiles. These antigens are not tumor specific but are termed *tumor-associated antigens* (TAAs) (Table 24.4). *Oncofetal antigens* are one prime example of a TAA. These antigens are encoded by genes expressed during embryogenesis and fetal development but are transcriptionally silent in the adult. These genes encode proteins that likely play a role in the rapid growth of embryonic cells and have been reactivated to perform the same function in the rapidly growing tumor. The most prominent group of oncofetal antigens are known as the cancer-testis antigens because in addition to being expressed by cancer cells, they are also expressed in the testis in normal males. Examples include the MAGE superfamily (made up of family members designated MAGE-A, MAGE-B, MAGE-C, MAGE-D, and necdin) whose members were first described in melanoma but later shown to be expressed by numerous cancers, including lung, head and neck, and bladder tumors. There are over 50 cancer-testis antigens known, with the T-cell epitopes for many of them identified.

Another class of TAAs are *tissue-specific differentiation antigens*, proteins that are normally expressed in the cells from which the cancer arises and that continue to be expressed following neoplastic transformation. Thus these antigens identify the tissue of origin of the tumor. The best-characterized examples of these are represented by the melanoma differentiation antigens gp100, Melan-A/MART-1, and tyrosinase. These genes encode proteins that function within the melanin biosynthetic pathway of skin cells and are also expressed by many pigmented melanoma tumors. Other examples of tissue-specific differentiation antigens include prostate-specific antigen (PSA) expressed by normal and cancerous prostate tissues as well as the carcinoembryonic antigen (CEA), which can be overexpressed in colon carcinomas. Her-2/Neu and MUC-1, both of which are expressed on breast carcinomas and other epithelial tumors, are also representatives of the tissue-specific differentiation antigens.

Mature, functional lymphocytes that recognize TAAs exist in the host, despite the fact that the TAAs are self proteins that are encoded by normal genes. The existence of these self-reactive lymphocytes seems to contradict the notion of self-tolerance. The reason that these TAA-specific lymphocytes exist in the host is most likely due to the anatomic constraints of central tolerance. As B cells and T cells mature in the bone marrow and thymus, respectively, lymphocytes that are able to bind and recognize self antigens are induced to undergo apoptosis. For this to happen, the self antigen must be expressed at the site where negative selection is occurring. However, many self proteins are not expressed in the bone marrow or thymus. Central deletion is therefore an incomplete process, and self-reactive lymphocytes that recognize antigens not expressed in the bone marrow or thymus are frequently not responsive to self antigens because they are maintained in a state of anergy. It is unclear why these autoreactive cells are maintained in an inactive state. It is possible that immune responses to TAAs are the reason: anergic lymphocytes may be incapable of responding to the levels of self antigen normally expressed by healthy cells, but responsive to the increased expression of these antigens in tumor cells. Research has demonstrated that under certain conditions anergy may be broken, resulting in reactivation of the self-reactive lymphocytes.

Methods for the Identification of Tumor Antigens

Although the existence of tumor antigens had been demonstrated in experiments showing it was possible to vaccinate against tumors, it took the tools of modern immunology and molecular biology to allow their identification at the molecular level (Table 24.5). Through techniques developed for identifying TSAs in animal models, a variety of human cancers have been shown to express antigens that may serve as useful targets for immunotherapy. The majority of these have been identified through their recognition by T cells raised through in vitro restimulation of a patient's peripheral lymphocytes with tumor cells. Most tumor antigens recognized by T cells have been identified using either a genetic or a biochemical approach. Both methods begin with a T-cell population that

Table 24.4 Comparison of TSAs and TAAs

Feature	TSAs	TAAs
Expressed by normal cells	No	Yes
Self or nonself protein	Nonself or altered-self	Self
Result of mutation	Usually	No
Role of tumor viruses in antigen production	TSA itself can be of viral origin	Viral promoter can enhance expression of host gene

Table 24.5 Examples of TSAs

Source of TSA	Example(s)	Notes
TSAs arising from mutation		
Point-mutated genes	Any gene	TSA is unique to each tumor
Fusion proteins	BCR-Abl oncogene, IgH–c-*myc* fusion	Frequently the result of chromosomal translocation; can be used as a marker for diagnosis
TSAs arising from viruses		
Viral proteins	Nucleocapsid, viral analog of host signaling molecule	Can be useful as a diagnostic marker; also attractive targets for immunotherapy if viral infection correlates well with transformation
Fusion of viral gene with host gene	c-*src*–provirus fusion	Can be useful as a diagnostic marker; also attractive targets for immunotherapy if viral infection correlates well with transformation

recognizes a specific tumor. In the genetic approach (Fig. 24.7), a cDNA library is prepared from the tumor and then small pools of these cDNAs are transfected into a target cell expressing the relevant MHC molecule. These transfected cells are then screened for their ability to stimulate tumor-specific T cells. Once a positive pool is iden-

tified, it is further subdivided until single cDNAs able to stimulate the tumor-reactive T cells can be identified and isolated. This expression cloning technique has been used primarily to identify cDNAs encoding antigens recognized by MHC class I-restricted CD8$^+$ T lymphocytes. A variation of this approach also has been used to clone

Figure 24.7 Genetic approach to identifying TSAs. Tumor cells are isolated from a tumor-bearing mouse and are used to prepare a tumor cell cDNA library. This library is then cloned into a cell line. Any cell that receives cDNA encoding a TSA (red squiggle) will express that TSA. TSA-expressing cells can be identified as being susceptible to killing by CTLs isolated from a vaccinated mouse that is resistant to tumor growth.

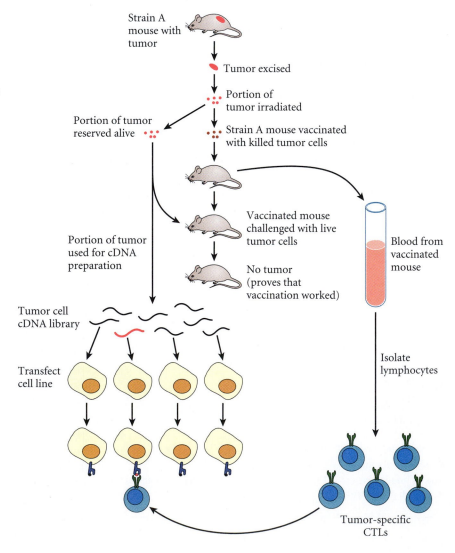

antigens recognized by CD4$^+$ T lymphocytes. In this method, tumor-derived cDNAs are expressed in bacteria that are then fed to macrophages. Following processing and MHC class II-restricted presentation of the encoded antigens, the macrophages are assayed for their ability to stimulate tumor-specific CD4$^+$ T cells until single cDNAs encoding the antigen can be isolated.

The biochemical approach to identifying tumor antigens relies on sequencing of peptides eluted from MHC molecules on the surface of tumor cells. This involves isolating MHC molecules from tumor cells and treating the cells with acid to release the bound peptides. The peptides are fractionated by high-pressure liquid chromatography and then tested for their ability to be recognized by tumor-reactive T cells. Peptide fractions found to stimulate the T cells are characterized by mass spectroscopy and direct sequencing. Once a full or partial amino acid sequence is obtained, it can be used to search DNA and protein databases to determine whether a match can be found with a known protein.

Direct analysis of peptides bound to MHC molecules has revealed motifs that reflect the binding preferences of different MHC molecules. These binding motifs, characterized by the presence of anchor residues at specific positions within 8 to 10 residue peptides, can be used to search for candidate peptides within the sequences of known oncogenes or tumor-associated proteins. This method is known as "reverse immunology" and has been used to deduce MHC-binding peptides from a variety of target antigens known to be associated with the transformed phenotype, such as specific oncogenes or differentiation antigens.

The latest approach to the identification of tumor antigens involves the serological analysis of cDNA expression libraries. This method, called SEREX (an acronym for serological analysis of autologous tumor antigens by recombinant cDNA expression and cloning), uses a patient's antibodies to probe cDNA expression libraries derived from the patient's own tumor (Fig. 24.8) and may identify antigens that have induced not only an antibody response but also the T-cell response needed to provide help to the B cell. It is hoped that such antigens that induce a coordinated response from T and B cells will prove to be useful in clinical immunotherapy.

Immune Cell Types Important in Antitumor Immunity

CTLs

Many studies have demonstrated that tumors expressing unique antigens are capable of eliciting tumor-specific CTLs that can eradicate the tumor by their inherent effector functions inducing cell lysis by CD95-CD95L interac-

tions and through release of vesicles containing proteases, perforin, granzymes, etc. Induction of memory T cells by tumors recognizing these tumor antigens may result in eradication of subsequent occurrences of the same tumor (Fig. 24.6B). These CTLs generally recognize peptides derived from the TSA bound to MHC class I proteins on the tumor cells' plasma membranes. Although tumor-specific CTLs are an efficient way of destroying tumors in a way that spares surrounding normal tissue, such CTLs do not always arise during the immune response to a tumor.

Several factors can impede the development of CTL-mediated immunity. Most tumors become genetically unstable at some point in their progression, and this instability results in rapid, random changes in the physiology of tumor cells. As tumor-specific CTLs become activated in the early stages of an immune response, those tumor cells that possess a unique antigen that CTLs can target, express high levels of MHC class I to present this antigen, and possess a functional apoptotic mechanism will be quickly killed by the newly activated CTLs. Unfortunately, this response can select for tumor-cell variants that lack one or more of these essential features, leading to their destruction. Thus, CTL-mediated immunity is usually marked by an early period of tumor remission, followed by relapses as CTL-resistant tumor variants expand. Specific changes commonly observed among tumor *escape variants* include loss of expression of the tumor-specific antigen, reduction or loss of MHC class I expression, loss of expression of the CD95 protein that binds the CTL protein CD95L to initiate apoptosis of the tumor cell, and overexpression of antiapoptotic proteins such Bcl-2 (Fig. 24.9). These escape mechanisms may also affect the effectiveness of antitumor vaccines.

Natural Killer Cells

Natural killer (NK) cells are granular, cytotoxic lymphoid cells that recognize their target cells in a manner that is neither antigen specific nor MHC restricted. NK cells were first identified as a type of lymphocyte able to kill heterologous tumor cells in the absence of any evidence that the individual providing the NK cell had ever had a tumor. NK-cell-mediated cytotoxicity is unaffected by tumor cell loss of MHC class I expression or by the lack of a TSA. To the contrary, one mechanism by which NK cells recognize target cells is by lack of expression of MHC class I by the target (see Fig. 1.19). It is thus possible that antitumor immunity is one of the primary functions of this leukocyte lineage. NK cells also express a low-affinity immunoglobulin G (IgG) receptor that allows them to kill target cells that are bound by antibody (antibody-dependent cell-mediated cytotoxicity [ADCC]). As NK-cell function is generally unchanged as a result of an immune

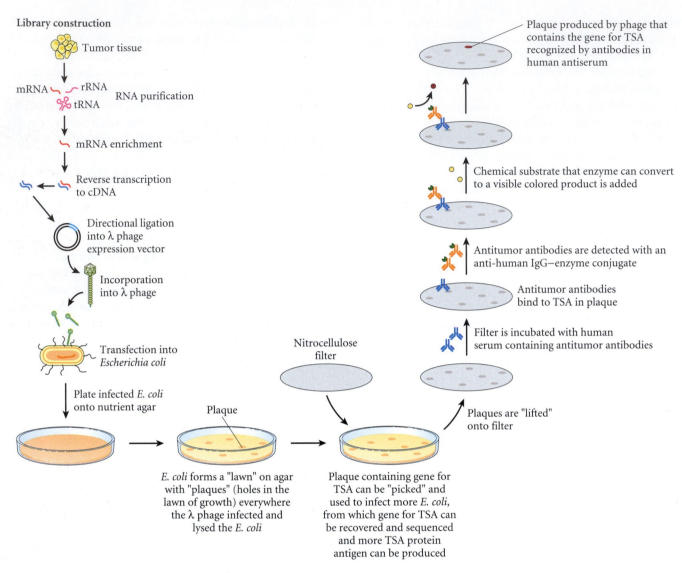

Figure 24.8 Method for SEREX detection of tumor antigens. A cDNA library is prepared from a human tumor and is used to transfect bacteria. These bacteria are then lysed on a filter, and the filter is then probed with the serum of the same patient from which the tumor was taken. A bacterial clone that is positively detected by the patient's serum contains tumor cDNA encoding a TSA. Adapted from O. Tureci et al., *Mol. Med. Today* **3**:342–349, 1999.

response, it may represent a major component of innate immunity targeting tumor cells that arise throughout life but never develop into a clinically detected state because the tumor cells are destroyed before they progress to become pathologic.

Macrophages

Macrophages also possess cytotoxic function mediated by lytic enzymes and oxidative mediators such as superoxide and nitric oxide. In addition, macrophages are capable of synthesizing and secreting the cytokine tumor necrosis factor alpha (TNF-α), which initiates the apoptotic pathway independently of the CD95-CD95L path-

way. Macrophages probably recognize tumor targets via their low-affinity IgG receptor, which would bind to antitumor antibodies bound to the tumor cell surface. Macrophages are also capable of ingesting antigens from killed tumor cells and presenting them to CD4[+] T cells. Therefore, macrophages can function as both initiators and effectors of the antitumor immune response.

Tumor Surveillance Theory

First proposed by Paul Ehrlich at the turn of the 20th century, the *tumor surveillance theory* was intended to explain the role of the immune system in preventing cancer. The theory states that mammalian cells undergo transformation to cancerous or precancerous states very frequently, but that the immune system successfully recognizes and destroys these transformed cells in most cases. Supporters of this theory hold that tumor initiation events are extremely common due to the harsh physical conditions and abundance of mutagenic substances in our environment. Even many nonmutagenic substances, in fact, are converted to mutagenic intermediates during their catabolism following ingestion or absorption into a mammalian organism. The host is continuously bombarded with mutagenic insults, whereas tumors are only clinically observed in the relatively rare cases where a tumor escapes recognition and killing by the immune system.

On the basis of tumor surveillance theory, one would predict that immune suppression or immunodeficiency would lead to an increased incidence of cancer. Although

Figure 24.9 Emergence of tumor variants that escape T-cell-mediated cytotoxicity. Tumor cells can evade recognition or killing if they reduce their expression of TSAs (**A**), reduce their expression of MHC class I (**B**), or stop expressing CD95L that initiates the apoptosis pathway upon CTL recognition (**C**). Last, tumor cells can escape cytotoxicity by overexpression of the antiapoptotic protein Bcl-2 (**D**).

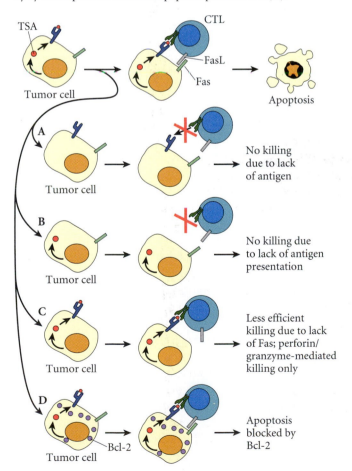

true in some cases, mostly involving leukemias, lymphomas, and other tumors of lymphoid or myeloid origin, such increases in tumor occurrence are not always observed, casting doubt on the validity of this theory. Because of the known importance of cytotoxic immune responses against tumor cells, genetic defects that negatively affect these responses have been studied as systems for testing the tumor surveillance theory. Chediak-Higashi syndrome (CHS) is a congenital defect in the gene encoding the protein LYST required for degranulation of macrophages, NK cells, neutrophils, and mast cells. In affected individuals, these cell types develop to maturity, although their cytoplasmic granules are enlarged. The cells are capable of recognizing target cells, but cytotoxic function is inhibited by an inability to mobilize their granules. Thus, bacteria are phagocytosed by macrophages but are not killed after phagocytosis, and cytotoxic function that requires degranulation does not occur. Individuals with CHS are at an increased risk for some types of cancer, as predicted by the tumor surveillance theory. However, patients with CHS do not have an increased risk of all types of cancer. Overall, there is probably some truth to the tumor surveillance theory, but the importance of tumor surveillance in host defense probably varies from case to case, depending on the type of tumor and other susceptibility factors possessed by the individual in question.

Tumor Immunotherapy

Over the past several decades, numerous strategies have been attempted to elicit protective antitumor immunity. These strategies include both active and passive immunization techniques. In some strategies, steps are taken to assist the host's normal immune response and to maximize its effectiveness. In other cases, highly specific antitumor agents are designed in the laboratory and introduced to the host to determine their effect on tumor growth. Although many of these strategies have yielded promising results, protection provided by the treatments is incomplete or functions well against some types of tumor, but not others. This inability to design a treatment that is effective against all types of tumor is probably related to the diverse cell types from which tumors are derived and to the extreme heterogeneity of cells that comprise each tumor (arising from the genetic instability that is an inherent trait of most tumor cells).

TILs and LAKs

Histological examination of the solid tumors reveals that they contain numerous leukocytes infiltrating the cell mass, including macrophages and lymphocytes. The lymphocytes among these cells are termed *tumor-infiltrating lymphocytes* (TILs) and comprise NK cells and tumor-specific CTLs that are activated and are presumably in the process of mounting an antitumor response. Numerous studies were carried out in the 1980s to examine the potency of these cells in killing tumor cells and the feasibility of applying these cells to antitumor therapies. Clinical trials have been performed where TILs were isolated from solid tumors, expanded in culture in the presence of exogenous growth factors, and then reintroduced into the patient. In some cases, transfusion of expanded TIL populations did succeed in reducing tumor burden. However, the general applicability of this therapy has not yet been established.

Cytotoxic antitumor leukocytes similar to TILs can also be derived in the laboratory by treating heterogeneous populations of leukocytes with interleukin-2 (IL-2) in culture. The IL-2 causes activation and proliferation of a subset of cells that are mostly NK cells, with smaller amounts of CTLs. Since they mostly comprise NK cells, these *lymphokine-activated killer* (LAK) cells kill their tumor-cell targets in a predominantly antigen-nonspecific manner.

Cytokine Therapy

CTLs, NK cells, and macrophages require certain combinations of cytokines for activation and acquisition of cytotoxic function. In the normal immune response, these cytokines are produced locally by helper T cells, antigen-presenting cells, and epithelial cells. Immune responses can be enhanced through the addition of exogenous cytokines introduced by a variety of methods. Purified recombinant cytokines can be injected intravenously into a patient. Alternatively, leukocytes can be isolated from a cancer patient and treated with cytokines in vitro, and the activated cells reintroduced into the patient. The first of these strategies has the advantage that the exogenous cytokines can affect all leukocytes in the patient, even those that have infiltrated a solid tumor, while in vitro cytokine treatment only helps activate circulating leukocytes that can be easily obtained via venipuncture. Despite this advantage, intravenous cytokine therapy has fallen out of favor due to the risk of *vascular leak syndrome*, which is associated with this practice. When high concentrations of cytokines are administered systemically, changes in vascular permeability that occur at very confined locations during normal immune responses can occur widely throughout the entire body, resulting in seepage of blood plasma from the vasculature into the interstitial tissues. The resulting edema and reduction in blood pressure can be fatal. Combination treatment regimens, where leukocytes are treated with high concentrations of cytokines in vitro followed by transfusion into a patient in combination with intravenous cytokines, have allowed lower concentrations of cytokines to be administered intravenously, partially alleviating the risk of vascular leak syndrome.

Several cytokines have been tested in this type of strategy, each for its ability to augment different aspects of the antitumor immune response. IL-2 is a potent paracrine T-cell growth factor, and its use can augment the antitumor T-cell response. In addition, IL-2 appears to improve the function of LAK cells. It has been used in patients with melanoma or renal cell carcinoma and induced an antitumor response in approximately 20% of patients and a complete response in 3 to 5% of patients. IL-12 skews T-cell responses toward the cell-mediated, T helper type 1 (TH1) pathway. IL-12 also has been used as therapy both systemically and locally with encouraging results; however, severe toxicities have limited its use and need to be addressed before extensive human clinical trials. Type I interferons (IFN-α and IFN-β) enhance expression of MHC class I on tumor cells, while type II interferon (IFN-γ) enhances expression of MHC class II on macrophages. IFN therapy has been used for treatment of melanoma, renal cell carcinoma, acquired immunodeficiency syndrome-related Kaposi's sarcoma, follicular lymphoma, hairy cell leukemia, and chronic myelogenous leukemia. Unfortunately, IFN therapy is associated with significant toxicity, including constitutional, neuropsychiatric, hematologic, and hepatic effects. As noted, the significant level of systemic toxicities upon cytokine treatment and the limited therapeutic window of dosing (the difference in effective levels versus toxic levels) being relatively small have limited the use of cytokines as adjuvant therapy for many of these tumors. Finally, cytokines have been used as vaccine adjuvants in antitumor vaccines. Both IL-2 and IL-12 have been promising in this respect in inducing improved TH1-type immune responses to various tumor antigens. In addition, dendritic cells pulsed with tumor antigens for use as cell-based vaccines have been treated with granulocyte-macrophage colony-stimulating factor, which can affect maturation and activation of dendritic cells (DCs).

Nonspecific Immune Stimulation and Adjuvants

In the 1890s, the physician William Coley observed tumor regression in a patient who developed a systemic bacterial infection (see http://www.cancerguide.org/coley.html for more information). He reasoned that the immune response initiated against the bacterial pathogen had somehow targeted the tumor. He began treating cancer patients with bacterial extracts (which were called *Coley's toxins*) in hopes of activating the immune system to attack their tumors. Although he reported some positive responses, they were sporadic, and this approach was largely discontinued in clinical practice in the 1920s although investigative uses of this preparation continue today in some parts of the world. This practice is not entirely without merit, however. Indeed, extracts from the bacterium bacillus Calmette-Guérin (BCG), a vaccine strain of *Mycobacterium bovis*, are presently used to treat a premalignant form of bladder cancer. In an early stage of disease, precancerous polyps begin forming that require surgical excision before they become metastatic. The polyps continually reemerge, necessitating repeated surgical procedures. In many patients, formation of these polyps ceases after several administrations of BCG extract into the bladder. Although the local immune response to these bacterial extracts is intense and can be painful, remission from the polyps is usually permanent, suggesting the formation of protective immunological memory against the precancerous epithelium.

Antitumor Vaccines

In cases where TAAs or TSAs can be identified, it may be feasible to create an antitumor vaccine. Evidence from studies utilizing immune adjuvant therapy TAA-specific monoclonal antibodies (MAbs) demonstrates that induction of an antitumor immune response could be potentially beneficial and may aid in treatment for certain cancers, especially those in which TAA have been identified. Antitumor vaccines range in complexity from whole, killed tumor cells to antigens identified and cloned by molecular methods. Since experimental evidence supports a role for both CTLs and antibodies in antitumor immunity, vaccine strategies are usually designed with the intention of generating a broad-based immune response eliciting many effector mechanisms.

There are a number of different approaches for developing antitumor vaccines. First and foremost is the identification of specific TAA that has minimal cross-reactivity with self antigens to decrease the possibility of inducing potential autoimmune reactions upon vaccination. In addition, the antigen itself needs to be immunogenic to be able to induce potentially protective antitumor antibodies that can elicit ADCC and to induce antitumor-specific CTL responses. If the TAA is too close in structure to a self antigen, it will be less immunogenic.

These difficulties are circumvented if the vaccine is to a known pathogen that can cause malignant transformation of cells. Over the past decades it has become increasingly apparent that a variety of microbial pathogens in addition to classic oncogenic viruses can cause cancer. For example, human papillomavirus is the main cause of cervical carcinoma, and a number of vaccine trials targeting human papillomavirus are currently ongoing that could potentially protect women from this disease. In addition, hepatitis B infection is a major cause of liver cancer, and the currently available hepatitis B vaccine can decrease the incidence of hepatic carcinomas. Other potential vaccines that are in development that protect against infectious causes of cancers include vaccines against *Helicobacter pylori* (gastric carcinoma), hepatitis C virus (hepatic carcinoma), human T-lymphotropic virus type 1 (adult T-cell leukemia), and Epstein-Barr virus (Burkitt's lymphoma and nasopharyngeal carcinoma).

The first generation of tumor-specific vaccines was relatively crude and consisted of whole cancer cells that were either irradiated or lysed. These vaccines were generally unsuccessful, but some evidence for optimism was seen as small but significant differences in recurrence rates were observed in trials targeting melanoma and renal and colorectal carcinomas. The next generation of vaccines relied on targeting defined TAAs that are designated by an alphabet soup nomenclature. Examples include the use of protein-based TAAs such as Her2/Neu expressed on breast carcinoma tissues and MAGE-1 and -3 expressed in melanoma cells. Carbohydrate-based antimelanoma vaccines are currently in development, as melanoma cells overexpress some specific gangliosides, namely GD3, GM2, and GD2, and early results using conjugate vaccines consisting of these gangliosides covalently linked to keyhole limpet hemocyanin, diphtheria toxin, or neisserial major outer membrane protein have been encouraging. Two somewhat related approaches currently being investigated are the use of viral vectors or naked DNA containing the gene for specific protein-based TAAs to induce immunity to the TAA. Such an approach may increase MHC class I presentation of the TAA. Examples of viral vectors include the use of adenovirus, vaccinia virus, or canarypox or fowlpox viruses expressing TAAs such as MART-1 and gp100 found on metastatic melanoma cells, CEA and p53 found on colorectal carcinoma cells, and PSA for prostate cancer. Recombinant TAAs have also been tested in humans, including MUC-1, a lipopeptide associated with breast tumor cells, KSA (colorectal carcinoma), and CEA. One promising set of potential antitumor vaccines is the use of DCs pulsed with TAAs or with cells from the specific tumor from each patient as the "vaccine delivery system." This method exploits the extremely potent ability of DCs to present antigen and elicit both humoral and CTL responses.

Upon successful vaccination or elicitation of an immune response, it is possible that tumor escape variants emerge that are resistant to the immune effectors (Fig. 24.9). This can arise due to alteration or loss of expression of the protective TAAs; overexpression of the CD95L to induce apoptosis of tumor-specific CTLs; loss of expression of the CD95 on the tumor cell, thereby decreasing the ability of tumor-specific CTLs to induce apoptosis; reduction or loss of MHC class I expression; and overexpression of antiapoptotic proteins such Bcl-2. Obviously, with immune pressure being exerted to eliminate the rapidly growing cancer cells, those that undergo a genetic variation due to mutation or altered expression of a gene involved in making the tumor susceptible to immunologic killing are going to survive and outgrow the more susceptible cells.

Genetic Modification of Tumor Cells To Improve Antitumor Immune Responses

T-cell activation is a multistep process requiring several positive signals in the form of antigen recognition, costimulatory signals, and stimulatory/growth-promoting cytokines. It is likely that this complex, multistep process evolved as a regulatory mechanism ensuring that T cells do not become activated inappropriately. The inability of most host cells to directly activate T cells, while important for preventing autoimmune reactions, works against the host when combating tumor cells that closely resemble the normal cells of the host. Most tumor cells do not produce the costimulatory signal or cytokines needed to activate T cells. One strategy in the development of antitumor vaccines has, therefore, been to genetically modify tumor cells to be capable of producing costimulatory signals and/or cytokines (Fig. 24.10). This is usually carried out by growing the tumor cells in the laboratory, then transfecting them with a gene encoding a costimulatory molecule such as IL-2 or CD80, then reinfusing the cells into the patients. This should make the TSAs or TAAs more immunogenic. Another means to enhance tumor antigen immunogenicity is to add a gene to the tumor cells that helps activate antigen-presenting cells, enhancing their ability to stimulate tumor-specific immune responses. Although such approaches have been successful in animals, their use in humans presents much greater complication, not the least of which is having to infuse cancer patients with their own tumor cells, which could exacerbate the tumor burden and allow for additional metastases to occur.

MAbs

MAbs first became available with the advent of hybridoma technology in 1975. MAbs recognize one specific epitope on an antigen, which on protein antigens usually

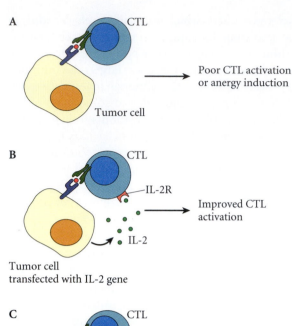

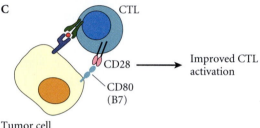

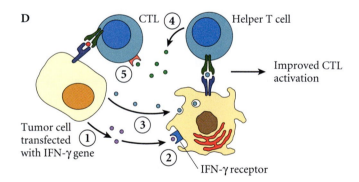

Figure 24.10 Tumor cells can be genetically engineered to make them more effective at CTL activation. (**A**) The original tumor cell may express a TSA, but with low or no expression of costimulatory activity; CTLs that recognize the tumor cell are not efficiently activated and may even be anergized. (**B and C**) If the tumor cell is transfected with the gene for IL-2 (**B**) or B7 (**C**), then the engineered tumor cell can effectively activate tumor-specific CTLs. (**D**.) Alternatively, the tumor cell can be engineered to express cytokines that recruit and activate professional antigen-presenting cells, for example, IFN-γ (**1**). The IFN-γ binds to a receptor on a macrophage (**2**), activating the macrophage and making it more effective at capturing and presenting (**3**) tumor antigens to helper T cells. The activated helper T cells secrete other cytokines such as IL-2 (**4**) that then help stimulate tumor-specific CTLs (**5**).

has only one of these epitopes per molecule. This technology made it possible to isolate antibodies that were specific for a single antigenic epitope, as opposed to polyclonal antibodies obtained from immune serum that recognize multiple epitopes. With this higher degree of specificity and lower probability of undesirable cross-reactivity, MAbs soon drew the attention of cancer researchers for their promise of being able to target tumor cells specifically. MAbs that bind to the surface of tumor cells are capable of activating ADCC reactions mediated by macrophages or NK cells and are also capable of activating the classical pathway of complement to lyse the tumor cells. Although there have been numerous instances of success with these reagents, in most cases MAbs achieve only temporary remission of the tumor.

The low level of effectiveness of most MAb therapeutics is due to loss of antigen on tumor surface. This loss can occur over the long term by mutation of the tumor cells followed by growth selection in favor of those tumors that lost antigen expression (Fig. 24.11), but it can occur in the short term by endocytosis of antigen-antibody complexes on the tumor cell surface. One way that researchers have attempted to get around this obstacle is to create MAbs that are specific for antigens that the tumor cell requires for its aberrant growth characteristics. One such TSA is the Her-2/Neu protein, a modified form of the epidermal growth factor receptor that is expressed by many carcinomas, especially metastatic breast carcinoma. The amplified growth-promoting signals transmitted by the modified gene product are thought to be required for one of the earliest stages of tumorigenesis. Epidermal growth factor receptor signaling by the modified oncogene is increased by at least two mechanisms: gene amplification and truncation of the receptor's intracellular tail to remove an inhibitory domain. A MAb specific for Her-2/Neu (Herceptin or trastuzumab) has been used successfully for the treatment of breast cancer in combination with other standard therapies. Exploration of Her-2/Neu synthesis and function has led to the discovery of yet a third mechanism whereby a tumor cell many evade the action of antitumor antibodies: synthesis of a splice variant of Her-2/Neu that comprises only the extracellular domain and is secreted rather than being membrane bound. This soluble Her-2/Neu is thought to favor tumor cell survival by competing with membrane-bound Her-2/Neu for binding by antibodies.

Heteroconjugate MAbs

Heteroconjugate MAbs are antibody reagents designed to have a dual antigenic specificity. One specificity of the heteroconjugate is against a tumor cell antigen, while the sec-

Tumor cells expressing various amounts of TSA

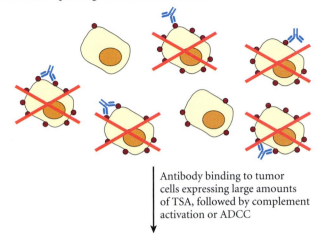

Antibody binding to tumor cells expressing large amounts of TSA, followed by complement activation or ADCC

Tumor cells expressing small and medium amounts of TSA
Replication of surviving tumor cells

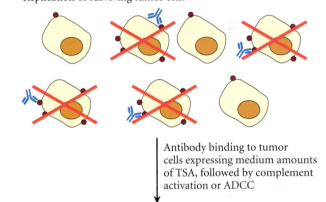

Antibody binding to tumor cells expressing medium amounts of TSA, followed by complement activation or ADCC

Tumor cells expressing small amounts of TSA
Replication of surviving tumor cells

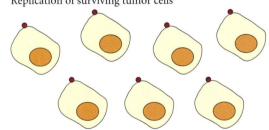

Figure 24.11 Loss of TSAs during an immune response is attributable to a stochastic variability of TSA expression and selection against those tumor cells that express higher amounts of the TSA.

ond specificity is against a leukocyte antigen. The goal is to physically cross-link an effector leukocyte such as a CTL to the tumor cell to facilitate target-cell recognition and killing. Heteroconjugates are generated by two different methods. In the first method (Fig. 24.12C), hybridomas producing each MAb are fused to each other. The resulting *quadroma* cell line produces heavy chains and light chains for both MAbs and assembles them into antibodies con-

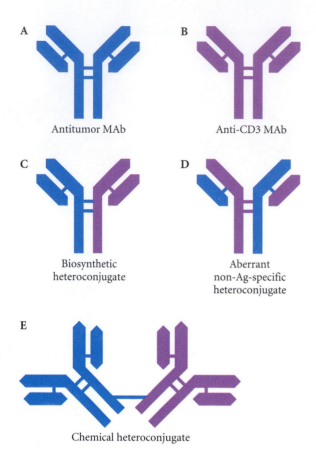

A

Antitumor MAb

B

Anti-CD3 MAb

C

Biosynthetic
heteroconjugate

D

Aberrant
non-Ag-specific
heteroconjugate

E

Chemical heteroconjugate

Figure 24.12 Production of bispecific heteroconjugate antibodies as antitumor reagents. If MAbs specific for a tumor (**A**) and for the CTL antigen CD3 (**B**) are synthesized in the same cell, the resulting heteroconjugate (**C**) is specific for both cell types, and can help CTLs attach to tumor cell targets. One drawback of this approach is that some of the antibodies are assembled into hybrid antibodies (**D**) that recognize neither antigen. One solution to this problem is to purify both MAbs and then chemically conjugate them (**E**).

taining one variable region against the tumor antigen, and a second variable region against the leukocyte antigen. This strategy is not favored because the quadroma is genetically unstable and has a tendency to lose expression of one or the other antibody. Also, the quadroma assembles some of the antibody chains into hybrid antibodies, which recognize neither antigen (Fig. 24.12D). A second method of making bispecific antibodies is to individually purify the two different MAbs and then chemically couple them to each other after purification (Fig. 24.12E).

Bispecific heteroconjugate antibodies have several advantages over "monospecific" antitumor antibodies. First, bispecific antibodies can serve to tether an effector leukocyte to a tumor cell, making leukocyte activation more likely and increasing the efficiency of other nonspecific cytotoxic functions. Second, if the leukocyte-specific portion of the heteroconjugate binds to an activation receptor on the leukocyte surface (such as the CD3 complex on T cells),

then binding of the heteroconjugate to the leukocyte can trigger leukocyte activation while tethering the leukocyte to a tumor cell target. Heteroconjugate antibodies tested to date have been directed against both protein (Her-2/Neu) and carbohydrate (Lewis^{x}) tumor antigens and against leukocyte antigens such as CD3 (on T cells) and FcγRII (on NK cells and macrophages). These trials have verified that heteroconjugates are capable of activating leukocytes and directing them to tumor cell targets.

Immunotoxins

Originally heralded as the long sought *magic bullet* to end the scourge of cancer, immunotoxin derivatives of MAbs were an intense focus of cancer research in the early 1990s. Immunotoxins are translational fusions of MAbs and bacterial exotoxins. The toxins commonly used in this strategy act by modifying and inactivating their target cell's protein synthesis machinery, and include ricin toxin, diphtheria toxin, and shiga toxin. The normal mechanism of action of these toxins includes a binding or internalization event mediated by the toxin's B subunit, followed by inhibition of protein synthesis mediated by the toxin's A subunit (Fig. 24.13A and B). The B subunit has a binding specificity that determines what type of cell is targeted by the toxin. A/B toxins include diphtheria toxin, cholera toxin, and pertussis toxin. In an immunotoxin, the DNA encoding the B subunit is typically removed from the toxin gene and replaced with the gene encoding an antibody (Fig. 24.13C). The antibody gene used for the immunotoxin is specific for a tumor cell antigen, ensuring that the immunotoxin will preferentially target tumor cells. Immunotoxins have met with limited success in cases where a tumor-specific antigen can be identified. However, this approach has recently been used successfully in treatment of B-cell lymphomas that overexpress CD20. Anti-CD20 MAbs linked to the A subunit (enzymatic subunit) of diphtheria toxin have been shown to decrease tumor size and increase survival in a small set of patients.

Summary

Cancer cells are altered cells of the host that acquire the ability to divide and expand in a dysregulated fashion. Their overall similarity to the host's normal healthy cells makes them difficult targets for the acquired immune response, and their rapid proliferation, paired with their genetic instability, greatly increases the likelihood that resistant escape variants of the tumor will emerge that are resistant to any therapy, whether it be a drug or an immune effector cell. Several components of the immune system have the ability to target and destroy tumor cells. These in-

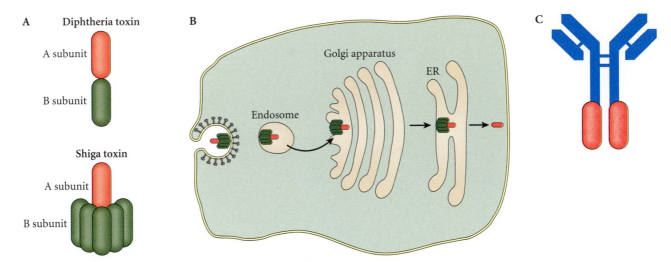

Figure 24.13 Immunotoxins are derived from MAbs and bacterial toxins. **(A)** Diagram of two prototypical two-subunit toxins, diphtheria toxin and Shiga toxin. Both have active (A) subunits that contain their enzymatic activity as well as binding (B) subunits that allow the toxin to specifically associate with, and enter, its target cell. **(B)** Mode of action of Shiga toxin. Shiga toxin enters cells by recruiting clathrin on the membrane of its target cell to form coated pits. The toxin is then trafficked through the Golgi apparatus and endoplasmic reticulum (ER). During this transport, the toxin is cleaved by the enzyme furin to liberate the A subunit. The A subunit translocates to the cytoplasm where it cleaves the 5'-terminal adenine from the 28S rRNA, preventing its assembly with the 60S ribosomal subunit. **(C)** In an immunotoxin, the B subunit of the bacterial toxin is removed and replaced with a monoclonal antibody recognizing a tumor antigen. In the example shown, the A subunit of Shiga toxin is fused to the heavy chain of an antitumor antibody.

clude antibodies, which can target tumor cells for complement-mediated damage or ADCC reactions; CTLs, which can directly kill tumor cells in an antigen-specific fashion; and NK cells, which can kill tumor cells that reduce their expression of MHC class I to evade CTL-mediated killing. Many immunotherapeutic strategies have been tested, ranging from nonspecific stimulation of the host's immune response to highly engineered multicomponent vaccines. In many cases, the development of tumor-specific vaccines is hindered by the lack of a tumor-specific antigen that would allow CTLs, TH cells, and B cells to attack the tumor while sparing normal healthy cells of the host. Nevertheless, several strategies have been developed that are effective in treating some forms of cancer. It is hoped that further research into the mechanisms of antitumor immunity will lead to additional treatment strategies, perhaps effective at killing a broader range of tumor types.

Suggested Readings

Foss, F. M. 2002. Immunologic mechanisms of antitumor activity. *Semin. Oncol.* **29**(3 Suppl. 7):5–11.

Hanahan, D., and R. A. Weinberg. 2000. The hallmarks of cancer. *Cell* **100**:57–70.

Helder, M.N., G. B. Wisman, and G. J. van der Zee. 2002. Telomerase and telomeres: from basic biology to cancer treatment. *Cancer Investig.* **20**:82–101.

Homey, B., A. Muller, and A. Zlotnik. 2002. Chemokines: agents for the immunotherapy of cancer? *Nat. Rev. Immunol.* **2**:175–184.

Knudson, A. G. 2001. Two genetic hits (more or less) to cancer. *Nat. Rev. Cancer* **1**:157–162.

Moingen, P. 2001. Cancer vaccines. *Vaccine* **19**:1305–1326.

Perez-Diez, A., and F. M. Marincola. 2002. Immunotherapy against antigenic tumors: a game with a lot of players. *Cell Mol. Life Sci.* **59**:230–240.

Reff, M. E., K. Hariharan, and G. Braslawsky. 2002. Future of monoclonal antibodies in the treatment of hematologic malignancies. *Cancer Control* **9**:152–166.

Ribas, A., L. H. Butterfield, J. A. Glaspy, and J. S. Economou. 2002. Cancer immunotherapy using gene-modified dendritic cells. *Curr. Gene Ther.* **2**:57–78.

Rosenberg, S. A. 2001. Progress in the development of immunotherapy for the treatment of patients with cancer. *J. Intern. Med.* **250**:462–475.

Tindle, R. W. 2002. Immune evasion in human papillomavirus-associated cervical cancer *Nat. Rev. Cancer* **2**:59–65.

Wang, S. C., L. Zhang, G. N. Hortobagyi, and M. C. Hung. 2001. Targeting HER2: recent developments and future directions for breast cancer patients. *Semin. Oncol.* **28**:21–29.

IMMUNE SYSTEM DYSFUNCTION: OVERACTIVITY

SECTION **VI**

chapter 25

Hypersensitivity

J. Patrick Whelan and Carolyn L. Cannon

The words "hypersensitivity" and "allergy" are broad terms for health problems ranging from the merely irritating, like the itching of eczema, to the life-threatening, as in asthma or anaphylactic shock. These conditions are of increasing importance in health and medicine, in part because of the significant increases in the prevalence and severity of asthma in recent years. Since 1984 in the United States, the number of childhood deaths due to asthma has increased by 300%, and a similar trend is seen in urban areas all over the world (Table 25.1). This field of study is usually referred to as allergy, and 100 years of research suggest that the pain and the peril of these conditions are a result of the overactivity of the body's own cells and chemical mediators, mostly produced in the skin and in mucous membranes. Why have humans evolved such a network of potentially lethal components, and why are some people so much more affected than others?

Perhaps more mysterious are a set of related conditions, also thought of as hypersensitivity disorders, that result from the binding of antibody to one's own tissues. These conditions are grouped together as "rheumatologic disorders," and many of the same cells and mediators are involved. The relationship of these diseases to normal immune function is still a source of considerable controversy.

Table 25.1 Trends in allergy[a]

Burden of asthma in the United States

6.8 million cases in 1980; 17.3 million in 2000

Prevalence increasing 5% per yr

500,000 new cases every yr

No. 1 reason for hospitalization of children

No. 1 reason for days lost from school

Estimated direct and indirect costs in 1998: $12.7 billion

3,850 deaths among persons aged 0–24 yr from 1980 through 1993

[a]The prevalence of atopic diseases, primarily bronchial asthma, atopic dermatitis (eczema), and allergic rhinoconjunctivitis (hay fever) is increasing.

Historical Understanding of the Concept of Hypersensitivity

Molecular and Cellular Factors in Hypersensitivity Reactions

The allergic diseases have been known since antiquity, but there was little insight into their causes until the late 19th century, when advances in histology led to the early delineation of the hematopoietic and mesenchymal cell lineages at the heart of all allergic reactions. At that time, three broad classes of cells were identified—mast cells, granulocytes, and mononuclear cells—that play different roles in hypersensitivity diseases (Fig. 25.1). Later on, molecular factors such as immunoglobulin E (IgE) antibodies also were shown to mediate many of the immunologic aspects of hypersensitivity reactions. The full picture of the molecular and cellular factors that mediate hypersensitivity is still not complete. One reason is that hypersensitivity reactions are a collection of immunologic disorders carried out by a diverse variety of effectors. Another is that clinical presentations of different hypersensitivity reactions, such as asthma, may be due to more than one immunologic mechanism. Overall, while there is a fairly sophisticated understanding of many of the means by which hypersensitivity reactions occur, there is ongoing study into this area to further delineate the contributions of various immunologic factors to the clinical signs and symptoms of hypersensitivity diseases.

Three Types of Hypersensitivity

The early 20th century brought about intense interest in these diseases, which were variously described at the time as "hypersensitiveness" or "hypersusceptibility." Sir William Osler fostered an early appreciation of the connection between the allergic symptoms of the nasal passages and those of the lungs in young people with his textbook on internal medicine published in 1892: "...the so-called hay fever is an affection which has many resemblances to bronchial asthma, with which the attacks may alternate. In the suddenness of onset and in many of their features these diseases have the same origin and differ only in site." During the ensuing years three fundamental types of hypersensitivity were delineated and classified: immediate, intermediate or serum sickness type, and delayed.

The first to be understood in any detail was *immediate-type hypersensitivity*, allergic reactions that emerge in a matter of minutes after exposure to a provocative substance. In 1912, Charles Richet and Paul Portier found that dogs given a first injection of an inactivated jellyfish toxin appeared healthy and had no obvious response to

Figure 25.1 Cellular actors in hypersensitivity reactions. (**A**) A mast cell. The German immunologist Paul Ehrlich first coined the term "Mastzellen," German for "well-fed cells," to describe the granule-laden appearance of these cells, which reside in the dermal layer of the skin and in the connective tissues of the mucous membranes. (**B**) Granulocytes. Similar granules are found in the cytoplasm of granulocytes, which circulate in the blood and are capable of entering sites of infection or inflammation as they are needed. Granulocytes of particular interest in the study of hypersensitivity are the eosinophils and basophils, which are distinguished by their respective affinities for acidic and basic dyes under microscopic examination. Neutrophils, also known as PMNs, are a third type of granulocyte with an important role in hypersensitivity reactions. They are perhaps better known for their role in antibacterial immune responses. (**C**) Mononuclear cells. These cells are central to virtually all acquired immune responses and play a more subtle part in allergic diseases. Molecular techniques have shown that the class of mononuclear cells can be further divided into monocytes and the diverse lymphocytic lineages.

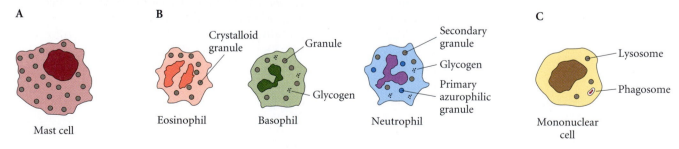

the injection. However, when given a second injection of the same inactivated toxin, the dogs developed acute shortness of breath and often died within minutes, illustrating an extreme type of immediate hypersensitivity known as *anaphylaxis*. Anaphylaxis is now appreciated to be a manifestation of what are most accurately called immediate-type hypersensitivity diseases.

Over the next 25 years, the several different forms of hypersensitivity were studied and differentiated, identifying a role for soluble factors (including antibodies) that would prove as essential as cells in mediating hypersensitivity. In 1906, the Austrian pediatrician Clemens von Pirquet coined the term *allergy* after noticing that some people given a second injection of horse serum for passive immunization against infection or smallpox vaccine developed reactions that were more dramatic than those following their first exposure. The term *serum sickness* entered the lexicon to describe this reaction to reexposure to foreign antigens, such as those in the horse serum, manifested by rash, arthritis, and blood in the urine.

An essential ingredient in the recipe for hypersensitivity is the presence of a precipitating agent. The field of hypersensitivity has its own vocabulary. The foreign substances that stimulate immune responses of other types, often referred to as *complete antigens* or *immunogens,* are called *allergens* when their recognition results in an allergic response. Allergy encompasses two different kinds of responses: immunity and hypersensitivity. *Immunity* is what usually happens after a vaccination: a response by the body that protects prophylactically against disease. In other circumstances, however, the vaccination causes an undesirable physical reaction, or anaphylaxis ("against protection"), indicative of a state of hypersensitivity. To make matters a little more confusing, the term "immunity" is also used to describe a type of hypersensitivity reaction in which the body reacts against itself without any clear prior provocation. Termed *autoimmunity*, this phenomenon encompasses a family of diseases such as rheumatoid arthritis, in which inflammation erupts in the joints and other tissues. Some have proposed calling these rheumatic diseases "auto-allergic diseases" to reflect their departure from the normal, protective function of the immune system, but autoimmunity is the commonly used term for hypersensitivity reactions directed at one's own tissues and organs.

During the middle years of the 20th century, allergy became synonymous with hypersensitivity. Allergic responses in their most typical form elicit symptoms in the respiratory and gastrointestinal tracts and the skin, the most common points of contact with allergens. These symptoms include sneezing, wheezing, nasal discharge, vomiting, diarrhea, itching, and rashes. Allergic disorders are diagnosed on the basis of both their symptoms and their dependence on specific precipitating factors in the environment. However, symptoms that are typical of allergies are also typical of other diseases. For example, wheezing in older individuals can result from fluid accumulation in the lungs secondary to failure of the heart or of the kidneys.

Although the factors initiating an allergic response may be identifiable, there is still considerable uncertainty as to why a particular person develops an allergic response to materials to which everyone is commonly exposed. Genetics plays a significant role. A word frequently used in place of "allergy" is *atopy* (pronounced ay'-top-ee), which represents the familial predisposition of certain individuals to react against common foreign substances in an uncommonly excessive way. The appropriateness of such a term may come into question as these diseases become more common: almost 25% of the U.S. population is affected by allergies or asthma. Osler noted in 1892 that no deaths had yet been attributed to asthma. In modern times, aside from the threefold increase in asthma-related deaths during the past 15 years, asthma is now the leading reason for hospitalization during childhood, with 164,000 children hospitalized for asthma in 1998 in the United States.

Mechanisms of Allergy

In addition to identifying the serum sickness reaction, von Pirquet subsequently identified a form of hypersensitivity associated with the skin test he developed for tuberculosis infection. Robert Koch in Germany had shown previously that reexposure of animals to tuberculosis injections into the skin resulted in a pronounced reaction, with its onset measured in days rather than in minutes (the hallmark of immediate-type) or hours (the hallmark of intermediate-type hypersensitivity or serum sickness). This *delayed-type hypersensitivity* (DTH) reaction was later distinguished from immediate hypersensitivity at a mechanistic level when it was observed that immediate hypersensitivity reactions required a soluble factor present in the serum, whereas DTH reactions were mediated primarily by cells. The true distinction awaited identification of that soluble factor by Kimishige and Teruko Ishizaka in the 1960s, who identified a new isotype of antibody called *IgE*, for which they won the Nobel Prize. Understanding of the DTH reaction advanced considerably when the T-cell antigen receptors were discovered and the role of CD4$^+$ T cells in the DTH reaction was appreciated.

With these developments in recent years, the definition of allergy has narrowed further. The term allergen is now used to describe only those antigens that provoke atopic, or

IgE-mediated, responses of immediate-type hypersensitivity. The biology of hypersensitivity is generally conceptualized now in terms of four categories, in addition to atopy, that were first set forth in the 1960s by Robert Coombs and Philip G. H. Gell. The first four "Gell and Coombs" reactions, called type I to type IV hypersensitivity, are characterized by a dependence on a preceding antigenic stimulus. The fifth, namely autoimmunity, has a more obscure etiology. All five differ in their specific clinical manifestations, the relative timing of the responses, the cells involved, and their variable dependence on immunoglobulin molecules.

As indicated in Fig. 25.2, type I reactions start within seconds following allergen exposure and are usually resolved within 2 hours after removal of the stimulus. Mast cells are the primary effector cells, and the response is triggered by the interaction of antigen with IgE antibodies bound to IgE receptors on the mast-cell surface. Type II and III responses constitute the intermediate-type hypersensitivity responses. They commence within hours after exposure to antigen and can resolve within 24 hours or persist for longer periods. Type II and III responses are initiated by IgG, and damage to host tissues is caused by cells such as neutrophils or natural killer (NK) cells. From a mechanistic standpoint, type II reactions occur when the antibodies bind to tissue-fixed antigens. In contrast, type III reactions occur when IgG antibodies to soluble self antigens form immune complexes that lodge in tissues. In both of these situations, local inflammatory responses that damage the tissue are activated. The type IV reaction, or DTH, is not seen until almost 48 hours after exposure to antigen. These reactions are mediated by helper T cells although new evidence suggests that IgM antibodies may be important for the recruitment of T cells to the site of antigen exposure. At the heart of the DTH reaction are T-cell-secreted cytokines that recruit and activate macrophages, the true foot soldiers that attempt to dispose of the antigen. These reaction types are not mutually exclusive, and some compounds can induce more than one kind of reactivity depending on the circumstances of the exposure.

Figure 25.2 Types of hypersensitivity responses. (**Top**) Salient features of immediate, intermediate, and delayed-type hypersensitivity responses. (**Middle**) Gell and Coombs classification of hypersensitivity responses. (**Bottom**) Typical manifestations of each response.

Immediate	Intermediate		Delayed
Start within seconds, resolve within 2 hours.	Start within hours, may resolve within 24 hours.		Start ~48 hours after antigen exposure.
Ag cross-linking of IgE on surface of mast cells induces release of vasoactive mediators.	Both involve IgG immune complex formation and cell damage through complement activation and either NK cells (type II) or neutrophils (type III).		T cells release cytokines that activate macrophages, resulting in cell damage.
Mast cell degranulation Type I: anaphylactic	Type II: cytotoxic	Type III: immune complex	Activated macrophage Type IV: cell mediated
Manifestations: systemic anaphylaxis or local anaphylaxis, such as hay fever, asthma, hives, food allergies, and eczema	Manifestations: blood transfusion reactions, erythroblastosis fetalis, and autoimmune hemolytic anemia	Manifestations: localized Arthus reactions and generalized reactions such as serum sickness, necrotizing vasculitis, glomerulonephritis, rheumatoid arthritis, and systemic lupus erythematosus	Manifestations: contact dermatitis, reactions to *Mycobacterium tuberculosis* and graft rejection

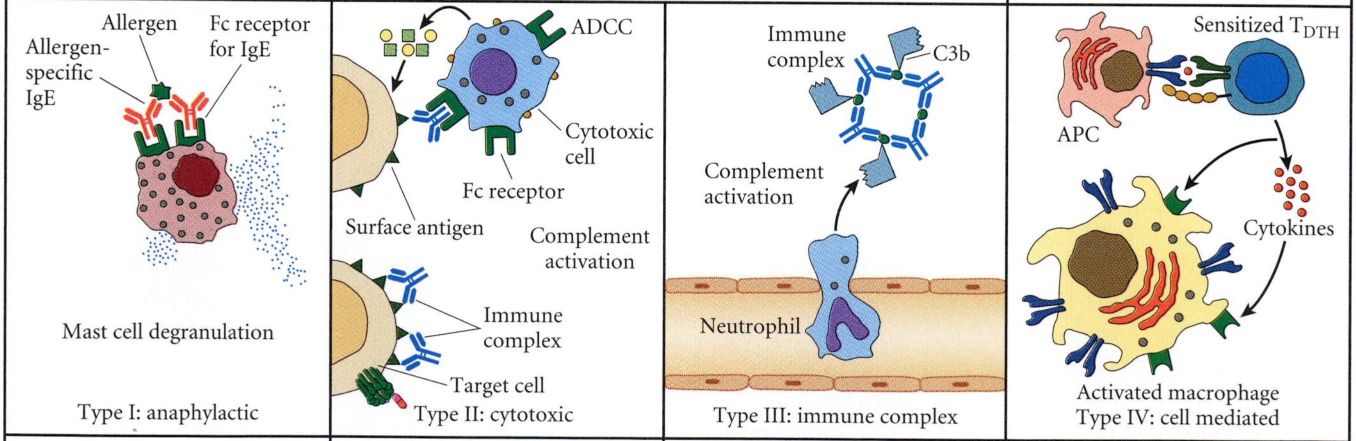

Subtypes of Allergic Responsiveness
Type I Immediate Hypersensitivity

Type I hypersensitivity responses occur within seconds to minutes of antigen exposure, leading to the designation of type I hypersensitivity as "immediate hypersensitivity" (Fig. 25.3). For example, when a mosquito bites a person, a series of 3 to 16 different salivary compounds are injected to prevent blood from clotting. Mast cells that line dermal veins recognize the mosquito proteins as foreign. The first time a mosquito bites, nothing happens; there is no immunity to the salivary proteins. However, if an immune response is generated, leading to the production of IgE antibodies, then subsequent mosquito bites elicit a

rapid response in the skin. The IgE produced to the initial bite is immobilized on the mast-cell surface due the presence of high-affinity receptors for IgE, termed $Fc\varepsilon 1$ receptor type I ($Fc\varepsilon RI$) in the plasma membrane. When the IgE on the mast-cell surface is cross-linked by antigen, the mast cell reacts by releasing histamine and serotonin (Table 25.2) into the connective tissue. The nearby capillary endothelial cells activate their intracellular actin scaffolding, pulling the endothelial cells apart. This increased capillary permeability allows the plasma component of the blood to seep into the tissues, bringing with it complement proteins and other soluble mediators of the innate immune response. This is how redness and swelling due to the mosquito bite come about.

The histamine also binds to local type c nerve fibers that sense pain and initiate the itching sensation. The most obvious result of the increased vascular permeability and nerve stimulation is the formation of a "wheal," or fluid-filled itchy bump. Within a few minutes, a neural arc is completed from the spinal cord that reacts to stimulation of the type c fiber by inducing dilation of the local capillaries to provide a better blood supply to a perceived site of infection. As a result, a vascular "flare" reaction develops that is characterized by increased redness surrounding the bite. The itching often provokes a scratching response from the sufferer, leading to even more extensive dilation of the local blood vessels.

The influx of plasma and its protein mediators of inflammation, such as immunoglobulin and complement factors, helps the local tissue decipher the nature and extent of the insult. Complement binds to the invading proteins or organisms and serves as a handle for local phagocytic cells, including the Langerhans cells of the skin. In the absence of further damage, the remaining complement-tagged antigens are drained from the tissue via the lymphatics. As the C3 component of complement is activated and the C3b fragment binds to the foreign proteins, the C3a fragment serves an important feedback regulatory function. C3a binds to certain populations of mast cells and inhibits further IgE-mediated degranulation, thus indicating their adequate recruitment of the plasma factors (such as complement) necessary to clear the perceived infection (Fig. 25.4). The most visible signs of the reaction then subside within a matter of minutes.

The immediate release of histamine is followed by a second wave of important immune mediators: the cysteinyl leukotriene class of arachidonic acid derivatives made by the mast cells (Fig. 25.5). These fatty acid-derived substances serve a variety of functions, including the recruitment of cells into the injured area. After the wheal-and-flare response disappears, many people will develop a

Figure 25.3 Immediate hypersensitivity. Exposure to allergen activates B cells to become IgE-secreting plasma cells. The IgE molecules from multiple plasma cell clones bind to IgE-specific receptors on mast cells and basophils. A second exposure to the allergen results in cross-linking of the bound IgE and the release of mediators, including vasoactive amines such as histamine. The mediators cause the contraction of smooth muscle, vasodilation, and increased vascular permeability that underlie, for example, hay fever symptoms.

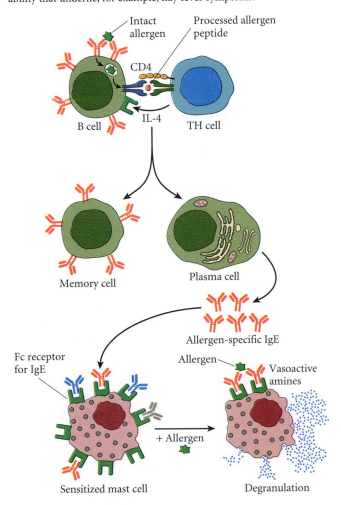

Table 25.2 Mediators of type I hypersensitivity reactions[a]

Mediator	Effects
Granule content release (immediate)	
Histamine	Increased vascular permeability, smooth-muscle contraction
Serotonin	Increased vascular permeability, smooth-muscle contraction
Eosinophil chemotactic factor	Eosinophil chemotaxis
Neutrophil chemotactic factor	Eosinophil chemotaxis
Proteases	Bronchial mucus secretion, degradation of blood vessel basement membrane, generation of complement split products
Membrane-derived lipid mediators (released over minutes)	
Prostaglandins	Vasodilation, contraction of pulmonary smooth muscle, platelet aggregation
Leukotrienes	Increased vascular permeability, contraction of pulmonary smooth muscle
Platelet-activating factor	Platelet aggregation and degranulation, contraction of pulmonary smooth muscle
Bradykinin	Increased vascular permeability, smooth-muscle contraction
Cytokine production (released over hours)	
IL-1, TNF-α	Systemic anaphylaxis, increased ICAM expression on endothelium
IL-3	Stimulates mast-cell growth and histamine secretion
IL-4	Stimulates mast-cell growth, induces activated B cells to class switch to IgG1 and IgE
IL-5	Promotes growth and differentiation of eosinophils
TGF-β	Chemotactically attracts monocytes and macrophages, induces IL-1 production by activated macrophages

[a]TGF, transforming growth factor; ICAM, intercellular adhesion molecule.

Figure 25.4 The dual role of complement in mast cell activation. (**A**) In serosal mast cell populations found in skin, muscle, and the peritoneal cavity, binding by the anaphylatoxins C3a and C5a to receptors specific for these complement cleavage factors on the cell surface results in degranulation even in the absence of IgE cross-linking. (**B**) In mucosal mast cell populations found, for example, in the intestine, C3a binds to a different receptor, the β chain of the FcϵRI receptor, blocking IgE binding and, hence, cross-linking and degranulation even in the presence of allergen.

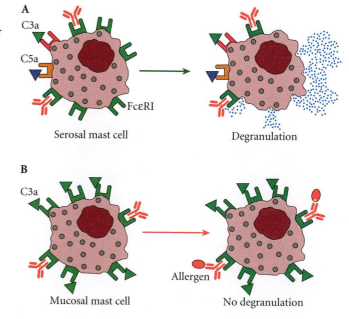

small bump, or papule, that lasts for hours or days. This is due to the influx of polymorphonuclear leukocytes (PMNs) and eosinophils during the first 2 hours to deal with infectious organisms injected by the mosquito (e.g., *Plasmodium* species that cause malaria, the yellow fever virus, or other mosquito-borne viruses). Over the next few hours, an ordered arrival of mononuclear cells, including CD4$^+$ T lymphocytes, contributes to maintaining the reaction.

IgE-mediated mast-cell degranulation plays a significant part in diverse hypersensitivity diseases, including asthma, hay fever, eczema, and food allergies (Table 25.3). The different clinical symptoms of these allergic diseases generally reflect the site of introduction of the allergen. In the upper respiratory tract hay fever symptoms are provoked when pollen, dust, etc., are inhaled. Asthma is a manifestation of allergic responses going on in the lower airways where wheezing can take place. Vomiting and

Table 25.3 Type I hypersensitivity responses

Asthma
   Wheezing
   Cough
   Chest tightness
Atopic rhinoconjunctivitis (hay fever)
   Runny, itchy nose and eyes
Atopic urticaria (hives)
Atopic dermatitis (eczema)
   Dry, itchy skin
Food allergies
   Acute
      Hives
      Anaphylaxis
      Flushing
      Angioedema
      Oral itching
   Chronic (not all are type I responses)
      Eczema
      Asthma
      Diarrhea
      Vomiting

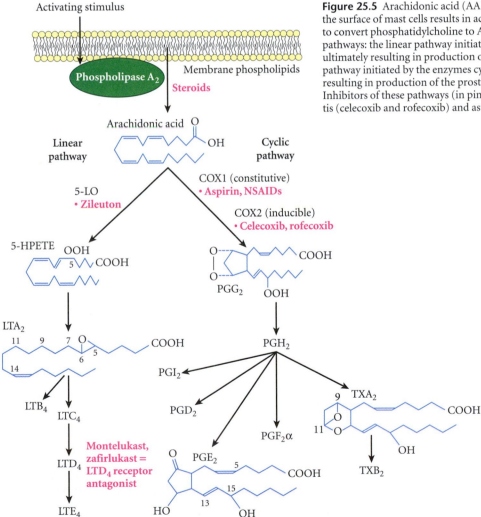

Figure 25.5 Arachidonic acid (AA) metabolites. Cross-linking of FcεRI on the surface of mast cells results in activation of phospholipase A$_2$, which acts to convert phosphatidylcholine to AA. AA serves as the precursor in two pathways: the linear pathway initiated by the enzyme 5-lipoxygenase (5-LO), ultimately resulting in production of the leukotrienes (LT); and the cyclic pathway initiated by the enzymes cyclooxygenase 1 and 2 (COX1 and COX2), resulting in production of the prostaglandins (PG) and thromboxanes (TX). Inhibitors of these pathways (in pink type) include drugs used to treat arthritis (celecoxib and rofecoxib) and asthma (montelukast and zafirlukast).

diarrhea are manifestations of food allergies, although in some cases food antigens are transported via the blood to lodge in the skin capillaries where they can cause rashes and hives. Skin contact with allergens leads to local rashes. Anaphylactic shock is thought to be due to triggering by IgE of the release of histamine-containing granules by basophils in the circulation. This leads to a generalized immediate-type hypersensitivity reaction and, if untreated, can proceed to shock wherein the dilation of blood vessels and subsequent fall in blood pressure can be lethal. Genetic and environmental factors both clearly play a role in determining whether an individual reacts disproportionately to a given stimulus and develops a hypersensitivity state (Tables 25.4 and 25.5).

Given the destructive and even potentially lethal nature of an IgE response, it is often asked why type I reactions occur at all, and why a harmful antibody isotype like IgE either evolved or persisted. It is not clear how and why an allergen elicits a harmful IgE response instead of a protective antibody response. And what keeps B cells from reacting similarly against all antigens? It is also not known how IgE antibodies travel back to the site of inoculation

Table 25.4 Genes associated with an increased risk of atopy[a]

Gene or protein	Location	Function	Notes on link to atopy
Mutations or polymorphisms in specific genes			
IL-13	5q31	Enhances bronchial mucus secretion and upregulates IgE production	Several polymorphisms are associated with variation in IgE levels
Esterase D	13q14	Found on RBC membranes	Polymorphism shows linkage to asthma and AD
SPINK5	5q32	SPINK5, the gene underlying Netherton disease, encodes a 15-domain serine proteinase inhibitor (LEKTI) expressed in epithelial and mucosal surfaces and the thymus	Rare, autosomal recessive disorder universally associated with atopy and AD; one of the six polymorphisms of SPINK5 significantly associated with atopy and AD in patients with Netherton disease
IL-12Rβ2	1p31.2	IL-12 induces IFN-γ, which downregulates IL-4 and ultimately IgE production	In one study, PBMCs of 10 of 75 atopic patients tested carried mutations in the IL-12β2 gene and had no IFN-γ response to IL-12
Polymorphisms in promoter genes			
IL-4Rα	16p12	A component of the receptor for both IL-4 and IL-13	Several of eight described promoter polymorphisms have been linked to asthma
MCP-1	17q11	Provokes mast-cell activation and increased expression of histidine decarboxylase mRNA in a dose-dependent manner; causes mast-cell, eosinophil, and macrophage recruitment and PGE$_2$ generation	Polymorphism in the gene regulatory region associated with asthma susceptibility and severity; frequency of −2518G polymorphism in the gene-regulatory region of MCP-1 significatly higher in asthmatic than in control children
FcεRIB	11q13	The high-affinity IgE receptor acts in antigen-induced mast-cell degranulation and in the release of cytokines that enhance IgE production	−109C/T promoter polymorphism at FcεRIB is a genetic factor that affects total serum IgE level
CTLA-4 (CD152)	2q33	B7-CD28–CTLA-4 interaction can promote the differentiation and development of the TH2 lymphocyte subset	Patients with −318C allele at the CTLA-4 promoter region had higher total serum IgE; presence of both the CTLA-4 and FcεRIB polymorphisms is correlated in patients with asthma
CD14	5q31	A high-affinity ligand for bacterial lipopolysaccharide that initiates an innate immune response to bacterial infection	The C-to-T transition in the promoter region of the CD14 gene on chromosome 5q31.1 associated with atopic phenotypes in a population study of schoolchildren in the United States

[a]AD, atopic dermatitis; MCP-1, monocyte chemoattractant protein 1; PBMC, peripheral blood mononuclear cell.

Table 25.5 Loci associated with an increased risk of atopy[a]

Locus	Candidate genes	Notes on links to atopy
5q31	Region contains IL-4, IL-13, IL-5, CD14, and GM-CSF	
6p	Near MHC	MHC region has shown consistent linkage to asthma
12q	No candidate genes	Consistently found linked to asthma in several studies
13q14	Other than ESD, no candidate genes	Linked to total serum IgE, asthma, and total serum IgA; low IgA concentrations occur more frequently in atopic children
7q and 14q	TCR genes	Linkage reported between specific IgE responses and the TCR α/β locus on 14q

[a]ESD, esterase D; TCR, T-cell receptor.

and to other areas of the body to bind to tissue-fixed mast cells. What mechanisms serve to keep the mast-cell system in balance as it is bombarded perpetually with a torrent of foreign substances?

Biology of IgE and how the immune system recognizes allergens

The existence of IgE was postulated long before the molecule itself was identified. In 1921, Karl Prausnitz gave himself a local injection of serum from his friend Heinz Kustner, who was allergic to fish. Injecting a fish extract before injecting the serum induced no reaction in Prausnitz's arm, but exposure to fish induced a typical wheal-and-flare response when Kustner's serum was injected first. This reaction demonstrated specificity for the offending allergen and was not induced by the serum of a nonallergic person. Subsequently referred to as Prausnitz-Kustner antibody, its molecular identity was the subject of a long search. In the end, identification of IgE proved elusive because serum normally contains minute quantities of IgE compared with the quantities of other antibody isotypes (IgE comprises about 0.004% of serum antibody). Like other antibodies, IgE is a protein composed of two heavy and two light chains. The heavy chains, designated ε chains, are similar to the heavy chains of other immunoglobulins, with a variable antigen-binding domain at the amino-terminal end of the protein. The antigen-binding domain of the ε heavy chain is connected to four constant domains, structurally more similar to μ heavy chains than to γ, α, or δ heavy chains, which have three constant domains. As with other immunoglobulin molecules, the heavy and light chains are attached to one another via multiple disulfide bonds. The Fc region of IgE has a high affinity for FcεRI expressed prominently on mast cells (Fig. 25.6).

Like other Ig molecules, the IgE ε heavy chain is transcribed into mRNA, encoding synthesis of two different protein isoforms: a membrane-bound and a secreted form. The membrane-bound form is expressed only on the surface of mature B lymphocytes that have undergone a class switch to the IgE locus and serves as an antigen receptor. The IgE-secreting plasma cells make soluble IgE molecules that travel through the interstitial tissues until they find the high-affinity FcεRI on mast cells or basophils. The difference between the IgE on the B-cell membrane and the IgE on the surface of the mast cell or basophil is a crucial one. Whereas the B cell will express only IgE with a single specificity for an allergen, a mast cell or basophil can potentially have different IgE molecules from different plasma cells specific for thousands of different allergens. One or a few antigenic specificities often predominate among the IgE molecules on a given mast cell, depending on the intensity of the antigen exposure in the tissue where the mast cell resides. For instance, mast cells in the small intestine will be more likely to bear IgE molecules specific for peanut proteins, whereas mast cells in the lungs may be more responsive to ragweed pollen, since these are where exposure to these particular allergens is most likely to occur.

Cells participating in the origins of allergic responses

One of the central questions in the allergy field is why certain animal or plant products—and in many cases some very specific proteins from pets, parasites, and plants—induce an allergic response when most other antigens are not allergens. The antigen specificity of IgE antibodies cannot account for this phenomenon, since the specificity is exactly the same as that of the original IgM molecule from the responsible B cell before the class switch to IgE production. It is not the shape or charge of a particular

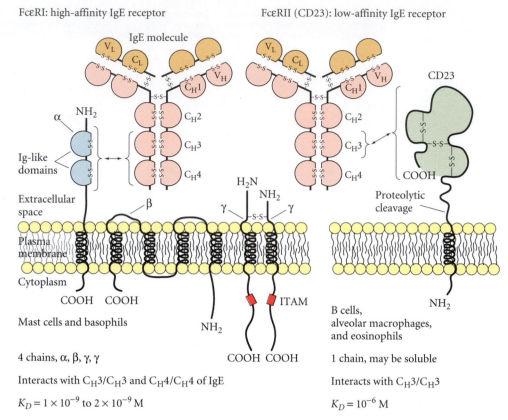

FcεRI: high-affinity IgE receptor

FcεRII (CD23): low-affinity IgE receptor

IgE molecule

CD23

Mast cells and basophils

ITAM

B cells, alveolar macrophages, and eosinophils

4 chains, α, β, γ, γ

Interacts with C_H3/C_H3 and C_H4/C_H4 of IgE

$K_D = 1 \times 10^{-9}$ to 2×10^{-9} M

1 chain, may be soluble

Interacts with C_H3/C_H3

$K_D = 10^{-6}$ M

Figure 25.6 Properties of the IgE-binding Fc receptors. (**Left**) The high-affinity receptor (FcεRI) present on mast cell and basophils. This receptor consists of four chains: an α chain with two 90-amino-acid domains homologous to the immunoglobulin-fold structure; a β chain that links the α chain to a γ homodimer, each chain of which has an immunoreceptor tyrosine-based activation motif (ITAM) important for cell activation through interaction with tyrosine kinases. The immunoglobulin-like folds of the α chain interact with the C_H3/C_H3 and C_H4/C_H4 domains of the IgE molecule. (**Right**) The low-affinity receptor (FcεRII) found on B cells, alveolar macrophages, and eosinophils. This receptor appears to play a role in regulating the intensity of the IgE response. The soluble form, generated by proteolysis, enhances IgE production by B cells.

allergen that makes it induce IgE, since under the right conditions the same structure can induce production of different types of immunoglobulins. Several factors seem to determine whether the body makes an IgE response. The route of exposure is important, with antigens given intravenously being much less likely than inhaled antigens to induce an allergic response. Dose of antigen exposure is also influential, with very low or high doses usually resulting in nonallergic responses.

New research in this field focuses attention on the way in which T cells are stimulated by allergens. One critical issue that has not been well defined has been how very large allergens such as pollen grains actually penetrate the body's external defenses to stimulate an immune response. It appears that eosinophils can function as scavenger cells that pick up allergens in the alveoli of the lung and then transport them specifically to the T-cell areas of the draining paratracheal lymph nodes. Eosinophils express major histocompatibility complex (MHC) class II molecules and the T-cell costimulatory molecules CD80 and CD86, properties of antigen-presenting cells (APCs). Eosinophils that take up allergen in the airways, and subsequently present it to T cells in the neighboring lymph nodes, may have a propensity to activate immune responses geared toward production of IgE. Classic research in the allergy field has

treated the eosinophil solely as an effector cell. However, newer data suggest the eosinophil also has a role in initiating the response (i.e., an *afferent* role).

How do eosinophils get recruited to sites of allergen exposure? Three components of the innate immune system appear to be important in deciding when eosinophil infiltration is necessary. First, epithelial cells that line the air spaces of the lung express at least three chemoattractive proteins that can mobilize eosinophils: RANTES, interleukin-16 (IL-16), and eotaxin. Injury to the surface epithelium may be one signal that initiates eosinophilic responses. Mast cells are another early source of chemical mediators that can recruit eosinophils. Mast cells are equipped not only with surface IgE that may be specific for allergens but also with complement receptors and pattern-recognition molecules that can trigger the mast cell to release cytokines and chemokines. Mice that are engineered to be deficient in mast cells have a significantly decreased ability to mobilize eosinophils in response to aerosolized allergens. A third type of cell that is important in the initiation of allergic responses is the γδ T lymphocyte. These cells line the subcutaneous and mucosal surfaces of the body. Mice lacking γδ T cells have decreased infiltration of eosinophils and αβ T cells in response to allergen exposure in the respiratory tract (Fig. 25.7).

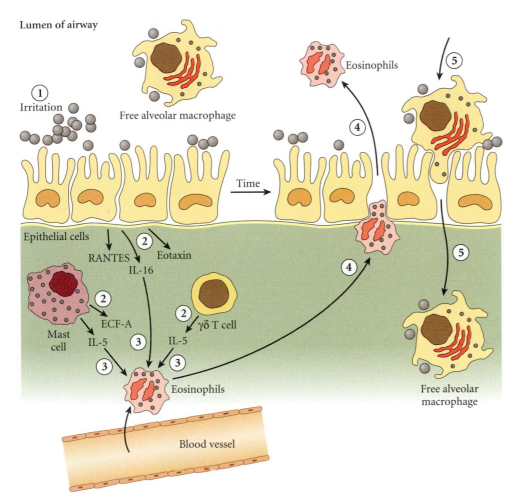

Lumen of airway

Figure 25.7 Recruitment of eosinophils in the early response to allergen. After irritation by allergens or injury (1), respiratory epithelial cells express the chemoattractive proteins RANTES, IL-16, and eotaxin (2). Tissue damage or antigen exposure causes cells lining the mucosal surface to release cytokines, including ECF-A and IL-5 released by mast cells and IL-5 released by neighboring γδ T lymphocytes (2). These cytokines act in concert to recruit eosinophils from the circulation (3), and eosinophils are then mobilized into the airways (4). Free alveolar macrophages in the airspaces, like eosinophils, are scavengers for particles, such as pollen grains. Free alveolar macrophages and eosinophils are capable of trafficking back into the tissues (5), although their role in triggering the IgE response is uncertain.

Model for the generation of IgE immunity

With each breath, we inhale large numbers of particles, including viruses coughed or sneezed out by other people, pollen grains (like ragweed, oak tree, or grass), and mold spores (Fig. 25.8). Much of this material sticks to the moist respiratory epithelium that lines the trachea and the bronchi and is passed back up by the coordinated motion of the cilia that compose the mucociliary escalator in the respiratory tract. Passageways that conduct air from the upper respiratory tract (where it is breathed in) to the terminal alveoli (where gas exchange takes place) divide or bifurcate at many levels to form smaller-diameter passages, which are named based on the relative diameter of the lumen. The bronchioles begin after 9 to 12 divisions of the airways and are about 5 millimeters (mm) or less in diameter. Typical allergen-bearing particles have a diameter 1/100 to 1/1,000 this size, but only those less than about 5 micrometers (μm) in diameter penetrate in substantial numbers past the terminal bronchioles into the air spaces. Pollen grains are typically 15 to 50 μm across, so they are much less likely to travel all the way through the 23 gen-

erations of bronchial divisions and into the alveoli. Rather, the size of pollen grains appears to limit them more to the upper airways, and it is perhaps not surprising that pollen has a greater association with "hay fever" (an upper respiratory disease) than with allergic asthma (a lower respiratory disease). The somewhat smaller allergens, such as cat dander particles and fecal matter from dust mites and cockroaches, can better travel the entire distance to the alveolar air spaces. These particles are much more likely to elicit asthma than are larger particles.

How do allergens come to the attention of the immune system? It is widely assumed that dendritic cells are the earliest messengers, carrying antigens to the lymph nodes that line the bronchial tree. However, a role for dendritic cells in induction of allergic responses is not established, and these cells are rarely found in the airways. Due to their potency as APCs, the rarity of dendritic cells does not exclude them as potential agents for initiating allergic responses. The very first exposure of the naive respiratory immune system to an allergen may also involve other phagocytic cells, such as alveolar macrophages. These cells

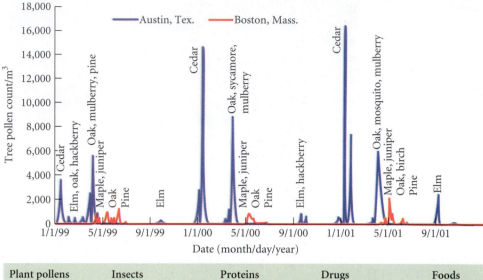

Figure 25.8 Common allergens. (**Top**) Exposure to environmental allergens may vary dramatically according to the season and location, as shown in the chart depicting pollen-count data compiled by the American Academy of Allergy, Asthma, and Immunology (http://www.aaaai.org). (**Bottom**) A partial listing of allergens associated with type I hypersensitivity reactions.

Plant pollens	Insects	Proteins	Drugs	Foods
Trees, as above	Cockroach calyx	Foreign serum	Penicillin	Nuts
Ragweed	Dust mites	Vaccines	Sulfonamides	Shellfish
Rye grass	Bee venom		Salicylates	Eggs
Timothy grass	Wasp venom	**Animals**	Local anesthetics	Milk
	Ant venom	Cat dander		
Mold spores		Dog dander		
		Horse hair		
		Mice		

are capable of shuttling from the air spaces back into the subepithelial tissues. Some workers have described a specialized "plasmacytoid" dendritic cell that can migrate to the T-cell areas of the bronchopulmonary lymph nodes, and stimulate T cells to proliferate and differentiate. These dendritic cells have the capability of steering CD4[+] T cells toward the type 2 helper T-cell (TH2) phenotype characterized by the propensity to make type II cytokines (IL-4, IL-5, and IL-13).

TH2 cells migrate from their characteristic location in the paracortical region of the lymph node to the interface of the T-cell region with the B-cell-rich cortex. Simultaneously, IgM-positive naive B cells in the primary follicles of the cortex use their IgM receptors to snag allergen molecules out of the afferent lymphatic flow entering the lymph node nearby. Little is known about how the allergen travels from the airways to the lymph node cortex where the B cells reside, but it is likely that the allergen is shuttled through the bronchiolar or alveolar lymphatics into the lymph node, where millions of B cells, each with a specific antigen-binding IgM receptor, are waiting for the opportunity to find an epitope on the antigen for which they have an affinity.

Binding of allergen to the surface IgM activates these B cells, which then travel to the edge of the cortex to meet the newly activated T cells. The initial interaction of the T cell and B cell at the cortex-paracortex interface leads both to migrate again, this time back into the B-cell-rich cortex. Together, the activated B cells and T cells launch the formation of a germinal center. Activated B cells produce two of their own cytokines: tumor necrosis factor alpha (TNF-α) and/or lymphotoxin. These factors stimulate a network of neighboring cells, the follicular dendritic cells (FDCs), found in the cortex of the lymph node. The FDCs respond to TNF-α by secreting a chemokine, *B-lymphocyte chemoattractant* (BLC, or CXCL13), which is essential for the homing of B cells to secondary lymphoid organs and the development of B-cell follicles. B cells have receptors for BLC that entice them to travel from their first interaction with T cells at the cortex-paracortex interface into proximity of the FDC.

Upon arriving back in the cortex, activated B cells proliferate in the *germinal center dark zone*. B cells then move into juxtaposition with the FDCs in an adjacent area of the germinal center called the *basal light zone*. There the B cells are positively selected by exposure to specific complement-coated antigen immobilized on the surface of complement receptor-bearing FDCs. In the first two germinal center stages, the B cells undergo *somatic hypermutation,* during which their Ig genes mutate and the resulting receptors are selected for the highest antigen affinity. Cells whose receptors mutate to a lower affinity then undergo apoptosis.

Activated high-affinity B cells that survive the basal light zone are reunited in the germinal center with the activated TH2 cells in the *apical light zone*. When an activated CD4$^+$ T cell has been induced to differentiate into a TH2 cell, it produces IL-4 and IL-13, which bind to receptors on the B cell. These cytokines induce class switch recombination, leading to IgE expression on the B-cell surface. The class-switched B cells undergo a final differentiative step, becoming IgE-secreting plasma cells or surface IgE-receptor-positive memory B cells that reside in the *mantle zone* surrounding the germinal center.

Thus, a cascade proceeds from initial antigen exposure of B cells and T cells and their subsequent interaction. The activated B cell signals its presence to the FDC, which summons the B cell into a complex in the cortex that becomes a new germinal center. B cells proliferate, undergo affinity maturation through somatic hypermutation, and complete the class switch process to IgE expression. Like other class-switched mature B cells, IgE-positive B lymphocytes then differentiate into IgE memory cells or IgE-secreting plasma cells.

Mechanics of immediate hypersensitivity responses

Once plasma cells begin making IgE, the atopic individual is considered to be "sensitized" to a particular allergen. Using their FcεRI, mast cells that line all the epithelial surfaces of the body avidly take up IgE of multiple allergenic specificities from the surrounding fluid and are then "armed" to recognize allergens for which the IgE is specific. This binding of IgE to its high-affinity receptor on mast cells is distinct from other Ig-FcR interactions, since most FcRs bind to antibody with moderate or low affinity. IgG FcRs, for instance, are capable of binding antibody only when the IgG is present as part of a large "immune complex" consisting of antibody and antigen. In contrast, the mast-cell IgE receptor, FcεRI, binds IgE with high affinity (K_d, $\sim 10^{-10}$ M) and can therefore bind soluble IgE in the absence of antigen. This binding of IgE to FcεRI, however, does not cause mast-cell activation; activation only occurs after subsequent binding of FcεRI-bound IgE to antigen. The transport route of the IgE is something of a mystery, since so little IgE circulates in the blood. IgE-secreting plasma cells are thought to be located primarily in the pharyngeal tonsils, but IgE sensitizing mast cells are found throughout the body. Mast cells circulate from the bone marrow to the peripheral tissues, where they differentiate into highly granular cells with receptors for IgE. Positioned strategically next to blood vessels at all the gateways to the body, mast cells can exert immediate effects on the permeability of blood vessels and the recruitment of other cellular reinforcements following allergen or antigen penetration of the epithelial layer that overlays the mast-cell-rich areas of the submucosa.

The cross-linking of the IgE-bearing FcεRI by an allergen results in a biochemical cascade in the mast cell involving multiple second-messenger systems (Fig. 25.9). The end result is the release of three different classes of compounds, each with distinct physicochemical properties and timing of their secretion, that work in a coordinated way to propel the hypersensitivity response. The best-studied events of FcεRI-initiated signal transduction include the activation of tyrosine kinases that trigger phospholipase Cγ1, an enzyme that causes the release of inositol phosphates such as inositol 1,4,5-trisphosphate (IP$_3$) (Fig. 25.10A). The appearance of IP$_3$ and sphingosine derivatives contributes to a sudden rush of calcium into the cytoplasm of the mast cell. The calcium flux is a critical trigger for the mobilization of the cellular cytoskeleton and a resultant release of the cell's histamine granules to the outside of the cell (Fig. 25.10C). Second, the initial activation of tyrosine kinase also turns on the Ras–mitogen-activated protein kinase pathway, which in turn activates phospholipase A$_2$ and commences the second wave of mediator release from the mast cell: the arachidonic acid metabolic cascade (Fig. 25.10B). Arachidonic acid is converted in the endoplasmic reticulum into vasoactive and chemotactic prostaglandins and leukotrienes. Last, the mitogen-activated protein kinase initiates transcriptional activation of important cytokine genes, resulting in the late synthesis and release of proteins such as IL-4 and IL-5. The sequential release of these vasoactive amines, then the lipid leukotrienes and prostaglandins, and finally the protein cytokines leads to the dramatic influx of fluid and cells that are the hallmark of the immediate hypersensitivity response.

Asthma as an important type I hypersensitivity disease

Asthma was recognized as long ago as 1892 by Sir William Osler as an inflammatory disease of the small bronchioles. Dramatic increases in the occurrence of asthma have been noted, particularly in industrialized countries. There is much speculation about the reason for this surprising observation, since many other types of illnesses affect residents of less industrialized countries disproportionately. With asthma as a major cause of illness particularly affecting young children, its immunologic basis is being studied in great detail to gain insight into the cellular and molecular factors that cause asthma to develop, with the expectation this will lead to new and improved treatments for this disease.

Pathologic examination of the airways from patients with advanced asthma demonstrates infiltration by eosinophils and monocytes, increased size and number of the mucus-producing goblet cells, and damage to the protective epithelial lining of the airway. Therefore the physiologic factors that maintain normal airway integrity are not performing their usual job. A number of factors contribute to maintaining the airways in their normal open configuration and the mast cells in a state of quiet readiness. Prostaglandin E_2 (PGE_2) (Fig. 25.5), for example, is produced both by airway epithelial cells and by the smooth muscle and, when inhaled, can protect people with asthma against allergen- or exercise-induced bronchospasm. PGE_2

blocks the release of acetylcholine from peribronchiolar nerve endings and helps maintain a relaxed tone for the smooth muscle, hence keeping the small airways open. Smooth-muscle cells also have β-adrenergic receptors that when occupied by an agonist, such as epinephrine (commonly known as adrenalin), signal the muscle cells to relax. PGE_2 has also been shown experimentally to block several aspects of the inflammatory cascade, including mast-cell degranulation, eosinophil chemotaxis, and activation of both B cells and T cells.

The lungs of people with asthma have significant inflammation affecting all layers of the bronchiolar tissue and involving multiple cell types. The surface epithelium is

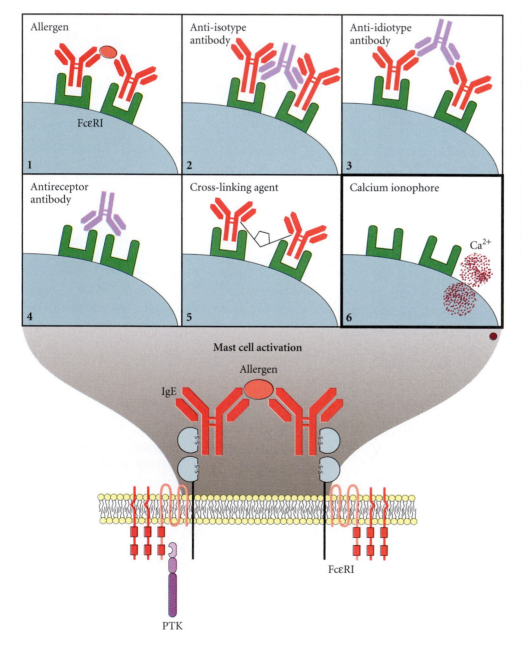

Figure 25.9 Initial step in mast cell activation. Cross-linking of the high-affinity IgE receptor (FcεRI) on the surface of the mast cell by rough allergen binding or any of numerous other methods (**1 to 5**) leads to activation of protein tyrosine kinases associated with the cytoplasmic domains of the β and γ chains of the receptor complex. The signaling cascade ultimately results in a sustained elevation in the intracellular calcium concentration, a step necessary for degranulation. Elevating the intracellular calcium concentration through incorporation of calcium ionophores into the mast-cell plasma membrane drives degranulation without the need for receptor cross-linking (**6**).

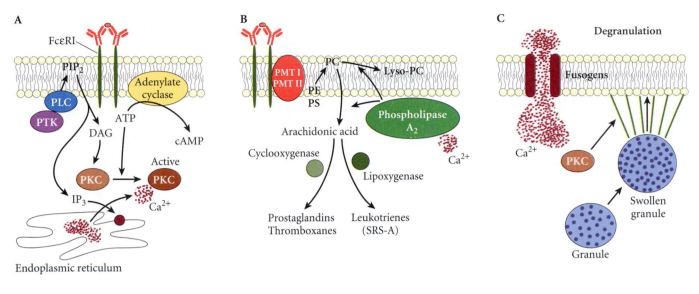

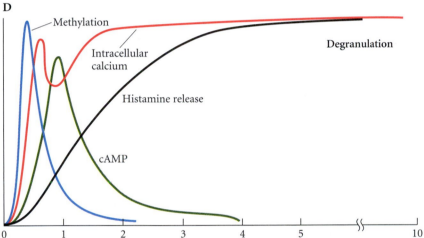

Figure 25.10 Mast cell activation and degranulation. (**A**) Cross-linking of FcεRI by allergen-bound IgE results in activation of adenylate cyclase, resulting in transient elevation of cyclic adenosine monophosphate (cAMP) and activation of protein kinase A. Cross-linking also activates protein tyrosine kinases (PTK) that, in turn, activate phospholipase C (PLC). PLC converts phosphatidylinositol 4,5-bisphosphate (PIP$_2$) into diacylglycerol (DAG) and IP$_3$. DAG activates protein kinase C (PKC), necessary for microtubule assembly and granule fusion. IP$_3$ mobilizes calcium from internal stores, which opens calcium channels in the plasma membrane to allow sustained elevation of intracellular calcium concentrations. (**B**) Cross-linking also activates an enzyme that converts phosphatidylserine (PhS) to phosphatidylethanolamine (PE), which is then methylated by the phospholipid methyl transferase enzymes I and II (PMT I and II) to form phosphatidylcholine (PC). Influx of calcium activates phospholipase A$_2$, which converts PC into lyso-PC and arachidonic acid. Arachidonic acid is the precursor for a variety of mediators. (**C**) PKC phosphorylates proteins on the membrane of the granule, changing the permeability to water and calcium. The granules swell and, through the action of microtubules and microfilaments, are pulled to the surface, fuse, and release their contents. (**D**) Time course of mast cell activation events.

coated by a layer of mucus thicker than that seen in the normal situation. The epithelium itself is punctuated by large numbers of goblet cells producing the extra mucus. The underlying lamina propria is thickened and packed with eosinophils and several different types of activated lymphocytes. Finally, the underlying smooth muscle that controls the diameter of the airway is now thickened and hyperreactive. In contrast to normal airways from nonasthmatics, the

bronchioles now contain high densities of mast cells that are armed with allergen-specific IgE.

An asthma attack is initiated when a sensitized individual is exposed to the allergen that binds to IgE on mast cells. A bronchiolar constrictive response begins within minutes of exposure, initiated by the release from the mast cells of the vasoactive amines such as histamine and the arachidonic acid derivatives. Mast-cell activation causes rapid

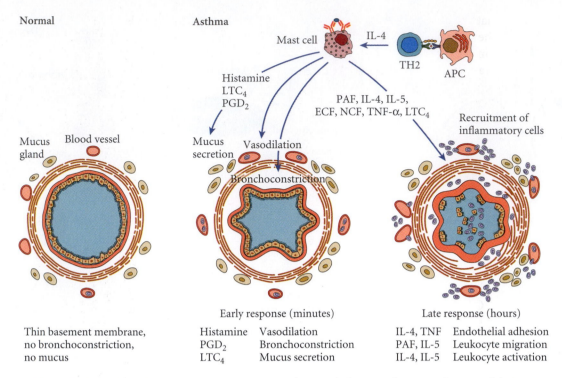

Normal   Asthma

Figure 25.11 Asthma. Cross-sectional representations of airways before an asthma exacerbation and during the early and the late inflammatory response are shown. In the early response, note the vasodilation, increased secretion of mucus by glands and goblet cells, and bronchoconstriction. The late response is characterized by worsening bronchoconstriction and remodeling of the airways with thickened lamina propria packed with eosinophils and lymphocytes. LTC_4, leukotriene; PAF, platelet-activating factor; PGD_2, prostaglandin D_2.

degranulation and release of histamine, which binds to smooth-muscle cells surrounding the airway and initiates a contractile response that can significantly narrow the lumen and restrict the passage of the air (Fig. 25.11).

The histamine release is followed very soon by the arachidonic acid cascade, particularly the release of prostaglandin D_2 and leukotriene C_4, which triggers a second wave of airway constriction, beginning about 12 hours after exposure and lasting up to 24 hours. This second wave is characterized by an acute mobilization of neutrophils into the airways about 2 hours into the attack; the neutrophils release their granules in an attempt to disable the perceived pathogen that triggered the initial response. Subsequently, there is a depletion of circulating blood eosinophils, which redistribute into the submucosal tissues and airways. In its extreme form, this "status asthmaticus" can severely compromise the ability to exchange oxygen for carbon dioxide and other waste products in the air spaces distal to the obstructed bronchioles. Death may result if these patients do not have access to timely intervention with steroids and β-agonists (e.g., epinephrine) and, occasionally, artificial respiratory support.

Other clinical manifestations of type I hypersensitivity

Food allergies can be the result of sensitization of the immune system through any of the four Gell and Coombs types of hypersensitivity, but IgE-mediated immediate hypersensitivity is probably involved in most cases (Table 25.3). The symptoms may be local and confined to the gastrointestinal tract, beginning with swelling of the lips on first contact with the allergen. This reaction may be followed by tingling and itching in the throat, nausea and vomiting, abdominal cramps, and diarrhea. But food allergens also can provoke more systemic reactions, including itching and generalized rash, diffuse swelling (angioedema), runny nose (rhinorrhea), shortness of breath and wheezing, and even shock.

The most common offending foods are peanuts and other nuts, shellfish, and eggs. Children also can suffer from sensitization to cow's milk and soy proteins, in part because newborns frequently are exposed to these in infant formulas (Fig. 25.8). One major reason for encouraging breast feeding in newborns is that it reduces the rate of development of food allergies.

Atopic urticaria, also called hives, is an IgE-mediated

response to allergens that either enter the skin from outside or travel through the circulation and manifest the allergic response in the skin. The most common inducers of these reactions are certain drugs and additives in processed foods. In a previously sensitized individual, the ingestion of an offending drug can cause itchy raised welts all over the body within a matter of minutes or hours after ingestion of the drug. These reactions often respond quickly to oral antihistamines or, in the more dramatic cases, can be suppressed by oral steroids.

Atopic eczema, also called atopic dermatitis, is a more involved inflammatory condition of the skin that is the epidermal equivalent of chronic asthma in the respiratory tract. These itchy, often painful and red areas of skin usually first appear during early childhood. With time, the skin thickens in response to scratching (a process known as "lichenification," akin to the appearance of lichen growing on a wet rock). Often the affected individual has other allergic problems, such as asthma or allergic rhinitis, and frequently other members of the family have them as well. Early in the disease, the epidermis shows swelling (or "spongiosis," like a sponge filled with water) and the underlying dermis is rich in activated CD4$^+$ memory TH cells. Interestingly, few eosinophils or mast cells are evident in the skin of these individuals, but they tend to have high concentrations of eosinophils in their blood. Their IgE levels in the blood also are elevated, and frequently they demonstrate allergic reactivity to a variety of foods. Giving children foods to which they have specific IgE antibodies may lead to exacerbation of their eczema.

As the disease progresses, affected individuals develop fibrosis (scarring) of the dermis and thickening of the basement membrane surrounding blood vessels in this layer of the skin. Langerhans cells in the skin typically express high levels of high-affinity IgE receptors. Many people with eczema have demonstrable infections with bacteria such as *Staphylococcus aureus*, fungi (e.g., *Candida*, *Pityrosporum*, and *Rhizopus* species), or viruses such as herpes simplex. The normal immune response to many of these organisms involves the production of cytokines characterized as part of the TH1 response, namely, interferon-γ (IFN-γ) and IL-2. Researchers have speculated that individuals with atopic disease may have immune systems that take a wrong turn in response to infection with any of a variety of organisms and mistakenly produce the TH2 set of cytokines. These chemical cues trigger an immune response that is incapable of clearing the infection that initiated this chain of events. In the process, the surrounding tissues are damaged by immune cells and effector molecules that are relatively ineffective against the microbial perpetrators. Application of steroid preparations to the skin in patients with eczema is often the only treatment available to calm this process. Steroids are potent immunosuppressive agents but have serious side effects that must be carefully monitored.

Determinants of susceptibility to atopic allergy

The large increase in the incidence and severity of asthma over the past 40 years serves to emphasize how little is known about why some persons have the propensity to respond adversely, sometimes fatally, to compounds in the environment that have no clear effect on others. Two major predisposing factors have been the focus of attention: genetics and exposure (Tables 25.4 and 25.5).

Although it is accepted that genetic susceptibility to asthma involves many genetic loci, one clear molecular correlate of the genetic predisposition to atopic disease is the increased risk of asthma in people with high basal levels of circulating IgE. The strongest genetic determinant of this IgE elevation so far is linked to a region of human chromosome 5q31–33 that holds a dense cluster of genes involved in immediate hypersensitivity. Among these genes are those encoding IL-3, IL-4, IL-5, and IL-13, granulocyte-macrophage colony-stimulating factor (GM-CSF), a β$_2$-adrenergic receptor, fibroblast growth factor, platelet-derived growth factor receptor, and a lymphocyte-specific glucocorticoid receptor. The IL-4 gene, or a closely linked gene, was identified with increased susceptibility to asthma in a large analysis of Amish families, each including more than one sibling affected by asthma. IL-4 polymorphisms associated with asthma susceptibility to date are limited to the promoter, where they can cause increased production of IL-4 with resultant asthma and higher total serum IgE. A gain-of-function mutation in the IL4-Rα gene is associated with severe atopic dermatitis and a disease called *hyper-IgE syndrome*. Other genes not linked to IL-4 are thought to be important as well. Nocturnal asthma correlates with the expression of a particular allele of the β$_2$-adrenergic receptor. A second significant genetic locus is on chromosome 11q13, which includes the FcεRI genes. A third genetic link is with the MHC class II gene cluster on chromosome 6p21. The complete sequencing of 5q31 and several other loci by the Human Genome Project is expected to enhance significantly the general understanding of these genetic susceptibility factors and how they lead to disease.

The second key determinant in susceptibility to asthma and other atopic disease is exposure to specific allergens. Respiratory allergens are frequently divided into two broad classes: outdoor and indoor allergens. Outdoor allergens tend to be seasonal, plant-derived compounds with a relatively large diameter and a propensity to cause symptoms of the hay fever type. Indoor allergens are more likely to be related to factors such as exposure to pets, cleanliness (presence of dust mites or cockroaches), and possibly exposure to urban air pollution. Many scientists have suggested that the very significant increase in asthma rates and severity is perhaps due to an increasing prevalence of some significant allergen(s) in the environment of cities worldwide. But different cities around the world have experienced the dramatic increases in association with sensitivity to a wide range of allergens.

Each April in the Northern Hemisphere, tree pollen is the principal cause of atopic rhinitis and conjunctivitis—inflammation, respectively, of the nasal mucosa and of the eye surface (Fig. 25.8). In May and June, grasses take over as the major irritant. By late summer, this "hay fever" is mostly caused by ragweed. A bad allergy season typically begins with a wet early spring that contributes to germination of trees and grasses. If the spring turns windy, warm, and dry, the conditions become ideal for the propagation and spread of pollen through the air. Thus, hay fever might be thought of as a consequence of external factors imposed on genetically susceptible individuals. One significant socioepidemiologic piece of the asthma puzzle has been the disproportionate effect in the United States on African Americans. This may represent a complex mixture of geographic, genetic, economic, and lifestyle factors and early-childhood exposure factors.

Type II Cytotoxicity Reactions

Type II hypersensitivity reactions are fundamentally different from immediate-type sensitivity, in that they can represent an attack by the immune system on the body's own tissues. Type II reactions were first appreciated as immune responses against a variety of drugs such as penicillin. These small molecules occasionally adhere to the surfaces of cells such as platelets and erythrocytes, creating so-called neo-self antigens on the cell surface. IgG antibodies that recognize the drug moiety then initiate an inflammatory cascade that results in the destruction of these cells, with resultant bleeding problems or anemia, respectively (Fig. 25.12). Type II reactions can also occur when self-tolerance is broken and an inappropriate immune response is made to self antigens on tissues.

Two principal factors distinguish type II reactions from immediate-type hypersensitivity. Type II reactions result from the action of the IgG class of immunoglobulin rather than that of IgE, and type II reactions occur when antibody to self proteins or carbohydrates binds to self tissues, with subsequent direct damage to the involved tissue. These reactions are most frequent in four sets of cir-

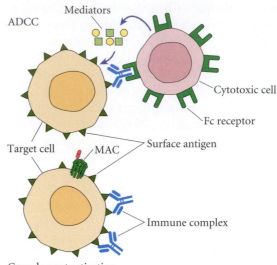

Figure 25.12 Intermediate type II (cytotoxic) hypersensitivity. Antibodies to self proteins or altered self proteins allow cells such as NK cells, macrophages, monocytes, neutrophils, and eosinophils to release a variety of mediators, including lytic enzymes, perforin, tumor necrosis factor, or granzymes to mediate target-cell killing. Alternatively, complement is activated and cells are lysed via the membrane attack complex. Two examples of type II hypersensitivity are as follows. Autoantibodies to pancreatic beta cells may contribute to insulin-dependent diabetes mellitus through destruction of the insulin-producing cells via antibody-dependent cell-mediated cytotoxicity. Hemolytic anemia is caused by adsorption of antibiotics, such as penicillin and certain cephalosporins, to proteins on RBC membranes, followed by IgM and IgG antibody production and complement lysis of the RBC.

cumstances: (i) a person receives antibodies from another individual (e.g., mother to child across the placenta) that bind to the recipient's tissues and cause damage; (ii) a person makes antibodies to the cells they received from another individual (e.g., erythrocytes in a blood transfusion or hyperacute rejection of a kidney transplant); (iii) a person has an antibody response to a foreign substance that has adhered to his or her own cells (e.g., the penicillin reaction); and (iv) a person makes antibodies to his or her own tissues (e.g., autoimmune skin diseases that result in the formation of blisters).

A classic, although now preventable, example of a type II reaction is the disease of newborn babies called *erythroblastosis fetalis* or, in the vernacular, "blue baby disease." All blood cells carry proteins decorated with complex carbohydrate structures that often vary among individuals and are the antigenic basis for different blood-group antigens. If the blood-group antigens the baby inherits from the father are different from those on the cells of the mother, the mother can be inoculated with these "foreign" blood groups on the baby's cells during delivery and produce antibodies. This will occur during delivery of a firstborn, usually with no consequences. However, for subsequent fetuses, an immune response may develop as a result of IgG antibodies that cross the placenta, enter the fetal circulation, and destroy fetal red cells. In erythroblastosis fetalis, a mother who is negative for expression of the Rh carbohydrate antigen on her red blood cells (Rh-negative RBCs) can be sensitized to make IgG antibodies to Rh if the baby's cells express it (Rh-positive RBCs). This IgG is not deleterious to the mother's health but will likely cause trouble for any subsequent Rh-positive baby by binding to the baby's RBCs and activating the classical complement cascade. The deposition of the classical C3

convertase on the RBC surface serves as a handle that is seized by phagocytic cells in the fetal spleen that destroy the baby's RBCs. In those RBCs not culled from the circulation, the convertase activity leads ultimately to deposition of the complement membrane attack complex on the remaining RBCs, leading to membrane disruption and cell death (Fig. 25.13).

Consequently, this reaction is called *antibody-dependent cytotoxic hypersensitivity*. The antibody involved may occasionally be of the IgM class rather than IgG. An example of this is a transfusion reaction against the ABO blood-group antigens. Individuals with type A blood express this

Figure 25.13 Development of erythroblastosis fetalis or hemolytic disease of the newborn results when an Rh$^-$ mother carries an Rh$^+$ fetus and becomes sensitized to the Rh factor antigen at delivery. (**A**) During a subsequent pregnancy with another Rh$^+$ fetus, maternal antibodies to Rh cross the placenta and destroy fetal red blood cells. (**B**) Sensitization can be blocked if the mother receives anti-Rh antibodies, Rhogam, within 24 to 48 hours after the first delivery.

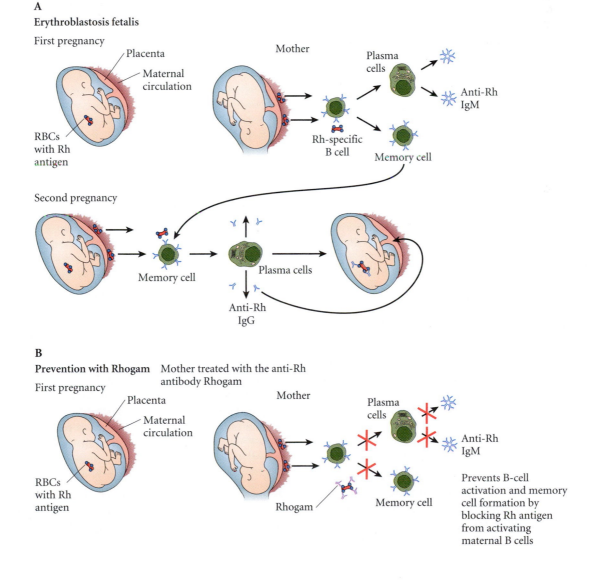

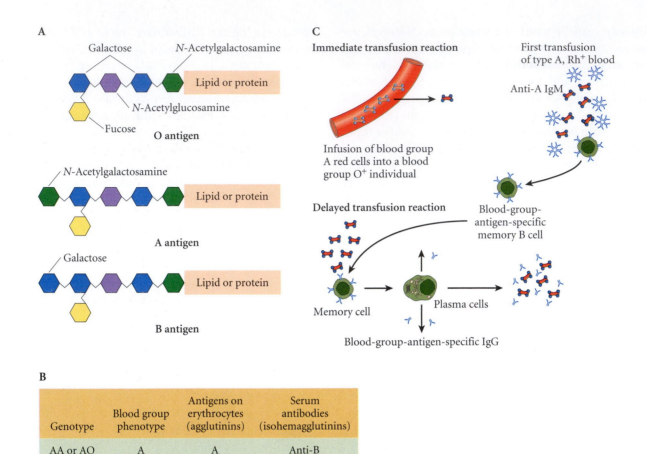

A

Galactose N-Acetylgalactosamine

Lipid or protein

N-Acetylglucosamine

Fucose

O antigen

N-Acetylgalactosamine

Lipid or protein

A antigen

Galactose

Lipid or protein

B antigen

C

Immediate transfusion reaction

Infusion of blood group A red cells into a blood group O⁺ individual

Delayed transfusion reaction

Memory cell   Plasma cells

Blood-group-antigen-specific IgG

First transfusion of type A, Rh⁺ blood

Anti-A IgM

Blood-group-antigen-specific memory B cell

B

Genotype	Blood group phenotype	Antigens on erythrocytes (agglutinins)	Serum antibodies (isohemagglutinins)
AA or AO	A	A	Anti-B
BB or BO	B	B	Anti-A
AB	AB	A and B	None
OO	O	None	Anti-A and anti-B

Figure 25.14 ABO blood groups and transfusion reactions. (**A**) Structure of the terminal sugars of the A, B, and O blood antigens, which constitute the distinguishing epitopes. (**B**) ABO genotype, phenotypes, agglutinins, and isoagglutinins. (**C**) Examples of immediate and delayed hemolytic transfusion reactions caused by transfusion of blood incompatible with major ABO blood-group and incompatible with minor blood-group antigen. The most common blood-group antigens that produce delayed transfusion reactions are Rh, Kidd, Kell, and Duffy. Symptoms of immediate reactions result from massive intravascular hemolysis of the transfused cells by IgM plus complement. The delayed reaction results from incomplete extravascular hemolysis mediated primarily by IgG.

antigen on their RBCs. Those with type B blood express this distinct antigen on their RBCs, those who are AB express both, and individuals who are type O express neither. For unknown reasons, everyone is sensitized early in life to make "natural" IgM antibodies to those ABO carbohydrate structures they do not possess. Thus, type O individuals have IgM antibodies to both A and B antigens, whereas AB individuals have neither antibody. Since IgM does not cross the placenta, it is not a problem for a mother to give birth to a baby with a different ABO blood group than her own. In a transfusion reaction between individuals with mismatched blood-group antigens, lysis of the transfused RBCs results in the rapid release into the serum of free hemoglobin, which is subsequently converted into

the toxic metabolite bilirubin. Thus, a person who has the A blood type and receives B-type blood will experience not only the death of the transfused cells by complement-dependent lysis but also will develop fever and chills caused by the massive activation of his or her immune system and the formation of bilirubin (Fig. 25.14).

The truly perplexing cytotoxicity reactions are those caused by antibodies produced by the body to its own tissues. This results in one form of autoimmune disease. For example, some individuals make IgG antibodies directed against different domains of the type VII collagen protein. This anchoring fibril protein helps hold the protective epidermis down to the blood vessel- and nerve-rich dermis beneath it. Antibodies reactive to type VII collagen cause the epidermis to separate from the dermis, with the formation of large blisters. Some of the antigens involved in type II hypersensitivity reactions are not limited to the tissues of one organ. Goodpasture disease, for example, affects two disparate organs, the lung and the kidney, as a consequence of the deposition of IgG antibody directed to type IV collagen in the basement membrane of both the kidney glomerulus and the thin-walled capillaries of the lung. In this case, the offending antibody binds to a protein in the extracellular matrix but damages the neighboring cells (Fig. 25.15). A similar effect on the kidney is seen in a related condition involving recognition of a cellular protein called the Heymann antigen. In both cases, binding of antibody to specific antigen results in the deposition of the complement-cascade components, with resultant damage to the affected cells.

Figure 25.15 Goodpasture disease. Deposition of IgG directed at the type IV collagen found in the kidney glomeruli and capillaries of the lung results in complement activation and influx of neutrophils. Neutrophil destruction of both tissues ultimately leads to respiratory and renal failure. The bottom left photo shows green fluorescent labeling of anti-basement membrane antibodies on a kidney glomerulus, highlighting the extensive pathology of the disease. Lung micrographs courtesy of Martha Warnock.

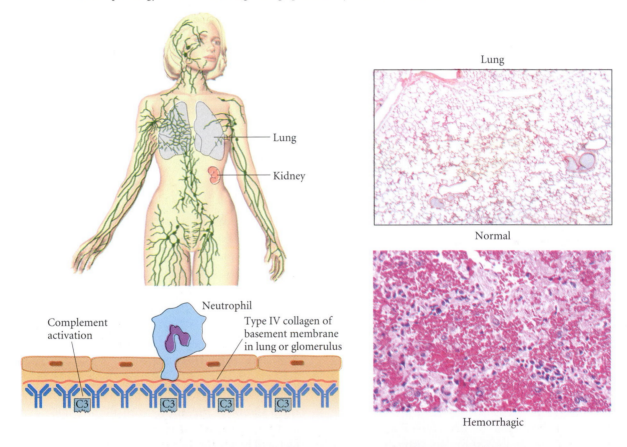
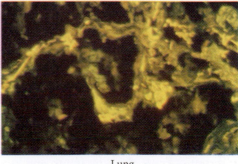
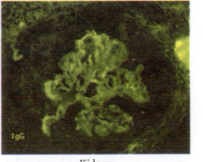

When the tissue recognized is an immobile structure such as the kidney glomerulus, another set of immune effector cells come into play. Complement activation by these antibody-antigen pairings effectively attract PMNs through the production of the C5a anaphylatoxin. These PMNs rush into the site of inflammation and respond to the immune complexes by releasing two forms of granules that bear different antimicrobial mediators. PMNs also activate their oxidative machinery in response to immune complexes, releasing significant amounts of reactive oxygen intermediates capable of damaging cells such as those in the glomerulus. Thus the tissue is inadvertently damaged as an innocent bystander following the binding of the IgG to the self antigen.

The antibodies also can bind to Fc receptors on the surface of NK cells, leading to tissue damage via antibody-dependent cell-mediated cytotoxicity. NK cells act like cytotoxic CD8$^+$ T cells, capable of lysing cells adjacent to those that have been targeted by the antibody affixed to the NK cell surface. Presumably, this system benefits the individual when the bound cell is cancerous or infected with a virus. But in persons with Goodpasture disease, the release of cytotoxic granules by NK cells may be detrimental to the normal glomerular epithelium and supporting mesangial cells.

Type III "Immune Complex" Hypersensitivity Reactions

A form of immunization devised in the late 19th century involved the transfer of antibodies from tetanus-inoculated horses to prevent tetanus in people exposed to the *Clostridium tetanus* bacterium and its toxin. Soon it was noted that some individuals given this horse serum developed rashes, arthritis, and even kidney failure. This serum sickness represents a form of hypersensitivity similar to the type II cytotoxicity reaction (Fig. 25.16). Both are caused by IgG antibodies made by the exposed person's immune system, in this case directed against soluble proteins in the horse serum. The distinction between type II and type III reactions lies fundamentally in the relationship of the antigen-antibody complex to the tissue where destruction occurs. In type II reactions, a tissue is damaged when antibody binds it directly and initiates the complement and other cytotoxic cascades. In type III reactions, the damaged tissues are innocent bystanders to destruction initiated when a soluble immune complex becomes deposited in these tissues. Certain organs are more sensitive to the deposition of immune complexes containing many different kinds of antigens or allergens and consequently are more likely to be affected in type III reactions. As in the example of serum sickness, the skin, joints, and kidneys are

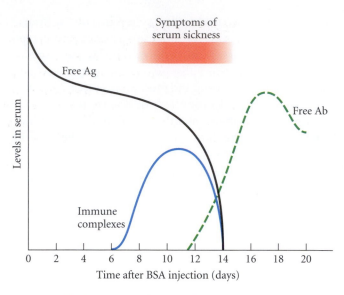

Figure 25.16 Time course of serum sickness. After antigen (bovine serum albumin [BSA]) is injected into a rabbit at day 0, antibody forms and complexes with the antigen to form immune complexes. The immune complexes are deposited in joints, kidneys, and capillaries, initiating the symptoms of serum sickness. Note that the serum sickness symptoms correspond with the peak of immune complex formation. As the immune complexes are cleared, free antibody appears in the blood and symptoms resolve. Based on F. G. Germuth, Jr., *J. Exp. Med.* **97**:257, 1953.

particularly sensitive to the trapping of immune complexes and thus are more susceptible to their deleterious consequences. Other organs that can be affected in more severe disease include the respiratory and gastrointestinal tracts, occasionally all in the same patient. The central role of antibodies other than IgE distinguishes both type II and type III reactions from type I hypersensitivity.

Basis for type III reactions

Two classes of type III reactions have received extensive study: those in which a clear precipitating antigen is identified and those presenting with all the clinical symptoms of a type III reaction but lacking any obvious initiating factor. The prototype of the first group is the reaction to many drugs, as typified by the formation of a response to therapeutic horse serum given to fight tetanus. Patients presenting to the emergency room with a generalized itchy rash, aches and pains, and microscopic blood in the urine, are usually asked whether they are taking any medications or health-food supplements. If so, simply discontinuing these drugs or food additives usually halts the reaction after a period of days, depending on its severity if it is due to type III hypersensitivity.

Routes of exposure other than the oral or intravenous routes (used for most medications) can lead to immune complex-mediated allergy. Inhalation of any of a great variety of foreign substances can produce a type III hypersensitivity reaction. Similar to the case of IgE-mediated type I hypersensitivity, the provoking substance is often one that is not obviously deleterious to the host, as an uncontrolled infection might be. Referred to as *hypersensitivity pneumonitis* or the *pneumoconioses*, these diseases are mostly occupational hazards of exposure to particular kinds of substances that lead to antibody formation and deposition of immune complexes in the lung parenchyma. These complexes initiate complement activation and produce a clinical syndrome featuring a chronic cough, shortness of breath, and often a low-grade fever.

An important difference between type III and type I reactions, aside from the isotype of the responsible antibody, is the anatomy: the pneumoconioses occur primarily in the alveolar air spaces whereas the IgE-mediated type I reactions appear to affect primarily the bronchiolar airways leading to the alveoli. The pneumoconioses include a carnival of colorful appellations: pigeon fanciers' lung, paprika splitters' lung, cork dust lung, duck fever, mushroom pickers' lung, maple bark disease, and farmers' lung (exposure to mold-like *Actinomycetes* bacteria from hay). Type III reactions may underlie the so-called sick-building syndrome caused by exposure to mold species including *Penicillium*, *Aspergillus*, and *Stachybotrys* spp. that grow in water-damaged buildings.

The type III reactions without an obvious provoking antigen are more difficult to understand. These conditions are typically described as rheumatologic diseases and can present with the same clinical symptoms as a drug reaction. Furthermore, when the affected tissues are examined under a microscope, antibody-containing immune complexes and other pathologic hallmarks are easily identified. The prototype for these diseases is systemic lupus erythematosus (SLE), in which the immune system makes antibodies to its own proteins, nucleic acids, and polysaccharides for no obvious reason. In many respects, the pathologic hallmark of SLE is the destruction of blood vessels to which these immune complexes bind. The true destruction of blood vessels in immune reactions is referred to as *vasculitis* (inflammation of the vascular system). Vasculitis itself represents a whole class of diseases, often catastrophic ones, that can damage any organ in the body, including the liver, brain, and heart. Most forms of vasculitis, those in fact that result from the deposition of immune complexes in the blood vessel walls, are consequently referred to as *hypersensitivity vasculitis*. The worst cases of SLE, rheumatoid arthritis, and even diseases of childhood such as Henoch-Schönlein purpura, are manifested in classic type III hypersensitivity vasculitis reactions.

Biology of type III reactions

Antibody-antigen complexes are constantly being formed in the body, both as a means of protecting against foreign invaders and of clearing normal senescent cells of all types. Apoptotic cells in particular are bound up by an array of highly cationic antibodies, forming immune complexes that must be cleared quickly from the body. RBCs and platelets are not often thought of as cells important to the immune system, but their surfaces are covered with Fc receptors that bind to nascent immune complexes in the circulation and pull them out of solution. When the RBCs and platelets travel into the liver and spleen, the immune complexes are stripped off their surfaces by macrophages that are part of the *reticuloendothelial system*, which is designed to capture and digest obsolete or deleterious compounds that have bound antibody or other opsonins.

Immune complexes begin to cause problems when they evade capture by the RBC and platelet Fc receptors. In the soluble form, immune complexes are able to lodge in the walls of diverse blood vessels around the body. Certain capillary networks appear to be particularly susceptible, namely the dermis layer of the skin, the synovium of the joints, and the kidney glomeruli. Not surprisingly, these are the tissues most affected by type III hypersensitivity, presenting typically with a rash, arthritis or other joint pain, and blood or protein in the urine.

When antigen-antibody complexes lodge in the basement membrane of a susceptible capillary, two important things happen. First, complement proteins are triggered into action. Release of C3a increases vascular permeability and allows more complement components to leave the circulation and localize at the site of immune complex deposition. A critical mass of deposited C3b results in activation of C5, with deposition of C5b on the antigen or neighboring tissue and release of C5a. Deposition of C5b triggers the formation of the membrane attack complex. Like C3a, C5a makes the capillary endothelium more sieve-like. But C5a and its by-products also function to recruit an array of immune cells to the site of the deposited immune complexes, the second important consequence of the deposition of immune complexes.

With the recruitment of PMNs and macrophages in response to the immobilized antigen-antibody complexes comes a new potential for collateral damage to the tissues. Binding of immune complexes to the Fc receptors on PMNs and macrophages initiates the release of reactive oxygen intermediates (e.g., hydrogen peroxide) and digestive enzyme-containing granules that can cause extensive damage to the capillary wall to which the immune complex is attached. The resulting destruction of the capillary has two principal effects. First, blood can leak out of the circulation; consequently, many drug reactions or diseases such as Henoch-Schönlein purpura are associated with the eruption of tiny, dark purple bumps in the skin referred to as *palpable purpura*. The escape of the blood produces the purple discoloration, and the ensuing macrophage activation and release of fibrin cause the lesion to be raised and braille-like (i.e., palpable). The second effect is the loss of circulation to the area of tissue normally supplied by the capillary. If enough neighboring capillaries are affected, the tissues are deprived of nutrients and suffer a toxic buildup of metabolic wastes that can result in the death of the tissue (i.e., ischemic damage).

Consequences of type III reactions for specific tissues

The deposition of antibody-antigen complexes in the skin, first demonstrated at the turn of the 19th century by Maurice Arthus, is referred to as the *Arthus reaction* (Fig. 25.17). His experimental system in animals allowed careful delineation of the kinetics and histology of type III responses. Antigen injected into the epidermal layer of the skin in a previously sensitized individual (someone already with specific antibodies to the antigen) begins to seep into the vascular dermal layer and to initiate complement activation. By about 4 hours after the injection, a local inflammatory reaction with redness and slight warmth of the skin is seen. This delay of hours rather than minutes is one of the key characteristics distinguishing type III hypersensitivity reactions from IgE-mediated type I reactions. The tissue swells as a result of the complement-mediated increase in vascular permeability. Destruction of local capillaries produces small hemorrhages in the skin. The influx of PMNs and macrophages contributes to the formation of *boggy edema* in the tissue, which lasts a period of hours and distinguishes these reactions from the wheal and flare seen in the type I hypersensitivity reaction. The death of local blood vessels and the tissue damage that ensues can result in formation of a microscopic scar referred to as *fibrinoid necrosis*. The Arthus reaction is thought to underlie the pain and tenderness associated with booster doses of tetanus and diphtheria toxoids.

The kidney glomerulus poses a special problem when immune complexes, complement, and other associated proteins are deposited there. A physical obstruction of the filtering apparatus occurs that compromises the ability of the kidney to maintain electrolyte balance and to purge the body of waste products of metabolism excreted by the kidney. The subsequent cellular immune response and tissue injury can ultimately lead to total destruction of the glomerulus and a permanent loss of function.

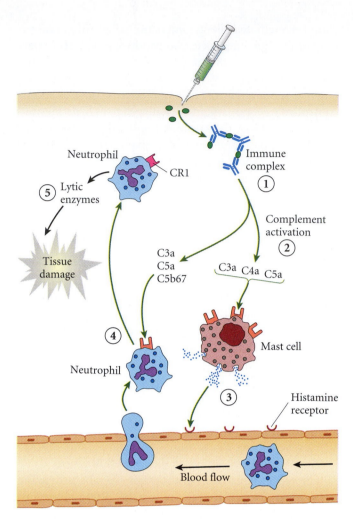

Figure 25.17 Immune complex hypersensitivity reaction (Arthus reaction). Injection of a medicine may induce immune complex formation (**1**), which results in complement activation via the classical pathway (**2**). The complement intermediates bind to mast cells (**3**), resulting in degranulation, and to neutrophils, mediating chemotaxis (**4**) and the release of lytic enzymes (**5**).

How do immune complexes become pathogenic?

Four factors appear to affect the likelihood of accumulation of immune complexes in a tissue: the size, charge, and concentration of the immune complexes and the relative ability of the reticuloendothelial macrophages to keep up with the rate of complex deposition (Table 25.6).

First, larger complexes appear to be cleared from the circulation much more easily than small complexes. A bacterium may have thousands of sites to which antibody and complement can bind, with a high likelihood of attachment of a macrophage to this opsonized organism. A smaller antigen, such as a nonrepetitive protein that has only one place capable of binding a particular antibody, presents a much more difficult target for capture by a macrophage.

Table 25.6 Factors influencing immune complex pathogenicity

Factor	Consequence(s)
Size	Smaller complexes cleared less readily than large
Charge	Positively charged immune complexes "stick" to negatively charged basement membranes
Concentration	Antibody-to-antigen ratio less than 1:1 is more difficult to clear than antibody excess
Macrophage phagocytic function	Genetic defects in genes encoding complement components limit ability of reticuloendothelial macrophages to clear complexes; intrinsic defect of macrophage phagocytic capacity also impairs immune complex clearance

Second, the charge on the complexes influences the ability of an immune complex to stick to certain types of capillary beds. For example, the kidney glomerulus has a highly anionic basement membrane, which functions by charge repulsion to keep most circulating proteins (themselves anionic) out of the urine. But an immune complex with a cationic character has a propensity to "stick" in the subendothelial space if the complex is not safely attached to the Fc receptors on the cellular components of the blood (e.g., RBCs).

Third, antibodies bind to antigens, like any other chemical reaction, with kinetics that depend on the relative concentrations of the two reactants. When antibodies are in great excess compared with the antigen for which they are specific, the typical polyvalent microbial antigen will probably have a large number of antibodies bound to it. These complexes then are cleared with relative ease by tissue macrophages. But as the antigen concentration increases and/or the antibody concentration declines, fewer antibody molecules will be bound to each antigen. Once the antibody-to-antigen ratio is 1:1, and especially if there is an excess of antigen, the likelihood increases that these complexes will not be captured by macrophages but will instead end up deposited in a susceptible capillary bed. In this respect, antigen excess has a tendency to be self-perpetuating, since smaller antigens with few attached antibodies will remain in circulation longer, heightening the antigen excess. This situation forms the basis of many type III hypersensitivity disorders such as farmers' lung, pigeon fanciers' lung, and sick-building syndrome. Also, complement deposition on circulating immune complexes can help promote physiologic clearance. Since complement component C1q cannot be activated by fewer than two IgG Fc regions, no classical complement activation occurs when there is a large excess of antigen. This exacerbates the persistence of the antigen complex in the circulation, since the opsonic and hence clearing abilities of complement cannot be used to enhance phagocytosis. However, when these complexes lodge in tissues and accumulate, then complement activation that is pathologic ensues, resulting in tissue damage.

Genetic disorders predisposing to type III hypersensitivity

The ability of the reticuloendothelial macrophages to clear immune complexes is essential for preventing type III hypersensitivity disorders. Individuals with a genetic deficiency of early components in the complement pathway have increased rates of type III hypersensitivity diseases. More than 90% of people deficient in component C1q develop a lupus-like syndrome with *glomerulonephritis* (inflammation of the kidney glomerulus) and severe skin disease. Likewise, deficiencies in complement components C4 and C2 lead to similar, although less severe, SLE. It is believed that these missing complement factors hinder clearance of immune complexes by preventing the reticuloendothelial system from clearing complement-opsonized immune complexes. In some autoimmune conditions, antibodies made to one's own complement proteins can block the biologic effects of these complement components, producing a syndrome very similar to that observed with complement deficiency.

Intrinsic inhibition of macrophage phagocytosis is another kind of defect predisposing to type III reactions. Even if their complement levels are normal, such individuals lack the mechanisms that promote ingestion of immune complexes. This defect results in the persistence of antigen exposure from apoptotic cells, which normally induce little or no inflammatory response.

DTH

DTH is the manifestation of CD4$^+$ T-cell immunity elicited by cytokine secretion from sensitized T cells that activates macrophages and other phagocytic cells in a tissue, initiating a local inflammatory response that ultimately results in the killing of intracellular microbes (see chapter 16 and Fig. 16.7). Prominent cytokines include IL-2, IFN-γ, macrophage inhibitory factor, and TNF-β. Type IV hypersensitivity is similarly mediated by immune CD4$^+$ T-cell secreting cytokines that activate phagocytic cells and initiate inflammation, but as a hypersensitivity reaction it is stimulated by what should otherwise be a harmless antigen. Classic examples of type IV hypersensitivity are skin reactions or contact hypersensitivities to poison oak, poison ivy, cosmetics, hair dyes, chemicals like turpentine and formaldehyde and substances like nickel. Type IV hypersensitivity reactions are delayed since it takes 12 to 48 hours for the reaction to become apparent. That is why exposure to poison ivy goes unnoticed until a day or two later, when the rash appears. Thus, in the same way that type I hypersensitivity reactions represent an inappropriate activation of the immune response that normally helps control eukaryotic parasites, type IV hypersensitivity reactions are inappropriate manifestations of the DTH response that normally protects against intracellular bacterial and fungal infections (Fig. 25.18).

Figure 25.18 DTH. (A) After initial contact with antigen, TH cells become sensitized, proliferate, and differentiate into T_{DTH} cells. (B) When these sensitized T_{DTH} cells come into contact with the same antigen again, they secrete cytokines that attract and activate macrophages, which function as the effector cell in the hypersensitivity reaction. MCAF, macrophage chemotactic and activating factor; MIF, macrophage-inhibition factor.

A Sensitization phase

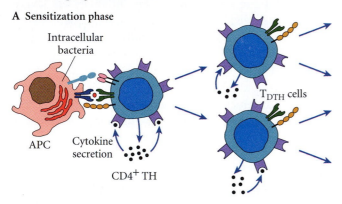

B Effector phase

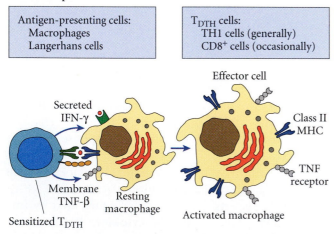

Thus, $CD4^+$ T cells are the critical recognition element in DTH and type IV hypersensitivity. Classically, DTH reactions were thought to stand in contrast to all other forms of hypersensitivity, in which antibodies are the key recognition element. The T-cell–antibody distinction for DTH was first proven by a simple experiment in the late 1950s. When a protein antigen is denatured (its conformation destroyed by heating or treatment with high salt concentrations), the antigen is perfectly capable of provoking a T-cell-dependent DTH reaction. In contrast, denaturation usually destroys the ability of antibodies to recognize their target antigens. This experiment was at the heart of understanding how T cells recognize their antigens, namely as digested pieces of larger proteins that are "presented" by MHC molecules on the surface of antigen-presenting cells. New experimental data indicate that DTH reactions and related "contact sensitivity" are not completely independent of humoral immunity, in that the recruitment of the effector T cells appears to depend on preceding complement activation by antigen-specific IgM antibodies.

Biology of DTH responses

A typical DTH reaction, like other specific immune responses, has two distinct phases: sensitization and the accelerated memory response (Fig. 25.18). The sensitization phase occurs with the first exposure to the antigen. When adsorbed onto the skin, those haptens capable of eventually activating a DTH first bind to skin proteins and create new epitopes. These proteins are ingested by local dendritic cells, processed, and presented to T cells in local lymph nodes or other areas of lymphocyte concentration. There, T cells differentiate into a TH1 subtype, in part as the result of the synthesis of IL-12 and other cytokines by the presenting APC. These T cells then proliferate and may differentiate into memory T cells (Fig. 25.19).

The clinically apparent response occurs a week or more later upon reexposure to the provoking antigen. This memory/effector phase of the response unfolds in a very predictable fashion. Recent research has shown that IgM antibodies to the sensitizing antigen are rapidly induced after reexposure on the skin. These antibodies activate complement, with C5a recruiting a population of PMNs that stay for only a few hours. Mast cells are also activated by C5a binding and produce TNF-α, which conditions the local vascular endothelium for recruitment of previously sensitized T cells. Within 12 hours, most of the PMNs are gone and are replaced by T cells and a monocyte infiltrate, accompanied by some basophils, that form cuffs around the local blood vessels. These activated T cells, because they are largely of the TH1 subtype, begin secreting large amounts of INF-γ upon restimulation by local APCs.

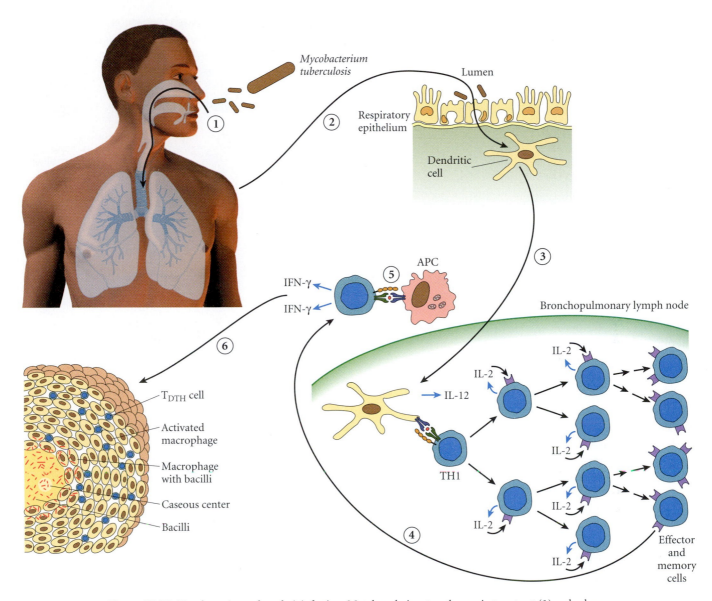

Figure 25.19 *Mycobacterium tuberculosis* infection. *M. tuberculosis* enters the respiratory tract (1) and subsequently the lamina propria of the respiratory bronchioles via M cells (2). Digested antigen is taken up by dendritic cells (3), which travel to regional lymph nodes and present *M. tuberculosis* antigens to TH1 cells. These TH1 cells proliferate (4) and may return to the site of initial infection. Restimulation by local APCs (5) results in production of IFN-γ and activation of macrophages. Failure to clear the organism results in granuloma formation (6).

A combination of increased vascular permeability and monocyte synthesis of fibrinogen results in the first vestiges of a fibrin "firewall" that will surround the perceived antigenic insult. This combination of cells and fibrin serves to create the clinical hallmark of a DTH reaction: the *indurated nodule* (from the Latin *durus,* meaning "hard"). The peak appearance of this firmness, at the center of an area of surrounding erythema in the skin or diffuse inflammation in other tissues, occurs at 2 to 3 days. Since most of the clinically problematic type IV hypersensitivities involve

the skin, the ultimate result is the formation of a rash, which usually fades in a matter of days.

In some cases the inciting material eludes simple degradation or, if the provoking antigen is a virulent microbe such as *Mycobacterium tuberculosis*, the response enters a third phase: *granuloma formation.* Granulomas are organized collections of immune cells, predominantly of the monocyte lineage, that functionally wall off a focus of inflammation from the surrounding tissues (see Fig. 16.9). These cells include monocytes that take on the appearance of epithelial cells (*epithelioid histiocytes*), macrophages, and multinucleated giant cells.

DTH in contact hypersensitivity and the pneumoconioses

Contact hypersensitivity (Fig. 25.20) is most commonly manifested as sensitivity to metals that provokes rashes from certain types of jewelry and the skin reaction to plants such as poison ivy. Many individuals experience rashes after exposure to some irritant. If the rash takes some time to develop, it could be mediated by type IV DTH. However, many rashes are initiated by chemical irritation to the skin but usually arise fairly soon after exposure to the irritant.

The small molecules eliciting these reactions, such as nickel sulfate or the plant compound urushiol, initiate the reaction by penetrating the epidermis (the outer layer of the skin). Plants of the genus *Rhus*, including poison sumac, poison ivy, and poison oak, contain urushiol. Closely related members of the same family include the cashew, mango, and pistachio trees; ingestion of their nuts or seeds can lead to systemic reactions in individuals previously sensitized to the resin of one of the *Rhus* plants. These small molecules first require chemical conjugation to a larger self protein in the skin. The altered self protein is then taken up by APCs, such as Langerhans cells in the dermis, and transported to local lymph nodes. Like other antigens, these altered self proteins are processed within the APC and presented on the surface of the cell in the context of an MHC class I or class II antigen-presenting molecule. CD4$^+$ or CD8$^+$ T cells in the vicinity with receptors specific for this neoepitope on the self protein will be stimulated to proliferate and differentiate into memory cells. The next exposure to the sensitizing agent results in local presentation by Langerhans cells and the eruption of small blisters (vesiculation) and/or formation of flaky irritation of the skin (eczema).

Other types of allergic reactions can involve more than one of the hypersensitivity mechanisms, since, in reality, the body frequently responds to allergic insults with a mixture of immune strategies. Pneumoconioses are pulmonary allergic responses that are first manifested as a type III reaction of immune complex deposition in the alveolar parenchyma of the lung. Ongoing antigen exposure, sometimes over a period of years in the case of an occupational exposure such as pitching hay or caring for pigeons, can eventually lead to a DTH-like response with T-cell activation and subsequent granuloma formation. The natural history of these lesions further illustrates a fourth stage of the evolution of DTH responses: the slow resolution of a granuloma often gives way to a *fibrosing reaction* akin to a scar laid down by fibroblasts after the de-

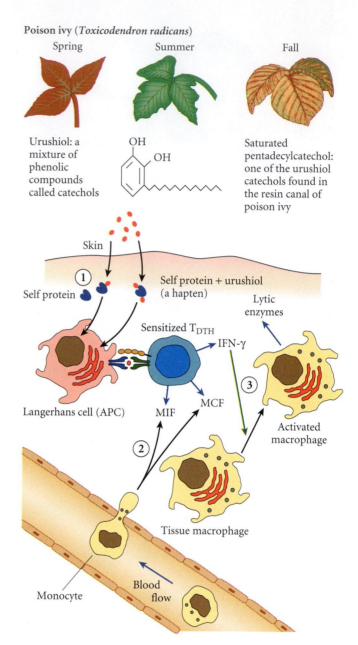

Figure 25.20 Contact sensitivity. Development of a DTH reaction after a second exposure to poison ivy occurs in 80 to 90% of Americans. Urushiol diffuses through the skin (**1**) and binds to self proteins that are engulfed by Langerhans cells. The Langerhans cell presents the hapten urushiol to a sensitized T$_{DTH}$ cell, which secretes a variety of cytokines (**2**). Approximately 48 to 72 hours after the exposure, macrophages accumulate at the site and release lytic enzymes, causing the characteristic rash and pustules (**3**).

struction of normal tissue. When the lung has been targeted, the progressive fibrosis can lead to progressive impairment of the oxygen- and carbon dioxide-exchanging capacity of the affected alveoli and the debilitating lung disease called *emphysema*.

Not all occupational exposure leads initially to an immune complex-type reaction. A syndrome similar to farmers' lung affects many individuals exposed to any of a variety of inorganic and relatively insoluble materials, e.g., coal miners' lung (anthracosis), silicosis, asbestosis, and iron workers' lung (siderosis). These nanometer-size particles clearly have access to the most distal parts of the lung in a way that larger organic molecules and particles do not. At autopsy, smokers, coal workers, and others repeatedly exposed to these particles are seen to have pigmented macrophages packed into their alveolar parenchyma and lining the parenchymal lymphatics. Clusters of these portly macrophages may be organized into granulomatous nodules, often with cavitation (the appearance of cavities) in the center. The process extends to local lymph nodes where T cells become activated. A TH1-type gene-activation pattern is observed in these lymph nodes, with IFN-γ and IL-12 produced and most likely contributing to the further activation of local macrophages. The lymph nodes themselves can progress to stone-like masses that evolve from pigmented granulomas to fibrosed scars visible on chest X rays, resulting from a fine deposition of calcium referred to as *eggshell calcification*. This is perhaps the fifth and final stage of granuloma evolution, as the body attempts to wall off the lesion more completely by the formation of a bone-like imprisonment of the original offending provocation.

Summary

IgE-mediated immunity is thought to have evolved as a means of protecting mammals against certain kinds of infections poorly controlled by other forms of adaptive immunity, such as infections with worms and parasitic protozoa. The ability to mount immediate hypersensitivity responses to an array of seemingly innocuous environmental proteins is thought to be an untoward consequence of hypervigilance of this system. Genetic and environmental factors interact to create this disease susceptibility, particularly in urban societies. For reasons that remain unclear, the incidence of asthmatic responsiveness to indoor allergens, in particular, increased dramatically during the second half of the 20th century.

Type II and type III reactions share some basic pathogenic mechanisms, both being mediated by antibody isotypes other than IgE. They both fall into a category of intermediate hypersensitivity, in that their onset and duration are measured in hours, rather than in minutes like the type I reactions, or in days, like the type IV reactions. The mediators of tissue destruction of type II and type III reactions are also similar, with early activation of complement proteins and, later, recruitment of granulocytes and macrophages.

The two forms of intermediate-type hypersensitivity differ in that the type II cytotoxicity reactions tend to be more organ specific, since they involve the binding of antibody directly to the cell or tissue that ultimately suffers the damage. Type III reactions involve the deposition of soluble antigen-antibody complexes that initiate a local inflammatory response in the vicinity of the otherwise innocent tissues that are ultimately damaged.

DTH stands apart from the other forms of hypersensitivity classified by Gell and Coombs, in that antibodies are not directly involved in the effector phase of the response. Rather, the activation of T lymphocytes through their antigen-specific cell surface receptors is the critical recognition event. DTH may represent a "last-stand" form of immunity that occurs primarily when antibodies or other immune elements have failed to recognize and clear a provocative antigen.

Many inflammatory diseases of unknown cause have pathology suggestive of a DTH mechanism. As more is understood about cytotoxic T lymphocytes, NK cells, γδ T cells, and other forms of T-cell immunity, the Gell and Coombs classification will need to be modified to continue its rich legacy as the framework for understanding many of the allergic and rheumatic diseases.

Suggested Reading

Burks, W. 2002. Current understanding of food allergy. *Ann. N. Y. Acad. Sci.* **964:**1–12.

Herz, U., P. Lacy, H. Renz, and K. Erb. 2000. The influence of infections on the development and severity of allergic disorders. *Curr. Opin. Immunol.* **12:**632–640.

James, D. G. 2000. A clinicopathological classification of granulomatous disorders. *Postgrad. Med. J.* **76:**457–465.

Kay, A. B. 2001. Allergic diseases and their treatment. *N. Engl. J. Med.* **344:**109–113.

Kobayashi, K., K. Kaneda, and T. Kasama. 2001. Immunopathogenesis of delayed-type hypersensitivity. *Microsc. Res. Tech.* **53:**241–245.

Repka-Ramirez, M. S., and J. N. Baraniuk. 2002. Histamine in health and disease. *Clin. Allergy Immunol.* **17:**1–25.

Sabroe, I., C. M. Lloyd, M. K. Whyte, S. K. Dower, T. J. Williams, and J. E. Pease. 2002. Chemokines, innate and adaptive immunity, and respiratory disease. *Eur. Respir. J.* **19:**350–355.

Toda, M., and S. J. Ono. 2002. Genomics and proteomics of allergic disease. *Immunology* **106:**1–10.

Umetsu, D. T., J. J. McIntire, O. Akbari, C. Macaubas, and R. H. DeKruyff. 2002. Asthma: an epidemic of dysregulated immunity. *Nat. Immunol.* **3:**715–720.

Wollenberg, A., S. Kraft, T. Oppel, and T. Bieber. 2000. Atopic dermatitis: pathogenetic mechanisms. *Clin. Exp. Dermatol.* **25:**530–534.

Yazdanbakhsh, M., P. G. Kremsner, and R. van Ree. 2002. Allergy, parasites, and the hygiene hypothesis. *Science* **296:** 490–494.

chapter 26

Autoimmunity and Disease

Harley Y. Tse and Michael K. Shaw

Autoimmunity and Autoimmune Diseases

The immune system has evolved out of the necessity to protect the host against foreign pathogens. To do this, the immune system must be able to distinguish foreign from self antigens. Higher animals use an elaborate antigen-recognition system involving receptors on both T and B cells. Gene rearrangement and somatic mutations generate a receptor repertoire capable of recognizing diverse and unpredictable pathogenic determinants. From this pool of specificities, it is necessary to sort out the receptors that are potentially reactive to self components. The immune system uses cell surface major histocompatibility complex (MHC) molecules as a tag of "selfness," such that antigens are not recognized singly but in association with self MHC class I or class II proteins. T lymphocytes bearing receptors that bind self peptide-MHC with high avidity are potentially autoreactive and are purged in the thymus during development. Low-affinity anti-self T cells, nevertheless, can emerge from this selection process. B lymphocytes also undergo negative selection. However, there is no equivalent of the thymus for containment of unselected, immature autoreactive B cells before their dispersion to the periphery. Thus, self-reactive B cells are found not only in the bone marrow but also in the white pulp of the spleen. Central tolerance is therefore by no means complete, and lymphocytes with receptor specificities for self antigens are readily detectable in healthy individuals. Normally, the presence of self-reactive (autoimmune) cells does not always lead to autoimmune diseases because their numbers are small and are kept in check by peripheral tolerance mechanisms. In this sense, autoimmunity should be distinguished from autoimmune diseases. Autoimmunity is a normal component of immune regulation as a consequence of MHC-restricted recognition. Low levels of autoreactive lymphocytes and autoantibodies are maintained in the body. Some of these entities may serve important physiologic functions. Rheumatoid factor (RF), which recognizes immunoglobulin G (IgG) antibodies, helps expedite the removal of harmful immune complexes from the circulation. Anti-idiotypic antibodies serve to regulate overactive immune responses. Recent research has also revealed beneficial roles of autoreactive T cells in neuroprotection and wound healing. Autoimmune diseases, on the other hand, are pathologic conditions resulting from failure of the tolerance mechanisms to specific self antigens. Some of these conditions can be severe and life-threatening. A great deal of insight has been derived regarding the common factors underlying autoimmune disease, which has provided important insights leading to development of different therapeutic approaches to treat these serious diseases.

Targets of Autoimmune Diseases

Self-reactive and foreign-reactive cells arise from the same pool of lymphocytes, and the two classes of cells are activated and proliferate to the same types of immune stimuli. Autoimmune responses can be mediated by both antibodies and T cells, although some diseases may lean more heavily toward one mediator than the other. Systemic lupus erythematosus (SLE), for example, is mediated primarily by IgG antibodies. Since production of IgG molecules requires class switching, there is evidence that T cells also play a role in the regulation of these antibodies. Multiple sclerosis (MS), on the other hand, a disease due to destruction of cells in the central nervous system, is clearly mediated by T cells. However, a contribution from antibodies to damage to neural cells has not been entirely ruled out.

Autoimmune diseases are traditionally grouped according to the targets of the attack. Immune responses to antigens expressed within a particular organ or gland are referred to as *organ-specific autoimmunity*. Common examples of organ-specific autoimmune diseases are diabetes mellitus (pancreatic beta-cells), myasthenia gravis (acetylcholine receptors), and thyroiditis (thyroid gland). Systemic autoimmunity, on the other hand, refers to conditions not limited to a single organ. These include rheumatoid arthritis (RA), MS, scleroderma, and SLE. For certain diseases, this classification may not be as clear-cut. MS, which is a disease of the central nervous system (CNS), appears to be more organ specific

than systemic, as lesions are normally focused in the brain and spinal cord. It is also interesting that individuals with one autoimmune disorder may be more susceptible to multiple autoimmune diseases. This points toward a possible common etiology for some of these ailments. A second feature of autoimmune diseases is the general predominance in females. In humans, women are at least 10 to 20 times more likely than men to develop SLE. Although the basis of this gender bias is not fully understood, there is evidence that the endocrine system plays an important regulatory role in autoimmune susceptibility.

Genetic Considerations

Many autoimmune diseases show increased prevalence among members of the same family. This observation provides hints that susceptibility to these diseases has a genetic basis. Studies in both human and animal models confirm that genetic predisposition is an important factor in disease susceptibility. How these genes contribute to the development of autoimmune diseases is still poorly understood. However, it is known that multiple genes are involved. As many as 12 genes are believed to contribute to disease expression in mouse models of SLE. To complicate matters, most of the "disease" genes have relatively low penetrance, such that no single gene can be used as a predictive marker for disease susceptibility. For example, certain MHC class I and class II genes show a strong association with autoimmune diseases, meaning individuals with the disease are more likely to have a certain HLA haplotype or allele than is generally found in the entire human population. However, it is not uncommon to find symptomatic individuals who lack expression of a disease-associated allele and individuals who express disease-associated alleles who do not show signs of the disease. The association of a particular allele with an autoimmune disease is thus expressed in terms of "relative risk." This relationship is obtained by calculating, in both normal and patient populations, the proportion that expresses a particular allele and the proportion that does not; these data are set up in a 2 × 2 contingency table (Table 26.1). The relative risk of disease association with a particular allele is the ratio of AD to BC. Relative risk measures how

Table 26.1 A 2 × 2 contingency table to calculate relative disease risk[a]

Disease expression	HLA allele expression	
	+	−
+	A	B
−	C	D

[a]Relative risk = AD/BC.

Table 26.2 Relative risk of some autoimmune diseases

Disease	Associated HLA	Relative risk
Addison disease	DR3/DQ	6.3
AS	B27	87.4
Behçet disease	B5	7.4
IDDM	DR3	5.3
MG	DR3	2.5
RA	DR4	4.2
SLE	DR3	5.8

many times more frequently a disease develops in individuals carrying the allele than in individuals lacking the allele. In general, a relative risk greater than 1 indicates an association between the disease and the allele in question. The greater the relative risk, the greater the association. As is true for all statistical evaluations, the significance of a reported relative risk will vary depending on the number of patients and control individuals tested in a particular study. Table 26.2 summarizes the relationship between HLA serotypes and the relative risk indices of some of the common autoimmune diseases. The most compelling correlation is between HLA-B27 and the pathogenesis of ankylosing spondylitis (AS), an inflammatory condition that affects joints of the spine.

Linkage disequilibrium, in which two or more genes are always inherited together because of their close proximity on the same chromosome, may result in errors in the identification of disease-associated alleles. For example, the relative risk between Sjögren syndrome and HLA-B8 that was originally reported ranged from 1.4 to 6.1 in a number of studies. An association of this disease with HLA-Dw3 had a relative risk of 6.9 to 19.2. Since a strong linkage disequilibrium between HLA-B8 and HLA-Dw3 exists, the apparent association of Sjögren syndrome with HLA-B8 could be due to its physical proximity to HLA-Dw3.

Environmental Factors and Autoimmune Diseases

Besides genetic factors, environmental agents may provoke or exacerbate a variety of autoimmune diseases. Notably, infection has been implicated as a direct precipitant of autoimmune diseases. Epidemiologic studies of MS have shown that the risk of developing the disease was higher in European residents of the northern latitudes than in those living in the southern latitudes. For reasons unknown, emigrants who moved from the north to the south before the age of 12 years assumed the risk level of the south and those who emigrated after the age of 12 years retained the risk level of the north. It is speculated that, in genetically susceptible individuals, contact with a pathologic agent during the early years may lead to development of MS later in life. Other factors affecting the development of autoimmune diseases include exposure to radiation, drugs, and toxins. The flares of SLE that follow exposure to ultraviolet light are a good example.

Cause-and-Effect Relationship of Autoimmunity and Autoimmune Diseases

Before labeling a clinical condition as an autoimmune disease, it is necessary to determine whether autoimmunity is actually the cause of the condition or a consequence of another pathologic process. This is not always an easy task. Determining an autoimmune pathology is usually based on finding autoreactive T lymphocytes and/or antibodies at the diseased tissues and organs. An ability to duplicate the clinical condition in animal models is also an important component. However, because of differences in genetics and cellular receptor repertoires, some of these animal models may not precisely duplicate the human disease. For example, experimental autoimmune encephalomyelitis (EAE) is often used as an animal model for MS in humans. This disease is induced in animals by immunizing them with an antigen from the myelin sheath of nerve fibers known as myelin basic protein (MBP). When administered with strong adjuvants, animals develop an acute hind-limb paralysis analogous to some degree to the muscle weakness experienced by patients with MS. Although MBP induces a clinical course and disease pathology in animals that is similar to that of human MS, MBP has not yet been conclusively identified as the autoantigen responsible for the development of MS in humans. Also, animals with EAE develop an acute disease that resolves quickly whereas human MS is a chronic and often progressive disease.

Pathogenesis of Autoimmune Diseases

Both cells and antibodies can mediate the tissue damage and pathology of autoimmune diseases. T cells can act as effector cells directly responsible for tissue destruction or as helper cells for the production of autoantibodies. Autoantibodies can attack target tissues and organs directly or diseases can result from the activation of the complement system by immune complexes that lodge in small blood vessels of tissues. Using the system that classifies autoimmune diseases into systemic or organ specific is helpful for relating immunologic mechanisms to disease manifestations. In the systemic or non-tissue-specific autoimmune diseases there is usually an antibody-mediated, immune complex-based pathology. In the organ-specific diseases there is either an antibody- or cell-mediated immune effector targeted to antigens expressed in a specific organ.

The biologic effectors that amplify many immunologic reactions that lead to important biologic outcomes of immune recognition, including complement, activated phagocytes, chemokine and cytokine production, and cellular cytotoxicity, are essential components of the pathology of autoimmunity. Thus the disease process involves not only a specific immune recognition step but also activation of effector functions that target self tissues much like the body targets harmful foreign microbes.

Systemic Immune Complex-Mediated Autoimmunity

SLE

SLE is a complex connective tissue disease with autoimmune characteristics affecting multiple organ systems. Clinical symptoms of SLE are highly variable among patients, ranging from mild skin lesions and arthritis to severe renal dysfunction, cardiomyopathy, and neuropsychiatric manifestations. Severity of the disease also tends to fluctuate over time. For these reasons, the American College of Rheumatology has set standard criteria for the classification of SLE, reserving the diagnosis of SLE for patients who have at least 4 of the 11 criteria.

SLE affects primarily young women between the ages of 20 and 40 years. Men are 10 times less likely than women to develop the disease. Arthritis and arthralgias are by far the most prevalent symptoms, affecting about 90% of patients. Arthritis involves primarily the small joints of the hands, the wrists, and the knees, but the inflammation in the joints (synovitis) is nonerosive. In addition, deposition of immune complexes containing autoantibodies with various nuclear antigens such as nucleic acids at the dermal-epidermal junction causes inflammation in the skin due to activation of the complement system. Patients develop a photosensitive rash over the bridge of the nose in a typical "butterfly" appearance (Fig. 26.1). Immune complexes can also be trapped in small arteries and arterioles, leading to vasculitis, or in the glomerular endothelium and epithelium, resulting in severe renal diseases. Glomerulonephritis occurs in more than 60% of SLE patients. Neuropsychiatric manifestation in the forms of fever, migraine headaches, and depression are also common. Other complications of SLE are hemolytic anemia and thrombocytopenia, resulting from lysis of red blood cells (RBCs) and platelets by autoantibodies specific for these cells.

The cause of SLE is not known, but more than 95% of patients with SLE have high titers of IgG antibodies to components of the cell nucleus (antinuclear antibodies [ANAs]) and an array of self molecules and cell surface

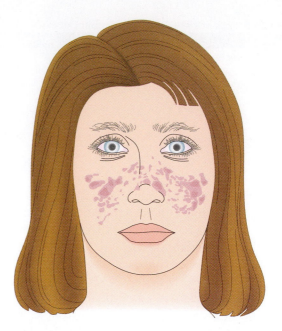

Figure 26.1 Patient with SLE with typical "butterfly" rash.

antigens (clotting factors, RBCs, platelets, and leukocytes). These ANAs most likely cause tissue damage via a mechanism similar to a type III hypersensitive reaction. Of the ANAs, two are characteristic of SLE and are used in diagnosis of the disease: antibodies to native double-stranded DNA (anti-dsDNA) and antibodies to small nuclear ribonucleoproteins, snRNP (anti-Sm). The levels of other autoantibodies, such as anti-DNA and antihistone, may also be greatly elevated, but these autoantibodies are not unique to SLE. The production of autoantibodies is related to polyclonal B-cell activation.

Most autoantibodies in SLE are of the high-affinity IgG type, pointing to the involvement of T cells in antibody class switching and affinity maturation. Indeed, treatment of SLE includes the use of cyclosporine A and cyclophosphamide, which inhibit the function of activated T cells. In mouse studies, depletion of T cells with antibodies to the Thy-1 T-cell antigen prevents autoantibody formation. Blocking CD40-CD40L interactions between T and B cells also ameliorates disease exacerbation. Despite the specificity of the autoantibodies in SLE for dsDNA, it is curious that immunization of animals with mammalian DNA does not usually elicit the production of autoantibodies. This has fueled speculation that the initiating nucleic acid antigens may be of viral or bacterial origin or might arise from chemical modification of nucleic acids that renders them immunogenic. This possibility lost some of its attractiveness when the circulating DNA in SLE patients was identified as being of endogenous, therefore human, origin.

As in many other autoimmune diseases, susceptibility to SLE has a genetic component. SLE affects especially African, Asian, and Hispanic ethnic groups. Concordance among monozygotic twins is between 30 and 60%, and disease has been associated with expression of HLA-DR2 and HLA-DR3 on chromosome 6. Relative risk for the HLA associations ranges from 2 to 5. Genes in the MHC class II region also influence disease susceptibility. Increased relative risk has recently been demonstrated in association with a polymorphism in tumor necrosis factor alpha (TNF-α) and with deficiency in complement components C2, C4, C5, and C8. A recent study found that patients with a deletion on one of the two genes encoding complement component 4 (the C4A gene dele-tion leading to a null allele) have an 80% chance of developing SLE.

RA

RA is a chronic inflammatory disease that has a systemic manifestation but affects primarily peripheral synovial joints (Fig. 26.2). Thus it is a hybrid of an immune complex-mediated autoimmune disease (similar to a type III hypersensitivity) localized to specific tissue types. The early phase of RA involves infiltration of lymphocytes and other mononuclear cells into the synovium, the area surrounding the joints. Most of the T cells are of the CD4$^+$ T helper (TH) cell type, although B cells also are present. Activated macrophages are responsible for secretion of in-

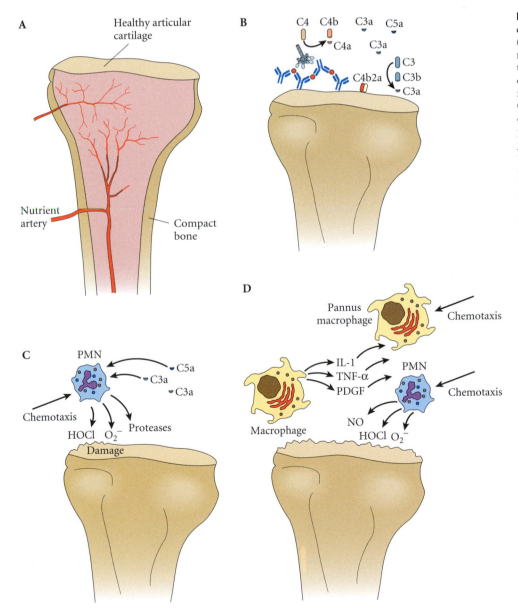

Figure 26.2 Immune-mediated joint damage in RA. (**A**) A healthy joint. (**B**) Persistent antigen-antibody immune complexes become lodged on the articular cartilage, leading to local complement activation. (**C**) Complement split products C3a, C4a, and C5a have chemotactic activity that draws leukocytes such as polymorphonuclear leukocytes (PMNs) to the joint. Proteases and reactive oxygen intermediates released from the PMN cause some joint damage. (**D**) Macrophages attracted to the joint by complement activation release cytokines that have further chemotactic activity, resulting in the formation of a vascularized granulation tissue called a pannus. Further release of proteases and reactive oxygen and nitrogen intermediates from leukocytes in the pannus causes more severe joint injury.

flammatory cytokines (interleukin-1 [IL-1], IL-8, and TNF-α) into the synovium. Chronic stages of the disease typically coincide with the formation of a structure known as a *pannus*. A pannus is a membrane of granulation tissue composed of mesenchyme- and bone marrow-derived cells. Formation of the pannus stimulates the release of IL-1, platelet-derived growth factor, prostaglandins, and substance P by macrophages, which ultimately cause cartilage destruction and bone erosion.

The etiology of RA remains unknown. T cells are thought to play a central role in the initiation and perpetuation of RA. They likely contribute to the production of autoantibodies as well as activation of cells within the synovium that can cause damage to the tissue. CD4$^+$ T cells are found to infiltrate the synovium during the early phase of RA, and most of these cells express the memory phenotype, indicating prior exposure to antigens. There is speculation that infectious agents or specific microbial components may provide the antigenic stimuli. Indeed, evidence of cross-reactivity between self proteins and microbial sequences (e.g., Epstein-Barr virus glycoprotein B) has been reported, and synovial T cells from rheumatoid joints give strong proliferative responses in vitro to heat shock proteins from *Escherichia coli*. There is also the possibility that subsets of T cells involved in RA are expanded by microbial superantigens. T cells with preferential expression of T-cell receptor (TCR) variable (V)-region genes have been isolated from the synovium of patients with RA. Autoreactive T cells specific for collagen and other synovial matrix components also may contribute to the disease.

In addition to T-cell reactivity, autoreactive antibodies referred to as RFs are also present in the synovium. RF autoantibodies are of the IgM, IgG, and IgA isotypes and are specific for the Fc portion of IgG molecules. How this situation comes about is unknown, but the genes encoding the V regions of RFs are not in the germ line configuration, indicating activation, somatic mutation, and class switching occur in those plasma cells producing RFs. This phenomenon requires T-cell help, and this may be one major role of the CD4$^+$ TH cells found in abundance in the RA synovium. Two types of RFs are known; one is produced by B cells using a limited amount of V-region diversity that preferentially precipitate with IgG at low pH and low temperatures. These *cold-reactive* RFs are not associated with RA but with other autoimmune diseases. The RFs found in RA patients are *warm reactive*, indicating a preference for binding to IgG at body temperature. The pathologic aspect of RF autoantibodies arises from their production within the synovium. In RA patients as much as 50% of the synovial tissues contain plasma cells

secreting RFs. This allows for the formation of immune complexes in the joint fluid, activation of complement, and an influx of neutrophils that are in a state of heightened activation. The neutrophils phagocytose the immune complexes but at the same time release destructive cytoplasmic factors that can harm the joint tissue. This leads to the chronic inflammation and swelling in the joints that result in stiffness and pain. In some cases the immune complexes of RFs and IgG enter the circulation and lodge in vascular tissue, leading to a vasculitis component of RA.

Rheumatoid arthritis has a worldwide distribution, with a frequency three to four times higher in women than in men. Sex hormones are implicated in the modulation of disease activities, as clinical symptoms of RA appear to remit during pregnancy and worsen during the postpartum period.

Susceptibility to RA is strongly influenced by genetic predisposition. Disease concordance between monozygotic twins is approximately 20% versus 5% in dizygotic twins. This low penetrance implies that the disease is multifactorial. RA has a strong association with expression of the MHC class II DR1 and DR4 alleles. Disease-associated alleles share sequences in the third hypervariable region at position 67 to 74 of the DR β-chain, which is likely to be involved in specific peptide binding of autoantigens. Whether this is the key to identification of the autoantigens involved remains to be seen.

MS

MS affects the proper functioning of the CNS and is representative of autoimmune diseases with tissue-specific etiology but systemic effects. Early descriptions of MS noted the formation of plaques in the tissues of the brain and spinal cord. These plaques are macroscopic areas of loss of myelin sheath covering the axons (axonal demyelination). Damage to the axons interferes with the transmission of nerve-signal impulses. As a result, patients with MS experience systemic loss of motor, sensory, bladder, and bowel functions. Clinical manifestation of MS takes two major forms: remitting/relapsing MS and progressive MS. In remitting/relapsing MS, disease onset is frequently followed by remission. In most cases, especially during the early stages of the disease, complete remission is attained. The duration of the remission period varies. About one-third of patients with MS experience relapse within a year. However, prolonged remitting/relapsing cycles eventually advance the disease into the secondary progressive form, in which patients no longer have distinctive periods of flare-ups and recovery but experience progressive worsening of their condition. In addition, a small percentage of patients with MS may develop a primary progressive disease course without a clearly detectable relapsing stage.

MS primarily results from T-cell-mediated attacks on the nerve tissues (Fig. 26.3). Histopathology shows heavy cellular infiltration of T cells, B cells, and macrophages into the CNS during the disease process. Subsequent local immune reactions induce the production of inflammatory cytokines and chemokines. It is not clear what ultimately causes demyelination of the axons. It is possible that myelin is damaged as a result of bystander effects in an inflammatory environment or that macrophages or even T cells directly attack myelin-producing oligodendrocytes and kill them. The role of B cells in MS remains undefined. Plasma cells are present in chronic plaques, and cerebrospinal fluid isolated from patients with MS contains increased levels of IgG antibodies. Some of these antibodies have antimyelin specificities, leading to the speculation that antibodies to myelin may participate in the destruction of oligodendrocytes.

The nature of the autoantigens responsible for initiating MS remains elusive. MBP has been suggested as the major autoantigen. In this respect, MBP-reactive T cells have been isolated from peripheral blood of patients with MS. There are also reports of restricted TCR V-region gene usage in T cells isolated from some MS patients, suggesting an antigen-specific immune response to processed and presented myelin antigens. The significance of these T cells has been debated because the frequency of MBP-specific T cells in patients with MS appears to be comparable to that in normal subjects. Some investigators even regard the autoimmune nature of MS as questionable. However, in animal models of EAE, myelin antigens have been used to induce pathology similar to that of MS.

MS has a distinct distribution pattern. It affects primarily North American and European whites. Prevalence generally increases with distance from the equator. The concordance rate for monozygotic twins is in the 25% range and only about 3% for dizygotic twins. Since migration from a region of high incidence to low incidence early in life reduces disease incidence, there is strong suspicion implicating environmental factors in determining susceptibility to MS. These data prompted extensive searches for possible infectious agents that trigger the development of MS. No definitive conclusions have been made from these studies, although links between MS and human herpesvirus 6, Epstein-Barr virus, and *Chlamydia pneumoniae* have been reported. MS also has a strong gender bias: 75% of patients with MS are female. Suppression of disease symptoms during pregnancy again provides evidence for the modulatory effects of hormones in MS.

The genetic basis of MS susceptibility also comes from familial studies. Relatives of patients are at higher risk than are members of the general population. MS is a complex disease, and multiple genetic loci are believed to be involved in disease susceptibility. Strong association has been shown for HLA-DQ6 and HLA-DR2 subgroups, the latter being expressed in 60% of patients with MS. So far, attempts to find a putative MS gene in the human genome have not been successful.

Organ-Specific Autoimmune Diseases

Myasthenia gravis

Myasthenia gravis (MG) is one of the few autoimmune diseases with a known autoantigen target. Muscle weakness and fatigability, the hallmarks of MG, are caused by

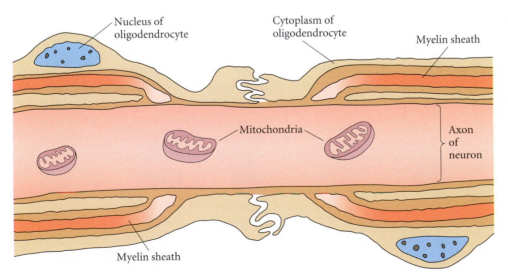

Figure 26.3 Cross section of a neuronal axon, highlighting the myelin sheath formed around the axon by the growth of Schwann cells. Myelin protein in the sheath is one of the principal targets of autoreactive T cells in human MS and mouse EAE.

Nucleus of oligodendrocyte

Cytoplasm of oligodendrocyte

Myelin sheath

Mitochondria

Axon of neuron

Myelin sheath

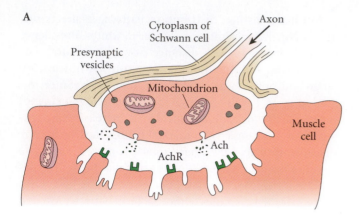

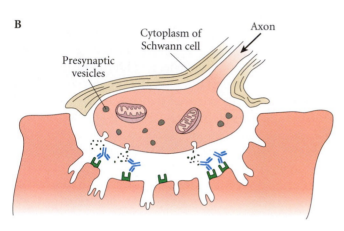

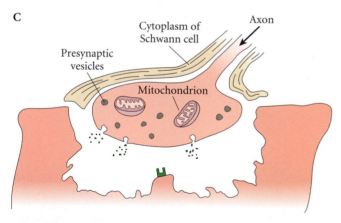

Figure 26.4 Autoimmune attack of the neuromuscular junction in MG. (**A**) An example of a normal neuromuscular junction. Nerve impulses are transmitted to skeletal muscle as the neurotransmitter (ACh) is released from vesicles in the neuron and binds to receptors (AChR) on the surface of the muscle cell. (**B**) The early stages of MG are attributable to blockage of AChR on muscle cells by antibodies generated against this receptor. (**C**) Later stages of disease are marked by antibody- and complement-mediated damage to the neuromuscular junction.

binding of antibody to nicotinic acetylcholine receptors (AChR) at the neuromuscular junction (Fig. 26.4). Nerve-signal transmission occurs with the release of ACh at the end of the nerve fiber propagating a signal and binding of the ACh to the AchR. In MG, high-affinity IgG autoantibodies reactive to AChR are found in the sera of 80 to 90% of patients. These IgG antibodies block the binding of ACh to AChR and prevent nerve-signal propagation.

The disease shows a bimodal gender and age distribution, affecting young women in their 20s and 30s and older men in their 60s and 70s. Initial clinical manifestations involve the extraocular muscles, the facial muscles, and the thymus gland. Patients commonly show weakness in eyelid movement and facial expression and also show generalized weakness involving limbs and the muscles. Thymic abnormality is another feature of MG; 60% of patients with MG have thymic hyperplasia and 10% have thymomas. Removal of an abnormal thymus has been shown to improve clinical conditions of MG.

There is abundant experimental evidence implicating autoantibodies in the development of MG. Antibodies to AChR are found at the neuromuscular junctions of patients with MG, and such antibodies can transfer characteristic features of MG into animals. There is also a direct correlation of clinical improvement with reduction in the level of antibodies to AChR. Binding of antibodies to AChR causes accelerated internalization and degradation of the receptors. Activation of complement components at neuromuscular junctions may also be part of the mechanism interfering with nerve-signal transmission.

The etiology of MG is less well understood. The disease has a strong genetic association with HLA-DR3, HLA-DQ2, and HLA-B8. MHC class II-restricted T cells specific for AChR have been demonstrated to be present in patients. T cells are not normally found in myasthenic muscle and function primarily to enhance antibody production. There are suggestions that environmental factors are involved in the induction of MG. Homology between AChR and peptides from infectious agents has been reported, suggesting that antibodies originally produced in response to an infectious agent may later cross-react with the AChR to cause MG pathology (a process known as "molecular mimicry"). However, what the eliciting event is that gives rise to the antibodies to AChR is not known and may be multifactoral.

Insulin-dependent diabetes mellitus (type 1 diabetes)

Insulin-dependent diabetes mellitus (IDDM or type 1 diabetes) is a cell-mediated autoimmune disease of the pancreas. It is caused by specific destruction of insulin-

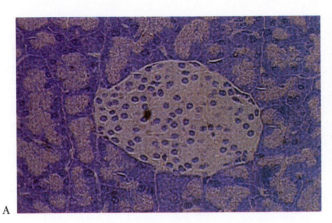
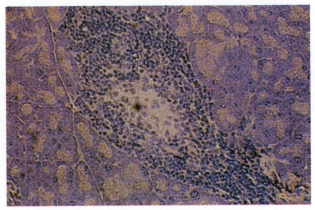

Figure 26.5 (A) Normal histology of pancreas, showing an islet of Langerhans that contains the insulin-producing beta cells. (B) IDDM is characterized by intense mononuclear cell infiltration of the islets and destruction of the beta cells. Reprinted from M. A. Atkinson and N. K. Maclaren, *Sci. Am.* 263(1):62–63, 66–71, with permission.

producing β cells of the islets of Langerhans (Fig. 26.5). Effects are systemic, however, due to the role of insulin in physiologic homeostasis. Lack of adequate production of insulin results in hyperglycemia (elevated blood sugar), hyperosmolality (elevated ionic strength), weight loss, and ketoacidosis (the presence of large quantities of acetoacetic acid, beta-hydroxybutyric acid, and acetone in body fluids). This produces chronic metabolic derangements that may lead to thickening of basement membranes in many tissues and affect blood flow to the extremities. There are many manifestations of diabetes, but these are generally not due to autoimmune mechanisms but rather to the loss of blood sugar regulation. Nerve-tissue destruction (neuropathy), leading to losses of limbs after nonhealing ulcers are formed, is a complication of diabetes. Kidney tissue destruction (nephropathy) is a severe complication of IDDM, and once nephropathy becomes severe enough to cause renal failure, patients are at high risk for cardiovascular diseases and death. Eye tissue abnormalities (retinopathies) potentially leading to blindness are another major complication of IDDM.

The infiltration of lymphocytes into the islets leads to a condition known as insulitis. This infiltration and the presence of autoantibodies are common features at the onset of IDDM and suggest an immune basis for the disease. There are indications that conditions of IDDM may exist in an asymptomatic preclinical stage for years, such that by the time of diagnosis, a majority of the beta cells are already destroyed. Lymphocytes found in insulitis consist of both CD4$^+$ and CD8$^+$ T cells and B cells. Macrophages activated by T cells play a major role in the pathogenesis of the disease. The T cells are reactive with several autoantigens, such as insulin, heat shock proteins, islet-cell antigens, and glutamic acid decarboxylase

(GAD). There is enhanced expression of MHC class I molecules on beta islets and increased CD8$^+$ T-cell-mediated cytotoxic activities at the lesion. Therefore, it is believed that CD8$^+$ cells can mediate cytotoxicity either directly or through inflammatory cytokines. CD4$^+$ T cells additionally contribute to the disease through release of the inflammatory cytokines interferon-gamma (IFN-γ) and TNF-α.

Although antibodies do not appear to be involved as a cause of the disease, autoantibodies reactive with cytoplasmic islet-cell antigens (islet-cell antibodies [ICAs]) are found in 80% of patients with newly diagnosed IDDM. ICAs are primarily IgG antibodies, and some of the target antigens include peripherin (an ocular glycoprotein), carboxypeptidase H, and islet-cell antigen 512. Because ICAs are also detected in the serum of prediabetic patients, these antibodies can be used as predictive markers for the development of IDDM. In addition, insulin autoantibodies also appear early and are present in 60% of patients with new-onset diabetes. Another important predictive autoantibody is antibody to GAD, which is present in 90% of patients with newly diagnosed IDDM. GAD is an enzyme involved in the biosynthesis of the inhibitory neurotransmitter γ-aminobutyric acid. The roles of autoantibodies in IDDM have not been defined, although in animal studies, diabetes does not occur in the absence of B cells.

IDDM is strongly correlated with the expression of HLA-DR3 (DRB1*0301, DRB1*0302) and HLA-DR4 (DRB1*0401, DRB1*0402); 90 to 95% of patients with IDDM have one or both of these alleles. Heterozygous individuals possessing both alleles have increased relative risk of diabetes. Disease association with HLA-DR3 and HLA-DR4, however, might be explained by their close linkage disequilibrium with another disease-correlated locus, HLA-DQ. In fact, it has been reported that the lack of an aspartic acid residue at position 57 of the DQ beta chain (e.g., DQB1*0201 and DQB1*0302, which have either a valine or a serine residue at position 57) confers susceptibility to IDDM. Conversely, the presence of an aspartic acid residue at this position (e.g., DQB1*0602) provides protection against IDDM. It appears that the charge of the amino acid at position 57 modifies the peptide-binding groove of the MHC molecule. Modification of the MHC groove may favor binding of certain self peptides or cross-reactive foreign peptides.

Viral infection has been implicated as the cause of IDDM, but a definitive cause remains elusive. There is possible sequence homology between the enzyme carboxypeptidase H, the coat protein of coxsackievirus, and the nucleoprotein of influenza virus. Antibodies to coxsackievirus are persistently increased in patients with IDDM. In some cases, congenital rubella infection has also been linked to IDDM. However, new-onset IDDM, which generally occurs in juveniles but can also occur in adults, appears to be acute, usually manifest as ketoacidosis. In some cases cerebral edema is present, and this is usually deadly. Viral infections may merely be the factor that brought the patient to a doctor to be examined. The complexity of the immunologic mechanisms associated with this disease points out the difficulty in finding a single factor provoking its onset.

Autoimmune thyroid diseases

Chronic autoimmune thyroiditis (Hashimoto's thyroiditis [HT]) and Graves' disease (GD) are two major pathologic manifestations of thyroid disorder. HT is an inflammatory condition of the thyroid characterized clinically by a goiter (enlargement of the thyroid gland) with or without decreased production of thyroid hormones (hypothyroidism). Cellular infiltration into the thyroid and circulation of autoantibodies are typically associated with

A

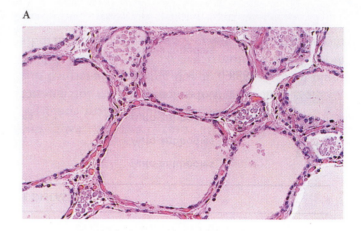

B

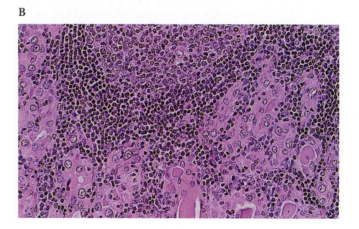

C

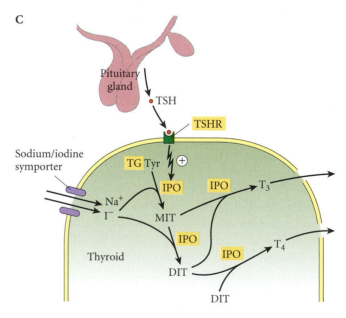

Figure 26.6 Thyroid destruction in the HT. (A) A normal thyroid. (B) Thyroid in HT, showing intense mononuclear cell infiltrate. (C) Diagram of a thyroid acinar cell showing the synthesis of thyroid hormones (T_3) and (T_4). Synthesis of T_3 and T_4 is stimulated by TSH released by the pituitary gland, which binds to a specific receptor (TSHR) on the acinar cell. Synthesis of T_3 and T_4 involves the modification of tyrosine amino acids (Tyr) of the protein thyroglobulin (TG) by covalent addition of iodine (I^-). This occurs by the action of the enzyme iodine peroxidase (IPO), and results in the formation of monoiodotyrosine (MIT) and diiodotyrosine (DIT). Further activity of the IPO enzyme causes a condensation reaction that combines MIT and DIT to form the hormones T_3 and T_4. The TSHR, IPO, and TG proteins are all targets of autoimmune responses during advanced HT, although the initial loss of thyroid activity is probably due to blockage of the TSHR by anti-TSHR antibodies. (A and B) Courtesy of Edward C. Klatt.

this disease (Fig. 26.6). Inflammation brought on by release of TH1 cytokines results in progressive cell-mediated destruction of the thyroid follicular cells. The normal function of the thyroid gland is to secrete the thyroid hormones thyroxine (tetraiodothyronine [T_4]) and triiodothyronine (T_3). These iodinated amino acids are released from the prohormone thyroglobulin. Reduction in thyroid hormone production in HT in turn leads to enhanced pituitary secretion of thyrotropin (or thyroid-stimulating hormone [TSH]), which stimulates thyroid cell growth. At later stages of HT, some patients may develop atrophy of the thyroid and symptoms of thyroid hormone deficiency. The actual mechanism of thyroid gland destruction is not clear. Cytokines, cytotoxic T cells, and Fas/FasL-mediated apoptosis all seem to be involved in this process.

Several candidate autoantigens are associated with HT. T cells and autoantibodies reactive with thyroglobulin have been identified. Enhanced circulating IgG autoantibodies to thyroglobulin are commonly found in the sera of 70% of patients with HT. In addition, almost all patients also have antibodies to thyroid peroxidase. Thyroid peroxidase is a membrane-bound enzyme catalyzing the iodination of the thyroglobulin tyrosine residues. Overall, autoantibodies do not appear to play a major role in the pathogenesis of autoimmune thyroiditis. The levels of autoantibodies to thyroglobulin do not usually correlate with severity of the disease, and in animal studies, transfer of antibodies to thyroglobulin does not lead to development of thyroiditis.

As with other autoimmune diseases, genetic and environmental factors are associated with HT. There is an increased incidence of disease among family members. However, association with HLA appears weak, and there are differences among ethnic groups. Some degrees of disease association with HLA-DR3 and HLA-DR5 have been reported. Women are affected more frequently than men (2:1 ratio). Concordance rates for monozygotic twins are low, again indicating a central role for environmental factors. Infection and molecular mimicry have been implicated, but data to support this contention are few.

In GD, clinical manifestations include development of hyperthyroidism and goiters. This is caused by stimulatory autoantibodies that bind to TSH receptors (TSHR) in the thyroid (Fig. 26.7). These antibodies are of the IgG isotype, and upon binding to TSHR stimulate thyroid follicle cell growth, uptake of iodine, and production of thyroid hormones. More than 90% of patients with GD have antibodies to TSHR in their serum. Evidence that autoantibodies may cause GD comes from the observation that children born to mothers with GD also develop signs of hyperthyroidism due to placental transfer of IgG antibodies. In addition to stimulatory autoantibodies, some patients have autoantibodies that bind TSHR but do not

Figure 26.7 GD is an autoimmune disease that results in overstimulation of the thyroid, not in its destruction. (**A**) Normal regulation of the production of thyroid hormones. Production of T_3 and T_4 is stimulated by TSH. Buildup of T_3 and T_4 has a feedback-inhibitory effect on the synthesis of TSH. (**B**) In GD, stimulatory anti-TSHR antibody binds to the TSHR, stimulating production of T_3 and T_4. While T_3 and T_4 negatively inhibit TSH production, the synthesis of T_3 and T_4 continues to be stimulated by the autoantibody in a completely unregulated fashion.

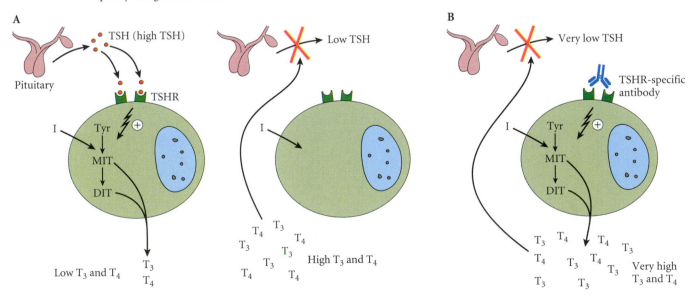

stimulate cellular activities. The mechanism by which these autoantibodies arise is not known. Viral infection is cited as one of the possible precipitants of the autoimmune response. GD strikes women 10 times more frequently than it does men. Association with HLA-DR3 is seen in 50% of patients with GD.

Animal Models of Autoimmune Diseases

In the past 30 years, animal studies have contributed extensively to the understanding of autoimmune diseases. These studies paved the way for development of some of the therapeutic remedies currently being used. In addition, animal models are important for furthering our understanding of the genetic, cellular, and molecular bases of autoimmune diseases.

Spontaneously Arising Autoimmune Diseases in Animals

Animal models for SLE

A number of murine models of SLE have been established during backcrosses to derive new inbred strains. In 1961, Mielschowsky et al. first reported the observation that New Zealand Black (NZB) strain mice uniformly developed symptoms of autoimmune hemolytic anemia early in life (Fig. 26.8). The disease was caused by antibodies specific for RBCs. In addition, the animals had low titers of autoantibodies to single-stranded DNA and dsDNA but rarely had glomerulonephritis. Crossing these mice with another strain, the New Zealand White (NZW), resulted in F1 animals (BWF1) that exhibited more severe

Figure 26.8 New Zealand Black/White progeny (BWF$_1$) mice are used as an experimental model of human SLE. BWF1 mice have many of the characteristics of human SLE. The data are from E. D. Dubois et al., *JAMA* **195**:285–289, 1966.

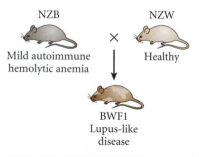

Symptom	% Positive BWF1 mice
Antinuclear antibodies	46
Proteinuria	80
Lupus nephropathy	75
Severe nephropathy	38

symptoms closely resembling human SLE: production of high titers of IgG autoantibodies to dsDNA, formation of immune complexes, development of fatal lupus nephritis, and a clear preponderance in females. Crossing of NZB mice with other normal strains, such as C57BL/6 and AKR, did not produce similar disease, thus indicating disease-contributing factors derived from the NZW parent. In this respect, the presence of NZW MHC genes enhances susceptibility and is associated with increased frequency of severe lupus nephritis. Genome-wide linkage analyses have allowed identification of at least 11 other non-MHC susceptibility loci. These are localized on chromosomes 1, 4, and 7 and control various disease traits ranging from B-cell hyperactivity to elevated serum levels of IgG antinuclear autoantibodies. The effects of hormones in the manifestation of lupus have also been elegantly demonstrated in animal studies. Castration of male mice renders them susceptible to development of SLE. Furthermore, direct administration of female sex hormones to female mice accelerates the disease, whereas male sex hormones inhibit disease. Similar effects have been seen in other autoimmune diseases.

The roles of T cells in lupus have been studied in BWF1 mice. Treatment with antibodies to T-cell markers, such as Thy-1 and CD4, abrogates the production of autoantibodies and the development of renal disease, demonstrating the requirement of the CD4 subset in disease development. Analysis of the T-cell repertoire, however, indicates that T-cell responses are polyclonal in nature and reveals no bias toward recognition of specific autoantigens. The TCR CDR3 region of anti-DNA T-cell clones displays charged motifs that may facilitate recognition and binding of autoantigens.

The lpr (lymphoproliferation) mutant of the MRL mouse strain represents another model for studying lupus. These mice were discovered because of apparent splenomegaly and lymphadenopathy. MRL/lpr mice have a shortened lifespan, produce antinuclear antibodies, and develop autoimmune glomerulonephritis. Further studies revealed that the lymphoproliferative phenotype is the result of a mutation in the gene encoding the Fas protein. Fas is a type I transmembrane protein, and binding of the Fas ligand (FasL) triggers cellular DNA fragmentation and apoptosis. Because of the mutation in the *Fas* gene, extrathymic autoreactive T cells and autoreactive B cells are allowed to accumulate instead of undergoing negative selection, subsequently leading to autoimmune attacks. Mutants of the *FasL* gene have also been identified. These mice are designated gld (generalized lymphoproliferative disease). This strain was originally derived in the C3H/HeJ strain but has now been backcrossed into various genetic backgrounds. The gld mice exhibit autoimmune phenotypes similar to those of lpr mice because of an inability to induce apoptosis in Fas-expressing T and B cells. In both strains of mice, lymphoproliferation and autoantibody production appear to be separate events and are regulated by different subsets of T cells. Elimination of CD4$^+$ T cells in lpr mice prevents autoantibody production whereas the absence of CD8$^+$ T cells inhibits lymphoproliferative responses. In addition to the *Fas* and *FasL* genes, background genes also are found to affect autoimmune manifestation. Breeding of the *lpr* gene onto C57BL/6 background produces only a mild autoimmune syndrome.

Another lupus-prone mouse strain, BXSB, presents a scenario different from that of other murine models of autoimmune diseases. These mice develop anti-dsDNA and immune complex glomerulonephritis, but more so in the male than in the female. A gene located in the Y chromosome (the *Yaa* gene) appears to provide an enhancing effect on disease development. T cells are primarily responsible for the disease pattern, as their elimination results in disease suppression. Although the BXSB system may seem unrelated to human SLE because more males than females are affected, it is interesting that male preponderance has been seen in some familial studies of human patients with SLE.

Animal models for IDDM

The nonobese diabetic (NOD) mouse strain, originally derived at the Shionogi Research Laboratories in Japan, has become the most extensively studied animal model of IDDM (Fig. 26.9). By 30 weeks of age, 80% of female mice and 30% of male mice of the NOD strain develop diabetes. Indications of insulitis can first be observed in NOD mice as young as 4 weeks old, with infiltration of dendritic cells, macrophages, and T and B cells into the pancreas. The severity of insulitis increases with age, and by 14 weeks animals begin to develop hyperglycemia. Although almost 100% of NOD mice develop insulitis, not all animals proceed to develop diabetes. The factors that precipitate the development of diabetes are still unknown. How-

ever, it is interesting that the incidence of disease is higher in mice maintained in sterile pathogen-free facilities than in those kept under conventional conditions.

The role of T cells in disease development has been extensively analyzed in NOD mice. Congenital athymic NOD mice do not develop insulitis or diabetes, and treatment of NOD mice with antibodies to T cells prevents disease (Fig. 26.9). Furthermore, transfer of spleen cells from diabetic NOD mice into irradiated recipients results in the development of disease in the recipient mice. The role of CD8$^+$ T cells in disease development is demonstrated in NOD beta$_2$-microglobulin-knockout mice and in NOD mice treated with antibodies to CD8, which develop neither insulitis nor diabetes. In addition, CD8$^+$ T-cell clones effectively transfer diabetes to SCID mice with matched MHC class I expression. All these results strongly suggest that CD8$^+$ T cells function as effector cells in mediating pancreatic beta-cell destruction. Indeed, CD8$^+$ diabetogenic T-cell clones that are cytotoxic to pancreatic beta cells in vitro have been isolated. However, the role of CD8$^+$ T cells is not absolute. Other studies indicate that CD4$^+$ T cells also have the capacity to function as effector cells. For example, some CD4$^+$ T-cell clones have been shown to adoptively transfer diabetes to recipients in the absence of endogenous CD8$^+$ T cells. TCR transgenic mice expressing TCRs derived from clone BDC 2.5, which is CD4$^+$ and diabetogenic, develop spontaneous insulitis and diabetes with kinetics similar to that in the natural NOD mice. It is suggested that CD8$^+$ T cells may initiate the disease and that CD4$^+$ T cells are recruited at a later stage.

Cross-breeding studies of NOD mice have identified at least 14 genetic loci that regulate the development of diabetes in these animals. Among these, the most extensively studied gene locus is *Idd1*, which maps to the MHC on chromosome 17. With respect to class II proteins, NOD mice only express one mouse MHC class II molecule, the IA molecule (IA^{g7}). They do not express the IE α chain because of a deletion in the promoter region of this gene. Expression of an E$_\alpha$ transgene, which allows expression of the whole IE molecule (equivalent of human HLA-DR),

Figure 26.9 (A) NOD mice are naturally prone to develop IDDM. (**B and C**) This disease is T cell mediated, since it can be prevented by either removal of a mouse's thymus at birth (**B**) or ablation of the mouse's T cells with a CD3-specific monoclonal antibody (**C**).

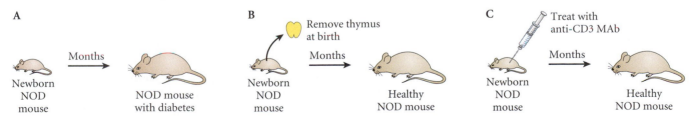

prevents the development of immune insulitis. IA^{g7} is unique in that it contains a serine at position 57 in the IA$_\beta$ molecule, whereas nondiabetic strains have aspartic acid in this position. This is reminiscent of the human HLA-DQ molecule in many patients with IDDM, which also exchanges an aspartic acid for a serine residue at position 57 of the beta chain. Taken together, the lack of IE expression and the unique sequence of IA^{g7} in NOD mice contribute to the development of diabetes in these mice. Replacement of aspartic acid in IA^{g7}, however, does not prevent development of the disease. Other gene loci must be analyzed to provide a better understanding of the mechanism of diabetes development.

Another animal model that has been extensively studied is the spontaneously diabetic BB rat isolated at the BioBreeding Laboratories in Canada. These animals exhibit insulitis and hyperglycemia similar to that seen in diabetic NOD mice. Development of the disease is T cell dependent, although multiple IgG autoantibodies also are detected during the prediabetic period. As in NOD mice, the MHC is shown to play an important role in the regulation of the disease.

Animal models for autoimmune thyroiditis

The obese strain of chicken spontaneously develops symptoms of autoimmune thyroiditis closely resembling HT. This strain was originally derived a half century ago from a C strain chicken bred at Cornell University in New York. Obese strain chickens start to show signs of hypothyroidism as early as the third week after hatching. The disease is characterized by cellular infiltration into the thyroid and the formation of germinal centers. The lymphoid compartments are generally hyperactive. Production of IL-2 is enhanced, and T cells express high levels of IL-2 receptors. Antibodies to thyroglobulin, T$_3$, and thyroxine are detected. Rapid iodine uptake also reflects changes in cellular activities in the target organ. As in HT, T cells play a major role in the disease, as thymectomy greatly reduces the formation of antibodies to thyroglobulin.

Spontaneous autoimmune thyroiditis is also seen in the Buffalo rat strain. NOD mice and BB rats, which spontaneously develop diabetes, also have a low incidence of autoimmune thyroiditis, bringing up the interesting possibility that some autoimmune diseases may have common pathologic mechanisms.

Experimentally Induced Animal Models

EAE as a model for MS
Historically, the origin of experimentally induced encephalomyelitis dates back to 1885, when Louis Pasteur administered patients an attenuated rabies vaccine derived from rabbit brain extracts in which the rabies virus was propagated. Some patients developed neurologic sequelae, which initially were attributed to the rabies virus itself. However, neurologic symptoms persisted in patients even after killed virus extracts were used. The discovery that patients also developed antibodies to the brain extracts strongly hinted at an immune response directed at antigens in the rabbit brain, a notion supported by the reproduction of similar symptoms in monkeys repeatedly injected with tissues from normal rabbit brain. The occurrence of disease was more consistent when the brain extracts were emulsified in complete Freund adjuvant. EAE has since been implemented in guinea pigs, rabbits, rats, and mice. EAE is most extensively analyzed in rats and mice because of the availability of genetically defined inbred strains. Rats with EAE exhibit only a monophasic disease with limited demyelination. In mice, some strains develop an acute disease phase followed by spontaneous remission and relapsing cycles (Fig. 26.10) more closely resembling the human condition. Although these animal models have been useful in advancing our understanding of MS, it should be recognized that MS is a clinically diverse syndrome, and no single experimental system can fully duplicate all the clinical and pathologic manifestations.

EAE is induced by immunization of animals with myelin proteins. The disease is characterized histopathologically by perivascular cellular infiltration of T cells, B cells, and macrophages into the brain and spinal cord and clinically by various degrees of paralysis (Fig. 26.11). Common myelin antigens include MBP, proteolipid protein, myelin oligodendrocyte glycoprotein, and defined encephalitogenic peptides of these proteins. Different mouse strains respond to distinct encephalitogenic epitopes, correlating with their MHC haplotypes. For example, PL and B10.PL mice (H-2^u) respond to MBP peptide 1–11, while SJL and B10.S mice (H-2^s) respond to MBP peptide 89–101. Experimental autoimmune encephalomyelitis is mediated by CD4$^+$ T cells, as demonstrated by the ability of CD4$^+$ T-cell clones to transfer disease adoptively to naive recipients. Heightened levels of TH1-type cytokines are associated with disease, implicating cell-mediated immunity in disease pathogenesis. Administration of IL-12 enhances disease because of its ability to induce production of IFN-γ. Conversely, TH2-type cytokines such as IL-4, IL-10, and transforming growth factor beta (TGF-β) are all effective in downregulating EAE.

Activated encephalitogenic T cells increase expression of adhesion molecules to facilitate their migration to the CNS. Once within the CNS, development of local inflammatory activities subsequently causes destruction of the myelin sheaths surrounding the axons. It is conceivable

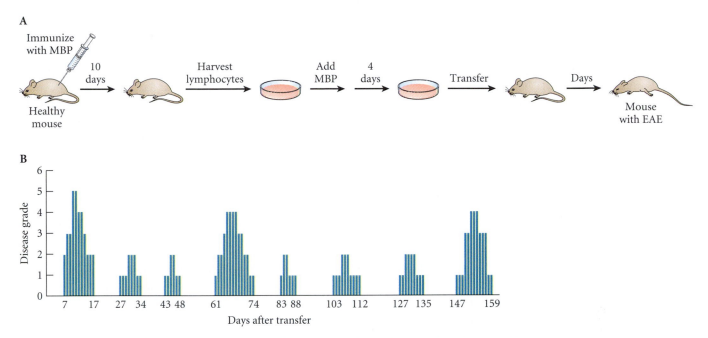

Figure 26.10 EAE is an animal model of the human disease MS. (**A**) EAE can be induced by vaccinating mice with MBP, expanding the MBP-specific lymphocytes in culture, and then introducing them into an isogenic mouse. (**B**) EAE follows a remitting/relapsing course similar to that observed in some humans with MS. Panel B is reproduced with permission from C. Kim and H. Y. Tse, *J. Neuroimmunol.* **46**:129–136, 1993.

that new sets of T cells specific for the various myelin antigens released from the damaged tissues would be sensitized, effectively broadening the overall specificities from the initial disease determinant to encompass a spectrum of other determinants. This process is referred to as *determinant spreading*. It is postulated that determinant spreading may account for the occurrence of disease relapses during the disease cycles.

Interestingly, encephalitogenic T-cell clones isolated from some rat strains (e.g., Lewis) and some mouse strains (e.g., PL and B10.PL) express a limited number of TCR V_β gene segments. More than 80% of encephalitogenic T-cell clones isolated from these rats and mice have TCR containing the $V_\beta 8.2$ gene segment. With this degree of homogeneity among encephalitogenic clones, it was once hoped that this phenomenon might provide a convenient target for immune intervention (e.g., the use of antibodies to $V_\beta 8.2$ to block or kill the disease-causing T cells). Unfortunately, dominant TCR gene segment usage has not been clearly demonstrated in other mouse strains or in human patients with MS. Nevertheless, transgenic mice expressing the encephalitogenic $V_\beta 8.2^+$ TCR have been constructed in the B10.PL strain. When housed in a conventional facility, 40 to 50% of these mice develop spontaneous EAE. This percentage is greatly reduced when the animals are housed in a pathogen-free environment. These results confirm the previous suspicion that

Figure 26.11 MBP-specific T cells in mice with EAE home to the brain, where they mediate destruction of the myelin sheath. The time course of lymphocyte homing to brain tissue correlates well with the onset of disease symptoms (bar at top of graph). Modified with permission from Y. Naparstek et al., *Eur. J. Immunol.* **13**:418–423, 1983.

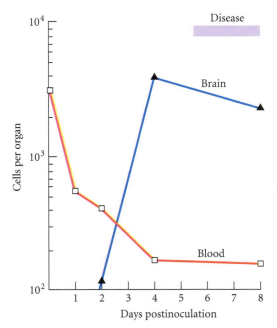

environmental factors such as infection can indeed influence the outcome of disease development.

Animal models for RA

Several animal models of RA have been widely studied. These include collagen-induced arthritis (CIA), adjuvant-induced arthritis, pristane-induced arthritis (PIA), and streptococcal cell wall arthritis. PIA is interesting because pristane is a synthetic paraffin oil and is unlikely to act as a specific antigen recognized immunologically by T and B cells. Rather, its effects are more likely related to its inflammatory activity acting as an adjuvant for certain unknown immunologic antigens. In this context, it is interesting to note that immunization with mycobacterial HSP65 in incomplete Freund adjuvant protects otherwise susceptible animals against PIA. In CIA, immunization of rats and mice with type II collagen (CII) provokes development of intense synovitis and joint destruction similar to that of RA. The disease is caused by T-cell immunity (Fig. 26.12) and antibody responses to CII, which is a major protein component of cartilage in the joints. As in RA, susceptibility to CIA is influenced by expression of MHC class II genes. H-2^q (DBA/1 and B10.Q) mice develop CIA when immunized with bovine, chick, or human CII. H-2^r (B10.RIII) mice respond to bovine and porcine CII but not to chick or human CII. CII is a large molecule consisting of 1,018 amino acids, and cyanogen bromide-cleaved fragments have been used to map the T-cell epitopes. H-2^q mice recognize as many as five determinants within cyanogen bromide fragment 11 (CB11), a large fragment spanning amino acid sequence 124–402, whereas H-2^r mice recognize one determinant (sequence 442–456) within the fragment CB8 (spanning residue 403–551). CD4$^+$ T cells and inflammatory cytokines are found to play an important role in mediating the autoimmune disease. Antibodies to CII contribute to injury by activating hemolytic complement.

A significant recent development is the successful expression of HLA class II molecules as a transgene in mice. When immunized with CII, transgenic mice expressing HLA-DQ8 (DQA1*0301 and DQB1*0302) developed a strong antibody response and severe polyarthritis similar to those developed in susceptible control mice, as demonstrated by G. H. Nabozny et al. in 1996. This novel animal model should prove very useful for study of human autoimmune diseases.

Experimental autoimmune MG

Myasthenia-like disease can be experimentally induced in animals immunized with AChR isolated from *Torpedo californica* (the Pacific electric ray). Experimental autoimmune MG (EAMG) has been established in rabbits, guinea pigs, rats, and mice. Initial studies focused on the effects of MHC haplotype and on mapping of the AChR immunogenic epitopes. AChR is a pentameric molecule consisting of two α subunits and one each of the β, δ, and

Figure 26.12 Vaccinating mice with CII induces autoimmune arthritis. This arthritis is mediated in large part by CD4$^+$ T cells, since destruction of these cells with an anti-CD4 monoclonal antibody both reduces the incidence of disease and slows its onset. From G. E. Ranges et al., *J. Exp. Med.* **162:**1105–1110, 1985, with permission.

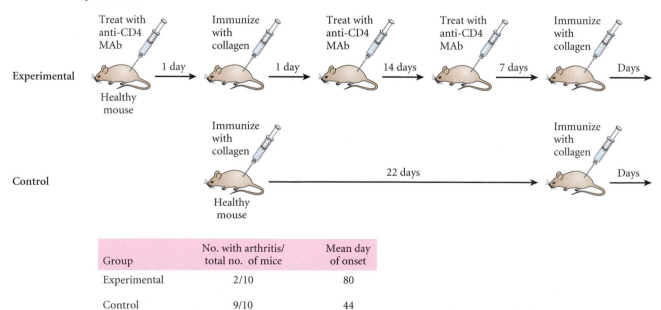

Group	No. with arthritis/ total no. of mice	Mean day of onset
Experimental	2/10	80
Control	9/10	44

ε subunits. The α subunits contain most immunogenic sequences. Like MG, EAMG is mediated by antibodies to AChR. Production of these antibodies also requires a contribution from CD4[+] TH cells. The T-cell epitope is nested within sequence 146–162 of the α subunit.

H-2[b] mice are highly susceptible to disease induction, and the genes regulating disease progression map to the IA region of the MHC. In the B6 mutant strain, B6.C-H2[bm12] (bm12), mutations in three amino acid residues in the β chain of the IA molecule result in reduced incidence of EAMG. Furthermore, as in NOD mice, B6 mice do not express the IE molecule on their cell surface because of a lack of expression of the IE α chain. Expression of an IE$_α$ transgene in these mice results in resistance to EAMG induction. These experiments provide direct evidence for the important roles played by MHC genes in autoimmune diseases.

Etiology of Autoimmunity

Despite the many studies in patients and animal models described in the previous sections, there is still no clear picture regarding the etiology of autoimmune diseases. It is evident that immunologic factors underlie these diseases, but the triggering factors have proven difficult to identify. Self-reactive lymphocytes are common in normal individuals, and their inappropriate activation and expansion may be responsible for initiating autoimmunity. These cells may have escaped negative selection because of low receptor affinity or recognition of cryptic determinants but then are stimulated in a way to make them pathologic. Both the TCR and gene products of the MHC assume important roles in determining if pathologic antigen presentation and T-cell activation will occur. It is conceivable that the nature of the antigen and antigenic stimulation leading to activation of the self-reactive cells may determine the mechanism of development of autoimmune diseases. There are many experimental observations to support a number of hypotheses about how autoimmune diseases arise.

Sequestered Antigens Not Exposed to Selection during Tolerance Induction

Tolerance induction to self antigens occurs when these antigens are encountered during lymphocyte development. Accordingly, self antigens that are not exposed to the immune system during this period, or that are present in low concentrations, cannot act during negative selection or during peripheral tolerance. Immunologically privileged sites, predominantly the brain, eye, testis, and ovary, are traditionally thought to be situated behind barriers that isolate them from exposure to the immune system. Sequestered proteins within these sites, if accidentally exposed to the immune system through injury or tissue damage, may be recognized as foreign. Examples cited by proponents of this mechanism include the formation of antibodies to spermatozoa following vasectomy in some men and the occasional development of sympathetic ophthalmia after ocular trauma. In a similar manner, autoimmunity can be induced by administration of autoantigens in many animal models of autoimmune diseases (e.g., EAE). On the other hand, data from recent research tend to argue against this hypothesis. First, the so-called blood-brain barrier is not as impermeable to cellular traffic in and out of the brain as originally thought. It has now been demonstrated that both naive and activated lymphoid cells routinely scout the CNS. Second, sequestration of proteins in immunologically privileged sites is not absolute. Transcripts of golli-MBP, a differentially spliced form of MBP normally present in the CNS, have been detected in non-neural tissues, including the thymus. In another series of experiments, transgenic mice expressing a transgene coding for hen egg lysozyme under the control of the αA crystallin promoter were created. Antigen expression is exclusively limited to the eye lens. When challenged with hen egg lysozyme, mice that express the transgene show complete tolerance to the antigen. These data imply that seemingly sequestered proteins, by as yet unknown mechanisms, are subjected to immune selection during development. Thus there is no clear evidence that exposure of a previously sequestered antigen may underlie some forms of autoimmunity.

Pathogens as Triggers of Autoimmunity

The idea that infectious agents may trigger activation of autoimmune mechanisms has persisted for over three decades, although investigators are still in search of direct proof. It is proposed that microbial determinants may possess sequences that are homologous or cross-reactive with host proteins (molecular mimicry), such that an immune response to the pathogen leads to activation of self-reactive lymphocytes. As more is learned about the mechanisms of lymphocyte activation, certain microbial proteins, such as enterotoxins, may also be found to have direct effects on immune cells.

Molecular mimicry between pathogen and host

The idea that a pathogen may trigger activation of autoimmune mechanisms is an attractive one because it provides a physiologic explanation for a pathologic state. According to this view, the microbial peptide has to be different enough immunologically to trigger an immune response and yet similar enough to cross-react with host proteins. It turns out that linear sequence homology between the microbial and host peptides is not even necessary. The TCR is degenerate enough to accommodate structurally related cross-reactive peptides. It is conceivable that some of these cross-reactive peptides may be derived from different microbes; thus, more than one pathogen may be involved in the triggering of a specific autoimmune disease.

In 1985, R. S. Fujinami and M. B. A. Oldstone reported that immunization of rabbits with a hepatitis B virus polymerase peptide that shares 6 of the 10 amino acid residues with an MBP sequence induced antibodies to MBP and disease symptoms resembling EAE in some animals. Similar observations have been made in IDDM, in which GAD65 and GAD67 share sequence homology with the coxsackievirus P2-C protein. These results suggest that an immune response to a viral epitope may cross-react with host proteins, leading to autoimmune diseases.

The concept that autoimmunity is a direct consequence of microbial infection, while attractive, is very difficult to prove. First, autoimmunity may develop years after the initial infection and when the pathogen is no longer around. Second, breaking of tolerance may have resulted from tissue injury and release of self proteins subsequent to microbial infection. In this scenario, inflammatory responses to the released self proteins would cause further tissue damage, which may make larger quantities and wider arrays of self-antigenic determinants available for lymphocyte stimulation (i.e., determinant spreading). These cycles can go on even in the absence of the initial pathogen. Thus, without the support of compelling evidence, firm conclusions cannot be drawn about the significance of molecular mimicry in autoimmune diseases.

Heat shock proteins as targets of autoimmune attack

Heat shock proteins (HSPs, or stress proteins) are a group of evolutionarily conserved proteins that are produced when cells respond to adverse changes in their environment and are immunodominant bacterial proteins. Among the T cells that respond to immunization with *Mycobacterium tuberculosis*, 20% are specific for HSP60. The reason for this high level of responses is not known. HSPs are also found in mammalian species. There is a 60% sequence homology between mycobacterial and human HSP60. For this reason, it is postulated that an immune response to mycobacterial HSP60 may lead to reactivity against endogenous host HSP60. HSP60 was first implicated in adjuvant-induced arthritis, when T cells from rats immunized with *M. tuberculosis* and specific for mycobacterial HSP60 were shown to transfer arthritis to naive recipients. Organs or tissues expressing the high levels of

host HSP60 will be affected most. The result may be secondary activation of resting autoimmune effector cells that cause the initiation of autoimmune diseases. However, direct evidence supporting this hypothesis is lacking, and further research is required to clarify these issues. HSP60 was initially reported to be a mitochondrial protein but has subsequently been shown also to be present in the cytoplasm and on the cell surface. Staining of frozen sections from patients with RA with antibodies to HSP60 shows high expression of the protein in the cartilage-pannus junction of the joint. However, expression of the protein is not correlated with inflammatory sites. Monocytes and macrophages appear to have the highest expression.

Superantigen as a polyclonal activator of autoreactive T cells

The term *superantigen* refers to several families of microbial toxins that have the ability to activate polyclonally subsets of T cells expressing certain TCR V_β genes. This activation usually requires presentation but not processing by antigen-presenting cells (APCs) and results in activation and massive proliferation of all T cells bearing the appropriate TCR V_β gene. It is estimated that some superantigens can activate as many as 20% of all T cells in a host organism, compared with only 0.0001 to 0.001% for a conventional peptide antigen. These observations immediately raise the possibility that some autoimmune diseases may be caused by encounters with superantigens. In this scenario, superantigens produced by infectious agents may polyclonally activate large subsets of T cells. If autoreactive T cells are among those being expanded, autoimmune attack on target organs may ensue. B cells, by virtue of their expression of MHC class II molecules, are able to present superantigens to T cells and in turn receive superantigen-induced T-cell help. The resulting autoantibody production may cause the formation of immune complexes and inflammatory reactivity resulting in tissue damage. Indirect support for this hypothesis comes from experiments indicating that mice recovering from acute EAE could be induced to redevelop disease by injection of the superantigen *Staphylococcus aureus* enterotoxin B (SEB). Administration of SEB to DBA/1 mice immunized with CII accelerated the onset of autoimmune disease with increased severity. However, data supporting the role of superantigens in human autoimmune diseases are lacking.

Therapy for Autoimmune Diseases

An ideal therapy for autoimmune diseases would selectively block the lymphocytes that cause autoimmunity without affecting the remainder of the immune system.

Although scientists have studied autoimmunity for more than a century, current therapies are far from ideal. To date, the only effective therapy consists of drugs that suppress the entire immune system. Many of the experimental systems currently used are aimed at the design of new strategies to specifically arrest autoimmune disease while leaving normal immune function unhindered.

Standard Therapies

At present there are two categories of therapy for autoimmune diseases that have been around for a while: *replacement therapies*, which provide relief from the symptoms of disease and hence better quality of life for the patients, and *immunosuppressive treatments*, which negatively regulate the immune responses that cause the disease symptoms. In addition, general therapies such as anti-inflammatory drugs for flare-ups in diseases such as arthritis are commonly used as first-line therapies until their efficacy diminishes. Usually with the more severe autoimmune diseases a more aggressive strategy must be pursued, and the anti-inflammatory drugs are combined with a more aggressive therapy.

Replacement therapies

While replacement therapies do little to stop the autoimmune process, they are effective in providing relief from the clinical sequelae of autoimmunity. The best known example of this type of treatment is the use of insulin by patients with IDDM. Injected insulin replaces the function of lost pancreatic beta cells, although side effects of this treatment can be severe, prompting research for alternative therapies. Replacement therapy also is used for the treatment of autoimmune thyroid disease. It is more effective than insulin therapy for IDDM because thyroid hormone treatment is inexpensive and relatively free of side effects. When thyroid function is lost as a result of autoimmune disease, as in HT, the lost hormones are replaced by synthetic analogs taken orally. Replacement therapy is also used to treat GD, in which thyroid function is increased because of autoimmune attack. In this case, the overactive thyroid is sacrificially destroyed (by either surgical removal or treatment with radiation) and thyroid function is then replaced with oral hormone therapy.

Immunosuppressive therapies

Immunosuppressive treatment of autoimmune disease has the advantage of halting the actual disease process rather than merely treating the end effect of the process. However, such treatments have the disadvantage of being fairly nonselective. Drugs such as corticosteroids or cyclophosphamide, for example, prevent lymphocyte prolif-

eration and thus block immune functions. While these drugs effectively suppress autoimmune diseases, they also block beneficial immune responses. This leaves the patients at increased risk for infection, necessitating careful regulation of drug dosage to balance beneficial and detrimental effects. Similarly, general immunosuppression can be achieved by using the drugs cyclosporine or FK506. These drugs block signal transduction cascades initiated by T-cell or IL-2-receptor engagement, preventing full T-cell activation (Fig. 26.13). The benefit of these drugs is that they spare beneficial T cells that are not activated at the time of drug administration. Nonsteroidal anti-inflammatory drugs in combination with a disease-modifying antirheumatic drug such as gold, hydroxychloroquine, sulfasalazine, methotrexate, leflunomide, or cyclosporine are another class of nonselective immunosuppressive agents used for the treatment of RA. The anti-inflammatory drugs inhibit inflammation by blocking the formation of cyclooxygenases, key mediators in the prostaglandin pathway, while the other drugs inhibit T-cell function in a variety of ways, some understood (e.g., cyclosporine) and others without a known molecular function (e.g., gold).

Cytokine/cytokine-inhibitor therapies

The newest forms of therapy for autoimmunity are directed at the specific cells or cytokines that contribute to or regulate the aberrant immune response. Cytokine therapy, the administration of cytokines or their inhibitors to modulate an immune response, is one of the more promising examples of this type of treatment. The pathogenic effects of inflammatory cytokines are blocked using one of three methods. First, anti-inflammatory cytokines can be administered to counter the effects of their inflammatory counterparts. For example, IL-4 can be used to inhibit the action of IFN-γ (see Fig. 15.16). Inflammatory cytokines can also be neutralized by the systemic administration of blocking monoclonal antibodies (Fig. 26.14). Last, antagonists of the cytokine can be administered. These antagonists can be either cytokine analogs that specifically bind to the cytokine receptor without triggering intracellular signaling or a soluble form of the cytokine receptor that competes with the cell surface receptor for cytokine binding (Fig. 26.14).

Recent clinical trials with systemic administration of IFN-β have demonstrated the immunomodulatory effects of this cytokine in patients with MS. The relapse rate over several years was much lower in patients treated with IFN-β than in control patients treated with placebo. Major advances in treatment of RA have recently come about with the introduction of therapies aimed at inhibiting the

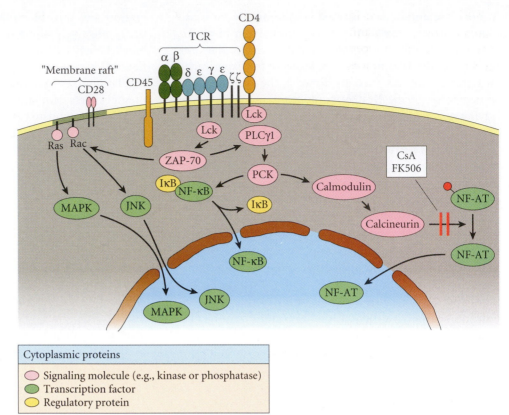

Figure 26.13 The immunosuppressants cyclosporin A (CsA) and FK506 inhibit the activation of T lymphocytes. T-cell activation requires nuclear translocation of several *transcription factors,* including NF-κB and NF-AT. To enter the nucleus, NF-AT must first be dephosphorylated by the phosphatase calcineurin. CsA and FK506 prevent T-cell activation by preventing calcineurin from dephosphorylating NF-AT.

Cytoplasmic proteins
● Signaling molecule (e.g., kinase or phosphatase)
● Transcription factor
● Regulatory protein

action of TNF-α. A chimeric mouse/human monoclonal antibody to TNF-α, called infliximab, has recently been licensed for use along with methotrexate (a general inhibitor of activated cells) for treatment of RA with outstanding success. Another approach has been to use a soluble TNF receptor (TNF-R) fusion protein, called etanercept, to reduce TNF-α levels. This protein works by blocking TNF-α from binding to membrane-anchored TNF-R. Etanercept has had clinical success similar to that of infliximab, but in RA it does not need to be used with methotrexate. These anti-TNF-α therapies are also showing efficacy in MG, AS, psoriatic arthritis, and other autoimmune and inflammatory diseases, but the extent of their efficacy is still under investigation. Furthermore, not all inflammatory diseases are treatable with anti-TNF-α therapies. In addition, these therapies are not without risk. Reports of increased susceptibility to infection, notably viral infections, histoplasmosis, and tuberculosis, have been published. These diseases likely involve TNF-α as a critical component of immunity. In an early trial of the TNF-R fusion protein for treatment of bacterial septic shock there was, in fact, an increase in mortality among patients given the highest doses of the drug compared with controls. Although TNF-α is a major factor in the severe complications of septic shock, if its levels are reduced too much, then the infection causing the shock cannot be adequately resisted.

Further enthusiasm for cytokine immunotherapy comes from animal models of autoimmune diseases, where systemic administration of anti-inflammatory cytokines such as IL-4, IL-10, IL-13, or TGF-β has been shown to protect animals from autoimmune disease.

Figure 26.14 Cytokine therapies for autoimmune disease. IFN-γ serves to activate macrophages and is a component of many autoimmune reactions. IFN-γ action can be blocked by either anti-IFN antibodies or a soluble *receptor decoy* that binds to the cytokine before the latter can bind a cell-surface IFN-γ receptor (IFN-R).

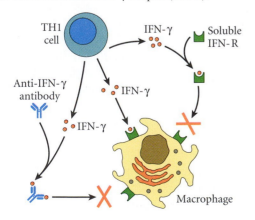

Compelling evidence for the efficacy of cytokine inhibitors comes from animal models in which treatment with soluble IFN-γ receptors neutralizes the effect of secreted IFN-γ and reduces disease severity.

Experimental Approaches

Treatment with monoclonal antibodies: blockade of accessory molecules

Advances in monoclonal antibody technology during the past two decades have made it possible for immunologists to produce antibodies to nearly any antigen, including those expressed on T cells. Through the use of so-called *depleting antibodies*, self-reactive T cells can be destroyed by complement-mediated lysis. Alternatively, the function of self-reactive T cells can be altered by the binding of *blocking antibodies* specific for TCR proteins crucial for delivering activating signals to the T cell. Pioneering studies used depleting antibodies directed at epitopes on autoreactive T cells, such as the CD4 molecule or the TCR. Most animal models of autoimmunity have been successfully treated by depleting T cells. Although these treatments are effective at suppressing disease, the result is general immunosuppression. More recently, administration of blocking or depleting antibodies directed to these same molecules has been shown to prevent the induction, and halt the progression, of autoimmune disease in models of MS, RA, SLE, and IDDM. Blocking the interaction of these key activation molecules can prevent the disease. Unfortunately, this effect is transient. When administration of antibody stops, activation of T cells can recur. One potential means to focus this therapy is to block only those T cells reacting to self antigens by administration of antibodies that bind to the autoreactive TCR. However, this therapy likely would need to be tailored to individual patients, making it impractical to carry out on a large scale with today's technology.

A more general approach might be to block the conserved molecules that contribute to the activation of T cells that provide the second costimulatory signal. A number of soluble and membrane-associated molecules are being investigated in this regard. The CD80-CD86 molecules that engage CD28 and CTLA-4 (CD152) receptors play a critical role in determining the fate of immune responses (activation versus inhibition). This costimulatory pathway is a highly promising therapeutic target for regulating immunopathologic immune responses (Fig. 26.15). In fact, inhibition of CD80-CD86/CD28 costimulation has been shown to have significant immunosuppressive effects: prolongation of the survival of organ transplants and inhibition of autoimmune disease in models of MS, IDDM, and SLE. The advantage of targeting these accessory acti-

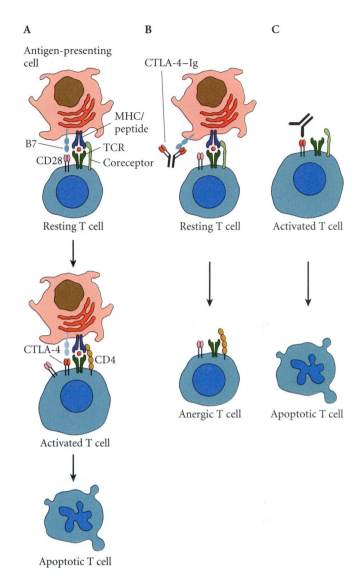

Figure 26.15 T-cell activation can be prevented by interfering with the CD28 and CTLA-4 costimulatory proteins of T cells. (**A**) Normal T-cell activation requires the delivery of one signal to the T cell via the TCR (green) binding to MHC-peptide complexes (either MHC class I or class II; class II is depicted) on an APC (the green curved shape is CD4 or CD8) and the delivery of a second signal to the T cell via an interaction between CD28 (pink) on the T cell with the B7 protein (blue) on the APC. After activation, the T cell increases its expression of the CTLA-4 protein (red). A subsequent interaction of CTLA-4 on the T cell with B7 on an APC (middle panel) turns off T-cell activation and leads to apoptosis of the T cell (bottom panel), thus ending the immune response. (**B**) The requirement of T-cell activation for the "second signal" can be used in therapy development. A soluble fusion protein of immunoglobulin and CTLA-4 (CTLA4-Ig) can bind to B7 on the APC and prevent B7 from binding to the T-cell CD28 protein. The T cell thus receives an incomplete signal and enters a state of unresponsiveness called *anergy*. (**C**) The role of CTLA-4 in terminating T-cell activation is also being studied as a possible therapy. An antibody to CTLA-4 can bind to CTLA-4 on activated self-reactive T cells, causing the T cell to inactivate and undergo apoptosis.

vation molecules is that the immunosuppressive effects appear to be long lasting, since treatment appears to induce a state of anergy in autoreactive T cells.

Altered peptide ligands

T cells recognize, via their TCR, antigenic peptides bound to MHC molecules on the cell surface of APCs. This interaction is highly specific, and subtle changes in the structure of the peptide epitope can affect recognition and T-cell activation (see Fig. 14.10). Studies in recent years have provided evidence that T-cell stimulation using variant synthetic peptides with amino acid substitutions at residues interacting with the TCR (TCR contact residues) can have differential effects on T-cell responsiveness (Fig. 26.16). Single amino acid substitutions of TCR contact residues in the peptide epitope can convert an immunogenic ("agonist") peptide into a tolerogenic ("antagonist") peptide, which is recognized by the antigen receptor of the T cell but inhibits activation and effector functions. The use of such altered peptide ligands (APLs) to modulate T-cell responses has been suggested as a means of treating T-cell-mediated autoimmune disorders.

Studies in the EAE model have shown the therapeutic potential of APLs as immunizing agents. The mechanism by which these APLs mediate tolerance to self is not well understood, but two mechanisms have been put forth. First, APLs may produce a state of clonal anergy in T cells that attack the nerves (referred to as encephalitogenic T cells). Second, APLs may function by generating regulatory T cells that modulate disease by a "bystander" suppression mechanism (see Fig. 14.17). The validity of this second mechanism is supported by the finding that APLs can block EAE induced by agonist self peptides that are totally unrelated to the antagonist peptide. APL treatment of autoimmune disease requires precise knowledge of the peptide epitopes recognized by autoreactive T cells. Because little is generally known of the nature of human disease epitopes, this type of therapy is still in the experimental phase.

Tolerance induction (oral tolerance)

Immunologic unresponsiveness to a specific antigen has been achieved by feeding the antigen to experimental animals. The resulting state, known as *oral tolerance*, has been proposed as a therapy for certain autoimmune diseases in which the antigen(s) that causes the disease has been presumptively identified. For instance, in the mouse model of MS, EAE, feeding animals myelin components results in immunologic hyporesponsiveness to the fed antigens. Furthermore, the animals are protected from disease induction if they are subsequently immunized with these same proteins. In the case of human MS, there is evidence that patients respond to at least one myelin component, MBP. These results have led to clinical trials in which patients with MS are fed myelin proteins. Although there is some evidence that the number of myelin-reactive T cells is reduced in these patients, to date this treatment does not appear to have an effect on clinical disease. It is possible, however, that these early clinical protocols need to be optimized before clinical suppression of disease can be realized.

Bone marrow transplantation

An emerging strategy for the treatment of autoimmune disease involves the transplantation of bone marrow to replace aberrant immune cells. This treatment is based on animal models that suggest that the autoimmune response arises from defects in hematopoietic stem cells. In theory, these defective stem cells mature into effector cells that escape negative selection processes in the thymus or

Figure 26.16 Altered peptide ligands are modified antigenic peptides that can exhibit antagonistic properties on T cells, inducing T-cell anergy instead of activation. These peptides offer promise as clone-specific reagents for preventing T-cell activation. The figure shows the HLA-DR4-presented peptide M12p54-68 derived from *Streptococcus M* protein. *(Top)* Amino acid substitutions at some positions resulted in T-cell antagonism. The size of each arrow corresponds to the relative percentage of substitutions at each position that resulted in antagonism. *(Bottom)* Of the antagonistic peptides, some of them cause antagonism along with partial activation (enlarged cell size, increased cytokine production without T-cell proliferation). Modified with permission from Y. Z. Chen et al., *J. Immunol.* **157**:3783–3790, 1996. Original figure in *J. Immunol.*: copyright 1996 The American Association of Immunologists, Inc.

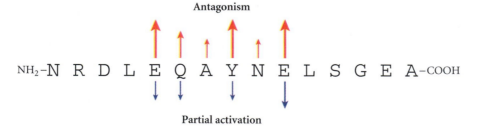

bone marrow. Autoimmune diseases in various animal models have been treated with bone marrow transplantation, including models of SLE, RA, and IDDM. This therapy requires the destruction of the animal's own immune system by treatment with high doses of chemotherapy or radiation. The host immune system is then reconstituted using allogeneic (not autologous) bone marrow that does not contain defective stem cells. A major drawback to this approach for human therapy is the induction of graft-versus-host disease, wherein mature immune cells that arise from the transferred bone marrow cells attack the genetically different host tissues, which they perceive as nonself.

Replacement transplantation therapies

A similar but less invasive transplantation strategy is the replacement of tissues lost due to disease pathology. The clearest success of this approach is seen in models of autoimmune diabetes. Here pancreatic beta cells are transplanted to provide insulin-secreting cells to the host. The transplants are noninvasive since donor beta cells are simply injected into the recipient. Transplant therapy of this type is effective in an animal model of IDDM and recently was found to be effective in human trials, completely relieving recipients of the obligatory use of insulin injections to regulate blood glucose levels. The success of this therapy depends on the survival of the allogeneic beta cells, which are often rejected by the host as foreign tissue. Thus means are needed to block rejection of the transplanted tissues. Immunosuppressive drugs can be used to block transplant rejection, but a more sophisticated strategy is being developed to protect the insulin-secreting beta cells. In experimental models, beta cells can be "hidden" from the host immune system by encapsulating them in synthetic membranes. Membrane sleeves are manufactured and placed under the skin of the host, and beta cells (or genetically engineered beta-cell lines) can be placed into the sleeve. The pores of the membrane allow diffusion of small molecules like glucose and insulin but prevent entry of destructive antibodies and T cells. Should complications occur, the beta cells can be easily removed. If beta-cell function diminishes, replacement cells are easily substituted in the sleeve.

Gene therapy

Although treatments with anti-inflammatory cytokines have therapeutic potential, the side effects inherent in their systemic administration can be severe, potentially limiting their utility. Delivering the cytokine only to the site(s) of inflammation would restrict these side effects. Recent work suggests that gene therapy techniques may now be

employed to this end. By isolating autoreactive lymphocytes and then engineering them to express a cytokine inhibitor (or an anti-inflammatory cytokine), the very cells that cause autoimmune disease can be used as "delivery vehicles" to shuttle regulatory cytokines to multiple sites of inflammation. Presumably, these cells would traffic to inflammatory sites because of the antigen receptor and other homing receptors displayed on their cell surface. This strategy has the advantage of allowing delivery of cytokine therapy to the tissue site of autoreactivity while limiting exposure of other (healthy) tissues to the cytokine.

Evidence of the therapeutic potential of this strategy comes from EAE experiments. In the laboratory, CNS antigen-specific T cells can be genetically engineered, using gene therapy techniques, to secrete anti-inflammatory cytokines or cytokine inhibitors (Fig. 26.17). When ad-

Figure 26.17 Diagram of a strategy to engineer self-reactive lymphocytes to perform regulatory functions. MBP-specific T cells from a mouse with EAE are isolated and transfected with a genetic construct directing overexpression of the regulatory cytokine IL-10. When reintroduced into the EAE mouse, these lymphocytes home to the area of autoimmune inflammation, where they exert negative regulatory effects on non-engineered self-reactive T cells.

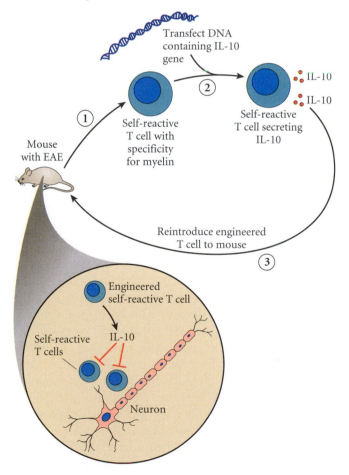

ministered to animals, the cells are found to traffic to sites of CNS inflammation or to lymph nodes draining a site of specific antigen immunization. When these modified cells are administered to animals before the induction of disease, onset is delayed and severity of clinical disease is reduced. Serum levels of the anti-inflammatory cytokine are not elevated, indicating that the therapeutic agent is delivered locally, rather than systemically. In another model, a gene therapy vector for producing a soluble IFN-γ receptor fused to the Fc portion of IgG was successful in preventing diabetes in animal models. Ultimately, the utility of gene therapy will be dependent on finding vectors that lead to the expression of the desired factor for long periods without untoward effects from the vector.

Summary

There exists a panoply of autoimmune diseases that may affect any of the organ systems in the body. Although the immune system exists to protect the host from multiple different types of pathogens and generally does not recognize or respond to self antigens, this self-tolerance is occasionally broken, resulting in autoimmunity. Self antigens can be recognized by the humoral or cellular immune system, resulting in a cascade of events that can damage local tissues or cells (e.g., IDDM), damage certain specific tissues (e.g., RA and MG), or elicit more systemic manifestations (SLE). Induction of antibodies or T-cell responses toward self antigens can occur due to escape and expansion of a small pool of lymphocytes that are normally present and can recognize, but usually not respond to, self antigens. In addition, induction of an immune response to some pathogens that contain antigens cross-reactive with self antigens may also induce an autoimmune phenotype (i.e., postinfectious reactive arthritis, rheumatic fever, etc.). Certain MHC types are associated with a greater incidence of autoimmune diseases, and this may be due to an enhanced ability to present and react to self antigens. In addition, females are generally more likely to get an autoimmune disease, indicating a role of sex steroids in the pathogenesis of many of these diseases. In animals, autoimmune diseases arise spontaneously (e.g., insulin-dependent diabetes in NOD mice) or can be induced by immunization with autoantigen (e.g., AChR for MG). These models have been extremely useful for unraveling the cellular and molecular basis for autoimmune disease. Treatments to attenuate autoimmune manifestations are mainly limited to drugs that decrease the intensity of the response by reducing inflammation or immune cell activation (e.g., steroids, cytoxan, methotrexate, etc.). Newer therapies include drugs that inhibit cytokine function (e.g., anti-TNF antibody, etc.), blockade of immune accessory molecules by monoclonal antibodies, use of APLs to bind to MHC that recognize self antigens and inhibit the immune response toward these antigens, transplantation therapies, gene therapy, and in severe cases, bone marrow transplants to replace cells that recognize self antigens with cells from a donor that does not.

Suggested Reading

Anderton, S. M., and D. C. Wraith. 2002. Selection and fine-tuning of the autoimmune T-cell repertoire. *Nat. Rev. Immunol.* 2:487–498.

Bendelac, A., M. Bonneville, and J. F. Kearney. 2001. Autoreactivity by design: innate B and T lymphocytes. *Nat. Rev. Immunol.* 1:177–186.

Bowness, P. 2002. HLA B27 in health and disease: a double-edged sword? *Rheumatology* (Oxford) 41:857–868.

Boyton, R. J., and D. M. Altmann. 2002. Transgenic models of autoimmune disease. *Clin. Exp. Immunol.* 127:4–11.

Brabb, T., P. von Dassow, N. Ordonez, B. Schnabel, B. Duke, and J. Goverman. 2000. In situ tolerance within the central nervous system as a mechanism for preventing autoimmunity. *J. Exp. Med.* 192:871–880.

Cohen, I. R. 2001. T-cell vaccination for autoimmune disease: a panorama. *Vaccine* 12:706–710.

Daikh, D. I., and Wofsy, D. 2001. Treatment of autoimmunity by inhibition of T cell costimulation. *Adv. Exp. Med. Biol.* 490:113–117.

Elenkov, I. J., and G. P. Chrousos. 2002. Stress hormones, proinflammatory and antiinflammatory cytokines, and autoimmunity. *Ann. N. Y. Acad. Sci.* 966:290–303.

Hemmer, B., S. Cepok, S. Nessler, and N. Sommer. 2002. Pathogenesis of multiple sclerosis: an update on immunology. *Curr. Opin. Neurol.* 15:227–231.

Kuchroo, V. K., A. C. Anderson, H. Waldner, M. Munder, E. Bettelli, and L. B. Nicholson. 2002. T cell response in experimental autoimmune encephalomyelitis (EAE): role of self and cross-reactive antigens in shaping, tuning, and regulating the autopathogenic T cell repertoire. *Annu. Rev. Immunol.* 20:101–123.

Liblau, R. S., F. S. Wong, L. T. Mars, and P. Santamaria. 2002. Autoreactive CD8 T cells in organ-specific autoimmunity: emerging targets for therapeutic intervention. *Immunity* 17:1–6.

Nabozny, G. H., J. M. Baisch, S. Cheng, D. Cosgrove, M. M. Griffiths, H. S. Luthra, and C. S. David. 1996. HLA-DQ8 transgenic mice are highly susceptible to collagen-induced arthritis: a novel model for human polyarthritis. *J. Exp. Med.* 183:27–37.

O'Shea, J. J., A. Ma, and P. Lipsky. 2002. Cytokines and autoimmunity. *Nat. Rev. Immunol.* 2:37–45.

Rosmalen, J. G., W. van Ewijk, and P. J. Leenen. 2002. T-cell education in autoimmune diabetes: teachers and students. *Trends Immunol.* 23:40–46.

Smith, J. B., and M. K. Haynes. 2002. Rheumatoid arthritis—a molecular understanding. *Ann. Intern. Med.* 136:908–922.

Townsend, S. E., C. W. Bennett, and C. C. Goodnow. 1999. Growing up on the streets: why B cell development differs from T cell development. *Immunol. Today* 20:217–220.

chapter 27

Transplantation Immunology

Anil Chandraker and Mohamed H. Sayegh

From time to time, injury or disease may render one or more of an individual's organs or tissues nonfunctional. In some instances, loss of function can be life-threatening, while in others it can result in a great reduction in quality of life. In such cases, it is desirable to replace the damaged organ or tissue with a functional one by a process known as *transplantation* (the transplanted organ or tissue is referred to as a *transplant* or a *graft*). From an immunological standpoint, transplantation is an interesting scenario. Its success requires that transplanted tissue, which is usually genetically different from the graft recipient (that is, immunologically *foreign*), be tolerated by the recipient's immune system so that it can continue to function.

The rate and diversity of solid-organ transplantation have increased dramatically over recent years. Early success in this field was first with transplantation of organs from one site to another within the same individual (a transplant referred to as an *autograft*) and then between different individuals who were genetically identical to each other (referred to as an *isograft*). A practical example of an autograft is transplantation of skin from one site on a person's body to another site, as is commonly done to repair large lesions on the skin of burn victims. Immunologically, these transplants are always successful since the transplanted tissue is *self tissue* that does not provoke an immune response (termed a *rejection reaction*). Practical examples of isografts are organ transplants performed between identical twins. Once again, such transplants are almost always successful, owing to the genetic similarity between the recipient and the transplanted tissue, which makes the graft *appear* to the recipient's immune system as self tissue. Although

649

usually successful, isografts are performed infrequently because of the rarity of patients who have an identical twin. Because of these factors, transplantation in the practical sense usually refers to grafting of tissue between genetically nonidentical individuals (a transplant referred to as an *allograft*). In such cases, the genetic dissimilarity between the donor and the recipient usually causes the transplanted tissue to be recognized as nonself by the immune system of the recipient. This usually results in the recipient's immune system destroying the transplanted tissue (*rejection*). Although early attempts at allogeneic tissue transplantation almost invariably ended in failure, short-term (and in some cases, long-term) success has now become achievable for many types of transplants. Current research in the field of *xenotransplantation* (transplantation from one species to another) is abun-

Figure 27.1 The time frame of graft acceptance and graft rejection. When a graft is accepted (left column), plasmin activation, a normal part of the wound healing process, results in low levels of complement (C′) activation. Relatively small numbers of white blood cells (WBC) are drawn to the site of engraftment by complement anaphylatoxins C3a, C5a, and C4a and assist the wound healing process. When a graft is rejected in a nonsensitized recipient (called a "first-set rejection"; middle column), small numbers of leukocytes are drawn to the site of engraftment by complement anaphylatoxins, but these lymphocytes recognize the graft as nonself tissue. T cells react to the foreign MHC antigens and produce cytokines that draw other immune cell types to the site. B cells can also be induced to produce antibodies (Ab) specific for donor antigens. These antibodies may contribute to graft destruction by triggering classical pathway complement activation as well as mediating antibody-dependent cell-mediated cytotoxicity (ADCC). The resultant activated macrophages and neutrophils produce reactive oxygen intermediates (ROIs), which further damage the engrafted tissue. Together, these immune mechanisms bring about the destruction of the donor tissue in about 2 weeks. If this same recipient receives a subsequent graft from the same donor or a donor whose tissues express MHC antigens substantially the same as those on the first donated organ, a similar graft rejection process (called a "second-set rejection"; right column) occurs, but the rejection happens much more quickly due to the presence of memory lymphocytes specific for donor antigens.

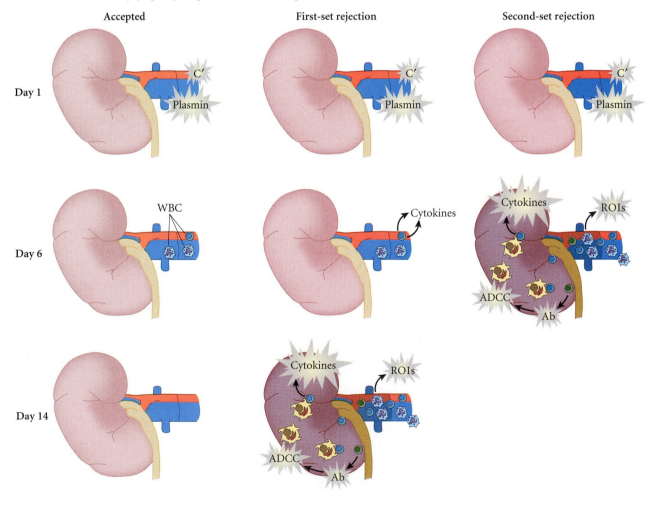

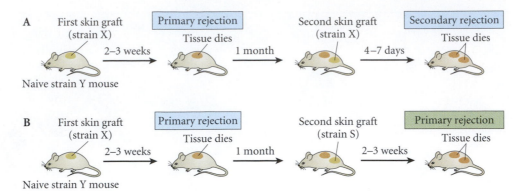

Figure 27.2 The antigen specificity of a secondary or second-set rejection can be demonstrated experimentally. (**A**) Two consecutive skin grafts from a strain X donor onto a strain Y recipient result in a secondary rejection. (**B**) If the second graft is taken from a donor that is genetically different from the first donor, the second rejection has primary rejection kinetics.

dant, and it is an intriguing possibility that future reference to a "transplant" may refer to a xenograft. If perfected, xenograft techniques hold the promise of alleviating the current shortages in our supply of donor organs.

Transplant rejection is primarily mediated by cellular factors of the immune system, such as T lymphocytes (Fig. 27.1). Cytotoxic T cells can directly kill the nonself cells of the graft, while helper T cells can secrete cytokines that support the subsequent activation of other immune cell types such as B cells, neutrophils, and macrophages. This central involvement of T lymphocytes in initiation of graft rejection explains why similarity in major histocompatibility complex (MHC) alleles between the donor and recipient is so crucial to graft acceptance. In a naive recipient without immunosuppression the antigens of the transplant will be recognized and responded to within 2 weeks, leading to a *first-set rejection* of the transplant (Fig. 27.1 and 27.2). This type of rejection can be accelerated in individuals previously exposed to the antigens of the donor tissue, leading to a *second-set rejection*. The more rapid immune response during a second-set rejection is attributable to immunological memory of the recipient to antigens of donor origin. Under normal circumstances of modern medicine, recipients of transplants receive a variety of drugs to suppress their immune system's response to the foreign antigens. However, this therapy must balance the need to suppress responses to the transplant with the host's need to have an immune system that can effectively fight off infectious agents. In situations where the immunosuppression is insufficient to fully prevent responses to the transplant, a form of rejection known as *chronic rejection* can take place. Chronic rejection involves both antibody and cellular immune effectors and may be unavoidable in some instances. In some rare cases a recipient might have high titers of preformed antibody to the

antigens of the transplanted tissue, and in concert with complement can lead to a very active and rapid rejection known as *hyperacute rejection* (Fig. 27.3 and 27.4). This is a major barrier for xenotransplantation since all humans have natural antibodies directed to various antigens commonly found on tissues of animal organs. Xenograft rejection also is due to a less well understood, slower reaction known as *delayed xenograft rejection*. In the different forms of tissue rejection most of the usual mediators of immune reactions play some kind of role.

Many of the recent improvements in the success rates of solid-organ transplantation are attributable to the advances in the understanding of the cellular and molecular mechanisms of the immune response to grafted tissues (Fig. 27.3). These mechanisms are all shaped by the genetics of transplantation, the immune mechanisms of graft rejection, current immunosuppressive therapy in solid-organ transplantation, and the possibility of inducing transplantation tolerance.

The Role of Major Histocompatibility Antigens versus Minor Histocompatibility Antigens in Transplantation

Major Histocompatibility Antigens

Early experiments in transplantation were the experimental basis for identifying the MHC antigens. The key conclusions were based on the observations that it was possible to transplant tissues from one site to another on the same individual (autograft) whereas tissue transplanted from one individual to another (allograft) was inevitably destroyed or rejected by the recipient. Early work conducted by Peter Gorer in the 1930s demonstrated that four groups of antigens on the transplanted tissue were

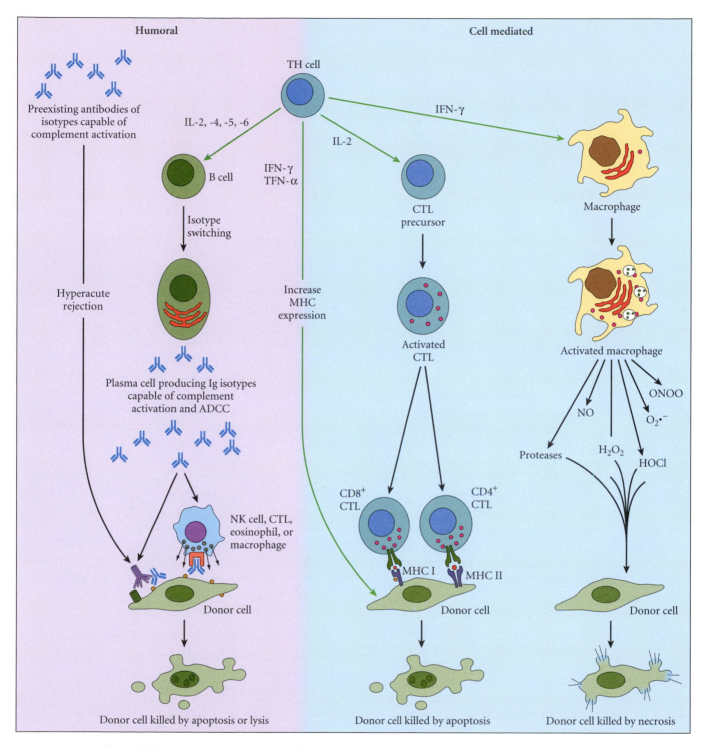

Figure 27.3 A summary of the immune effector mechanisms that can bring about graft rejection. Humoral mechanisms are shown on the left; cell-mediated mechanisms are on the right.

important determinants of graft acceptance or rejection. Later work demonstrated that one of these four groups was a particularly important determinant in tissue compatibility. This group of proteins was therefore designated as the MHC because these proteins seemed to be the most

important factors in determining the compatibility of a transplanted tissue (i.e., likely to be accepted by a transplant recipient). MHC is a generic name that refers to these compatibility proteins in all species, but for some species their MHC is given a specific designation. In hu-

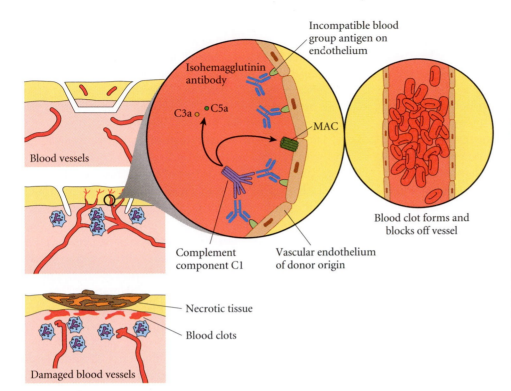

Isohemagglutinin antibody

Incompatible blood group antigen on endothelium

C3a C5a

MAC

Complement component C1

Vascular endothelium of donor origin

Blood vessels

Necrotic tissue

Blood clots

Damaged blood vessels

Blood clot forms and blocks off vessel

Figure 27.4 Hyperacute rejection occurs if the recipient has preexisting antibodies specific for donor antigens. In earlier days, this was most commonly caused by incompatibility of the ABO blood-group antigens between the donor and recipient (this has been averted by routine screening of ABO antigens before transplantation). ABO antigens are expressed on vascular endothelial cells and will be quickly bound by recipient *isohemagglutinin* antibodies, resulting in complement activation, membrane attack complex (MAC) formation, and the generation of complement anaphylatoxins that draw leukocytes such as neutrophils to the site. The clotting system is activated, and blood clots form and block off the blood supply to the engrafted tissue. Rejection can be so fast that the graft never becomes completely revascularized.

mans this family of proteins is called HLA (human leukocyte antigens) because they were found to be expressed on white blood cells. In mice, the MHC proteins are collectively referred to as the H-2 proteins (H for histocompatibility, and 2 referring to Gorer's original nomenclature), since the MHC turned out to be identical to the proteins Gorer classified as *type 2 histocompatibility antigens*. MHC molecules bind antigenic peptides to present them to T cells. However, when a transplant is performed between genetically nonidentical individuals, the nonself MHC proteins on the surface of the engrafted cells can result in T-cell activation. Since MHC class I products (see Fig. 11.2, top) are expressed on the surface of all nucleated cells, virtually any transplanted tissue is capable of triggering T-cell activation in this way. Usually MHC class II proteins (see Fig. 11.2, bottom) are expressed only on B lymphocytes, monocytes, macrophages, dendritic cells, and activated T lymphocytes; however, endothelial and epithelial cells are also capable of expressing MHC class II during intense or prolonged inflammation. Therefore, both MHC class I and class II proteins can stimulate rejection reactions.

Minor Histocompatibility Antigens

Although MHC proteins are certainly the main molecular determinants of graft acceptance or rejection, both clinical and experimental observations of outcomes of transplants have frequently indicated that other molecular de-

terminants exist that provoke immune rejection. For example, when a transplant is carried out between two animals with identical MHC alleles but with genetic differences in the remainder of their genomes (*MHC-congenic animals*) (see Fig. 11.5), the graft is still rejected. In these cases, the graft is rejected more slowly and the rejection reactions that occur are usually less destructive to the target tissue than when the donor and recipient have different MHC alleles. Because of the apparently less dramatic role these antigens have in graft acceptance or rejection, the antigens have been termed *minor histocompatibility antigens*. There are multiple minor histocompatibility antigens; in fact, almost any gene product that exists in multiple alleles can function as a minor histocompatibility antigen. Minor histocompatibility antigens initially were described in the mouse as antigens encoded by the Y chromosome in males and that elicited a rejection reaction of male tissues transplanted into females. These Y-chromosome-encoded antigens are presented to the T cells of the transplant recipient as antigenic peptides bound to the host's own MHC, eliciting an alloimmune response known as the *indirect pathway of allorecognition*.

Tissue Typing

The first major tissue typing system was the definition of the ABO blood group antigens by Karl Landsteiner in 1930. This led to the first successful type of transplantation, which was blood transfusion. Blood-group matching is a critical part of identifying compatible donors and recipients in all transplants. Since individuals lacking either group A, group B, or both (type O individuals) antigens make natural immunoglobulin M antibodies to the nonself antigens, these antibodies can potentially attack the foreign tissue and destroy via complement activation. ABO blood-group antigens are not only expressed on red blood cells but also on epithelial cells and endothelial cells that line the blood vessels of the transplanted tissue.

The best way to minimize the rejection response of the graft recipient is to match as many of the MHC antigens as possible. In the case of humans this requires HLA matching. The closer the HLA match, the longer the tissue survives (Fig. 27.5). Furthermore, the better the match in the class II antigens, particularly the DRB locus, the better the survival. However, HLA matching is not always feasible. In the cases where there is limited donor organ survival once removed from a body, the organ must be quickly transplanted into an available recipient. Other than ABO blood-group typing, other typing may not be practical.

HLA typing is carried out by the microlymphocytotoxicity assay (Fig. 27.6). Lymphocytes from the donor and recipient are obtained from the blood by differential centrifugation or other techniques and further purified. Specific numbers of cells are then dispensed into microtiter plates already loaded with antibodies to known HLA antigens. The antibody-cell mixtures are incubated, then rabbit

complement is added to lyse cells bound by the antibody. Dead cells are then stained with the dye trypan blue, and the microtiter wells are observed under a phase-contrast microscope. The amount of cytotoxicity is scored on a scale of 0 to 8, and the wells with the highest percentage of dead cells are considered to be indicative of expression of the HLA antigen to which the antibody was directed.

Difficulties with the microlymphocytotoxicity assay are principally based on the use of a rapid and necessary serologic assay to infer the degree of relatedness of HLA proteins. However, because HLA antigens share epitopes (public epitopes) as well as express restricted, private determinants (see chapter 11) the ability of a given antibody to determine adequately the closeness of individual HLA proteins is limited. Genetic typing is also revealing differences at the amino acid level that may or may not be important in tissue typing for transplantation. Correlations of serologic and genetic types of HLA proteins can be found at http://www.worldmarrow.org/Dictionary/Dict2001Table2.html. Finally, it is not clear which mismatches are important and which are trivial. Some antibodies indicate a difference in HLA antigens that are of no consequence for the outcome of a transplant. Finally, the importance of tissue typing and matching is not going to be the same for all organ and tissue transplants. Therefore, the utility of tissue typing, while of obvious benefit in many ways, is still not sufficiently well understood to know the degree to which matching must occur in a given transplant situation for this method to optimally minimize problems with transplant rejection.

Initiation of a Graft Rejection Response

Most grafts undergo an early period of acceptance without attack from the immune system. During the first-set rejection (Fig. 27.1) there is an early period of tissue survival. This is occurring during the sensitization phase of graft rejection, when the immune response is developing. Here the lymphocytes that will ultimately produce the effectors that destroy the transplanted tissues are undergoing antigen recognition, activation, proliferation, and differentiation. This is usually occurring in a local lymph node or area of lymphocyte maturation associated with the tissue. Following this sensitization phase the lymphocytes must migrate back to the donated tissue and initiate destruction during the effector phase. For the sensitization phase to be initiated, the recipient's T cells must recognize the antigens on the transplant as foreign. This occurs in a process termed *allorecognition*, which takes into account the ability of T cells to react to foreign MHC anti-

Figure 27.5 Graft acceptance is most successful when there are few genetic mismatches between the donor and recipient at the MHC locus. Redrawn from T. Moen et al., *N. Engl. J. Med.* **303:**850–854, 1980, with permission.

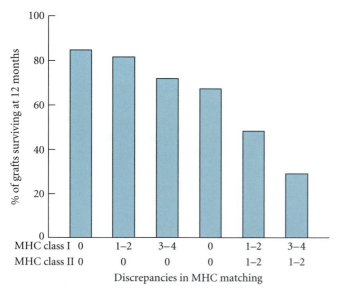

| MHC class I | 0 | 1–2 | 3–4 | 0 | 1–2 | 3–4 |
| MHC class II | 0 | 0 | 0 | 0 | 1–2 | 1–2 |

Discrepancies in MHC matching

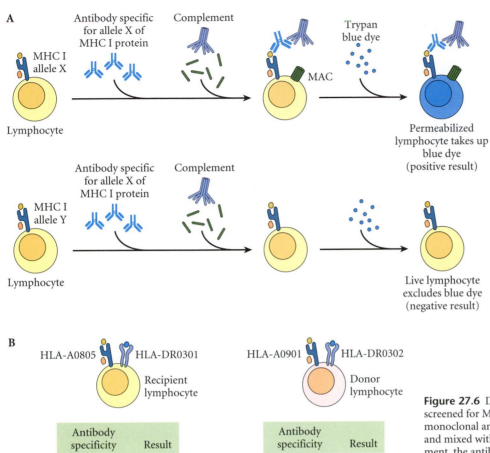

Figure 27.6 Donor and recipient lymphocytes can be screened for MHC alleles by the use of allele-specific monoclonal antibodies. (**A**) If lymphocytes are isolated and mixed with MHC-specific antibodies and complement, the antibodies can recognize the cognate MHC allotype and trigger complement activation and MAC formation. The MAC-permeabilized cells can be identified microscopically by their inability to exclude the dye trypan blue from their cytoplasm. (**B**) A sample tissue typing carried out a small panel of MHC allele-specific antibodies. Note that in this simplified example, only one MHC I and one MHC II protein are shown, and each cell is assumed to be homozygous for the alleles encoding these MHC proteins.

gens presenting peptides derived either from their own cytoplasm (MHC class I) or obtained exogenously and presented by MHC class II.

Mechanisms of Allorecognition

T-cell recognition of alloantigens is the central event in graft rejection. In the classic T-cell response to foreign antigen, T cells recognize foreign antigen through interaction of the T-cell receptor (TCR) with peptide bound to self MHC on antigen-presenting cells (APCs) (see chapter 14 for a complete description of T-cell activation). In graft rejection this "classical" mechanism of T-cell activation involves presentation of alloantigens taken or released from the transplant tissue by the recipient's APCs to the recipient's T cells. However, this is but one of two ways the T cell can recognize the foreign antigens of the graft.

In the second mechanism APCs that are transplanted along with the tissue directly activate recipient T cells by the mechanism of allorecognition (see Fig. 14.14). Both of these pathways seem to play roles in the problem of transplant rejection.

Indirect allorecognition

One way that alloantigens of the graft can stimulate the recipient's T cells is by the presentation of proteolytically processed (nonself) alloantigen by the recipient's own (self) MHC. Because the alloantigens are not being bound directly by the recipient's TCR but are instead being processed and presented to the TCR as a peptide-MHC complex, this mechanism of alloantigen recognition is called the *indirect pathway* (Fig. 27.7). This mechanism of antigen recognition is similar to that used by T cells to recognize most protein antigens, except that in this case the antigens are proteins derived from the grafted tissue. For this pathway to be operative, there must be some mechanism whereby the recipient's APCs acquire antigens from the transplanted tissue. The alloantigens that stimulate such T-cell responses can be any of the minor histocompatibility antigens, and shedding of these antigens from donor tissue results in immune recognition by the recipient. Indeed, antigenic peptides derived from allo-MHC, which are shed from donor APCs that are carried along in the transplanted tissue, are taken up by the recipient's own APCs, proteolytically processed, and bound to intact self MHC expressed on the surface of the recipient's APCs. Overall, the immune response to the foreign antigens in this case follows the usual routes of antigen processing, presentation, and recognition by T cells.

Direct allorecognition

Indirect allorecognition is generally thought to be the weaker of the two mechanisms of T-cell activation during graft rejection. The more potent means of T-cell activation during rejection is thought to occur via the binding to the transplant recipient's TCRs of intact (i.e., not processed or presented) allo-MHC that is on the surface of APCs of donor origin (Fig. 27.7). In this case the allo-MHC containing the self peptide from the transplant tissue is recognized as if it were self MHC presenting processed foreign peptide. Thus, the recipient's T cells respond to the allo-MHC–allopeptide complex as if it were the same as self MHC presenting foreign peptide.

Figure 27.7 Direct versus indirect allorecognition. In indirect allorecognition, donor antigens (which may be donor MHC or any other donor protein that differs from recipient proteins) are proteolytically processed and presented to the recipient's T cells by the recipient's own (self) MHC. Direct allorecognition is the binding of recipient TCRs to intact allo-MHC on the surface of cells APCs of donor origin. These TCRs are binding directly to the foreign MHC without the need for processing of the foreign MHC.

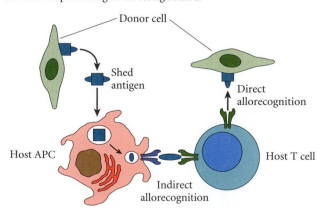

Since the recipient's TCRs bind directly to the foreign MHC without the foreign MHC having to be processed and presented, this mechanism of T-cell activation is termed *direct allorecognition*.

Immature T cells (thymocytes) undergo the process of negative selection as a normal part of T-cell maturation in the thymus. Negative selection destroys thymocytes that bear self-reactive TCRs, thus ensuring that the T cells of an individual organism are *tolerant* of self antigens. However, an individual's T cells are not tolerant of any antigenic peptide (self or nonself) presented on foreign MHC. Thus, the nonself MHC present on the surface of engrafted tissue can activate T cells by binding to the TCR. This mechanism of allorecognition is much more potent than the indirect pathway of recognition and involves an estimated 100- to 1,000-fold greater number of T-cell clones responding to the transplant than does the indirect alloresponse. Since this scenario only occurs in vivo when a T cell of one MHC haplotype encounters a target cell (or APC) of a different haplotype, direct allorecognition is generally considered to be unique to organ transplantation.

The Roles of Direct and Indirect Allorecognition in Graft Rejection

The exact roles of direct and indirect allorecognition in graft rejection have yet to be determined. Regardless, it is important to note that these two pathways of T-cell stimulation have different consequences for the immune response. The direct pathway usually elicits a cytotoxic response involving both cytotoxic T lymphocytes (CTLs) and helper T (TH) cells specific for the graft-derived cells (Fig. 27.8). In contrast, the indirect response is capable of recognizing allopeptides only in the context of self MHC (usually MHC class II) and is therefore more likely to generate a CD4$^+$ TH cell response. Therefore, indirect allorecognition is more likely to initiate delayed-type hypersensitivity (DTH) reactions (when TH1 cells predominate) and B-lymphocyte responses (when TH2 cells predominate). Primarily because of these differences, it has been suggested that the direct response is more important in mediating rapid (acute) rejection and that the indirect response mediates longer-term (chronic) allograft rejection. However, the two pathways are not mutually exclusive, and the relative contribution of each to the processes of acute and chronic rejection remains unclear.

Although both the direct and the indirect pathways of allorecognition have been shown to contribute to allograft rejection, precisely *where* T cells encounter alloantigen is not as clear. The donor-derived leukocytes are thought to act as stimulators of the direct pathway of allorecognition,

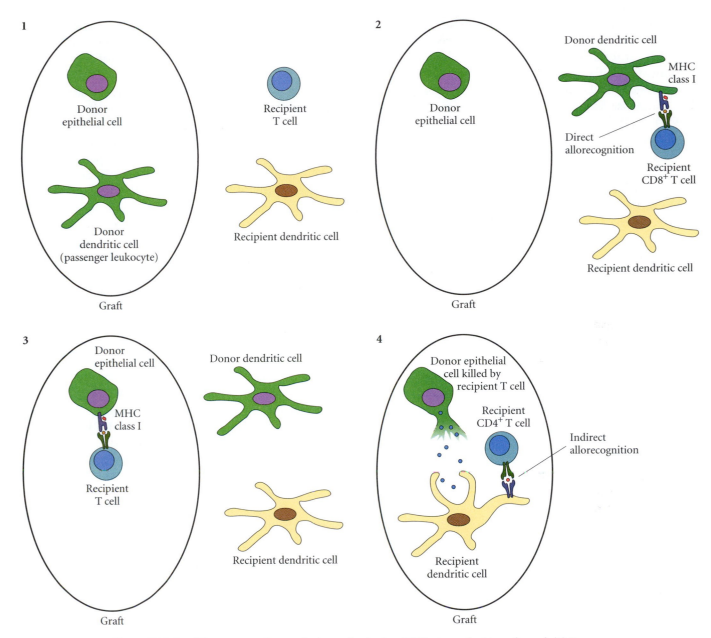

Figure 27.8 Possible sequence of events during graft rejection. (1) The transplant is performed. (2) Donor dendritic cells or macrophages present within the graft (*passenger leukocytes*) leave the graft and stimulate recipient T cells by direct allorecognition. (3) Recipient T cells activated in this way recirculate throughout the recipient and enter the graft, where they kill donor cells in the graft. (4) Donor cells killed in this way release donor antigens, which can be phagocytosed by recipient APCs and presented to recipient T-cells on MHC II in a manner that is restricted by the recipient's self MHC (indirect allorecognition).

possibly within the graft itself. Certainly, organs depleted of donor-derived professional APCs have been shown in some cases not to induce an immune response. Donor-derived APCs also are known to circulate to regional lymphoid tissue in the recipient, although whether they induce a direct response or provide alloantigen that feeds into the indirect response is not known with certainty.

T-Cell Activation

For a T cell to be activated, it must receive several signals from the APC/target cell and from its immediate environment (see Fig. 14.21 and 14.22). Knowledge of these interactions is crucial for designing drugs that could be used to inhibit immune responses to transplanted tissues, hence the emphasis on studying these interactions in detail. Although the chief interactions are between the TCR and MHC and CD28-CD80 or CD86, newly recognized costimulatory pathways could also be targets of inhibition to interfere with the undesired response to transplantation antigens. These include inducible costimulator (ICOS)-ICOS ligand, CD27-CD70, OX40-OX40L, 4-1 BB–4-1 BBL (members of the tumor necrosis factor [TNF] receptor–TNF family), heat-stable antigen (ligand unknown), and ICAM-1–LFA-1. It is likely that these molecules have different functions, including costimulation of memory versus effector cells or the ability to interact with different types of APCs. One goal is to determine if any of these are more active in responding to transplanted tissues, which would make them attractive targets for inhibition in transplant recipients.

The TH1-TH2 polarity of the T-cell response determines which cytokines are produced during the response (see Fig. 3.1) and appears to have an impact on the rejection response made to transplanted tissues. This, in turn, will strongly influence which effector arms of the immune system are recruited to take part in the response. TH1 cells produce interleukin-2 (IL-2), interferon-gamma (IFN-γ), and transforming growth factor beta and are involved in the cell-mediated immune response that likely mediates most of the more severe rejection reactions. Polarization of the TH cell population to a TH2 subset has been associated with induction of tolerance to transplants; however, causality between tolerance and TH cell polarization toward the TH2 phenotype still has to be established. Nonetheless, one strategy to pursue in managing transplants is to direct immune responses to the TH2 phenotype with the expectation this will be less harmful to the transplanted tissue. TH2 cells produce IL-4, IL-5, IL-10, and IL-13 and classically provide help for a B-cell response. Although antibodies can cause tissue damage in a transplant recipient, they may be less harmful than cellular responses, allowing for better management of the transplant.

Effector Mechanisms of Allograft Rejection

An allograft induces a variety of immune effector mechanisms (Fig. 27.3), making it difficult to determine which specific ones are involved in damaging transplanted tissue. Furthermore, the role of CD4$^+$ T cells as helper cells makes it likely that these cells are central to generating graft-rejection responses but may not be the final mediators of rejection. Controversy remains about the exact role of the CTL responses mediated by CD8$^+$ T cells in graft rejection. Presumably these cells could directly bind to

foreign MHC class I on target cells in the transplant and try to destroy the target cell by secretion of perforins and granzymes, activation of the Fas death pathway, or production of TNF-α. However, the role of CD8$^+$ T cells in transplant rejection is more circumstantial than directly supported by experimental evidence. Evidence for involvement of CTLs in rejection includes the recovery of these cells from allografts undergoing rejection and the ability of CTL clones to produce organ injury when injected into experimental animals. However, experiments conducted with CD8-knockout mice indicate that these animals are still capable of rejecting both skin and vascularized allografts such as heart tissues, despite their lack of CD8$^+$ CTLs (Fig. 27.9). Similar results were obtained when antibodies to CD8 were used to deplete CD8$^+$ T cells before transplantation. On the other hand, CD4-knockout mice have been shown to be incapable of rejecting allografts, indicating a central role for CD4$^+$ TH cells in this process.

CD4$^+$ TH cells can be critical to transplant rejection through a variety of mechanisms. They can provide help to produce CD8$^+$ CTLs, initiate macrophage-induced DTH reactions, and augment production of antibodies by B lymphocytes. Whereas the macrophages that take part in DTH reactions are directed to respond by antigen-activated T cells, the ensuing injury (caused by local production of a variety of different molecules, including TNF-α, oxygen-free radicals, and reactive nitrogen) affects self and foreign cells equally that are in the vicinity of the activated macrophage. DTH effector responses can therefore be considered somewhat nonspecific despite the fact that the initial activation event (CD4$^+$ T-cell activation) is antigen specific. This reaction could damage self tissue at sites where there is close interaction of the donor and recipient tissues, such as the anastamosis of donor and recipient blood vessels. Also, over time, host cells may migrate into transplant tissue. There is some evidence that the DTH response may be important in the development of chronic rejection.

Antibodies can also play a role in transplant rejection. By providing CTLs with antigenic specificity, an antibody-dependent cell-mediated cytotoxic response against the antigen-bearing transplanted cells can be elicited. Antibody-mediated rejection is particularly important in patients who have been sensitized by previous exposure to alloantigens. Although antibody-mediated rejection has been rare since the advent of serologic cross-matching, which is designed specifically to detect preformed antibodies in the recipient by the addition of recipient serum to donor cells, an allograft can be rejected in minutes to hours through preformed antibodies directed to the allograft (hyperacute rejection).

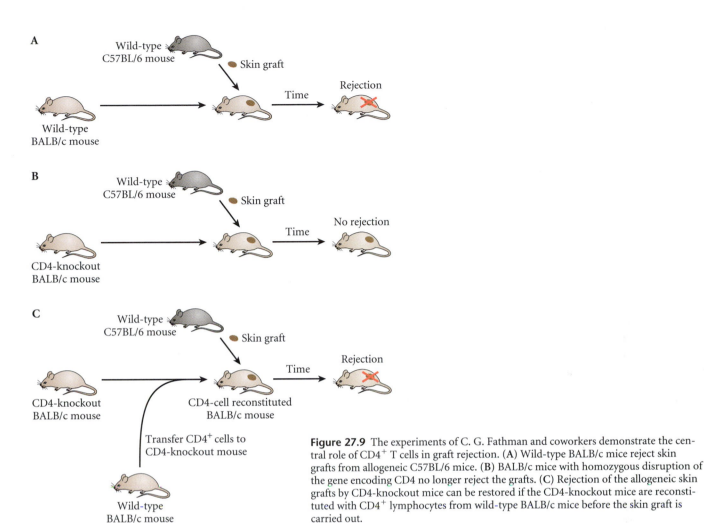

Figure 27.9 The experiments of C. G. Fathman and coworkers demonstrate the central role of CD4$^+$ T cells in graft rejection. (**A**) Wild-type BALB/c mice reject skin grafts from allogeneic C57BL/6 mice. (**B**) BALB/c mice with homozygous disruption of the gene encoding CD4 no longer reject the grafts. (**C**) Rejection of the allogeneic skin grafts by CD4-knockout mice can be restored if the CD4-knockout mice are reconstituted with CD4$^+$ lymphocytes from wild-type BALB/c mice before the skin graft is carried out.

The role of natural killer (NK) cells is not well understood in the context of allograft rejection. NK cells do not need to interact with antigen to induce cytokine-mediated cell lysis. On the contrary, NK cells possess inhibitory receptors that recognize self HLA and prevent them from killing cells that bear self MHC. However, if donor cells can express NK-cell inhibitory receptors, then the host's NK cells would ignore them. Alternately, lack of recognition of donor MHC by the NK-cell inhibitory pathway could lead to NK-cell-mediated tissue destruction. Because the exact combinations of NK-cell inhibitors and inhibitory receptors are not defined, it is conceivable that in some situations these cells play a role in destruction of donor tissues whereas in other individuals the NK cell is not a major participant.

Chemokines

An essential component of the immune response to allografts is the mechanism by which T cells, among other effector leukocytes, find their way to (and into) the trans-planted organs. This occurs as the result of interactions between signaling molecules and their receptors on endothelial cells and leukocytes. Chemokines are key to this process and are produced by endothelial cells or activated platelets during injury or infection. Since chemokines enhance the effect of adhesion molecules expressed on activated endothelium, increasing the efficiency of leukocyte recruitment to the site of injury, they provide a mechanism for translation of a nonspecific injury into a specific immune response directed against an allograft.

The importance of chemokines in transplantation has been demonstrated in an investigation of kidney graft function in patients homozygous for a null allele of *CCR5*. The CCR5 protein is a coreceptor for entry of human immunodeficiency virus (HIV) into macrophages (see chapter 22), and individuals homozygous for the null allele are highly resistant to HIV infection. About 1 to 2% of Caucasians are homozygous for this *CCR5* null allele. The CCR5 chemokine receptor is expressed by large numbers of infiltrating leukocytes in both acute and chronic graft rejection. In a study of 1,200 recipients of kidney transplants, 22 were homozygous for this allele. Only one of the grafts among *CCR5*-null patients was lost during the follow-up period, with an allograft half-life of 60 years (compared with 17 years for *CCR5*-heterozygous patients and for patients homozygous for the wild-type *CCR5* allele). These data highlight the importance of chemokines and their receptors in graft rejection reactions and suggest potential targets for therapeutic interventions.

Graft-versus-Host Disease

Oftentimes a transplanted graft will contain donor immunocompetent cells. This is going to be an obvious problem when tissues that contain high levels of donor lymphocytes, such as bone marrow, are transplanted. Under these circumstances the immunocompetent cells of the donor will recognize the recipient's cells as foreign and mount an immune response against these tissues, resulting in *graft-versus-host disease* (GVHD) (Fig. 27.10). Donor lymphocytes can recognize both major and minor histocompatibility antigens as foreign and respond to them. Patients with GVHD experience many clinical symptoms as the cells of mucosal surfaces, such as epithelial cells, are attacked and die. Symptoms such as weight loss, diarrhea, skin lesions and rashes, liver destruction, lung destruction, and even death can occur. In a procedure such as bone marrow transplantation the donor tissue is usually treated to remove mature donor lymphocytes. But this must be done as a careful balancing act; if the mature cells are depleted in too great a degree, the transplanted cells will not engraft and restore an immune system to the recipient. Also, when bone marrow transplantation is carried out in patients with diseases such as leukemia, there is a desirable effect from GVHD wherein the donor cells attack the leukemic cells of the recipient. In this graft-versus-leukemia reaction there can be substantial benefit in eliminating leukemic cells. Indeed,

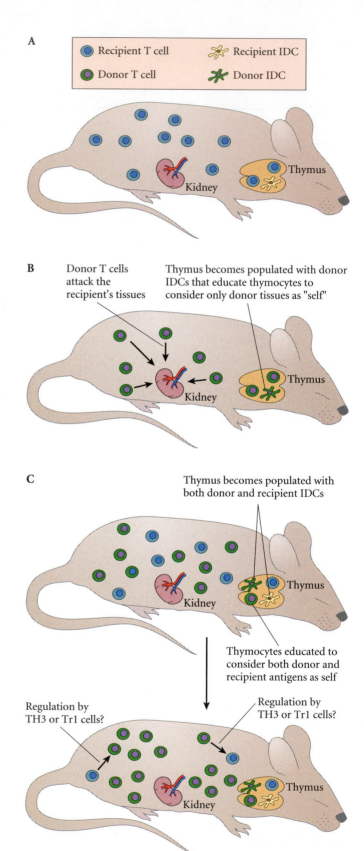

Figure 27.10 Bone marrow transplantation. (A) Mouse before experimental transplant. (B) The mouse's own hematopoietic system is ablated by radiation, followed by transplant of heterologous marrow. The thymus becomes colonized with interdigitating dendritic cells (IDCs) of donor origin. The donor MHC molecules on these IDCs are the basis of negative selection of new thymocytes maturing in the thymus. New T cells that are selected on these donor MHC proteins will regard the recipient's MHC proteins as nonself and attack the recipient's tissues (a phenomenon called GVHD). (C) If the recipient is irradiated and then reconstituted with a mixture of donor and recipient marrow, the thymus will be colonized by IDCs of both donor and recipient origin, and new T cells will be educated to regard both donor and recipient MHC as self. Tolerance may also be maintained by a small population of regulatory T cells such as TH3 or Tr1 cells.

when donor bone marrow to be given to a leukemic patient has been too depleted of mature T cells, the leukemia is more likely to relapse.

The immunologic manifestations of GVHD are due to cell-mediated cytotoxicity engendered by the donor lymphocytes against the recipient's tissues. An allogeneic recognition of the recipient's cells by the donor lymphocytes results in the development of both CD4$^+$ and CD8$^+$ cells that attack recipient tissues. It is often difficult to prevent and treat GVHD, and attempts to find tissue matches to eliminate or reduce the intensity of the disease involve sophisticated laboratory tests. Since bone marrow transplantation, a major cause of GVHD, does not usually have to be done on an immediate basis, time is available to use tests such as the mixed-lymphocyte reaction (see Fig. 11.16) to minimize responses of donor T cells to recipient cells. However, a more accurate measure than just whether or not the donor T cells respond to the recipient's cells can be obtained with an assay referred to as a *limiting dilution assay*. Here different amounts of donor T cells are added to constant amounts of recipient cells in a mixed-lymphocyte reaction and after several days the wells are scored for the presence or absence of cytotoxicity. Obviously, the more donor T cells that are reactive with recipient cells, the higher proportion of wells with cytotoxicity will be seen when fewer donor T cells are added. Through statistical analysis the frequency of donor T cells reactive with recipient cells can be counted, and bone marrow used that has the lowest number of reactive T cells.

Tolerance

Tolerance is the outcome of the process whereby self-reactive T-cell clones are eliminated (clonal deletion) or maintained in a prolonged state of functional inactivity (clonal anergy) (see Fig. 14.15). When this process occurs during the maturation of T-cell precursors, it is referred to as *central tolerance*; when it occurs after T-cell development, it is referred to as *peripheral tolerance*. From the standpoint of transplantation immunology, graft-specific tolerance can be viewed as the ultimate goal of transplantation as a clinical practice, since successful induction of such tolerance theoretically should lead to complete acceptance of any tissue or organ graft. Tolerance induction has, therefore, become a major focus of transplantation research.

Experimental central tolerance can be achieved by the reprogramming of the immune system through ablation of the T-cell repertoire, followed by the infusion of a mixture of donor and syngeneic bone marrow, which then reconstitutes the T-cell repertoire in the presence of both donor and native antigens (Fig. 27.10). Whereas experimental ablation of recipient T cells was originally accomplished through the use of ionizing radiation or chemical regimens, immunosuppression can now be achieved by using monoclonal antibodies targeted at T-cell antigens. Other mechanisms of inducing central tolerance include microchimerism and the activation of so-called veto cells, a type of regulatory T cell (see Fig. 14.17). *Microchimerism* refers to the persistence of small numbers of donor-derived cells in the recipient and has been shown to occur in both experimental models and humans (Fig. 27.11). This is particularly notable in recipients of allogeneic bone marrow, where persistence of donor cells can be easily tracked. It has been suggested that the low-level persistence of donor-derived antigens prevents the recipient's T cells from mounting a response to alloantigens. The exact mechanisms by which this occurs remain to be defined; indeed, the persistence of microchimerism may be the re-

Figure 27.11 Microchimerism. After a solid-organ transplant, small numbers of donor-derived leukocytes can be established throughout the body of the graft recipient. These donor cells persist for years and may aid in the establishment of central tolerance and in the maintenance of peripheral tolerance.

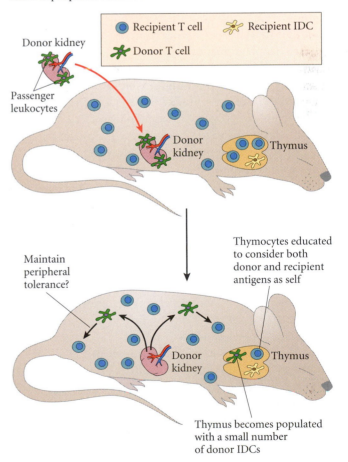

sult rather than the cause of tolerance induction. *Veto cells* are donor-derived regulatory T cells that express MHC class I on their surface and interact with donor T cells, inducing death of the T cells. The action of the regulatory veto cells results in clonal deletion (see chapter 14 and Fig. 14.17). Their exact role in tolerance induction remains to be defined, but their activity seems to be relevant only in the case of the T-cell response to target cells bearing the MHC class I.

Peripheral tolerance is a much more complex situation, with multiple strategies shown to be capable of inducing long-term survival of allografts in the experimental setting. The mechanisms involved in the development of peripheral tolerance include clonal anergy, clonal deletion, and clonal regulation by the regulatory and suppressor T-cell subpopulations. Each of these mechanisms can be induced through multiple pathways. Anergy is a state of unresponsiveness in which T cells specifically recognize antigen but do not respond to it. It is known that not all forms of anergy are the same; some forms can be reversed by exogenous cytokines such as IL-2, whereas others cannot. The fate of anergic T cells also may differ, as variable degrees of clonal deletion have been documented with the induction of anergy in different experimental situations. Some anergic T cells have also been shown experimentally to be able to transfer tolerance from one individual to another. This phenomenon, also known as *infectious tolerance*, is one of the key pieces of evidence suggesting the existence of regulatory T cells capable of suppressing or inhibiting a T-cell response. Other evidence includes the need for donor antigen to maintain a tolerant state and the large proportion of T cells found in tolerant grafts. Regulation of T-cell responses by cell types other than T cells also has been observed in some states of experimental transplantation tolerance. The identity of these regulatory cells has been hard to determine, possibly because a number of different cells may be capable of suppressing or regulating an antigen-specific T-cell response, depending on the circumstances of T-cell recognition of antigen.

A newer form of tolerance induction involves alloantigen administration before transplantation. While perhaps counterintuitive, alloantigen administration along with an appropriate set of modifying drugs can induce tolerance instead of immune activation in experimental animals. When given along with low doses of the T-cell inhibitor cyclosporin, alloantigens either induce regulatory T cells that inhibit effector T cells or prevent the development of effector T-cell responses directly. Pretransplantation alloantigen tolerization would be possible when the donor can be identified ahead of time, such as in living kidney donors or bone marrow transplantation. Although

any donor cell expressing MHC antigens could theoretically stimulate tolerance, the particular cell types from the donors that need to be used are not well defined nor is the route of administration. Soluble forms of MHC antigens given by a mucosal route have led to transplant tolerance in animal models.

Some lines of experimental evidence suggest that the TH2 phenotype is inherently capable of inducing tolerance. TH2 cytokines have been shown to be associated with a "regulatory" phenomenon, but causality between secretion of TH2 cytokines and tolerance remains to be fully established. Some studies have shown that infusion of the TH2 cytokines IL-4, IL-10, and IL-13 prolongs allograft survival, but this finding has been refuted by others. Evidence against the tolerogenicity of TH2 cells includes the ability to induce tolerance in IL-4-knockout mice, the finding that IL-2-knockout mice do not develop tolerance to islet-cell transplants, and the finding that graft rejection occurs in IFN-γ-knockout mice just as rapidly as in wild-type mice. Another study has shown that the transfer of TH2-like alloreactive cells into immunodeficient severe combined immunodeficiency (SCID) mice resulted in rapid allograft rejection. However, a more recent study has indicated that TH2 clones are capable of regulating immune responses to allopeptides both in vitro and in vivo. In summary, data to support the hypothesis that the TH2 response is inherently tolerogenic are still lacking, and the exact role of TH1 and TH2 cytokines in rejection or tolerance remains controversial. Since the development of T cells into TH1 or TH2 phenotypes is usually mutually exclusive, it has been argued that the predominance of TH2 cells in situations of tolerance induction may merely indicate lack of a dominant TH1 response. Despite the remaining uncertainty, however, there is a consensus that TH1 cytokines are important in rejection but are necessary for tolerance induction and that TH2 cytokines may facilitate tolerance induction but are not always necessary.

Immunosuppression

One of the key advances responsible for increasing the success of solid-organ transplantation has been the development of more-powerful immunosuppressive drugs. Although many experimental methods of immunosuppression were tested in the early days of transplantation, the first widely used regimen consisted of a combination of steroids and the nucleotide analog azathioprine, which inhibited cellular proliferation. Even though steroids are still widely used in the vast majority of immunosuppressive regimens, one of the biggest challenges in transplantation today is to find an efficacious regimen of immuno-suppression that does not include steroids, with their plethora of adverse side effects. Until recently, basic immunosuppressive protocols consisted of triple therapy: steroids, cyclosporine, and azathioprine. Over the past few years, a number of newer immunosuppressive drugs have been introduced, and clinicians are evaluating new combinations in order to understand how to use them effectively together to gain maximal benefit and minimal side effects. Indeed, the main reason for using multiple drugs is to target different aspects of the immune response that will allow the lowest possible dose of individual drugs and to capitalize on potential synergistic effects of these drugs.

Another major consideration in immunosuppressive therapy is the balance of immunosuppressive strategies with tolerogenic therapies when the latter are available. A number of immunosuppressive drugs, including calcineurin inhibitors such as cyclosporine and tacrolimus (FK506) and (possibly) steroids, interfere with induction of transplantation tolerance. In certain scenarios, therefore, it may be necessary not only to use immunosuppression when needed but also to do so with "tolerance-

friendly" regimens. The large number of molecular interactions and cellular activation pathways involved in immune responses provide many potential places where selective immunosuppression might be used to enhance graft survival (Fig. 27.12).

Classes of Immunosuppressive Drugs

Corticosteroids

Corticosteroids were the first drugs to be used for immunosuppression in transplantation, and unlike the majority of drugs currently used, they were not designed specifically to be immunosuppressive agents. They inhibit the expression of a number of cytokines, including IL-1, IL-2, IL-3, IL-6, TNF-α, and IFN-γ. IL-2 plays a central role in stimulating the cascade of events leading to the activation and proliferation of T lymphocytes. Corticosteroids inhibit both direct and indirect expression of IL-2. The administration of these medications therefore leads to decreased activation of T cells. IL-1 and IL-6 have also been shown to have important roles in the activation of T cells. Since some of the cytokines inhibited by corticosteroids have chemoattractant activity, corticosteroids

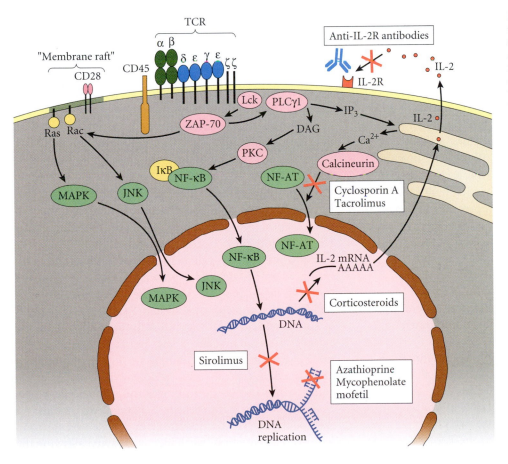

Figure 27.12 A simplified diagram of the central molecular events necessary for T-cell activation, highlighting the steps that are interrupted by various immunosuppressive drugs. Cyclosporine and tacrolimus complex with an immunophilin protein, and this complex prevents the dephosphorylation and activation of the transcription factor NF-AT. Corticosteroids inhibit the transcription of numerous cytokine genes, including the IL-2 gene, and reduce the stability of cytokine mRNAs. IL-2 action can also be inhibited through the use of IL-2 receptor (IL-2R)-specific monoclonal antibodies. Sirolimus (rapamycin) complexes with an immunophilin, and this complex inhibits the activity of proteins that regulate the entry of cells into the cell-division cycle. Azathioprine and mycophenolate mofetil prevent DNA synthesis by inhibiting purine biosynthesis.

also have nonspecific immunosuppressive effects, including the inhibition of the migration of monocytes to areas of inflammation.

Steroids are used in both induction (used at high doses in the perioperative period) and maintenance therapy, and doses are increased for the treatment of acute rejection. The side effects of steroids are numerous and diverse and are particularly worrisome in children, in whom they cause growth retardation. They also cause osteoporosis, hyperlipidemia, hypertension, diabetes, avascular necrosis, and cataracts and increase the risks of bacterial and fungal infection. Several transplant centers have introduced regimens of low-dose steroids and early withdrawal of steroid therapy, while other centers have stopped using steroids completely. To date, none of these protocols have proven to be entirely successful, usually because of the increased risk of rejection, but it is hoped that the use of the newer immunosuppressive drugs will help eliminate the need for corticosteroids in immunosuppressive regimens.

Azathioprine

Azathioprine is a prodrug of 6-mercaptopurine, a purine analog. It is metabolized in the liver to 6-mercaptopurine and 6-thioinosinic acid. In lymphocytes, 6-mercaptopurine is incorporated into cellular DNA, where it inhibits purine nucleotide synthesis and interferes with the synthesis and metabolism of RNA. Unlike other immunosuppressive agents (e.g., steroids and calcineurin inhibitors), azathioprine does not prevent gene activation. It works to inhibit gene replication and resultant T-cell activation. This mechanism allows azathioprine to be an effective agent in preventing acute rejection; however, it is ineffective in treating chronic rejection. Although azathioprine has been replaced by another drug, mycophenolate mofetil, at many centers, azathioprine is still commonly used because it is inexpensive. Its main side effect is dose-dependent bone marrow suppression, especially if it is used in combination with allopurinol, which potentiates the toxicity of azathioprine by inhibiting the enzyme xanthine oxidase.

Mycophenolate Mofetil

Mycophenolate mofetil is one of the new generation of synthetic drugs designed especially for use in transplantation. Like azathioprine, which it has come to replace in many transplant centers, mycophenolate mofetil is a prodrug; it is metabolized to mycophenolic acid and prevents proliferation of lymphocytes rather than their activation. Mycophenolic acid is a reversible inhibitor of inosine monophosphate dehydrogenase, which is the rate-limiting enzyme in the de novo synthesis of guanosine nucleotide and nucleosides. It thus interferes with purine synthesis. Unlike other cell types, lymphocytes do not possess a functional salvage pathway to recycle purine bases. A second purported mechanism of action for mycophenolate mofetil is the prevention of peptide glycosylation, which is required for the efficient trafficking of growth factors and their receptors from the endoplasmic reticulum to the cell surface. Because of its effect on B lymphocytes, mycophenolate mofetil, unlike most other immunosuppressive drugs, is an effective treatment for antibody-mediated tissue rejection.

There is increasing evidence for another role of antibodies in some forms of acute rejection and chronic rejection, in that B cells may be able to act as highly efficient APCs for T-cell activation, using their cell surface antibody to capture alloantigens efficiently even when quantities of these antigens are very low. Clinically, mycophenolate mofetil, although not useful in most types of acute rejection, has proved to be effective as rescue therapy in some forms of refractory rejection, especially when used with tacrolimus. The major side effects of mycophenolate mofetil are gastrointestinal toxicity, especially dose-dependent diarrhea, esophagitis, and gastritis. Bone marrow toxicity in the form of leukopenia and anemia is also relatively common but usually also responds to dose reduction.

Calcineurin Inhibitors

Calcineurin inhibitors prevent T-cell activation by interfering with signal 1 transduction. There are currently two drugs in this class, cyclosporine and tacrolimus (FK506); cyclosporine is now available in a variety of different generic formulations.

Cyclosporine

Cyclosporine was the first of the calcineurin inhibitors to be used in transplantation. It combines with its cytoplasmic receptor protein, cyclophilin. This complex of cyclophilin and cyclosporine then binds the cytoplasmic phosphatase enzyme, calcineurin. This results in the inhibition of calcineurin phosphatase activity, preventing both the dephosphorylation of the transcription factor NF-AT (nuclear factor of activated T cells) and the subsequent translocation of this transcription factor from the cytoplasm to the nucleus, a key step in IL-2 gene activation. The net result is a reduction in IL-2 synthesis and a cessation of T-cell activation. Clinically, reduction in the concentration of IL-2 minimizes the immune response associated with allograft rejection. Patients maintained on therapeutic levels of cyclosporine experience an approximately 50% reduction in calcineurin activity, allowing the patient to retain a degree of immune responsiveness sufficient to maintain host defenses against common environmental pathogens. After its discovery, cyclosporine was used along with steroids and azathioprine as one of the key immunosuppressive agents and contributed to a substantial improvement in early graft survival after transplantation. However, it has also raised concerns because of the nephrotoxic potential of cyclosporine (especially to native kidneys in heart and lung transplant recipients) and its possible contribution to chronic allograft dysfunction in renal transplant recipients. Among its side effects are lipid abnormalities, hypertension, neurotoxicity, gum hyperplasia, and hirsutism, most of which are dose dependent.

Tacrolimus

Tacrolimus, although it bears little structural resemblance to cyclosporine, is also a calcineurin inhibitor. Tacrolimus interacts with an intracellular immunophilin-binding protein (FK-binding protein) and this complex binds to calcineurin, inhibiting its action. In addition to suppressing IL-2, tacrolimus hinders the transcription of other cytokines, including IL-3, IL-4, INF-γ, granulocyte-macrophage colony-stimulating factor, and TNF-α, activities that may add to its potent immunosuppressive actions. On a weight basis, tacrolimus is a much more powerful immunosuppressive agent than cyclosporine and has been shown to be effective as "rescue therapy" in some patients not responding to cyclosporine. Tacrolimus has become the calcineurin inhibitor of choice in liver and pancreas transplantation. Tacrolimus has some of the same side effects as cyclosporine, namely nephrotoxicity and induction of hypertension, but, unlike cyclosporine, it does not induce gum hyperplasia and hirsutism. It can, however, cause greater neurologic side effects and induce posttransplantation diabetes.

Sirolimus

Structurally like tacrolimus, sirolimus (also called rapamycin) is a macrolide antibiotic that also binds to FK-binding protein, but their mechanisms of action are very different. Sirolimus interferes with late T-cell function and is classified as a target of rapamycin inhibitor. The interaction of sirolimus with the target of rapamycin results in impairment in the ability of IL-2 to trigger T cells to enter the division cycle. Early studies have shown that sirolimus and calcineurin inhibitors are actually synergistic. Using sirolimus along with cyclosporine without azathioprine results in better outcomes in transplantation. Combinations of tacrolimus and sirolimus have shown early promise in clinical trials, but further studies are required to establish sirolimus's place in clinical transplantation.

Polyclonal Antibodies

Currently, two polyclonal antibodies, lymphocyte immune globulin and antithymocyte globulin, are commonly used in clinical transplantation. Both are used to lyse peripheral T cells. These antibodies can be used as induction therapy, with the expectation of leading to graft tolerance once the immune system recovers in the presence of the graft, or for the treatment of resistant acute rejection. They are powerful agents that can effectively reduce the circulating T-cell population to very low levels and are administered for short courses.

Monoclonal Antibodies

Monoclonal antibodies have been designed to target specific antigens on human T cells. The first monoclonal antibody to be used clinically was OKT3 (called muromonab-CD3), a mouse monoclonal antibody that binds to the CD3 complex on T cells and impedes the ability of these cells to become stimulated by foreign antigens. This monoclonal antibody was introduced into clinical transplantation in the early 1980s and, along with cyclosporine, resulted in 1-year kidney transplant survival rates increasing from about 60% to almost 90%. During OKT3 therapy, CD3-positive cells are depleted, but T cells with other surface markers, such as CD2, CD4, and CD11, reappear. Within 24 to 48 hours after the discontinuation of therapy, CD3 cells return to circulation; therefore, alternative immunosuppressants must be at therapeutic levels before OKT3 therapy is discontinued. OKT3 has been used successfully for the treatment of acute rejection episodes. It can cause a cytokine-release syndrome due to release of T-cell-derived cytokines, including TNF-α, IL-2, and INF-γ, with the first couple of doses, which can result in fever, chills, and severe pulmonary edema. However, as a mouse monoclonal antibody it elicits human-anti-mouse antibodies (so-called HAMA response) so its utility is limited until a recipient makes a HAMA response.

Interleukin-2 Receptor Antagonists

Two IL-2 receptor antagonists, basiliximab and daclizumab, are now available and are used in induction therapy. Both are based on murine antibodies directed at the IL-2 receptor and block IL-2 activation through its receptor. The original mouse antibodies have been modified to make them less antigenic by substituting elements of human antibodies. They bind to the α subunit of the high-affinity IL-2 receptor, CD25, which is expressed only on activated lymphocytes, and when bound competitively inhibit the IL-2 activation of lymphocytes. Unlike other immunosuppressive drugs, the side-effect profile of IL-2 receptor antagonists is relatively benign, leading to some questioning about their efficacy. However, clinical trials have shown that these antagonists, when used with standard therapies to induce immunosuppression, reduce the rate of acute rejection. The role in the treatment of acute rejection has not been defined.

Summary

Immune recognition of allogeneic antigens on donor tissues is the main cause for rejection of transplants. Rejection of these allografts is either by direct means through immune recognition of the foreign cells by CD8[+] CTLs and CD4[+] TH cells or indirectly by presentation of nonself peptides derived from the transplant presented by the host MHC molecules. Immune mediators of graft rejection include antibody-dependent cytotoxicity in hyperacute rejection, CD8[+] CTL cytolytic activity in acute rejection, and CD4[+] DTH responses in chronic rejection. Many of the treatments to prevent transplant rejection today are based on suppressing these types of responses. Categories of immunosuppressants include corticosteroids, which can inhibit the expression of a number of cytokines, including IL-1, IL-2, IL-3, IL-6, TNF-α, and IFN-γ, and subsequently inhibit activation and proliferation of T lymphocytes; nucleoside analogs such as azathioprine or inhibitors of nucleoside synthesis such as mycophenolic compounds; calcineurin inhibitors, like cyclosporine; and monoclonal and polyclonal antibodies that recognize T cells and inhibit their function either by direct lysis or by inhibiting activating cytokines such as IL-2. With greater understanding of the immune mechanisms that effect transplant rejection, better modalities of treatment can be developed with fewer side effects.

Suggested Reading

Fox-Marsh, A., and L. C. Harrison. 2002. Emerging evidence that molecules expressed by mammalian tissue grafts are recognized by the innate immune system. *J. Leukoc Biol.* **71:**401–409.

Hall, B. M. 2000. Mechanisms of induction of tolerance to organ allografts. *Crit. Rev. Immunol.* **20:**267–324.

Le Moine, A., M. Goldman, and D. Abramowicz. 2002. Multiple pathways to allograft rejection. *Transplantation* **73:** 1373–1381.

Li, X. C., T. B. Strom, L. A. Turka, and A. D. Wells. 2001. T-cell death and transplantation tolerance. *Immunity* **14:**407–416.

Martelli, M. F., F. Aversa, E. Bachar-Lustig, A. Velardi, S. Reich-Zelicher, A. Tabilio, H. Gur, and Y. Reisner. 2002. Transplants across human leukocyte antigen barriers. *Semin. Hematol.* **39:**48–56.

Pascual, M., T. Theruvath, T. Kawai, N. Tolkoff-Rubin, and A. B. Cosimi. 2002. Strategies to improve long-term outcomes after renal transplantation. *N. Engl. J. Med.* **346:**580–590.

Rotrosen, D., J. B. Matthews, and J. A. Bluestone. 2002. The immune tolerance network: a new paradigm for developing tolerance-inducing therapies. *J. Allergy Clin. Immunol.* **110:**17–23.

Teshima, T., and J. L. Ferrara. 2002. Understanding the alloresponse: new approaches to graft-versus-host disease prevention. *Semin. Hematol.* **39:**15–22.

Womer, K. L., M. K. Nadim, and M. H. Sayegh. 2000. T-cell recognition of allograft target antigens. *Curr. Opin. Organ Transplant.* **5:**23–28.

Yamada, A., and M. H. Sayegh. 2002. The CD154-CD40 costimulatory pathway in transplantation. *Transplantation.* **73:** S36–S39.

APPENDIX A
CD Antigens

Antigen	Other name(s)	Expressed on:	Function(s)
CD1	T6		Presentation of lipid or heat shock antigens to T cells
CD1a	R4, HTA1	Thymocytes, dendritic cells	
CD1b	R1	Thymocytes, dendritic cells	
CD1c	M241, R7	B cells	
CD1d	R3	Intestinal epithelium	
CD1e	R2	Thymocytes, dendritic cells	
CD2	LFA-2, T11, E-rosette receptor; CD58-binding adhesion molecule	T cells, thymocytes, NK cells	Adhesion molecule; T-cell activation
CD3 δ subunit γ subunit ε subunit	TCR complex, T3	T cells, thymocytes, NK-1 T cells	T-cell maturation; antigen- dependent T-cell activation
CD4	L3T4, T4, W3/25	MHC class II-restricted T cells, thymocytes, monocytes/ macrophages, granulocytes	Coreceptor for MHC class II-restricted T-cell activation; receptor for HIV; receptor for IL-16
CD5	Leu1, T1, Ly-1, Tp67	T cells, thymocytes, some mature B cells	Modulation of TCR and BCR signaling; ligand for CD72
CD6	T12	Most peripheral T cells, thymocytes, some B cells	Adhesion molecule; possible costimulatory molecule for mature T cells
CD7	gp40	Pluripotent hematopoietic cells, T cells, thymocytes	Regulation of apoptosis
CD8 α subunit β subunit	 Leu2, Lyt2, T8 Leu2, Lyt3	T cells, thymocytes	MHC class I-restricted T-cell activation
CD9	MRP-1 p24, DRAP-27	Platelets, B cells, activated T cells, eosinophils, basophils	Regulates cell adhesion and migration; trigger for platelet activation
CD10	Common acute lymphoblastic leukemia antigen (CALLA), EC 3.4.24.11 (neprilysin), enkephalinase, gp100, metalloendopeptidase, neutral endopeptidase (NEP)	B-cell precursors, T-cell precursors, bone marrow stromal cells	Protease
CD11a	α-L integrin chain, LFA-1 (leukocyte function-associated molecule 1) α chain	Monocytes, macrophages, granulocytes, lymphocytes	Cell adhesion; ligand for ICAM-1 (CD54)
CD11b	iC3bR, complement receptor 3 (CR3); α chain of MAC-1 integrin; α_M integrin chain	Granulocytes, monocytes, NK cells, some T cells, some B cells	Mediates interactions of neutrophils and monocytes with activated endothelium; phagocytosis of complement-coated antigens; chemotaxis of leukocytes

(continued)

Antigen	Other name(s)	Expressed on:	Function(s)
CD11c	α-X integrin chain, αxβ₂, CR4, leukocyte surface antigen, p150,95	Monocytes, macrophages, NK cells, granulocytes, some T cells, some B cells	Cell-cell adhesion; phagocytosis of complement-coated antigens
CD12w	p90-120	Monocytes, granulocytes, platelets	Not known
CD13	Aminopeptidase N (APN), EC 3.4.11.2, gp150	Progenitors of granulocytes and monocytes (CFU-GM), granulocytes, monocytes, bone marrow stromal cells, osteoclasts	Cell maturation?; cell migration
CD14	LPS receptor (LPS-R)	Monocytes, macrophages	Receptor for lipopolysaccharide (LPS); coreceptor for Toll-like receptors TLR2 and TLR4
CD15	Lewis X, Lex, SSEA-1, 3-FAL, 3-FL, LNFP III (lacto-*N*-neo-fucopentose III), X-hapten	Monocytes, neutrophils, eosinophils	Cell adhesion; phagocytosis?
CD15s	Sialyl Lewis X, sLex, sialylated Lewis X	Neutrophils, lymphocytes, immature type I dendritic cells	Cell adhesion; phagocytosis
CD16a	FcγRIIIA	Macrophages, NK cells, neutrophils	Low-affinity IgG receptor; opsonized phagocytosis; antibody-dependent cellular cytotoxicity (ADCC)
CD16b	FcγRIIIB	Neutrophils	Inhibits activation; extends survival; induces cytokine production
CDw17	Lactosylceramide (LacCer)	Monocytes, granulocytes, basophils, platelets, some peripheral B cells (CD19⁺), tonsillar dendritic cells	Phagocytosis?
CD18	β₂ integrin chain	All leukocytes	Cell adhesion
CD19	B4	Follicular dendritic cells, B cells (except plasma cells)	Part of B-cell coreceptor with CD21 and CD81
CD20	B1, Bp35	B cells	B-cell activation
CD21	C3d receptor, CR2, Epstein-Barr virus receptor (EBV-R)	B cells, follicular dendritic cells, some immature thymocytes	Receptor for EBV, C3d, C3dg, and iC3b; part of the B-cell coreceptor with CD19 and CD81
CD22	BL-CAM, Lyb8	Surface of mature B cells, cytoplasm of late pro- and early pre-B cells	B-cell–B-cell adhesion; ligand for CD75
CD23	B6, BLAST-2, FcεRII, Leu-20; low-affinity IgE receptor	B cells, monocytes, follicular dendritic cells, eosinophils	Regulation of IgE synthesis; trigger for TNF, IL-1, IL-6, and GM-CSF synthesis by monocytes
CD24	BA-1, heat-stable antigen (HSA)	B-cells, granulocytes	Cell adhesion
CD25	IL-2 receptor α chain, IL-2R, Tac antigen	Activated T cells; stimulated monocytes/macrophages	α subunit of IL-2 receptor
CD26	EC 3.4.14.5, adenosine deaminase-binding protein (ADA-binding protein), dipeptidylpeptidase IV (DPP IV ectoenzyme)	T cells, B cells, NK cells, macrophages	Costimulatory in T-cell activation
CD27	S152, T14	Thymocytes, T cells, B cells, NK cells, macrophages	Costimulatory signal for T- and B-cell activation and T-cell development
CD28	T44, Tp44	Thymocytes, T cells, plasma cells	Costimulation in T-cell activation
CD29	β₁ integrin chain, GP, platelet GPIIa, VLA-β chain	Leukocytes	β subunit of VLA-1 integrin
CD30	Ber-H2 antigen, Ki-1 antigen	Activated T cells, activated B cells, activated NK cells, monocytes	Stimulation of proliferation or cell death
CD31	GPIIa′, endocam, platelet endothelial cell adhesion molecule (PECAM-1)	Endothelial cells, platelets, monocytes, neutrophils, NK cells, T cells	Adhesion molecule
CD32	FcγRII	B cells, granulocytes, monocytes	Receptor for Fc portion of antigen-IgG immune complexes
CD33	gp67, p67	Monocytes, myeloid precursors	Adhesion molecule

Antigen	Other name(s)	Expressed on:	Function(s)
CD34	gp105–120	Hematopoietic stem and progenitor cells; endothelial cells	Adhesion molecule
CD35	C3bR, C4bR, CR1, immune adherence receptor	Erythrocytes, neutrophils, monocytes, eosinophils, B cells	Receptor for C4b/C3b-coated particles; cofactor for C3b and C4b cleavage
CD36	GPIIIb, GPIV, OKM5-antigen, PASIV	Platelets, monocytes, macrophages, endothelial cells	Adhesion molecule in platelet adhesion and recognition of apoptotic neutrophils
CD37	gp52-40	B cells, T cells, neutrophils, granulocytes, monocytes	Signal transduction
CD38	T10, ADP ribosyl cyclase, cADP ribosyl hydrolase	B cells, T cells, plasma cells	NAD glycohydrolase
CD39	Bp50	B cells, T cells, neutrophils, granulocytes, monocytes	Signal transduction
CD40	Bp50	B cells, macrophages, follicular dendritic cells, endothelial cells, fibroblasts, keratinocytes, hematopoietic cell progenitors	B-cell growth, differentiation, and isotype switching; stimulates cytokine production in macrophages and dendritic cells; stimulates production of adhesion molecules on dendritic cells
CD41	Glycoprotein IIb (GPIIb), αIIb integrin chain; forms platelet fibrinogen receptor by associating with GPIIIa	Platelets, megakaryocytes	Subunit of platelet fibrinogen receptor, platelet aggregation
CD42		Megakaryocytes, platelets	Adhesion to endothelium, activates clotting cascade
CD42a	GPIX		
CD42b	GPIb-α, glycocalicin		
CD42c	GPIb-β		
CD42d	GPV		
CD43	gpL115, leukocyte sialoglycoprotein, leukosialin, sialophorin	All leukocytes	Anti-cell adhesion molecule?
CD44	ECMR III, H-CAM, HUTCH-1, Hermes, Lu In-related, Pgp-1, gp85	Most cell types	Adhesion molecule for leukocyte homing
CD44R	CD44v, CD44v9	Epithelial cells and monocytes	Adhesion molecule for leukocyte homing
CD45	Leukocyte common antigen (LCA), T200, EC 3.1.3.4, B220, Ly5	All hematopoietic cells	T- and B-cell activation; receptor-mediated activation of other leukocytes
CD45R			
CD45RA			
CD45RB			
CD45RC			
CD45RO			
CD46	Membrane cofactor protein (MCP)	Lymphocytes	Negative regulator of complement activation and deposition on plasma membranes
CD47	Rh-associated protein, gp42, integrin-associated protein (IAP), neurophilin, ovarian carcinoma antigen 3 (OA3), MEM-133, CDw149	Most cell types	Adhesion molecule
CD48	BCM1, Blast-1, Hu Lym3, OX-45	All leukocytes except neutrophils	Adhesion molecule
CD49a	α_1 integrin chain, very late antigen 1 α chain (VLA-1 α chain)	Activated T cells, monocytes, neuronal cells, smooth muscle	Adhesion molecule
CD49b	α_2 integrin chain, GPIa VLA-2 α chain	B cells, monocytes, platelets, megakaryocytes; neuronal cells, epithelial and endothelial cells; osteoclasts	Adhesion molecule
CD49c	α_3 integrin chain, VLA-3 α chain	B cells	Adhesion molecule

(continued)

Antigen	Other name(s)	Expressed on:	Function(s)
CD49d	α_4 integrin chain, VLA-4 α chain	T cells, B cells, monocytes, eosinophils, basophils, mast cells, thymocytes, NK cells, dendritic cells	Adhesion molecule for lymphocyte migration; costimulatory molecule for T-cell activation
CD49e	α_5 integrin chain, FNR α chain, VLA-5 α chain	Many cell types	Adhesion molecule
CD49f	α_6 integrin chain, platelet gpI, VLA-6 α chain	T cells, monocytes, platelets, megakaryocytes	Adhesion molecule
CD50	Intercellular adhesion molecule 3 (ICAM-3)	All leukocytes	Costimulatory molecule; adhesion molecule
CD51	VNR-α chain, α V integrin chain, vitronectin receptor	Platelets, megakaryocytes	Adhesion molecule
CD52	CAMPATH-1, HE5	Thymocytes, lymphocytes, monocytes, macrophages	Complement activation; cell aggregation?
CD53	MRC OX44	Leukocytes	Signal transduction; activation of B cells
CD54	Intercellular adhesion molecule 1 (ICAM-1)	Endothelial cells, T cells, B cells, monocytes	Adhesion molecule; receptor for rhinoviruses; ligand for CD11a/CD18 and CD11b/CD18
CD55	Decay-accelerating factor (DAF)	Most cells	Regulator of complement activation and deposition on plasma membranes
CD56	Leu-19, NKH1, neural cell adhesion molecule (NCAM)	NK cells, T cells	Immune function not known; adhesion molecule for neuronal cells
CD57	HNK1, Leu-7	NK cells; T cells, B cells, monocytes	Associated with regulatory lymphocytic subpopulations
CD58	Lymphocyte function-associated antigen 3 (LFA-3)	Many cell types	Adhesion molecule
CD59	IF-5Ag, H19, HRF20, MACIF, MIRL, P-18, protectin	Most cell types	Inhibitor of complement-mediated lysis; costimulator of T-cell activation; cell adhesion
CDw60	9-*O*-Acetyl-ganglioside D3	T cells, platelets, thymic epithelium, keratinocytes, fibroblasts, smooth muscle cells	Costimulatory for T cells
CD61	CD61A, GPIIb/IIIa, β_3 integrin chain	Platelets, megakaryocytes, macrophages	Adhesion molecule
CD62E	E-selectin, ELAM-1, LECAM-2	Activated endothelium	Adhesion molecule
CD62L	L-selectin, LAM-1, LECAM-1, Leu-8, MEL-14, TQ-1	B cells, T cells, monocytes, granulocytes, NK cells, thymocytes	Adhesion molecule for lymphocyte homing
CD62P	P-selectin, granule membrane protein 140 (GMP-140), platelet activation-dependent granule-external membrane protein (PADGEM)	Endothelium, platelets, megakaryocytes	Adhesion molecule
CD63	LIMP, MLA1, PTLGP40, gp55, granulophysin, lysosome-associated membrane glyco-protein 3 (LAMP-3), melanoma-associated antigen (ME491), neuroglandular antigen (NGA)	Platelets, endothelium, degranulated neutrophils, monocytes, macrophages, endothelium	Adhesion molecule
CD64	FcγRI	Monocytes, macrophages, dendritic cells, activated neutrophils	Receptor for IgG-antigen complexes; mediates phagocytosis, ADCC
CD65	Ceramide-dodecasaccharide, VIM-2	Myeloid cells	Adhesion molecule?
CD65s	Sialylated-CD65, VIM-2	Granulocytes, monocytes	Adhesion molecule
CD66a	NCA-160, biliary glycoprotein (BGP)	Granulocytes, epithelial cells	Adhesion molecule; receptor for *Neisseria gonorrheae* and *N. meningitidis*
CD66b	CD67, CGM6, nonspecific cross-reactive antigen 95 (NCA-95)	Granulocytes	Adhesion molecule

Antigen	Other name(s)	Expressed on:	Function(s)
CD66c	NCA, NCA-50/90	Granulocytes, epithelial cells	Adhesion molecule
CD66d	CGM1	Granulocytes	Receptor for *N. gonorrheae* and *N. meningitidis*
CD66e	Carcinoembryonic antigen (CEA)	Epithelial cells	Adhesion molecule
CD66f	Pregnancy-specific b1 glycoprotein, SP-1, pregnancy-specific glycoprotein (PSG)	Fetal liver, placenta	Protection of fetus from maternal immune system
CD68	gp110, macrosialin	Monocytes, macrophages, dendritic cells, neutrophils, basophils, mast cells, hematopoietic progenitor cells, activated T cells, some B cells	Not known
CD69	Activation-inducer molecule (AIM), EA 1, MLR3, gp34/28, very early activation (VEA)	Activated T cells, thymocytes, B cells, NK cells, neutrophils, eosinophils, thymocytes	Lymphocyte, monocyte, and platelet activation; role in lysis mediated by activated NK cells
CD70	CD27-ligand, Ki-24 antigen	Activated T and B cells, macrophages	Costimulation of B and T cells
CD71	T9, transferrin receptor (TfR)	All proliferating cells	Iron uptake by cells; iron sequestration
CD72	Ly-19.2, Ly-32.2, Lyb-2	B cells	B-cell costimulation; ligand for CD5
CD73	Ecto-5′-nucleotidase	T cells, B cells, follicular dendritic cells, epithelial cells, endothelial cells	Dephosphorylation of ribo- and deoxyribonucleoside monophosphates; allows nucleoside uptake
CD74	MHC class II-specific chaperone, Ii, invariant chain	B cells, activated T cells, macrophages, endothelial cells, epithelial cells	Intracellular trafficking of MHC class II proteins
CD75		B cells, T cells, erythrocytes	B-cell–B-cell adhesion; ligand for CD22
CD76		B cells, T cells	Not known
CD77	PK blood group antigen, Burkitt's lymphoma antigen (BLA), ceramide trihexoside (CTH), globotriaosylceramide (Gb3)	Germinal center B cells	Regulation of T-cell–B-cell collaboration; regulation of B-cell activation
CDw78	Ba	B cells	Unknown
CD79a	Ig-α, MB1	B cells	Component of B-cell antigen receptor (BCR); required for cell surface expression and signal transduction through BCR
CD79b	Ig-β, B29	B cells	Component of B-cell antigen receptor (BCR); required for cell surface expression and signal transduction through BCR
CD80	B7, B7-1, BB1	Activated B and T cells; macrophages	Regulation of T-cell activation
CD81	Target for anti-proliferative antigen 1 (TAPA-1)	Many hematopoietic cells; endothelial and epithelial cells	Part of B-cell coreceptor with CD19 and CD21
CD82	4F9, C33, IA4, KAI1, R2	Activated cells	Signal transduction in T cells; activation of monocytes
CD83	HB15	Dendritic cells, activated B and T cells	Not known
CD84 CD84a CD84b CD84c CD84d	MAX.3, GR6	B cells, monocytes, platelets, macrophages, dendritic cells	Adhesion, stimulation of cytokine secretion
CD85	LIR-1, ILT2, GR4	Monocytes, macrophages, B cells, dendritic cells, NK cells, T cells	T-cell activation Regulation of T-cell activation; ligand for CD28 and CD152
CD86	B7-2, B70	Dendritic cells, B cells, monocytes	Receptor for uPA, cell adhesion
CD87	Urokinase plasminogen activator receptor (uPAR)	T cells, NK cells, monocytes, neutrophils, endothelial cells, fibroblasts, smooth muscle cells, keratinocytes, hepatocytes	

(continued)

Antigen	Other name(s)	Expressed on:	Function(s)
CD88	C5a receptor (C5aR)	Granulocytes, monocytes, dendritic cells	Initiation of inflammation; activation of granulocytes
CD89	Fcα receptor (Fcα-R), IgA Fc receptor, IgA receptor	Neutrophils, monocytes, eosinophils, macrophages, some B cells, some T cells	Activation of phagocytosis, degranulation, respiratory burst
CD90	Thy-1	Hematopoietic stem cells, thymocytes, T cells, lymph node HEV	Lymphocyte costimulation?
CD91	α_2-Macroglobulin receptor (alpha 2M-R); low-density lipoprotein-receptor-related protein (LRP)	Monocytes, many nonhematopoietic cells	α_2-Macroglobulin receptor
CDw92	GR9	Monocytes, granulocytes, lymphocytes	Not known
CDw93	GR11	Monocytes, granulocytes, endothelial cells	Not known
CD94	Kp43	NK cells, γδ T cells	Inhibition of NK-cell activation
CD95	APO-1, Fas antigen (Fas)	Activated T and B cells	Mediation of apoptosis-inducing signals
CD96	T-cell activation increased late expression (TACTILE)	Activated T cells, NK cells	Not known
CD97	BL-KDD/F12, GR1	Activated B and T cells, monocytes, granulocytes	Binding to CD55
CD98	4F2, FRP-1, RL-388	Many types of activated cells	Regulation of cellular activation; amino acid transporter
CD99	CD99R, E2, *MIC2* gene product	Lymphocytes, thymocytes	Induces programmed cell death
CD100	GR3	Many hematopoietic cell types	T-cell activation and adhesion
CD101	P126, V7, immunoglobulin superfamily member 2	Monocytes, granulocytes, dendritic cells, T cells	T-cell activation
CD102	Intercellular adhesion molecule 2 (ICAM-2)	Vascular endothelial cells, monocytes, platelets	Adhesion molecule; ligand for CD11a/CD18
CD103	Integrin αE chain; human mucosal lymphocytic antigen 1 (HML-1)	Intraepithelial lymphocytes, lamina propria T cells	Adhesion molecule for tissue-specific homing; activation of intraepithelial lymphocytes
CD104	β_4 integrin chain, tumor-specific protein 180 (TSP-180)	Thymocytes; neuronal, epithelial, and endothelial cells; Schwann cells	Adhesion molecule
CD105	Endoglin	Endothelial cells, monocytes, macrophages, bone marrow stroma	Regulates responses to TGF-β_1
CD106	INCAM-110, vascular cell adhesion molecule 1 (VCAM-1)	Endothelial cells	Adhesion molecule
CD107a	Lysosome-associated membrane protein (LAMP-1)	Activated platelets, activated T cells, activated endothelium, activated neutrophils	Protein degradation?
CD107b	Lysosome-associated membrane protein 2 (LAMP-2)	Activated platelets, activated endothelium, activated neutrophils	Protein degradation?
CDw108	John-Milton-Hagen (JMH) human blood group antigen, GR2	Lymphocytes	Adhesion molecule
CD109	8A3, E123, 7D1	Activated T cells, activated platelets, vascular endothelium, megakaryocyte progenitors	Not known
CD114	CSF3R, HG-CSFR, granulocyte colony-stimulating factor receptor (G-CSFR)	Granulocytes, monocytes, platelets, endothelial cells, placenta	Regulator of myeloid proliferation and differentiation
CD115	c-fms, colony-stimulating factor 1R (CSF-1R), macrophage colony-stimulating factor receptor (M-CSFR)	Monocytes, macrophages	Regulator of myeloid proliferation and differentiation

Antigen	Other name(s)	Expressed on:	Function(s)
CD116	GM-CSF receptor α chain	Macrophages, neutrophils, eosinophils, dendritic cells	Subunit of the GM-CSF receptor
CD117	c-kit, stem cell factor receptor (SCFR)	Hematopoietic stem cells and progenitor cells, mast cells	Growth factor receptor
CD119	IFN-γR, IFN-γRa	Macrophages, monocytes, B cells, endothelium	Interferon receptor
CD120a	TNFRI, p55	Many cell types	TNF receptor
CD120b	TNFRII, p75, TNFRp80	Many cell types	TNF receptor
CD121a	IL-1R, type 1 IL-1R	Thymocytes, T cells	Type 1 interleukin-1 receptor
CDw121b	Type 2 IL-1R	B cells, macrophages, monocytes	Type 2 interleukin-1 receptor
CD122	Interleukin-2 receptor β chain (IL-2Rβ)	T cells, B cells, NK cells, monocytes, macrophages	Subunit of IL-2 and IL-15 receptors
CD123	IL-3 receptor α subunit (IL-3Rα)	Hematopoietic stem cells, granulocytes, monocytes, megakaryocytes	Subunit of IL-3 receptor
CD124	IL-4R	Many cell types	Subunit for IL-4 and IL-13 receptors
CD125	IL-5Rα	Eosinophils, B cells, basophils	Subunit of IL-5 receptor
CD126	Interleukin-6 receptor (IL-6R)	T cells, monocytes, B cells, hepatocytes	Subunit of IL-6 receptor
CD127	IL-7 receptor (IL-7R), IL-7 receptor α (IL-7Rα), P90 117 R	B-cell precursors, T cells	Subunit of IL-7 receptor
CD128a	CXCR1, interleukin-8 receptor A (IL-8RA)	Neutrophils, basophils, lymphocytes	Chemotaxis, neutrophil activation; IL-8 receptor; also binds chemokines CXCL2, -3, -5, -6, -7, and -8
CD128b	CXCR2, interleukin-8 receptor B (IL-8RB)	Not known	IL-8 receptor; also binds chemokines CXCL2, -3, -5, -6, -7, and -8
CD130	gp130	Almost all cell types	Signaling subunit of receptors for interleukin-6, interleukin-11, leukemia inhibitory factor, ciliary neurotrophic factor, oncostatin M
CD131	Common beta subunit	Myeloid cells; early B cells	Signaling subunit of IL-3, GM-CSF, and IL-5 receptors
CD132	Common cytokine receptor γ chain, common γ chain, γc	T cells, B cells, NK cells, monocytes, macrophages, neutrophils	Subunit of IL-2, IL-4, IL-7, IL-9, and IL-15 receptors
CD134	OX40	T cells	Adhesion molecule; costimulation
CD135	FMS-like tyrosine kinase 3 (flt3), Flk-2, STK-1	Myeloid progenitors, B-cell progenitors, monocytic progenitors	Growth factor receptor
CDw136	Macrophage-stimulating protein receptor (MSP receptor), ron (p158^{ron})	Monocytes, epithelial cells, neural cells	Activates migration
CDw137	4-1BB, induced by lymphocyte activation (ILA)	T cells, B cells, monocytes, some epithelial cells	Costimulator of T-cell activation
CD138	Heparin sulfate proteoglycan, syndecan-1	B cells	Binding to collagen type 1
CD139		B cells, monocytes, granulocytes, follicular dendritic cells	Not known
CD140a	Platelet-derived growth factor receptor (PDGF-R), PDGFR, α platelet-derived growth factor receptor (PDGFRα)	Endothelial cells	Subunit of PDGF receptor
CD140b	β platelet-derived growth factor receptor (PDGFRβ)	Endothelial cells	Subunit of PDGF receptor
CD141	Fetomodulin, thrombomodulin (TM)	Endothelial cells, megakaryocytes, platelets, monocytes, neutrophils	Anticoagulant
CD142	Coagulation factor III, thromboplastin, tissue factor (TF)	Monocytes, endothelial cells	Part of coagulation pathway

(continued)

Antigen	Other name(s)	Expressed on:	Function(s)
CD143	EC 3.4.15.1, angiotensin-converting enzyme (ACE), peptidyl dipeptidase A, kininase II	Endothelial cells, macrophages, T cells	Regulation of blood pressure via vasoactive peptides, angiotensin II, and bradykinin
CD144	Cadherin-5, VE-cadherin	Endothelium	Adhesion molecule
CDw145		Epithelial cells	Not known
CD146	A32, MCAM, MUC18, mel-CAM, S-endo	Endothelial cells, T cells	Adhesion molecule
CD147	5A11, basigin, CE9, HT7, M6, neurothelin, OX-47, extracellular-matrix metalloproteinase inducer (EMMPRIN), gp42	Leukocytes, red blood cells, platelets, endothelial cells	Adhesion molecule
CD148	HPTP-eta, high-cell-density-enhanced PTP1 (DEP-1), p260	Granulocytes, monocytes, T cells, dendritic cells, platelets	Contact inhibition of cell division
CDw149	MEM-133, CD47, Rh-associated protein, gp42	Lymphocytes, monocytes, neutrophils, eosinophils, platelets	Not known
CDw150	IPO-3, signaling lymphocyte activation molecule (SLAM)	Thymocytes, some T cells, B cells, dendritic cells, endothelial cells	B-cell costimulation
CD151	PETA-3, SFA-1	Platelets, megakaryocytes, endothelial cells	Adhesion molecule; ligand for β_1 integrins
CD152	Cytotoxic T lymphocyte-associated protein 4 (CTLA-4)	T cells, some B cells	Negative regulator of T-cell activation; ligand for C80 and CD86
CD153	CD30 ligand (CD30L)	T cells, macrophages, neutrophils, B cells	Ligand for CD30, costimulates T-cell activation
CD154	CD40 ligand (CD40L), T-BAM, TNF-related activation protein (TRAP), gp39	Activated CD4$^+$ T cells	Ligand for CD40, B-cell activation
CD155	Poliovirus receptor (PVR)	Monocytes, macrophages, thymocytes, neurons	Cell-to-matrix adhesion; germinal center organization receptor for poliovirus
CD156	A disintegrin and metalloprotease (ADAM8), MS2	Neutrophils, monocytes	Extravasation of leukocytes
CD157	BP-3/IF-7, BST-1, Mo5	Granulocytes, monocytes, B-cell progenitors, T-cell progenitors, follicular dendritic cells	Stimulates growth of lymphocyte progenitors; ADP-ribosyl cyclase; cADP-ribose hydrolase
CD158a	EB6, MHC class I-specific receptors, p50.1, p58.1	NK cells, some T cells	Regulates NK cell cytolytic activity upon binding MHC class I
CD158b	GL183, MHC class I-specific receptors, p50.2, p58.2	NK cells, some T cells	Regulates NK cell cytolytic activity upon binding MHC class I
CD161	NKR-PIA, killer cell lectin-like receptor subfamily B member 1	NK cells, T cells, thymocytes	Regulates NK cell cytotoxicity; thymocyte proliferation
CD162	PSGL-1	T cells, monocytes, granulocytes. B cells	Adhesion molecule
CD163	GH1/61, M130, RM3/1	Monocytes, macrophages	Regulation of inflammation
CD164	MUC-24, multiglycosylated core protein 24 (MGC-24v)	Hematopoietic progenitor cells	Adhesion; regulator of proliferation
CD165	AD2, gp37	Lymphocytes, thymocytes, monocytes, platelets	Adhesion molecule
CD166	BEN, DM-GRASP, KG-CAM, neurolin, SC-1, activated leukocyte cell adhesion molecule (ALCAM)	T cells, monocytes, epithelium, neurons, fibroblasts	Adhesion molecule
CD168	RHAMM	Neural cells	Cell motility
CD173	Blood group O	Erythrocytes, lymphocytes	Cell-cell interactions, cell-bacterial interactions
CD174	Lewis Y (LeY), blood group H	Erythrocytes, lymphocytes	Cell-cell interactions, cell-bacterial interactions
CD177	Neutrophil glycoprotein NB1	Neutrophils	Unknown
CD178	FasL	CTLs	Activator of Fas-mediated apoptosis
CD180	RP105	B cells	B-cell activation

Antigen Names with CD Designation Equivalents

Pre-CD name	CD designation	Pre-CD name	CD designation
1F-5Ag	CD59	B4	CD19
3-FAL	CD15	B6	CD23
3-FL	CD15	B7-1	CD80
4-1BB	CDw137	B7-2	CD86
4-F2	CD98	B29	CD79b
4F9	CD82	B70	CD86
5A11	CD147	B220	CD45
7D1	CD109	Ba	CDw78
8A3	CD109	BA-1	CD24
9-*O*-Acetyl-ganglioside D3	CDw60	Basigin	CD147
A32	CD146	BB1	CD80
Activated leukocyte cell adhesion molecule (ALCAM)	CD166	BCM1	CD48
		BEN	CD166
Activation inducer molecule (AIM)	CD69	Ber-H2 antigen	CD30
AD2	CD165	β_1 integrin chain	CD29
ADAM8	CD156	β_2 integrin chain	CD18
Adenosine deaminase (ADA)-binding protein	CD26	β_3 integrin chain	CD61
		β_4 integrin chain	CD104
ADP-ribosyl cyclase/cyclic ADP hydrolase	CD38	β platelet-derived growth factor receptor (PDGFRβ)	CD140b
α IIb integrin chain	CD41		
α platelet-derived growth factor receptor	CD140a	Biliary glycoprotein (BGP)	CD66a
α_1 integrin chain	CD49a	Blast-1	CD48
α_2 integrin chain	CD49b	Blast-2	CD23
α_2-macroglobulin receptor (α_2 MR)	CD91	BL-CAM	CD22
α_3 integrin chain	CD49c	BL-KDD/F12	CD97
α_4 integrin chain	CD49d	Blood group antigen H	CD174
α_5 integrin chain	CD49e	Blood group antigen O	CD173
α_6 integrin chain	CD49f	BP-3/IF-7	CD157
α_L integrin chain	CD11a	Bp35	CD20
α_M integrin chain	CD11b	Bp50	CD39, CD40
α_V integrin chain	CD51	BST-1	CD157
α_X integrin chain	CD11c	Burkitt's lymphoma antigen (BLA)	CD77
Aminopeptidase N (APN)	CD13	c-kit	CD117
Angiotensin-converting enzyme (ACE)	CD143	C33	CD82
APO-1	CD95	C3bR	CD35
Axb2	CD11c	C3d receptor	CD21
B1	CD20	C4bR	CD35

(continued)

Pre-CD name	CD designation	Pre-CD name	CD designation
C5a receptor (C5aR)	CD88	EC 3.4.15.1	CD143
Cadherin-5	CD144	EC 3.4.24.11	CD10
Carcinoembryonic antigen (CEA)	CD66e	ECMR III	CD44
CD2R	CD2	Ecto-5′-nucleotidase	CD73
CD11a β subunit	CD18	ELAM-1	CD62E
CD11b β subunit	CD18	Endocam	CD31
CD11c β subunit	CD18	Endoglin	CD105
CD27 ligand	CD70	Enkephalinase	CD10
CD30 ligand (CD30L)	CD153	Epstein-Barr virus receptor (EBV-R)	CD21
CD40 ligand (CD40L)	CD154	Extracellular matrix metalloproteinase inducer (EMMPRIN)	CD147
CD44v	CD44R		
CD44v9	CD44R	Fas	CD95
CD45R	CD45	Fas antigen	CD95
CD67	CD66b	Fas ligand (FasL)	CD178
CD74 p35	CD74	Fcα receptor	CD89
CD99R	CD99	Fcε receptor II	CD23
CE9	CD147	Fcγ receptor I	CD64
Ceramide-dodecasaccharide	CD65	Fcγ receptor II	CD32
Ceramide trihexoside (CTH)	CD77	Fcγ receptor IIIA	CD16a
CGM1	CD66d	Fcγ receptor IIIB	CD16b
CGM6	CD66b	FcRI	CD64
Class II-specific chaperone	CD74	FcRII	CD32
Coagulation factor III	CD142	FcRIIIA	CD16a
Colony-stimulating factor 1R (CSF-1R)	CD115	FcRIIIB	CD16b
Colony-stimulating factor 3R (CSF-3R)	CD114	Fetomodulin	CD141
Common acute lymphoblastic leukemia antigen (CALLA)	CD10	Flk-2	CD135
		flt3	CD135
Common β subunit	CDw131	FMS-like tyrosine kinase	CD135
Common cytokine receptor γ chain	CD132	FNR α chain	CD49e
Common γ chain	CD132	FRP-1	CD98
Complement receptor type 1 (CR1)	CD35	γc	CD132
Complement receptor type 2 (CR2)	CD21	GHI/61	CD163
Complement receptor type 3 (CR3)	CD11b	GL183	CD158b
Complement receptor type 4 (CR4)	CD11c	Globotriaosylceramide (Gb3)	CD77
CXCR1	CDw128a	Glycocalicin	CD42b
CXCR2	CDw128b	Glycoprotein IIb	CD41
Cytotoxic T lymphocyte-associated protein 4 (CTLA-4)	CD152	GM-CSF receptor α chain	CD116
		GP	CD29
Decay-accelerating factor (DAF)	CD55	gp34/28	CD69
Dipeptidylpeptidase IV	CD26	gp37	CD165
DM-GRASP	CD166	gp39	CD154
DPP IV ectoenzyme	CD26	gp40	CD7
DRAP-27	CD9	gp42	CD47
E-rosette receptor	CD2	gp52-40	CD37
E-selectin	CD62E	gp55	CD63
E2	CD99	gp67	CD33
E123	CD109	gp85	CD44
EA 1	CD69	gp100	CD10
EB6	CD158a	gp105-120	CD34
EC 3.1.3.4	CD45	gp110	CD68
EC 3.4.11.2	CD13	gp130	CD130
EC 3.4.14.5	CD26	gp150	CD13

Pre-CD name	CD designation	Pre-CD name	CD designation
GPIa	CD49b	Intercellular adhesion molecule 1 (ICAM-1)	CD54
GPIba	CD42b	Intercellular adhesion molecule 2 (ICAM-2)	CD102
GPIbα	CD42b	Intercellular adhesion molecule 3 (ICAM-3)	CD50
GPIbb	CD42c	Interferon-γ receptor (IFN-γ-R)	CDw119
GPIbβ	CD42c	Interferon-γ receptor a	CDw119
GPIIa'	CD31	Interleukin-1 receptor (IL-IR)	CD121a
GPIIb	CD41	Interleukin-1 receptor, type 1	CD121a
GPIIb/IIIa	CD61	Interleukin-1 receptor, type 2	CDw121b
GPIIIb	CD36	Interleukin-2 receptor	CD25
GPIV	CD36	Interleukin-2 receptor α chain (IL-2Rα)	CD25
GPIX	CD42a	Interleukin-2 receptor β chain (IL-2Rβ)	CD122
gpL115	CD43	Interleukin-3 receptor α chain	CD123
GPV	CD42d	Interleukin-4 receptor α chain	CD124
GR1	CD97	Interleukin-5 receptor α chain	CDw125
GR2	CDw108	Interleukin-6 receptor subunit	CD126
GR3	CD100	Interleukin-7 receptor	CD127
GR4	CD85	Interleukin-7 receptor α chain	CD127
GR6	CD84	Interleukin-8 receptor, type A	CDw128a
GR9	CDw92	Interleukin-8 receptor, type B	CDw128b
GR11	CD93	Interleukin-16 receptor	CD4
Granule membrane protein 140 (GMP-140)	CD62P	Immunoglobulin α (Ig-α)	CD79a
		Immunoglobulin β (Ig-β)	CD79b
Granulocyte colony-stimulating factor receptor (G-CSFR)	CD114	Immunoglobulin A (IgA) Fc receptor	CD89
		Immunoglobulin A (IgA) receptor	CD89
Granulophysin	CD63	John-Milton-Hagen human blood group antigen (JMH)	CDw108
H19	CD59		
HB15	CD83	KAI1	CD82
H blood group antigen	CD174	KG-CAM	CD166
H-CAM	CD44	Ki-1 antigen	CD30
Heat-stable antigen (HSA)	CD24	Ki-24 antigen	CD70
Heparan sulfate proteoglycan	CD138	Killer cell lectin-like receptor subfamily B member 1	CD161
Hermes	CD44		
HG-CSFR	CD114	Kininase II	CD143
High-cell-density-enhanced protein tyrosine phosphatase 1 (DEP-1)	CD148	Kp43	CD94
		L3T4	CD4
HNK1	CD57	Lacto-*N*-neo-fucopentaose III	CD15
HPTP-eta	CD148	Lactosylceramide (LacCer)	CDw17
HRF20	CD59	LECAM-1	CD62L
HT7	CD147	LECAM-2	CD62E
HTA1	CD1a	L-selectin	CD62L
Hu Lym3	CD48	Leu-1	CD5
Human mucosal lymphocyte antigen 1 (HML-1)	CD103	Leu-2	CD8
		Leu-7	CD57
HUTCH-1	CD44	Leu-8	CD62L
IA4	CD82	Leu-19	CD56
iC3bR	CD82	Leu-20	CD23
INCAM-110	CD106	Leukocyte common antigen (LCA)	CD45
Induced by lymphocyte activation (ILA)	CDw137	Leukocyte function-associated antigen 1 (LFA-1)	CD11a
In-related	CD44		
Integrin α E chain	CD103	Leukocyte function-associated antigen 1α (LFA-1α)	CD11a
Integrin-associated protein (IAP)	CD47		

(continued)

Pre-CD name	CD designation	Pre-CD name	CD designation
Leukocyte function-associated antigen 2 (LFA-2)	CD2	MHC-class I-specific receptor	CD158b
		MIC2 gene-product	CD99
Leukocyte function-associated antigen 3 (LFA-3)	CD58	MLA1	CD63
		MLR3	CD69
Leukocyte sialoglycoprotein	CD43	Mo1	CD11b
Leukocyte surface antigen	CD11c	Mo5	CD157
Leukocyte surface antigen α	CD11a	MRP-1	CD9
Leukosialin	CD43	MS2	CD156
Lewis X (Lex)	CD15	MUC18	CD146
LIMP	CD63	MUC-24	CD164
Lipoarabinomannan-1 (LAM-1)	CD62L	Multiglycosylated core protein 24 (MGC-24)	CD164
Lipopolysaccharide receptor (LPS-R)	CD14		
LNFP III	CD15	NB1	CD177
Low-affinity IgE receptor	CD23	NCA	CD66c
Low-density lipoprotein receptor-related protein (LRP)	CD91	NCA-50/90	CD66c
		NCA-95	CD66b
Lu	CD44	NCA-160	CD66a
Ly-1	CD5	Neprilysin	CD10
Ly5	CD45	Neural cell adhesion molecule (NCAM)	CD56
Ly-19.2	CD72	Neuroglandular antigen (NGA)	CD63
Ly-32.2	CD72	Neurolin	CD166
Lyb-2	CD72	Neurophilin	CD47
Lyb8	CD22	Neurothelin	CD147
Lysosome-associated membrane glycoprotein 1 (LAMP-1)	CD107a	Neutral endopeptidase (NEP)	CD10
		Neutrophil glycoprotein NB1	CD177
Lysosome-associated membrane glycoprotein 2 (LAMP-2)	CD107b	NKH1	CD56
		NKR-P1A	CD161
Lysosome-associated membrane glycoprotein 3 (LAMP-3)	CD63	O blood group antigen	CD173
		OKM5 antigen	CD36
Lyt2	CD8α	Ovarian carcinoma antigen 3 (OA3)	CD47
Lyt3	CD8β	OX40	CD134
M6	CD147	OX-45	CD48
M130	CD163	OX-47	CD147
M241	CD1c	P18	CD59
Mac-1	CD11b	P126	CD101
MACIF	CD59	p150,95	CD11c
Macrophage colony-stimulating factor receptor (M-CSFR)	CD115	p158^{ron}	CDw136
		p24	CD9
Macrophage-stimulating protein receptor (msp receptor)	CDw136	p260	CD148
		p50.1	CD158a
Macrosialin	CD68	p50.2	CD158b
MB1	CD79a	p55	CD120a
ME491	CD63	p58.1	CD158a
MEL-14	CD62L	p58.2	CD158b
Melanoma-associated antigen	CD63	p67	CD33
Mel-CAM	CD146	p75	CD120b
MEM-133	CD47	p90 II7 R	CD127
Membrane cofactor protein (MCP)	CD46	p90-120	CDw12
Membrane inhibitor of reactive lysis (MIRL)	CD59	PASIV	CD36
		PDGFRa	CD140a
Metalloendopeptidase	CD10	Peptidyl dipeptidase A	CD143
MHC-class I-specific receptor	CD158a		

Pre-CD name	CD designation	Pre-CD name	CD designation
PETA-3	CD151	T9	CD71
Pgp-1	CD44	T10	CD38
Pk blood group	CD77	T11	CD2
P-selectin	CD62P	T12	CD6
Platelet activation-dependent granule external membrane protein (PADGEM)	CD62P	T14	CD27
		T44	CD28
Platelet endothelial cell adhesion molecule (PECAM-1)	CD31	T200	CD45
		Tac antigen	CD25
Platelet gpI	CD49f	Target for antiproliferative antigen 1 (TAPA-1)	CD81
Platelet GPIIa	CD29		
Platelet-derived growth factor receptor (PDGF-R)	CD140a	T-BAM	CD154
		T-cell activation increased late expression (TACTILE)	CD96
Poliovirus receptor (PVR)	CD155		
Pregnancy-specific glycoprotein (PSG)	CD66f	Thrombomodulin (TM)	CD141
Pregnancy-specific b1 glycoprotein	CD66f	Thromboplastin	CD142
Protectin	CD59	Thy-1	CD90
PSGL	CD162	Tissue factor (TF)	CD142
PSGL-1	CD162	TNFR p80	CD120b
PTLGP40	CD63	Tp44	CD28
R1	CD1b	Tp67	CD5
R2	CD1e	TQ-1	CD62L
R3	CD1d	Transferrin receptor (TfR)	CD71
R4	CD1a	Tumor necrosis factor receptor (TNFR), type I	CD120a
R7	CD1c		
RHAMM	CD168	Tumor necrosis factor receptor (TNFR), type II	CD120b
Rh-associated protein	CD47		
RL-388	CD98	Tumor necrosis factor-related activation protein (TRAP)	CD154
RM3/1	CD163		
ron	CDw/136	Tumor-specific protein 180 antigen (TSP-1180)	CD104
RP105	CD180		
S152	CD27	Urokinase plasminogen activator receptor (uPAR)	CD87
SC-1	CD166		
S-endo	CD146	V7	CD101
SFA-1	CD151	Vascular cell adhesion molecule 1 (VCAM-1)	CD106
Sialophorin	CD43		
Sialylated CD65	CD65s	VE-cadherin	CD144
Sialyl Lewis X	CD15s	Very early activation (VEA)	CD69
Signaling lymphocyte activation molecule (SLAM)	CDw150	Very late antigen α 1 chain (VLA-α1)	CD49a
		Very late antigen α 2 chain (VLA-α2)	CD49b
SLe-x	CD15s	Very late antigen α 3 chain (VLA-α3)	CD49c
sLex	CD15s	Very late antigen α 4 chain (VLA-α4)	CD49d
SP-1	CD66f	Very late antigen α 5 chain (VLA-α5)	CD49e
SSEA-1	CD15	Very late antigen α 6 chain (VLA-α6)	CD49f
Stem cell factor receptor (SCFR)	CD117	Very late antigen β chain (VLA-β)	CD29
STK-1	CD135	VIM-2	CD65
Syndecan-1	CD138	VIM2	CD65s
T1	CD5	Vitronectin receptor (VNR)	CD51
T6	CD1	VNR α chain	CD51
T8	CD8α	W3/25	CD4
		X-hapten	CD15

Cytokines, Chemokines, and Their Receptors

Cytokine	Other name(s)	Produced by:	Activities
Growth factors			
EGF	Epidermal growth factor, β-urogastrone	Monocytes, kidneys	Stimulates growth of epithelial cells of epidermis
EGF-R	EGF receptor	Most cell types	
Epo	Erythropoietin	Kidneys, liver	Stimulates maturation of red blood cells
Epo-R	Epo receptor	Erythroid progenitor cells	
aFGF	Acidic fibroblast growth factor, heparin-binding growth factor, endothelial cell growth factor, embryonic kidney-derived angiogenesis factor I, retina-derived growth factor, prostatropin	Brain, osteoblasts, kidneys, endothelial cells, smooth muscle, retinas	Regulates cell proliferation, differentiation, and motility; regulates angiogenesis
bFGF	Basic fibroblast growth factor, leukemia growth factor, macrophage growth factor, many other names	Brain, retinas, pituitary, kidneys, testes, monocytes, epithelial cells, endothelial cells	Regulates cell proliferation, differentiation, and motility; regulates angiogenesis
FGFR-1	Fibroblast growth factor receptor 1, flg	Fetal brain, skin	
FGFR-2	bek	Bone, brain, intestine, kidneys, liver, lungs, skin	
FGFR-3		Bone, brain, intestine, kidneys, lungs, skin	
FGFR-4		Fetal adrenal glands, intestine, kidneys, liver, lungs	
G-CSF	Granulocyte colony-stimulating factor, colony-stimulating factor β, pluripoietin	Bone marrow, stroma, macrophages, endothelial cells	Stimulates development of neutrophils; stimulates proliferation and migration of endothelial cells
G-CSFR	G-CSF receptor	Neutrophils, neutrophil progenitors, endothelial cells, platelets	
GM-CSF	Granulocyte-macrophage colony-stimulating factor, colony-stimulating factor α, pluripoietin-α	T cells, macrophages, endothelial cells, fibroblasts	Stimulates differentiation of granulocyte and monocyte progenitors; stimulates growth of endothelial cells
GM-CSFR	GM-CSF receptor, CDw116/KH97	Granulocyte progenitors, monocyte progenitors, endothelial cells, fibroblasts	
LIF	Leukemia inhibitory factor, hepatocyte-stimulating factor, human interleukin for DA cells (HILDA)	T cells, monocytes, fibroblasts	Stimulates proliferation of hematopoietic stem cells; stimulates platelet formation; regulates acute-phase response
LIFR	LIF receptor	Monocytes, liver	

(continued)

Cytokine	Other name(s)	Produced by:	Activities
M-CSF	Monocyte colony-stimulating factor, colony-stimulating factor 1	B cells, T cells, monocytes, epithelial cells, endothelial cells, fibroblasts, osteoblasts	Stimulates differentiation of monocyte/macrophage progenitors
M-CSFR	M-CSF receptor, CD115, c-Fms	Macrophages, monocyte and macrophage progenitors	
NGF	Nerve growth factor, β-NGF	Brain, prostate	Growth factor for neurons; stimulates differentiation of B cells
LNGFR	Low-affinity NGF receptor, p75^{LNGF}	Brain, epithelial cells, endothelial cells, neurons	
trkA	High-affinity NGF receptor, p140^{Trk}	Brain, B cells, some epithelial lineages	
PDGF	Platelet-derived growth factor, glioma-derived growth factor, osteosarcoma-derived growth factor	Platelets, macrophages, endothelial cells, some epithelial cells, fibroblasts, megakaryocytes, kidneys	Stimulates growth of fibroblasts
PDGFR	PDGF receptor	Chondrocytes, fibroblasts	
SCF	Stem cell factor, Steel factor (SLF), Kit ligand, mast cell growth factor	Bone marrow, stroma, fibroblasts, kidneys, liver, lungs	Regulates early stages of hematopoiesis
SCFR	SCF receptor, CD117, c-Kit	Most hematopoietic progenitors	
TGF-α	Transforming growth factor α, sarcoma growth factor	Monocytes, keratinocytes	Stimulates differentiation of epithelial cells
TGFαR	TGF-α receptor, c-*erbB*	Epithelial cells	
TGF-β	Differentiation inhibiting factor, cartilage-inducing factor, glioblastoma-derived T-cell suppressor factor	Most cell types	Regulates hematopoiesis and wound repair by inhibiting cell proliferation; regulates B-cell isotype switching
TGFβRI	TGF-β receptor I	Most cell types	High-affinity TGF-β receptor
TGFβRII		Most cell types	High affinity TGF-β receptor
TGFβRIII		Most cell types	Low-affinity TGF-β receptor
Interleukins			
IL-1	Interleukin-1, lymphocyte-activating factor, endogenous pyrogen, leukocyte endogenous mediator, mononuclear cell factor, catabolin	Monocytes, macrophages, dendritic cells, T cells, B cells, NK cells, endothelium, smooth muscle, fibroblasts, keratinocytes, chondrocytes	Induction of acute-phase response
IL-1R	IL-1 receptor	T cells, B cells, monocytes, NK cells, basophils, neutrophils, eosinophils, dendritic cells, fibroblasts, endothelial cells	
Type I	CD121a		
Type II	CDw121b	T cells, B cells, monocytes, keratinocytes	
IL-2	T-cell growth factor	T cells	Stimulates growth of T cells, B cells, NK cells, monocytes, macrophages
IL-2R			
Low-affinity (α chain)	CD25	Activated T cells, activated B cells	
Intermediate-affinity (βγ chains)	CD122/CD132	T cells, B cells, NK cells, monocytes, macrophages	
High-affinity (αβγ chains)		Activated T cells, activated B cells	

Cytokine	Other name(s)	Produced by:	Activities
IL-3	Mast cell growth factor, multi-colony-stimulating factor, eosinophil colony-stimulating factor, hematopoietic cell growth factor, burst-promoting activity, P-cell-stimulating factor activity, Thy-1-inducing factor, WEHI-2 growth factor	T cells, mast cells, eosinophils	Stimulates early stages of hematopoiesis; promotes growth of monocytes and B cells
IL-3R	CD123	Hematopoietic stem cells and progenitor cells, pre-B cells, B cells, monocytes	
IL-4	B-cell-stimulating factor 1	T cells, mast cells	Regulates TH1-TH2 axis; induces antibody isotype switching in B cells, favoring production of IgE and IgG4 in humans (or of IgE and IgG1 in mice); regulates some stages of hematopoiesis
IL-4R	CD124	Hematopoietic progenitor cells, pre-B cells, B cells, macrophages, T cells, mast cells, fibroblasts, endothelial cells, epithelial cells	
IL-5	Eosinophil differentiation factor, eosinophil colony-stimulating factor, B-cell growth factor II, IgA-enhancing factor, T-cell-replacing factor	T cells, mast cells, eosinophils	Stimulates eosinophil growth
IL-5R	CDw125	Eosinophils, basophils	
IL-6	Hepatocyte-stimulating factor, B-cell stimulatory factor 2, interferon-β_2 hybridoma/plasmacytoma growth factor, hepatocyte-stimulating factor, monocyte-granulocyte inducer 2, thrombopoietin	B cells, T cells, macrophages, fibroblasts, keratinocytes, endothelial cells	Regulates acute-phase response; regulates inflammation
IL-6R	CD126	T cells, activated B cells, monocytes, fibroblasts	
IL-7	Lymphopoietin	Bone marrow stroma, thymic stroma	Regulates early stages of lymphoid cell development
IL-7R	CD127	B-cell progenitors, T-cell progenitors, monocytes	
IL-8	Granulocyte chemotactic protein, neutrophil-activating factor (protein), monocyte-derived neutrophil-activating peptide, leukocyte adhesion inhibitor, CXCL8	B cells, T cells, monocytes, fibroblasts, endothelial cells, epithelial cells, keratinocytes, hepatocytes, chondrocytes	Regulates inflammation by serving as a chemotactic signal; stimulates angiogenesis
IL-8R	CXCR1, CXCR2	Neutrophils, lymphocytes, monocytes, basophils, eosinophils, endothelial cells	
IL-9	Mast-cell growth-enhancing activity, T-cell growth factor III, p40	T cells	Stimulates activation of T cells and mast cells
IL-9R		T cells, mast cells, macrophages	

(continued)

Cytokine	Other name(s)	Produced by:	Activities
IL-10	Cytokine synthesis inhibitory factor	T cells, monocytes, macrophages, keratinocytes	Regulates TH1-TH2 axis
IL-10R		Many hematopoietic cells	
IL-11	Adipogenesis inhibitory factor	Bone marrow stroma, fibroblasts	Stimulates growth of monocyte/macrophage progenitors; inhibits development of adipocytes
IL-11R		Hematopoietic progenitors	
IL-12	NK cell stimulatory factor, cytotoxic T lymphocyte maturation factor	B cells, monocytes, macrophages	Regulates TH1-TH2 axis; stimulates activity of NK cells and TH1 cells
IL-12R		T cells, NK cells	
IL-13	P600	T cells	Anti-inflammatory; enhances B-cell activation
IL-13R		Activated B cells, monocytes, keratinocytes, epithelial cells, smooth and cardiac muscle, hepatocytes	
IL-14	High-molecular-weight B-cell growth factor	T cells	Stimulates B-cell proliferation; inhibits antibody secretion
IL-14R		B cells	
IL-15		Monocytes, epithelial cells, skeletal muscle, bone marrow stromal cells, placenta	Stimulates cytotoxic T lymphocytes; stimulates mast-cell cytokine production; stimulates B-1-cell development; regulates apoptosis of keratinocytes; stimulates T-cell development
IL-15R		B-1 B cells, thymocytes, mast cells, keratinocytes	
IL-16	Lymphocyte chemoattractant factor	T cells	Serves as a chemotactic signal for T cells, monocytes, and eosinophils; enhances activation of T cells
IL-16R	CD4	T cells, monocytes, eosinophils	
IL-17		T cells	Enhances cytokine expression; induces expression of cell adhesion molecules on fibroblasts; regulates expression of complement proteins
IL-17B		Pancreas, small intestine, stomach	Stimulates monocyte cytokine secretion
IL-17C		Undetectable	Stimulates monocyte cytokine secretion
IL-17E			Proinflammatory
IL-17R		Many cell types	
IL-17BR	IL-17 receptor homolog 1, IL-17Rh1, EVI27	Kidneys, pancreas, liver, brain	Receptor of IL-17B, IL-17E
IL-18		B cells, T cells, monocytes, dendritic cells, keratinocytes, osteoblasts	Proinflammatory; induces activation of T cells, NK cells, and neutrophils
IL-18R		T cells, NK cells, neutrophils	
IL-19	ZMDA1	T cells	Regulation of skin inflammation (part of IL-19 activity)
IL-19R	Binds to type I IL-20R		
IL-20		Keratinocytes	Induces proliferation of keratinocytes

Cytokine	Other name(s)	Produced by:	Activities

IL-20R
  Type I IL-20R
    α chain (IL-20R α)
    β chain (IL-20R β)
 	
  Type II IL-20R
    α chain (IL-20R α)
    β chain (IL-20R β)
	ZCYTO10
	
	DIRS1
	
	DIRS1
		Keratinocytes
		
		Skin, testes, heart,
		placenta, salivary gland
		
		Skin, testes
			Binds both IL-19 and IL-20

IL-21	IL-10-related T-cell inducible factor (IL-TIF)	T cells, mast cells	Induces acute-phase response
IL-21R		Hepatocytes	
IL-22	IL-TIF	Activated T cells	Induces acute-phase response; modulates cytokine production
IL-22R	CRF2-4	Hepatocytes, kidneys, pancreas, intestine	
IL-23	IL-12p40/IL-12p35, IL-12p40/p19	Dendritic cells	
IL-23R	IL-12Rβ1/IL-23R	Memory T cells	T-cell activation
IL-24	Melanoma differentiation-associated antigen 7 (MDA-7), suppressor of tumorigenicity protein 16 (ST16)	Monocytes, T cells	
IL-24R	IL-20RA/IL-20RB		Antitumor cytotoxicity
IL-25		TH2 cells	Type I hypersensitivity
IL-25R			
IL-26	AK155	T cells, NK cells	
IL-26R			
IL-27	EBI3/P28	Antigen-presenting cells	
IL-27R	WSX-1/TCCR	Naive T cells	T-cell activation
Interferons			
IFN-α	Leukocyte interferon, B-cell interferon, lymphoblast interferon, Namalwa interferon, buffy coat interferon, IFNα(I) Note: More than 24 nonallelic IFN-α genes have been discovered in humans. These genes include IFNα4B, IFNα7 (IFNαJ1), IFNα8 (IFNαB2), IFNαA (IFNα2), IFNαB, IFNαC, IFNαD (IFNα1), IFNαF, IFNαG (IFNα5), IFNαH (IFNα14), IFNαI, IFNαK (IFNα6), and IFNαM1.	Lymphocytes, monocytes, macrophages	Resistance to viral infection; regulation of MHC class I expression
IFN-β	Fibroblast interferon, interferon-β1	Fibroblasts, epithelial cells	Resistance to viral infection; regulation of MHC class I expression
IFN-γ	Immune interferon, type II interferon	T cells, NK cells	Macrophage activation
IFN-ω	IFNα(II), IFNα(II)-1	Lymphocytes, monocytes, macrophages	Resistance to viral infection; regulation of MHC class I expression
IFN-κ		Keratinocytes	Resistance to viral infection; regulation of MHC class I expression
IFNαBR		Most cell types	Receptor for IFN-α, IFN-β
IFNα/βR	Type I interferon receptor	Most cell types	Receptor for all IFN-α, IFN-ω, and IFN-β
IFNγR	Type II interferon receptor, CDw119	B cells, T cell, macrophages, neutrophils, platelets	Receptor for IFN-γ

(continued)

Cytokine	Other name(s)	Produced by:	Activities
Tumor necrosis factors			
TNF-α	Tumor necrosis factor alpha, cachectin, macrophage cytotoxin, hemorrhagic factor, necrosin, cytotoxin, macrophage cytotoxic factor	B cells, T cells, monocytes, macrophages, fibroblasts	Regulator of inflammation; cytotoxic for transformed cells
TNF-β	Cytotoxin, lymphotoxin (LT), differentiation-inducing factor	B cells, T cells, monocytes, macrophages, fibroblasts	Regulator of inflammation; cytotoxic for transformed cells
TNFRI	Type I TNF receptor, CD120a, p55	Most cell types	Binds both TNF-α and TNF-β
TNFRII	Type II TNF receptor, CD120b, p75	Most cell types	Binds both TNF-α and TNF-β
Chemokines			
CCL1	TCA-3, P500, I-309	T cells, mast cells	Chemoattractant for monocytes
CCL2	Macrophage chemoattractant protein 1 (MCP-1), monocyte chemoattractant and activating factor, lymphocyte-derived chemotactic factor, glioma-derived monocyte chemotactic factor	T cells, monocytes, fibroblasts, endothelial cells, keratinocytes, smooth muscle	Chemoattractant for monocytes; activates monocytes and basophils
CCL3	MIP-1α, GOS19, pAT464, pLD78, TY5	B cells, T cells, macrophages, neutrophils	Chemoattractant for B cells, CTLs, eosinophils
CCL4	Macrophage inflammatory protein 1β (MIP-1β), ACT-2, G26, HC21, H400, HIMAP, SISγ, MAD-5, pAT744	B cells, T cells, macrophages	Chemoattractant for monocytes and lymphocytes
CCL5	RANTES, SISδ	T cells, macrophages	Chemoattractant for monocytes, T cells, eosinophils; activates basophils and eosinophils
CCL6	MIP-related protein 1 (MRP-1)		
CCL7	Macrophage chemotactic protein 3, MARC	T cells	Chemoattractant for many cell types
CCL8	MCP-2	Many connective tissues	Inflammation
CCL9	MRP-2, MIP-1γ	T cells	Inflammation
CCL10	CCF18	Macrophages	T-cell activation
CCL11	Eotaxin	Epithelial cells, fibroblasts	Chemoattractant for monocytes, eosinophils
CCL12	MCP-5, Scya12	Macrophages	Chemoattractant for monocytes
CCL13	MCP-4	Bronchoepithelium	Chemoattractant for monocytes, T cells, eosinophils, basophils
CCL14	CKβ1, hemofiltrate CC chemokine 1 (HCC-1)	Many tissues	Monocyte activation
CCL15	HCC-2, leukotactin-1, MIP-5	Intestine, liver	Chemoattractant for monocytes, neutrophils, eosinophils, lymphocytes
CCL16	HCC-4, Mtn-1, liver-expressed chemokine (LEC)	Hepatocytes	Chemoattractant for monocytes
CCL17	Thymus and activation regulated chemokine (TARC)	Dendritic cells	Chemoattractant for T cells
CCL18	DC-CK1, pulmonary and activation regulated chemokine (PARC), MIP-4, Scya18	Macrophages	T-cell activation
CCL19	ELC, EBI-1 ligand chemokine, CKβ11, MIP-3β	Dendritic cells	Chemoattractant for lymphocytes mediating homing to lymph nodes
CCL20	Liver- and activation-regulated chemokine (LARC)	Liver	Chemoattractant for lymphocytes
CCL21	6Ckine, secondary lymphoid tissue chemokine (SLC), exodus2	Spleen, lymph nodes	Chemoattractant for lymphocytes

Cytokine	Other name(s)	Produced by:	Activities
CCL22	Macrophage-derived chemokine (MDC), stimulated T-cell chemoattractant protein 1 (STCP1)	Dendritic cells	Chemoattractant for dendritic cells, NK cells, TH2 cells
CCL23	CKβ8	Bone	Chemoattractant for osteoclast precursors
CCL24	Eotaxin-2	Skin	Chemoattractant for eosinophils, basophils, neutrophils, macrophages
CCL25	TECK, CKβ15	Thymus, intestinal epithelium	Homing of lymphocytes to lymphoid tissues
CCL26	Eotaxin-3, MIP-4a	Endothelial cells, fibroblasts	Eosinophil homing
CCL27	ALP (an abbreviation of its amino-terminal amino acid sequence), cutaneous T-cell-attracting chemokine (CTACK), ES cell chemokine (ESkine), interleukin-11 receptor-locus chemokine (ILC)	Keratinocytes	Homing of memory lymphocytes to skin
CXCL1	MIP-2, GROα, MGSA, KC	Monocytes, epithelial cells, endothelial cells, fibroblasts	Chemoattractant for neutrophils
CXCL2	MIP-2α, GROβ, KC	Monocytes, epithelial cells, endothelial cells, fibroblasts	Chemoattractant for neutrophils
CXCL3	MIP-2β, GROγ, KC	Monocytes, epithelial cells, endothelial cells, fibroblasts	Chemoattractant for neutrophils
CXCL4	Platelet factor 4	Platelets	Inducible hematopoiesis
CXCL5	ENA-78, LIX	Epithelial cells	Neutrophil activation, angiogenesis
CXCL6	GCP-2, CKα-3	Fibroblasts	Chemoattractant for neutrophils, neutrophil activation, angiogenesis
CXCL7	Platelet basic protein (PBP), CTAP-III low-affinity platelet factor 4, NAP-2 (CTAP-III and NAP-2 are proteolytic cleavage products of PBP precursor)	Platelets	Chemoattractant for neutrophils
CXCL8	IL-8, granulocyte chemotactic protein, neutrophil-activating factor (protein), monocyte-derived neutrophil-activating peptide, leukocyte adhesion inhibitor	B cells, T cells, monocytes, fibroblasts, endothelial cells, epithelial cells, keratinocytes, hepatocytes, chondrocytes	Chemoattractant for neutrophils
CXCL9	IFN-γ-inducible protein 10, CRG-2, C7, Mig, γIP-10	T cells, monocytes, endothelial cells, fibroblasts	Chemoattractant for monocytes and activated T cells
CXCL10	IP-10, CRG-2	Macrophages, keratinocytes	T-cell inflammation
CXCL11	I-TAC, IP-9, SCYB9B	Macrophages, fibroblasts, multiple tissues	T-cell inflammation
CXCL12	Stromal cell-derived factor 1α, SDF-1	Bone marrow stroma, fibroblasts	Stimulates growth of B-cell progenitors
CXCL13	BLC, BCA-1	Dendritic cells	B-cell homing to follicles
CXCL14	BRAK	Epithelial cells, B cells, monocytes	Chemoattractant for monocytes, macrophage maturation
CXCL15	Lungkine	Bronchoepithelium	Inflammation
CXCL16		B cells, macrophages	T-cell inflammation
CX$_3$CL1	Fractalkine, neurotactin	Neuronal cells	Maintaining survivability of microglial macrophages?
XCL1	ATAC, lymphotactin	NK cells, T cells	Chemoattractant for lymphocytes

(continued)

Cytokine	Other name(s)	Produced by:	Activities
CCR1		T cells, platelets, monocytes, granulocyte progenitors, macrophage progenitors, mast cells, neutrophils, NK cells	Receptor for CCL3, -5, -7, -14, -15, -16, -23
CCR2		Monocytes, mast cells, T cells, NK cells, basophils, neutrophils	Receptor for CCL2, -7, -12, -13
CCR3		TH2 cells, mast cells, eosinophils, platelets, basophils	Receptor for CCL5, -7, -8, -13, -15, -24, -26
CCR4		TH2 cell, platelets, NK cells	Receptor for CCL17, -22
CCR5		Monocytes, TH1 cells, dendritic cells, macrophages, mast cells	Receptor for CCL3, -4, -5
CCR6	GPR-CY4	Lymphocytes, dendritic cells	Receptor for CCL20
CCR7	EBI-1, BLR-2	Lymphocytes, dendritic cells	Receptor for CCL19, -20
CCR8		NK cells, TH2 cells	Receptor for CCL1, -4
CCR9		T cells, thymocytes, macrophages, dendritic cells	Receptor for CCL25
CCR10		Cutaneous T cells	Receptor for CCL27
CCR11		Heart, intestine, lungs	Receptor for CCL2, -8, -13
CXCR1	IL-8 receptor	Neutrophils, lymphocytes, monocytes, basophils, eosinophils, endothelial cells, mast cells	Receptor for CXCL2, -3, -5, -6, -7, -8
CXCR2	IL-8 receptor	Neutrophils, lymphocytes, monocytes, basophils, eosinophils, endothelial cells, mast cells	Receptor for CXCL1, -2, -3, -5, -6, -7, -8
CXCR3		TH1 cells, endothelial cells, B cells, NK cells	Receptor for CXCL9, -10, -11
CXCR4		Platelets, endothelial cells, lymphocytes, monocytes, dendritic cells	Receptor for CXCL12
CXCR5		Lymphocytes	Receptor for CXCL13
CXCR6		Memory T cells	Receptor for CXCL16
CX_3CR1		Microglial macrophages, T cells, NK cells, neutrophils	Receptor for CX_3CL1
XCR1		T cells	Receptor for XCL1

APPENDIX D
Cell Types and Immune-Related Functions

Cell type	Lineage	Principal anatomic location(s)	Normal concentration	Immune-related function(s)
B cell	Lymphoid	Blood, spleen, lymph nodes	$8 \times 10^2/\text{mm}^3$	Antibody production, antigen presentation
Basophil	Myeloid	Blood	$8 \times 10^1/\text{mm}^3$	Type 1 hypersensitivity
Dendritic cell (DC)				
DC1	Myeloid	Blood and many tissues		Antigen presentation for type 1 helper T cells
DC2	Lymphoid	Blood and many tissues		Antigen presentation for type 2 helper T cells
Eosinophil	Myeloid	Blood	$2 \times 10^2/\text{mm}^3$	Defense against eukaryotic parasites, late phase of type 1 hypersensitivity
Erythrocyte	Erythroid	Blood	$5 \times 10^6/\text{mm}^3$	Removal of antigen-antibody complexes from blood
Macrophage	Myeloid	Many tissues		Phagocytosis, antigen presentation
Mast cell	Myeloid	Many tissues		Regulation of inflammation, type 1 hypersensitivity
Monocyte	Myeloid	Blood	$4 \times 10^2/\text{mm}^3$	Antigen presentation
Natural killer cell	Lymphoid	Blood	$2 \times 10^2/\text{mm}^3$	Cytotoxicity against virally infected, cancerous cells
Neutrophil	Myeloid	Blood	$6 \times 10^3/\text{mm}^3$	Phagocytosis, antibacterial innate defense
Megakaryocyte	Myeloid	Bone marrow		Production of platelets
Platelet	Myeloid	Blood	$2 \times 10^5/\text{mm}^3$	Clotting, defense against eukaryotic parasites
T cell	Lymphoid	Blood, spleen, lymph nodes	$2 \times 10^3/\text{mm}^3$	
Helper T cell	Lymphoid	Blood, spleen, lymph nodes	$15 \times 10^2/\text{mm}^3$	Regulation of acquired response, cytokine production
Cytotoxic T cell	Lymphoid	Blood, spleen, lymph nodes	$6 \times 10^2/\text{mm}^3$	Cytotoxicity against altered self cells

APPENDIX E
Historical Timeline of Immunology

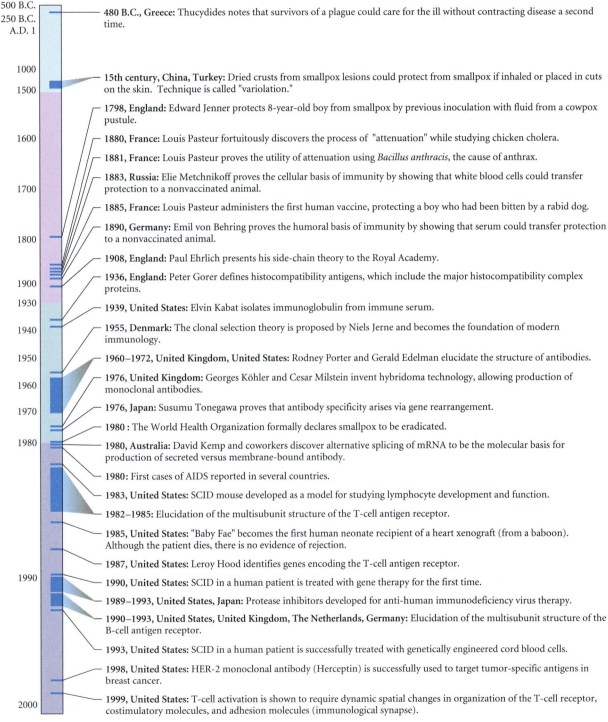

500 B.C.
250 B.C.
A.D. 1

480 B.C., Greece: Thucydides notes that survivors of a plague could care for the ill without contracting disease a second time.

1000

1500

15th century, China, Turkey: Dried crusts from smallpox lesions could protect from smallpox if inhaled or placed in cuts on the skin. Technique is called "variolation."

1798, England: Edward Jenner protects 8-year-old boy from smallpox by previous inoculation with fluid from a cowpox pustule.

1600

1880, France: Louis Pasteur fortuitously discovers the process of "attenuation" while studying chicken cholera.

1881, France: Louis Pasteur proves the utility of attenuation using *Bacillus anthracis*, the cause of anthrax.

1883, Russia: Elie Metchnikoff proves the cellular basis of immunity by showing that white blood cells could transfer protection to a nonvaccinated animal.

1700

1885, France: Louis Pasteur administers the first human vaccine, protecting a boy who had been bitten by a rabid dog.

1890, Germany: Emil von Behring proves the humoral basis of immunity by showing that serum could transfer protection to a nonvaccinated animal.

1800

1908, England: Paul Ehrlich presents his side-chain theory to the Royal Academy.

1936, England: Peter Gorer defines histocompatibility antigens, which include the major histocompatibility complex proteins.

1900

1930

1939, United States: Elvin Kabat isolates immunoglobulin from immune serum.

1940

1955, Denmark: The clonal selection theory is proposed by Niels Jerne and becomes the foundation of modern immunology.

1950

1960–1972, United Kingdom, United States: Rodney Porter and Gerald Edelman elucidate the structure of antibodies.

1976, United Kingdom: Georges Köhler and Cesar Milstein invent hybridoma technology, allowing production of monoclonal antibodies.

1960

1976, Japan: Susumu Tonegawa proves that antibody specificity arises via gene rearrangement.

1970

1980 : The World Health Organization formally declares smallpox to be eradicated.

1980

1980, Australia: David Kemp and coworkers discover alternative splicing of mRNA to be the molecular basis for production of secreted versus membrane-bound antibody.

1980: First cases of AIDS reported in several countries.

1983, United States: SCID mouse developed as a model for studying lymphocyte development and function.

1982–1985: Elucidation of the multisubunit structure of the T-cell antigen receptor.

1985, United States: "Baby Fae" becomes the first human neonate recipient of a heart xenograft (from a baboon). Although the patient dies, there is no evidence of rejection.

1987, United States: Leroy Hood identifies genes encoding the T-cell antigen receptor.

1990

1990, United States: SCID in a human patient is treated with gene therapy for the first time.

1989–1993, United States, Japan: Protease inhibitors developed for anti-human immunodeficiency virus therapy.

1990–1993, United States, United Kingdom, The Netherlands, Germany: Elucidation of the multisubunit structure of the B-cell antigen receptor.

1993, United States: SCID in a human patient is successfully treated with genetically engineered cord blood cells.

1998, United States: HER-2 monoclonal antibody (Herceptin) is successfully used to target tumor-specific antigens in breast cancer.

2000

1999, United States: T-cell activation is shown to require dynamic spatial changes in organization of the T-cell receptor, costimulatory molecules, and adhesion molecules (immunological synapse).

Changes in color of vertical bar denote changes in time scale.
*In some cases, no location is given. This denotes that the advance was the result of work performed in many laboratories in many nations.

APPENDIX F
Time Course of a Typical Immune Response

Each horizontal black bar shows the range of time after an injury or infection where each immunological event first takes place. The top two entries illustrate events that occur locally at the actual site of injury or infection, while the remainder of the entries show systemic immunological events. It is important that these are only typical values; actual immune responses offer many exceptions to these "typical" values.

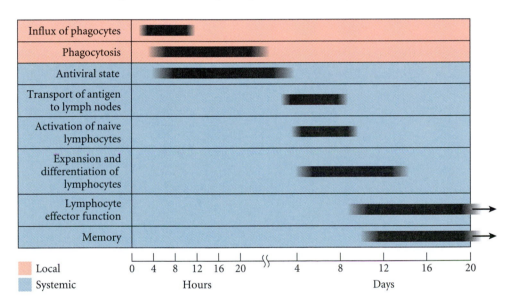

APPENDIX G

Comparison of Relative Sizes of Cells, Structures, and Molecules That Are Relevant to Infection and Immunity

The sizes of larger cells and structures are given in linear measures of micrometers (μm) and nanometers (nm), while molecule sizes are given in relative molecular weight (MW). The sizes of IgM and IgG are given in both nanometers and relative molecular weight.

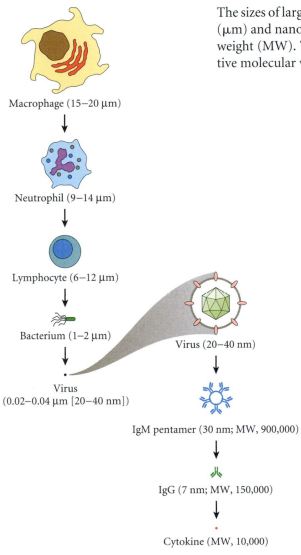

Macrophage (15–20 μm)

Neutrophil (9–14 μm)

Lymphocyte (6–12 μm)

Bacterium (1–2 μm)

Virus
(0.02–0.04 μm [20–40 nm])

Virus (20–40 nm)

IgM pentamer (30 nm; MW, 900,000)

IgG (7 nm; MW, 150,000)

Cytokine (MW, 10,000)

Index

Page numbers followed by the letter f indicate information found in figures; page numbers followed by the letter t indicate information found in tables.